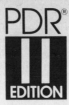

PHYSICIANS' DESK REFERENCE®

CONSUMERS' GUIDE TO NONPRESCRIPTION DRUGS

The same reference that doctors use...now in an
expanded paperback version for the general reader!

Publisher: Edward R. Barnhart

Director of Production: MARJORIE A. DUFFY

Production Manager: CARRIE HENWOOD

Manager of Production Services:
ELIZABETH H. CARUSO

Format Editor: MILDRED M. SCHUMACHER

Index Editor: ADELE L. DOWD

Medical Consultant:
GERALD F. DEDERICK JR. M.D.

Art Associate: JOAN AKERLIND

Editorial Assistant: CATHLEEN BUNNELL

Editorial Consultant: DAVID W. SIFTON

Administrative Assistants: SONIA C. RYAN
HELENE WATTMAN

National Sales Manager: KEVIN D. MILLER

Account Managers: JEFFERY J. BONISTALLI
CHARLIE J. MEITNER
JOANNE C. TERZIDES

Marketing and Circulation Director:
ROBIN B. BARTLETT

Assistant Circulation Director:
ANNETTE G. VERNON

Fulfillment Manager: ANITA H. MOORE

Professional Relations Manager:
ANNA E. BARBAGALLO

Marketing Administrator: DAWN TERRANOVA

Circulation Coordinator: MARY J. CADLEY

Senior Research Analyst: PATRICIA DeSIMONE

ISBN 0-87489-713-0

Foreword

Responsible self-medication is becoming ever more important in the health care of Americans. Self-medication continues to offer quick and inexpensive relief for minor health discomforts. Consumers have found the convenient availability and low cost of over-the-counter medications(OTCs) an invaluable adjunct to the professional health care system. Many medications formerly available by prescription can now be purchased over-the-counter, without prescription.

Nonprescription drugs can be safely and efficiently used as long as the directions on the label are followed. These instructions include the medical indications for the product along with dosage, side effects and suggestions when professional help may be indicated prior to taking the drug.

The fact that these medications are obtainable without a prescription does not mean they are not effective remedies. Product labels should be carefully read so that each ingredient is known. This is especially important if one is taking other over-the-counter or prescription drugs with the same ingredients. Failure to observe this can lead to overdosage. Never take a larger dose than directed on the package without advice from a physician or pharmacist. Knowing the ingredients is very important for those who have allergies or side effects from various medications. Observe warnings about interactions with other drugs. If side effects such as drowsiness or lightheadedness occur, do not continue to take the medication but contact the physician or pharmacist. There are also medical conditions that can be aggravated by certain drugs, so observe all warnings carefully and when in doubt contact the proper professional.

Physicians' Desk Reference® Consumers' Guide to Nonprescription Drugs is published annually by Medical Economics Company Inc., with the cooperation of the manufacturers whose products are described in the Product Information and Diagnostics, Devices and Medical Aids Sections. Its purpose is to make available essential information on nonprescription products.

The function of the Publisher is the compilation, organization, and distribution of this information. Each product description has been prepared by the manufacturer, and edited and approved by the manufacturer's medical department, medical director, and/or medical consultant. In organizing and presenting the material, the Publisher does not warrant or guarantee any of the products described or perform any independent analysis in connection with any of the product information contained herein. PHYSICIANS' DESK REFERENCE® CONSUMERS' GUIDE TO NONPRESCRIPTION DRUGS does not assume, and expressly disclaims, any obligation to obtain and include information other than that provided to it by the manufacturer. In making this material available it should be understood that the Publisher is not advocating the use of any product described. Besides the information given here, additional information on any product may be obtained through the manufacturer.

EDWARD R. BARNHART
Publisher

HOW TO USE THIS EDITION

If you want to find . . .	And you already know . . .	Here's where to look . . .
the brand name of a product	the manufacturer's name	White Section: Manufacturers' Index
	its generic name	Yellow Section: Active Ingredients Index*
the manufacturer's name	the product's brand name	Pink Section: Product Name Index*
	the product's generic name	Yellow Section: Active Ingredients Index*
essential product information, such as: active ingredients indications actions warnings drug interaction precautions symptoms & treatment of oral overdosage dosage & administration how supplied	the product's brand name	Pink Section: Product Name Index*
	the product's generic name	Yellow Section: Active ingredients Index*
a product with a particular chemical action	the chemical action	Yellow Section: Active Ingredients Index*
a product with a particular active ingredient	the active ingredient	Yellow Section: Active Ingredients Index*
a similar acting product	the product classification	Blue Section: Product Category Index*
generic name of a brand name product	the product's brand name	Pink Section: Product Name Index. Generic name will be found under "Active Ingredients" in Product Information Section.

In the Pink, Blue and Yellow Sections, the page numbers following the product name refer to the pages in the Product Identification Section where the product is pictured and the Product Information Section where the drug is comprehensively described.

Contents

Continued on next page

Contents

Common Health Problems

A Guide to Self-Treatment

Most common ailments are uncomfortable and inconvenient but not serious or disabling. You can treat many of them, such as colds, athlete's foot, and diarrhea, by using products you can obtain without a prescription. If you are careful to follow the instructions drug companies put in their packages to guide you, these products may relieve your symptoms and will have no harmful effects. If relief doesn't occur within a reasonable time, do what the package instructions advise: consult your doctor.

ACNE—*See also Product Category Index (blue section) under Dermatologicals, Acne Preparations*

Acne is an inflammatory skin disease characterized by pimples, blackheads, and whiteheads. It is caused by increased activity of the sebaceous glands in the skin that normally produce the oils for the proper lubrication of the skin and hair. Teenagers are the most frequent victims of this condition, because the large amounts of hormones their bodies produce during this period of growth cause an excess production of oils that become blocked in the pores.

Except in cases of severe acne, which should be treated by a dermatologist, most teenagers treat themselves with one or more of the many products available. These remedies include keratolytic drying and peeling preparations, plain skin cleansers, antibacterials, and vitamin A. Caution: Vitamin A used in heavy doses can cause toxic reactions.

ALLERGY—*See also Product Category Index (blue section) under Allergy Relief Products and Dermatologicals*

Another word for allergy is hypersensitivity. The body's immune system, which is supposed to make antibodies to destroy bacteria or viruses, sometimes becomes sensitive to harmless substances (called allergens) and makes antibodies against them. Foods can be allergens, as can inhalants (pollens, molds, dust, animal dander) and the secretions of plants like poison ivy. Immune cells in the blood and body tissues secrete a chemical called histamine, which causes the symptoms: itching eyes, nose, throat, and skin; runny nose, coughing, and sneezing; wheezing and asthma; headaches; rashes and hives.

Foods that cause allergies can be avoided, once they have been identified, and your exposure to allergens in the air can be minimized, as by staying away from cats and dogs and by vacuuming often to get rid of dust. However, it is hard to avoid airborne allergens altogether.

Mild allergic symptoms can be controlled by taking antihistamines and decongestants. For serious allergies, you'll need to enlist a doctor's help. He or she may prescribe prescription drugs or recommend a series of injections, which will help block the allergic reaction by desensitizing you to the substance or substances that are causing your problem.

ANEMIA—*See also Product Category Index (blue section) under Hematinics. See your physician.*

Anemia is a disease that affects the red cells in the blood. The job of these cells is to carry oxygen from the lungs to the tissues all through the body. To achieve this, a chemical in the cells called hemoglobin combines with the oxygen picked up in the lungs. Either too few red blood cells or not enough hemoglobin can cause anemia.

Iron deficiency anemia, the most common type is usually simple to treat. It results when dietary intake of iron is insufficient for the body's needs, as in pregnancy, or when there is excessive loss of iron, during heavy menstrual periods. Occasionally, however, it is a sign of slow internal bleeding in the intestines or other organs. Your doctor can rule out occult bleeding and perform blood tests that will identify the kind of supplement you need to take.

Other anemias are far more serious. In hemolytic anemia, the red blood cells are destroyed faster than the body can make them. Sickle cell anemia is an inherited disease in which the shape of the red cells is distorted, so that they rupture and get stuck in the small capillaries, causing pain and other serious side effects.

Symptoms of anemia include fatigue, pallor, easy bruising, weakness, and breathlessness. A doctor's diagnosis is a must; do not self-treat without his or her advice.

ARTHRITIS—*See also Product Category Index (blue section) under Analgesics and Arthritis Medications*

This term covers a multitude of ailments that have some symptoms in common. Pain or swelling of a joint and the tissues around it is the most common. It's never a good idea to treat such symptoms for more than a few days before consulting a doctor, as the exact type of arthritis must be determined for proper therapy.

Osteoarthritis is a very common joint disease. Its symptoms of pain, swelling, and stiffness of one or more joints may come and go over months, even years. Gradually, the pain may lessen while stiffness increases. In older people, the condition is caused by wear and tear, and it usually is found in the hips, knees, and spine. It can also occur in young adults as the result of athletic injuries or accidents.

What happens inside the joint is that the

smooth lining begins to break down, and the bone gradually becomes thick and misshapen. Because it hurts to move the joint, the muscles around it aren't used and start to waste away. Once your doctor has ordered x-rays and told you that you have osteoarthritis, you can treat it with warm, wet heat (hot baths, compresses). Rubbing the affected joint with a compound containing oil of wintergreen, menthol, camphor, or turpentine oil often brings relief. If you use one of these medications, be sure not to cover it with a bandage; if you do, a blister may form. Aspirin or another analgesic will help relieve the pain.

Other forms of arthritis are rheumatoid, gout, pseudogout, and various joint diseases due to infections. These all require professional help.

ASTHMA—*See also Product Category Index (blue section) under Asthma Preparations*
Asthma is an ailment caused by swelling of the lining of the bronchial tubes and contraction of the muscles in the walls of the bronchi. Asthma attacks are accompanied by wheezing and difficult breathing. They may be caused by an allergy—to pollen, house dust, feathers, cat or dog hairs, and occasionally foods or medications. Some persons have asthma that is not related to a specific allergy but triggered by an infection or other factor. Even exercise can start an attack, and emotional stress can aggravate if not actually cause one. For a start, try to ferret out the cause of the attacks. Do they usually come while you are jogging, or visiting a friend who owns a cat?

There are many new medications that help control asthma attacks, such as antihistamines and brochodilators, which act by relaxing the bronchial muscles and opening the blocked bronchial tubes. Pills, sprays, and liquids are available. A doctor's help and advice are usually needed to control this distressing problem.

ATHLETE'S FOOT—*See also Product Category Index (blue section) under Dermatologicals, Fungicides*
The symptoms of athlete's foot are redness, flakiness, itching, and cracking of the skin between the toes. The condition is caused by a fungus and is contagious. The fungus thrives on damp floors, particularly around swimming pools and in dressing rooms and showers.

Dry carefully between your toes before applying one of the many available antifungal creams, sprays, or powders. Do everything you can to prevent your feet from becoming damp with perspiration: wear cotton socks or sandals and shoes that allow air to circulate, expose your shoes to the air when you're not wearing them, and put on clean socks every day.

BAD BREATH (halitosis)—*See also Product Category Index (blue section) under Oral Hygiene Aid and Mouthwashes*
There are many causes for bad breath. If the unpleasant smell comes from decaying bits of food stuck between your teeth, washing them away will certainly help, although brushing and flossing are more effective. However, there are many other causes. Perhaps a decaying tooth, not bits of food, is to blame.

Bad breath can also be the result of smoking, gum inflammation or infection, or an ulcer in your mouth. Certain lung ailments can cause you to cough up phlegm that has an unpleasant smell.

Some foods and drinks are absorbed into the bloodstream, and these will cause bad breath. Alcohol, onions, and garlic are well-known offenders.

People who wear dentures need to be especially careful about bad breath, which results when bits of food stick to the dentures. Be sure to clean them thoroughly on both sides everyday.

If simple measures do not work and the odor persists, check with your dentist or with a physician. Occasionally, an infection or tumor of the nose, throat, or sinuses may be responsible.

BODY LICE—*See also Product Category Index (blue section) under Antiparasitics*
These tiny insects live in the hairs, feeding on blood they suck from the skin. They may be found in the scalps of school children. Their eggs, which are called nits, look like little white dots. If you find nits in your child's hair, report it to the teacher. Washing with ordinary soap won't remove the nits, as they are firmly attached to the hair. A medicated shampoo designed for the purpose will kill the insects and their eggs. Be sure to follow package instructions carefully.

BURNS—*See also Product Category Index (blue section) under Dermatologicals, Burn Relief*
Damage to the skin may be caused by heat,

electricity, or chemicals. If only the superficial (top) layer of the skin is damaged, the skin will become red and may eventually blister. Such minor injuries should be cared for immediately, by immersing the burned skin in cold or iced water, or holding it under the cold water faucet. After 10 minutes, cover the area with an ointment or spray. Some products contain a local anesthetic to relieve pain, while others also contain an antiseptic that is useful for preventing blisters from becoming infected. You should never break a blister; open blisters are much more likely to become infected.

For more serious burns, get professional help right away. Don't put ointments, creams, or anything greasy on a serious burn, because it will have to be removed before proper treatment can be started.

BURSITIS—*See also Product Category Index (blue section) under Analgesics, Internal and Topical*
This painful condition is the result of an inflammation of the bursae, small sacs located near joints. They contain fluid that serves to lessen friction of parts that must move against each other all the time. When a bursa is irritated, it becomes swollen and painful. The joints most often affected are the shoulder, knee, elbow, and big toe.

The best treatment for bursitis is to rest the joint. Pain relief medications may moderate the discomfort while you wait for the inflammation to subside. If pain is severe or recurs, injections of steroids into the sac can be performed by the doctor. At times the bursa must be surgically removed to get permanent relief.

CANKER SORES—*See also Product Category Index (blue section) under Canker Sore Preparations*
Canker sores look very much like cold sores, but they are not caused by a virus. Although the precise cause is unknown, vitamin deficiencies and stress may increase a person's susceptibility. They may also occur along with some illness that lowers your resistance. While they clear up without treatment, the druggist can supply preparations to speed healing and give relief.

COLDS—*See also Product Category Index (blue section) under Cold Preparations*
Colds are viral infections common to the entire human race. Antibiotics, which are effective only against bacterial infections, do not cure them. However, many products now available on pharmacists' shelves can reduce discomforting symptoms. Decongestants will help clear your clogged nose and may help prevent sinusitis. They also make breathing easier, particularly at night. An expectorant cough medicine will loosen the phlegm or mucus and help you bring it up. Plenty of fluids are also important as they keep the mucus from thickening.

While colds are a nuisance and uncomfortable, they are not serious in themselves. However, more serious ailments, such as tonsillitis, strep throat, and influenza, may seem at first to be "just a cold," and other complications, such as bronchitis, sinusitis, or even pneumonia, may follow a cold. Check with a physician if your symptoms are severe, if you run a significant fever, if the cold "hangs on," or if it gets worse after starting to get better.

COLD SORES (herpes simplex)—*See also Product Category Index (blue section) under Herpes Treatment*
Cold sores are blisters on the lips or inside the mouth caused by a virus called herpes simplex. In the mouth, the blisters develop into ulcers, causing the surrounding gum tissue to become red and swollen. At times a fever may go along with this infection. In due course, it will clear up without any treatment. However, the virus remains in the body at the same site, and later on, when you catch a cold or are exposed to strong sunlight or wind, it may cause a fresh attack. A mild mouthwash and medication for the fever are the usual forms of treatment. A soothing ointment may help the sores on the lip heal and make them less uncomfortable.

There is one real danger from a herpes infection: if you touch the sores and then rub your eye, you might develop a corneal ulcer, which can be very serious. So be careful to wash your hands frequently and keep them away from your eyes.

CONSTIPATION—*See also Product Category Index (blue section) under Laxatives*
Often, people worry about being constipated when what they really mean is that they do not have as many bowel movements as other family members or friends. Some individuals have one movement a day, but others have them more often, while still others have as few as two or three a week. Each body has its own rhythm, and as long as it causes no prob-

lems, that's the normal pattern for that particular body.

However, if your pattern changes, and you start having irregular, more infrequent, or difficult bowel movements, you may consider yourself constipated. The problem can be the result of diet, some medicine you have been taking, or hemorrhoids. If you don't take time to go to the bathroom and stay there long enough, constipation can be the result.

If diet is the problem, try to eat more raw fruits, vegetables, salads, and whole-grain cereals. Bran is helpful. Drink plenty of liquids, and exercise regularly. If none of this works, there are many laxatives on the market, but try not to let taking them become a habit as this can be very difficult to change. Don't take laxatives for abdominal pain, nausea, or vomiting. These can be symptoms of appendicitis, for which you should see your doctor.

CORNS AND CALLUSES—*See also Product Category Index (blue section) under Corn and Callus Removers*
Corns and calluses are caused by pressure on the skin, usually from a shoe that is new or doesn't fit properly. The result is a thickening of the skin.

Calluses are not usually painful; corns have a hard center and may hurt. Treat corns and calluses with some bland ointment, and rub off dead skin with a pumice stone. Wear corn plasters to protect the corn from pressure. Preparations containing salicylic acid can be used to soften the layers of skin so that a corn or callus can be peeled off. At times what appears to be a callus on the bottom of the foot may actually be due to a plantar wart. If simple remedies do not help, get professional advice.

COUGHS—*See also Product Category Index (blue section) under Cough Preparations*
Coughing is the body's way of freeing the airways of foreign matter of any sort, from a morsel of food to a fragment of mucus or phlegm. Coughing is also a sign of irritation, either from something inhaled, such as paint or tobacco smoke; from an illness, such as TB; occasionally, from a tumor. What you should do about it depends on the cause of the cough.

Coughs that produce phlegm or mucus help clear the lungs and passageways of the offending substance. Cough medicines

known as expectorants loosen the phelgm, making it easier to cough up. Coughing should gradually diminish as less phlegm is produced. A medicine containing a cough suppressant will help soothe the irritation left by coughing at the end of a cold. Suppressants should not be used until you have stopped producing phlegm.

A cough with cold symptoms and fever that persists for several days could be a symptom of bronchitis or pneumonia, and you should see your doctor. Blood in the phlegm is also a sign of trouble that warrants a physician's attention.

A dry cough, or one that has continued for several weeks or months, can be a sign of allergy, chronic irritation, tuberculosis, or lung cancer. The sooner you consult a doctor, the better.

Directions that accompany cough preparations always give careful instructions about the size of the dose. Be especially sure not to give children more medicine than the instructions advise.

Because of early vaccination, very few children catch whooping cough, a disease that produces paroxysms of coughing ending in a whoop. Every child should be inoculated against it in the first year of life.

CRADLE CAP—*See also Product Category Index (blue section) under Dermatologicals, Cradle Cap Agent, Seborrhea Treatment, Shampoos*
Cradle cap is a form of eczema that afflicts babies. It usually begins with scales on the scalp. Later, the scales may spread, forming yellow, greasy patches. Sometimes the eczema extends and patches appear on the face, behind the ears, or in the folds of the neck, armpits, and groin. Cradle cap goes away by itself. Just keep the areas clean and dry. You may also rub them gently with a nonperfumed baby oil or a cream. If infection occurs, you will see redness in or around the eczema. Ask your doctor for an antibiotic cream.

CROUP—*Call your physician*
Croup is an inflammatory disease of the respiratory tract that occurs in early childhood and is caused by viruses. The child gasps for breath, and the cough sounds like the barking of a small dog. The quickest way to stop it is to sit with the child in the bathroom, with hot water running in the shower. Usually, as the room fills with steam, the cough will subside. If it doesn't, or if the child has a fever along

with the croup, call your doctor. If you find it necessary to take the child to the hospital emergency room, bundle him or her up warmly and try to keep cold air away from nose and mouth.

CUTS AND SCRAPES—*See also Product Category Index (blue section) under Analgesics, Topical; Antibacterials and Antiseptics; Dermatologicals, Anesthetics and Antibacterial; Skin Wound Preparations*
Minor cuts and scrapes should be washed thoroughly with soap and water. An antiseptic can be applied to help kill any remaining germs, and bandages are available in all shapes and sizes to protect the wound and keep it clean. Don't disturb the bandage or let it get wet for 24 hours. Then take it off and examine the wound. If a dry scab hasn't formed yet, wash with soap and water again and rebandage. After a scab forms, it's best to leave the area unbandaged. Wash it as usual, but don't apply any product likely to keep the scab wet or soft.

With a serious cut, the first order or business is to stop or slow heavy bleeding. Apply firm pressure directly over the cut, preferably with clean padding such as a towel between your hand and the wound but if necessary with your hand alone. The bleeding should stop or slow substantially within a few minutes.

Cuts that spurt or gush blood are an emergency—apply pressure and get help right away. Other wounds that need a doctor's attention promptly are large scrapes, especially if dirt is embedded in them; deep cuts and puncture wounds, which may require a tetanus shot; gaping wounds, which may need stitches; and animal bites.

DANDRUFF—*See also Product Category Index (blue section) under Dermatologicals, Dandruff Medications, Coal Tar and Sulfur, Shampoos*
Dandruff consists of scales or small flakes of dead skin. They appear on the scalp when its cells are growing too fast. This scaling, sometimes accompanied by itching or inflammation, is caused by oversecretion of the oil-producing glands of the scalp.

Several medicated shampoos are available for treatment of dandruff. They may contain tar, zinc pyrithione, selenium sulfide, or other ingredients. If they fail to clear up the condition, better see a physician.

DENTAL HYGIENE—*See also Product Category Index (blue section) under Dental Preparations, Mouthwashes, Oral Hygiene Aid, Tooth Desensitizers*
If you wish to avoid extra trips to the dentist without losing any of your teeth, you must spend a reasonable amount of time caring for them.

Use a toothbrush at least twice a day, in the morning and at bedtime.

Use dental floss between your teeth daily; it will remove bits of food that escape your toothbrush and plaque along your gum-line, which can cause chronic inflammation.

Eat sensibly: don't consume too much sugar, which damages tooth enamel.

Eat plenty of foods that need to be chewed, such as crisp apples; these act as cleaners.

Make sure your tooth enamel is strengthened with fluoride. We now know that this mineral prevents decay. Most toothpastes contain fluoride. You can also use fluoride mouthwash or tablets, or a fluoride gel. If your water supply is fluoridated, check with your dentist to find out whether additional fluoride is advisable.

Fluoride treatments for children under twelve are a yearly must. While the enamel is still forming on the teeth is the best time to build healthy teeth.

Pay two visits a year to your dentist. Should a cavity form despite all your care, catching it early can save the tooth. The dentist will also check your gums. Untreated gum disease can damage the underlying bone and is a common cause of tooth loss in middle-aged and older people.

DIAGNOSTIC PRODUCTS AND DEVICES—*See also Product Category Index (blue section) under Diagnostics*
Many home devices and kits are available. The following are some of the most popular.

Blood pressure kits
These kits include a cloth cuff containing an inflatable bag with a rubber bulb and a valve for inflating and deflating the bag, and a gauge that registers pressure. Most kits also contain a stethoscope.

Three types of kits are available. The mercury type is the most accurate. Instead of a column of mercury, the aneroid type uses a needle that moves clockwise on a dial as pressure is increased and counterclockwise as it is decreased. The electronic aneroid type gives you a digital readout of your blood pressure and is easiest to use, though not always dependable.

Blood sugar tests

For many years, diabetics have used home tests to measure the amount of sugar in the urine. Now home tests are also available for measuring the amount of sugar in the blood. The tests are useful for people with hypoglycemia as well as diabetics. They are marketed as kits that contain a meter—about the size of a tape recorder—plus alcohol wipes, insulin syringes, blood lancets, and reagent strips. The procedure is to prick the finger and transfer the blood to a reagent strip, place the strip in the meter, and wait for the glucose-level readout.

Occult blood tests

Some physicians suggest that everyone over 50 have an annual test to spot minute amounts of blood in the bowel movements, which can be a sign of cancer of the colon. Several types of home test are available. Most are very simple and can be interpreted right away; some require mailing specimens to a lab or to the doctor for analysis.

Poison safeguard kits

These kits usually contain ipecac (to induce vomiting) and activated charcoal (used as an antidote). They also include printed information about safeguards, symptoms, and procedures for various common poisons.

Pregnancy tests

These tests work by combining a few drops of urine with antibodies to a hormone, human chorionic gonadotropin (hCG), found in the urine of pregnant women. If you are pregnant, the hCG in your urine will combine with the antibodies, changing the color on a paper strip or forming a brown ring at the bottom of the test tube. The kits are reasonably accurate, but far from 100%.

Thermometers

The standard mercury-in-glass thermometer is one of several devices for taking temperatures. Chemical thermometers, which are disposable, look like tongue depressors. A series of dots containing the chemical change color to indicate the temperature. Disposable thermometers have the advantage as they are not fragile like glass. In addition, because they are not used a second time, there is no danger of reinfection.

Liquid crystal thermometers are made of aluminum or plastic. To take a patient's temperature, simply place it on the forehead. These reusable devices can be washed in warm water with a disinfectant soap; boiling or alcohol may spoil them.

Electronic thermometers give readings in 30 to 60 seconds. Some even offer a digital readout. The disadvantage is that they are fairly expensive.

Tests for urinary tract infection

Those who know they are susceptible to these infections, which can lead to kidney damage, can detect a transient infection by using one of these kits. They are also helpful for people with diabetes or hypertension, who are susceptible to urinary tract infection.

DIAPER RASH—*See also Product Category Index (blue section) under Dermatologicals, Dermatitis Relief; Diaper Rash Relief*
Diaper rash is an acute inflammation of the skin of the buttocks, groin, or genitals. Several factors contribute to the development of diaper rash. Urine trapped in the diaper keeps the skin moist. Moist skin is more susceptible to abrasion or chafing than dry skin. It's also more easily irritated by enzymes found in the stool. The interaction of urine and feces compound the problem by producing ammonia. Ammonia raises the pH of the area which increases the activity of fecal enzymes and makes the skin more susceptible to their irritating effects.

Changing diapers frequently and keeping the skin clean and dry will generally solve the problem. Disposable diapers with an absorbent gel material (AGM) can help reduce wetness and contact with irritants. Soothing creams and oils can help speed healing.

Diaper rash usually clears in two or three days. If you think your child's rash is taking too long to heal, contact your pediatrician for further advice and treatment.

DIARRHEA—*See also Product Category Index (blue section) under Diarrhea Preparations*
This condition—the frequent passage of unformed, watery stools—may be accompanied by crampy pains in the abdomen, nausea and vomiting, headache, or other symptoms. A single bout of diarrhea can be caused by eating spoiled food; by a bacterial or viral infection; by a medication, such as an antibiotic; or

by an emotional upset.

Most products used to treat diarrhea contain an adsorbant, which binds the bacteria or toxins causing the symptoms and transports them through the intestines to be excreted. Along with the medication you choose, be sure to drink plenty of fluids to replace the body fluid you are losing in the diarrhea.

You should call the doctor if the pain in your abdomen continues or recurs; if you find blood in a bowel movement; or if your attack of diarrhea goes away but returns after a few days. Chronic diarrhea can be a sign of serious illness.

Diarrhea in infants may be caused by sugar added to juice or formula, or even by sweets eaten by a nursing mother. Adding solids to a baby's diet while he or she is still too young to digest solid food also causes diarrhea, as do food allergies. If the baby has a fever, or if the symptoms continue, call your doctor. Dehydration can develop quickly, especially in very young babies.

EARWAX—*See also Product Category Index (blue section) under Cerumenolytics*
It's normal for the glands in the outer ear canal to produce wax. However, some people's ears produce so much wax that it blocks the canal, making the ear feel plugged up. It may even make hearing difficult.

Serious damage can be done to the ear drum by poking into your ear with a stick or swab. However, it is safe to use one of the preparations made to drop into the ear to soften the wax, after which it can be irrigated with a soft rubber syringe. It is not safe to use any of these products if you know that your ear drum is perforated. If there is any doubt about this, have a doctor check your ear before you put anything into it.

EYE IRRITATION—*See also Product Category Index (blue section) under Ophthalmologicals*
For minor irritation, there are three kinds of eye drops: artificial tears, eye washes, and decongestants. If you have glaucoma, it's important to avoid decongestants.

Swelling and redness of the eyelid, along with red streaks in the eye itself, is called conjunctivitis or pink eye. It can be caused by viruses or bacteria, an allergy, or irritation. Often, symptoms include a yellowish discharge and a sensation of sand under the lid.

If you have these symptoms, or pain or blurred vision, see your eye doctor.

FLEAS
These creatures lay their eggs on animals, and in rugs, mattresses, and the like. The eggs hatch after about seven days. Flea bites cause irritation as well as itching. Repellants, sprays, powders, and fumigants are available for destroying these pests. If the fleas are coming from a pet dog or cat, spray the animal's bedding as well as the animal.

HEADACHE—*See also Product Category Index (blue section) under Analgesics*
Everyone gets a headache from time to time. Common headaches are caused by tension of the muscles of the neck and scalp. They may be brought on by emotional stress, lack of sleep, or occasionally by eye strain or noise. Taking a warm bath helps relaxation, and massage of neck muscles can be soothing. Also, many headache remedies are available.

Severe or unusual headaches or ones associated with other symptoms, such as nausea and vomiting, may be a sign of a serious illness for which you should see a doctor. Among the causes are migraine, allergies, injuries, severe high blood pressure, brain tumors, infection, and hemorrhages. When in doubt, seek immediate medical assistance.

HEMORRHOIDS—*See also Product Category Index (blue section) under Anorectal Products. See your physician.*
Hemorrhoids are small veins in (or just outside) the rectum that have become swollen and inflamed. Usually, they are caused by straining during constipated bowel movements; other causes are abdominal pressure that accompanies advancing pregnancy, diarrhea, and prolonged standing or sitting. The veins, which have become swollen, can rupture and bleed when you move your bowels. Hemorrhoids can become very painful, may itch, and may protrude outside the rectum. This protrusion is know as prolapse.

While varicose veins are not dangerous, they are not the only cause of rectal bleeding; another serious one is cancer of the rectum or large intestine. For this reason, it's important to see your doctor, to make sure it's hemorrhoids that are responsible for the blood you are noticing on the toilet paper or in the toilet bowl.

Once you know for sure your problem is hemorrhoids, you can do a great deal to alleviate the symptoms. Wash with soap and warm water after every bowel movement, and dry carefully with soft paper. Eat foods that help avoid constipation, such as fresh fruits, vegetables, and bread and cereals made of whole grains or bran. Many products are available to ease your discomfort. Rectal suppositories and ointments can help shrink the hemorrhoids and soothe the pain.

HERPES GENITALIS—*See your physician.*
This infection of the genitals is caused by herpes simplex virus type 2. (This is not to be confused with herpes simplex virus type 1, a related virus that causes cold sores.) Herpes genitalis is a painful infection that is usually sexually transmitted. The hands can also convey it from one person to another.

Symptoms begin about six days after contact with someone who has the infection. They include pain, tenderness, or itching around the penis or vulva. Often, but not always, there may be a general feeling of illness, fever, or headache. Later, blisters form on the penis or vulva, in the vagina or on the cervix, and sometimes on the thighs or buttocks. When they break, painful ulcers are formed. These open sores last from one to three weeks. The virus often stays in the body, so the symptoms may recur months or even years later.

Since the condition is infectious, it is important to avoid sexual intercourse until the symptoms have cleared. Medications that can control this illness should be prescribed by a doctor. One self-treatment that helps is to take frequent warm baths followed by drying. A hair dryer is the best way to do this as no rubbing of the painful areas takes place.

INDIGESTION—*See also Product Category Index (blue section) under Antacids and Flatulence Relief*
This common complaint refers to various symptoms, from a bad taste in the mouth, heartburn, hiccuping, discomfort in the chest, or feelings of nausea, to the need to belch or pass gas. You may have one, several, or all these symptoms.

There are as many causes as there are symptoms. Some people have indigestion whenever they get upset; some have it after eating certain foods; some when they eat too fast; some when they drink more than usual.

It's particularly common in women who are pregnant and in anyone who is obese or constipated, or who smokes heavily. Some people swallow air when drinking fluids, and this fills up the stomach.

Acid indigestion can often be relieved by antacids. Severe or recurrent indigestion should be evaluated by a doctor, as should "indigestion" that comes on after exercise or causes pain or pressure in the chest, which can be a sign of heart problems.

INSECT BITES AND STINGS—*See also Product Category Index (blue section) under Insect Bite and Sting Preparations; Insect Sting Emergency Kit*
Most insect bites are a nuisance and can be alleviated by various creams, ointments, and lotions, which cut down on the inflammation, itching, and swelling. But some people have severe allergic reactions, especially to yellow jacket stings. Rather than just local swelling and pain, they quickly develop general symptoms, such as hives and swelling of the face and throat and difficulty breathing. Such a reaction should prompt immediate trip to the emergency room. Those people who are aware of their allergy can carry an emergency kit, prescribed by a physician, which contains antihistamines, steroids, and prefilled syringes containing adrenalin that they can use themselves to prevent severe reactions. For those who are not allergic, ammonia applied to the bite area may give quick relief after stings of yellow jackets or bees.

INSOMNIA—*See also Product Category Index (blue section) under Sleep Aids*
While it's said that the average adult needs seven to eight hours of sleep, there is no such thing as "the average adult." You may need nine hours of sleep to feel well, while another person may get along well with only five hours. It won't harm you to sleep less than usual, unless you find yourself feeling overtired and are unable to sleep when you do go to bed.

There are many reasons people have trouble getting to sleep and staying asleep. Some are easily discovered. If you have been taking sleeping pills or tranquilizers and then stopped, you'll be wakeful for a few weeks until you get used to doing without them. Eating too much or drinking too much coffee, tea, or alcohol late in the afternoon or in the evening can cause wakefulness. One common cause of insomnia is anxiety. If you have trouble sleeping only occasionally, one of the many products available without a prescription will probably help you become drowsy and drop off. Most such medications contain antihistamines and aren't habit-forming. Stronger medicines usually are habit-forming, and can be taken only under a doctor's supervision.

MENSTRUAL PROBLEMS—*See also Product Category Index (blue section) under Menstrual Preparations*
Before menstruation begins each month, many women have various unpleasant symptoms known as premenstrual syndrome (PMS). These include breast tenderness, fluid retention, irritability, and tension. When menstruation actually begins, it may be accompanied by cramping pains, which can be severe. Mild PMS and cramps can be relieved by one of the many products available for these problems. They contain analgesics and some also have agents to decrease bloating, cramping, and tension. Prescription drugs are also available to treat PMS.

Severe cramps that are not relieved by any of these products may be caused by endometriosis, a pelvic infection, a fibroid tumor, or an intrauterine device (IUD). A doctor will be able to diagnose the cause.

MOTION SICKNESS—*See also Product Category Index (blue section) under Motion Sickness Remedies*
No one who has ever been seasick needs to be told what a miserable experience it can be. The same symptoms—nausea and vomiting—also are caused by the motion of an airplane, train, car, or even a swing. The first symptoms are often yawning, a need to swallow frequently, and a cold sweat. Headache and dizziness are also common.

If you are susceptible to motion sickness, don't drink any alcohol or eat too much before starting on a trip. Try to sit over the wing (in a plane) or in the front seat (in a car). Don't try to read. It's best not to eat or drink during short trips. Nonprescription medications, taken about an hour before starting out, can help; prescription medications for motion sickness are also available.

PAIN—*See also Product Category Index (blue section) under Analgesics*
Pain is nature's way of protecting you from the hazards of your environment. Without this warning signal, you wouldn't snatch your hand away from a hot stove, know when you had torn a ligament in your ankle, or suspect that you might have appendicitis. For example, in some diabetic patients, the nerves of the feet deteriorate, and the person does not feel areas of pressure or small injuries. Because no pain is felt, a deep ulcer can develop before the person realizes something is happening. Fortunately, pain by its nature and severity will also tell you when to go to a doctor.

Sometimes pain comes from things that are annoying but not too serious. A headache, toothache, or minor arthritic or muscular ache will generally be temporarily relieved by an analgesic.

There are four basic analgesics available, alone or in combination—acetaminophen, aspirin, ibuprofen, and salicylamide. Some products also contain caffeine, which is not an analgesic. Caffeine is thought to be of value because it constricts dilated blood vessels that may be contributing to the pain.

Besides the analgesics you take internally to treat arthritic and muscle pain, there are those that can be rubbed on the skin for relief of local pain. They are counterirritants that dilate the small blood vessels and bring blood closer to the skin's surface, producing increased circulation and warmth. The increase in blood flow to the joint or muscle below speeds up the healing process.

Most of these compounds are "volatile oils" that have a familiar and pleasant odor. Oil of wintergreen, menthol, camphor, and turpentine are the most commonly used.

Some products contain ingredients that soothe pain and irritation by local anesthetic action.

You must be careful when using these products not to cover them with bandages, because this might cause the skin to blister.

PERSPIRATION PROBLEMS—*See also Product Category Index (blue section) under Deodorants; Dermatologicals, Antiperspirants*
Excessive perspiration, or hyperhidrosis, is a troubling problem for some people. It is caused by overactive sweat glands, usually in the armpits, on the palms of the hands or soles of the feet, in the groin, or beneath the breasts. In some cases, the skin may scale and split. The accompanying unpleasant odor is produced by bacteria and yeasts, which

break down the moistened and dead skin cells.

Antiperspirants containing aluminum hydrochloride control perspiration in most people. If they don't work, or if you develop a painful or persistent rash, see your doctor. Don't put antiperspirant on a rash; just keep it clean and as dry as possible for a few days to see whether it will clear up on its own.

POISON IVY—*See also Product Category Index (blue section) under Dermatologicals, Poison Ivy, Oak or Sumac; Poison Ivy and Oak Preparations*
Poison ivy causes an allergic reaction about two days after the oil on the leaves come in contact with the skin. The longer the oil remains on the skin, the more severe the rash.

At first redness and itching appear, followed by blisters. If there is oil underneath the fingernails, it can be carried from one part of the body to another by scratching. Washing thoroughly with soap and water soon after exposure may prevent the rash from developing or reduce its severity.

Many products containing steroids, calamine, zinc oxide, local anesthetics, and anti-itching medications are available from the pharmacist. Poison oak and sumac, as well as other plants, can cause similar problems and are treated the same.

PRICKLY HEAT—*See also Product Category Index (blue section) under Dermatologicals*
This rash, which occurs mostly during hot, humid weather, is caused by blocked sweat glands. The rash consists of clusters of pin-head-size bumps, which burn and itch. Adults have it as well as infants.

A variety of products can be used to relieve the itching and speed healing. Avoidance of wool products that cover the skin will greatly help in providing relief.

PUBIC LICE—*See also Product Category Index (blue section) under Antiparasitics*
These miniature, crab-like, blood-sucking insects live in the pubic hair and the hair around the anus. They may sometimes be found on other body hair as well as on the eyebrows and eyelashes. They are very small (1 to 2 millimeters across), but they can be seen with the naked eye if you look closely. The female lays white eggs, called nits. Washing will not remove them, as they are firmly attached to the hairs. To kill the lice and their eggs, use a special lotion or shampoo.

Pubic lice may be caught by sexual contact with someone who has them. They often cause itching, especially at night. If you also note any symptoms of more serious sexually transmitted disease, such as a genital discharge or sore, check with your physician without delay.

RINGWORM—*See Your Physician*
This skin disease is not caused by a worm at all, but by a fungus infection called tinea. It causes scaly, round, itchy patches on the skin. It often affects the scalp, where it produces bald patches.

Ringworm is contagious and can be caught from a pet dog or cat. However, it is most common among children of school age. If your child has ringworm of the scalp you'll need a doctor's help as soon as possible. The doctor will prescribe an oral medication to kill the fungus. Destroy the brushes, combs, and hats the child has been using recently. As this is contagious, contact the school to inquire as to how long the child should stay at home before returning to class.

Tinea may also be found on other parts of the body, such as the trunk, the crotch, and the foot (see Athlete's Foot). On the trunk and crotch, it starts as a small, itchy, red patch, which gets gradually bigger. The center of the patch heals, leaving a red ring on the skin.

SPRAINS—*See also Product Category Index (blue section) under Analgesics*
The acronym for treatment of a sprained ankle, knee, or wrist is RICE: Rest, Ice, Compression, and Elevation. Have the victim sit or lie down. Fill an icebag or plastic bag with ice and wrap it in a towel. Put it on the injured part for about 15 minutes, then take it off for about the same amount of time. Keep doing this off and on for 24-36 hours, to reduce swelling and pain. If the injury aches, an analgesic can be taken. Some sprains benefit from being wrapped, firmly but not tightly, with an elastic bandage for a week or so, starting about 24 hours after the injury.

Signs of a possible break or torn ligament include severe pain, swelling, and bruising at the site of the injury. Sprains cause swelling, too, so it can be hard to be sure. If you think a bone may be broken, go for an x-ray promptly; don't "Wait overnight to be sure."

SUNBURN PREVENTION—*See also Product Category Index (blue section) under Dermatologicals, Sunscreens*
A burn caused by too much exposure of your skin to the sun's ultraviolet rays (or those of a sunlamp) can damage your skin, causing it to grow red or blister. If you know from past experience that you burn easily, take proper precautions. Use a sunscreen before going out into bright sunlight. These products contain chemicals that filter out the burning rays. After you swim, or if you have been perspiring heavily, be sure to put on more sunscreen. Some sunscreens offer partial protection; others filter out all the ultraviolet rays. The degree of protection is always plainly marked on the package.

Skin cancers related to sun exposure and sunburn are becoming more common. As a preventive measure, many doctors recommend the regular use of a sunscreen with an SPF (Sun Protection Factor) of 15 or higher.

VITAMINS AND MINERALS—*See also Product Category Index (blue section) under Dietary Supplements & Vitamins*
Vitamins are chemical compounds found in plants and animals that are necessary to maintain normal growth and metabolism of the body. Most vitamins cannot be manufactured by the body, so they have to be obtained from the food you eat or from vitamin supplements. The same is true for minerals. Minerals play an important role in fluid and chemical balance. They are involved in maintaining the proper body acidity and are essential for glandular function, blood clotting, and muscle activity. Calcium and phosphorus in proper proportions are needed for good bone development. Iron is a component of blood hemoglobin, as is zinc in insulin and iodine in thyroid secretions. Many other minerals such as copper, magnesium, fluorine, chromium, and selenium are essential in very small amounts.

Most experts agree that the best way to get the proper vitamin and mineral intake is to eat a balanced diet. This is easier said than done, however. Some people do not or cannot plan and prepare a proper diet. In addition, vitamin requirements increase during certain events in life such as pregnancy, illness, or dieting. When the diet is inadequate, necessary nutrients can be obtained from vitamin-mineral supplements.

Vitamins
Vitamin A is essential for healthy skin and hair, and necessary for adequate vision.
Vitamin B_1 (thiamine) is essential for normal digestion of food, because it helps digest carbohydrates into energy and fat. It is also essential for nerve cell, heart, and muscle function.
Vitamin B_2 (riboflavin) helps maintain healthy skin and body tissues.
Vitamin B_3 (niacin) helps keep the body tissues in healthy condition, and the central nervous system functioning.
Vitamin B_5 (pantothenic acid) is involved in the metabolism of carbohydrates, fats, and proteins. It also aids energy production, keeps the nervous system and gastrointestinal tract in healthy condition, and plays a role in immunity.
Vitamin B_6 (pyridoxine) aids the metabolism of proteins and fats, and is essential for proper cell function.
Vitamin B_9 (folic acid) helps in the manufacture of red blood cells and metabolism of food to energy.
Vitamin B_{12} (cyanocobalamin) is needed to synthesize hemoglobin and the development of healthy red blood cells. It is also essential for nerve cell function and helps prevent certain forms of anemia.
Vitamin C (ascorbic acid) is essential for normal teeth, bones, blood vessels, formation of collagen (a protein that helps support body structures), and wound healing. It also helps the body absorb and use iron from food.
Vitamin D (calciferol) promotes absorption of calcium and phosphorus to make strong bones and teeth.
Vitamin E (alpha-tocopherol) helps prevent oxygen from destroying other substances in the body and is needed for stability of muscle, red blood cell tissue, and membranes.
Vitamin H (biotin) is necessary for the body in manufacturing certain fat-like substances essential for metabolism.
Vitamin K is essential for the formation of prothrombin, a substance necessary for normal blood clotting.

Dosage recommendations
A term you see on vitamin and mineral product labels is RDA (Recommended Daily Dietary Allowances). The RDA was established by the National Research Council as a guide to the amounts of vitamins needed for maintenance of good nutrition. Vitamin and mineral amounts are expressed as milligrams

(mg.), micrograms (mcg.), or International Units (I.U.).

High doses of vitamins—well over 100% RDA—can cause problems. Some vitamins are water-soluble, so that excessive amounts are easy to excrete; others are oil-soluble and tend to be retained in the body. It's best to stay away from excessive amounts of vitamins except under special circumstances or with professional advice.

WARTS—*See also Product Category Index (blue section) under Dermatologicals, Wart Removers*

These lumps on the skin are caused by viruses that live in the skin cells and hasten the cells' growth. The common wart is a small, hard, horny, white or pink lump with an uneven surface. Less common are the smooth, brown variety and the small, white ones with a depression in the middle. Warts on the bottom of the foot are called plantar warts. Unlike other warts, they can be painful because the pressure of walking pushes them into the foot.

Most warts eventually disappear without treatment. However, if you don't want to wait for this to happen, use one of the many preparations that are available. It's perfectly safe to treat warts with home remedies, except for those on the face or the genitals since the skin in these areas is too sensitive. Be sure to follow package directions carefully as these medications are irritating to the surrounding skin just as they are to the wart.

If you have what appears to be a rapidly growing wart or one that is not uniform in color, show it to a doctor as soon as possible as it may actually be a tumor that requires urgent treatment. Genital warts should be removed by a doctor.

WEIGHT REDUCTION—*See also Product Category Index (blue section) under Appetite Suppressants; Foods, Dietetic*

If you eat more food over an extended period of time than your body requires for producing energy, it will be stored as fat and you will become overweight. To curb the appetite or reduce the amount of food you eat, there are several classes of products that can help. Bulk formers make you feel full, so that you eat less. Glucose preparations raise your blood glucose levels and make you feel as though you don't need as much to eat. Artificial sweeteners give you that sweet taste without the calories of sugar. These and other products can be used as aids in a weight reduction plan.

Such a plan should rely mainly on a balanced, reduced-calorie diet and on increasing exercise. The body breaks down subcutaneous fat to provide the fuel that makes the muscles work. The best exercises are those that are enjoyable. Some people like to walk briskly, others jog or ride a bicycle, swim, or play games such as tennis, racquetball, etc. Vigorous exercise several times a week is good for the cardiovascular system, too.

WORMS—*See Your Physician*

Pinworms, which look like white threads, are very tiny worms that infest small children. They catch them by swallowing the worm's eggs in contaminated food or by touching the clothing or toys of a child who has worms. The eggs can also be acquired in a sandbox where an infected child has been playing.

Once inside the body, the eggs hatch. After about two weeks, adult females come out and lay their eggs during the night around the child's anus. This causes itching and when the child scratches, some eggs stick to the fingers. The next time the fingers go into the mouth, more eggs are swallowed.

The worms can often be seen in bowel movements or around the child's anus at night. If you see no worms but have reason to suspect their presence, put a strip of adhesive tape across the anus in the morning where eggs can stick to it. Give the tape to your doctor.

Because these worms are so contagious every member of the family can catch them. Careful handwashing and changing and washing sheets, pillow cases, and night things help prevent spread. The doctor can prescribe a drug that kills the parasites in the intestines.

Tapeworms get into the human body via pork or beef that hasn't been cooked sufficiently. The worm embeds its head in the wall of the intestine and starts to grow. Pieces of the worm break off from time to time and can be seen in bowel movements; they look like pieces of narrow white ribbon.

Symptoms of tapeworms include weight loss, some pain in the abdomen, loss of appetite, and irritation around the anus. Your doctor will do a microscopic examination of a stool sample and prescribe a medication that will kill the worm.

Guidelines for using drugs

Nonprescription or over-the-counter (OTC) drugs are available without a doctor's prescription. These drugs can be used safely and without medical supervision by most people as long as label directions are followed.

Label instructions provide very important information to the consumer. They tell how to use the product for best results and how to avoid misusing it. Many labels include warnings that: (1) suggest limits on the length of use; (2) discuss side effects; and (3) detail conditions that may require a physician's advice before taking the drug.

Following are a few specific suggestions for using nonprescription drugs.
1. Read the product label thoroughly each time you purchase a nonprescription drug. Watch for label "flags." They draw your attention to important changes in labeling information.

2. Become familiar with the ingredients in each product you take. If you take more than one medicine containing the same ingredient, you may be taking an overdose. If taking a prescription drug, ask the pharmacist whether the OTC product you have in mind can be taken at the same time.

3. Be aware of any nonprescription drugs you should not take. Make a list of those drugs you should avoid.

4. Follow label directions carefully. Never take a larger dose than directed on the package labeling, unless on the recommendation of your doctor or pharmacist.

5. Observe all warnings carefully especially as to drowsiness, dizziness, and drug interactions. Patients with certain conditions should consult with their physician or pharmacist before taking some nonprescription drugs. When in doubt, ask.

6. If your instructions are to take the medication once daily, you should take it at the same time each day. One suggestion is to try taking the medicine with a daily ritual, such as brushing your teeth. Certain drugs are best taken at certain times. Diuretics, for example, should be taken in the morning, unless your doctor directs you otherwise.
   If the medication is to be taken twice daily, take each dose 12 hours apart. Drugs prescribed for three times daily should be taken every 8 hours, unless otherwise directed. Certain medications should be taken with each meal. Be sure to read the label carefully or check with your pharmacist. If the instructions are "as needed," ask your pharmacist to specify how long you should wait between doses.

Consult your doctor or pharmacist if you feel uncomfortable with a drug you are taking, or if you experience any adverse reactions. Don't make decisions on drug use without the advice of these health professionals. Know the names of all medications you take, what they are for, and how you should take them. Don't hesitate to question your doctor or pharmacist about your medications.

SECTION 1
Manufacturers' Index

The manufacturers whose names appear in this index have provided information concerning their products in either the Product Information Section, Product Identification Section, or the Diagnostics, Devices and Medical Aids Section.

Included in this index are the names and addresses of manufacturers, individuals or departments to whom you may address inquiries, a partial list of products as well as emergency telephone numbers wherever available.

The symbol ◆ indicates that the product is shown in the Product Identification Section.

PAGE

ABBOTT LABORATORIES   **502**
For Medical Information
  Pharmaceutical Products Division
      (312) 937-7069
  Hospital Products Division
      (312) 937-3806
Order Entry/Customer Service Inquiries
  Pharmaceutical Products Division
      (800) 255-5162
  Hospital Products Division
      (800) 222-6883
OTC Products Available
Dayalets Filmtab
Dayalets Plus Iron Filmtab
Optilets-500 Filmtab
Optilets-M-500 Filmtab
Surbex
Surbex with C
Surbex-750 with Iron
Surbex-750 with Zinc
Surbex-T

ADRIA LABORATORIES   **403, 503**
Division of Erbamont Inc.
Administrative Offices
7001 Post Road
Dublin, OH 43017
Mailing Address
P.O. Box 16529
Columbus, OH 43216-6529

Address inquiries to:
Medical Dept.   (614) 764-8100
OTC Products Available
◆Emetrol
Evac-Q-Kit
Evac-Q-Kwik
◆Modane Plus Tablets
Modane Soft Capsules
◆Modane Tablets

Modane Versabran
Taloin Ointment
Xylo-Pfan

PAGE

ALLERGAN   **403, 504**
PHARMACEUTICALS
A Division of Allergan, Inc.
2525 Dupont Drive
Irvine, CA 92715
Address Inquiries to:
Product Information Services
      (800) 433-8871
      (714) 752-4500
For Medical Emergencies Contact:
Product Information Services
      (714) 752-4500
OTC Products Available
◆Celluvisc Lubricant Ophthalmic Solution
Lacril Lubricant Ophthalmic Solution
◆Lacri-Lube S.O.P.
Liquifilm Forte
◆Liquifilm Tears
◆Prefrin Liquifilm
◆Refresh Lubricant Ophthalmic Solution
◆Refresh P.M.
◆Relief Eye Drops for Red Eyes
◆Tears Plus Lubricant Ophthalmic
  Solution

B. F. ASCHER & COMPANY,   **403, 506**
INC.
15501 West 109th Street
Lenexa, KS 66219
Mailing Address: P.O. Box 717
Shawnee Mission, KS 66201-0717
Address inquiries to:
Joan F. Bowen   (913) 888-1880
For Medical Emergencies Contact:
Dan Henry
      (913) 888-1880

PAGE

OTC Products Available
◆Ayr Saline Nasal Drops
◆Ayr Saline Nasal Mist
◆Mobigesic Analgesic Tablets
◆Mobisyl Analgesic Creme
◆Pen•Kera Creme
  Soft 'N Soothe Anti-Itch Creme
◆Unilax Stool Softener/Laxative Softgel
  Capsules

ASTRA PHARMACEUTICAL   **403, 508**
PRODUCTS, INC.
50 Otis Street
Westboro, MA 01581-4428
Address inquiries to:
Roy E. Hayward, Jr.   (508) 366-1100
For Medical Emergencies Contact:
Dr. William Gray   (508) 366-1100
OTC Products Available
◆Xylocaine Ointment 2.5%

AU PHARMACEUTICALS   **508**
P.O. Box 811233
Dallas, TX 75381-1000
Address inquiries to:
Michael Vick   (800) 232-2246
For Medical Emergencies Contact
Rita Gates, PhD   (214) 340-1503
OTC Products Available
Aurum the Gold Lotion
TheraGold
Therapeutic Gold

AYERST LABORATORIES   **508**
Division of American Home Products
Corporation
685 Third Avenue
New York, NY 10017-4071
For information for Ayerst's consumer
products, see product listings under

    (◆ Shown in Product Identification Section)

Whitehall Laboratories.
Please turn to Whitehall Laboratories,
page 743.

BAKER CUMMINS **404, 508**
DERMATOLOGICALS, INC.
8800 NW 36th Street
Miami, FL 33178
Address inquiries to:
(305) 590-2200
For Medical Emergencies Contact:
Medical Dept. (305) 590-2200
OTC Products Available
Acno Cleanser
Acno Lotion
◆Aqua-A Cream
◆Aquaderm Therapeutic Cream
◆Aquaderm Therapeutic Lotion
◆P & S Liquid
◆P & S Plus Tar Gel
◆P & S Shampoo
Panscol Medicated Lotion and Ointment
Phacid Shampoo
Ultra Derm Bath Oil
Ultra Derm Moisturizer
Ultra Mide 25
◆X-Seb Shampoo
◆X-Seb Plus Conditioning Shampoo
◆X-Seb T Shampoo
◆X-Seb T Plus Conditioning Shampoo

BAKER CUMMINS **404, 511**
PHARMACEUTICALS, INC.
8800 NW 36th Street
Miami, FL 33178
Address inquiries to:
(305) 590-2200
For Medical Emergencies Contact:
Medical Dept. (305) 590-2200
OTC Products Available
◆Snaplets-D
◆Snaplets-DM
◆Snaplets-EX
◆Snaplets-FR
◆Snaplets-Multi

BAUSCH & LOMB **404, 512**
PERSONAL PRODUCTS
DIVISION
1400 North Goodman Street
Rochester, NY 14692-0450
OTC Products Available
◆Allergy Drops
◆Duolube Eye Ointment
◆Eye Wash
◆Moisture Drops

BEACH PHARMACEUTICALS **513**
Division of Beach Products, Inc.
Executive Office
5220 S. Manhattan Ave.
Tampa, FL 33611 (813) 839-6565
Manufacturing and Distribution
Main St. at Perimeter Rd.
Conestee, SC 29605
Toll Free 1-(800) 845-8210
Address inquiries to:
Victor De Oreo, R Ph, V.P., Sales
(803) 277-7282
Richard Stephen Jenkins, Exec. V.P.
(813) 839-6565
OTC Products Available
Beelith Tablets

BECTON DICKINSON CONSUMER **513**
PRODUCTS
One Becton Drive
Franklin Lakes, NJ 07417-1883
Address inquiries to:
Consumer Service (201) 848-6574
OTC Products Available
B-D Glucose Tablets

BEECHAM PRODUCTS
See SMITHKLINE BEECHAM
CONSUMER BRANDS

BEIERSDORF INC. **404, 514**
P.O. Box 5529
Norwalk, CT 06856-5529

Address inquiries to:
Medical Division (203) 853-8008
OTC Products Available
◆Aquaphor Healing Ointment
◆Basis Soap-Combination Skin
◆Basis Soap-Extra Dry Skin
◆Basis Soap-Normal to Dry Skin
◆Basis Soap-Oily Skin
◆Basis Soap-Sensitive Skin
◆Eucerin Moisturizing Cleansing Bar
◆Eucerin Moisturizing Creme
(Unscented)
◆Eucerin Moisturizing Lotion (Unscented)
Nivea Bath Silk Bath Oil
Nivea Bath Silk Bath & Shower Gel
(Extra-Dry Skin)
Nivea Bath Silk Bath & Shower Gel
(Normal-to-Dry Skin)
◆Nivea Moisturizing Creme
◆Nivea Moisturizing Lotion (Extra
Enriched)
◆Nivea Moisturizing Lotion (Original
Formula)
◆Nivea Moisturizing Oil
Nivea Sun After Sun Lotion
Nivea Sun SPF 15
Nivea Visage Creme
Nivea Visage Lotion

BENSON PHARMACAL COMPANY **517**
Division of American Victor Co., Inc.
431 Hempstead Avenue
West Hempstead, NY 11552
Address inquiries to:
Sami K. Moukaddem, RPh
(516) 486-5560
OTC Products Available
Altocaps-400 Capsules
Combi-Cap Capsules
Roygel 25 mg Capsules
Roygel 50 mg Capsules
Roygel 100 mg Capsules
Roygel Ultima Capsules
Toco-A-Benson Capsules
Vit "A" Capsules

BLAINE COMPANY, INC. **517**
2700 Dixie Highway
Fort Mitchell, KY 41017
Address inquiries to:
Mr. Alex M. Blaine (606) 341-9437
OTC Products Available
Mag-Ox 400
Uro-Mag

BLISTEX INC. **404, 517**
1800 Swift Drive
Oak Brook, IL 60521
(312) 571-2870
(800) 323-7343
Address inquiries to:
Vice President, Technical Services
For Medical Emergencies Contact:
Manager, Quality Control
OTC Products Available
Blistex Daily Conditioning Treatment for
Lips
Blistex Medicated Lip Ointment
Blistik Medicated Lip Balm
◆Dyprotex Diaper Rash Pads
Foille First Aid Liquid, Ointment &
Spray
Ivarest Medicated Cream & Lotion
Kank-a Medicated Formula
Lip Medex

BLOCK DRUG COMPANY, INC. **518**
257 Cornelison Avenue
Jersey City, NJ 07302
Address inquiries to:
Steve Gattanella (201) 434-3000
For Medical Emergencies Contact:
James Gingold (201) 434-3000
OTC Products Available
Arthritis Strength BC Powder
BC Powder
BC Cold Powder Multi-Symptom
Formula
BC Cold Powder Non-Drowsy Formula
Nytol Tablets
Promise Toothpaste
Mint Gel Sensodyne
Mint Sensodyne Toothpaste
Original Sensodyne Toothpaste

Tegrin for Psoriasis Lotion, Cream &
Soap
Tegrin Medicated Shampoo

BOEHRINGER INGELHEIM **404, 520**
PHARMACEUTICALS, INC.
90 East Ridge
P.O. Box 368
Ridgefield, CT 06877
Address inquiries to:
Medical Services Dept.
(203) 798-9988
OTC Products Available
◆Dulcolax Suppositories
◆Dulcolax Tablets
Nōstril Nasal Decongestant
Nōstrilla Long Acting Nasal
Decongestant

BOIRON-BORNEMAN, INC. **405, 522**
1208 Amosland Road
Norwood, PA 19074
Address inquiries to:
Robert Matsuk, R.Ph.
National Sales Manager
(215) 532-2035
For Medical Emergencies Contact:
Technical Services Department
(215) 532-2035
OTC Products Available
◆Oscillococcinum

BRISTOL LABORATORIES **522**
A Bristol-Myers Company
2400 W. Lloyd Expressway
Evansville, IN 47721
(812) 429-5000
OTC Products Available
Naldecon CX Adult Liquid
Naldecon DX Adult Liquid
Naldecon DX Children's Syrup
Naldecon DX Pediatric Drops
Naldecon EX Children's Syrup
Naldecon EX Pediatric Drops
Naldecon Senior DX Cough/Cold Liquid
Naldecon Senior EX Cough/Cold Liquid

BRISTOL-MYERS PRODUCTS **405, 525**
(Division of Bristol-Myers Company)
345 Park Avenue
New York, NY 10154
Address Product Inquiries to:
Products Division
Public Affairs Department
345 Park Avenue
New York, NY 10154
Address Medical Inquiries about
OTC Products to:
Department of Medical Services
1350 Liberty Avenue
Hillside, NJ 07207
In Emergencies Call:
(212) 546-4616 (9 AM-5 PM)
(212) 546-4700 (Other times)
OTC Products Available
Ammens Medicated Powder
B.Q. Cold Tablets
Ban Antiperspirant Cream Deodorant
Ban Basic Non-aerosol Antiperspirant
Spray
Ban Roll-On Antiperspirant
Ban Solid Antiperspirant Deodorant
◆Arthritis Strength Tri-Buffered Bufferin
Analgesic Caplets
◆Extra Strength Tri-Buffered Bufferin
Analgesic Tablets
◆Tri-Buffered Bufferin Analgesic Tablets
and Caplets
◆Allergy Sinus Comtrex Multi-Symptom
Allergy/Sinus Formula Tablets &
Caplets
Cough Formula Comtrex
◆Comtrex Multi-Symptom Cold Reliever
Tablets/Caplets/Liquid/Liquigels
◆Congespirin For Children Aspirin Free
Chewable Cold Tablets
◆Datril Extra-Strength Analgesic Tablets
& Caplets

(◆ Shown in Product Identification Section)

◆Excedrin Extra-Strength Analgesic
Tablets & Caplets
◆Excedrin P.M. Analgesic/Sleeping Aid
Tablets and Caplets
◆Sinus Excedrin Analgesic, Decongestant
Tablets & Caplets
◆4-Way Cold Tablets
◆4-Way Fast Acting Nasal Spray (regular
& mentholated) & Metered Spray
Pump (regular)
◆4-Way Long Lasting Nasal Spray &
Metered Spray Pump
Minit-Rub Analgesic Ointment
Mum Antiperspirant Cream Deodorant
◆No Doz Fast Acting Alertness Aid
Tablets
◆Nuprin Ibuprofen/Analgesic Tablets and
Caplets
◆Pazo Hemorrhoid Ointment &
Suppositories
◆Therapeutic Mineral Ice
Tickle Antiperspirant
Ultra Ban Aerosol Antiperspirant
Ultra Ban Roll-on Antiperspirant
Ultra Ban Solid
Antiperspirant/Deodorant

BURROUGHS WELLCOME CO. 406, 533
3030 Cornwallis Road
Research Triangle Park, NC 27709
(800) 722-9292
For Medical or Drug Information:
Contact Drug Information Service
Business hours only
(8:15 AM to 4:15 PM EST)
(800) 443-6763
For 24-hour Medical Emergency
Information, call (800) 443-6763
For Sales Information:
Contact Sales Distribution
Department
Address Other Inquiries to:
Consumer Products Division
Branch Office
Burlingame, CA 94010
1760 Rollins Road (415) 697-5630
OTC Products Available
Actidil Syrup
◆Actidil Tablets
◆Actifed Capsules
◆Actifed Plus Caplets
◆Actifed Plus Tablets
◆Actifed Syrup
◆Actifed Tablets
◆Actifed 12-Hour Capsules
◆AllerAct Decongestant Caplets
◆AllerAct Decongestant Tablets
◆AllerAct Tablets
Ammonia Aromatic, Vaporole
Borofax Ointment
◆Empirin Aspirin
Lubafax Surgical Lubricant, Sterile
◆Marezine Tablets
◆Neosporin Cream
◆Neosporin Ointment
◆Neosporin Maximum Strength Ointment
◆Polysporin Ointment
◆Polysporin Powder
◆Polysporin Spray
◆Sudafed Children's Liquid
◆Sudafed Cough Syrup
◆Sudafed Plus Liquid
◆Sudafed Plus Tablets
◆Sudafed Sinus Caplets
◆Sudafed Sinus Tablets
◆Sudafed Tablets, 30 mg
◆Sudafed Tablets, Adult Strength, 60
mg
◆Sudafed 12 Hour Capsules
Wellcome Lanoline

CAMPBELL LABORATORIES INC. 541
Address Inquiries to:
Richard C. Zahn, President
P.O. Box 812, FDR Station
New York, NY 10150-0812
(212) 688-7684
OTC Products Available
Herpecin-L Cold Sore Lip Balm

CARNATION NUTRITIONAL PRODUCTS 408, 541
5045 Wilshire Boulevard
Los Angeles, CA 90036
Address inquiries to:
Steve Witherly, PhD (213) 932-6125
For Medical Emergencies Contact:
Russell Merritt, MD (213) 932-6659
OTC Products Available
Follow-Up Formula
◆Good Start

CHATTEM INC., CONSUMER PRODUCTS DIVISION 542
Division of Chattem, Inc.
1715 West 38th Street
Chattanooga, TN 37409
Address Inquiries to:
David Robb (615) 821-4571
For Medical Emergencies Contact:
Walt Ludwig (615) 821-4571
OTC Products Available
Black-Draught Granulated
Black-Draught Lax-Senna Tablets
Black-Draught Syrup
Blis-To-Sol Liquid
Blis-To-Sol Powder
Flex-all 454 Pain Relieving Gel
Norwich Extra-Strength Aspirin
Norwich Regular Strength Aspirin
Nullo Deodorant Tablets
Pamprin Multi-Symptom Extra-Strength
Pain Relief Formula Tablets
Pamprin Maximum Cramp Relief
Formula Tablets, Caplets & Capsules
Pamprin-IB
Prēmsyn PMS Capsules & Caplets
Soltice Quick-Rub

CHURCH & DWIGHT CO., INC. 407, 543
469 North Harrison Street
Princeton, NJ 08540
Address inquiries to:
Mr. Stephen Lajoie (609) 683-5900
For Medical Emergencies Contact:
Mr. Stephen Lajoie (609) 683-5900
OTC Products Available
Arm & Hammer Pure Baking Soda
◆OTIX Drops Ear Wax Removal Aid

CIBA CONSUMER PHARMACEUTICALS 408, 544
Division of CIBA-GEIGY Corporation
Raritan Plaza III
Edison, NJ 08837
Address inquiries to:
(201) 906-6000
For Medical Emergencies Contact:
(201) 277-5000
OTC Products Available
◆Acutrim 16 Hour Appetite Suppressant
◆Acutrim Late Day Appetite Suppressant
◆Acutrim II Maximum Strength Appetite
Suppressant
◆Doan's - Extra-Strength Analgesic
◆Doan's - Regular Strength Analgesic
Fiberall Chewable Tablets, Lemon
Creme Flavor
◆Fiberall Fiber Wafers - Fruit & Nut
◆Fiberall Fiber Wafers - Oatmeal Raisin
◆Fiberall Powder Natural Flavor
◆Fiberall Powder Orange Flavor
◆Nupercainal Cream and Ointment
◆Nupercainal Pain Relief Cream
◆Nupercainal Suppositories
◆Otrivin Nasal Spray & Nasal Drops
◆Otrivin Pediatric Nasal Drops
◆Privine Nasal Solution
◆Privine Nasal Spray
◆Q-vel Muscle Relaxant Pain Reliever
◆Slow Fe Tablets
◆Sunkist Children's Chewable
Multivitamins - Complete
◆Sunkist Children's Chewable
Multivitamins - Plus Extra C
◆Sunkist Children's Chewable
Multivitamins - Plus Iron
◆Sunkist Children's Chewable
Multivitamins - Regular
◆Sunkist Vitamin C - Chewable
◆Sunkist Vitamin C - Easy to Swallow

COLGATE-PALMOLIVE COMPANY 409, 549
A Delaware Corporation
300 Park Avenue
New York, NY 10022
Address inquiries to:
Consumers:
Consumer Affairs
300 Park Avenue
New York, NY 10022
(212) 310-2000
Physicians:
Medical Director
909 River Road
Piscataway, NJ 08854
(201) 878-7500
For Medical Emergencies Contact:
9 AM to 5 PM (201) 878-7500
5 PM to 9 AM (201) 547-2500
OTC Products Available
Colgate Dental Cream
◆Colgate Junior Fluoride Gel Toothpaste
◆Colgate MFP Fluoride Gel
◆Colgate MFP Fluoride Toothpaste
◆Colgate Mouthwash Tartar Control
Formula
◆Colgate Tartar Control Formula
◆Colgate Tartar Control Gel
Colgate Toothbrushes
Curad Bandages
Dermassage Dish Liquid
◆Fluorigard Anti-Cavity Fluoride Rinse
Mersene Denture Cleanser
Ultra Brite Toothpaste

COLUMBIA LABORATORIES, INC. 408, 550
16400 N.W. 2nd Avenue
Miami, FL 33169
Address inquiries to:
Professional Services Dept.
(305) 944-3666
For Medical Emergencies Contact
(305) 944-3666
OTC Products Available
◆Replens

COMMERCE DRUG COMPANY, INC. 550
Division Del Laboratories, Inc.
565 Broad Hollow Road
Farmingdale, NY 11735
Address inquiries to:
Donna Coughlin
Regulatory Manager
(516) 293-7070, Ext. 3275
For Medical Emergencies Contact:
Harry Gordon, Ph.D.
(516) 293-7070, Ext. 2068
Donna Coughlin
(516) 293-7070, Ext. 3275
OTC Products Available
Boil•Ease
Dermarest
Diaper Guard
Off•Easy Wart Removal Kit
Baby Orajel
Baby Orajel Nighttime Formula
Orajel Maximum Strength
Orajel Mouth-Aid
Pronto Lice Killing Shampoo Kit
Pronto Lice Killing Spray
Propa pH Cleanser for
Normal/Combination Skin
Propa pH Cleanser for Sensitive Skin
Stye Ophthalmic Ointment
Tanac Liquid
Tanac Roll-on
Tanac Stick

CUMBERLAND-SWAN, INC. 409, 553
Corporate Headquarters:
Cumberland-Swan, Inc.
One Swan Drive
Smyrna, TN 37167
(615) 459-8900
Watts: (800) 251-3068
Address inquiries to:
Vice President, Regulatory Affairs
Vice President of Marketing
Regional Sales Office
Cumberland-Swan, Inc., West Coast
9817 7th Street
Rancho, Cucamonga, CA 91730

(◆ Shown in Product Identification Section)

(714) 980-5522
Watts: (800) 624-9137
OTC Products Available
Swan Acetaminophen Tablets, Caplets
Swan Antacids
Swan Aspirin Tablets, Coated Tablets,
Caplets
Swan Calamine Lotion
◆Swan Citroma (Citrate of Magnesia)
Swan Cough/Cold/Allergy Preparations
Swan Epsom Salt
Swan Hydrogen Peroxide Solution (3%)
Swan Ibuprofen Coated Tablets, Caplets
Swan Isopropyl and Ethyl Rubbing
Alcohol
Swan Milk of Magnesia
Swan Mineral Oil

"ESPECIALLY" PRODUCTS INC. 554
4300 Via Dolce, #202
Marina Del Rey, CA 90292
Address inquiries to:
P.O. Box 4577
Playa Del Rey, CA 90296
(213) 823-2873
For Medical Emergencies Contact:
Marilynn Pratt, MD
(213) 823-2873
OTC Products Available
Crème de la Femme

FISONS CONSUMER 409, 554
HEALTH GROUP
Fisons Pharmaceuticals
P.O. Box 1212
Rochester, NY 14603
Address inquiries to:
Product Service Department
P.O. Box 1212
Rochester, NY 14603
(716) 475-9000
FAX (716) 383-1637
For Medical Emergencies Contact
Fisons Pharmaceuticals
(716) 475-9000
OTC Products Available
◆Allerest Allergy Tablets
Allerest Children's Chewable Tablets
Allerest Eye Drops
Allerest Headache Strength Tablets
Allerest 12 Hour Caplets
Allerest 12 Hour Nasal Spray
◆Allerest No Drowsiness Tablets
Allerest Sinus Pain Formula
◆Americaine Hemorrhoidal Ointment
◆Americaine Topical Anesthetic Ointment
◆Americaine Topical Anesthetic Spray
Bacid Capsules
◆CaldeCORT Anti-Itch Hydrocortisone
Cream
◆CaldeCORT Anti-Itch Hydrocortisone
Spray
◆CaldeCORT Light Cream
◆Caldesene Medicated Ointment
◆Caldesene Medicated Powder
Cholan HMB
◆Cruex Antifungal Powder, Spray Powder
& Cream
◆Desenex Antifungal Cream
Desenex Antifungal Foam
◆Desenex Antifungal Liquid
◆Desenex Antifungal Ointment
◆Desenex Antifungal Powder
◆Desenex Antifungal Spray Powder
◆Desenex Foot & Sneaker Deodorant
Spray
Desenex Soap
Emul-O-Balm
Isoclor Liquid and Tablets
Isoclor Timesule Capsules
Kondremul
Neo-Cultol
Sinarest Nasal Spray
Sinarest No Drowsiness Tablets
Sinarest Tablets & Extra Strength
Tablets
◆Ting Antifungal Cream
◆Ting Antifungal Powder
◆Ting Antifungal Spray Liquid
◆Ting Antifungal Spray Powder

Vaponefrin
Vitron-C and Vitron-C Plus
FLEMING & COMPANY 557
1600 Fenpark Dr.
Fenton, MO 63026
Address inquiries to:
John J. Roth, M.D. (314) 343-8200
For Medical Emergencies Contact:
John R. Roth, M.D. (314) 343-8200
OTC Products Available
Chlor-3 Condiment
Impregon Concentrate
Magonate Tablets and Liquid
Marblen Suspension Peach/Apricot
Marblen Suspension Unflavored
Marblen Tablets
Nephrox Suspension
Nicotinex Elixir
Ocean Nasal Mist
Ocean-A/S Nasal Spray
Ocean-Plus Mist
Purge Concentrate

GLENBROOK 410, 558
LABORATORIES
Division of Sterling Drug Inc.
90 Park Avenue
New York, NY 10016
Address inquiries to:
Medical Director (212) 907-2764
OTC Products Available
◆Children's Bayer Chewable Aspirin
◆Bayer Children's Cold Tablets
◆Bayer Children's Cough Syrup
◆Genuine Bayer Aspirin Tablets &
Caplets
◆Maximum Bayer Aspirin Tablets &
Caplets
◆Therapy Bayer Aspirin Caplets
◆8 Hour Bayer Timed-Release Aspirin
◆Haley's M-O, Regular & Flavored
◆Midol 200 Advanced Pain Formula
◆Maximum Strength Midol
Multi-Symptom Formula
◆Maximum Strength Midol PMS
Premenstrual Syndrome Formula
◆Regular Strength Midol Multi-Symptom
Formula
◆Children's Panadol Chewable Tablets,
Liquid, Infants' Drops
◆Junior Strength Panadol
◆Maximum Strength Panadol Tablets
and Caplets
◆Phillips' LaxCaps
◆Phillips' Milk of Magnesia Liquid
◆Phillips' Milk of Magnesia Tablets
◆Stri-Dex Maximum Strength Pads
◆Stri-Dex Regular Strength Pads
◆Vanquish Analgesic Caplets

GOLDLINE LABORATORIES 567
THE WELLSPRING DIVISION
1900 West Commercial Blvd.
Ft. Lauderdale, FL 33309-3018
OTC Product Available
Nose Better Nasal Gel
Nose Better Nasal Spray

HERALD PHARMACAL, INC. 567
6503 Warwick Road
Richmond, VA 23225
Address inquiries to:
Henry H. Kamps
(804) 745-3400
For Medical Emergencies Contact:
Henry H. Kamps
(804) 745-3400
OTC Products Available
Aqua Glycolic Lotion
Aqua Glycolic Shampoo
Aqua Glyde Cleanser
Aquaray 20 Sunscreen
Cam Lotion

HERBERT LABORATORIES 567
2525 Dupont Drive
Irvine, CA 92715
Address inquiries to:
Product Information Services
(714) 955-6200
For Medical Emergencies Contact:
Product Information Services
(714) 955-6200

OTC Products Available
AquaTar Therapeutic Tar Gel
Bluboro Powder Astringent Soaking
Solution
Danex Protein Enriched Dandruff
Shampoo
Photoplex Broad Spectrum Sunscreen
Lotion
Vanseb Cream and Lotion Dandruff
Shampoos
Vanseb-T Cream and Lotion Tar
Dandruff Shampoos

HOECHST-ROUSSEL 411, 568
PHARMACEUTICALS INC.
Routes 202-206
P.O. Box 2500
Somerville, NJ 08876-1258
Address medical inquiries to:
Scientific Services Dept.
(800) 445-4774
(8:30 AM-5:00 PM EST)
For medical emergency information
only, after hours and on weekends,
call: (201) 231-2000
OTC Products Available
◆Doxidan Liquigels
◆Festal II Digestive Aid
◆Surfak Liquigels

HYGEIA SCIENCES, INC. 411, 771
Newton, MA 02160
OTC Products Available
◆First Response Ovulation Predictor Test
◆First Response Pregnancy Test

ICN PHARMACEUTICALS, 411, 569
INC.
ICN Plaza
3300 Hyland Avenue
Costa Mesa, CA 92626
Address inquiries to:
Karen Chapman
Professional Service Dept.
(714) 545-0100
For Medical Emergencies Contact:
Medical Department
(800) 548-5100
OTC Products Available
◆Insta-Glucose

INTER-CAL CORPORATION 569
421 Miller Valley Road
Prescott, AZ 86301
Address inquiries to:
Gerald W. Elders (602) 445-8063
OTC Products Available
Ester-C Tablets

JACKSON-MITCHELL 570
PHARMACEUTICALS, INC.
1485 East Valley Road, Suite C
P.O. Box 5425
Santa Barbara, CA 93108
Address inquiries to:
Carol Jackson (805) 565-1538
For Medical Emergencies Contact:
Carol Jackson (805) 565-1538
Branch Offices
Turlock, CA 95380
P.O. Box 934 (209) 667-2019
OTC Products Available
Meyenberg Evaporated Goat Milk - 12
1/2 fl. oz.
Meyenberg Powdered Goat Milk - 4 oz.
& 14 oz.

JOHNSON & JOHNSON 411, 570
CONSUMER PRODUCTS,
INC.
Grandview Road
Skillman, NJ 08558
Address inquiries to:
(800) 526-3967
For Medical Emergencies Contact:
(800) 526-3967
OTC Products Available
Johnson & Johnson First Aid Cream
◆JOHNSON'S Baby Sunblock Cream
(SPF 15)
◆JOHNSON'S Baby Sunblock Lotion
(SPF 15)
◆JOHNSON'S Baby Sunblock Lotion
(SPF 30+)
K-Y Brand Lubricating Jelly

PURPOSE Dual Treatment Moisturizer (SPF 12)
PURPOSE Soap
◆SUNDOWN Sunblock Combi Pack, Ultra Protection (SPF 15)
SUNDOWN Sunblock Cream, Ultra Protection (SPF 15)
◆SUNDOWN Sunblock Stick, Ultra Protection (SPF 15)
SUNDOWN Sunblock Stick, Ultra Protection (SPF 30+)
SUNDOWN Sunscreen Lotions Maximal Protection (SPF 8)
◆ Ultra Protection Sunblock (SPF 15)
Ultra Protection Sunblock (SPF 20)
Ultra Protection Sunblock (SPF 25)
Ultra Protection Sunblock (SPF 30+)

KREMERS URBAN COMPANY
See SCHWARZ PHARMA

LACTAID INC. 411, 571
P.O. Box 111
Fire Road and Lister Lane
Pleasantville, NJ 08232-0111
Address inquiries to:
Alan E. Kligerman (609) 653-6100
(800) 257-8650
Canada (800) 387-5711
OTC Products Available
◆Lactaid Caplets
◆Lactaid Drops

LAKESIDE 412, 572
PHARMACEUTICALS
Division of Merrell Dow
Pharmaceuticals Inc.
Cincinnati, OH 45242-9553
(513) 948-9111
Address inquiries to:
Professional Information Department
Business hours only
(8:15 AM to 5:00 PM EST)
(800) 552-3656
For Medical Emergency Information
Only after hours or on weekends
(513) 948-9111
OTC Products Available
◆Cēpacol Anesthetic Lozenges (Troches)
◆Cēpacol/Cēpacol Mint Mouthwash/Gargle
◆Cēpacol Throat Lozenges
◆CĒPASTAT Cherry Flavor Sore Throat Lozenges
◆CĒPASTAT Sore Throat Lozenges
◆Citrucel Orange Flavor
◆Citrucel Regular Flavor
◆Novahistine DMX
◆Novahistine Elixir
Simron Capsules
Simron Plus Capsules
Singlet Tablets

LAVOPTIK COMPANY, INC. 576, 771
661 Western Avenue North
St. Paul, MN 55103
Address inquiries to:
661 Western Avenue North
St. Paul, MN 55103 (612) 489-1351
For Medical Emergencies Contact:
B. C. Brainard (612) 489-1351
OTC Products Available
Lavoptik Eye Cup
Lavoptik Eye Wash

LEDERLE LABORATORIES 412, 576
Division of American Cyanamid Co.
One Cyanamid Plaza
Wayne, NJ 07470
Address inquiries on medical matters to:
Professional Services Dept.
Lederle Laboratories
Pearl River, NY 10965
8 AM to 4:30 PM EST
(914) 735-2815
All other inquiries and after hours emergencies
(914) 732-5000
Distribution Centers
ATLANTA
Contact EASTERN (Philadelphia)
Distribution Center

CHICAGO
Bulk Address
1100 East Business Center Drive
Mt. Prospect, IL 60056
Mail Address
P.O. Box 7614
Mt. Prospect, IL 60056-7614
(800) 533-3753
DALLAS (312) 827-8871
Bulk Address
7611 Carpenter Freeway
Dallas, TX 75247
Mail Address
P.O. Box 655731
Dallas, TX 75265 (800) 533-3753
(214) 631-2130
LOS ANGELES
Bulk Address
2300 S. Eastern Ave.
Los Angeles, CA 90040
Mail Address
T.A. Box 2202
Los Angeles, CA 90051
(800) 533-3753
(213) 726-1016
EASTERN (Philadelphia)
Bulk Address
202 Precision Drive
Horsham, PA 19044
Mail Address
P.O. Box 933
Horsham, PA 19044 (800) 533-3753
(215) 672-5400
OTC Products Available
Acetaminophen Capsules, Tablets, Elixir, Liquid
Aureomycin Ointment 3%
◆Caltrate 600
◆Caltrate 600 + Iron
◆Caltrate, Jr.
◆Caltrate 600 + Vitamin D
◆Centrum
◆Centrum, Jr. (Children's Chewable) + Extra C
◆Centrum, Jr. (Children's Chewable) + Extra Calcium
◆Centrum, Jr. (Children's Chewable) + Iron
Docusate Sodium (DSS) USP Capsules, Syrup
Docusate Sodium (DSS) w/Casanthranol Capsules, Syrup
◆Ferro-Sequels
Ferrous Gluconate Iron Supplement
Ferrous Sulfate
◆FiberCon
Filibon Prenatal Vitamin Tablets
Gevrabon Liquid
Gevral Protein Powder
Gevral T Tablets
Gevral Tablets
Guaifenesin w/D-Methorphan Hydrobromide Syrup
Guaifenesin Syrup
Incremin w/Iron Syrup
Lederplex Capsules and Liquid
Neoloid Emulsified Castor Oil
Peritinic Tablets
Pseudoephedrine HCl Syrup & Tablets
Quinine Capsules
Stresscaps Capsules
◆Stresstabs
◆Stresstabs + Iron, Advanced Formula
◆Stresstabs + Zinc
Triprolidine HCl with Pseudoephedrine HCl Syrup & Tablets
◆Zincon Dandruff Shampoo

LEEMING DIVISION 413, 583
Pfizer Inc.
100 Jefferson Rd.
Parsippany, NJ 07054
Address inquiries to:
Research and Development Dept.
(201) 887-2100
OTC Products Available
Ben-Gay External Analgesic Products
Bonine Tablets
◆Desitin Ointment
RID Lice Control Spray
RID Lice Killing Shampoo

Rheaban Maximum Strength Tablets
Unisom Dual Relief Nighttime Sleep Aid/Analgesic
Unisom Nighttime Sleep Aid
◆Visine A.C. Eye Drops
◆Visine Extra Eye Drops
◆Visine Eye Drops
◆Visine L.R. Eye Drops
Wart-Off Wart Remover

LEHN & FINK 413, 587
Division of Sterling Drug Inc.
Personal Products Division
225 Summit Avenue
Montvale, NJ 07645
Address inquiries to:
(201) 573-5700
OTC Products Available
◆Diaparene Baby Powder
◆Diaparene Cradol
◆Diaparene Medicated Cream
◆Diaparene Peri-Anal Medicated Ointment
Diaparene Supers Baby Wash Cloths

LIFESCAN INC. 771
1051 South Milpitas Blvd.
Milpitas, CA 95035
For the name of your local representative, call toll-free:
In the US: (800) 227-8862
In Canada: (800) 663-5521
OTC Products Available
One Touch Blood Glucose Monitoring System

LOMA LINDA FOODS INC. 588
Address inquiries to:
Marketing Office
11503 Pierce Street
Riverside, CA 92505 (714) 687-7800
(800) 932-5525
CA only (800) 442-4917
OTC Products Available
I-Soyalac: Liquid Concentrate and Ready-to-Use
Soyalac: Liquid Concentrate, Ready-to-Use and Powder

LUYTIES PHARMACAL COMPANY 589
P. O. Box 8080
St. Louis, MO 63156
Address Inquiries to:
Customer Service (800) 325-8080
OTC Products Available
Yellolax

MACSIL, INC. 589
1326 Frankford Avenue
Philadelphia, PA 19125
(215) 739-7300
OTC Products Available
Balmex Baby Powder
Balmex Emollient Lotion
Balmex Ointment

MARION LABORATORIES, 413, 590
INC.
Pharmaceutical Products Division
Marion Industrial Park
Marion Park Drive
Kansas City, MO 64137
Address inquiries to:
Product Surveillance Dept.
P.O. Box 9627
Kansas City, MO 64134
(816) 966-5000
OTC Products Available
◆Debrox Drops
◆Gaviscon Antacid Tablets
◆Gaviscon-2 Antacid Tablets
◆Gaviscon Extra Strength Relief Formula Liquid Antacid
◆Gaviscon Extra Strength Relief Formula Antacid Tablets
◆Gaviscon Liquid Antacid
◆Gly-Oxide Liquid
◆Os-Cal 500 Chewable Tablets
◆Os-Cal 250+D Tablets
◆Os-Cal 500+D Tablets
◆Os-Cal Fortified Tablets
◆Os-Cal Plus Tablets
◆Os-Cal 500 Tablets
◆Throat Discs Throat Lozenges

(◆ Shown in Product Identification Section)

MARLYN HEALTH CARE   **593**
6324 Ferris Square
San Diego, CA 92121
                              (800) 462-7596
OTC Products Available
4-Hair
4-Nails
Hep-Forte Capsules
Marlyn Formula 50
Marlyn Formula 50 Mega Forte
Marlyn PMS
Osteo Fem
Pro-Skin-E (Face Capsule)
Pro-Skin Nutribloxx

McNEIL CONSUMER   **414, 593**
PRODUCTS CO.
Division of McNeil-PPC, Inc.
Camp Hill Road
Fort Washington, PA 19034
                              (215) 233-7000
Address inquiries to:
Consumer Affairs Department
Fort Washington, PA 19034
Manufacturing Divisions
Fort Washington, PA 19034
Southwest Manufacturing Plant
4001 N. I-35
Round Rock, TX 78664
OTC Products Available
◆Imodium A-D Caplets and Liquid
◆Medipren ibuprofen Caplets and
   Tablets
◆Pediacare Cold Formula Liquid
◆Pediacare Cough-Cold Formula Liquid
   and Chewable Tablets
◆Pediacare Infants' Oral Decongestant
   Drops
◆Pediacare Night Rest Cough-Cold
   Formula Liquid
◆Sine-Aid Maximum Strength Sinus
   Headache Caplets
◆Sine-Aid Maximum Strength Sinus
   Headache Tablets
◆Tylenol acetaminophen Children's
   Chewable Tablets & Elixir
◆Tylenol Allergy Sinus Medication
   Caplets, Maximum Strength
◆Children's Tylenol Cold Liquid Formula
   and Chewable Cold Tablets
◆Tylenol Cold Medication Caplets and
   Tablets
◆Tylenol Cold Medication Liquid
◆Tylenol Cold Medication No Drowsiness
   Formula Caplets
   Tylenol, Extra-Strength, acetaminophen
   Adult Liquid Pain Reliever
◆Tylenol, Extra-Strength, acetaminophen
   Caplets, Gelcaps, Tablets
◆Tylenol, Infants' Drops
◆Tylenol, Junior Strength,
   acetaminophen Coated Caplets
◆Tylenol, Maximum Strength, Sinus
   Medication Tablets and Caplets
◆Tylenol, Regular Strength,
   acetaminophen Tablets and Caplets

MEAD JOHNSON NUTRITIONALS   **605**
A Bristol-Myers Company
2400 W. Lloyd Expressway
Evansville, IN 47721
                              (812) 429-5000
Address inquiries to:
Scientific Information Section
Medical Department
OTC Products Available
Enfamil Full-Year Formula
Enfamil With Iron Full-Year Formula
Enfamil Full-Year Formula Nursette
HIST 1
HIST 2
HOM 1
HOM 2
LYS 1
LYS 2
Lofenalac
Low Methionine Diet Powder (Product
   3200 K)
Low PHE-TYR Diet Powder (Product
   3200 AB)
Lytren Oral Electrolyte Solution
MSUD Diet Powder
MSUD 1

MSUD 2
Moducal
Mono- and Disaccharide-Free Diet
   Powder (Product 3232 A)
Nutramigen Protein Hydrolysate
   Formula
OS 1
OS 2
PKU 1
PKU 2
PKU 3
Phenyl-Free
Pregestimil
ProSobee Soy Isolate Formula
ProSobee Soy Isolate Formula Nursette
Protein-Free Diet Powder (Product
   80056)
TYR 1
TYR 2
UCD 1
UCD 2

MEAD JOHNSON   **416, 605**
PHARMACEUTICALS
A Bristol-Myers Comapny
2400 W. Lloyd Expressway
Evansville, IN 47721-0001
                              (812) 429-5000
Address Inquiries to:
Scientific Information Section
   Medical Department
OTC Products Available
◆Colace
◆Peri-Colace

MEDICONE COMPANY   **416, 606**
225 Varick St.
New York, NY 10014
Address inquiries to:
Medical Director   (212) 924-5166
OTC Products Available
◆Medicone Derma Ointment
◆Medicone Dressing Cream
◆Medicone Rectal Ointment
◆Medicone Rectal Suppositories
◆Mediconet Cleansing Cloths

MERICON INDUSTRIES, INC.   **607**
8819 North Pioneer Rd.
Peoria, IL 61615
Address inquiries to:
Thomas P. Morrissey (800) 242-6464
   In IL Collect (309) 693-2150
OTC Products Available
Delacort
Orazinc Capsules
Orazinc Lozenges

MILES INC.   **416, 607**
CONSUMER HEALTHCARE
DIVISION
1127 Myrtle Street
Elkhart, IN 46514
Address inquiries to:
Manager, Consumer Affairs Dept.
                              (219) 264-8955
OTC Products Available
◆Alka-Mints Chewable Antacid
◆Alka-Seltzer Advanced Formula Antacid
   & Non-Aspirin Pain Reliever
◆Alka-Seltzer Effervescent Antacid
◆Alka-Seltzer Effervescent Antacid and
   Pain Reliever
◆Alka-Seltzer Extra Strength
   Effervescent Antacid and Pain
   Reliever
◆Alka-Seltzer (Flavored) Effervescent
   Antacid and Pain Reliever
◆Alka-Seltzer Plus Cold Medicine
◆Alka-Seltzer Plus Night-Time Cold
   Medicine
◆Bactine Antiseptic/Anesthetic First Aid
   Spray
◆Bactine First Aid Antibiotic Ointment
◆Bactine Hydrocortisone Skin Care
   Cream
◆Biocal 500 mg Tablet Calcium
   Supplement

◆Bugs Bunny Children's Chewable
   Vitamins + Minerals with Iron and
   Calcium (Sugar Free)
◆Bugs Bunny Children's Chewable
   Vitamins (Sugar Free)
◆Bugs Bunny With Extra C Children's
   Chewable Vitamins (Sugar Free)
◆Bugs Bunny Plus Iron Children's
   Chewable Vitamins (Sugar Free)
◆Flintstones Children's Chewable
   Vitamins
◆Flintstones Children's Chewable
   Vitamins With Extra C
◆Flintstones Children's Chewable
   Vitamins Plus Iron
◆Flintstones Complete With Calcium, Iron
   & Minerals Children's Chewable
   Vitamins
◆Miles Nervine Nighttime Sleep-Aid
◆One-A-Day Essential Vitamins
◆One-A-Day Maximum Formula Vitamins
   and Minerals
◆One-A-Day Plus Extra C Vitamins
◆Stressgard Stress Formula Vitamins
◆Within Multivitamin for Women with
   Calcium, Extra Iron and Zinc

MORE DIRECT HEALTH   **614**
PRODUCTS
6351-E Yarrow Drive
Carlsbad, CA 92009
Address inquiries to:
                              (619) 438-1935
For Medical Emergencies Contact:
                              (619) 438-1935
OTC Products Available
CigArrest Tablets

MURDOCK   **417, 615**
PHARMACEUTICALS, INC.
1400 Mountain Springs Park
Springville, UT 84663
Address inquiries to:
Shawna D. Otte   (801) 489-3631
For Medical Emergencies Contact:
Michael D. Corrigan (801) 489-3631
OTC Products Available
◆Lactase
◆SinuStat Nasal Decongestant

MURO PHARMACEUTICAL, INC.   **615**
890 East Street
Tewksbury, MA 01876-9987
Address inquiries to:
Professional Service Dept.
                              (800) 225-0974
                              (508) 851-5981
OTC Products Available
Bromfed Syrup
Salinex Nasal Mist and Drops

NATREN, INC.   **616**
3105 Willow Lane
Westlake Village, CA 91361
Address inquiries to:
                    Toll-Free (800) 992-3323
                    CA Only (800) 992-9393
OTC Products Available
Bifido Factor (Bifidobacterium bifidum)
Bulgaricum I.B. (L. Bulgaricus)
Life Start (Bifidobacterium infantis)
M.F.A. (Milk Free Acidophilus)
Superdophilus (L. acidophilus)

NATURE'S BOUNTY, INC.   **418, 616**
90 Orville Drive
Bohemia, NY 11716
Address inquiries to:
Professional Service Dept.
                              (516) 567-9500
                              (800) 645-5412
OTC Products Available
ABC to Z
Acidophilus
B-Complex +C (Long Acting) Tablets
B-6 50 mg., 100 mg., 200 mg.
B-12 & B-12 Sublingual Tablets
B-50 Tablets
B-100 Tablets-Ultra B Complex
Beta-Carotene Capsules
Bounty Bears (Children's Chewables)

(◆ Shown in Product Identification Section)

Bounty Bears with Iron (Children's Chewables)
C-500 mg., C-1000 mg., C-1500 mg. & Time Release Formulas
CRP Cholesterol Reducing Plan
Calciday-667 Tablets
Calmtabs Tablets
Cod Liver Oil
E-400 (Natural d-alpha)
E-Oil
◆Ener-B Vitamin B$_{12}$ Nasal Gel Dietary Supplement
Garlic Oil 15 gr. & 77 gr.
KLB6 Capsules
KLB6 Complete Tablets
KLB6 Grapefruit Diet
l-Lysine 500 mg. Tablets
Lecithin 1200 mg. Capsules
M-KYA
Nature's Bounty 1 Tablets
Nature's Bounty Slim Quick
Niacin 500 mg.
Oat Bran 850 mg.
Oyster Calcium Tablets
Oystercal-500
Oystercal-D 250
Potassium Tabs
Slim with Fiber
Stress "1000" Tablets
l-Tryptophan (200 mg. & 667 mg.)
Ultra Vita-Time Tablets
Vitamin A 10,000 I.U. & 25,000 I.U.
Vitamin C with Rose Hips
Vitamin E (d-alpha tocopheryl)
Water Pill (Natural Diuretic)
Water Pill with Potassium (Natural Diuretic)
Zacne Tablets
Zinc 10 mg., 25 mg., 50 mg. Tablets

NEUTROGENA   **418, 616**
CORPOPRATION
5760 West 96th Street
Los Angeles, CA 90045
Address inquiries to:
Mitchell S. Wortzman (213) 642-1150
For Medical Emergencies Contact:
Mitchell S. Wortzman
9:00AM to 5PM-PCT (213) 642-1150
After Hours (213) 670-8421
OTC Products Available
◆Neutrogena Cleansing Wash
◆Neutrogena Moisture
◆Neutrogena Moisture SPF 15 Untinted
◆Neutrogena Moisture SPF 15 with Sheer Tint
◆Neutrogena Sunblock

NEW LIFE HEALTH   **420, 617**
PRODUCTS CORP.
P. O. Box 9157
Morris Plains, NJ 07950-9157
Address inquiries to:
Dr. Michael S. Fey
(201) 989-7500
24 Hour FAX (201) 989-7911
OTC Products Available
◆New Life Smoking Deterrent Lozenges

NORCLIFF THAYER INC.
See SMITHKLINE BEECHAM
CONSUMER BRANDS

NOXELL CORPORATION   **418, 617**
11050 York Road
Hunt Valley MD 21030-2098
For Medical Emergencies Contact:
Edward M. Jackson, Ph.D.
(301) 785-4397
OTC Products Available
◆Noxzema Antiseptic Skin Cleanser-Extra Strength Formula
◆Noxzema Antiseptic Skin Cleanser-Regular Formula
◆Noxzema Antiseptic Skin Cleanser-Sensitive Skin Formula
◆Noxzema Clear-Ups Anti-Acne Gel

◆Noxzema Clear-Ups Maximum Strength Lotion, Vanishing
◆Noxzema Clear-Ups Medicated Pads-Maximum Strength 2.0% Salicylic Acid
◆Noxzema Clear-Ups Medicated Pads-Regular Strength 0.5% Salicyclic Acid
◆Noxzema Clear-Ups On-the-Spot Treatment, Tinted & Vanishing
Noxzema Clear-Ups Peel-Off Mask
Noxzema Medicated Shave Cream
◆Noxzema Medicated Skin Cream

NUAGE LABORATORIES, LTD.   **619**
4200 Laclede Avenue
St. Louis, MO 63108
Address inquiries to:
Customer Service   (314) 533-9600
OTC Products Available
Biochemic Tissue Salts
Bioplasma
Calcium Fluoride
Calcium Phosphate
Calcium Sulfate
Ferrous Phosphate
Magnesium Phosphate
Potassium Chloride
Potassium Phosphate
Potassium Sulfate
Silica
Sodium Chloride
Sodium Phosphate
Sodium Sulfate
Tissue A
Tissue B
Tissue C
Tissue D
Tissue E
Tissue G
Tissue H
Tissue I
Tissue J
Tissue K
Tissue M
Tissue N
Tissue O
Tissue P

NUMARK LABORATORIES,   **418, 619**
INC.
P. O. Box 6321
Edison, NJ 08818
Address inquiries to:
Susan Wilson   (800) 338-8079
OTC Products Available
◆Certain Dri Antiperspirant

O'CONNOR PHARMACEUTICALS   **619**
16400 N.W. 2nd Avenue
Miami, FL 33169
Address inquiries to:
Richard B. Seymour   (305) 944-3666
For Medical Emergencies Contact:
Richard B. Seymour   (305) 944-3666
OTC Products Available
Diasorb Liquid (4 oz.)
Diasorb Tablets (24)
Legatrin Night Leg Cramp Relief
Vaporizer in a Bottle Nasal Decongestant

OHM LABORATORIES, INC.   **418, 620**
P.O. Box 279
Franklin Park, NJ 08823
Address inquiries to:
Arun Heble   (201) 297-3030
For Medical Emergencies Contact:
(201) 297-3030
OTC Products Available
Bisacodyl Tablets 5 mg.
◆Ibuprofen Tablets
◆Ibuprohm Caplets
Ohmni-Scon Chewable Tablets
Pseudoephedrine Hydrochloride Tablets
Trisudrine Tablets

ORTHO PHARMACEUTICAL
CORPORATION   **418, 620, 772**
Advanced Care Products
Route #202
Raritan, NJ 08869   (201) 524-0400

For Medical Emergencies Contact:
Dr. B. Malyk   (201) 524-1305
OTC Products Available
◆Advance Pregnancy Test
◆Conceptrol Contraceptive Inserts
◆Conceptrol Gel • Single Use Contraceptives
◆Daisy 2 Pregnancy Test
◆Delfen Contraceptive Foam
◆Fact Plus Pregnancy Test
◆Gynol II Extra Strength Contraceptive Jelly
◆Gynol II Original Formula Contraceptive Jelly
◆Massé Breast Cream
◆Micatin Antifungal Cream
◆Micatin Antifungal Deodorant Spray Powder
◆Micatin Antifungal Powder
◆Micatin Antifungal Spray Liquid
◆Micatin Antifungal Spray Powder
Micatin Jock Itch Cream
Micatin Jock Itch Spray Powder
◆Ortho Personal Lubricant
Ortho-Creme Contraceptive Cream
◆Ortho-Gynol Contraceptive Jelly

P & S LABORATORIES
210 West 131st Street
Los Angeles, CA 90061
See STANDARD HOMEOPATHIC COMPANY

PADDOCK LABORATORIES, INC.   **623**
3101 Louisiana Ave. North
Minneapolis, MN 55427
Address inquiries to:
Jerry A. Ellinghuysen
(612) 546-4676
Roscoe D. Heim   (800) 328-5113
For Medical Emergencies Contact:
Bruce G. Paddock   (800) 328-5113
OTC Products Available
Actidose with Sorbitol
Actidose-Aqua, Activated Charcoal
Emulsoil
Glutose
Ipecac Syrup, USP

PARKE-DAVIS   **419, 624, 772**
Consumer Health Products Group
Division of Warner-Lambert Company
201 Tabor Road
Morris Plains, New Jersey 07950
See also Warner-Lambert Company
(201) 540-2000
For product information call:
1-(800) 223-0432
For medical information call:
(201) 540-3950
Regional Sales Offices
Atlanta, GA 30328
1140 Hammond Drive
(404) 396-4080
Baltimore (Hunt Valley), MD 21031
11350 McCormick Road
(301) 666-7810
Chicago (Schaumburg), IL 60195
1111 Plaza Drive   (312) 884-6990
Dallas (Grand Prairie), TX 75234
12200 Ford Road   (214) 484-5566
Detroit (Troy), MI 48084
500 Stephenson Highway
(313) 589-3292
Los Angeles (Tustin), CA 92680
17822 East 17th Street
(714) 731-3441
Memphis, TN 38119
1355 Lynnfield Road
(901) 767-1921
New York (Paramus, NJ) 07652
12 Route 17 North
(201) 368-0733
Pittsburgh, PA 15220
1910 Cochran Road
(412) 343-9855
Seattle (Bellevue), WA 98004
301 116th Avenue, SE
(206) 451-1119
OTC Products Available
Agoral
Agoral, Marshmallow Flavor
Agoral, Raspberry Flavor

(◆ Shown in Product Identification Section)

Alcohol, Rubbing (Lavacol)
Alophen Pills
◆Anusol Hemorrhoidal Suppositories
◆Anusol Ointment
◆Benadryl Anti-Itch Cream
◆Benadryl Decongestant Elixir
◆Benadryl Decongestant Kapseals
◆Benadryl Decongestant Tablets
◆Benadryl Elixir
◆Benadryl 25 Kapseals
◆Benadryl Plus
◆Benadryl Plus Nighttime
◆Benadryl Spray
◆Benadryl 25 Tablets
◆Benylin Cough Syrup
◆Benylin Decongestant
◆Benylin DM
◆Benylin Expectorant
◆Caladryl Cream, Lotion
•◆e.p.t. plus In-Home Early Pregnancy
    Test
◆e.p.t Stick Test
◆Gelusil Liquid & Tablets
Gelusil-II Liquid & Tablets
Gelusil-M Liquid & Tablets
Geriplex-FS Kapseals
Geriplex-FS Liquid
Hydrogen Peroxide Solution
Lavacol
◆Myadec
Natabec Kapseals
Peroxide, Hydrogen
◆Promega
◆Promega Pearls
Rubbing Alcohol (Lavacol)
Siblin Granules
◆Sinutab Allergy Formula Sustained
    Action Tablets
◆Sinutab Maximum Strength Caplets
◆Sinutab Maximum Strength Tablets
◆Sinutab Maximum Strength Without
    Drowsiness Tablets & Caplets
◆Sinutab Regular Strength Without
    Drowsiness Formula
Thera-Combex H-P Kapseals
Tucks Cream
Tucks Ointment
◆Tucks Premoistened Pads
Tucks Take-Alongs
◆Ziradryl Lotion

PHARMAFAIR, INC.   633
205-C Kelsey Lane
Silo Bend
Tampa, FL 33619
    Address inquiries to:
Saul Schwartz, National Field Manager
                (800) 227-1427
                (813) 972-7705
    OTC Products Available
Benzoyl Peroxide Gel 5% and 10%
Cortifair Cream 0.5%
Cortifair Lotion 0.5%
Ear Drops
Eye Drops
Eye Wash
Lubrifair Ophthalmic Ointment
Lubrifair Ophthalmic Solution
Meclizine HCl Chewable Tablets 25 mg
Ocugestrin Solution
Petrolatum Ophthalmic Ointment
Pseudoephedrine HCl Tablets 30mg
Tearfair Dry Eyes Solution
Tearfair Ointment
Tolnaftate 1% Cream and 1% Solution
Topisporin Ointment

PLOUGH, INC.   421, 633
3030 Jackson Avenue
Memphis, TN 38151
    Address inquiries to:
Consumer Relations Dept.
                (901) 320-2386
    For Medical Emergencies Contact:
Clinical Affairs Dept.
                (901) 320-2011
    OTC Products Available
◆Aftate for Athlete's Foot
◆Aftate for Jock Itch
Aspergum
Coppertone Sun Spray Mist SPF 10
◆Coppertone Sunblock Lotion SPF 15
Coppertone Sunblock Lotion SPF 25

◆Coppertone Sunblock Lotion SPF 30
Coppertone Sunblock Lotion SPF 45
◆Coppertone Sunscreen Lotion SPF 6
◆Coppertone Sunscreen Lotion SPF 8
◆Correctol Laxative Tablets
Cushion Grip Denture Adhesive
◆Di-Gel Antacid/Anti-Gas
◆Duration 12 Hour Mentholated Nasal
    Spray
◆Duration 12 Hour Nasal Spray
◆Duration 12 Hour Nasal Spray Pump
◆Duration Long Acting Nasal
    Decongestant Tablets
◆Feen-A-Mint Gum
◆Feen-A-Mint Pills and Chocolated Pills
Muskol Insect Repellent Aerosol Liquid
Muskol Insect Repellent Lotion
Muskol Insect Repellent Pump Spray
Muskol Insect Repellent Roll-on
◆Regutol Stool Softener
◆Shade Oil-Free Gel SPF 15
Shade Oil-Free Gel SPF 25
◆Shade Sunblock Lotion SPF 15
Shade Sunblock Lotion SPF 30
◆Shade Sunblock Lotion SPF 45
Shade Sunblock Stick SPF 30
◆Solarcaine
St. Joseph Adult Aspirin (325 mg.)
◆St. Joseph Adult Chewable Aspirin (81
    mg.)
St. Joseph Anti-Diarrheal for Children
◆St. Joseph Aspirin-Free Fever Reducer
    for Children Chewable Tablets, Liquid
    & Infant Drops
St. Joseph Cold Tablets for Children
◆St. Joseph Cough Suppressant for
    Children
◆St. Joseph Measured Dose Nasal
    Decongestant
◆St. Joseph Nighttime Cold Medicine
◆Stay Trim Diet Gum
◆Stay Trim Diet Mints
◆Water Babies by Coppertone Sunblock
    Cream SPF 25
◆Water Babies by Coppertone Sunblock
    Lotion SPF 15
◆Water Babies by Coppertone Sunblock
    Lotion SPF 30
◆Water Babies by Coppertone Sunblock
    Lotion SPF 45

PROCTER & GAMBLE   422, 638
P.O. Box 599
Cincinnati, OH 45201
Also see Richardson-Vicks Inc.

    Address inquiries to:
Arnold P. Austin   (800) 358-8707
    For Medical Emergencies Contact:
J.B. Lucas, M.D.   (513) 626-3350
After hours, call Collect
                        (513) 751-5525
    OTC Products Available
Denquel Sensitive Teeth Toothpaste
◆Head & Shoulders
◆Metamucil Effervescent Sugar Free,
    Lemon-Lime Flavor
◆Metamucil Effervescent Sugar Free,
    Orange Flavor
◆Metamucil Powder, Orange Flavor
◆Metamucil Powder, Regular Flavor
◆Metamucil Powder, Strawberry Flavor
◆Metamucil Powder, Sugar Free, Orange
    Flavor
◆Metamucil Powder, Sugar Free, Regular
    Flavor
◆Maximum Strength Pepto-Bismol Liquid
◆Pepto-Bismol Liquid & Tablets

REED & CARNRICK   422, 642
1 New England Avenue
Piscataway, NJ 08854
    Address Inquiries to:
Professional Service Dept.
                (201) 981-0070
    For Medical Emergencies Contact:
Medical Director   (201) 981-0070
    OTC Products Available
Alphosyl Lotion
Phazyme Drops Liquid Simethicone
◆Phazyme-125 Softgels Maximum
    Strength
Phazyme Tablets

◆Phazyme-95 Tablets
◆proctoFoam/non-steroid
◆R&C Lice Treatment Kit
◆R&C Shampoo
◆R&C Spray III
Trichotine Liquid, Vaginal Douche
Trichotine Powder, Vaginal Douche

THE REESE CHEMICAL   423, 643
COMPANY
10617 Frank Avenue
Cleveland, OH 44106
    Address inquiries to:
George W. Reese, III
                    (216) 231-6441
    OTC Products Available
◆Reese's Pinworm Medicine

REID-ROWELL   423, 643
901 Sawyer Road
Marietta, GA 30062
and
210 Main Street W.
Baudette, MN 56623
    Address Inquiries to:
Medical Services Department
                    (404) 578-9000
    For Medical Emergencies Contact:
Medical Services Department
                    (404) 578-9000
    OTC Products Available
◆Balneol
◆Hydrocil Instant

REQUA, INC.   644
Box 4008
1 Seneca Place
Greenwich, CT 06830
    Address inquiries to:
Geoffrey Geils   (203) 869-2445
    OTC Products Available
Charcoaid
Charcoal Tablets
Charcocaps

RICHARDSON-VICKS INC.   423, 644
One Far Mill Crossing
Shelton, CT 06484
    Address inquiries to:
Associate Director of Professional
    and Regulatory Services
Vicks Research Center
                    (203) 925-6000

    For Medical Emergencies Contact
Medical Director
Vicks Research Center
                    (203) 925-6000

    OTC Products Available
◆Children's Chloraseptic Lozenges
◆Chloraseptic Liquid, Cherry, Menthol or
    Cool Mint
◆Chloraseptic Liquid - Nitrogen Propelled
    Spray
◆Chloraseptic Lozenges, Cherry, Menthol
    or Cool Mint
◆Clearasil Adult Care Medicated Blemish
    Cream
Clearasil Adult Care Medicated Blemish
    Stick
Clearasil Antibacterial Soap
Clearasil 10% Benzoyl Peroxide
    Medicated Anti-Acne Lotion
◆Clearasil Doubleclear Pads - Regular
    and Maximum Strength
◆Clearasil Maximum Strength Medicated
    Anti-Acne Cream, Tinted
◆Clearasil Maximum Strength Medicated
    Anti-Acne Cream, Vanishing
◆Clearasil Medicated Astringent
Cremacoat 1
Cremacoat 2
Cremacoat 3
Cremacoat 4
◆Dramamine Chewable Tablets
◆Dramamine Liquid
◆Dramamine Tablets
Head & Chest Cold Medicine
◆Icy Hot Balm
◆Icy Hot Cream
◆Icy Hot Stick
◆Percogesic Analgesic Tablets
Vicks Children's Cough Syrup
◆Vicks Children's NyQuil

(◆ Shown in Product Identification Section)

Vicks Cough Silencers Cough Drops
◆Vicks Daycare Colds Caplets
◆Vicks Daycare Colds Liquid
Vicks Formula 44 Cough Control Discs
◆Vicks Formula 44 Cough Medicine
◆Vicks Formula 44D Decongestant
   Cough Medicine
◆Vicks Formula 44M Multi-Symptom
   Cough Medicine
Vicks Inhaler
◆Vicks NyQuil Nighttime Colds
   Medicine-Original & Cherry Flavor
Vicks Oracin Cherry Flavor Cooling
   Throat Lozenges
Vicks Oracin Cooling Throat Lozenges
◆Vicks Pediatric Formula 44 Cough
   Medicine
◆Vicks Pediatric Formula 44 Cough &
   Cold Medicine
◆Vicks Pediatric Formula 44 Cough &
   Congestion Medicine
◆Vicks Sinex Decongestant Nasal Spray
◆Vicks Sinex Decongestant Nasal Ultra
   Fine Mist
◆Vicks Sinex Long-Acting Decongestant
   Nasal Spray
◆Vicks Sinex Long-Acting Decongestant
   Nasal Ultra Fine Mist
Vicks Throat Drops
   Cherry Flavor
   Ice Blue
   Lemon Flavor
   Regular Flavor
Vicks Throat Lozenges
◆Vicks Vaporub
Vicks Vaposteam
Vicks Vatronol Nose Drops
Victors Menthol-Eucalyptus Vapor
   Cough Drops
   Cherry Flavor
   Regular

ORAL HEALTH PRODUCTS
Benzodent Analgesic Denture Ointment
Complete Denture Cleanser and
   Toothpaste in One
Extra Hold Fasteeth for Lowers Denture
   Adhesive Powder
Fixodent Denture Adhesive Cream
Fasteeth Denture Adhesive Powder
Kleenite Denture Cleanser

**A. H. ROBINS COMPANY,   424, 654
INC.
CONSUMER PRODUCTS
DIVISION**
3800 Cutshaw Avenue
Richmond, VA 23230
   Address inquiries to:
The Medical Department
                    (804) 257-2000
   For Medical Emergencies Contact:
Medical Department   (804) 257-2000
(day or night)
If no answer, call answering service
                    (804) 257-7788
   OTC Products Available
◆Allbee with C Caplets
◆Allbee C-800 Plus Iron Tablets
◆Allbee C-800 Tablets
◆Chap Stick Lip Balm
◆Chap Stick Petroleum Jelly Plus
◆Chap Stick Petroleum Jelly Plus with
   Sunblock 15
◆Chap Stick Sunblock 15 Lip Balm
Cough Calmers Lozenges
◆Dimacol Caplets
◆Dimetane Decongestant Caplets
◆Dimetane Decongestant Elixir
◆Dimetane Elixir
◆Dimetane Extentabs 8 mg
◆Dimetane Extentabs 12 mg
◆Dimetane Tablets
◆Dimetapp Elixir
◆Dimetapp Extentabs
◆Dimetapp Plus Caplets
◆Dimetapp Tablets
◆Donnagel
◆Robitussin
◆Robitussin Night Relief
◆Robitussin-CF
◆Robitussin-DM
◆Robitussin-PE
◆Z-Bec Tablets

**RORER CONSUMER   425, 662
PHARMACEUTICALS**
a division of
Rorer Pharmaceutical Corporation
500 Virginia Drive
Fort Washington, PA 19034
   *For Medical Emergencies/
   Product Information Contact:*
Medical Services
                    (215) 628-6627
                    (215) 628-6065
   *For Reports of Adverse Drug
   Experiences Contact:*
Product Surveillance (215) 956-5136
   *For Quality Assurance
   Questions Contact:*
John Chiles
Complaint Coordinator
                    (215) 628-6416
   *For Regulatory
   Questions Contact:*
Margaret Masters
Assoc. Director, Regulatory Control
                    (215) 628-6085
   For Product Information Contact:
Medical Services
                    (215) 628-6627
                    (215) 628-6065
   OTC Products Available
◆Ascriptin A/D Caplets
◆Extra Strength Ascriptin Caplets
◆Regular Strength Ascriptin Tablets
◆Camalox Suspension
◆Camalox Tablets
Fermalox Tablets
◆Extra Strength Maalox Plus Suspension
◆Extra Strength Maalox Tablets
◆Maalox Plus Tablets
◆Maalox Suspension
◆Maalox Tablets
◆Maalox TC Suspension
◆Maalox TC Tablets
◆Myoflex Creme
◆Perdiem Fiber Granules
◆Perdiem Granules

ROSS LABORATORIES   426, 668
Division of Abbott Laboratories USA
P.O. Box 1317
Columbus, OH 43216-1317
   Address Inquiries to:
Medical Director   (614) 227-3333
   OTC Products Available
Advance Nutritional Beverage With Iron
Alimentum Protein Hydrolysate Formula
   With Iron
◆Clear Eyes Lubricating Eye Redness
   Reliever
◆Ear Drops by Murine—(See Murine Ear
   Wax Removal System/Murine Ear
   Drops)
Isomil Soy Protein Formula With Iron
Isomil SF Sucrose-Free Soy Protein
   Formula With Iron
◆Murine Ear Drops
◆Murine Ear Wax Removal System
◆Murine Eye Lubricant
◆Murine Plus Lubricating Eye Redness
   Reliever
Pedialyte Oral Electrolyte Maintenance
   Solution
RCF Ross Carbohydrate Free Low-Iron
   Soy Protein Formula Base
Rehydralyte Oral Electrolyte
   Rehydration Solution
◆Selsun Blue Dandruff Shampoo
◆Selsun Blue Dandruff Shampoo-Extra
   Medicated
◆Selsun Blue Extra Conditioning
   Dandruff Shampoo
Similac Low-Iron Infant Formula
Similac PM 60/40 Low-Iron Infant
   Formula
Similac Special Care With Iron 24
   Premature Infant Formula
Similac With Iron Infant Formula
◆Tronolane Anesthetic Cream for
   Hemorrhoids
◆Tronolane Anesthetic Suppositories for
   Hemorrhoids

**RYDELLE LABORATORIES,   427, 675
INC.**
Subsidiary of S.C. Johnson & Son, Inc.
1525 Howe Street
Racine, WI 53403
   Address inquiries to:
Carol Hansen
Consumer Affairs Director
                    (414) 631-4000
   For Medical Emergencies Contact:
Richard D. Stewart M.D., M.P.H.,
F.A.C.P.
                    (414) 631-2111
   OTC Products Available
◆Aveeno Bath Oilated
◆Aveeno Bath Regular
◆Aveeno Cleansing Bar for Acne
◆Aveeno Cleansing Bar for Dry Skin
◆Aveeno Cleansing Bar for Normal to
   Oily Skin
◆Aveeno Lotion
◆Aveeno Shower and Bath Oil
◆Rhulicream
◆Rhuligel
◆Rhulispray

**SANDOZ   427, 676
PHARMACEUTICALS/
CONSUMER DIVISION**
59 Route 10
East Hanover NJ 07936
   Address Medical Inquiries To:
Medical Department
Sandoz Pharmaceuticals Corporation
East Hanover, NJ 07936
                    (201) 503-7500
   Address Other Inquiries To:
Drug Regulation and Regulatory
Affairs Department
Sandoz Pharmaceuticals Corporation
East Hanover, NJ 07936
                    (201) 503-6462
   OTC Products Available
Acid Mantle Creme
◆BiCozene Creme
Cama Arthritis Pain Reliever
◆Dorcol Children's Cough Syrup
◆Dorcol Children's Decongestant Liquid
◆Dorcol Children's Fever & Pain Reducer
◆Dorcol Children's Liquid Cold Formula
◆Ex-Lax Chocolated Laxative
◆Ex-Lax Pills, Unflavored
◆Extra Gentle Ex-Lax
◆Extra Strength Gas-X Tablets
◆Gas-X Tablets
◆Gentle Nature Natural Vegetable
   Laxative
◆TheraFlu Flu and Cold Medicine
Triaminic Allergy Tablets
Triaminic Chewables
◆Triaminic Cold Tablets
◆Triaminic Expectorant
◆Triaminic Nite Light
◆Triaminic Syrup
◆Triaminic-12 Tablets
◆Triaminic-DM Syrup
◆Triaminicin Tablets
◆Triaminicol Multi-Symptom Cold Tablets
◆Triaminicol Multi-Symptom Relief
Ursinus Inlay-Tabs

SCHERING CORPORATION   428, 683
Galloping Hill Road
Kenilworth, NJ 07033
   Address inquiries to:
Professional Services Department
   9:00 AM to 5:00 PM EST
                    (800) 526-4099
   After regular hours and on weekends:
                    (201) 298-4000
   OTC Products Available
◆A and D Ointment*
◆Afrin Cherry Scented Nasal Spray
   0.05%
◆Afrin Children's Strength Nose Drops
   0.025%
◆Afrin Menthol Nasal Spray, 0.05%
◆Afrin Nasal Spray 0.05% and Nasal
   Spray Pump
◆Afrin Nose Drops 0.05%

(◆ **Shown in Product Identification Section**)

◆Afrinol Repetabs Tablets Long-Acting Nasal Decongestant
◆Chlor-Trimeton Allergy Syrup, Tablets & Long-Acting Repetabs Tablets
◆Chlor-Trimeton Decongestant Tablets
◆Chlor-Trimeton Long Acting Decongestant Repetabs Tablets
◆Chlor-Trimeton Maximum Strength Timed Release Allergy Tablets
◆Chlor-Trimeton Sinus Caplets
Cod Liver Oil Concentrate Capsules*
Cod Liver Oil Concentrate Tablets*
Cod Liver Oil Concentrate Tablets w/Vitamin C*
Complex 15 Hand & Body Moisturizing Cream
Complex 15 Hand & Body Moisturizing Lotion
Complex 15 Moisturizing Face Cream
◆Coricidin 'D' Decongestant Tablets
Coricidin Decongestant Nasal Mist
◆Coricidin Demilets Tablets for Children
◆Coricidin Maximum Strength Sinus Headache Caplets
◆Coricidin Tablets
Demazin Nasal Decongestant/ Antihistamine Repetabs Tablets & Syrup
Dermolate Anti-Itch Cream
Disophrol Chronotab Sustained-Action Tablets*
Disophrol Tablets*
◆Drixoral Antihistamine/Nasal Decongestant Syrup
◆Drixoral Non-Drowsy Extended-Release Tablets
◆Drixoral Plus Extended-Release Tablets
◆Drixoral Sustained-Action Tablets
◆Emko Because Contraceptor Vaginal Contraceptive Foam
◆Emko Vaginal Contraceptive Foam
Mol-Iron Tablets*
Mol-Iron w/Vitamin C Tablets*
◆OcuClear Eye Drops (See PDR For Ophthalmology)
◆Tinactin Aerosol Liquid 1%
◆Tinactin Aerosol Powder 1%
◆Tinactin Antifungal Cream, Solution & Powder 1%
◆Tinactin Jock Itch Cream 1%
◆Tinactin Jock Itch Spray Powder 1%
*Schering/White Product Line

SCHWARZ PHARMA   430, 693
Kremers Urban Company
P.O. Box 2038
Milwaukee, WI 53201
Address inquiries to:
Technical Services Department
(414) 354-4300
(800) 558-5114
For Medical Emergencies Contact:
(414) 354-4300
(800) 558-5114
OTC Products Available
Calciferol Drops
◆Fedahist Decongestant Syrup
◆Fedahist Expectorant Pediatric Drops
◆Fedahist Expectorant Syrup
◆Fedahist Tablets
Gemnisyn Tablets
Kudrox Suspension
◆Lactrase Capsules
Milkinol

**SCOT-TUSSIN PHARMACAL   694
COMPANY, INC.**
P.O. Box 8217
50 Clemence Street
Cranston, RI 02920-0217
Address inquiries to:
Professional Service Department
(800) 638-SCOT
(401) 942-8555
OTC Products Available
Febrol Liquid Sugar-Free, Dye-Free & Alcohol-Free
Ferro-Bob Tablets
Hayfebrol Liquid Allergy Relief Formula, Sugar-Free, Dye-Free, Cholesterol-Free, Alcohol-Free & Sodium-Free
Scot-Tussin DM 2 Syrup (with sugar)

Scot-Tussin Sugar-Free DM Cough & Cold Medicine (No Sorbitol, Sodium, Alcohol or Cholesterol)
Scot-Tussin Sugar-Free Expectorant (No Sugar, Sodium, Dye or Cholesterol)
Scot-Tussin Sugar-Free Original 5-Action Cold Formula (No Alcohol or Cholesterol)
Scot-Tussin Syrup (with sugar) Original 5-Action Cold Formula (No Alcohol)
Vita-Bob Softgels Multivitamins
Vitalize Stress Formula with Iron, Sugar-Free, Alcohol-Free, Cholesterol-Free, Dye-Free, Sodium-Free Liquid
Vita-Plus E Softgels Natural 400 I.U.
Vita-Plus G (geriatric) Softgels
Vita-Plus H (hematinic) Softgels

**SMITHKLINE BEECHAM   430, 695
CONSUMER BRANDS**
P.O. Box 1467
Pittsburgh, PA 15230
Address inquiries to:
Professional Services Dept.
(800) BEECHAM
(412) 928-1050
OTC Products Available
◆A-200 Pediculicide Shampoo & Gel
AsthmaHaler Mist Epinephrine Bitartrate Bronchodilator
AsthmaNefrin Solution "A" Bronchodilator
Esotérica Medicated Fade Cream
FemIron Multi-Vitamins and Iron
Geritol Complete Tablets
Geritol Liquid - High Potency Iron & Vitamin Tonic
Hold Cough Suppressant Lozenges
◆Liquiprin Children's Elixir
◆Liquiprin Infants' Drops
Massengill Baby Powder Soft Cloth Towelette and Unscented Soft Cloth Towelette
Massengill Disposable Douche
Massengill Liquid Concentrate
Massengill Medicated Disposable Douche
Massengill Medicated Liquid Concentrate
Massengill Medicated Soft Cloth Towelette
Massengill Powder
◆Nature's Remedy Natural Vegetable Laxative
N'ICE Medicated Sugarless Sore Throat and Cough Lozenges
N'ICE Sore Throat Spray
◆Oxy Clean Lathering Facial Scrub
◆Oxy Clean Medicated Cleanser
◆Oxy Clean Medicated Pads - Regular, Sensitive Skin, and Maximum Strength
◆Oxy Clean Medicated Soap
◆Oxy Night Watch
◆Oxy 10 Daily Face Wash
◆Oxy-5 and Oxy-10 Tinted and Vanishing Formulas with Sorboxyl
S.T.37 Antiseptic Solution
Serutan Natural-Fiber Laxative Toasted Granules
Sominex
Sominex Liquid
Sominex Pain Relief Formula
Sucrets (Regular and Mentholated)
Sucrets Children's Cherry Flavored Sore Throat Lozenges
Sucrets Cold Relief Formula
Sucrets Cough Control Formula
Sucrets Maximum Strength and Sucrets Wild Cherry (Regular Strength) Sore Throat Lozenges
Sucrets Maximum Strength Sprays
Thermotabs
◆Tums Antacid Tablets
◆Tums E-X Antacid Tablets
◆Tums Liquid Extra-Strength Antacid
◆Tums Liquid Extra-Strength Antacid with Simethicone
Vivarin Stimulant Tablets

**SMITHKLINE CONSUMER   430, 705
PRODUCTS**
a SmithKline Beckman Company
One Franklin Plaza
P.O. Box 8082
Philadelphia, PA 19101
Address inquiries to:
Medical Department   (215) 751-5000
OTC Products Available
◆A.R.M. Allergy Relief Medicine Caplets
◆Acnomel Cream
◆Aqua Care Cream
◆Aqua Care Lotion
◆Benzedrex Inhaler
◆Clear by Design Medicated Acne Gel
◆Clear By Design Medicated Cleansing Pads
◆Congestac Caplets
◆Contac Continuous Action Decongestant Capsules
◆Contac Cough Formula
◆Contac Cough & Sore Throat Formula
◆Contac Jr. Children's Cold Medicine
◆Contac Maximum Strength Continuous Action Decongestant Caplets
◆Contac Nighttime Cold Medicine
◆Contac Severe Cold Formula Caplets
◆Contac Sinus Caplets Maximum Strength Non-Drowsy Formula
◆Contac Sinus Tablets Maximum Strength Non-Drowsy Formula
◆Ecotrin Enteric Coated Aspirin Maximum Strength Tablets and Caplets
◆Ecotrin Enteric Coated Aspirin Regular Strength Tablets and Caplets
◆Feosol Capsules
◆Feosol Elixir
◆Feosol Tablets
◆Ornex Caplets
◆Sine-Off Maximum Strength Allergy/Sinus Formula Caplets
◆Sine-Off Maximum Strength No Drowsiness Formula Caplets
◆Sine-Off Sinus Medicine Tablets-Aspirin Formula
◆Teldrin Timed-Release Allergy Capsules, 12 mg.
◆Troph-Iron Liquid
◆Trophite Liquid

E. R. SQUIBB & SONS, INC.   433, 717
General Offices
P.O. Box 4000
Princeton, NJ 08540 (609) 921-4000
Address Inquiries to:
Squibb Professional Services Dept.
P.O. Box 4000
Princeton, NJ 08540 (609) 921-4006
Distribution Centers
ATLANTA, GEORGIA
P.O. Box 16503
Atlanta, GA 30321
All Customers Call   (800) 241-5364
CHICAGO, ILLINOIS
P.O. Box 788
Arlington Heights, IL 60006
State of IL Customers Call
(800) 942-0674
All Others Call   (800) 323-0665
DALLAS, TEXAS
Mail or telephone orders and customer service inquiries should be directed to Atlanta, GA (see above)
State of MS Customers Call
(800) 241-1744
All others call   (800) 241-5364
LOS ANGELES, CALIFORNIA
P.O. Box 428
La Mirada, CA 90638
State of CA Customers Call
(800) 422-4254
State of HI Customers Call
(714) 521-7050
All Others Call   (800) 854-3050
SEATTLE, WASHINGTON
Mail or telephone orders and customer service inquiries should be directed to Los Angeles, CA (see above)
States of AK and MT Customers Call
(714) 521-7050

(◆ **Shown in Product Identification Section**)

State of CA Customers Call
(800) 422-4254
All Others Call   (800) 854-3050
NEW YORK AREA
P.O. Box 2013
New Brunswick, NJ 08903
State of NJ Customers Call
(800) 352-4865
State of ME Customers Call
(201) 469-5400
All Others Call   (800) 631-5244
OTC Products Available
Engran-HP Tablets
Proto-Chol Natural Fish Oil Gelcaps
Spec-T Sore Throat Anesthetic
Lozenges
Spec-T Sore Throat/Cough Suppressant
Lozenges
Spec-T Sore Throat/Decongestant
Lozenges
Spectrocin Plus Ointment
Theragran Jr. Chewable Tablets
Theragran Jr. Chewable Tablets with
Extra Vitamin C
Theragran Jr. Chewable Tablets with
Iron
◆Theragran Liquid
◆Theragran Stress Formula
◆Theragran Tablets
◆Theragran-M Tablets
Trigesic Tablets
Valadol Liquid
Valadol Tablets
Vigran Plus Iron Tablets
Vigran Tablets

**STANDARD HOMEOPATHIC   718
COMPANY**
210 West 131st Street
Box 61067
Los Angeles, CA 90061
OTC Products Available
Hyland's Bed Wetting Tablets
Hyland's Calms Forté Tablets
Hyland's Colic Tablets
Hyland's Cough Syrup with Honey
Hyland's C-Plus Cold Tablets
Hyland's Teething Tablets
Hyland's Vitamin C for Children

**STELLAR PHARMACAL   433, 719
CORPORATION**
1990 N.W. 44th Street
Pompano Beach, FL 33064-8712
Address inquiries to:
Scott L. Davidson   (305) 972-6060
Customer Service & Order Department
(800) 845-7827
OTC Products Available
◆Star-Otic Ear Solution

**STUART   433, 719
PHARMACEUTICALS**
a business unit of ICI Americas Inc.
Wilmington, DE 19897 USA
Address inquiries to:
Yvonne A. Graham, Manager
Professional Services
(302) 886-2231
For Medical Emergencies:
After hours & on weekends
(302) 886-3000
OTC Products Available
◆ALternaGEL Liquid
◆Dialose Capsules
◆Dialose Plus Capsules
◆Effer-Syllium Natural Fiber Bulking
Agent
Ferancee Chewable Tablets
◆Ferancee-HP Tablets
◆HIBICLENS Antimicrobial Skin Ckeanser
HIBISTAT Germicidal Hand Rinse
HIBISTAT Towelette
◆Kasof Capsules
◆Mylanta Liquid
◆Mylanta Tablets
◆Mylanta-II Liquid
◆Mylanta-II Tablets
◆Mylicon Drops
◆Mylicon Tablets
◆Mylicon-80 Tablets
◆Mylicon-125 Tablets
◆Orexin Softab Tablets

◆Probec-T Tablets
◆STUART PRENATAL Tablets
◆The Stuart Formula Tablets
◆Stuartinic Tablets

SYNTEX LABORATORIES, INC.   726
3401 Hillview Avenue
P.O. Box 10850
Palo Alto, CA 94304
*Direct General/Sales/Order inquiries
for U.S. Marketed products to:*
Marketing Information Department
Specify product   (415) 855-5050
*Direct Medical inquiries on
U.S. marketed products to:*
Medical Services Department
General Medical Inquiries
(415) 855-5545
Adverse Reactions Inquiries
(415) 852-1386
OTC Products Available
Carmol 20 Cream
Carmol 10 Lotion

**THOMPSON MEDICAL   434, 727
COMPANY, INC.**
919 Third Avenue
New York, NY 10022
Address inquiries to:
Medical Services   (212) 688-4420
OTC Products Available
Appedrine, Maximum Strength Tablets
Aqua-Ban, Maximum Strength Plus
Tablets
Aqua-Ban Tablets
Aspercreme Creme & Lotion
Control Capsules
◆Cortizone-5 Creme & Ointment
Dexatrim Capsules
Dexatrim Maximum Strength
Caffeine-Free Caplets
Dexatrim Maximum Strength
Caffeine-Free Capsules
◆Dexatrim Maximum Strength Plus
Vitamin C/Caffeine-free Caplets
◆Dexatrim Maximum Strength Plus
Vitamin C/Caffeine-free Capsules
Dexatrim Maximum Strength Pre-Meal
Caplets
Diar Aid Tablets
Encare Vaginal Contraceptive
Suppositories
End Lice
Ibuprin
◆NP-27 Cream, Solution, Spray Powder
& Powder
Prolamine Maximum Strength Capsules
◆Sleepinal Night-time Sleep Aid Capsules
Slim-Fast
Sportscreme
Tempo Antacid with Antigas Action
◆Ultra Slim Fast

**TRITON CONSUMER PRODUCTS,   730
INC.**
5105-190 Tollview Drive
Rolling Meadows, IL 60008
Address inquiries to:
Karen Shrader   (708) 577-5900
For Medical Emergencies Contact
(708) 577-5900
OTC Products Available
MG 217 Psoriasis Ointment and Lotion
MG 217 Psoriasis Shampoo and
Conditioner
MG 400 Severe Dandruff Shampoo
ProTech First-Aid Stik
Skeeter Stik Insect Bite Medication
Skeeter Stop 100 Insect Repellent
Tick Away Insect Repellent

UAS LABORATORIES   730
9201 Penn Avenue South #10
Minneapolis, MN 55431
Address inquiries to:
Dr. S. K. Dash   (612) 881-1915
(800) 422-3371
OTC Products Available
DDS-Acidophilus

ULTRABALANCE PRODUCTS   731
5800 Soundview Drive
Gig Harbor, WA 98335

Address Inquiries to:
UltraBalance Products
Division of HealthComm
P.O. Box 1729
Gig Harbor, WA 98335
For Technical Assistance Contact:
(800) 648-5883
OTC Products Available
UltraBalance Weight Management
Products - Herbulk
UltraBalance Weight Management
Products - Protein Formula

THE UPJOHN COMPANY   434, 731
7000 Portage Road
Kalamazoo, MI 49001
*For Medical and Pharmaceutical
Information, Including Emergencies:*
(616) 329-8244
(616) 323-6615
*Pharmaceutical Sales Areas
and Distribution Centers*
Atlanta (Chamblee)
GA 30341-2626   (404) 451-4822
Boston (Wellesley)
MA 02181   (617) 431-7970
Buffalo (Amherst)
NY 14221   (716) 632-5942
Chicago (Oak Brook Terrace)
IL 60181   (708) 574-3300
Cincinnati, OH 45202
(513) 723-1010
Dallas (Irving)
TX 75062   (214) 256-0022
Denver, CO 80216   (303) 399-3113
Hartford (Enfield)
CT 06082   (203) 741-3421
Honolulu, HI 96818   (808) 422-2777
Kalamazoo, MI 49001
(616) 323-4000
Kansas City, MO 64131
(816) 361-2286
Los Angeles, CA 90038
(213) 463-8101
Memphis, TN 38119   (901) 685-8192
Minneapolis (Bloomington), MN 55437
(612) 921-8484
New York (Uniondale)
NY 11553   (516) 745-6100
Orlando, FL 32809   (407) 859-4591
Philadelphia (Berwyn)
PA 19312   (215) 993-0100
Pittsburgh (Bridgeville)
PA 15017   (412) 257-0200
Portland, OR 97232   (503) 232-2133
St. Louis, MO 63146   (314) 872-8626
San Francisco (Palo Alto)
CA 94306-2117   (415) 493-8080
Shreveport, LA 71129
(318) 688-3700
Washington, DC 20011
(202) 882-6163
OTC Products Available
Alkets Tablets
Baciguent Antibiotic Ointment
Calcium Gluconate Tablets, USP
Calcium Lactate Tablets, USP
Cheracol Cough Syrup
◆Cheracol D Cough Formula
◆Cheracol Plus Head Cold/Cough
Formula
Citrocarbonate Antacid
Clocream Skin Cream
◆Cortaid Cream with Aloe
◆Cortaid Lotion
◆Cortaid Ointment with Aloe
◆Cortaid Spray
Cortef Feminine Itch Cream
Diostate D Tablets
◆Haltran Tablets
◆Kaopectate Concentrated Anti-Diarrheal,
Peppermint Flavor
◆Kaopectate Concentrated Anti-Diarrheal,
Regular Flavor
◆Kaopectate Chewable Tablets
◆Maximum Strength Kaopectate Tablets
Anti-Diarrhea Medicine
Lipomul Oral Liquid
◆Motrin IB Caplets and Tablets
Myciguent Antibiotic Cream
Myciguent Antibiotic Ointment
◆Mycitracin Triple Antibiotic Ointment
Orthoxicol Cough Syrup

(◆ Shown in Product Identification Section)

P-A-C Revised Formula Analgesic
  Tablets
Phenolax Wafers
Progaine Shampoo
◆Pyrroxate Capsules
Sigtab Tablets
Super D Perles
Unicap Capsules & Tablets
Unicap Jr Chewable Tablets
◆Unicap M Tablets
Unicap Plus Iron Vitamin Formula
  Tablets
◆Unicap Sr. Tablets
◆Unicap T Therapeutic Potency Vitamin
  & Mineral Formula Tablets
Zymacap Capsules

**WAKUNAGA OF AMERICA   435, 735
CO., LTD.**
Subsidiary of Wakunaga Pharmaceutical
Co., Ltd.
23501 Madero
Mission Viejo, CA 92691
          Address inquires to:
                    (714) 855-2776
          OTC Products Available
◆Kyolic
  Kyo-Dophilus, Capsules: Acido-
    philus, Bifidus, S. Faecalis
  Kyo-Green, Powder: Barley &
    Wheat Grass, Chlorella,
    Brown Rice, Kelp
  Kyolic Formula 106 Capsules:
    Aged Garlic Extract Powder
    (300 mg) & Vitamin E
  Kyolic Super Formula 104
    Capsules: Aged Garlic Extract
    Powder (300 mg)
  Kyolic Super Formula 105
    Capsules: Aged Garlic Extract
    Powder (200 mg)
  Kyolic Super Formula 100
    Capsules & Tablets: Aged Garlic
    Extract Powder (300 mg)
  Kyolic Super Formula 100 Tablets:
    Aged Garlic Extract Powder
    (270 mg)
◆ Kyolic-Aged Garlic Extract Flavor &
    Odor Modified Enriched with
    Vitamins B_1 & B_{12}
  Kyolic-Aged Garlic Extract Flavor &
    Odor Modified Plain
  Kyolic-Aged Garlic Extract Liquid
    Enriched with Vitamin B, & B_{12}
  Kyolic-Aged Garlic Extract Liquid
    Plain
  Kyolic-Formula 101 Capsules:
    Aged Garlic Extract (270 mg)
  Kyolic-Formula 103 Capsules:
    Aged Garlic Extract Powder
    (220 mg)
  Kyolic-Formula 101 Tablets: Aged
    Garlic Extract Powder (270 mg)
  Kyolic-Super Formula 104,
    Aged Garlic Extract
    Powder (300 mg) with
    Lecithin
  Kyolic-Super Formula 103,
    Capsules: Aged Garlic Extract
    Powder (220 mg) with Vitamin C,
    Astragalus, Calcium
  Kyolic-Super Formula 105,
    Capsules: Aged Garlic Extract
    Powder (250 mg) with
    Selenium, Vitamins A & E
  Kyolic-Super Formula 106,
    Capsules: Aged Garlic Extract
    Powder (300 mg) with Vitamin
    E, Cayenne Pepper, Hawthorn
    Berry
◆ Kyolic-Super Formula 101, Tablets
    & Capsules: Aged Garlic
    Extract Powder (270 mg)
    with Brewer's Yeast, Kelp & Algin
  Kyolic-Super Formula 102, Tablets
    & Capsules: Aged
    Garlic Extract Powder
    (350 mg) with Enzyme Complex

WALKER, CORP & CO., INC.   435, 736
203 E. Hampton Place
Syracuse, NY 13206

          Address inquiries to:
P.O. Box 1320
Syracuse, NY 13201 (315) 463-4511
          For Medical Emergencies Contact:
Robert G. Long   (315) 638-4763
          OTC Products Available
◆Evac-U-Gen Mild Laxative

WALKER PHARMACAL COMPANY   736
4200 Laclede
St. Louis, MO 63108
          Address Inquiries to:
Customer Service   (314) 533-9600
          OTC Products Available
HIKE Antiseptic Ointment
PRID Salve

WALLACE LABORATORIES   435, 736
Half Acre Road
Cranbury, NJ 08512
          Address inquiries to:
Wallace Laboratories
Div. of Carter-Wallace, Inc.
P.O. Box 1001
Cranbury, NJ 08512 (609) 655-6000
          For Medical Emergencies:
                    (609) 799-1167
          OTC Products Available
◆Maltsupex Liquid, Powder & Tablets
◆Ryna Liquid
◆Ryna-C Liquid
◆Ryna-CX Liquid
◆Syllact Powder

**WARNER-LAMBERT   435, 738, 775
COMPANY**
Consumer Health Products Group
201 Tabor Road
Morris Plains, NJ 07950
See also Parke-Davis
          Address Inquiries to:
Robert Kirpitch   (201) 540-3204
          For Medical Emergencies Call:
                    (201) 540-2000
          OTC Products Available
Bromo-Seltzer
Corn Husker's Lotion
◆Early Detector
Efferdent Extra Strength Denture
  Cleanser
◆Professional Strength Efferdent
Halls Cough Formula
◆Halls Mentho-Lyptus Cough
  Suppressant Tablets
Halls Vitamin C Drops
Listerex Lotion
◆Listerine Antiseptic
◆Listerine Antiseptic Lozenges Regular
  Strength
◆Listerine Maximum Strength Antiseptic
  Lozenges
◆Listermint with Fluoride
◆Lubriderm Cream
◆Lubriderm Lotion
◆Lubriderm Skin Conditioning Oil
◆Rolaids
◆Rolaids (Calcium Rich)
◆Rolaids (Sodium Free)
◆Extra Strength Rolaids
Sloan's Linament
Super Anahist Tablets

**WESTWOOD   436, 741
PHARMACEUTICALS INC.**
100 Forest Avenue
Buffalo, NY 14213

                    (716) 887-3400
*Address inquiries on Alpha Keri,
  Fostex, Keri, and PreSun
  products to:*
Consumer Affairs Department
                    (800) 468-7746
Address all other inquiries to:
Consumer Affairs Department
                    (716) 887-3773
          OTC Products Available
◆Alpha Keri Moisture Rich Body Oil
◆Alpha Keri Moisture Rich Cleansing Bar
Balnetar
Estar Gel
Fostex 10% Benzoyl Peroxide
  Cleansing Bar
Fostex 5% Benzoyl Peroxide Gel
Fostex 10% Benzoyl Peroxide Gel

Fostex 10% Benzoyl Peroxide Tinted
  Cream
Fostex 10% Benzoyl Peroxide Wash
Fostex Medicated Cleansing Bar
Fostex Medicated Cleansing Cream
Fostril Lotion
Keri Creme
Keri Facial Soap
◆Keri Lotion-Herbal Scent
◆Keri Lotion-Original Formula
◆Keri Lotion-Silky Smooth Formula
◆Lac-Hydrin Five
Lowila Cake
◆Moisturel Cream
◆Moisturel Lotion
◆Moisturel Sensitive Skin Cleanser
Pernox Lotion
Pernox Medicated Scrub
Pernox Shampoo
PreSun 15 Facial Stick/Lip Protector
  Sunscreen
PreSun 15 Facial Sunscreen
PreSun for Kids
PreSun 8, 15 and 39 Creamy
  Sunscreens
◆PreSun 15 and 29 Sensitive Skin
  Sunscreen
PreSun 23 Sunscreen Sprays
Sebucare Lotion
Sebulex & Sebulex Cream Shampoo
Sebulex Shampoo with Conditioners
Sebulon Dandruff Shampoo
Sebutone and Sebutone Cream
  Shampoos

**WHITEHALL LABORATORIES
INC.   436, 743, 777**
Division of American Home Products
  Corporation
685 Third Avenue
New York, NY 10017
          Address Professional Inquiries to:
                    (800) 343-0856
          Address Consumer Inquiries to:
                    (212) 878-5503
          OTC Products Available
◆Advil Ibuprofen Caplets and Tablets
◆Anacin Analgesic Coated Caplets
◆Anacin Analgesic Coated Tablets
Anacin-3 Children's Acetaminophen
  Chewable Tablets, Alcohol-Free Liquid
  and Infants' Drops
◆Anacin-3 Maximum Strength
  Acetaminophen Film Coated Caplets
◆Anacin-3 Maximum Strength
  Acetaminophen Film Coated Tablets
Anacin Maximum Strength Analgesic
  Coated Tablets
◆Anacin-3 Regular Strength
  Acetaminophen Film Coated Tablets
◆Anbesol Baby Teething Gel Anesthetic
◆Anbesol Gel Antiseptic-Anesthetic
◆Anbesol Gel Antiseptic-Anesthetic -
  Maximum Strength
◆Anbesol Liquid Antiseptic-Anesthetic
◆Anbesol Liquid Antiseptic-Anesthetic -
  Maximum Strength
Arthritis Pain Formula Aspirin-Free by
  the Makers of Anacin Analgesic
  Tablets
◆Arthritis Pain Formula by the Makers of
  Anacin Analgesic Tablets and Caplets
Beminal Forte
Beminal Stress Plus with Iron
Beminal Stress Plus with Zinc
Beminal 500 Tablets
Bisodol Antacid Powder
Bisodol Antacid Tablets
Bronitin Asthma Tablets
Bronitin Mist
◆Clearblue Easy
◆Clearplan Easy Ovulation Predictor
Clusivol Capsules and Syrup
◆CoAdvil Caplets
Compound W Gel
Compound W Solution
Denalan Denture Cleanser

(◆ **Shown in Product Identification Section**)

◆Denorex Medicated Shampoo and
  Conditioner
◆Denorex Medicated Shampoo, Extra
  Strength
  Denorex Medicated Shampoo, Extra
  Strength With Conditioners
◆Denorex Medicated Shampoo, Regular
  & Mountain Fresh Herbal Scent
◆Dermoplast Anesthetic Pain Relief
  Lotion
◆Dermoplast Anesthetic Pain Relief
  Spray
◆Dristan Decongestant/Antihistamine/
  Analgesic Coated Caplets
◆Dristan Decongestant/Antihistamine/
  Analgesic Coated Tablets
  Dristan Inhaler
◆Dristan Long Lasting Menthol Nasal
  Spray
◆Dristan Long Lasting Nasal Spray,
  Regular
◆Maximum Strength Dristan
  Decongestant/Analgesic Coated
  Caplets
◆Dristan Nasal Spray, Regular & Menthol
  Dristan Room Vaporizer
  Dristan-AF Decongestant/
  Antihistamine/Analgesic Tablets
  Dry and Clear Acne Medicated Lotion &
  Double Strength Cream

Enzactin Cream
Fiber Guard
Freezone Solution

Heather Feminine Deodorant Spray
Heet Analgesic Liniment
Heet Analgesic Spray
InfraRub Analgesic Cream
Kerodex Cream 51 (for dry or oily
  work)
Kerodex Cream 71 (for wet work)
Larylgan Throat Spray
Medicated Cleansing Pads by the
  Makers of Preparation H
  Hemorrhoidal Remedies
Momentum Muscular Backache
  Formula

Neet Bikini Line Hair Remover
Neet Depilatory Cream
Neet Depilatory Lotion

Outgro Solution
Oxipor VHC Lotion for Psoriasis

Posture 300 mg
◆Posture 600 mg
  Posture-D 300 mg
◆Posture-D 600 mg
◆Preparation H Hemorrhoidal Cream
◆Preparation H Hemorrhoidal Ointment
◆Preparation H Hemorrhoidal
  Suppositories
◆Primatene Mist
◆Primatene Mist Suspension
◆Primatene Tablets-M Formula
◆Primatene Tablets-P Formula
◆Primatene Tablets-Regular Formula

Quiet World Nighttime Pain Formula
Riopan Antacid Chew Tablets
Riopan Antacid Chew Tablets in
  Rollpacks
◆Riopan Antacid Suspension
  Riopan Antacid Swallow Tablets
  Riopan Plus Chew Tablets
  Riopan Plus Chew Tablets in Rollpacks
  Riopan Plus 2 Chew Tablets
◆Riopan Plus Suspension
◆Riopan Plus 2 Suspension

◆Semicid Vaginal Contraceptive Inserts
  Sleep-eze 3 Tablets
  Sudden Action Breath Freshener
  Sudden Beauty Country Air Mask
  Sudden Beauty Hair Spray

Today Personal Lubricant
◆Today Vaginal Contraceptive Sponge
  Trendar Ibuprofen Tablets
  Viro-Med Tablets
  Youth Garde Moisturizer Plus PABA

WINTHROP CONSUMER   **438, 755**
PRODUCTS
Division of Sterling Drug Inc.
90 Park Avenue
New York, NY 10016
Address inquiries to:
Winthrop Consumer Products
For Medical Emergencies Contact:
Medical Department   (212) 907-3027
                      (212) 907-3029
OTC Products Available
◆Bronkaid Mist
  Bronkaid Mist Suspension
◆Bronkaid Tablets
◆Campho-Phenique Cold Sore Gel
◆Campho-Phenique Liquid
◆Campho-Phenique Triple Antibiotic
  Ointment Plus Pain Reliever
  Fergon Elixir
◆Fergon Tablets
  NTZ Long Acting Nasal Spray & Drops
  0.05%
◆NāSal Moisturizing Nasal Spray
◆NāSal Moisturizing Nose Drops
  Neo-Synephrine 12 Hour Adult Nose
  Drops
  Neo-Synephrine 12 Hour Nasal Spray
◆Neo-Synephrine 12 Hour Nasal Spray
  Pump
  Neo-Synephrine 12 Hour Vapor Nasal
  Spray
  Neo-Synephrine Jelly
◆Neo-Synephrine Nasal Sprays
◆Neo-Synephrine Nose Drops
◆pHisoDerm For Baby
◆pHisoDerm Skin Cleanser and
  Conditioner - Regular and Oily
◆pHisoPUFF
  WinGel Liquid & Tablets

WINTHROP PHARMACEUTICALS   **760**
90 Park Avenue
New York, NY 10016
Address Medical Inquiries to:
Professional Services Department
                      (800) 446-6267
All Other Information:
90 Park Avenue
New York, NY 10016
                      (212) 907-2000
OTC Products Available
Anti-Rust Tablets
Bronkolixir
Bronkotabs Tablets
Drisdol
pHisoDerm (see Winthrop Consumer
  Products)
Pontocaine Cream
Pontocaine Ointment
Zephiran Chloride Aqueous Solution
Zephiran Chloride Concentrate Solution
Zephiran Chloride Spray
Zephiran Chloride Tinted Tincture
Zephiran Towelettes

WYETH-AYERST   **438, 763**
LABORATORIES
Division of American Home Products
Corporation
P.O. Box 8299
Philadelphia, PA 19101
Address inquiries to:
Professional Service   (215) 688-4400
For EMERGENCY Medical Information
Day or night call   (215) 688-4400

WYETH-AYERST DISTRIBUTION
CENTERS
Atlanta, GA—P.O. Box 1773
  Paoli, PA 19301-1773
                      (800) 666-7248
  Freight address:
  221 Armour Drive NE
  Atlanta, GA 30324
  Mail DEA order forms to:
  P.O. Box 4365
  Atlanta, GA 30302
Boston MA—P.O. Box 1773
  Paoli, PA 19301-1773
                      (800) 666-7248

Freight address:
7 Connector Road
Andover, MA 01810
Mail DEA order forms to:
P.O. Box 1776
Andover, MA 01810
Chamblee, GA—P.O. Box 1773
  Paoli, PA 19301-1773
                      (800) 666-7248

Freight address:
3600 American Drive
Chamblee, GA 30341
Chicago, IL—P.O. Box 1773
  Paoli, PA 19301-1773
                      (800) 666-7248

Freight address:
745 N. Gary Avenue
Carol Stream, IL 60188
Mail DEA order forms to:
P.O. Box 140
Wheaton, IL 60189-0140
Dallas, TX—P.O. Box 1773
  Paoli, PA 19301-1773
                      (800) 666-7248

Freight address:
11240 Petal Street
Dallas, TX 75238
Mail DEA order forms to:
P.O. Box 650231
Dallas, TX 75265-0231
Foster City, CA—P.O. Box 1773
  Paoli, PA 19301-1773
                      (800) 666-7248

Freight address:
1147 Chess Drive
Foster City, CA 94404
Hawaii—P.O. Box 1773
  Paoli, PA 19301-1773
                      (800) 666-7248
Mail DEA order forms to:
96-1185 Waihona, Street, Unit C1
Pearl City, HI 96782
Kansas City, MO—P.O. Box 1773
  Paoli, PA 19301-1773
                      (800) 666-7248

Freight address:
1340 Taney Street
North Kansas City, MO 64116
Mail DEA order forms to:
P.O. Box 7588
North Kansas City, MO 64116
Los Angeles, CA—P.O. Box 1773
  Paoli, PA 19301-1773
                      (800) 666-7248

Freight address:
6530 Altura Blvd.
Buena Park, CA 90620
Mail DEA order forms to:
P.O. Box 5000
Buena Park, CA 90622-5000
Philadelphia, PA—P.O. Box 1773
  Paoli, PA 19301-1773
                      (800) 666-7248

Freight address:
31 Morehall Road
Frazer, PA 19355
Mail DEA order forms to:
P.O. Box 61
Paoli, PA 19301
Seattle, WA—P.O. Box 1773
  Paoli, PA 19301-1773
                      (800) 666-7248

Freight address:
19255 80th Ave. South
Kent, WA 98032
Mail DEA order forms to:
P.O. Box 5609
Kent, WA 98064-5609

South Plainfield, NJ—P.O. Box 1773
  Paoli, PA 19301-1773
                      (800) 666-7248
Freight address:
4000 Hadley Road
South Plainfield, NJ 07080

(◆ Shown in Product Identification Section)

OTC Products Available
◆Aludrox Oral Suspension
◆Amphojel Suspension
◆Amphojel Suspension without Flavor
◆Amphojel Tablets
◆Basaljel Capsules
◆Basaljel Suspension
◆Basaljel Tablets
◆Cerose-DM
◆Collyrium for Fresh Eyes
◆Collyrium Fresh

◆Nursoy, Soy Protein Isolate Formula for Infants, Concentrated Liquid, Ready-to-Feed, and Powder
◆Resol Oral Electrolyte Rehydration & Maintenance Solution
◆SMA Iron Fortified Infant Formula, Concentrated, Ready-To-Feed & Powder
◆SMA lo-iron
◆Wyanoids Relief Factor Hemorrhoidal Suppositories

ZILA PHARMACEUTICALS,   439, 766 INC.
777 East Thomas Road
Phoenix, AZ 85014
Address inquiries to:
Ed Pomerantz,
Vice President, Marketing
(602) 957-7887
OTC Products Available
ZilaBrace Oral Analgesic Gel
◆Zilactin Medicated Gel
ZilaDent Oral Analgesic Gel

SECTION 2

Product Name Index

In this section only described products are listed in alphabetical sequence by brand name or generic name. They have page numbers to assist you in locating the descriptions. For additional information on other products, you may wish to contact the manufacturer directly. The symbol ◆ indicates the product is shown in the Product Identification Section.

(◆ **Shown in Product Identification Section**)

(◆ Shown in Product Identification Section)

(◆ Shown in Product Identification Section)

(◆ Shown in Product Identification Section)

(◆ Shown in Product Identification Section)

(◆ Shown in Product Identification Section)

(◆ Shown in Product Identification Section)

(◆ Shown in Product Identification Section)

SECTION 3
Product Category Index

Products described in the Product Information (White) Section are listed according to their classifications. The headings and subheadings have been determined by the OTC Review process of the U.S. Food and Drug Administration. Classification of products have been determined by the Publisher with the cooperation of individual manufacturers. In cases where there were differences of opinion or where the manufacturer had no opinion, the Publisher made the final decision.

ANALGESICS

ACETAMINOPHEN

ACETAMINOPHEN & COMBINATIONS

Noxzema Antiseptic Skin Cleanser-Sensitive Skin Formula (Noxell) p 418, 618

S.T.37 Antiseptic Solution (SmithKline Beecham) p 702

Sucrets Maximum Strength Sprays (SmithKline Beecham) p 703

Zephiran Chloride Aqueous Solution (Winthrop Pharmaceuticals) p 760

Zephiran Chloride Spray (Winthrop Pharmaceuticals) p 760

Zephiran Chloride Tinted Tincture (Winthrop Pharmaceuticals) p 760

OPHTHALMIC

Stye Ophthalmic Ointment (Commerce) p 553

TOPICAL

Anbesol Gel Antiseptic-Anesthetic (Whitehall) p 437, 745

Anbesol Gel Antiseptic-Anesthetic - Maximum Strength (Whitehall) p 437, 745

Anbesol Liquid Antiseptic-Anesthetic (Whitehall) p 437, 745

Anbesol Liquid Antiseptic-Anesthetic - Maximum Strength (Whitehall) p 437, 745

Bactine Antiseptic/Anesthetic First Aid Spray (Miles Consumer) p 417, 611

Hibiclens Antimicrobial Skin Cleanser (Stuart) p 433, 721

Hibistat Germicidal Hand Rinse (Stuart) p 723

Impregon Concentrate (Fleming) p 557

Noxzema Antiseptic Skin Cleanser-Extra Strength Formula (Noxell) p 418, 617

Noxzema Antiseptic Skin Cleanser-Regular Formula (Noxell) p 418, 617

Noxzema Antiseptic Skin Cleanser-Sensitive Skin Formula (Noxell) p 418, 618

Orajel Mouth-Aid (Commerce) p 552

Sucrets Maximum Strength Sprays (SmithKline Beecham) p 703

Zephiran Chloride Aqueous Solution (Winthrop Pharmaceuticals) p 760

Zephiran Chloride Spray (Winthrop Pharmaceuticals) p 760

Zephiran Chloride Tinted Tincture (Winthrop Pharmaceuticals) p 760

ANTIBIOTICS

TOPICAL

Baciguent Antibiotic Ointment (Upjohn) p 731

Myciguent Antibiotic Ointment (Upjohn) p 733

Mycitracin Triple Antibiotic Ointment (Upjohn) p 435, 733

Neosporin Cream (Burroughs Wellcome) p 407, 537

Neosporin Ointment (Burroughs Wellcome) p 407, 537

Neosporin Maximum Strength Ointment (Burroughs Wellcome) p 407, 537

Polysporin Ointment (Burroughs Wellcome) p 407, 537

Polysporin Powder (Burroughs Wellcome) p 407, 538

Polysporin Spray (Burroughs Wellcome) p 407, 538

ANTIDOTES

ACUTE TOXIC INGESTION

Charcoaid (Requa) p 644

ANTIEMETICS
(see under NAUSEA MEDICATIONS)

ANTIHISTAMINES

Actifed Plus Caplets (Burroughs Wellcome) p 407, 534

Actifed Plus Tablets (Burroughs Wellcome) p 407, 535

BC Cold Powder Multi-Symptom Formula (Block) p 518

Isoclor Timesule Capsules (Fisons Consumer) p 556

Pediacare Night Rest Cough-Cold Formula Liquid (McNeil Consumer Products) p 415, 594

ANTI-INFLAMMATORY AGENTS

SALICYLATES

Aurum the Gold Lotion (Au Pharmaceuticals) p 508

TheraGold (Au Pharmaceuticals) p 508

Therapeutic Gold (Au Pharmaceuticals) p 508

OTHER

Herpecin-L Cold Sore Lip Balm (Campbell) p 541

ANTIPARASITICS

ARTHROPODS

LICE

A-200 Pediculicide Shampoo & Gel (SmithKline Beecham) p 430, 695

Pronto Lice Killing Shampoo Kit (Commerce) p 552

Pronto Lice Killing Spray (Commerce) p 552

R&C Shampoo (Reed & Carnrick) p 422, 642

R&C Spray III (Reed & Carnrick) p 422, 643

RID Lice Control Spray (Leeming) p 584

RID Lice Killing Shampoo (Leeming) p 584

HELMINTHS

ASCARIS (ROUNDWORM)

Reese's Pinworm Medicine (Reese Chemical) p 423, 643

ENTEROBIUS (PINWORM)

Reese's Pinworm Medicine (Reese Chemical) p 423, 643

ANTIPERSPIRANTS
(see under DEODORANTS & DERMATOLOGICALS, ANTIPERSPIRANTS)

ANTIPYRETICS

Advil Ibuprofen Caplets and Tablets (Whitehall) p 436, 743

BC Cold Powder Multi-Symptom Formula (Block) p 518

BC Cold Powder Non-Drowsy Formula (Block) p 518

Ibuprofen Tablets (Ohm Laboratories) p 418, 620

Ibuprohm Caplets (Ohm Laboratories) p 418, 620

Snaplets-FR (Baker Cummins Pharmaceuticals) p 404, 511

ANTITUSSIVES
(see under COUGH & COLD PREPARATIONS)

APPETITE SUPPRESSANTS

Acutrim 16 Hour Appetite Suppressant (CIBA Consumer) p 408, 544

Acutrim Late Day Appetite Suppressant (CIBA Consumer) p 408, 544

Acutrim II Maximum Strength Appetite Suppressant (CIBA Consumer) p 408, 544

Dexatrim Capsules (Thompson Medical) p 727

Dexatrim Maximum Strength Caffeine-Free Caplets (Thompson Medical) p 727

Dexatrim Maximum Strength Caffeine-Free Capsules (Thompson Medical) p 727

Dexatrim Maximum Strength Plus Vitamin C/Caffeine-free Caplets (Thompson Medical) p 434, 727

Dexatrim Maximum Strength Plus Vitamin C/Caffeine-free Capsules (Thompson Medical) p 434, 727

Dexatrim Maximum Strength Pre-Meal Caplets (Thompson Medical) p 727

ARTHRITIS MEDICATIONS

NSAIDS

Ibuprofen Tablets (Ohm Laboratories) p 418, 620

Ibuprohm Caplets (Ohm Laboratories) p 418, 620

SALICYLATES

Therapy Bayer Aspirin Caplets (Glenbrook) p 410, 561

Norwich Extra-Strength Aspirin (Chattem) p 542

Norwich Regular Strength Aspirin (Chattem) p 542

ARTIFICIAL TEARS PREPARATIONS

Celluvisc Lubricant Ophthalmic Solution (Allergan Pharmaceuticals) p 403, 504

Lacril Lubricant Ophthalmic Solution (Allergan Pharmaceuticals) p 505

Liquifilm Forte (Allergan Pharmaceuticals) p 505

Liquifilm Tears (Allergan Pharmaceuticals) p 403, 505

Prefrin Liquifilm (Allergan Pharmaceuticals) p 403, 505

Refresh Lubricant Ophthalmic Solution (Allergan Pharmaceuticals) p 403, 506

Relief Eye Drops for Red Eyes (Allergan Pharmaceuticals) p 403, 506

Tears Plus Lubricant Ophthalmic Solution (Allergan Pharmaceuticals) p 403, 506

ASTHMA PREPARATIONS

AsthmaHaler Mist Epinephrine Bitartrate Bronchodilator (SmithKline Beecham) p 695

AsthmaNefrin Solution "A" Bronchodilator (SmithKline Beecham) p 695

Bronkaid Mist (Winthrop Consumer Products) p 438, 755

Bronkaid Mist Suspension (Winthrop Consumer Products) p 756

Bronkaid Tablets (Winthrop Consumer Products) p 438, 756

Bronkolixir (Winthrop Pharmaceuticals) p 760

Bronkotabs Tablets (Winthrop Pharmaceuticals) p 760

Primatene Mist (Whitehall) p 437, 751

Primatene Mist Suspension (Whitehall) p 437, 752

Primatene Tablets-M Formula (Whitehall) p 437, 752

Primatene Tablets-P Formula (Whitehall) p 437, 752

Primatene Tablets-Regular Formula (Whitehall) p 437, 752

ASTRINGENTS
(see under DERMATOLOGICALS, ASTRINGENTS)

ATHLETE'S FOOT TREATMENT
(see under DERMATOLOGICALS, FUNGICIDES)

B

BABY PRODUCTS

Caldesene Medicated Ointment (Fisons Consumer) p 409, 555

Caldesene Medicated Powder (Fisons Consumer) p 409, 555

Desitin Ointment (Leeming) p 413, 583

Diaper Guard (Commerce) p 551

Dyprotex Diaper Rash Pads (Blistex) p 404, 517

Johnson's Baby Sunblock Lotion (SPF 15) (Johnson & Johnson Consumer) p 411, 570

Massengill Baby Powder Soft Cloth Towelette and Unscented Soft Cloth Towelette (SmithKline Beecham) p 698

Baby Orajel (Commerce) p 551

Baby Orajel Nighttime Formula (Commerce) p 551

pHisoDerm For Baby (Winthrop Consumer Products) p 438, 759

Triaminic-12 Tablets (Sandoz Consumer) p 427, 682

Triaminicin Tablets (Sandoz Consumer) p 428, 682

Triaminicol Multi-Symptom Cold Tablets (Sandoz Consumer) p 428, 682

Triaminicol Multi-Symptom Relief (Sandoz Consumer) p 428, 683

Children's Tylenol Cold Liquid Formula and Chewable Cold Tablets (McNeil Consumer Products) p 415, 600

Tylenol Cold Medication Caplets and Tablets (McNeil Consumer Products) p 415, 601

Tylenol Cold Medication Liquid (McNeil Consumer Products) p 415, 601

Vicks Children's NyQuil (Richardson-Vicks Inc.) p 423, 651

Vicks Formula 44 Cough Medicine (Richardson-Vicks Inc.) p 423, 649

Vicks NyQuil Nighttime Colds Medicine-Original & Cherry Flavor (Richardson-Vicks Inc.) p 423, 652

Vicks Pediatric Formula 44 Cough & Cold Medicine (Richardson-Vicks Inc.) p 423, 650

DECONGESTANTS

ORAL & COMBINATIONS

Actifed Capsules (Burroughs Wellcome) p 406, 533

Actifed Plus Caplets (Burroughs Wellcome) p 407, 534

Actifed Plus Tablets (Burroughs Wellcome) p 407, 535

Actifed Syrup (Burroughs Wellcome) p 406, 534

Actifed Tablets (Burroughs Wellcome) p 407, 535

Actifed 12-Hour Capsules (Burroughs Wellcome) p 406, 534

Afrinol Repetabs Tablets Long-Acting Nasal Decongestant (Schering) p 428, 684

Alka-Seltzer Plus Cold Medicine (Miles Consumer) p 416, 610

Alka-Seltzer Plus Night-Time Cold Medicine (Miles Consumer) p 416, 611

AllerAct Decongestant Caplets (Burroughs Wellcome) p 407, 536

AllerAct Decongestant Tablets (Burroughs Wellcome) p 407, 536

Allerest No Drowsiness Tablets (Fisons Consumer) p 409, 554

BC Cold Powder Multi-Symptom Formula (Block) p 518

BC Cold Powder Non-Drowsy Formula (Block) p 518

Bayer Children's Cold Tablets (Glenbrook) p 410, 559

Benadryl Decongestant Elixir (Parke-Davis) p 419, 625

Benadryl Decongestant Kapseals (Parke-Davis) p 419, 625

Benadryl Decongestant Tablets (Parke-Davis) p 419, 625

Benylin Decongestant (Parke-Davis) p 420, 628

Benylin Expectorant (Parke-Davis) p 420, 628

Bromfed Syrup (Muro) p 615

Cerose-DM (Wyeth-Ayerst) p 439, 764

Cheracol Plus Head Cold/Cough Formula (Upjohn) p 434, 731

Chlor-Trimeton Decongestant Tablets (Schering) p 428, 685

Chlor-Trimeton Long Acting Decongestant Repetabs Tablets (Schering) p 428, 685

CoAdvil (Whitehall) p 436, 746

Allergy Sinus Comtrex Multi-Symptom Allergy/Sinus Formula Tablets & Caplets (Bristol-Myers Products) p 405, 528

Comtrex Multi-Symptom Cold Reliever Tablets/Caplets/Liquid/Liquigels (Bristol-Myers Products) p 405, 527

Congespirin For Children Aspirin Free Chewable Cold Tablets (Bristol-Myers Products) p 405, 529

Congestac Caplets (SmithKline Consumer) p 431, 707

Contac Continuous Action Decongestant Capsules (SmithKline Consumer) p 431, 708

Contac Jr. Children's Cold Medicine (SmithKline Consumer) p 431, 711

Contac Maximum Strength Continuous Action Decongestant Caplets (SmithKline Consumer) p 431, 707

Contac Nighttime Cold Medicine (SmithKline Consumer) p 431, 711

Contac Severe Cold Formula Caplets (SmithKline Consumer) p 431, 709

Contac Sinus Caplets Maximum Strength Non-Drowsy Formula (SmithKline Consumer) p 431, 707

Contac Sinus Tablets Maximum Strength Non-Drowsy Formula (SmithKline Consumer) p 431, 708

Coricidin 'D' Decongestant Tablets (Schering) p 429, 686

Coricidin Demilets Tablets for Children (Schering) p 429, 687

Coricidin Maximum Strength Sinus Headache Caplets (Schering) p 429, 688

Demazin Nasal Decongestant/Antihistamine Repetabs Tablets & Syrup (Schering) p 688

Dimacol Caplets (Robins) p 424, 656

Dimetane Decongestant Caplets (Robins) p 425, 657

Dimetane Decongestant Elixir (Robins) p 425, 657

Dimetapp Elixir (Robins) p 425, 658

Dimetapp Extentabs (Robins) p 425, 658

Dimetapp Plus Caplets (Robins) p 425, 659

Dimetapp Tablets (Robins) p 425, 658

Disophrol Chronotab Sustained-Action Tablets (Schering) p 689

Dorcol Children's Cough Syrup (Sandoz Consumer) p 427, 677

Dorcol Children's Decongestant Liquid (Sandoz Consumer) p 427, 677

Dorcol Children's Liquid Cold Formula (Sandoz Consumer) p 427, 678

Dristan Decongestant/Antihistamine/Analgesic Coated Caplets (Whitehall) p 437, 748

Dristan Decongestant/Antihistamine/Analgesic Coated Tablets (Whitehall) p 437, 748

Maximum Strength Dristan Decongestant/Analgesic Coated Caplets (Whitehall) p 437, 749

Drixoral Antihistamine/Nasal Decongestant Syrup (Schering) p 429, 689

Drixoral Plus Extended-Release Tablets (Schering) p 429, 690

Drixoral Sustained-Action Tablets (Schering) p 429, 690

Duration Long Acting Nasal Decongestant Tablets (Plough) p 421, 634

Sinus Excedrin Analgesic, Decongestant Tablets & Caplets (Bristol-Myers Products) p 405, 406, 531

4-Way Cold Tablets (Bristol-Myers Products) p 406, 531

Fedahist Decongestant Syrup (Schwarz Pharma) p 430, 693

Fedahist Tablets (Schwarz Pharma) p 430, 693

Hyland's C-Plus Cold Tablets (Standard Homeopathic) p 719

Naldecon CX Adult Liquid (Bristol Laboratories) p 522

Naldecon DX Adult Liquid (Bristol Laboratories) p 522

Naldecon DX Children's Syrup (Bristol Laboratories) p 523

Naldecon DX Pediatric Drops (Bristol Laboratories) p 523

Naldecon EX Children's Syrup (Bristol Laboratories) p 523

Naldecon EX Pediatric Drops (Bristol Laboratories) p 524

Novahistine DMX (Lakeside Pharmaceuticals) p 412, 574

Novahistine Elixir (Lakeside Pharmaceuticals) p 412, 575

Ornex Caplets (SmithKline Consumer) p 432, 715

Pediacare Cold Formula Liquid (McNeil Consumer Products) p 415, 594

Pediacare Cough-Cold Formula Liquid and Chewable Tablets (McNeil Consumer Products) p 415, 594

Pediacare Infants' Oral Decongestant Drops (McNeil Consumer Products) p 415, 594

Pyrroxate Capsules (Upjohn) p 435, 733

Robitussin Night Relief (Robins) p 425, 661

Robitussin-CF (Robins) p 425, 660

Robitussin-PE (Robins) p 425, 660

Ryna Liquid (Wallace) p 435, 737

Ryna-C Liquid (Wallace) p 435, 737

Ryna-CX Liquid (Wallace) p 435, 737

Sinarest No Drowsiness Tablets (Fisons Consumer) p 557

Sine-Aid Maximum Strength Sinus Headache Caplets (McNeil Consumer Products) p 415, 596

Sine-Aid Maximum Strength Sinus Headache Tablets (McNeil Consumer Products) p 415, 596

Sine-Off Maximum Strength Allergy/Sinus Formula Caplets (SmithKline Consumer) p 432, 715

Sine-Off Maximum Strength No Drowsiness Formula Caplets (SmithKline Consumer) p 432, 715

Sine-Off Sinus Medicine Tablets-Aspirin Formula (SmithKline Consumer) p 432, 716

Singlet Tablets (Lakeside Pharmaceuticals) p 576

SinuStat Nasal Decongestant (Murdock) p 417, 615

Sinutab Maximum Strength Caplets (Parke-Davis) p 420, 631

Sinutab Maximum Strength Tablets (Parke-Davis) p 420, 631

Sinutab Maximum Strength Without Drowsiness Tablets & Caplets (Parke-Davis) p 420, 632

Sinutab Regular Strength Without Drowsiness Formula (Parke-Davis) p 420, 631

Snaplets-D (Baker Cummins Pharmaceuticals) p 404, 511

Snaplets-Multi (Baker Cummins Pharmaceuticals) p 404, 512

St. Joseph Cold Tablets for Children (Plough) p 637

St. Joseph Nighttime Cold Medicine (Plough) p 421, 637

Sudafed Children's Liquid (Burroughs Wellcome) p 407, 538

Sudafed Cough Syrup (Burroughs Wellcome) p 407, 538

Sudafed Plus Liquid (Burroughs Wellcome) p 407, 539

Sudafed Plus Tablets (Burroughs Wellcome) p 407, 539

Sudafed Sinus Caplets (Burroughs Wellcome) p 407, 540

Sudafed Sinus Tablets (Burroughs Wellcome) p 407, 540

Sudafed Tablets, 30 mg (Burroughs Wellcome) p 407, 539

Sudafed Tablets, Adult Strength, 60 mg (Burroughs Wellcome) p 407, 539

Sudafed 12 Hour Capsules (Burroughs Wellcome) p 408, 540

TheraFlu Flu and Cold Medicine (Sandoz Consumer) p 427, 679

Triaminic Chewables (Sandoz Consumer) p 680

Triaminic Cold Tablets (Sandoz Consumer) p 427, 680

Triaminic Expectorant (Sandoz Consumer) p 427, 680

Triaminic Nite Light (Sandoz Consumer) p 428, 681

Triaminic Syrup (Sandoz Consumer) p 427, 681

Gynol II Original Formula Contraceptive Jelly (Ortho Pharmaceutical) p 419, 621

Ortho-Gynol Contraceptive Jelly (Ortho Pharmaceutical) p 419, 623

Semicid Vaginal Contraceptive Inserts (Whitehall) p 438, 754

CORN & CALLUS REMOVERS

Freezone Solution (Whitehall) p 749

COSMETICS

Herpecin-L Cold Sore Lip Balm (Campbell) p 541

COUGH PREPARATIONS

ANTITUSSIVES & COMBINATIONS

Bayer Children's Cough Syrup (Glenbrook) p 410, 559

Benylin Cough Syrup (Parke-Davis) p 420, 627

Benylin Decongestant (Parke-Davis) p 420, 628

Benylin DM (Parke-Davis) p 420, 627

Cerose-DM (Wyeth-Ayerst) p 439, 764

Cheracol D Cough Formula (Upjohn) p 434, 731

Cheracol Plus Head Cold/Cough Formula (Upjohn) p 434, 731

Comtrex Multi-Symptom Cold Reliever Tablets/Caplets/Liquid/Liquigels (Bristol-Myers Products) p 405, 527

Contac Cough Formula (SmithKline Consumer) p 431, 709

Contac Cough & Sore Throat Formula (SmithKline Consumer) p 431, 710

Contac Jr. Children's Cold Medicine (SmithKline Consumer) p 431, 711

Contac Nighttime Cold Medicine (SmithKline Consumer) p 431, 711

Contac Severe Cold Formula Caplets (SmithKline Consumer) p 431, 709

Dimacol Caplets (Robins) p 424, 656

Dorcol Children's Cough Syrup (Sandoz Consumer) p 427, 677

Halls Mentho-Lyptus Cough Suppressant Tablets (Warner-Lambert) p 435, 738

Hold (SmithKline Beecham) p 697

Hyland's Cough Syrup with Honey (Standard Homeopathic) p 718

Naldecon CX Adult Liquid (Bristol Laboratories) p 522

Naldecon DX Adult Liquid (Bristol Laboratories) p 522

Naldecon DX Children's Syrup (Bristol Laboratories) p 523

Naldecon DX Pediatric Drops (Bristol Laboratories) p 523

Naldecon Senior DX Cough/Cold Liquid (Bristol Laboratories) p 524

Novahistine DMX (Lakeside Pharmaceuticals) p 412, 574

Pediacare Cough-Cold Formula Liquid and Chewable Tablets (McNeil Consumer Products) p 415, 594

Pediacare Night Rest Cough-Cold Formula Liquid (McNeil Consumer Products) p 415, 594

Robitussin Night Relief (Robins) p 425, 661

Robitussin-CF (Robins) p 425, 660

Robitussin-DM (Robins) p 425, 660

Ryna-C Liquid (Wallace) p 435, 737

Ryna-CX Liquid (Wallace) p 435, 737

Snaplets-DM (Baker Cummins Pharmaceuticals) p 404, 511

Snaplets-Multi (Baker Cummins Pharmaceuticals) p 404, 512

St. Joseph Cough Suppressant for Children (Plough) p 421, 637

Sucrets Cough Control Formula (SmithKline Beecham) p 703

Sudafed Cough Syrup (Burroughs Wellcome) p 407, 538

TheraFlu Flu and Cold Medicine (Sandoz Consumer) p 427, 679

Triaminic Nite Light (Sandoz Consumer) p 428, 681

Triaminic-DM Syrup (Sandoz Consumer) p 427, 681

Triaminicol Multi-Symptom Cold Tablets (Sandoz Consumer) p 428, 682

Triaminicol Multi-Symptom Relief (Sandoz Consumer) p 428, 683

Tylenol Cold Medication No Drowsiness Formula Caplets (McNeil Consumer Products) p 415, 602

Vicks Children's Cough Syrup (Richardson-Vicks Inc.) p 648

Vicks Children's NyQuil (Richardson-Vicks Inc.) p 423, 651

Vicks Daycare Daytime Colds Medicine Caplets (Richardson-Vicks Inc.) p 423, 648

Vicks Daycare Multi-Symptom Colds Medicine Liquid (Richardson-Vicks Inc.) p 423, 648

Vicks Formula 44 Cough Control Discs (Richardson-Vicks Inc.) p 649

Vicks Formula 44 Cough Medicine (Richardson-Vicks Inc.) p 423, 649

Vicks Formula 44D Decongestant Cough Medicine (Richardson-Vicks Inc.) p 423, 649

Vicks Formula 44M Multi-Symptom Cough Medicine (Richardson-Vicks Inc.) p 423, 650

Vicks NyQuil Nighttime Colds Medicine-Original & Cherry Flavor (Richardson-Vicks Inc.) p 423, 652

Vicks Pediatric Formula 44 Cough Medicine (Richardson-Vicks Inc.) p 423, 650

Vicks Pediatric Formula 44 Cough & Cold Medicine (Richardson-Vicks Inc.) p 423, 650

Vicks Pediatric Formula 44 Cough & Congestion Medicine (Richardson-Vicks Inc.) p 423, 651

Vicks Vaporub (Richardson-Vicks Inc.) p 424, 653

Vicks Vaposteam (Richardson-Vicks Inc.) p 653

EXPECTORANTS & COMBINATIONS

Benylin Expectorant (Parke-Davis) p 420, 628

Cheracol D Cough Formula (Upjohn) p 434, 731

Cough Formula Comtrex (Bristol-Myers Products) p 528

Contac Cough Formula (SmithKline Consumer) p 431, 709

Contac Cough & Sore Throat Formula (SmithKline Consumer) p 431, 710

Dimacol Caplets (Robins) p 424, 656

Dorcol Children's Cough Syrup (Sandoz Consumer) p 427, 677

Fedahist Expectorant Pediatric Drops (Schwarz Pharma) p 430, 693

Fedahist Expectorant Syrup (Schwarz Pharma) p 430, 693

Naldecon CX Adult Liquid (Bristol Laboratories) p 522

Naldecon DX Adult Liquid (Bristol Laboratories) p 522

Naldecon DX Children's Syrup (Bristol Laboratories) p 523

Naldecon DX Pediatric Drops (Bristol Laboratories) p 523

Naldecon EX Children's Syrup (Bristol Laboratories) p 523

Naldecon EX Pediatric Drops (Bristol Laboratories) p 524

Naldecon Senior DX Cough/Cold Liquid (Bristol Laboratories) p 524

Naldecon Senior EX Cough/Cold Liquid (Bristol Laboratories) p 525

Novahistine DMX (Lakeside Pharmaceuticals) p 412, 574

Robitussin (Robins) p 425, 659

Robitussin-CF (Robins) p 425, 660

Robitussin-DM (Robins) p 425, 660

Robitussin-PE (Robins) p 425, 660

Ryna-CX Liquid (Wallace) p 435, 737

Snaplets-EX (Baker Cummins Pharmaceuticals) p 404, 511

Sudafed Cough Syrup (Burroughs Wellcome) p 407, 538

Triaminic Expectorant (Sandoz Consumer) p 427, 680

Vicks Children's Cough Syrup (Richardson-Vicks Inc.) p 648

Vicks Daycare Daytime Colds Medicine Caplets (Richardson-Vicks Inc.) p 423, 648

Vicks Daycare Multi-Symptom Colds Medicine Liquid (Richardson-Vicks Inc.) p 423, 648

Vicks Formula 44D Decongestant Cough Medicine (Richardson-Vicks Inc.) p 423, 649

Vicks Formula 44M Multi-Symptom Cough Medicine (Richardson-Vicks Inc.) p 423, 650

LOZENGES

N'ICE Medicated Sugarless Sore Throat and Cough Lozenges (SmithKline Beecham) p 699

Sucrets Cold Relief Formula (SmithKline Beecham) p 703

Vicks Cough Silencers Cough Drops (Richardson-Vicks Inc.) p 648

Vicks Formula 44 Cough Control Discs (Richardson-Vicks Inc.) p 649

Vicks Throat Lozenges (Richardson-Vicks Inc.) p 653

NON-NARCOTIC

Cough Formula Comtrex (Bristol-Myers Products) p 528

OTHER

N'ICE Medicated Sugarless Sore Throat and Cough Lozenges (SmithKline Beecham) p 699

N'ICE Sore Throat Spray (SmithKline Beecham) p 699

COUGH & COLD PREPARATIONS

NON-NARCOTIC

Isoclor Timesule Capsules (Fisons Consumer) p 556

Pediacare Night Rest Cough-Cold Formula Liquid (McNeil Consumer Products) p 415, 594

D

DANDRUFF & SEBORRHEA PREPARATIONS

(see under DERMATOLOGICALS, DANDRUFF MEDICATIONS & SEBORRHEA TREATMENT)

DECONGESTANTS

ORAL

Cough Formula Comtrex (Bristol-Myers Products) p 528

Isoclor Timesule Capsules (Fisons Consumer) p 556

Pediacare Night Rest Cough-Cold Formula Liquid (McNeil Consumer Products) p 415, 594

Snaplets-DM (Baker Cummins Pharmaceuticals) p 404, 511

Snaplets-EX (Baker Cummins Pharmaceuticals) p 404, 511

Tylenol Allergy Sinus Medication Caplets, Maximum Strength (McNeil Consumer Products) p 415, 603

DECONGESTANTS, EXPECTORANTS & COMBINATIONS

Cough Formula Comtrex (Bristol-Myers Products) p 528

DECONGESTANTS, OPHTHALMIC

DECONGESTANT COMBINATIONS

Prefrin Liquifilm (Allergan Pharmaceuticals) p 403, 505

Relief Eye Drops for Red Eyes (Allergan Pharmaceuticals) p 403, 506

Visine Extra Eye Drops (Leeming) p 413, 586

DECONGESTANT/ASTRINGENT COMBINATIONS

Visine A.C. Eye Drops (Leeming) p 413, 586

DECONGESTANTS

Clear Eyes Lubricating Eye Redness Reliever (Ross) p 426, 669

Collyrium Fresh (Wyeth-Ayerst) p 439, 764

Murine Plus Lubricating Eye Redness Reliever (Ross) p 426, 671

Visine Eye Drops (Leeming) p 413, 585

Visine L.R. Eye Drops (Leeming) p 413, 586

VASOCONSTRICTORS

Visine L.R. Eye Drops (Leeming) p 413, 586

DEMULCENT

Celluvisc Lubricant Ophthalmic Solution (Allergan Pharmaceuticals) p 403, 504

Lacril Lubricant Ophthalmic Solution (Allergan Pharmaceuticals) p 505

Liquifilm Forte (Allergan Pharmaceuticals) p 505

Liquifilm Tears (Allergan Pharmaceuticals) p 403, 505

Murine Eye Lubricant (Ross) p 426, 670

Murine Plus Lubricating Eye Redness Reliever (Ross) p 426, 671

Prefrin Liquifilm (Allergan Pharmaceuticals) p 403, 505

Refresh Lubricant Ophthalmic Solution (Allergan Pharmaceuticals) p 403, 506

Relief Eye Drops for Red Eyes (Allergan Pharmaceuticals) p 403, 506

Tears Plus Lubricant Ophthalmic Solution (Allergan Pharmaceuticals) p 403, 506

Visine Extra Eye Drops (Leeming) p 413, 586

DENTAL PREPARATIONS

CAVITY AGENTS

Colgate Junior Fluoride Gel Toothpaste (Colgate-Palmolive) p 409, 549

Colgate MFP Fluoride Gel (Colgate-Palmolive) p 409, 549

Colgate MFP Fluoride Toothpaste (Colgate-Palmolive) p 409, 549

Colgate Tartar Control Formula (Colgate-Palmolive) p 409, 550

Colgate Tartar Control Gel (Colgate-Palmolive) p 409, 550

Fluorigard Anti-Cavity Fluoride Rinse (Colgate-Palmolive) p 409, 550

Listermint with Fluoride (Warner-Lambert) p 436, 739

DENTIFRICES

Colgate Junior Fluoride Gel Toothpaste (Colgate-Palmolive) p 409, 549

Colgate MFP Fluoride Gel (Colgate-Palmolive) p 409, 549

Colgate MFP Fluoride Toothpaste (Colgate-Palmolive) p 409, 549

Colgate Tartar Control Formula (Colgate-Palmolive) p 409, 550

Colgate Tartar Control Gel (Colgate-Palmolive) p 409, 550

Denquel Sensitive Teeth Toothpaste (Procter & Gamble) p 638

Promise Toothpaste (Block) p 519

Mint Gel Sensodyne (Block) p 519

Mint Sensodyne Toothpaste (Block) p 519

Original Sensodyne Toothpaste (Block) p 519

RINSES

Chloraseptic Liquid, Cherry, Menthol or Cool Mint (Richardson-Vicks Inc.) p 423, 645

Chloraseptic Liquid - Nitrogen Propelled Spray (Richardson-Vicks Inc.) p 423, 645

Colgate Mouthwash Tartar Control Formula (Colgate-Palmolive) p 409, 549

Fluorigard Anti-Cavity Fluoride Rinse (Colgate-Palmolive) p 409, 550

Listerine Antiseptic (Warner-Lambert) p 435, 739

Listermint with Fluoride (Warner-Lambert) p 436, 739

TARTAR AGENT

Colgate Mouthwash Tartar Control Formula (Colgate-Palmolive) p 409, 549

Colgate Tartar Control Formula (Colgate-Palmolive) p 409, 550

Colgate Tartar Control Gel (Colgate-Palmolive) p 409, 550

OTHER

Anbesol Gel Antiseptic-Anesthetic (Whitehall) p 437, 745

Anbesol Gel Antiseptic-Anesthetic - Maximum Strength (Whitehall) p 437, 745

Anbesol Liquid Antiseptic-Anesthetic (Whitehall) p 437, 745

Anbesol Liquid Antiseptic-Anesthetic - Maximum Strength (Whitehall) p 437, 745

Chloraseptic Lozenges, Cherry, Menthol or Cool Mint (Richardson-Vicks Inc.) p 423, 645

Gly-Oxide Liquid (Marion) p 414, 591

ZilaBrace Oral Analgesic Gel (Zila Pharmaceuticals) p 766

Zilactin Medicated Gel (Zila Pharmaceuticals) p 439, 766

ZilaDent Oral Analgesic Gel (Zila Pharmaceuticals) p 766

DENTURE PREPARATIONS

Anbesol Gel Antiseptic-Anesthetic (Whitehall) p 437, 745

Anbesol Gel Antiseptic-Anesthetic - Maximum Strength (Whitehall) p 437, 745

Anbesol Liquid Antiseptic-Anesthetic (Whitehall) p 437, 745

Anbesol Liquid Antiseptic-Anesthetic - Maximum Strength (Whitehall) p 437, 745

Professional Strength Efferdent (Warner-Lambert) p 435, 738

Medicone Derma Ointment (Medicone) p 416, 606

DEODORANTS

Certain Dri Antiperspirant (Numark) p 418, 619

Nullo Deodorant Tablets (Chattem) p 542

DERMATOLOGICALS

ABRADANT

Oxy Clean Lathering Facial Scrub (SmithKline Beecham) p 430, 700

pHisoPUFF (Winthrop Consumer Products) p 438, 759

ACNE PREPARATIONS

Acno Cleanser (Baker Cummins Dermatologicals) p 508

Acno Lotion (Baker Cummins Dermatologicals) p 508

Acnomel Cream (SmithKline Consumer) p 430, 705

Aqua Glyde Cleanser (Herald Pharmacal) p 567

Aveeno Cleansing Bar for Acne (Rydelle) p 427, 675

Biochemic Tissue Salts (NuAGE Laboratories) p 619

Clear by Design Medicated Acne Gel (SmithKline Consumer) p 431, 706

Clear By Design Medicated Cleansing Pads (SmithKline Consumer) p 431, 706

Clearasil Adult Care Medicated Blemish Cream (Richardson-Vicks Inc.) p 424, 645

Clearasil 10% Benzoyl Peroxide Medicated Anti-Acne Lotion (Richardson-Vicks Inc.) p 646

Clearasil Doubleclear Pads - Regular and Maximum Strength (Richardson-Vicks Inc.) p 424, 645

Clearasil Maximum Strength Medicated Anti-Acne Cream, Tinted (Richardson-Vicks Inc.) p 424, 646

Clearasil Maximum Strength Medicated Anti-Acne Cream, Vanishing (Richardson-Vicks Inc.) p 424, 646

Clearasil Medicated Astringent (Richardson-Vicks Inc.) p 424, 646

DDS-Acidophilus (UAS Laboratories) p 730

Noxzema Antiseptic Skin Cleanser-Extra Strength Formula (Noxell) p 418, 617

Noxzema Antiseptic Skin Cleanser-Regular Formula (Noxell) p 418, 617

Noxzema Clear-Ups Anti-Acne Gel (Noxell) p 418, 618

Noxzema Clear-Ups Maximum Strength Lotion, Vanishing (Noxell) p 418, 618

Noxzema Clear-Ups Medicated Pads-Maximum Strength 2.0% Salicylic Acid (Noxell) p 418, 618

Noxzema Clear-Ups Medicated Pads-Regular Strength 0.5% Salicylic Acid (Noxell) p 418, 618

Noxzema Clear-Ups On-the-Spot Treatment, Tinted & Vanishing (Noxell) p 418, 618

Oxy Clean Medicated Cleanser (SmithKline Beecham) p 430, 700

Oxy Clean Medicated Pads - Regular, Sensitive Skin, and Maximum Strength (SmithKline Beecham) p 430, 700

Oxy Clean Medicated Soap (SmithKline Beecham) p 430, 700

Oxy Night Watch (SmithKline Beecham) p 430, 701

Oxy 10 Daily Face Wash (SmithKline Beecham) p 430, 701

Oxy-5 and Oxy-10 Tinted and Vanishing Formulas with Sorboxyl (SmithKline Beecham) p 430, 699

Propa pH Cleanser for Normal/Combination Skin (Commerce) p 553

Propa pH Cleanser for Sensitive Skin (Commerce) p 553

Stri-Dex Maximum Strength Pads (Glenbrook) p 411, 566

Stri-Dex Regular Strength Pads (Glenbrook) p 411, 566

ANALGESIC

Americaine Topical Anesthetic Ointment (Fisons Consumer) p 409, 554

Americaine Topical Anesthetic Spray (Fisons Consumer) p 409, 554

Aspercreme Creme & Lotion (Thompson Medical) p 727

Benadryl Anti-Itch Cream (Parke-Davis) p 419, 625

Benadryl Spray (Parke-Davis) p 419, 627

Boil•Ease (Commerce) p 550

Campho-Phenique Triple Antibiotic Ointment Plus Pain Reliever (Winthrop Consumer Products) p 438, 757

Icy Hot Balm (Richardson-Vicks Inc.) p 423, 647

Icy Hot Cream (Richardson-Vicks Inc.) p 423, 647

Icy Hot Stick (Richardson-Vicks Inc.) p 423, 647

Therapeutic Mineral Ice (Bristol-Myers Products) p 406, 533

ANESTHETICS, TOPICAL

Americaine Topical Anesthetic Ointment (Fisons Consumer) p 409, 554

Americaine Topical Anesthetic Spray (Fisons Consumer) p 409, 554

Bactine Antiseptic/Anesthetic First Aid Spray (Miles Consumer) p 417, 611

Boil•Ease (Commerce) p 550

Campho-Phenique Triple Antibiotic Ointment Plus Pain Reliever (Winthrop Consumer Products) p 438, 757

Dermoplast Anesthetic Pain Relief Lotion (Whitehall) p 437, 747

Dermoplast Anesthetic Pain Relief Spray (Whitehall) p 437, 748

Medicone Derma Ointment (Medicone) p 416, 606

Solarcaine (Plough) p 421, 637

ANTIBACTERIAL

Anbesol Gel Antiseptic-Anesthetic (Whitehall) p 437, 745

Anbesol Gel Antiseptic-Anesthetic - Maximum Strength (Whitehall) p 437, 745

Anbesol Liquid Antiseptic-Anesthetic (Whitehall) p 437, 745

Anbesol Liquid Antiseptic-Anesthetic - Maximum Strength (Whitehall) p 437, 745

Keri Lotion-Silky Smooth Formula (Westwood) p 436, 741

Massengill Medicated Soft Cloth Towelette (SmithKline Beecham) p 698

Medicone Derma Ointment (Medicone) p 416, 606

Moisturel Cream (Westwood) p 436, 741

Moisturel Lotion (Westwood) p 436, 741

Noxzema Medicated Skin Cream (Noxell) p 418, 619

Rhulicream (Rydelle) p 427, 676

Rhuligel (Rydelle) p 427, 676

Rhulispray (Rydelle) p 427, 676

Tucks Cream (Parke-Davis) p 633

Tucks Ointment (Parke-Davis) p 633

Tucks Premoistened Pads (Parke-Davis) p 420, 632

Tucks Take-Alongs (Parke-Davis) p 632

Xylocaine 2.5% Ointment (Astra) p 403, 508

Ziradryl Lotion (Parke-Davis) p 420, 633

PSORIASIS AGENTS

Aveeno Bath Oilated (Rydelle) p 427, 675

Aveeno Bath Regular (Rydelle) p 427, 675

Cortizone-5 Creme & Ointment (Thompson Medical) p 434, 727

Denorex Medicated Shampoo and Conditioner (Whitehall) p 437, 747

Denorex Medicated Shampoo, Extra Strength (Whitehall) p 437, 747

Denorex Medicated Shampoo, Extra Strength With Conditioners (Whitehall) p 747

Denorex Medicated Shampoo, Regular & Mountain Fresh Herbal Scent (Whitehall) p 437, 747

MG 217 Psoriasis Ointment and Lotion (Triton Consumer Products) p 730

MG 217 Psoriasis Shampoo and Conditioner (Triton Consumer Products) p 730

P & S Liquid (Baker Cummins Dermatologicals) p 404, 509

Oxipor VHC Lotion for Psoriasis (Whitehall) p 750

P & S Plus Tar Gel (Baker Cummins Dermatologicals) p 404, 509

P & S Shampoo (Baker Cummins Dermatologicals) p 404, 509

Panscol Medicated Lotion and Ointment (Baker Cummins Dermatologicals) p 509

Tegrin for Psoriasis Lotion, Cream & Soap (Block) p 520

Tegrin Medicated Shampoo (Block) p 519

X-Seb T Shampoo (Baker Cummins Dermatologicals) p 404, 510

X-Seb T Plus Conditioning Shampoo (Baker Cummins Dermatologicals) p 404, 510

SEBORRHEA TREATMENT

Denorex Medicated Shampoo and Conditioner (Whitehall) p 437, 747

Denorex Medicated Shampoo, Extra Strength (Whitehall) p 437, 747

Denorex Medicated Shampoo, Extra Strength With Conditioners (Whitehall) p 747

Denorex Medicated Shampoo, Regular & Mountain Fresh Herbal Scent (Whitehall) p 437, 747

Diaparene Cradol (Lehn & Fink) p 413, 587

Head & Shoulders (Procter & Gamble) p 422, 638

Tegrin Medicated Shampoo (Block) p 519

Zincon Dandruff Shampoo (Lederle) p 413, 582

SHAMPOOS

Aqua Glycolic Shampoo (Herald Pharmacal) p 567

Danex Protein Enriched Dandruff Shampoo (Herbert) p 568

Denorex Medicated Shampoo and Conditioner (Whitehall) p 437, 747

Denorex Medicated Shampoo, Extra Strength (Whitehall) p 437, 747

Denorex Medicated Shampoo, Extra Strength With Conditioners (Whitehall) p 747

Denorex Medicated Shampoo, Regular & Mountain Fresh Herbal Scent (Whitehall) p 437, 747

Diaparene Cradol (Lehn & Fink) p 413, 587

Head & Shoulders (Procter & Gamble) p 422, 638

MG 217 Psoriasis Shampoo and Conditioner (Triton Consumer Products) p 730

P & S Shampoo (Baker Cummins Dermatologicals) p 404, 509

Phacid Shampoo (Baker Cummins Dermatologicals) p 509

R&C Shampoo (Reed & Carnrick) p 422, 642

Selsun Blue Dandruff Shampoo (Ross) p 426, 672

Selsun Blue Dandruff Shampoo-Extra Medicated (Ross) p 426, 672

Selsun Blue Extra Conditioning Dandruff Shampoo (Ross) p 426, 672

Tegrin Medicated Shampoo (Block) p 519

Vanseb Cream and Lotion Dandruff Shampoos (Herbert) p 568

Vanseb-T Cream and Lotion Tar Dandruff Shampoos (Herbert) p 568

X-Seb Shampoo (Baker Cummins Dermatologicals) p 404, 510

X-Seb Plus Conditioning Shampoo (Baker Cummins Dermatologicals) p 404, 510

X-Seb T Shampoo (Baker Cummins Dermatologicals) p 404, 510

X-Seb T Plus Conditioning Shampoo (Baker Cummins Dermatologicals) p 404, 510

Zincon Dandruff Shampoo (Lederle) p 413, 582

SKIN BLEACHES

Esotérica Medicated Fade Cream (SmithKline Beecham) p 696

SKIN PROTECTANT

Caldesene Medicated Ointment (Fisons Consumer) p 409, 555

Caldesene Medicated Powder (Fisons Consumer) p 409, 555

Chap Stick Petroleum Jelly Plus (Robins) p 424, 655

Desitin Ointment (Leeming) p 413, 583

Diaparene Baby Powder (Lehn & Fink) p 413, 587

Diaparene Medicated Cream (Lehn & Fink) p 413

Diaparene Peri-Anal Medicated Ointment (Lehn & Fink) p 413

Diaper Guard (Commerce) p 551

Wellcome Lanoline (Burroughs Wellcome) p 540

SOAPS & CLEANSERS

Alpha Keri Moisture Rich Cleansing Bar (Westwood) p 436, 741

Aqua Glyde Cleanser (Herald Pharmacal) p 567

Aveeno Bath Oilated (Rydelle) p 427, 675

Aveeno Bath Regular (Rydelle) p 427, 675

Aveeno Cleansing Bar for Acne (Rydelle) p 427, 675

Aveeno Cleansing Bar for Dry Skin (Rydelle) p 427, 675

Aveeno Cleansing Bar for Normal to Oily Skin (Rydelle) p 427, 675

Aveeno Shower and Bath Oil (Rydelle) p 427, 676

Basis Soap-Combination Skin (Beiersdorf) p 404, 514

Basis Soap-Extra Dry Skin (Beiersdorf) p 404, 514

Basis Soap-Normal to Dry Skin (Beiersdorf) p 404, 514

Basis Soap-Sensitive Skin (Beiersdorf) p 404, 514

Cam Lotion (Herald Pharmacal) p 567

Clear By Design Medicated Cleansing Pads (SmithKline Consumer) p 431, 706

Desenex Soap (Fisons Consumer) p 556

Diaparene Supers Baby Wash Cloths (Lehn & Fink) p 587

Eucerin Moisturizing Cleansing Bar (Beiersdorf) p 404, 514

Lubriderm Skin Conditioning Oil (Warner-Lambert) p 436, 739

Massengill Baby Powder Soft Cloth Towelette and Unscented Soft Cloth Towelette (SmithKline Beecham) p 698

Moisturel Sensitive Skin Cleanser (Westwood) p 436, 742

Neutrogena Cleansing Wash (Neutrogena) p 418, 616

Nivea Bath Silk Bath & Shower Gel (Extra-Dry Skin) (Beiersdorf) p 515

Nivea Bath Silk Bath & Shower Gel (Normal-to-Dry Skin) (Beiersdorf) p 515

Noxzema Antiseptic Skin Cleanser-Extra Strength Formula (Noxell) p 418, 617

Noxzema Antiseptic Skin Cleanser-Regular Formula (Noxell) p 418, 617

Noxzema Antiseptic Skin Cleanser-Sensitive Skin Formula (Noxell) p 418, 618

Noxzema Clear-Ups Medicated Pads-Maximum Strength 2.0% Salicylic Acid (Noxell) p 418, 618

Noxzema Clear-Ups Medicated Pads-Regular Strength 0.5% Salicyclic Acid (Noxell) p 418, 618

Noxzema Medicated Skin Cream (Noxell) p 418, 619

Oxy Clean Lathering Facial Scrub (SmithKline Beecham) p 430, 700

Oxy Clean Medicated Cleanser (SmithKline Beecham) p 430, 700

Oxy Clean Medicated Pads - Regular, Sensitive Skin, and Maximum Strength (SmithKline Beecham) p 430, 700

Oxy Clean Medicated Soap (SmithKline Beecham) p 430, 700

Oxy Night Watch (SmithKline Beecham) p 430, 701

Oxy 10 Daily Face Wash (SmithKline Beecham) p 430, 701

pHisoDerm For Baby (Winthrop Consumer Products) p 438, 759

pHisoDerm Skin Cleanser and Conditioner - Regular and Oily (Winthrop Consumer Products) p 438, 759

Purpose Soap (Johnson & Johnson Consumer) p 571

STEROIDS & COMBINATIONS

Massengill Medicated Soft Cloth Towelette (SmithKline Beecham) p 698

SULFUR & SALICYLIC ACID

Aveeno Cleansing Bar for Acne (Rydelle) p 427, 675

Vanseb Cream and Lotion Dandruff Shampoos (Herbert) p 568

SUNBURN PREPARATIONS

Americaine Topical Anesthetic Ointment (Fisons Consumer) p 409, 554

Americaine Topical Anesthetic Spray (Fisons Consumer) p 409, 554

Aveeno Bath Oilated (Rydelle) p 427, 675

Aveeno Bath Regular (Rydelle) p 427, 675

Bactine Antiseptic/Anesthetic First Aid Spray (Miles Consumer) p 417, 611

Balmex Ointment (Macsil) p 590

BiCozene Creme (Sandoz Consumer) p 427, 676

Dermarest (Commerce) p 551

Dermoplast Anesthetic Pain Relief Lotion (Whitehall) p 437, 747

INSECT BITE & STING PREPARATIONS

Americaine Topical Anesthetic Ointment (Fisons Consumer) p 409, 554
Americaine Topical Anesthetic Spray (Fisons Consumer) p 409, 554
Aveeno Bath Oilated (Rydelle) p 427, 675
Bactine Antiseptic/Anesthetic First Aid Spray (Miles Consumer) p 417, 611
Bactine Hydrocortisone Skin Care Cream (Miles Consumer) p 417, 612
BiCozene Creme (Sandoz Consumer) p 427, 676
Delacort (Mericon) p 607
Medicone Derma Ointment (Medicone) p 416, 606
Nupercainal Cream and Ointment (CIBA Consumer) p 408, 546
Nupercainal Pain Relief Cream (CIBA Consumer) p 408, 546
Rhulicream (Rydelle) p 427, 676
Rhuligel (Rydelle) p 427, 676
Rhulispray (Rydelle) p 427, 676
Solarcaine (Plough) p 421, 637

IRON DEFICIENCY PREPARATIONS
(see under HEMATINICS)

IRRIGATING SOLUTION, OPHTHALMIC
FOR EXTERNAL USE
Collyrium for Fresh Eyes (Wyeth-Ayerst) p 439, 764
Lavoptik Eye Wash (Lavoptik) p 576

L

LAXATIVES
BULK
Citrucel Orange Flavor (Lakeside Pharmaceuticals) p 412, 574
Citrucel Regular Flavor (Lakeside Pharmaceuticals) p 412, 573
Effer-Syllium Natural Fiber Bulking Agent (Stuart) p 433, 720
Fiberall Chewable Tablets, Lemon Creme Flavor (CIBA Consumer) p 545
Fiberall Fiber Wafers - Fruit & Nut (CIBA Consumer) p 408, 545
Fiberall Fiber Wafers - Oatmeal Raisin (CIBA Consumer) p 408, 545
Fiberall Powder Natural Flavor (CIBA Consumer) p 408, 545
Fiberall Powder Orange Flavor (CIBA Consumer) p 408, 546
FiberCon (Lederle) p 412, 578
Hydrocil Instant (Reid-Rowell) p 423, 644
Maltsupex Liquid, Powder & Tablets (Wallace) p 435, 736
Metamucil Effervescent Sugar Free, Lemon-Lime Flavor (Procter & Gamble) p 422, 640
Metamucil Effervescent Sugar Free, Orange Flavor (Procter & Gamble) p 422, 640
Metamucil Powder, Orange Flavor (Procter & Gamble) p 422, 639
Metamucil Powder, Regular Flavor (Procter & Gamble) p 422, 638
Metamucil Powder, Strawberry Flavor (Procter & Gamble) p 422, 639
Metamucil Powder, Sugar Free, Orange Flavor (Procter & Gamble) p 422, 640
Metamucil Powder, Sugar Free, Regular Flavor (Procter & Gamble) p 422, 639
Perdiem Fiber Granules (Rorer Consumer) p 426, 667
Perdiem Granules (Rorer Consumer) p 426, 667
Serutan Natural-Fiber Laxative Toasted Granules (SmithKline Beecham) p 701
Syllact Powder (Wallace) p 435, 738
UltraBalance Weight Management Products - Herbulk (UltraBalance Products) p 731

COMBINATIONS
Correctol Laxative Tablets (Plough) p 421, 634
Dialose Plus Capsules (Stuart) p 433, 720
Doxidan Liquigels (Hoechst-Roussel) p 411, 568
Extra Gentle Ex-Lax (Sandoz Consumer) p 427, 679
Feen-A-Mint Pills and Chocolated Pills (Plough) p 421, 635
Nature's Remedy Natural Vegetable Laxative (SmithKline Beecham) p 430, 699
Perdiem Granules (Rorer Consumer) p 426, 667
Peri-Colace (Mead Johnson Pharmaceuticals) p 416, 605
Unilax Stool Softener/Laxative Softgel Capsules (Ascher) p 403, 507

FECAL SOFTENERS
Biochemic Tissue Salts (NuAGE Laboratories) p 619
Colace (Mead Johnson Pharmaceuticals) p 416, 605
Correctol Laxative Tablets (Plough) p 421, 634
Dialose Capsules (Stuart) p 433, 720
Dialose Plus Capsules (Stuart) p 433, 720
Extra Gentle Ex-Lax (Sandoz Consumer) p 427, 679
Feen-A-Mint Pills and Chocolated Pills (Plough) p 421, 635
Kasof Capsules (Stuart) p 433, 723
Modane Plus Tablets (Adria) p 403, 504
Perdiem Fiber Granules (Rorer Consumer) p 426, 667
Perdiem Granules (Rorer Consumer) p 426, 667
Phillips' LaxCaps (Glenbrook) p 411, 565
Surfak Liquigels (Hoechst-Roussel) p 411, 569
Unilax Stool Softener/Laxative Softgel Capsules (Ascher) p 403, 507

MINERAL OIL
Agoral, Plain (Parke-Davis) p 624
Haley's M-O, Regular & Flavored (Glenbrook) p 411, 563

SALINE
Haley's M-O, Regular & Flavored (Glenbrook) p 411, 563
Phillips' Milk of Magnesia Liquid (Glenbrook) p 411, 565
Phillips' Milk of Magnesia Tablets (Glenbrook) p 411, 566
Swan Citroma (Citrate of Magnesia) (Cumberland-Swan) p 409, 553

STIMULANT
Agoral, Marshmallow Flavor (Parke-Davis) p 624
Agoral, Raspberry Flavor (Parke-Davis) p 624
Correctol Laxative Tablets (Plough) p 421, 634
Dialose Plus Capsules (Stuart) p 433, 720
Dulcolax Suppositories (Boehringer Ingelheim) p 404, 520
Dulcolax Tablets (Boehringer Ingelheim) p 404, 520
Emulsoil (Paddock) p 623
Evac-U-Gen Mild Laxative (Walker, Corp) p 435, 736
Ex-Lax Chocolated Laxative (Sandoz Consumer) p 427, 678
Ex-Lax Pills, Unflavored (Sandoz Consumer) p 427, 678
Extra Gentle Ex-Lax (Sandoz Consumer) p 427, 679
Feen-A-Mint Gum (Plough) p 421, 635
Feen-A-Mint Pills and Chocolated Pills (Plough) p 421, 635
Gentle Nature Natural Vegetable Laxative (Sandoz Consumer) p 427, 679

Modane Plus Tablets (Adria) p 403, 504
Modane Tablets (Adria) p 403, 504
Nature's Remedy Natural Vegetable Laxative (SmithKline Beecham) p 430, 699
Neoloid (Lederle) p 581
Perdiem Granules (Rorer Consumer) p 426, 667
Phillips' LaxCaps (Glenbrook) p 411, 565
Purge Concentrate (Fleming) p 558
Unilax Stool Softener/Laxative Softgel Capsules (Ascher) p 403, 507
Yellolax (Luyties) p 589

LEG MUSCLE CRAMP PREPARATIONS
Q-vel Muscle Relaxant Pain Reliever (CIBA Consumer) p 408, 548

LICE TREATMENTS
(see under ANTIPARASITICS, ARTHROPODS)

LIP BALM
Campho-Phenique Cold Sore Gel (Winthrop Consumer Products) p 438, 756
Campho-Phenique Liquid (Winthrop Consumer Products) p 438, 757
Chap Stick Lip Balm (Robins) p 424, 655
Chap Stick Sunblock 15 Lip Balm (Robins) p 424, 655
Herpecin-L Cold Sore Lip Balm (Campbell) p 541
ZilaBrace Oral Analgesic Gel (Zila Pharmaceuticals) p 766
Zilactin Medicated Gel (Zila Pharmaceuticals) p 439, 766
ZilaDent Oral Analgesic Gel (Zila Pharmaceuticals) p 766

LUBRICANTS
Ortho Personal Lubricant (Ortho Pharmaceutical) p 419, 623

LUBRICANTS, OPHTHALMIC
Celluvisc Lubricant Ophthalmic Solution (Allergan Pharmaceuticals) p 403, 504
Clear Eyes Lubricating Eye Redness Reliever (Ross) p 426, 669
Collyrium Fresh (Wyeth-Ayerst) p 439, 764
Duolube Eye Ointment (Bausch & Lomb Personal) p 404, 512
Lacril Lubricant Ophthalmic Solution (Allergan Pharmaceuticals) p 505
Lacri-Lube S.O.P. (Allergan Pharmaceuticals) p 403, 505
Liquifilm Forte (Allergan Pharmaceuticals) p 505
Liquifilm Tears (Allergan Pharmaceuticals) p 403, 505
Moisture Drops (Bausch & Lomb Personal) p 404, 513
Murine Eye Lubricant (Ross) p 426, 670
Murine Plus Lubricating Eye Redness Reliever (Ross) p 426, 671
Prefrin Liquifilm (Allergan Pharmaceuticals) p 403, 505
Refresh Lubricant Ophthalmic Solution (Allergan Pharmaceuticals) p 403, 506
Refresh P.M. (Allergan Pharmaceuticals) p 403, 506
Relief Eye Drops for Red Eyes (Allergan Pharmaceuticals) p 403, 506
Tears Plus Lubricant Ophthalmic Solution (Allergan Pharmaceuticals) p 403, 506
Visine Extra Eye Drops (Leeming) p 413, 586

M

MENSTRUAL PREPARATIONS
Haltran Tablets (Upjohn) p 434, 732
Ibuprofen Tablets (Ohm Laboratories) p 418, 620

P

PAIN RELIEVERS
(see under ANALGESICS)

PEDICULICIDES
(see under ANTIPARASITICS)

PLATELET INHIBITORS
Therapy Bayer Aspirin Caplets
(Glenbrook) p 410, 561

POISON IVY & OAK PREPARATIONS
Aveeno Bath Oilated (Rydelle) p 427,
675
Aveeno Bath Regular (Rydelle) p 427,
675
Bactine Hydrocortisone Skin Care
Cream (Miles Consumer) p 417, 612
Caladryl Cream & Lotion (Parke-Davis)
p 420, 628
CaldeCORT Anti-Itch Hydrocortisone
Cream (Fisons Consumer) p 409,
555
CaldeCORT Anti-Itch Hydrocortisone
Spray (Fisons Consumer) p 409, 555
CaldeCORT Light Cream (Fisons
Consumer) p 409, 555
Cortaid Cream with Aloe (Upjohn)
p 434, 731
Cortaid Lotion (Upjohn) p 434, 731
Cortaid Ointment with Aloe (Upjohn)
p 434, 731
Cortaid Spray (Upjohn) p 434, 731
Cortizone-5 Creme & Ointment
(Thompson Medical) p 434, 727
Delacort (Mericon) p 607
Dermolate Anti-Itch Cream (Schering)
p 689
Rhulicream (Rydelle) p 427, 676
Rhuligel (Rydelle) p 427, 676
Rhulispray (Rydelle) p 427, 676
Ziradryl Lotion (Parke-Davis) p 420,
633

PREGNANCY TESTS
(see under DIAGNOSTICS,
PREGNANCY TESTS)

PREMENSTRUAL THERAPEUTICS
(see under MENSTRUAL
PREPARATIONS)

PRICKLY HEAT AIDS
(see under DERMATOLOGICALS,
DERMATITIS RELIEF & POWDERS)

PYRETICS
(see under ANTIPYRETICS)

S

SALT SUBSTITUTES
Chlor-3 Condiment (Fleming) p 557

SALT TABLETS
Thermotabs (SmithKline Beecham)
p 704

SCABICIDES
(see under ANTIPARASITICS)

SHAMPOOS
(see under DERMATOLOGICALS,
SHAMPOOS)

SHINGLES RELIEF
(see under ANALGESICS)

SINUSITIS AIDS
(see under COLD PREPARATIONS)

SKIN BLEACHES
(see under DERMATOLOGICALS, SKIN
BLEACHES)

SKIN CARE PRODUCTS
(see under DERMATOLOGICALS)

SKIN PROTECTANTS
Caldesene Medicated Ointment (Fisons
Consumer) p 409, 555
Caldesene Medicated Powder (Fisons
Consumer) p 409, 555

Chap Stick Lip Balm (Robins) p 424,
655
Chap Stick Petroleum Jelly Plus
(Robins) p 424, 655
Chap Stick Petroleum Jelly Plus with
Sunblock 15 (Robins) p 424, 656
Chap Stick Sunblock 15 Lip Balm
(Robins) p 424, 655
Impregon Concentrate (Fleming) p 557

SKIN WOUND PREPARATIONS
CLEANSERS
(see under DERMATOLOGICALS,
WOUND CLEANSER)
HEALING AGENTS
Medicone Dressing Cream (Medicone)
p 416, 606
PRID Salve (Walker Pharmacal) p 736
PROTECTANTS
Medicone Dressing Cream (Medicone)
p 416, 606
S.T.37 Antiseptic Solution (SmithKline
Beecham) p 702

SLEEP AIDS
(see also under HYPNOTICS;
SEDATIVES)
Biochemic Tissue Salts (NuAGE
Laboratories) p 619
Excedrin P.M. Analgesic/Sleeping Aid
Tablets and Caplets (Bristol-Myers
Products) p 405, 530
Hyland's Calms Forté Tablets (Standard
Homeopathic) p 718
Magonate Tablets and Liquid (Fleming)
p 557
Miles Nervine Nighttime Sleep-Aid
(Miles Consumer) p 417, 613
Nytol Tablets (Block) p 518
Sleep-eze 3 Tablets (Whitehall) p 754
Sleepinal Night-time Sleep Aid Capsules
(Thompson Medical) p 434, 729
Sominex (SmithKline Beecham) p 701
Sominex Liquid (SmithKline Beecham)
p 702
Unisom Nighttime Sleep Aid (Leeming)
p 585

SMOKING CESSATION AID
CigArrest Tablets (More Direct Health
Products) p 614
New Life Smoking Deterrent Lozenges
(New Life Health Products) p 420,
617

SORE THROAT PREPARATIONS
(see under COLD PREPARATIONS,
LOZENGES & THROAT LOZENGES)

STIFF NECK RELIEF
(see under ANALGESICS)

STIMULANTS
No Doz Fast Acting Alertness Aid
Tablets (Bristol-Myers Products)
p 406, 532
Vivarin Stimulant Tablets (SmithKline
Beecham) p 705

SUNSCREENS
(see under DERMATOLOGICALS,
SUNSCREENS)

SUPPLEMENTS
(see under DIETARY SUPPLEMENTS)

SWIMMERS'S EAR PREVENTION
Star-Otic Ear Solution (Stellar) p 433,
719

T

TEETHING REMEDIES
Anbesol Baby Teething Gel Anesthetic
(Whitehall) p 437, 745
Anbesol Gel Antiseptic-Anesthetic
(Whitehall) p 437, 745
Anbesol Gel Antiseptic-Anesthetic -
Maximum Strength (Whitehall) p 437,
745
Anbesol Liquid Antiseptic-Anesthetic
(Whitehall) p 437, 745

Anbesol Liquid Antiseptic-Anesthetic -
Maximum Strength (Whitehall) p 437,
745
Hyland's Teething Tablets (Standard
Homeopathic) p 719
Baby Orajel (Commerce) p 551
Baby Orajel Nighttime Formula
(Commerce) p 551

TENNIS ELBOW RELIEF
(see under ANALGESICS)

THROAT LOZENGES
Cēpacol Anesthetic Lozenges (Troches)
(Lakeside Pharmaceuticals) p 412,
573
Cēpacol Throat Lozenges (Lakeside
Pharmaceuticals) p 412, 572
Cēpastat Cherry Flavor Sore Throat
Lozenges (Lakeside Pharmaceuticals)
p 412, 573
Cēpastat Sore Throat Lozenges
(Lakeside Pharmaceuticals) p 412,
573
Children's Chloraseptic Lozenges
(Richardson-Vicks Inc.) p 423, 644
Chloraseptic Lozenges, Cherry, Menthol
or Cool Mint (Richardson-Vicks Inc.)
p 423, 645
Hold (SmithKline Beecham) p 697
Listerine Antiseptic Lozenges Regular
Strength (Warner-Lambert) p 435,
739
Listerine Maximum Strength Antiseptic
Lozenges (Warner-Lambert) p 435,
739
N'ICE Medicated Sugarless Sore Throat
and Cough Lozenges (SmithKline
Beecham) p 699
Sucrets (Regular and Mentholated)
(SmithKline Beecham) p 702
Sucrets Children's Cherry Flavored
Sore Throat Lozenges (SmithKline
Beecham) p 703
Sucrets Cold Relief Formula
(SmithKline Beecham) p 703
Sucrets Cough Control Formula
(SmithKline Beecham) p 703
Sucrets Maximum Strength and Sucrets
Wild Cherry (Regular Strength) Sore
Throat Lozenges (SmithKline
Beecham) p 703
Throat Discs Throat Lozenges (Marion)
p 414, 593
Vicks Formula 44 Cough Control Discs
(Richardson-Vicks Inc.) p 649
Vicks Throat Lozenges
(Richardson-Vicks Inc.) p 653

TOOTH DESENSITIZERS
Promise Toothpaste (Block) p 519
Mint Gel Sensodyne (Block) p 519
Mint Sensodyne Toothpaste (Block)
p 519
Original Sensodyne Toothpaste (Block)
p 519

U

UNIT DOSE SYSTEMS
Allbee with C Caplets (Robins) p 424,
654
Dimetapp Elixir (Robins) p 425, 658
Dimetapp Extentabs (Robins) p 425,
658
Peri-Colace (Mead Johnson
Pharmaceuticals) p 416, 605
Z-Bec Tablets (Robins) p 425, 661

V

VAGINAL PREPARATIONS
CONTRACEPTIVES
(see under CONTRACEPTIVES)
DOUCHES
Massengill Disposable Douche
(SmithKline Beecham) p 698
Massengill Liquid Concentrate
(SmithKline Beecham) p 698
Massengill Medicated Disposable
Douche (SmithKline Beecham) p 698

VITAMINS

Altocaps-400 Capsules (Benson Pharmacal) p 517

Drisdol (Winthrop Pharmaceuticals) p 760

Ester-C Tablets (Inter-Cal) p 569

OTHER

Beelith Tablets (Beach) p 513

Cod Liver Oil Concentrate Capsules (Schering) p 686

Cod Liver Oil Concentrate Tablets (Schering) p 686

Halls Vitamin C Drops (Warner-Lambert) p 738

Mol-Iron w/Vitamin C Tablets (Schering) p 692

Nicotinex Elixir (Fleming) p 558

Orexin Softab Tablets (Stuart) p 434, 725

Sunkist Vitamin C - Chewable (CIBA Consumer) p 409, 549

Sunkist Vitamin C - Easy to Swallow (CIBA Consumer) p 409, 549

W

WART REMOVERS
(see under DERMATOLOGICALS, WART REMOVERS)

WEIGHT CONTROL PREPARATIONS
(see under APPETITE SUPPRESSANTS OR FOODS)

WET DRESSINGS
(see under DERMATOLOGICALS, WET DRESSINGS)

SECTION 4

Active Ingredients Index

In this section the products described in the Product Information (White) Section are listed under their chemical (generic) name according to their principal ingredient(s). Products have been included under specific headings by the Publisher with the cooperation of individual manufacturers.

Singlet Tablets (Lakeside Pharmaceuticals) p 576
Sinutab Maximum Strength Caplets (Parke-Davis) p 420, 631
Sinutab Maximum Strength Tablets (Parke-Davis) p 420, 631
Sinutab Maximum Strength Without Drowsiness Tablets & Caplets (Parke-Davis) p 420, 632
Sinutab Regular Strength Without Drowsiness Formula (Parke-Davis) p 420, 631
Snaplets-FR (Baker Cummins Pharmaceuticals) p 404, 511
Sominex Pain Relief Formula (SmithKline Beecham) p 702
St. Joseph Aspirin-Free Fever Reducer for Children Chewable Tablets, Liquid & Infant Drops (Plough) p 421, 636
St. Joseph Cold Tablets for Children (Plough) p 637
St. Joseph Nighttime Cold Medicine (Plough) p 421, 637
Sudafed Sinus Caplets (Burroughs Wellcome) p 407, 540
Sudafed Sinus Tablets (Burroughs Wellcome) p 407, 540
TheraFlu Flu and Cold Medicine (Sandoz Consumer) p 427, 679
Triaminicin Tablets (Sandoz Consumer) p 428, 682
Tylenol acetaminophen Children's Chewable Tablets & Elixir (McNeil Consumer Products) p 415, 596
Tylenol Allergy Sinus Medication Caplets, Maximum Strength (McNeil Consumer Products) p 415, 603
Children's Tylenol Cold Liquid Formula and Chewable Cold Tablets (McNeil Consumer Products) p 415, 600
Tylenol Cold Medication Caplets and Tablets (McNeil Consumer Products) p 415, 601
Tylenol Cold Medication Liquid (McNeil Consumer Products) p 415, 601
Tylenol Cold Medication No Drowsiness Formula Caplets (McNeil Consumer Products) p 415, 602
Tylenol, Extra-Strength, acetaminophen Adult Liquid Pain Reliever (McNeil Consumer Products) p 599
Tylenol, Extra-Strength, acetaminophen Caplets, Gelcaps, Tablets (McNeil Consumer Products) p 414, 598
Tylenol, Infants' Drops (McNeil Consumer Products) p 414, 596
Tylenol, Junior Strength, acetaminophen Coated Caplets (McNeil Consumer Products) p 415, 597
Tylenol, Maximum Strength, Sinus Medication Tablets and Caplets (McNeil Consumer Products) p 415, 604
Tylenol, Regular Strength, acetaminophen Tablets and Caplets (McNeil Consumer Products) p 414, 598
Unisom Dual Relief Nighttime Sleep Aid/Analgesic (Leeming) p 585
Vanquish Analgesic Caplets (Glenbrook) p 411, 567
Vicks Daycare Daytime Colds Medicine Caplets (Richardson-Vicks Inc.) p 423, 648
Vicks Daycare Multi-Symptom Colds Medicine Liquid (Richardson-Vicks Inc.) p 423, 648
Vicks Formula 44M Multi-Symptom Cough Medicine (Richardson-Vicks Inc.) p 423, 650
Vicks NyQuil Nighttime Colds Medicine-Original & Cherry Flavor (Richardson-Vicks Inc.) p 423, 652

ACETIC ACID
Star-Otic Ear Solution (Stellar) p 433, 719

**ACETYLSALICYLIC ACID
(see under ASPIRIN)**

ACONITE
Hyland's Cough Syrup with Honey (Standard Homeopathic) p 718

ALLANTOIN
Aveeno Lotion (Rydelle) p 427, 676
Herpecin-L Cold Sore Lip Balm (Campbell) p 541
Nose Better Nasal Gel (Goldline) p 567
Tegrin for Psoriasis Lotion, Cream & Soap (Block) p 520

ALOE
Cortaid Cream with Aloe (Upjohn) p 434, 731
Cortaid Ointment with Aloe (Upjohn) p 434, 731
Nature's Remedy Natural Vegetable Laxative (SmithKline Beecham) p 430, 699
Nivea Bath Silk Bath & Shower Gel (Extra-Dry Skin) (Beiersdorf) p 515
Nivea Bath Silk Bath & Shower Gel (Normal-to-Dry Skin) (Beiersdorf) p 515
Nivea Sun After Sun Lotion (Beiersdorf) p 516
Nivea Visage Creme (Beiersdorf) p 516
Nivea Visage Lotion (Beiersdorf) p 516

**ALPHA TOCOPHERAL ACETATE
(see under VITAMIN E)**

ALUMINUM ACETATE
Acid Mantle Creme (Sandoz Consumer) p 676

ALUMINUM CARBONATE
Basaljel Capsules (Wyeth-Ayerst) p 438, 763
Basaljel Suspension (Wyeth-Ayerst) p 439, 763
Basaljel Tablets (Wyeth-Ayerst) p 438, 763

ALUMINUM CHLORIDE
Certain Dri Antiperspirant (Numark) p 418, 619

ALUMINUM CHLOROHYDRATE
Desenex Foot & Sneaker Deodorant Spray (Fisons Consumer) p 410, 556

ALUMINUM HYDROXIDE
Extra Strength Ascriptin Caplets (Rorer Consumer) p 426, 663
Cama Arthritis Pain Reliever (Sandoz Consumer) p 677
Camalox Suspension (Rorer Consumer) p 426, 663
Camalox Tablets (Rorer Consumer) p 426, 663
Gaviscon Extra Strength Relief Formula Liquid Antacid (Marion) p 413, 591
Gaviscon Extra Strength Relief Formula Antacid Tablets (Marion) p 413, 590
Gaviscon Liquid Antacid (Marion) p 414, 591
Gelusil Liquid & Tablets (Parke-Davis) p 420, 629
Gelusil-II Liquid & Tablets (Parke-Davis) p 629
Extra Strength Maalox Plus Suspension (Rorer Consumer) p 426, 664
Extra Strength Maalox Tablets (Rorer Consumer) p 426, 664
Maalox Plus Tablets (Rorer Consumer) p 426, 664
Maalox Suspension (Rorer Consumer) p 426, 664
Maalox Tablets (Rorer Consumer) p 426, 664
Maalox TC Suspension (Rorer Consumer) p 426, 665
Maalox TC Tablets (Rorer Consumer) p 426, 665
Nephrox Suspension (Fleming) p 558
WinGel Liquid & Tablets (Winthrop Consumer Products) p 760

ALUMINUM HYDROXIDE GEL
ALternaGEL Liquid (Stuart) p 433, 719
Aludrox Oral Suspension (Wyeth-Ayerst) p 438, 763
Amphojel Suspension (Wyeth-Ayerst) p 438, 763
Amphojel Suspension without Flavor (Wyeth-Ayerst) p 438, 763
Mylanta Liquid (Stuart) p 433, 723
Mylanta-II Liquid (Stuart) p 433, 724

ALUMINUM HYDROXIDE GEL, DRIED
Amphojel Tablets (Wyeth-Ayerst) p 438, 763
Ascriptin A/D Caplets (Rorer Consumer) p 425, 662
Regular Strength Ascriptin Tablets (Rorer Consumer) p 425, 662
Gaviscon Antacid Tablets (Marion) p 413, 590
Gaviscon-2 Antacid Tablets (Marion) p 414, 591
Mylanta Tablets (Stuart) p 433, 723
Mylanta-II Tablets (Stuart) p 433, 724

ALUMINUM SULFATE
Bluboro Powder Astringent Soaking Solution (Herbert) p 567

AMMONIUM ALUM
Massengill Powder (SmithKline Beecham) p 698

AMYLASE
Festal II Digestive Aid (Hoechst-Roussel) p 411, 568

**ASCORBIC ACID
(see under VITAMIN C)**

ASPIRIN
Alka-Seltzer Effervescent Antacid and Pain Reliever (Miles Consumer) p 416, 608
Alka-Seltzer Extra Strength Effervescent Antacid and Pain Reliever (Miles Consumer) p 416, 610
Alka-Seltzer (Flavored) Effervescent Antacid and Pain Reliever (Miles Consumer) p 416, 609
Alka-Seltzer Plus Cold Medicine (Miles Consumer) p 416, 610
Alka-Seltzer Plus Night-Time Cold Medicine (Miles Consumer) p 416, 611
Anacin Analgesic Coated Caplets (Whitehall) p 436, 744
Anacin Analgesic Coated Tablets (Whitehall) p 436, 744
Anacin Maximum Strength Analgesic Coated Tablets (Whitehall) p 744
Arthritis Pain Formula by the Makers of Anacin Analgesic Tablets and Caplets (Whitehall) p 437, 746
Arthritis Strength BC Powder (Block) p 518
Ascriptin A/D Caplets (Rorer Consumer) p 425, 662
Extra Strength Ascriptin Caplets (Rorer Consumer) p 426, 663
Regular Strength Ascriptin Tablets (Rorer Consumer) p 425, 662
BC Powder (Block) p 518
BC Cold Powder Multi-Symptom Formula (Block) p 518
BC Cold Powder Non-Drowsy Formula (Block) p 518
Children's Bayer Chewable Aspirin (Glenbrook) p 410, 558
Bayer Children's Cold Tablets (Glenbrook) p 410, 559
Genuine Bayer Aspirin Tablets & Caplets (Glenbrook) p 410, 559
Maximum Bayer Aspirin Tablets & Caplets (Glenbrook) p 410, 560
Therapy Bayer Aspirin Caplets (Glenbrook) p 410, 561
8 Hour Bayer Timed-Release Aspirin (Glenbrook) p 410, 561
Arthritis Strength Tri-Buffered Bufferin Analgesic Caplets (Bristol-Myers Products) p 405, 526

Extra Strength Tri-Buffered Bufferin Analgesic Tablets (Bristol-Myers Products) p 405, 527
Tri-Buffered Bufferin Analgesic Tablets and Caplets (Bristol-Myers Products) p 404, 525
Cama Arthritis Pain Reliever (Sandoz Consumer) p 677
Ecotrin Enteric Coated Aspirin Maximum Strength Tablets and Caplets (SmithKline Consumer) p 432, 712
Ecotrin Enteric Coated Aspirin Regular Strength Tablets and Caplets (SmithKline Consumer) p 432, 712
Empirin Aspirin (Burroughs Wellcome) p 407, 536
Excedrin Extra-Strength Analgesic Tablets & Caplets (Bristol-Myers Products) p 405, 530
4-Way Cold Tablets (Bristol-Myers Products) p 406, 531
Momentum Muscular Backache Formula (Whitehall) p 750
Norwich Extra-Strength Aspirin (Chattem) p 542
Norwich Regular Strength Aspirin (Chattem) p 542
Sine-Off Sinus Medicine Tablets-Aspirin Formula (SmithKline Consumer) p 432, 716
St. Joseph Adult Chewable Aspirin (81 mg.) (Plough) p 421, 635
Ursinus Inlay-Tabs (Sandoz Consumer) p 683
Vanquish Analgesic Caplets (Glenbrook) p 411, 567

ASPIRIN BUFFERED

Arthritis Pain Formula by the Makers of Anacin Analgesic Tablets and Caplets (Whitehall) p 437, 746
Ascriptin A/D Caplets (Rorer Consumer) p 425, 662
Extra Strength Ascriptin Caplets (Rorer Consumer) p 426, 663
Regular Strength Ascriptin Tablets (Rorer Consumer) p 425, 662
Arthritis Strength Tri-Buffered Bufferin Analgesic Caplets (Bristol-Myers Products) p 405, 526
Extra Strength Tri-Buffered Bufferin Analgesic Tablets (Bristol-Myers Products) p 405, 527
Tri-Buffered Bufferin Analgesic Tablets and Caplets (Bristol-Myers Products) p 404, 525

ASPIRIN MICRONIZED

Arthritis Pain Formula by the Makers of Anacin Analgesic Tablets and Caplets (Whitehall) p 437, 746

ASPIRIN, ENTERIC COATED

Therapy Bayer Aspirin Caplets (Glenbrook) p 410, 561

ATROPINE SULFATE

Donnagel (Robins) p 425, 659

ATTAPULGITE

Kaopectate Concentrated Anti-Diarrheal, Peppermint Flavor (Upjohn) p 434, 732
Kaopectate Concentrated Anti-Diarrheal, Regular Flavor (Upjohn) p 434, 732
Kaopectate Chewable Tablets (Upjohn) p 434, 732
Maximum Strength Kaopectate Tablets Anti-Diarrhea Medicine (Upjohn) p 434, 733

ATTAPULGITE, ACTIVATED

Diasorb Liquid (4 oz.) (O'Connor) p 619
Diasorb Tablets (24) (O'Connor) p 619
Rheaban Maximum Strength Tablets (Leeming) p 584

AVOBENZONE

Photoplex Broad Spectrum Sunscreen Lotion (Herbert) p 568

B

BACITRACIN

Baciguent Antibiotic Ointment (Upjohn) p 731
Bactine First Aid Antibiotic Ointment (Miles Consumer) p 417, 612
Campho-Phenique Triple Antibiotic Ointment Plus Pain Reliever (Winthrop Consumer Products) p 438, 757
Mycitracin Triple Antibiotic Ointment (Upjohn) p 435, 733

BACITRACIN ZINC

Neosporin Ointment (Burroughs Wellcome) p 407, 537
Neosporin Maximum Strength Ointment (Burroughs Wellcome) p 407, 537
Polysporin Ointment (Burroughs Wellcome) p 407, 537
Polysporin Powder (Burroughs Wellcome) p 407, 538
Polysporin Spray (Burroughs Wellcome) p 407, 538
Topisporin Ointment (Pharmafair) p 633

BALSAM PERU

Anusol Hemorrhoidal Suppositories (Parke-Davis) p 419, 624
Anusol Ointment (Parke-Davis) p 419, 624
Medicone Rectal Ointment (Medicone) p 416, 606
Medicone Rectal Suppositories (Medicone) p 416, 606

BALSAM PERU, SPECIAL FRACTION OF

Balmex Baby Powder (Macsil) p 589
Balmex Ointment (Macsil) p 590

BELLADONNA ALKALOIDS

Hyland's Bed Wetting Tablets (Standard Homeopathic) p 718

BENZALKONIUM CHLORIDE

Bactine Antiseptic/Anesthetic First Aid Spray (Miles Consumer) p 417, 611
Mediconet Cleansing Cloths (Medicone) p 416, 607
Noxzema Antiseptic Skin Cleanser-Sensitive Skin Formula (Noxell) p 418, 618
Orajel Mouth-Aid (Commerce) p 552
Tanac Liquid (Commerce) p 553
Tanac Roll-on (Commerce) p 553
Tanac Stick (Commerce) p 553
Zephiran Chloride Aqueous Solution (Winthrop Pharmaceuticals) p 760
Zephiran Chloride Spray (Winthrop Pharmaceuticals) p 760
Zephiran Chloride Tinted Tincture (Winthrop Pharmaceuticals) p 760

BENZOCAINE

Americaine Hemorrhoidal Ointment (Fisons Consumer) p 409, 554
Americaine Topical Anesthetic Ointment (Fisons Consumer) p 409, 554
Americaine Topical Anesthetic Spray (Fisons Consumer) p 409, 554
Anbesol Baby Teething Gel Anesthetic (Whitehall) p 437, 745
Anbesol Gel Antiseptic-Anesthetic (Whitehall) p 437, 745
Anbesol Gel Antiseptic-Anesthetic - Maximum Strength (Whitehall) p 437, 745
Anbesol Liquid Antiseptic-Anesthetic (Whitehall) p 437, 745
Anbesol Liquid Antiseptic-Anesthetic - Maximum Strength (Whitehall) p 437, 745
BiCozene Creme (Sandoz Consumer) p 427, 676
Boil•Ease (Commerce) p 550
Cēpacol Anesthetic Lozenges (Troches) (Lakeside Pharmaceuticals) p 412, 573
Children's Chloraseptic Lozenges (Richardson-Vicks Inc.) p 423, 644

Dermoplast Anesthetic Pain Relief Lotion (Whitehall) p 437, 747
Dermoplast Anesthetic Pain Relief Spray (Whitehall) p 437, 748
Medicone Derma Ointment (Medicone) p 416, 606
Medicone Dressing Cream (Medicone) p 416, 606
Medicone Rectal Ointment (Medicone) p 416, 606
Medicone Rectal Suppositories (Medicone) p 416, 606
Baby Orajel (Commerce) p 551
Baby Orajel Nighttime Formula (Commerce) p 551
Orajel Maximum Strength (Commerce) p 552
Orajel Mouth-Aid (Commerce) p 552
Oxipor VHC Lotion for Psoriasis (Whitehall) p 750
Pazo Hemorrhoid Ointment & Suppositories (Bristol-Myers Products) p 406, 533
Rhulicream (Rydelle) p 427, 676
Rhulispray (Rydelle) p 427, 676
Solarcaine (Plough) p 421, 637
Tanac Liquid (Commerce) p 553
Tanac Roll-on (Commerce) p 553
Tanac Stick (Commerce) p 553
Vicks Cough Silencers Cough Drops (Richardson-Vicks Inc.) p 648
Vicks Formula 44 Cough Control Discs (Richardson-Vicks Inc.) p 649
Vicks Throat Lozenges (Richardson-Vicks Inc.) p 653
ZilaBrace Oral Analgesic Gel (Zila Pharmaceuticals) p 766
ZilaDent Oral Analgesic Gel (Zila Pharmaceuticals) p 766

BENZOPHENONE-3

Neutrogena Moisture SPF 15 Untinted (Neutrogena) p 418, 616
Neutrogena Moisture SPF 15 with Sheer Tint (Neutrogena) p 418, 616
Neutrogena Sunblock (Neutrogena) p 418, 617
Nivea Visage Creme (Beiersdorf) p 516
Nivea Visage Lotion (Beiersdorf) p 516

BENZOYL PEROXIDE

Benzoyl Peroxide Gel 5% and 10% (Pharmafair) p 633
Clear by Design Medicated Acne Gel (SmithKline Consumer) p 431, 706
Clearasil 10% Benzoyl Peroxide Medicated Anti-Acne Lotion (Richardson-Vicks Inc.) p 646
Clearasil Maximum Strength Medicated Anti-Acne Cream, Tinted (Richardson-Vicks Inc.) p 424, 646
Clearasil Maximum Strength Medicated Anti-Acne Cream, Vanishing (Richardson-Vicks Inc.) p 424, 646
Noxzema Clear-Ups Maximum Strength Lotion, Vanishing (Noxell) p 418, 618
Noxzema Clear-Ups On-the-Spot Treatment, Tinted & Vanishing (Noxell) p 418, 618
Oxy 10 Daily Face Wash (SmithKline Beecham) p 430, 701
Oxy-5 and Oxy-10 Tinted and Vanishing Formulas with Sorboxyl (SmithKline Beecham) p 430, 699

BENZYL ALCOHOL

Cēpacol Throat Lozenges (Lakeside Pharmaceuticals) p 412, 572
Rhuligel (Rydelle) p 427, 676

BETA CAROTENE

UltraBalance Weight Management Products - Protein Formula (UltraBalance Products) p 731
Within Multivitamin for Women with Calcium, Extra Iron and Zinc (Miles Consumer) p 417, 614

BIFIDOBACTERIA

Bifido Factor (Bifidobacterium bifidum) (Natren) p 616
Life Start (Bifidobacterium infantis) (Natren) p 616

BISABOLOL

Basis Soap-Sensitive Skin (Beiersdorf) p 404, 514

BISACODYL

Dulcolax Suppositories (Boehringer Ingelheim) p 404, 520
Dulcolax Tablets (Boehringer Ingelheim) p 404, 520

BISMUTH SUBGALLATE

Anusol Hemorrhoidal Suppositories (Parke-Davis) p 419, 624

BISMUTH SUBNITRATE

Balmex Ointment (Macsil) p 590

BISMUTH SUBSALICYLATE

Maximum Strength Pepto-Bismol Liquid (Procter & Gamble) p 422, 641
Pepto-Bismol Liquid & Tablets (Procter & Gamble) p 422, 641

BONESET

Hyland's C-Plus Cold Tablets (Standard Homeopathic) p 719

BORIC ACID

Borofax Ointment (Burroughs Wellcome) p 536
Collyrium for Fresh Eyes (Wyeth-Ayerst) p 439, 764
Collyrium Fresh (Wyeth-Ayerst) p 439, 764
Eye Wash (Bausch & Lomb Personal) p 404, 512
Star-Otic Ear Solution (Stellar) p 433, 719

BORNYL ACETATE

Vicks Inhaler (Richardson-Vicks Inc.) p 651

BROMPHENIRAMINE MALEATE

Bromfed Syrup (Muro) p 615
Dimetane Decongestant Caplets (Robins) p 425, 657
Dimetane Decongestant Elixir (Robins) p 425, 657
Dimetane Elixir (Robins) p 424, 656
Dimetane Extentabs 8 mg (Robins) p 424, 656
Dimetane Extentabs 12 mg (Robins) p 425, 656
Dimetane Tablets (Robins) p 424, 656
Dimetapp Elixir (Robins) p 425, 658
Dimetapp Extentabs (Robins) p 425, 658
Dimetapp Plus Caplets (Robins) p 425, 659
Dimetapp Tablets (Robins) p 425, 658
Drixoral Antihistamine/Nasal Decongestant Syrup (Schering) p 429, 689

BUROW'S SOLUTION

Star-Otic Ear Solution (Stellar) p 433, 719

C

CAFFEINE

Anacin Analgesic Coated Caplets (Whitehall) p 436, 744
Anacin Analgesic Coated Tablets (Whitehall) p 436, 744
Anacin Maximum Strength Analgesic Coated Tablets (Whitehall) p 744
Excedrin Extra-Strength Analgesic Tablets & Caplets (Bristol-Myers Products) p 405, 530
No Doz Fast Acting Alertness Aid Tablets (Bristol-Myers Products) p 406, 532
Vanquish Analgesic Caplets (Glenbrook) p 411, 567
Vivarin Stimulant Tablets (SmithKline Beecham) p 705

CALAMINE

Caladryl Cream & Lotion (Parke-Davis) p 420, 628
Rhulicream (Rydelle) p 427, 676
Rhulispray (Rydelle) p 427, 676

CALCIUM

Bugs Bunny Children's Chewable Vitamins + Minerals with Iron and Calcium (Sugar Free) (Miles Consumer) p 417, 613
Flintstones Complete With Calcium, Iron & Minerals Children's Chewable Vitamins (Miles Consumer) p 417, 613
One-A-Day Maximum Formula Vitamins and Minerals (Miles Consumer) p 417, 614
Within Multivitamin for Women with Calcium, Extra Iron and Zinc (Miles Consumer) p 417, 614

CALCIUM ACETATE

Bluboro Powder Astringent Soaking Solution (Herbert) p 567

CALCIUM ASCORBATE

Ester-C Tablets (Inter-Cal) p 569

CALCIUM CARBONATE

Alka-Mints Chewable Antacid (Miles Consumer) p 416, 607
Alka-Seltzer Advanced Formula Antacid & Non-Aspirin Pain Reliever (Miles Consumer) p 416, 607
Ascriptin A/D Caplets (Rorer Consumer) p 425, 662
Extra Strength Ascriptin Caplets (Rorer Consumer) p 426, 663
Regular Strength Ascriptin Tablets (Rorer Consumer) p 425, 662
Balmex Baby Powder (Macsil) p 589
Biocal 500 mg Tablet Calcium Supplement (Miles Consumer) p 417, 612
Tri-Buffered Bufferin Analgesic Tablets and Caplets (Bristol-Myers Products) p 404, 525
Caltrate 600 (Lederle) p 412, 576
Caltrate 600 + Iron (Lederle) p 412, 577
Caltrate, Jr. (Lederle) p 412, 576
Caltrate 600 + Vitamin D (Lederle) p 412, 577
Camalox Suspension (Rorer Consumer) p 426, 663
Camalox Tablets (Rorer Consumer) p 426, 663
Centrum, Jr. (Children's Chewable) + Extra Calcium (Lederle) p 412, 578
Di-Gel Antacid/Anti-Gas (Plough) p 421, 634
Marblen Suspension Peach/Apricot (Fleming) p 558
Marblen Suspension Unflavored (Fleming) p 558
Marblen Tablets (Fleming) p 558
Os-Cal 500 Chewable Tablets (Marion) p 414, 592
Os-Cal 250+D Tablets (Marion) p 414, 592
Os-Cal 500+D Tablets (Marion) p 414, 592
Os-Cal 500 Tablets (Marion) p 414, 592
Rolaids (Calcium Rich) (Warner-Lambert) p 436, 740
Rolaids (Sodium Free) (Warner-Lambert) p 436, 740
Extra Strength Rolaids (Warner-Lambert) p 436, 740
Thermotabs (SmithKline Beecham) p 704
Tums Liquid Extra-Strength Antacid (SmithKline Beecham) p 430, 704
Tums Liquid Extra-Strength Antacid with Simethicone (SmithKline Beecham) p 430, 704

CALCIUM CARBONATE, PRECIPITATED

Tums Antacid Tablets (SmithKline Beecham) p 430, 704

Tums E-X Antacid Tablets (SmithKline Beecham) p 430, 704

CALCIUM CHLORIDE

Resol Oral Electrolyte Rehydration & Maintenance Solution (Wyeth-Ayerst) p 439, 765

CALCIUM (OYSTER SHELL)

Os-Cal 250+D Tablets (Marion) p 414, 592
Os-Cal Fortified Tablets (Marion) p 414, 592
Os-Cal Plus Tablets (Marion) p 414, 592
Os-Cal 500 Tablets (Marion) p 414, 592

CALCIUM PHOSPHATE

Hyland's Teething Tablets (Standard Homeopathic) p 719

CALCIUM PHOSPHATE, DIBASIC

Centrum, Jr. (Children's Chewable) + Extra Calcium (Lederle) p 412, 578

CALCIUM PHOSPHATE, TRIBASIC

Posture 600 mg (Whitehall) p 437, 750
Posture-D 600 mg (Whitehall) p 437, 751

CALCIUM POLYCARBOPHIL

FiberCon (Lederle) p 412, 578

CALCIUM UNDECYLENATE

Caldesene Medicated Powder (Fisons Consumer) p 409, 555
Cruex Antifungal Powder, Spray Powder & Cream (Fisons Consumer) p 409, 555

CAMPHOR

Afrin Menthol Nasal Spray (Schering) p 428, 684
Aurum the Gold Lotion (Au Pharmaceuticals) p 508
Caladryl Cream & Lotion (Parke-Davis) p 420, 628
Campho-Phenique Cold Sore Gel (Winthrop Consumer Products) p 438, 756
Campho-Phenique Liquid (Winthrop Consumer Products) p 438, 757
Nose Better Nasal Gel (Goldline) p 567
Noxzema Clear-Ups Medicated Pads-Maximum Strength 2.0% Salicylic Acid (Noxell) p 418, 618
Noxzema Clear-Ups Medicated Pads-Regular Strength 0.5% Salicyclic Acid (Noxell) p 418, 618
Noxzema Medicated Skin Cream (Noxell) p 418, 619
Rhulicream (Rydelle) p 427, 676
Rhuligel (Rydelle) p 427, 676
Rhulispray (Rydelle) p 427, 676
TheraGold (Au Pharmaceuticals) p 508
Therapeutic Gold (Au Pharmaceuticals) p 508
Vicks Inhaler (Richardson-Vicks Inc.) p 651
Vicks Vaporub (Richardson-Vicks Inc.) p 424, 653
Vicks Vaposteam (Richardson-Vicks Inc.) p 653

CAPRYLIC/CAPRIC TRIGLYCERIDE

Aqua-A Cream (Baker Cummins Dermatologicals) p 404, 508
Aquaderm Therapeutic Cream (Baker Cummins Dermatologicals) p 404, 509
Aquaderm Therapeutic Lotion (Baker Cummins Dermatologicals) p 404, 509

CARBAMIDE PEROXIDE

Debrox Drops (Marion) p 413, 590
Ear Drops (Pharmafair) p 633
Ear Drops by Murine—(See Murine Ear Wax Removal System/Murine Ear Drops) (Ross) p 426, 669
Gly-Oxide Liquid (Marion) p 414, 591

2-ETHYLHEXYL SALICYLATE

Coppertone Sun Spray Mist SPF 10 (Plough) p 634
Coppertone Sunblock Lotion SPF 25 (Plough) p 633
Coppertone Sunblock Lotion SPF 30 (Plough) p 421, 633
Coppertone Sunblock Lotion SPF 45 (Plough) p 633
Shade Oil-Free Gel SPF 15 (Plough) p 422, 637
Shade Oil-Free Gel SPF 25 (Plough) p 637
Shade Sunblock Lotion SPF 30 (Plough) p 637
Shade Sunblock Lotion SPF 45 (Plough) p 422, 637
Shade Sunblock Stick SPF 30 (Plough) p 637
Water Babies by Coppertone Sunblock Cream SPF 25 (Plough) p 422, 638
Water Babies by Coppertone Sunblock Lotion SPF 30 (Plough) p 422, 638
Water Babies by Coppertone Sunblock Lotion SPF 45 (Plough) p 422, 638

EUCALYPTOL
(see also under EUCALYPTUS, OIL OF)

Afrin Menthol Nasal Spray (Schering) p 428, 684
Noxzema Clear-Ups Medicated Pads-Maximum Strength 2.0% Salicylic Acid (Noxell) p 418, 618
Noxzema Clear-Ups Medicated Pads-Regular Strength 0.5% Salicylic Acid (Noxell) p 418, 618
Noxzema Medicated Skin Cream (Noxell) p 418, 619

EUCALYPTUS, OIL OF

Halls Mentho-Lyptus Cough Suppressant Tablets (Warner-Lambert) p 435, 738
Listerine Antiseptic (Warner-Lambert) p 435, 739
Noxzema Clear-Ups Medicated Pads-Maximum Strength 2.0% Salicylic Acid (Noxell) p 418, 618
Noxzema Clear-Ups Medicated Pads-Regular Strength 0.5% Salicyclic Acid (Noxell) p 418, 618
Noxzema Medicated Skin Cream (Noxell) p 418, 619
Vicks Vaporub (Richardson-Vicks Inc.) p 424, 653
Vicks Vaposteam (Richardson-Vicks Inc.) p 653

EUCERITE

Eucerin Moisturizing Cleansing Bar (Beiersdorf) p 404, 514
Nivea Bath Silk Bath & Shower Gel (Extra-Dry Skin) (Beiersdorf) p 515
Nivea Bath Silk Bath & Shower Gel (Normal-to-Dry Skin) (Beiersdorf) p 515
Nivea Moisturizing Creme (Beiersdorf) p 404, 515
Nivea Moisturizing Lotion (Extra Enriched) (Beiersdorf) p 404, 515
Nivea Moisturizing Lotion (Original Formula) (Beiersdorf) p 404, 516
Nivea Moisturizing Oil (Beiersdorf) p 404, 516
Nivea Sun After Sun Lotion (Beiersdorf) p 516
Nivea Sun SPF 15 (Beiersdorf) p 516
Nivea Visage Creme (Beiersdorf) p 516
Nivea Visage Lotion (Beiersdorf) p 516

F

FERRIC PYROPHOSPHATE

Troph-Iron Liquid (SmithKline Consumer) p 432, 717

FERROUS FUMARATE

Bugs Bunny Plus Iron Children's Chewable Vitamins (Sugar Free) (Miles Consumer) p 417, 612
Caltrate 600 + Iron (Lederle) p 412, 577
Centrum, Jr. (Children's Chewable) + Iron (Lederle) p 412, 578
FemIron Multi-Vitamins and Iron (SmithKline Beecham) p 696
Ferancee Chewable Tablets (Stuart) p 720
Ferancee-HP Tablets (Stuart) p 433, 721
Ferro-Sequels (Lederle) p 413, 578
Flintstones Children's Chewable Vitamins Plus Iron (Miles Consumer) p 417, 612
One-A-Day Maximum Formula Vitamins and Minerals (Miles Consumer) p 417, 614
Stressgard Stress Formula Vitamins (Miles Consumer) p 417, 614
Stresstabs + Iron, Advanced Formula (Lederle) p 413, 582
Stuartinic Tablets (Stuart) p 434, 726
Theragran-M Tablets (Squibb) p 433, 717
Within Multivitamin for Women with Calcium, Extra Iron and Zinc (Miles Consumer) p 417, 614

FERROUS GLUCONATE

Fergon Elixir (Winthrop Consumer Products) p 757
Fergon Tablets (Winthrop Consumer Products) p 438, 757

FERROUS SULFATE

Dayalets Plus Iron Filmtab (Abbott) p 502
Feosol Capsules (SmithKline Consumer) p 432, 714
Feosol Elixir (SmithKline Consumer) p 432, 714
Feosol Tablets (SmithKline Consumer) p 432, 714
Fermalox Tablets (Rorer Consumer) p 664
Mol-Iron Tablets (Schering) p 692
Mol-Iron w/Vitamin C Tablets (Schering) p 692
Similac Special Care With Iron 24 Premature Infant Formula (Ross) p 674
Slow Fe Tablets (CIBA Consumer) p 409, 548

FISH OILS

Promega (Parke-Davis) p 420, 630
Promega Pearls (Parke-Davis) p 420, 630

FOLIC ACID

Allbee C-800 Plus Iron Tablets (Robins) p 424, 654
Bugs Bunny Children's Chewable Vitamins (Sugar Free) (Miles Consumer) p 417, 612
Bugs Bunny With Extra C Children's Chewable Vitamins (Sugar Free) (Miles Consumer) p 417, 613
Bugs Bunny Plus Iron Children's Chewable Vitamins (Sugar Free) (Miles Consumer) p 417, 612
Flintstones Children's Chewable Vitamins (Miles Consumer) p 417, 612
Flintstones Children's Chewable Vitamins With Extra C (Miles Consumer) p 417, 613
Flintstones Children's Chewable Vitamins Plus Iron (Miles Consumer) p 417, 612
One-A-Day Essential Vitamins (Miles Consumer) p 417, 613
One-A-Day Maximum Formula Vitamins and Minerals (Miles Consumer) p 417, 614
One-A-Day Plus Extra C Vitamins (Miles Consumer) p 417, 614
Stressgard Stress Formula Vitamins (Miles Consumer) p 417, 614

Stuart Prenatal Tablets (Stuart) p 434, 726
The Stuart Formula Tablets (Stuart) p 434, 725
Theragran Stress Formula (Squibb) p 433, 718
Within Multivitamin for Women with Calcium, Extra Iron and Zinc (Miles Consumer) p 417, 614

G

GARLIC EXTRACT

Kyolic (Wakunaga) p 435, 735

GELATIN A

Lacril Lubricant Ophthalmic Solution (Allergan Pharmaceuticals) p 505

GINSENG

Roygel Ultima Capsules (Benson Pharmacal) p 517

GLUCOSE, LIQUID

Insta-Glucose (ICN Pharmaceuticals) p 411, 569

GLYCERIN

Aqua Care Cream (SmithKline Consumer) p 431, 706
Basis Soap-Normal to Dry Skin (Beiersdorf) p 404, 514
Clear Eyes Lubricating Eye Redness Reliever (Ross) p 426, 669
Collyrium Fresh (Wyeth-Ayerst) p 439, 764
Diaparene Medicated Cream (Lehn & Fink) p 413
Lac-Hydrin Five (Westwood) p 436, 741
P & S Liquid (Baker Cummins Dermatologicals) p 404, 509
Mediconet Cleansing Cloths (Medicone) p 416, 607
Moisture Drops (Bausch & Lomb Personal) p 404, 513
Replens (Columbia) p 408, 550
S.T.37 Antiseptic Solution (SmithKline Beecham) p 702
Tucks Premoistened Pads (Parke-Davis) p 420, 632
Tucks Take-Alongs (Parke-Davis) p 632
Ultra Mide 25 (Baker Cummins Dermatologicals) p 510

GLYCERIN ANHYDROUS

Otix Drops Ear Wax Removal Aid (Church & Dwight) p 407, 543

GLYCERYL GUAIACOLATE
(see under GUAIFENESIN)

GLYCERYL STEARATE

Aqua-A Cream (Baker Cummins Dermatologicals) p 404, 508
Aquaderm Therapeutic Cream (Baker Cummins Dermatologicals) p 404, 509
Aquaderm Therapeutic Lotion (Baker Cummins Dermatologicals) p 404, 509
Diaparene Cradol (Lehn & Fink) p 413, 587

GLYCOLIC ACID

Aqua Glycolic Lotion (Herald Pharmacal) p 567
Aqua Glycolic Shampoo (Herald Pharmacal) p 567
Aqua Glyde Cleanser (Herald Pharmacal) p 567

GOAT MILK

Meyenberg Evaporated Goat Milk - 12 1/2 fl. oz. (Jackson-Mitchell) p 570
Meyenberg Powdered Goat Milk - 4 oz. & 14 oz. (Jackson-Mitchell) p 570

GUAIFENESIN

Benylin Expectorant (Parke-Davis) p 420, 628
Bronkaid Tablets (Winthrop Consumer Products) p 438, 756

Phillips' Milk of Magnesia Tablets
(Glenbrook) p 411, 566
Rolaids (Sodium Free)
(Warner-Lambert) p 436, 740
WinGel Liquid & Tablets (Winthrop
Consumer Products) p 760

MAGNESIUM OXIDE

Beelith Tablets (Beach) p 513
Tri-Buffered Bufferin Analgesic Tablets
and Caplets (Bristol-Myers Products)
p 404, 525
Cama Arthritis Pain Reliever (Sandoz
Consumer) p 677
Mag-Ox 400 (Blaine) p 517
Uro-Mag (Blaine) p 517

MAGNESIUM SALICYLATE

Doan's - Extra-Strength Analgesic (CIBA
Consumer) p 408, 544
Doan's - Regular Strength Analgesic
(CIBA Consumer) p 408, 544
Mobigesic Analgesic Tablets (Ascher)
p 403, 507

MAGNESIUM TRISILICATE

Gaviscon Antacid Tablets (Marion)
p 413, 590
Gaviscon-2 Antacid Tablets (Marion)
p 414, 591

MALT SOUP EXTRACT

Maltsupex Liquid, Powder & Tablets
(Wallace) p 435, 736

MECLIZINE HYDROCHLORIDE

Bonine Tablets (Leeming) p 583
Meclizine HCl Chewable Tablets 25 mg
(Pharmafair) p 633

MENTHOL

Afrin Menthol Nasal Spray (Schering)
p 428, 684
Aurum the Gold Lotion (Au
Pharmaceuticals) p 508
Ben-Gay External Analgesic Products
(Leeming) p 583
Cēpastat Cherry Flavor Sore Throat
Lozenges (Lakeside Pharmaceuticals)
p 412, 573
Cēpastat Sore Throat Lozenges
(Lakeside Pharmaceuticals) p 412,
573
Denorex Medicated Shampoo and
Conditioner (Whitehall) p 437, 747
Denorex Medicated Shampoo, Extra
Strength (Whitehall) p 437, 747
Denorex Medicated Shampoo, Extra
Strength With Conditioners
(Whitehall) p 747
Denorex Medicated Shampoo, Regular
& Mountain Fresh Herbal Scent
(Whitehall) p 437, 747
Dermoplast Anesthetic Pain Relief
Lotion (Whitehall) p 437, 747
Dermoplast Anesthetic Pain Relief
Spray (Whitehall) p 437, 748
Flex-all 454 Pain Relieving Gel
(Chattem) p 542
Halls Mentho-Lyptus Cough
Suppressant Tablets
(Warner-Lambert) p 435, 738
Icy Hot Balm (Richardson-Vicks Inc.)
p 423, 647
Icy Hot Cream (Richardson-Vicks Inc.)
p 423, 647
Icy Hot Stick (Richardson-Vicks Inc.)
p 423, 647
Listerine Antiseptic (Warner-Lambert)
p 435, 739
Medicone Derma Ointment (Medicone)
p 416, 606
Medicone Dressing Cream (Medicone)
p 416, 606
Medicone Rectal Ointment (Medicone)
p 416, 606
Medicone Rectal Suppositories
(Medicone) p 416, 606
N'ICE Medicated Sugarless Sore Throat
and Cough Lozenges (SmithKline
Beecham) p 699
N'ICE Sore Throat Spray (SmithKline
Beecham) p 699

Nose Better Nasal Gel (Goldline) p 567
Noxzema Clear-Ups Medicated
Pads-Maximum Strength 2.0%
Salicylic Acid (Noxell) p 418, 618
Noxzema Clear-Ups Medicated
Pads-Regular Strength 0.5%
Salicyclic Acid (Noxell) p 418, 618
Noxzema Medicated Skin Cream
(Noxell) p 418, 619
Rhuligel (Rydelle) p 427, 676
Selsun Blue Dandruff Shampoo-Extra
Medicated (Ross) p 426, 672
Sucrets Cold Relief Formula
(SmithKline Beecham) p 703
TheraGold (AU Pharmaceuticals) p 508
Therapeutic Gold (AU Pharmaceuticals)
p 508
Therapeutic Mineral Ice (Bristol-Myers
Products) p 406, 533
Vicks Formula 44 Cough Control Discs
(Richardson-Vicks Inc.) p 649
Vicks Inhaler (Richardson-Vicks Inc.)
p 651
Vicks Vaporub (Richardson-Vicks Inc.)
p 424, 653
Vicks Vaposteam (Richardson-Vicks
Inc.) p 653
X-Seb T Plus Conditioning Shampoo
(Baker Cummins Dermatologicals)
p 404, 510

METHIONINE

Geritol Liquid - High Potency Iron &
Vitamin Tonic (SmithKline Beecham)
p 697

METHYL GLUCETH-20

Basis Soap-Extra Dry Skin (Beiersdorf)
p 404, 514

METHYL SALICYLATE

Aurum the Gold Lotion (Au
Pharmaceuticals) p 508
Ben-Gay External Analgesic Products
(Leeming) p 583
Icy Hot Balm (Richardson-Vicks Inc.)
p 423, 647
Icy Hot Cream (Richardson-Vicks Inc.)
p 423, 647
Icy Hot Stick (Richardson-Vicks Inc.)
p 423, 647
Listerine Antiseptic (Warner-Lambert)
p 435, 739
TheraGold (Au Pharmaceuticals) p 508
Therapeutic Gold (Au Pharmaceuticals)
p 508

METHYLBENZETHONIUM CHLORIDE

Diaparene Baby Powder (Lehn & Fink)
p 413, 587
Diaparene Cradol (Lehn & Fink) p 413,
587
Diaparene Medicated Cream (Lehn &
Fink) p 413
Diaparene Peri-Anal Medicated
Ointment (Lehn & Fink) p 413

METHYLCELLULOSE

Citrucel Orange Flavor (Lakeside
Pharmaceuticals) p 412, 574
Citrucel Regular Flavor (Lakeside
Pharmaceuticals) p 412, 573

METHYLPARABEN

Noxzema Clear-Ups Maximum Strength
Lotion, Vanishing (Noxell) p 418,
618

MICONAZOLE NITRATE

Micatin Antifungal Cream (Ortho
Pharmaceutical) p 419, 622
Micatin Antifungal Deodorant Spray
Powder (Ortho Pharmaceutical)
p 419, 622
Micatin Antifungal Powder (Ortho
Pharmaceutical) p 419, 622
Micatin Antifungal Spray Liquid (Ortho
Pharmaceutical) p 419, 622
Micatin Antifungal Spray Powder (Ortho
Pharmaceutical) p 419, 622
Micatin Jock Itch Cream (Ortho
Pharmaceutical) p 622

Micatin Jock Itch Spray Powder (Ortho
Pharmaceutical) p 622

MINERAL OIL

Agoral, Plain (Parke-Davis) p 624
Agoral, Marshmallow Flavor
(Parke-Davis) p 624
Agoral, Raspberry Flavor (Parke-Davis)
p 624
Aqua Care Cream (SmithKline
Consumer) p 431, 706
Aqua Care Lotion (SmithKline
Consumer) p 431, 706
Aqua-A Cream (Baker Cummins
Dermatologicals) p 404, 508
Aquaderm Therapeutic Cream (Baker
Cummins Dermatologicals) p 404,
509
Aquaderm Therapeutic Lotion (Baker
Cummins Dermatologicals) p 404,
509
Aquaphor Healing Ointment
(Beiersdorf) p 404, 514
Aveeno Shower and Bath Oil (Rydelle)
p 427, 676
Balneol (Reid-Rowell) p 423, 643
Creme de la Femme ("Especially"
Products) p 554
Diaparene Cradol (Lehn & Fink) p 413,
587
Diaparene Medicated Cream (Lehn &
Fink) p 413
Diaparene Peri-Anal Medicated
Ointment (Lehn & Fink) p 413
Duolube Eye Ointment (Bausch & Lomb
Personal) p 404, 512
Eucerin Moisturizing Creme
(Unscented) (Beiersdorf) p 404, 514
Eucerin Moisturizing Lotion (Unscented)
(Beiersdorf) p 404, 515
Haley's M-O, Regular & Flavored
(Glenbrook) p 411, 563
Keri Lotion-Original Formula
(Westwood) p 436, 741
Lacri-Lube S.O.P. (Allergan
Pharmaceuticals) p 403, 505
Lubrifair Ophthalmic Ointment
(Pharmafair) p 633
P & S Liquid (Baker Cummins
Dermatologicals) p 404, 509
Nephrox Suspension (Fleming) p 558
Nivea Bath Silk Bath Oil (Beiersdorf)
p 515
Pen•Kera Creme (Ascher) p 403, 507
Refresh P.M. (Allergan
Pharmaceuticals) p 403, 506
Replens (Columbia) p 408, 550
Tearfair Ointment (Pharmafair) p 633
Ultra Derm Bath Oil (Baker Cummins
Dermatologicals) p 509
Ultra Mide 25 (Baker Cummins
Dermatologicals) p 510

MINERAL WAX

Aquaphor Healing Ointment
(Beiersdorf) p 404, 514
Eucerin Moisturizing Creme
(Unscented) (Beiersdorf) p 404, 514

MULTIVITAMINS

Dayalets Filmtab (Abbott) p 502

MULTIVITAMINS WITH MINERALS

Centrum, Jr. (Children's Chewable) +
Extra C (Lederle) p 412, 577
Dayalets Plus Iron Filmtab (Abbott)
p 502
Optilets-500 Filmtab (Abbott) p 502
Optilets-M-500 Filmtab (Abbott) p 502
Sunkist Children's Chewable
Multivitamins - Complete (CIBA
Consumer) p 409, 548
Sunkist Children's Chewable
Multivitamins - Plus Extra C (CIBA
Consumer) p 409, 548
Sunkist Children's Chewable
Multivitamins - Plus Iron (CIBA
Consumer) p 409, 548
Sunkist Children's Chewable
Multivitamins - Regular (CIBA
Consumer) p 409, 548
Surbex-750 with Iron (Abbott) p 503
Surbex-750 with Zinc (Abbott) p 503
Theragran-M Tablets (Squibb) p 433,
717

Johnson's Baby Sunblock Lotion (SPF 15) (Johnson & Johnson Consumer) p 411, 570

Johnson's Baby Sunblock Lotion (SPF 30+) (Johnson & Johnson Consumer) p 411, 570

Nivea Sun SPF 15 (Beiersdorf) p 516

PreSun 15 Facial Sunscreen (Westwood) p 742

PreSun for Kids (Westwood) p 742

PreSun 8, 15 and 39 Creamy Sunscreens (Westwood) p 742

PreSun 15 and 29 Sensitive Skin Sunscreen (Westwood) p 436, 743

PreSun 23 Sunscreen Sprays (Westwood) p 742

Purpose Dual Treatment Moisturizer (SPF 12) (Johnson & Johnson Consumer) p 570

Shade Oil-Free Gel SPF 15 (Plough) p 422, 637

Shade Oil-Free Gel SPF 25 (Plough) p 637

Shade Sunblock Lotion SPF 15 (Plough) p 422, 637

Shade Sunblock Lotion SPF 30 (Plough) p 637

Shade Sunblock Lotion SPF 45 (Plough) p 422, 637

Shade Sunblock Stick SPF 30 (Plough) p 637

Sundown Sunblock Combi Pack Ultra Protection (SPF 15) (Johnson & Johnson Consumer) p 411, 571

Sundown Sunblock Cream, Ultra Protection (SPF 15) (Johnson & Johnson Consumer) p 411, 571

Sundown Sunblock Lotion, Ultra Protection (SPF 15) (Johnson & Johnson Consumer) p 411, 571

Sundown Sunblock Lotion, Ultra Protection (SPF 25) (Johnson & Johnson Consumer) p 571

Sundown Sunblock Lotion, Ultra Protection (SPF 20) (Johnson & Johnson Consumer) p 571

Sundown Sunblock Lotion, Ultra Protection (SPF 30+) (Johnson & Johnson Consumer) p 571

Sundown Sunblock Stick, Ultra Protection (SPF 15) (Johnson & Johnson Consumer) p 410, 571

Sundown Sunblock Stick, Ultra Protection (SPF 30+) (Johnson & Johnson Consumer) p 571

Sundown Sunscreen Lotion, Maximal Protection (SPF 8) (Johnson & Johnson Consumer) p 571

Water Babies by Coppertone Sunblock Cream SPF 25 (Plough) p 422, 638

Water Babies by Coppertone Sunblock Lotion SPF 15 (Plough) p 422, 638

Water Babies by Coppertone Sunblock Lotion SPF 30 (Plough) p 422, 638

Water Babies by Coppertone Sunblock Lotion SPF 45 (Plough) p 422, 638

OXYMETAZOLINE HYDROCHLORIDE

Afrin Cherry Scented Nasal Spray 0.05% (Schering) p 428, 684

Afrin Children's Strength Nose Drops 0.025% (Schering) p 428, 684

Afrin Menthol Nasal Spray (Schering) p 428, 684

Afrin Nasal Spray 0.05% and Nasal Spray Pump (Schering) p 428, 684

Afrin Nose Drops 0.05% (Schering) p 428, 684

Coricidin Decongestant Nasal Mist (Schering) p 686

Dristan Long Lasting Menthol Nasal Spray (Whitehall) p 437, 748

Dristan Long Lasting Nasal Spray, Regular (Whitehall) p 437, 748

Duration 12 Hour Mentholated Nasal Spray (Plough) p 421, 634

Duration 12 Hour Nasal Spray (Plough) p 421, 634

Duration 12 Hour Nasal Spray Pump (Plough) p 421, 635

4-Way Long Lasting Nasal Spray & Metered Spray Pump (Bristol-Myers Products) p 406, 532

NTZ Long Acting Nasal Spray & Drops 0.05% (Winthrop Consumer Products) p 758

Neo-Synephrine 12 Hour Adult Nose Drops (Winthrop Consumer Products) p 758

Neo-Synephrine 12 Hour Nasal Spray (Winthrop Consumer Products) p 758

Neo-Synephrine 12 Hour Nasal Spray Pump (Winthrop Consumer Products) p 438, 758

Neo-Synephrine 12 Hour Vapor Nasal Spray (Winthrop Consumer Products) p 758

Nostrilla Long Acting Nasal Decongestant (Boehringer Ingelheim) p 521

Vicks Sinex Long-Acting Decongestant Nasal Spray (Richardson-Vicks Inc.) p 424, 653

Vicks Sinex Long-Acting Decongestant Nasal Ultra Fine Mist (Richardson-Vicks Inc.) p 424, 653

Visine L.R. Eye Drops (Leeming) p 413, 586

P

PEG-7-GLYCERYL COCOATE

Nivea Bath Silk Bath & Shower Gel (Extra-Dry Skin) (Beiersdorf) p 515

Nivea Bath Silk Bath & Shower Gel (Normal-to-Dry Skin) (Beiersdorf) p 515

PADIMATE O (OCTYL DIMETHYL PABA)

Chap Stick Lip Balm (Robins) p 424, 655

Chap Stick Petroleum Jelly Plus with Sunblock 15 (Robins) p 424, 656

Chap Stick Sunblock 15 Lip Balm (Robins) p 424, 655

Nivea Sun SPF 15 (Beiersdorf) p 516

Photoplex Broad Spectrum Sunscreen Lotion (Herbert) p 568

PAMABROM

Maximum Strength Midol PMS Premenstrual Syndrome Formula (Glenbrook) p 410, 563

Premsyn PMS (Chattem) p 542

PANTHENOL

Geritol Liquid - High Potency Iron & Vitamin Tonic (SmithKline Beecham) p 697

PANTOTHENIC ACID

Allbee with C Caplets (Robins) p 424, 654

Allbee C-800 Plus Iron Tablets (Robins) p 424, 654

Allbee C-800 Tablets (Robins) p 424, 654

One-A-Day Essential Vitamins (Miles Consumer) p 417, 613

One-A-Day Maximum Formula Vitamins and Minerals (Miles Consumer) p 417, 614

One-A-Day Plus Extra C Vitamins (Miles Consumer) p 417, 614

Probec-T Tablets (Stuart) p 434, 725

Stressgard Stress Formula Vitamins (Miles Consumer) p 417, 614

Stuartinic Tablets (Stuart) p 434, 726

Within Multivitamin for Women with Calcium, Extra Iron and Zinc (Miles Consumer) p 417, 614

Z-Bec Tablets (Robins) p 425, 661

PECTIN

Donnagel (Robins) p 425, 659

PETROLATUM

A and D Ointment (Schering) p 428, 683

Aqua Care Cream (SmithKline Consumer) p 431, 706

Aqua Care Lotion (SmithKline Consumer) p 431, 706

Aquaphor Healing Ointment (Beiersdorf) p 404, 514

Basis Soap-Normal to Dry Skin (Beiersdorf) p 404, 514

Caldesene Medicated Ointment (Fisons Consumer) p 409, 555

Chap Stick Lip Balm (Robins) p 424, 655

Chap Stick Sunblock 15 Lip Balm (Robins) p 424, 655

Desitin Ointment (Leeming) p 413, 583

Dyprotex Diaper Rash Pads (Blistex) p 404, 517

Eucerin Moisturizing Creme (Unscented) (Beiersdorf) p 404, 514

Lac-Hydrin Five (Westwood) p 436, 741

Petrolatum Ophthalmic Ointment (Pharmafair) p 633

Preparation H Hemorrhoidal Cream (Whitehall) p 437, 751

Preparation H Hemorrhoidal Ointment (Whitehall) p 437, 751

PETROLEUM DISTILLATES

Pronto Lice Killing Spray (Commerce) p 552

PHENIRAMINE MALEATE

Dristan Nasal Spray, Regular & Menthol (Whitehall) p 437, 748

PHENOBARBITAL

Bronkolixir (Winthrop Pharmaceuticals) p 760

Bronkotabs Tablets (Winthrop Pharmaceuticals) p 760

Primatene Tablets-P Formula (Whitehall) p 437, 752

PHENOL

Anbesol Gel Antiseptic-Anesthetic (Whitehall) p 437, 745

Anbesol Liquid Antiseptic-Anesthetic (Whitehall) p 437, 745

Campho-Phenique Cold Sore Gel (Winthrop Consumer Products) p 438, 756

Campho-Phenique Liquid (Winthrop Consumer Products) p 438, 757

Cepastat Cherry Flavor Sore Throat Lozenges (Lakeside Pharmaceuticals) p 412, 573

Cepastat Sore Throat Lozenges (Lakeside Pharmaceuticals) p 412, 573

Chloraseptic Liquid, Cherry, Menthol or Cool Mint (Richardson-Vicks Inc.) p 423, 645

Chloraseptic Liquid - Nitrogen Propelled Spray (Richardson-Vicks Inc.) p 423, 645

Chloraseptic Lozenges, Cherry, Menthol or Cool Mint (Richardson-Vicks Inc.) p 423, 645

P & S Liquid (Baker Cummins Dermatologicals) p 404, 509

Noxzema Medicated Skin Cream (Noxell) p 418, 619

PRID Salve (Walker Pharmacal) p 736

Panscol Medicated Lotion and Ointment (Baker Cummins Dermatologicals) p 509

PHENOLPHTHALEIN

Agoral, Marshmallow Flavor (Parke-Davis) p 624

Agoral, Raspberry Flavor (Parke-Davis) p 624

Modane Plus Tablets (Adria) p 403, 504

Modane Tablets (Adria) p 403, 504

Phillips' LaxCaps (Glenbrook) p 411, 565

PHENOLPHTHALEIN, YELLOW

Correctol Laxative Tablets (Plough) p 421, 634

Doxidan Liquigels (Hoechst-Roussel) p 411, 568

Evac-U-Gen Mild Laxative (Walker, Corp) p 435, 736

Ex-Lax Chocolated Laxative (Sandoz Consumer) p 427, 678

ZINC OXIDE
Anusol Hemorrhoidal Suppositories (Parke-Davis) p 419, 624
Anusol Ointment (Parke-Davis) p 419, 624
Balmex Baby Powder (Macsil) p 589
Balmex Ointment (Macsil) p 590
Caldesene Medicated Ointment (Fisons Consumer) p 409, 555
Desitin Ointment (Leeming) p 413, 583
Diaparene Peri-Anal Medicated Ointment (Lehn & Fink) p 413
Dyprotex Diaper Rash Pads (Blistex) p 404, 517
Medicone Derma Ointment (Medicone) p 416, 606
Medicone Dressing Cream (Medicone) p 416, 606
Medicone Rectal Ointment (Medicone) p 416, 606
Medicone Rectal Suppositories (Medicone) p 416, 606
Nupercainal Suppositories (CIBA Consumer) p 408, 547
Pazo Hemorrhoid Ointment & Suppositories (Bristol-Myers Products) p 406, 533
Ziradryl Lotion (Parke-Davis) p 420, 633

ZINC PYRITHIONE
Zincon Dandruff Shampoo (Lederle) p 413, 582

ZINC SULFATE
Orazinc Capsules (Mericon) p 607
Surbex-750 with Zinc (Abbott) p 503
Visine A.C. Eye Drops (Leeming) p 413, 586

ZINC UNDECYLENATE
Desenex Antifungal Cream (Fisons Consumer) p 409, 556
Desenex Antifungal Ointment (Fisons Consumer) p 409, 556
Desenex Antifungal Powder (Fisons Consumer) p 409, 556
Desenex Antifungal Spray Powder (Fisons Consumer) p 409, 556

Certified
poison control centers

The regional poison control centers in the following list are certified by the American Association of Poison Control Centers. To receive certification, each center must meet certain criteria. It must, for example, serve a large geographic area; it must be open 24 hours a day and provide direct dialing or toll-free access; it must be supervised by a medical director; and it must have registered pharmacists or nurses available to answer questions from the public.

Staff members of these regional centers are trained to resolve toxicity situations in the home of the caller, but, in some instances, hospital referrals are given.

The regional centers have a wide variety of toxicology resources, including a computer capability covering some 350,000 substances that are updated quarterly. They also offer a range of educational services to the public as well as to the health-care professional. In some states, these large centers exist side by side with smaller poison control centers that provide more limited information.

AMERICAN ASSOCIATION OF POISON CONTROL CENTERS

ALABAMA

Alabama Poison Center
Alabama Poison Center
809 University Boulevard East
Tuscaloosa, AL 35401
Emergency Numbers
  800/462-0800 AL only
  205/345-0600
FAX: 205/759-7994
Director: Richard W. Looser, B.S.;
  205/345-0938
Medical Director: Perry L.
Lovely, M.D.; 205/345-0600

Children's Hospital of Alabama Regional Poison Control Center
1600 7th Avenue South
Birmingham, AL 35233
Emergency Numbers
  205/939-9201 AL only
  800/292-6678
  205/933-4050
Director: William D. King,
R. Ph., M.P.H.; 205/939-9720
Medical Director: Edward C.
Kohaut, M.D.; 205/939-9100

ARIZONA

Arizona Poison and Drug Information Center
Health Sciences Center,
Room 3204K
1501 North Campbell
Tucson, AZ 85724

Emergency Numbers
  602/626-6016 (Tucson)
  800/362-0101 (statewide)
FAX: 602/626-4063
Director: Theodore G. Tong,
Pharm. D.; 602/626-7899
Medical Director: John B.
Sullivan, Jr., M.D.;
  602/626-6312

Samaritan Regional Poison Center
Good Samaritan Medical
Center
1130 East McDowell, Suite A5
Phoenix, AZ 85006
Emergency Numbers
  602/253-3334
FAX: 602/239-4138
Director: Joyce M. Bradley,
R.N., M.S.; 602/253-0813
Medical Director: Donald B.
Kunkel, M.D.; 602/253-2314

CALIFORNIA

Fresno Regional Poison Control Center
Fresno Community Hospital
and Medical Center
Fresno and R Streets
Fresno, CA 93715
Emergency Numbers
  209/445-1222
  800/346-5922
FAX: 209/442-6483

Director: Brent R. Ekins,
Pharm. D.; 209/442-6479
Medical Director: Rick Geller,
M.D.; 209/442-6408

Los Angeles County Medical Association
Regional Poison Center
1925 Wilshire Bouevard
Los Angeles, CA 90057
Emergency Numbers
  213/664-2121
  213/484-5151
  800/777-6476
FAX: 213/413-5255
Director: Corrine Ray, R.N.,
B.S; 213/664-2121
Medical Director: Marc J.
Bayer, M.D.; 818/364-3107

San Diego Regional Poison Center
UCSD Medical Center
225 Dickinson Street
San Diego, CA 92103-1990
Emergency Numbers
  619/543-6000
  800/876-4766
FAX: 619/692-1867
Director: Anthony S.
Manoguerra, Pharm. D.;
  619/543-6010
Medical Director: George M.
Shumaik, M.D.; 619/543-3666

San Francisco Regional Poison Center
San Francisco General Hospital
1001 Potrero Avenue, Room IE86
San Francisco, CA 94110
Emergency Numbers
415/476-6600
800/523-2222
FAX: 415/821-8513
Director/Medical Director:
Kent R. Olson, M.D.;
415/821-5524

UC Davis Regional Poison Control Center
2315 Stockton Boulevard, Room 1511
Sacramento, CA 95817
Emergency Numbers
916/453-3692
800/342-9293 (Northern CA only)
FAX: 916/453-7796
Director: Judith Alsop, Pharm. D.; 916/453-3414
Medical Director: Timothy Albertson, M.D., Ph.D.;
916/453-5010

COLORADO

Rocky Mountain Poison and Drug Center
645 Bannock Street
Denver, CO 80204-4507
Emergency Numbers
303/629-1123 (CO)
FAX: 303/623-1119
Director: Barry H. Rumack, M.D.; 303/893-7774
Medical Director: Kenneth Kulig, M.D., F.A.C.E.P.;
303/893-7774

FLORIDA

Florida Poison Information Center
The Tampa General Hospital
Davis Islands
Post Office Box 1289
Tampa, FL 33601
Emergency Numbers
813/253-4444 (Tampa only)
800/282-3171 (Florida)
Director: Sven A. Normann, Pharm.D.; 813/251-7044
Co-Medical Directors: James V. Hilllman, M.D.; Gregory G. Gaar, M.D.; 813/251-6911

GEORGIA

Georgia Regional Poison Control Center
80 Butler Street, S.E.
Atlanta, GA 30335-3801
Emergency Numbers
404/589-4400
800/282-5846 (GA only)
FAX: 404/525-2816
Director: Gaylord P. Lopez, Pharm.D.; 404/589-4400
Medical Director: Robert J. Geller, M.D.; 404/589-4400

KENTUCKY

Kentucky Regional Poison Center of Kosair Chidren's Hospital
224 East Broadway, Suite 305
Louisville, KY 40202
Emergency Numbers
502/589-8222
800/722-5725 (KY Toll free)
Director: Nancy J. Matyunas, Pharm.D.; 502/562-7263
Medical Director: George C. Rodgers Jr, M.D., Ph.D.;
502/562-8837

MARYLAND

Maryland Poison Center
20 North Pine Street
Baltimore, MD 21201
Emergency Numbers
301/528-7701
800/492-2414 (MD only)
FAX: 301/328-7184
Director: Gary M. Oderda, Pharm.D., M.P.H.; 301/328-7604
Medical Director: Richard L. Gorman, M.D; 301/328-7604

MASSACHUSETTS

Massachusetts Poison Control System
300 Longwood Avenue
Boston, MA 02115
Emergency Numbers
617/232-2120 Boston Area
800/682-9211 Toll Free in MA
Director/Medical Director:
Alan Woolf, M.D., M.P.H.;
617/735-6609

MICHIGAN

Blodgett Regional Poison Center
1840 Wealthy Street S.E.
Grand Rapids, MI 49506
Emergency Numbers
800/632-2727 MI only
FAX: 616/774-7204
Director: Daniel J. McCoy, Ph.D.; 616/774-7851
Medical Director: John R. Mauer, M.D.; 616/774-7851

Poison Control Center
Children's Hospital of Michigan
3901 Beaubien Boulevard
Detroit, MI 48201
Emergency Numbers
313/745-5711 (Metro Detroit)
800/462-6642 (Rest of MI)
FAX: 313/745-5602
Director/Medical Director:
Regine Aronow, M.D.;
313/745-5335
Administrative Manager:
Richard Dorsch, M.D.;
313/745-5329

MINNESOTA

Hennepin Regional Poison Center
Hennepin County Medical Center
701 Park Avenue South
Minneapolis, MN 55415
Emergency Numbers
612/347-3141
FAX: 612/347-3968
Director: Michael J. Wieland, R.Ph.; 612/347-3144
Medical Director: Louis J. Ling, M.D.; 612/347-3174

Minnesota Regional Poison Center
St. Paul-Ramsey Medical Center
640 Jackson Street
St. Paul, MN 55101
Emergency Numbers
612/221-2113
800/222-1222 MN only
Director: Leo Sioris, Pharm.D.; 612/221-3192
Medical Director: Samuel Hall, M.D., A.B.M.T.;
612/221-3470

MISSOURI

Cardinal Glennon Children's Hospital
Regional Poison Center
1465 South Grand Boulevard
St. Louis, MO 63104
Emergency Numbers
800/392-9111 (MI only)
314/772-5200
800/366-8888
FAX: 314/577-5355
Director: Michael W.
Thompson, B.S. Pharm.;
314/772-8300
Medical Director: Anthony J.
Scalzo, M.D.; 314/772-8300

NEW JERSEY

New Jersey Poison Information and Education System
201 Lyons Avenue
Newark, NJ 07112
Emergency Numbers
800/962-1253 (NJ only)
201/923-0764 (Outside of NJ)
FAX: 201/926-0013
Director/Medical Director:
Steven M. Marcus, M.D;
201/926-7443

NEW MEXICO

New Mexico Poison and Drug Information Center
University of New Mexico
Albuquerque, NM 87131
Emergency Numbers
505/843-2551
800/432-6866 (NM only)
Director: William G.
Troutman, Pharm.D.;
505/277-4261
Medical Director: Dan
Tandberg, M.D.; 505/277-5064

NEW YORK

Long Island Regional Poison Control Center
2201 Hempstead Turnpike
East Meadow, NY 11554
Emergency Numbers
516/542-2323

Director/Medical Director:
Howard C. Mofenson, M.D.;
516/542-3707

New York City Poison Center
455 First Avenue, Room 123
New York, NY 10016
Emergency Numbers
212/340-4494
212/764-7667
FAX: 212/340-4525
Director: Richard S.
Weisman, Pharm.D.;
212/340-4497
Medical Director: Lewis
Goldfrank, M.D.; 212/561-3346

NORTH CAROLINA

Duke Regional Poison Control Center
Duke University Medical Center
Box 3007
Durham, NC 27710
Emergency Numbers
800/672-1697 (NC only)
Medical Director: Shirley
Osterhout, M.D.; 919/684-4438
Assistant Director: Chris
Rudd, Pharm.D.;
919/681-4574

OHIO

Central Ohio Poison Center
700 Children's Drive
Columbus, OH 43205
Emergency Numbers
614/228-1323
800/682-7625
Director: Judith G. D'Orsi,
B.A. 614/461-2717
Medical Director: Mary Ellen
Mortensen, M.D.;
614/461-2256

Regional Poison Control System and Cincinnati Drug and Poison Information Center
231 Bethesda Avenue, M.L., #144
Cincinnati, OH 45267-0144
Emergency Numbers
513/558-5111
FAX: 513/558-5301
Director: Leonard T. Sigell,
Ph.D.; 513/558-9182
Medical Director: Clifford G.
Grulee, Jr., M.D.;
513/558-7336

OREGON

Oregon Poison Center
Oregon Health Sciences University
3181 SW Sam Jackson Park Road
Portland, OR 97201
Emergency Numbers
503/279-8968;
800/452-7165 OR only
Director: Terry Putman, R.N.;
503/279-7799
Medical Director: Brent T.
Burton, M.D.; 503/279-7799

PENNSYLVANIA

Delaware Valley Regional Poison Control Center
One Children's Center
34th & Civic Center Boulevard
Philadelphia, PA 19104
Emergency Numbers
215/386-2100
FAX: 215/386-3692
Director: Thomas E.
Kearney, Pharm.D.; 215/823-7203
Medical Director: Fred M.
Henretig, M.D.; 215/596-8454

Pittsburgh Poison Center
One Children's Place
3705 5th Avenue at DeSoto
Pittsburgh, PA 15213
Emergency Numbers
412/681-6669
FAX: 412/692-5868
Director: Edward P.
Krenzelok, Pharm.D.;
412/692-5600
Assistant Director: Bonnie S.
Dean, R.N., B.S.N.;
412/692-5600
Medical Director: Sandra M.
Schneider, M.D.;
412/648-6000, ext. 3669

RHODE ISLAND

593 Eddy Street
Providence, RI 02903
Emergency Numbers
401/277-5727
401/277-8062 (TDD)
Director: Philip N. Johnson,
Ph.D.; 401/277-5906
Medical Director: William J.
Lewander, M.D.; 401/277-5906

TEXAS

North Texas Poison Center
5201 Harry Hines Boulevard
Dallas, TX 75235
Emergency Numbers
214/590-5000
800/441-0040 (TX only)
FAX: 214/590-8096,
Attention: Poison Center
Director: Lena C. Day, R.N.,
B.S.N., C.S.P.I.; 214/590-5625
Medical Director: Gary Reed,
M.D.; 214/688-2992
Assistant Medical Director:
Tom Kurt, M.D.; 214/590-6625

Texas State Poison Center
University of Texas Medical
Branch
Galveston, TX 77550-2780
Emergency Numbers
409/765-1420 (Galveston)
800/392-8548 (TX only)
713/654-1701 (Houston)
512/478-4490 (Austin)

Director: Michael D. Ellis,
M.S.; 409/761-3332
Medical Director: Wayne R.
Snodgrass, M.D., Ph.D.;
409/761-1561

UTAH

**Intermountain Regional
Poison Control Center**
50 North Medical Drive,
Building 528
Salt Lake City, UT 84132
Emergency Number
801/581-2151
Director: Joseph C. Veltri,
Pharm.D.; 801/581-7504
Medical Director: Douglas
Rollins, M.D., Ph.D.;
801/581-5117

WASHINGTON, D.C.

**National Capital Poison
Center**
Georgetown University
Hospital
3800 Reservoir Road, N.W.
Washington, DC 20007

Business/Emergency
Numbers
202/625-3333
202/784-4660 (TTY)
FAX: 202/784-2530
Director/Medical Director:
Toby Litovitz, M.D.;
202/784-2088

WEST VIRGINIA

West Virginia Poison Center
3110 MacCorkle Avenue, S.E.
Charleston, WV 25304
Emergency Numbers
304/348-4211 (local)
800/642-3625 (intrastate)
FAX: 304/348-9560
Director: Gregory P. Wedin,
Pharm.D.; 304/347-1212
Medical Director: David E.
Seidler, M.D.; 304/347-1212

SECTION 5
Product Identification Section

This section is designed to help you identify products and their packaging.

Participating manufacturers have included selected products in full color. Where capsules and tablets are included they are shown in actual size. Packages generally are reduced in size.

For more information on products included, refer to the description in the PRODUCT INFORMATION SECTION or check directly with the manufacturer.

While every effort has been made to reproduce products faithfully, this section should be considered only as a quick-reference identification aid.

INDEX BY MANUFACTURER

ADRIA

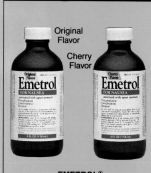

Original Flavor

Cherry Flavor

EMETROL®
(phosphorated carbohydrate solution)

Adria

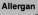

MODANE®
(phenolphthalein)

MODANE® PLUS
(phenolphthalein and docusate sodium)

ALLERGAN

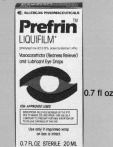

30 single-use containers
(0.01 fl oz each)

CELLUVISC™
Lubricant Ophthalmic
Solution

Allergan

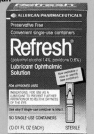

7 g   3.5 g

Also available:
0.7 g unit dose (24 pack)

LACRI-LUBE® S.O.P.®
Sterile Ophthalmic Ointment

Allergan

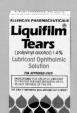

Liquifilm® Tears
(polyvinyl alcohol) 1.4%
Lubricant Ophthalmic Solution

1 fl oz

1 fl oz   sterile   30 mL

Also available: ½ fl oz

LIQUIFILM TEARS®
Lubricant Ophthalmic Solution

Allergan

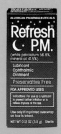

Prefrin™ LIQUIFILM®
(phenylephrine HCl 0.12%, polyvinyl alcohol 1.4%)
Vasoconstrictor (Redness Reliever)
and Lubricant Eye Drops

0.7 fl oz

0.7 FL OZ   STERILE   20 mL

PREFRIN™ LIQUIFILM®
Vasoconstrictor (Redness Reliever)
and Lubricant Eye Drops
(phenylephrine HCl 0.12%,
polyvinyl alcohol 1.4%)

Allergan

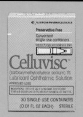

Refresh P.M.
(white petrolatum 56.8%, mineral oil 41.5%)
Lubricant Ophthalmic Ointment
Preservative Free

0.12 oz (3.5 g)

Preservative-free
Nighttime treatment for
dry eyes.

REFRESH® P.M.
Eye Lubricant

Allergan

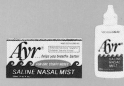

Refresh®
(polyvinyl alcohol 1.4%, povidone 0.6%)
Lubricant Ophthalmic Solution

50 single-use containers
(0.01 fl oz each)

Also available:
30 single-use containers

REFRESH®
Lubricant Ophthalmic Solution

Allergan

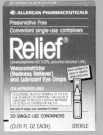

Relief®
(phenylephrine HCl 0.12%, polyvinyl alcohol 1.4%)
Vasoconstrictor
(Redness Reliever)
and Lubricant Eye Drops

30 single-use containers
(0.01 fl oz each)   STERILE

RELIEF®
Vasoconstrictor (Redness Reliever)
and Lubricant Eye Drops

Allergan

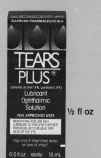

TEARS PLUS®
(polyvinyl alcohol 1.4%, povidone 0.6%)
Lubricant
Ophthalmic
Solution

½ fl oz

0.5 fl oz   sterile   15 mL

Also available: 1 fl oz

TEARS PLUS®
Lubricant Ophthalmic Solution

ASCHER

AYR® SALINE NASAL MIST

AYR® SALINE NASAL DROPS

B. F. Ascher & Co., Inc.

FOR GREATER PAIN RELIEF

Mobigesic®
Analgesic / Muscle Relaxant
Anti-inflammatory / Antipyretic

Available: 18's, 50's & 100's

MOBIGESIC®
ANALGESIC TABLETS

B. F. Ascher & Co., Inc.

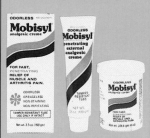

Mobisyl®
analgesic creme

ODORLESS Mobisyl
penetrating external analgesic creme

Mobisyl
analgesic creme

Net wt. 3.5 oz (100 g)

Also Available: 1.25 oz

MOBISYL®
ANALGESIC CREME

B. F. Ascher & Co., Inc.

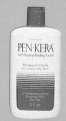

PEN·KERA®

Available in 8 oz bottle

PEN·KERA®

Therapeutic Creme
for Chronic Dry Skin

B. F. Ascher & Co., Inc.

CONSTIPATION?

UNILAX

Available in 15's
& 60's

CONSTIPATION?

UNILAX

UNILAX®
Softgel
Capsules

ASTRA

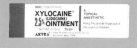

XYLOCAINE® 2.5% OINTMENT
A TOPICAL ANESTHETIC

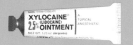

XYLOCAINE® 2.5% OINTMENT
A TOPICAL ANESTHETIC

Available in 35g Tube

XYLOCAINE® 2.5% OINTMENT
(lidocaine)

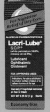

BAKER CUMMINS

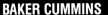

Baker Cummins Dermatologicals

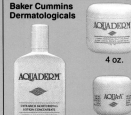

4 oz.

2 oz.
(contains the Vitamin A Derivative, Retinyl Palmitate)

7.5 fl. oz.

AQUADERM™ & AQUA-A®
Softens, Soothes & Protects Skin

Baker Cummins Dermatologicals

Controls dandruff & seborrheic dermatitis

X-SEB® SHAMPOO   **X-SEB® T SHAMPOO**

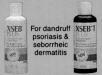

For dandruff psoriasis & seborrheic dermatitis

X-SEB® PLUS   **X-SEB® T PLUS**
CONDITIONING SHAMPOOS

Bausch & Lomb

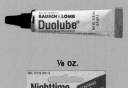

⅛ oz.

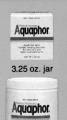

DUOLUBE®
Lubricant Eye Ointment
Nighttime Relief for Dry Eyes

Beiersdorf

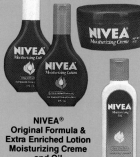

NIVEA®
Original Formula & Extra Enriched Lotion
Moisturizing Creme and Oil

For Very Dry Skin

Baker Cummins Dermatologicals

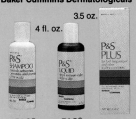

3.5 oz.

4 fl. oz.

P&S® Shampoo   **P&S® Liquid**   **P&S® Plus Tar Gel**

P&S Shampoo: controls seborrheic dermatitis & psoriasis of the scalp

P&S Liquid: helps remove scales of the scalp

P&S Plus Tar Gel: for psoriasis & other scaling conditions

BAUSCH & LOMB

0.5 fl. oz.

MOISTURE DROPS® ARTIFICIAL TEARS

Lubricant Eye Drops
Soothing Relief for Dry Eyes

BEIERSDORF

3.25 oz. jar

1.75 oz. tube

16 oz. jar

AQUAPHOR®
Healing Ointment
For dry skin, minor cuts and burns

BLISTEX, INC.

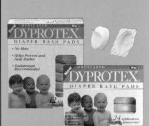

Available in boxes of 24 and 42 applications

DYPROTEX®
Diaper Rash Pads

Baker Cummins Pharmaceuticals

SNAPLETS-FR™
Pre-Measured Packs for Children's Fever & Pain Symptoms

SNAPLETS-MULTI™   **SNAPLETS-D™**

SNAPLETS-DM™   SNAPLETS-EX™

Pre-Measured Packs for Children's Cough & Cold Symptoms

Bausch & Lomb

0.5 fl. oz.

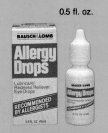

ALLERGY DROPS
Lubricant/Redness Reliever
Eye Drops

Bausch & Lomb

4 fl. oz.

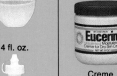

EYE WASH
Cleanses, Refreshes and Soothes
Irritated Eyes

Beiersdorf

BASIS
Normal to Dry Skin   Sensitive Skin

BASIS
Extra Dry Skin   Oily Skin

BASIS®
Facial Soap

Cleans and Softens the Skin

Beiersdorf

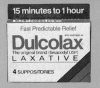

Creme

Cleansing Bar   Lotion

EUCERIN®
Unscented & Moisturizing
For Dry Skin Care

Boehringer Ingelheim

15 minutes to 1 hour

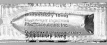

Dulcolax
The original brand (bisacodyl USP)
LAXATIVE
4 SUPPOSITORIES

Available in boxes of 4's, 8's, 16's and 50's

10 mg.
Dulcolax® Suppositories
(bisacodyl USP)

Boehringer Ingelheim

Overnight Relief

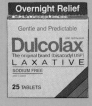

Gentle and Predictable

Dulcolax
The original brand (bisacodyl USP)
LAXATIVE
SODIUM FREE
25 TABLETS

Available in boxes of 10's, 25's, 50's and 100's

12  5 mg.

Dulcolax® Tablets
(bisacodyl USP)

BOIRON-BORNEMAN

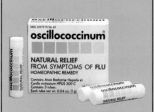

OSCILLOCOCCINUM®

Homeopathic remedy for relief of flu-like symptoms

Bristol-Myers Products

Bottles of 30, 60 and 100 coated tablets

EXTRA STRENGTH TRI-BUFFERED BUFFERIN® TABLET
(buffered aspirin)

Bristol-Myers Products

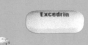
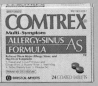

Available in blister packs of 24 and bottles of 50 tablets

COMTREX® A/S TABLETS MULTI-SYMPTOM ALLERGY-SINUS FORMULA
(acetaminophen, pseudoephedrine, chlorpheniramine)

Bristol-Myers Products

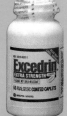

Bottles of 24, 50 & 80

EXCEDRIN® CAPLETS
Aspirin/Acetaminophen/Caffeine

Bristol-Myers Products

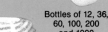

Bottles of 40 and 100 coated caplets

ARTHRITIS STRENGTH TRI-BUFFERED BUFFERIN® CAPLET
(buffered aspirin)

Bristol-Myers Products

Bottles of 6 & 10 oz.

COMTREX® LIQUID

Bristol-Myers Products

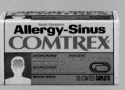

Available in blister packs of 24 and bottles of 36 caplets

COMTREX® A/S CAPLETS MULTI-SYMPTOM ALLERGY-SINUS FORMULA
(acetaminophen, pseudoephedrine, chlorpheniramine)

Bristol-Myers Products

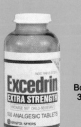

Bottles of 12, 30, 60, 100, 165, 225 & 375

EXCEDRIN® TABLETS
Aspirin/Acetaminophen/Caffeine

Bristol-Myers Products

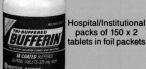

Bottles of 12, 36, 60, 100, 200 and 1000

Hospital/Institutional packs of 150 x 2 tablets in foil packets

TRI-BUFFERED BUFFERIN® TABLET
(buffered aspirin)

Bristol-Myers Products

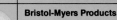

Blister packs of 24, bottles of 50

COMTREX® TABLETS

Bristol-Myers Products

Bottles of 24

ASPIRIN FREE CONGESPIRIN®
(acetaminophen 81 mg., phenylephrine 1.25 mg.)

Bristol-Myers Products

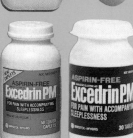

Bottles of 10, 30, 50 & 80

EXCEDRIN P.M.®

Bristol-Myers Products

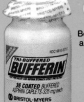

Bottles of 36, 60 and 100 coated caplets

TRI-BUFFERED BUFFERIN® CAPLET
(buffered aspirin)

Bristol-Myers Products

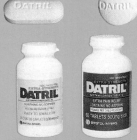

Carded 16 and bottles of 36

COMTREX® CAPLETS

Bristol-Myers Products

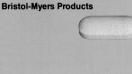
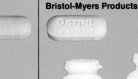

Bottles of 24 & 36 caplets   Bottles of 30, 60 & 100 tablets

EXTRA STRENGTH DATRIL® CAPLETS AND TABLETS
(acetaminophen)

Bristol-Myers Products

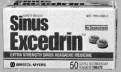
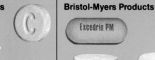

Available in blister packs of 24 and bottles of 50 tablets

SINUS EXCEDRIN® TABLETS
(acetaminophen, pseudoephedrine)

Bristol-Myers Products

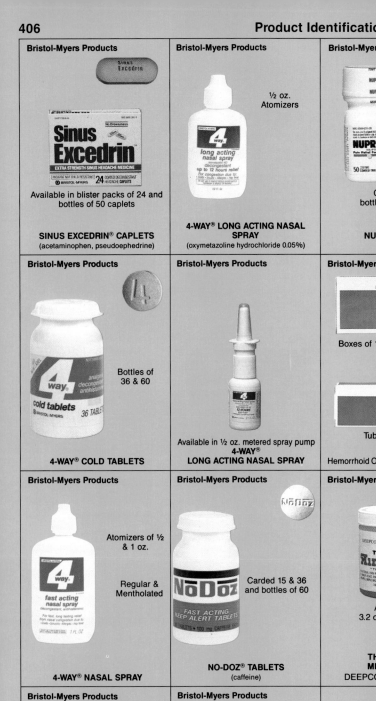

Available in blister packs of 24 and
bottles of 50 caplets

SINUS EXCEDRIN® CAPLETS
(acetaminophen, pseudoephedrine)

Bristol-Myers Products

½ oz.
Atomizers

**4-WAY® LONG ACTING NASAL
SPRAY**
(oxymetazoline hydrochloride 0.05%)

Bristol-Myers Products

200 mg.

Carded 8 and
bottles of 24, 50, 100
and 150

NUPRIN® TABLET
(ibuprofen)

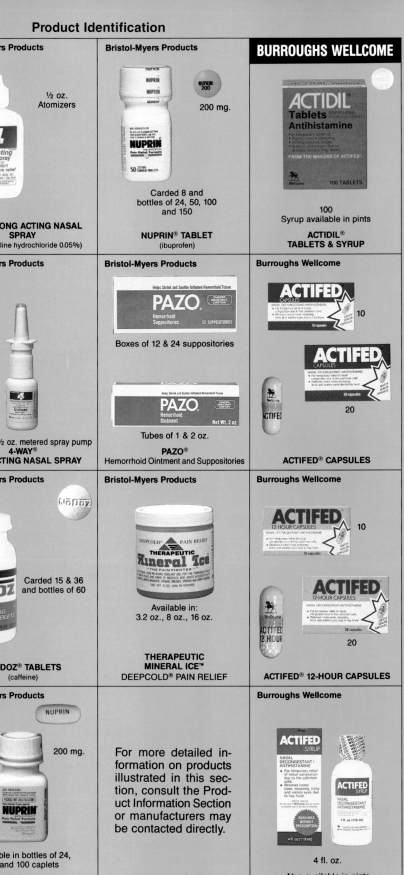

BURROUGHS WELLCOME

100
Syrup available in pints

**ACTIDIL®
TABLETS & SYRUP**

Bristol-Myers Products

Bottles of
36 & 60

4-WAY® COLD TABLETS

Bristol-Myers Products

Available in ½ oz. metered spray pump
**4-WAY®
LONG ACTING NASAL SPRAY**

Bristol-Myers Products

Boxes of 12 & 24 suppositories

Tubes of 1 & 2 oz.
PAZO®
Hemorrhoid Ointment and Suppositories

Burroughs Wellcome

10

20

ACTIFED® CAPSULES

Bristol-Myers Products

Atomizers of ½
& 1 oz.

Regular &
Mentholated

4-WAY® NASAL SPRAY

Bristol-Myers Products

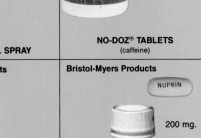

Carded 15 & 36
and bottles of 60

NO-DOZ® TABLETS
(caffeine)

Bristol-Myers Products

Available in:
3.2 oz., 8 oz., 16 oz.

**THERAPEUTIC
MINERAL ICE™**
DEEPCOLD® PAIN RELIEF

Burroughs Wellcome

10

20

ACTIFED® 12-HOUR CAPSULES

Bristol-Myers Products

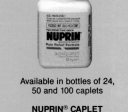

Available in ½ oz. metered spray pump
**4-WAY®
FAST ACTING NASAL SPRAY**

Bristol-Myers Products

200 mg.

Available in bottles of 24,
50 and 100 caplets

NUPRIN® CAPLET
(ibuprofen)

For more detailed in-
formation on products
illustrated in this sec-
tion, consult the Prod-
uct Information Section
or manufacturers may
be contacted directly.

Burroughs Wellcome

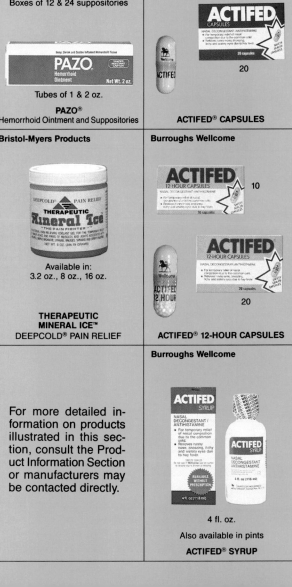

4 fl. oz.

Also available in pints

ACTIFED® SYRUP

Burroughs Wellcome

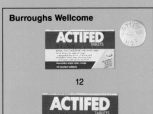

12

24

Also available in 48s and in bottles of 100

**ACTIFED®
TABLETS**

Burroughs Wellcome

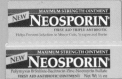

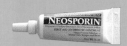

250

Also available in 50s and 100s

EMPIRIN® ASPIRIN TABLETS

Burroughs Wellcome

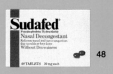

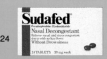

Available in ½ oz. tubes

**MAXIMUM STRENGTH
NEOSPORIN® FIRST AID
ANTIBIOTIC OINTMENT**

Burroughs Wellcome

100

48

24

SUDAFED® 30 mg TABLETS

Burroughs Wellcome

20

20

Also available in 40s

**ACTIFED® PLUS
CAPLETS & TABLETS**

Burroughs Wellcome

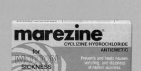

12

Also available in 100s

MAREZINE® TABLETS

Burroughs Wellcome

Powder, 0.35 oz. (10g)

Spray, 3 oz. (85g)

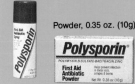

Ointment ½ oz.
1 oz.

**POLYSPORIN®
FIRST AID ANTIBIOTIC
SPRAY, POWDER & OINTMENT**

Burroughs Wellcome

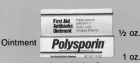

100

**SUDAFED®
60 mg TABLETS**

Burroughs Wellcome

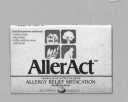

24

**ALLERACT™
TABLETS**

Burroughs Wellcome

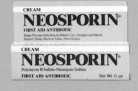

Available in ½ oz. tubes

**NEOSPORIN®
FIRST AID
ANTIBIOTIC CREAM**

Burroughs Wellcome

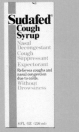

8 fl. oz.   4 fl. oz.

SUDAFED® COUGH SYRUP

Burroughs Wellcome

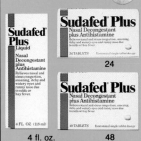

24

4 fl. oz.   48

**SUDAFED® PLUS
LIQUID & TABLETS**

Burroughs Wellcome

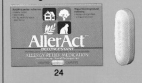

24

24

Also available in 48s

**ALLERACT™
DECONGESTANT CAPLETS & TABLETS**

Burroughs Wellcome

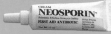

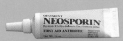

Available in ½ and 1 oz. tubes

**NEOSPORIN®
FIRST AID
ANTIBIOTIC OINTMENT**

Burroughs Wellcome

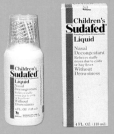

4 fl. oz.

CHILDREN'S SUDAFED® LIQUID

Burroughs Wellcome

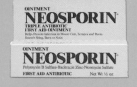

24

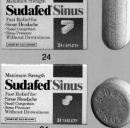

24

Also available in 48s

**SUDAFED® SINUS
CAPLETS & TABLETS**

Burroughs Wellcome

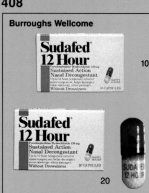

10

20

Also available in 40s

SUDAFED® 12 HOUR CAPSULES

CARNATION

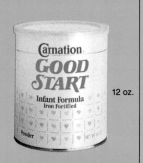

12 oz.

GOOD START™
Infant Formula Iron Fortified

CHURCH & DWIGHT

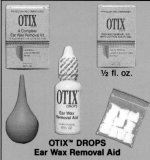

½ fl. oz.

OTIX™ DROPS
Ear Wax Removal Aid

Available: OTIX™ Drops with Cotton
Ear Plugs & Complete Wax Removal
Kit Including Bulb Irrigator

COLUMBIA

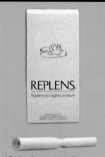

12 single-use applicators

REPLENS™
Replenishes vaginal moisture

CIBA CONSUMER

ACUTRIM®
Appetite Suppressants
Caffeine Free/Precision Release™

CIBA Consumer

REGULAR STRENGTH DOAN'S®

EXTRA STRENGTH DOAN'S®

DOAN'S®
Backache Analgesic
Relieves back pain
Available in packages of 24 & 48

CIBA Consumer

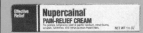

FIBERALL
Natural Fiber Therapy
for Regularity

Available in:
Powders: 10 and 15 oz. Natural, Orange
Wafers: 14 Fruit & Nut, Oatmeal Raisin
Tablets: 18

CIBA Consumer

Available in 2 oz and 1 oz tubes

Prompt, temporary relief of pain,
itching, and burning
due to painful hemorrhoids.

NUPERCAINAL®
Hemorrhoidal & Anesthetic
Ointment

CIBA Consumer

Available in boxes of
12 and 24 suppositories

Temporary relief of itching, burning,
and discomfort of hemorrhoids.

NUPERCAINAL®
Hemorrhoidal Suppositories

CIBA Consumer

1½ oz

Prompt, temporary relief of painful
sunburn, minor burns, scrapes,
scratches, and nonpoisonous
insect bites.

NUPERCAINAL®
Pain-Relief Cream

CIBA Consumer

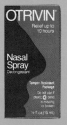

½ fl oz

OTRIVIN®
Nasal Decongestant Spray

CIBA Consumer

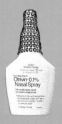

.66 fl oz

OTRIVIN®
Nasal Decongestant Drops

CIBA Consumer

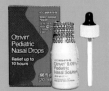

.66 fl oz

OTRIVIN®
Pediatric
Nasal Decongestant Drops

CIBA Consumer

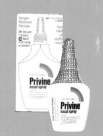

½ fl oz

PRIVINE®
Nasal Decongestant Spray

CIBA Consumer

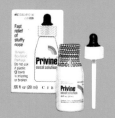

.66 fl oz

PRIVINE®
Nasal Decongestant Solution

CIBA Consumer

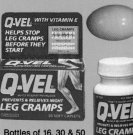 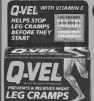

Bottles of 16, 30 & 50
Soft Gels
Q-vel®
Muscle Relaxant
Pain Reliever

CIBA Consumer

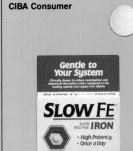

Available in packages of
30, 60 & 100 tablets
SLOW FE®
Slow Release Iron

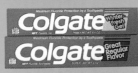

Available in
flip-top
tubes or in
pump dispensers

COLGATE® MFP®
FLUORIDE
TOOTHPASTE & GEL

Colgate-Palmolive

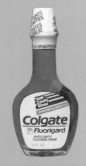

FLUORIGARD™
Anti-Cavity Fluoride Rinse

Fisons

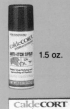

1.5 oz.

½ oz.

½ oz.

CaldeCORT Light™
CaldeCORT® CREAM and SPRAY
(hydrocortisone acetate, 5%)

CIBA Consumer

SUNKIST®
Vitamin C Citrus Complex
250 & 500 mg chewable tablets;
500 mg easy to swallow caplets;
60 mg chewable tablets
(11-tablet roll)

Colgate-Palmolive

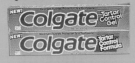

Available in
flip-top
tubes or in
pump dispensers

COLGATE®
TARTAR CONTROL
FORMULA & GEL

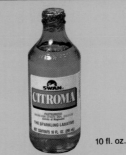

10 fl. oz.

CITROMA®
(citrate of magnesia)
The Sparkling Laxative

Fisons

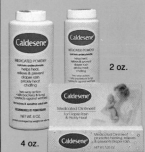

2 oz.

4 oz.

1.25 oz.

CALDESENE®
MEDICATED POWDER and OINTMENT

CIBA Consumer

Regular

+Extra C

+Iron

Complete

SUNKIST®
Children's Multivitamins

Colgate-Palmolive

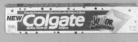 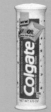

Available in
flip-top tubes
or in pump
dispensers

Flip-top tube
available in 2.7,
4.5, 6.4 and 8.2 oz.
Pump available
in 4.5 oz.

COLGATE® JUNIOR
Fluoride Gel Toothpaste

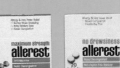

24 tablets

20 tablets

MAXIMUM
STRENGTH
ALLEREST®
TABLETS

NO
DROWSINESS
ALLEREST®
TABLETS

Allergy & Hay Fever Relief

Fisons

Spray Powder

Cream

CRUEX®
Antifungal Spray Powder & Cream
Relieves Itching, Chafing, Rash

Colgate-Palmolive

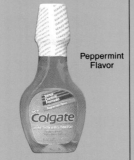

Peppermint
Flavor

COLGATE® MOUTHWASH
Tartar Control Formula

Fisons

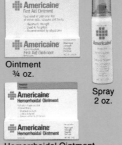

Ointment
¾ oz.

Spray
2 oz.

Hemorrhoidal Ointment
1 oz.

AMERICAINE®
(benzocaine)

Fisons

½ oz.

2.7 oz.

DESENEX®
Spray Powder, Powder, Cream &
Ointment
Relieves Symptoms of Athlete's Foot

Fisons

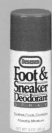

3 oz.

**DESENEX®
FOOT & SNEAKER
DEODORANT**

Soothes, Cools, Comforts
& Absorbs Moisture

Glenbrook

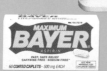
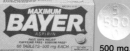

Available in bottles of 30 and 60

500 mg.

Available in boxes of
30, 60 and 100 tablets
MAXIMUM BAYER® ASPIRIN
Toleraid® Micro-Thin Coating
Sodium Free • Caffeine Free

Glenbrook

Available in bottle
of 30 tablets

**BAYER® CHILDREN'S
COLD TABLETS**

Glenbrook

Available in packages of 16 and 32
coated tablets

MIDOL® 200

Fisons

Cream

0.5 oz.

3 oz.

Powder

Spray
Liquid

Spray
Powder

TING®
For Athlete's Foot &
Jock Itch

Glenbrook

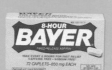

Available in bottles of
30, 72, and 125 caplets

**8-HOUR BAYER®
TIMED-RELEASE ASPIRIN**
Sodium Free • Caffeine Free

Glenbrook

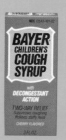

Available in 3 oz. cherry flavor

**BAYER® CHILDREN'S
COUGH SYRUP**

Glenbrook

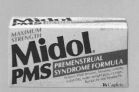

Available in bottles of
16 and 32 caplets

**MIDOL® PMS
MAXIMUM STRENGTH**

GLENBROOK

Division of Sterling Drug Inc.

Caplets available in bottles of
50, 100 and 200

Glenbrook

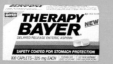

Available in bottles of
50 and 100 caplets

THERAPY BAYER®
Delayed Release Enteric Aspirin
Sodium Free • Caffeine Free

Glenbrook

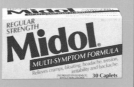

Available in packages of 12, 30
and 60 caplets®

MIDOL®

Glenbrook

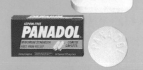
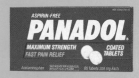

MAXIMUM STRENGTH PANADOL®
Coated Caplets and Tablets
Acetaminophen

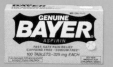

Available in packs of 12 tablets
and bottles of 24, 50,
100, 200, 300 and 365

GENUINE BAYER® ASPIRIN
Toleraid® Micro-Thin Coating
Sodium Free • Caffeine Free

Glenbrook

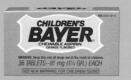

Available in bottle
of 36 tablets

**BAYER® CHILDREN'S
CHEWABLE ASPIRIN**

Glenbrook

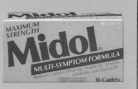

Available in packages of
8, 16 and 32 caplets®

**MIDOL®
MAXIMUM STRENGTH**

Glenbrook

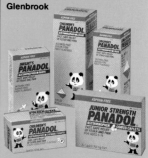

CHILDREN'S PANADOL®
Chewable Tablets, Caplets, Liquid
and Drops
Acetaminophen

Glenbrook

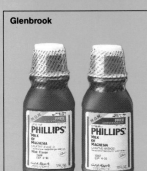

Available in regular and mint flavor
4 oz., 12 oz., 26 oz. plastic bottles

PHILLIPS'® MILK OF MAGNESIA

Glenbrook

Maximum
Strength
Pads

In containers of
12, 42 and 75 pads

Regular
Strength
Pads

In containers
of 42 pads

Maximum & Regular Strength BIG PADS
Available in containers of 42 pads

STRIDEX®

Hoechst-Roussel

50 mg
Packages of
30 and 100

240 mg
Packages of
7 and 30,
Bottles of 100

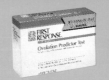
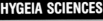

Stool Softener

SURFAK®
(docusate calcium USP)

Consumer Products Inc.

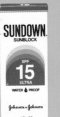

Also available
SPF 8, 20,
25 & 30+

Also available
SPF 24

**SUNDOWN® SUNBLOCK
Lotions and Creams**

Glenbrook

**PHILLIPS'® MILK OF MAGNESIA
TABLETS**
Available in mint flavored
chewable tablets in blister
packed 24 and bottles of
100 and 200

Glenbrook

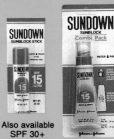

Available in packages
of 30, 60 and 100 caplets

**VANQUISH®
Extra-Strength Pain Formula
with Two Buffers**

Ovulation Predictor Test

Pregnancy
Test

FIRST RESPONSE®

Consumer Products Inc.

Also available
SPF 30+

**SUNDOWN® SUNBLOCK
Sticks and Combi™ Pack**

Glenbrook

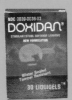

Available in regular and flavored
4 oz., 12 oz. and 26 oz. plastic bottles

HALEY'S M-O®

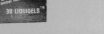

Packages
of 10 and 30,
Bottles of 100

Stimulant/Stool Softener Laxative

DOXIDAN®
(docusate calcium USP,
phenolphthalein USP)

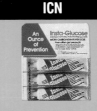

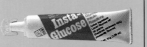

INSTA-GLUCOSE
For treatment of insulin
reaction/hypoglycemia

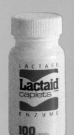

(Both sides of
caplet shown)

LACTAID® CAPLETS
(lactase enzyme tablets)

Glenbrook

24 capsules

**LAXCAPS®
Laxative Plus Softener
Combined Action Formula**

Hoechst-Roussel

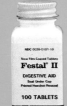

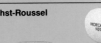

Bottles
of 100
Tablets

Digestive Aid

FESTAL® II
(digestive enzymes)

Consumer Products Inc.

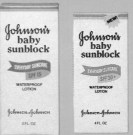

Waterproof Lotion
Also available in SPF 15 Cream
**JOHNSON'S BABY SUNBLOCK
Everyday Suncare**

Lactaid Inc.

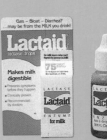

LACTAID®
(lactase enzyme)

Lakeside Pharmaceuticals

Cēpacol Gold

Available in 4, 12, 18, 24 and 32 fl. oz. bottles

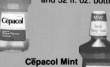

Cēpacol Mint

CĒPACOL®
Mouthwash/Gargle

Lakeside Pharmaceuticals

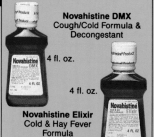

Novahistine DMX
Cough/Cold Formula & Decongestant

4 fl. oz.

4 fl. oz.

Novahistine Elixir
Cold & Hay Fever Formula

NOVAHISTINE® DMX & ELIXIR
Cough/Cold Products

Lederle

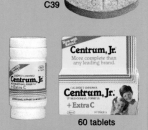

C45

For Calcium-Rich Bone and Iron-Rich Blood.

Bottles of 60

CALTRATE® 600+IRON+VITAMIN D
High Potency Calcium Supplement

Lederle

C39

Centrum, Jr.
More complete than any leading brand.

Centrum, Jr.
+Extra C

60 tablets

CENTRUM, JR.®
Children's Chewable Vitamin/Mineral Formula + Extra C

Lakeside Pharmaceuticals

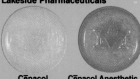

Cēpacol Throat Lozenges   **Cēpacol Anesthetic Lozenges (Troches)**

18 lozenges per package

CĒPACOL®
Throat Lozenges

LEDERLE

LEDERMARK®
Product Identification Code

Many Lederle tablets and capsules bear an identification code, and these codes are listed with each product pictured. A current listing appears in the Product Information Section of the 1990 Physicians' Desk Reference.

Lederle

C360

Helps Build Strong Bones and Teeth

NEW CHEWABLE

CALTRATE® JR.
Chewable Calcium Supplement For Children

Lederle

C60

Centrum, Jr.
More calcium than any leading brand.

Centrum, Jr.
+EXTRA CALCIUM

60 tablets

CENTRUM, JR® +Extra Calcium
Children's Chewable Vitamin/Mineral Formula

Lakeside Pharmaceuticals

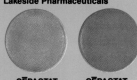

CĒPASTAT Regular   **CĒPASTAT Cherry**

18 lozenges per package

CĒPASTAT®
Sore Throat Lozenges

Lederle
Now available in smaller size tablet

C600

More calcium per tablet than a half-quart of milk.

Bottles of 60

Caltrate 600

Caltrate 600

CALTRATE® 600
High Potency Calcium Supplement

Lederle

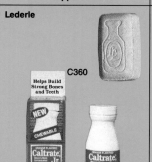

Centrum
From A to Zinc

Centrum
From A to Zinc

Bottles of 100 + 30
Bottles of 60

ADVANCED FORMULA
Centrum
From A to Zinc

30 TABLETS WITH 100

C1

Advanced Formula CENTRUM®
High Potency Multivitamin/Multimineral Formula

Lederle

F66

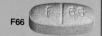

Helps Maintain Regularity for Good Digestive Health

FiberCon
Bulk-Forming Fiber Laxative

Natural Action of Fiber Easy-to-Swallow Tablets

Box of 36

Lakeside Pharmaceuticals

CITRUCEL

CITRUCEL Orange
Available in 16 oz. and 30 oz. containers

CITRUCEL Regular
Available in 7 oz. and 10 oz. containers

CITRUCEL

CITRUCEL®
Therapeutic Fiber for Regularity

Lederle
Now available in smaller size tablet

C40

More calcium per tablet than a half-quart of milk.

Bottles of 60

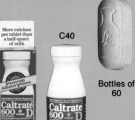
Caltrate 600 ± D   Caltrate 600 ± D

CALTRATE® 600+D
High Potency Calcium Supplement

Lederle

C2

60 tablets

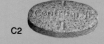

Centrum, Jr.
More complete than any leading brand.

Centrum, Jr.
+IRON

Centrum, Jr.

CENTRUM, JR.®
Children's Chewable Vitamin/Mineral Formula + Iron
More Essential Nutrients

Helps Maintain Regularity for Good Digestive Health

FiberCon
Bulk-Forming Fiber Laxative

Natural Action of Fiber Easy-to-Swallow Tablets

Box of 60

Helps Maintain Regularity for Good Digestive Health

FiberCon
Bulk-Forming Fiber Laxative

Natural Action of Fiber Easy-to-Swallow Tablets

NEW LARGER SIZE

Box of 90

Also available in bottles of 500 and unit dose
FIBERCON®
Calcium Polycarbophil
Bulk-Forming Fiber Laxative

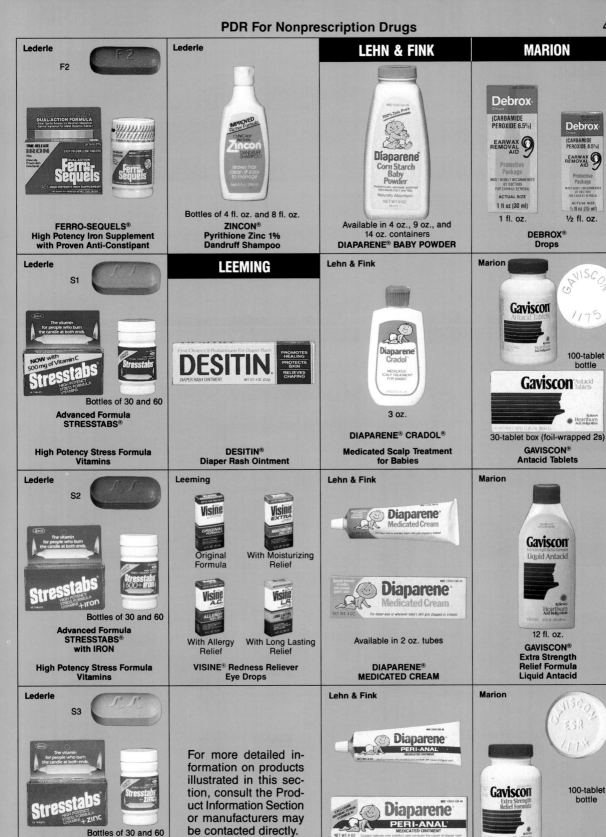

Lederle

F2

FERRO-SEQUELS®
High Potency Iron Supplement
with Proven Anti-Constipant

Lederle

Bottles of 4 fl. oz. and 8 fl. oz.
ZINCON®
Pyrithione Zinc 1%
Dandruff Shampoo

LEHN & FINK

Available in 4 oz., 9 oz., and
14 oz. containers
DIAPARENE® BABY POWDER

MARION

1 fl. oz.   ½ fl. oz.

DEBROX®
Drops

Lederle

S1

Advanced Formula
STRESSTABS®

High Potency Stress Formula
Vitamins

Bottles of 30 and 60

LEEMING

DESITIN®
Diaper Rash Ointment

Lehn & Fink

3 oz.

DIAPARENE® CRADOL®

Medicated Scalp Treatment
for Babies

Marion

100-tablet
bottle

30-tablet box (foil-wrapped 2s)

GAVISCON®
Antacid Tablets

Lederle

S2

Advanced Formula
STRESSTABS®
with IRON

High Potency Stress Formula
Vitamins

Bottles of 30 and 60

Leeming

Original   With Moisturizing
Formula   Relief

With Allergy   With Long Lasting
Relief   Relief

VISINE® Redness Reliever
Eye Drops

Lehn & Fink

Available in 2 oz. tubes

DIAPARENE®
MEDICATED CREAM

Marion

12 fl. oz.

GAVISCON®
Extra Strength
Relief Formula
Liquid Antacid

Lederle

S3

Advanced Formula
STRESSTABS®
with ZINC

High Potency Stress Formula
Vitamins

Bottles of 30 and 60

For more detailed in-
formation on products
illustrated in this sec-
tion, consult the Prod-
uct Information Section
or manufacturers may
be contacted directly.

Lehn & Fink

Available in 2 oz. tubes

DIAPARENE®
PERI-ANAL OINTMENT

Marion

100-tablet
bottle

GAVISCON®
Extra Strength
Relief Formula Antacid Tablets

Marion

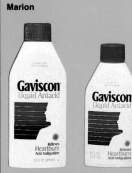

12 fl. oz.   6 fl. oz.

**GAVISCON®
Liquid Antacid**

Marion

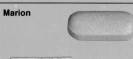
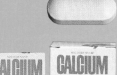

Bottle of
60 tablets

**OS-CAL® 500+D
Tablets**
(calcium with vitamin D)

Marion

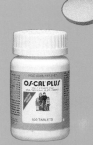

Bottle of 100 tablets

**OS-CAL® PLUS
Multivitamin and Multimineral
Supplement**

McNeil Consumer

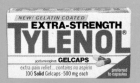

500 mg.

NEW! GELATIN COATED
**EXTRA-STRENGTH
TYLENOL®
GELCAPS**
extra pain relief...contains no aspirin
100 Solid Gelcaps - 500 mg each

Gelcaps available in
tamper-resistant bottles
of 24, 50, 100 and 150.

EXTRA-STRENGTH TYLENOL®
acetaminophen
GELCAPS®

Marion

GAVISCON 2 1172

Box of 48
foil-wrapped
tablets

Double Strength
Gaviscon-2
Antacid Tablets

**GAVISCON®-2
Antacid Tablets**

Marion

Bottles of 60 and 120 tablets

**OS-CAL® 500
Tablets**

Marion

MARION
**THROAT
DISCS**
THROAT LOZENGES

Box of 60 lozenges

**THROAT DISCS®
Throat Lozenges**

McNeil Consumer

500 mg.

THE PAIN RELIEVER HOSPITALS USE MOST
**EXTRA-STRENGTH
TYLENOL®
TABLETS**
acetaminophen
extra pain relief...contains no aspirin
100 tablets - 500 mg each

Tablets available in tamper-resistant
vials of 10 and bottles of 30, 60, 100
and 200. Liquid: 8 fl. oz.

EXTRA-STRENGTH TYLENOL®
acetaminophen
Tablets & Liquid

Marion

Gly-Oxide
(CARBAMIDE
PEROXIDE 10%)

CLEANSING ANTISEPTIC
for the MOUTH

Gly-Oxide
(CARBAMIDE
PEROXIDE 10%)

CLEANSING ANTISEPTIC
for the MOUTH

2 fl. oz.   ½ fl. oz.

GLY-OXIDE® Liquid

Marion

MARION
OS-CAL
1650

CALCIUM
WITH VITAMIN D ADDED

Bottles of 100 and 240 tablets

**OS-CAL® 250+D
Tablets**
(calcium with vitamin D)

McNEIL CONSUMER

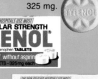

325 mg.

THE PAIN RELIEVER HOSPITALS USE MOST
**REGULAR STRENGTH
TYLENOL®
TABLETS**
acetaminophen
safe, fast pain relief...without aspirin
24 TABLETS - 325 mg each

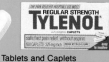

THE PAIN RELIEVER HOSPITALS USE MOST
**REGULAR STRENGTH
TYLENOL®**
acetaminophen
safe, fast pain relief...without aspirin
100 CAPLETS - 325 mg each

Tablets and Caplets
Available in 24's, 50's and 100's.

REGULAR STRENGTH TYLENOL®
acetaminophen   Tablets and Caplets

McNeil Consumer

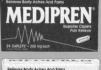

Relieves Body Aches And Pains
MEDIPREN®
Ibuprofen Caplets
Pain Reliever
24 CAPLETS - 200 mg each

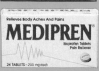

Relieves Body Aches And Pains
MEDIPREN®
Ibuprofen Tablets
Pain Reliever
24 TABLETS - 200 mg each

Caplets and Tablets available in
bottles of 24, 50 and 100.

MEDIPREN®
ibuprofen

Marion

OS-CAL

CALCIUM
HIGH POTENCY
500 MG SUPPLEMENT
CHEWABLE TABLETS

Bottle of
60 tablets

**OS-CAL® 500
Chewable Tablets**

Marion

MULTIVITAMIN
& MINERALS
WITH ADDED CALCIUM
OS-CAL
FORTIFIED

Bottle of 100 tablets

**OS-CAL® Fortified
Multivitamin and Minerals
With Added Calcium**

McNeil Consumer

500 mg.

THE PAIN RELIEVER HOSPITALS USE MOST
**EXTRA-STRENGTH
TYLENOL®
CAPLETS**
acetaminophen
extra pain relief...contains no aspirin
100 Caplets - 500 mg each

Caplets available in tamper-
resistant vials of 10 and
bottles of 24, 50, 100 and 175.

EXTRA-STRENGTH TYLENOL®
acetaminophen
Caplets

McNeil Consumer

SAFETY SEALED
INFANTS'
**TYLENOL®
DROPS**
Relieves infants'
fever and pain without
aspirin complications

Available in ½ fl. oz. bottle with
child-resistant safety cap and
calibrated dropper.

INFANTS' TYLENOL®
acetaminophen
Alcohol Free Drops

McNeil Consumer

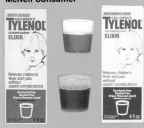

Available in cherry and grape flavors in 2 and 4 fl. oz. bottles with child-resistant safety cap and convenient dosage cup.
CHILDREN'S TYLENOL®
acetaminophen
Alcohol Free Elixir

McNeil Consumer

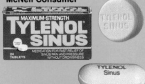
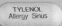

MAXIMUM-STRENGTH TYLENOL® SINUS MEDICATION
Caplets: Bottles of 24's and 50's.
Tablets: Bottles of 24's and 50's

McNeil Consumer

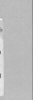

Available in blister-packs of 24 and bottles of 50.
TYLENOL® COLD
Medication
No Drowsiness
Formula Caplets

McNeil Consumer

Available in 4 fl. oz. bottle with child-resistant safety cap and convenient dosage cup.
PEDIACARE®
Cold Formula

McNeil Consumer

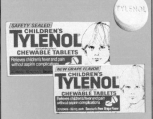

Fruit flavor: available in bottles of 30 with child-resistant safety cap and blister-packs of 48.

Grape flavor: available in bottles of 30 with child-resistant safety cap.

CHILDREN'S TYLENOL®
acetaminophen
Chewable Tablets

McNeil Consumer

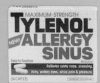

MAXIMUM-STRENGTH TYLENOL® ALLERGY SINUS MEDICATION

Caplets: Blister pack of 24's and bottles of 50's.

McNeil Consumer

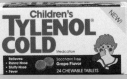

Available in bottles of 24 chewable tablets with child-resistant safety cap.
CHILDREN'S TYLENOL® COLD
Chewable Cold Tablets

McNeil Consumer

Bottles of 24 chewable tablets.

McNeil Consumer

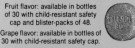

Available in child-resistant blister-pack of 30.
JUNIOR STRENGTH TYLENOL®
acetaminophen
Swallowable Tablets

McNeil Consumer

Available in blister-packs of 24 and bottles of 50.
TYLENOL® COLD
Medication
Tablets and Caplets

McNeil Consumer

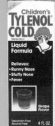

Available in 4 fl. oz. bottle with child-resistant safety cap and convenient dosage cup.
CHILDREN'S TYLENOL® COLD
Liquid Cold Formula

McNeil Consumer

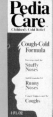

4 fl. oz. bottle with convenient dosage cup.

Both with child-resistant safety cap.

PEDIACARE®
Cough-Cold Formula

McNeil Consumer

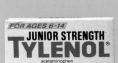

Available in blister packs of 24 and bottles of 50 and 100 tablets.

No Drowsiness Formula

McNeil Consumer

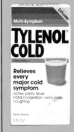

Available in 5 fl. oz. bottle with child-resistant safety cap and convenient dosage cup enclosed.

TYLENOL® COLD
Medication Liquid

McNeil Consumer

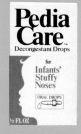

Available in ½ fl. oz. bottle with child-resistant safety cap and calibrated dropper.
PEDIACARE®
Oral Decongestant Drops

McNeil Consumer

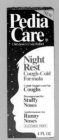

Available in 4 fl. oz. bottle with child-resistant safety cap and convenient dosage cup.
PEDIACARE® NIGHTREST
Cough-Cold Formula

MAXIMUM STRENGTH SINE-AID®
Relieves sinus headache and pressure

McNeil Consumer

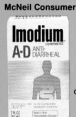

Available in 2, 3 and 4 fl. oz. bottles with a convenient dosage cup, and caplets in 6's and 12's.

IMODIUM® A-D
loperamide HCl
ANTI-DIARRHEAL

MEDICONE

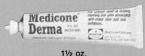

1½ oz.

MEDICONE® DERMA
Anesthetic/Astringent Ointment

MILES INC.

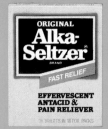

**ALKA-SELTZER® BRAND
EFFERVESCENT
ANTACID & PAIN RELIEVER**

**Miles Inc.
Consumer Healthcare Division**

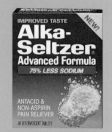

**ALKA-SELTZER®
ADVANCED FORMULA**

MEAD JOHNSON PHARM.

50 mg

100 mg

Bottles of 30, 60, 250 and 1000
Stool Softener

†COLACE®
(docusate sodium)

Medicone

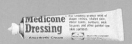

1½ oz.

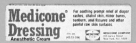

**MEDICONE® DRESSING
Anesthetic Cream**

**Miles Inc.
Consumer Healthcare Division**

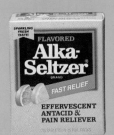

**ALKA-SELTZER® BRAND
FLAVORED EFFERVESCENT
ANTACID & PAIN RELIEVER**

**Miles Inc.
Consumer Healthcare Division**

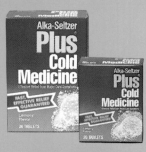

**ALKA-SELTZER PLUS®
COLD MEDICINE**

Mead Johnson Pharmaceuticals

Bottles of 30, 60, 250 and 1000
Laxative and Stool Softener

†PERI-COLACE®
(casanthranol and docusate sodium)

Medicone

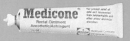

1½ oz.

MEDICONE® RECTAL OINTMENT

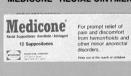

**MEDICONE®
RECTAL SUPPOSITORIES**

**Miles Inc.
Consumer Healthcare Division**

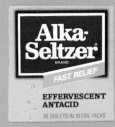

**ALKA-SELTZER® BRAND
EFFERVESCENT ANTACID**

**Miles Inc.
Consumer Healthcare Division**

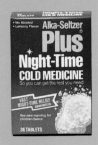

**ALKA-SELTZER PLUS®
NIGHT-TIME
COLD MEDICINE**

While every effort has been made to reproduce products faithfully, this section is to be considered a Quick-Reference identification aid.

Medicone

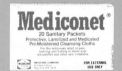

20 Packets

Moist Cleansing Cloths

**MEDICONET®
CLEANSING CLOTHS**

**Miles Inc.
Consumer Healthcare Division**

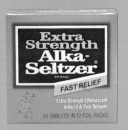

**ALKA-SELTZER® BRAND
EXTRA STRENGTH
EFFERVESCENT ANTACID &
PAIN RELIEVER**

**Miles Inc.
Consumer Healthcare Division**

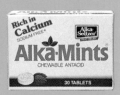

**ALKA-MINTS® CHEWABLE
ANTACID**
(Calcium Carbonate 850 mg)

Miles Inc.
Consumer Healthcare Division

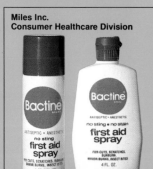

**BACTINE® BRAND
ANTISEPTIC • ANESTHETIC
FIRST AID SPRAY**
Aerosol and Liquid

Miles Inc.
Consumer Healthcare Division

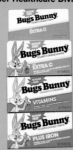

**BUGS BUNNY® BRAND SUGAR FREE
CHILDREN'S CHEWABLE VITAMINS
WITH EXTRA C, REGULAR,
AND PLUS IRON**

Miles Inc.
Consumer Healthcare Division

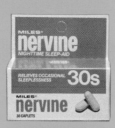

**MILES® NERVINE
NIGHTTIME SLEEP-AID**
(Diphenhydramine HCl 25 mg)

Miles Inc.
Consumer Healthcare Division

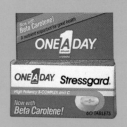

**STRESSGARD®
STRESS FORMULA VITAMINS**

Miles Inc.
Consumer Healthcare Division

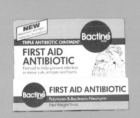

**BACTINE®
FIRST AID
ANTIBIOTIC OINTMENT**

Miles Inc.
Consumer Healthcare Division

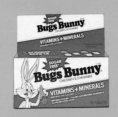

**BUGS BUNNY® BRAND SUGAR FREE
CHILDREN'S CHEWABLE
VITAMINS + MINERALS**

Miles Inc.
Consumer Healthcare Division

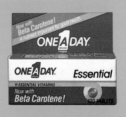

**ONE A DAY® BRAND
ESSENTIAL VITAMINS**

Miles Inc.
Consumer Healthcare Division

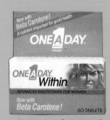

**ONE-A-DAY® WITHIN®
Advanced Multivitamin
For Women With Calcium &
Extra Iron**

Miles Inc.
Consumer Healthcare Division

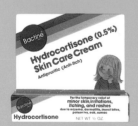

**BACTINE® BRAND
HYDROCORTISONE (0.5%)
SKIN CARE CREAM**

Miles Inc.
Consumer Healthcare Division

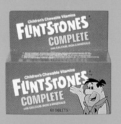

**FLINTSTONES® BRAND COMPLETE
CHILDREN'S CHEWABLE VITAMINS
WITH IRON, CALCIUM & MINERALS**

Miles Inc.
Consumer Healthcare Division

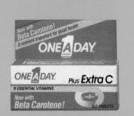

**ONE A DAY® BRAND PLUS EXTRA C
VITAMINS**
11 essential vitamins
with high potency
300 mg Vitamin C

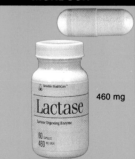

460 mg

LACTASE ENZYME
(3450 FCC units per capsule)
60 count bottle

Miles Inc.
Consumer Healthcare Division

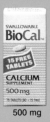

500 mg

**BIOCAL™
CALCIUM SUPPLEMENT**
(Calcium Carbonate)

Miles Inc.
Consumer Healthcare Division

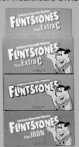

**FLINTSTONES® BRAND
CHILDREN'S CHEWABLE VITAMINS
WITH EXTRA C, REGULAR,
AND PLUS IRON**

Miles Inc.
Consumer Healthcare Division

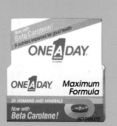

**ONE A DAY® BRAND
MAXIMUM FORMULA
THE MOST COMPLETE
ONE A DAY® BRAND**

Murdock

500 mg

SinuStat™
Contains naturally extracted
pseudoephedrine HCl

30 count bottle

NATURE'S BOUNTY

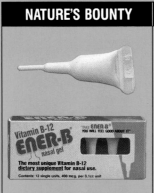

ENER-B®
Vitamin B-12 Nasal Gel

NEUTROGENA

NEUTROGENA® CLEANSING WASH

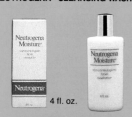

4 fl. oz.

NEUTROGENA MOISTURE®

4 fl. oz.

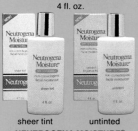

sheer tint   untinted

NEUTROGENA MOISTURE®
SPF 15 FORMULA

Non-Comedogenic
Facial Moisturizer

Neutrogena

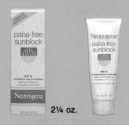

2¼ oz.

NEUTROGENA®
PABA-FREE SUNBLOCK
SPF 15
Maximum Sun Protection
Waterproof—Rubproof—
Sweatproof

NOXELL

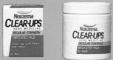

Regular Strength

Maximum Strength

CLEAR-UPS®
Medicated Cleansing Pads

Noxell

Vanishing   Concealing
(invisible)   (tinted)

CLEAR-UPS®
On-The-Spot
Acne Medicine

Noxell

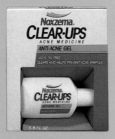

CLEAR-UPS®
Anti-Acne Gel
Acne Medicine

Noxell

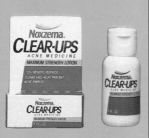

CLEAR-UPS®
Maximum Strength Lotion
Acne Medicine

Noxell

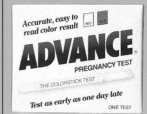

NOXZEMA®
Greaseless   Medicated
Skin Cream

Noxell

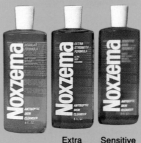

Regular   Extra   Sensitive
Formula   Strength   Skin
        Formula   Formula

NOXZEMA®
Antiseptic Skin Cleanser

NUMARK

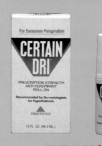

CERTAIN DRI®
Anti-Perspirant Roll-On

For Excessive Perspiration

OHM LABORATORIES

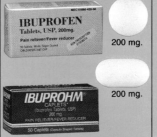

200 mg.

200 mg.

Tablets and Caplets available in
bottles of 24, 50 and 100

IBUPROFEN TABLETS
IBUPROHM CAPLETS

ORTHO

Ortho—Advanced Care Prods.

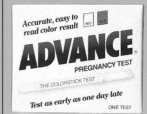

Test as early as one day late
ADVANCE®
Pregnancy Test

Ortho—Advanced Care Prods.

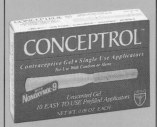

6's (6 easy-to-use prefilled applicators)
10's (10 easy-to-use prefilled applicators)

CONCEPTROL™
Contraceptive Gel
Single Use Contraceptives
[nonoxynol 9, 4% (100 mg)]

Ortho—Advanced Care Prods.

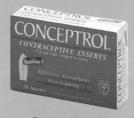

For use with condom
or alone.

CONCEPTROL™
Contraceptive Inserts

[nonoxynol 9, 8.34% (150 mg)]

Ortho—Advanced Care Prods.

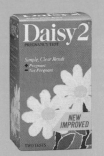

Two complete tests in each kit

DAISY 2®
Pregnancy Test

Ortho—Advanced Care Prods.

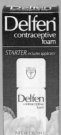

Starter (0.70 oz. vial w/applicator package)
Refill (0.70 oz. and 1.75 oz. vial only packages)
DELFEN® Contraceptive Foam
[nonoxynol 9, 12.5% (100 mg)]

Ortho—Advanced Care Prods.

2 oz. tube
MASSÉ® Breast Cream

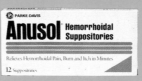

Available in boxes of 12, 24 and 48

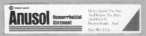

Available in 1 Oz. and 2 Oz. Tubes
ANUSOL®
Suppositories and Ointment

Parke-Davis

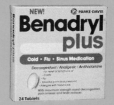

Available in boxes of 24 and 48
BENADRYL® PLUS
Decongestant/Analgesic/
Antihistamine

Ortho—Advanced Care Prods.

Fact PLUS

Unmistakable Result
FACT PLUS™
Pregnancy Test

Ortho—Advanced Care Prods.

Spray Powder and Spray Deodorant (3.0 oz.)
Cream (½ oz. and 1 oz.)
Spray Liquid (3.5 oz.)
MICATIN® Antifungal
For Athlete's Foot
(miconazole nitrate, 2%)

Parke-Davis

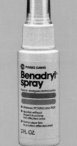

Available in Cream and Spray
BENADRYL®
Topical Antihistamine

Parke-Davis

Honey-Lemon Flavor

Available in 6 Fl. Oz. Bottles
BENADRYL® PLUS
NIGHTTIME

Ortho—Advanced Care Prods.

GYNOL II ORIGINAL FORMULA

Gynol II is intended for use with a diaphragm.

Starter (2.5 oz. tube with applicator package)
Refill (2.5 oz. and 3.8 oz. tube only packages)

GYNOL II®
Contraceptive Jelly
[nonoxynol 9, 2% (100 mg)]

Ortho—Advanced Care Prods.

ORTHO-GYNOL

Ortho-Gynol is intended for use with a diaphragm.

ORTHO-GYNOL®
Contraceptive Jelly
(diisobutylphenoxypolyethoxyethanol, 1.00%)

Parke-Davis

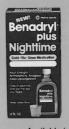

Available in boxes of 24
BENADRYL®
Decongestant

Parke-Davis

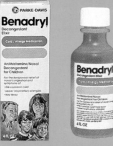

Available in 4 Oz. and 8 Oz. Bottles
BENADRYL®
Elixir

Ortho—Advanced Care Prods.

GYNOL II EXTRA STRENGTH

Contraceptive Jelly.
For use with condom, diaphragm or alone.

2.85 oz. tube with applicator
GYNOL II™
Extra Strength
[nonoxynol 9, 3% (150 mg)]

Ortho—Advanced Care Prods.

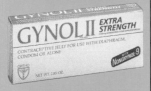

2 oz. and 4 oz. tubes

ORTHO® PERSONAL LUBRICANT

Parke-Davis

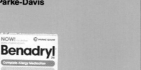

Kapseals available in boxes of 24 and 48

Tablets available in boxes of 24 and bottles of 100
BENADRYL® 25

Parke-Davis

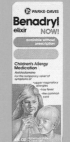

Available in 4 Oz. Bottles
BENADRYL®
Decongestant Elixir

Parke-Davis

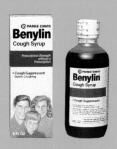

Available in 4 Oz. and 8 Oz. Bottles
BENYLIN®
Cough Syrup

Parke-Davis

Cream

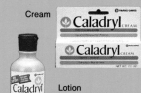

Lotion

For relief from itching due to:
Poison Ivy, Insect Bites, Poison Oak,
Skin Irritation
CALADRYL®
Topical Antihistamine/Skin Protectant

Parke-Davis

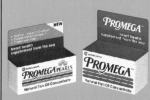

PROMEGA™
PEARLS
600 mg.
Soft Gels

PROMEGA™
1000 mg.
Soft Gels

Parke-Davis

10 Sustained
Action Tablets

12 Hour Relief of Nasal Congestion,
Runny Nose, Sneezing,
Itchy/Watery Eyes

ALLERGY FORMULA
SINUTAB®

Parke-Davis

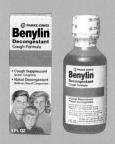

Available in 4 Oz. Bottles
BENYLIN®
Decongestant Cough Formula

Parke-Davis

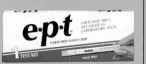

1 test kit

Stick test is simple to do and easy
to read. Instructions enclosed.

e•p•t®
STICK TEST
Early Pregnancy Test

Parke-Davis

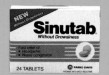

Easy-to-open package
(Non-child resistant)

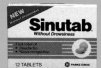

Child-resistant package
REGULAR SINUTAB®

Parke-Davis

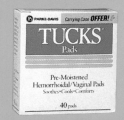

40 pads

Also available in 100 pad packages

TUCKS®
Pre-Moistened Pads

Parke-Davis

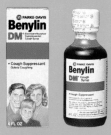

Available in 4 Oz. Bottles
BENYLIN DM®
Cough Syrup

Parke-Davis

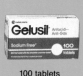

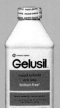

100 tablets
Also available:
50 tablets

GELUSIL®
Antacid-Anti-gas
Sodium Free

12 Fl. Oz.

Parke-Davis

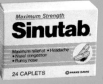

Caplets

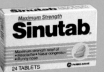

Tablets

MAXIMUM STRENGTH
SINUTAB®

Parke-Davis

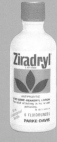

6 Fl. Oz.
ZIRADRYL® LOTION

Parke-Davis

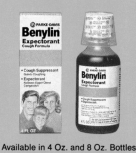

Available in 4 Oz. and 8 Oz. Bottles
BENYLIN® EXPECTORANT

Parke-Davis

Available in bottles of 130 Tablets
MYADEC®
Multivitamin-Multimineral
Supplement

Parke-Davis

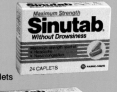

Caplets

Tablets

MAXIMUM STRENGTH
SINUTAB®
Without Drowsiness

NEW LIFE

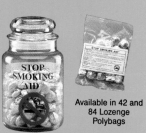

Available in 42 and
84 Lozenge
Polybags

STOP SMOKING AID™
BRAND SMOKING DETERRENT
LOZENGES

PLOUGH, INC.

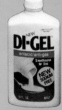

Aerosol Liquid

Gel

4.0 oz.   0.5 oz.

Also available in 3.5 oz. spray powder
and 2.25 oz. shaker powder.

AFTATE® FOR ATHLETE'S FOOT
(tolnaftate 1%)

Plough, Inc.

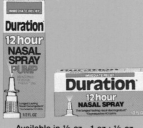

Available in ½ oz., 1 oz.; ½ oz.
measured dosage pump spray;
and ½ oz. mentholated.
(oxymetazoline HCl)

**DURATION®
NASAL SPRAY**

Plough, Inc.

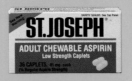

36 caplets

**ST. JOSEPH®
ADULT CHEWABLE ASPIRIN
Low Strength Caplets**

Each caplet contains 81 mg.
of aspirin

Plough, Inc.

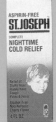

4 fl. oz.
bottle

Each 5 cc (average teaspoon) contains:
Chlorpheniramine maleate 1 mg.,
pseudoephedrine hydrochloride 15 mg.,
acetaminophen 160 mg., dextromethorphan
hydrobromide 5 mg.

**ST. JOSEPH®
NIGHTTIME COLD RELIEF**

Plough, Inc.

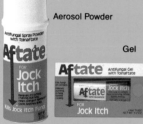

Aerosol Powder

Gel

3.5 oz.   0.5 oz.
Also available in 1.5 oz. shaker powder.

AFTATE® FOR JOCK ITCH
(tolnaftate 1%)

Plough, Inc.

Available in 10's or 20's

**DURATION®
DECONGESTANT TABLETS**
(pseudoephedrine sulfate)

Plough, Inc.

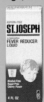

Available in 2 fl. oz. and 4 fl. oz.
sizes.

**ST. JOSEPH®
COUGH SUPPRESSANT
FOR CHILDREN**
(dextromethorphan hydrobromide)

Plough, Inc.

3 oz.
Lotion

3 oz.
Spray

(benzocaine and triclosan)

4.5 oz.
spray with
aloe

**SOLARCAINE® FIRST-AID
PRODUCTS**
For sunburns, minor burns,
cuts and scrapes

Plough, Inc.

Available in
15, 30, 60
and 90 tablet sizes.

CORRECTOL® LAXATIVE
(Tablet contains 100 mg. docusate sodium
and 65 mg. yellow phenolphthalein.)

Plough, Inc.

Laxative Gum   Laxative plus
Softener

Chocolated Mint Laxative

FEEN-A-MINT® LAXATIVE

Gum contains:
97.2 mg. phenolphthalein.
Pills contain: 100 mg. docusate
sodium and 65 mg. phenolphthalein.
Chocolate contains: 65 mg.
phenolphthalein.

Plough, Inc.

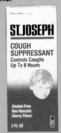

**ST. JOSEPH® ASPIRIN-FREE
Fever Reducers
Alcohol-Free, Sugar-Free
Infant Drops—Liquid and Tablets**

Plough, Inc.

Gum Available in
Spearmint, Peppermint
& Cinnamint

**STAY TRIM®
Appetite Suppressant Product**
(phenylpropanolamine HCl)

Plough, Inc.

Liquid   Tablets

Mint and Lemon/Orange flavors,
6 fl. oz. and 12 fl. oz. liquid plus 30
and 90 tablet sizes.
Now also available in 3-roll pack
and 60 tablet bottle (Mint only).

DI-GEL®

Plough, Inc.

Available in 30, 60 and 90
tablet sizes.

**REGUTOL®
STOOL SOFTENER**
(100 mg. docusate sodium per tablet)

Plough, Inc.

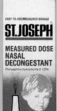

½ fl. oz.
bottle

**ST. JOSEPH® MEASURED DOSE
NASAL DECONGESTANT**
(phenylephrine HCl 0.125%)

Plough, Inc.

4 fl. oz.

SPF 15   SPF 6   SPF 8   SPF 30

New PABA-free ingredients:
SPF 6–15: Ethylhexyl
p-methoxycinnamate, oxbenzone
SPF 25, 30: Ethylhexyl p-methoxycinnamate,
2-ethylhexyl salicylate, homosalate,
oxybenzone
SPF 45: Ethylhexyl p-methoxycinnamate,
2-ethylhexyl salicylate, octocrylene,
oxybenzone.

Also available in SPF 4, SPF 25 and
SPF 45 Lotion.

**COPPERTONE® WATERPROOF
SUNSCREENS**

Plough, Inc.

SPF 15 Gel

SPF 15 Lotion

SPF 45 Lotion

4 fl. oz.

Also available in SPF 25 oil-free gel, SPF 30 lotion and SPF 30 sunblock stick.

**SHADE®
WATERPROOF SUNSCREENS**

Plough, Inc.

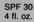

SPF 15
4 fl. oz.

SPF 25
3 fl. oz.

SPF 30
4 fl. oz.

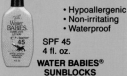

• Hypoallergenic
• Non-irritating
• Waterproof

SPF 45
4 fl. oz.

**WATER BABIES®
SUNBLOCKS**

PROCTER & GAMBLE

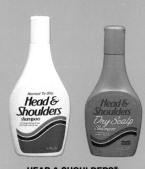

**HEAD & SHOULDERS®
Dandruff Care Shampoo**

Procter & Gamble

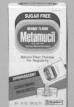
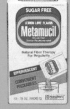

**EFFERVESCENT SUGAR FREE
METAMUCIL®
Natural Therapeutic Fiber
for Regularity**

Procter & Gamble

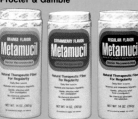

Available in Box of 30 Convenient Packets

METAMUCIL®

**Natural Therapeutic Fiber
for Regularity**

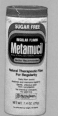
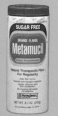

SUGAR FREE METAMUCIL®

**Natural Therapeutic Fiber
for Regularity**

Procter & Gamble

Liquid available in 4 oz., 8 oz., 12 oz. and 16 oz. plastic bottles

Tablets available in cartons of 24 and 42

PEPTO-BISMOL® LIQUID AND TABLETS

Procter & Gamble

Liquid available in 4 oz., 8 oz. and 12 oz. plastic bottles

**MAXIMUM STRENGTH
PEPTO-BISMOL®**

REED & CARNRICK

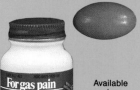

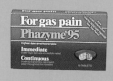

Available in 50s and 100s

PHAZYME® 95
An antiflatulent to alleviate or relieve symptoms of gas.

Reed & Carnrick

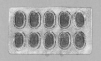

**PHAZYME® 95
Consumer 10 Packs**

An antiflatulent to alleviate or relieve symptoms of gas.

Reed & Carnrick

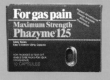

Available in 50s

**MAXIMUM STRENGTH
PHAZYME® 125**
An antiflatulent to alleviate or relieve symptoms of gas. Softgel capsule for ease of swallowing.

Reed & Carnrick

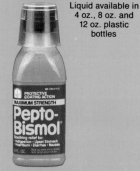

**MAXIMUM STRENGTH
PHAZYME® 125
Consumer 10 Packs**
An antiflatulent to alleviate or relieve symptoms of gas.

Reed & Carnrick

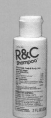

**Non-steroid
PROCTOFOAM®
Hemorrhoidal Foam**

Reed & Carnrick

Available in 2 and 4 fl. oz. sizes

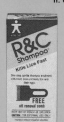

R&C SHAMPOO®
Kills head, crab and body lice and their eggs. Effective nit comb included.

Reed & Carnrick

Available in 5 and 10 oz. sizes

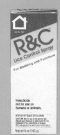
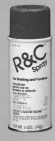

R&C SPRAY®
Controls lice and their eggs in the home. Insecticide: not for use on humans or animals.

Reed & Carnrick

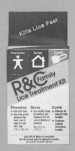

R&C LICE TREATMENT KIT
Contains 4 oz. R&C SHAMPOO, 5 oz. R&C SPRAY and nit comb.

REESE CHEMICAL CO.

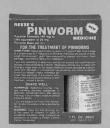

REESE'S PINWORM MEDICINE

Available in bottles of
1 fl. oz. with English
and Spanish directions

REID-ROWELL

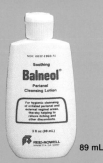

89 mL

BALNEOL®
Perianal Cleansing Lotion

Reid-Rowell

30 single-
dose packets

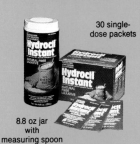

8.8 oz jar
with
measuring spoon

HYDROCIL® INSTANT
Bulk Forming Agent for
Constipation

RICHARDSON-VICKS INC.

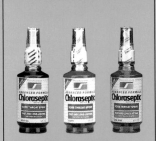

Available: Menthol, Cherry and Cool Mint
in 6 oz. spray. Menthol and Cherry in 12 oz.
gargle/refill and 1.5 oz. aerosol spray.
CHLORASEPTIC® LIQUID

Richardson-Vicks Inc.

Children's Grape

Cool Mint

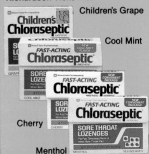

Cherry

Menthol

Available: Menthol and Cherry in
cartons of 18 and 36; Cool Mint and
Children's Grape in cartons of 18.

CHLORASEPTIC® LOZENGES

Richardson-Vicks Inc.

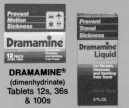

DRAMAMINE®
(dimenhydrinate)
Tablets 12s, 36s
& 100s

DRAMAMINE® LIQUID
(dimenhydrinate syrup USP)
Liquid 3 fl. oz.

**DRAMAMINE®
CHEWABLE**
(dimenhydrinate)
Tablets 8s & 24s

Richardson-Vicks Inc.

Bottles of 6 oz. and 10 oz.
and packets of 20 Caplets

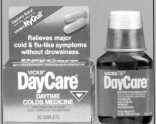

VICKS® DAYCARE®
Daytime Colds Medicine
(acetaminophen, pseudoephedrine
hydrochloride, dextromethorphan
hydrobromide, guaifenesin)

Richardson-Vicks Inc.

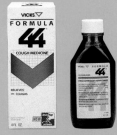

Available in 4 oz. and 8 oz.

**VICKS® FORMULA 44®
Cough Medicine**
(dextromethorphan hydrobromide,
chlorpheniramine maleate)

Richardson-Vicks Inc.

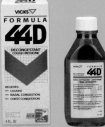

Available in 4 oz. and 8 oz.

**VICKS® FORMULA 44D®
Decongestant Cough Medicine**
(dextromethorphan hydrobromide,
pseudoephedrine hydrochloride,
guaifenesin)

Richardson-Vicks Inc.

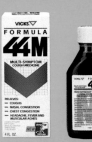

Available in 4 oz. and 8 oz.

VICKS® FORMULA 44M®
(dextromethorphan hydrobromide,
pseudoephedrine hydrochloride,
guaifenesin, acetaminophen)

Richardson-Vicks Inc.

Cough   Cough &   Cough &
      Congestion   Cold

Pediatric Formula 44®

Richardson-Vicks Inc.

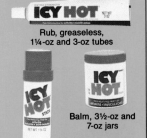

Rub, greaseless,
1¼-oz and 3-oz tubes

Balm, 3½-oz and
7-oz jars

Stick, 1¾ oz

ICY HOT®
Analgesic Balm, Rub and Stick for
Pain from Arthritis and Muscle Aches

Richardson-Vicks Inc.

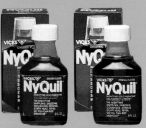

Original Flavor: 6 oz., 10 oz., 14 oz.
Cherry Flavor: 6 oz., 10 oz., 14 oz.

**VICKS® NYQUIL®
NIGHTTIME COLDS MEDICINE**
(acetaminophen, doxylamine succinate,
pseudoephedrine hydrochloride, dextromethorphan hydrobromide)

Richardson-Vicks Inc.

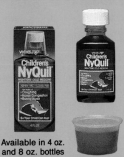

Available in 4 oz.
and 8 oz. bottles

VICKS® CHILDREN'S NYQUIL®
(chlorpheniramine maleate,
pseudoephedrine HCl, dextromethorphan
hydrobromide)

Richardson-Vicks Inc.

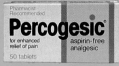

Available in bottles of
24, 50 and 90
PERCOGESIC®
analgesic
(acetaminophen and
phenyltoloxamine citrate)

Richardson-Vicks Inc.

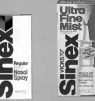

Sinex®   Sinex®
           Ultra Fine Mist

Available in ½ oz., 1 oz. squeeze bottles
and new ½ oz. measured dose atomizer.
VICKS® SINEX® ULTRA FINE MIST
Decongestant Nasal Spray
(phenylephrine hydrochloride,
cetylpyridinium chloride)

Richardson-Vicks Inc.

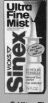

Sinex®
Long-Acting

Sinex® Ultra Fine
Mist 12 Hour

Available in ½ oz., 1 oz. squeeze bottles and
new ½ oz. measured dose atomizer.
VICKS® SINEX® LONG-ACTING
Decongestant Nasal Spray
(oxymetazoline hydrochloride)

Richardson-Vicks Inc.

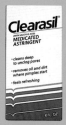

4 oz. size
CLEARASIL®
Medicated Astringent

For Oily Skin
(0.5% salicylic acid)

A. H. Robins

Available in bottles of 130 and 1000
ALLBEE® WITH C CAPLETS

A. H. Robins

Dimacol®
Expectorant/Nasal Decongestant/Cough Suppressant
COLD & COUGH CAPLETS
■ Relieves stuffy nose
■ Reduces chest congestion
■ Controls cough
■ Contains no sedatives

Available in consumer cartons of 12
and 24 and bottles of 100 and 500
DIMACOL® CAPLETS

Richardson-Vicks Inc.

2 oz. tube   1.5 oz., 3.0 oz.,
6 oz. jar

VICKS® VAPORUB®
Decongestant Cough Suppressant
(menthol, camphor, eucalyptus oil)

Richardson-Vicks Inc.

Regular   Maximum
32 pads

CLEARASIL®
Double Clear Dual Textured
Medicated Pads
(salicylic acid)

A. H. Robins

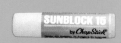

Ultra sunscreen protection (SPF-15)

Helps prevention and healing of dry,
chapped, sun- and windburned lips.

CHAP STICK®
SUNBLOCK 15 Lip Balm

A. H. Robins

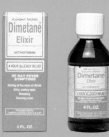

Available in bottles of 4 Fl. Oz.
and 16 Fl. Oz.

DIMETANE® ELIXIR
(Brompheniramine Maleate Elixir, USP)

Richardson-Vicks Inc.
Also Available: Clearasil
Medicated Anti-Acne Lotion

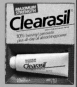
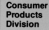

Vanishing   Tinted
Both available in .65 and 1.0 oz.
sizes

CLEARASIL®
Acne Treatment Cream
(10% benzoyl peroxide)

A. H. ROBINS

Consumer
Products
Division

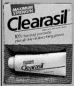

Available in bottles of 60
ALLBEE® C-800 TABLETS

A. H. Robins

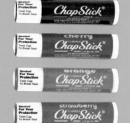

CHAP STICK®
Lip Balm

A. H. Robins

Dimetane
Tablets   **4 mg**
ANTIHISTAMINE

4 HOUR ALLERGY RELIEF
OF HAY FEVER SYMPTOMS
Itching of the nose or throat
Itchy, watery eyes
Sneezing   Running nose

24 TABLETS

Available in consumer cartons of
24 and bottles of 100 and 500

DIMETANE® TABLETS
(Brompheniramine Maleate Tablets, USP)

Richardson-Vicks Inc.
Also Available:
Clearasil Medicated Blemish Stick

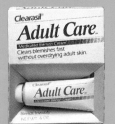

Clearasil
Adult Care
Medicated Blemish Cream
Clears blemishes fast
without overdrying adult skin.

.6 oz. size

CLEARASIL® ADULT CARE™
(sulfur, resorcinol)

A. H. Robins

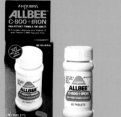

Available in bottles of 60
ALLBEE® C-800 PLUS IRON TABLETS

A. H. Robins

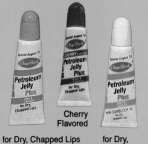

Cherry
Flavored

for Dry, Chapped Lips   for Dry,
Chapped Lips
with
SUNBLOCK 15

CHAP STICK® Petroleum Jelly Plus

A. H. Robins

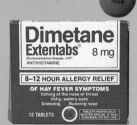

Dimetane
Extentabs®   **8 mg**
(Brompheniramine Maleate, USP)
ANTIHISTAMINE

8–12 HOUR ALLERGY RELIEF
OF HAY FEVER SYMPTOMS
Itching of the nose or throat
Itchy, watery eyes
Sneezing   Running nose

12 TABLETS

Available in consumer cartons of 12
and bottles of 100

DIMETANE EXTENTABS® 8 mg
(Brompheniramine Maleate, USP)

A. H. Robins

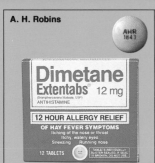

Dimetane
Extentabs® 12 mg
(Brompheniramine Maleate, USP)
ANTIHISTAMINE

12 HOUR ALLERGY RELIEF

OF HAY FEVER SYMPTOMS
Itching of the nose or throat
Itchy, watery eyes
Sneezing   Running nose

12 TABLETS

Available in consumer cartons of 12
and bottles of 100

DIMETANE EXTENTABS® 12 mg
(Brompheniramine Maleate, USP)

A. H. Robins

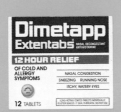

Dimetapp
Extentabs®

12 HOUR RELIEF

OF COLD AND
ALLERGY
SYMPTOMS

NASAL CONGESTION
SNEEZING   RUNNING NOSE
ITCHY, WATERY EYES

12 TABLETS

Available in consumer cartons of 12,
24 and 48 and bottles of 100 and 500

DIMETAPP EXTENTABS®

A. H. Robins

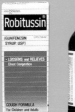

Robitussin
(GUAIFENESIN SYRUP, USP)

- LOOSENS and RELIEVES
Chest Congestion

COUGH FORMULA
For Children and Adults

Available in bottles of 4 Fl. Oz.,
8 Fl. Oz., 16 Fl. Oz. and 128 Fl. Oz.

ROBITUSSIN® SYRUP
(Guaifenesin Syrup, USP)

A. H. Robins

Robitussin
NIGHT RELIEF

- RELIEVES ALL MAJOR
COLD SYMPTOMS
So You Can Sleep
- ALCOHOL-FREE
- ASPIRIN-FREE

COLD FORMULA
For Children and Adults
CHERRY FLAVORED

Available in bottles of 4 Fl. Oz. and
8 Fl. Oz. with convenient dosage cup.

ROBITUSSIN NIGHT RELIEF®

A. H. Robins

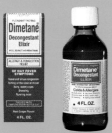

Dimetane
Decongestant
Elixir

ALLERGY & CONGESTION
RELIEF

OF HAY FEVER
SYMPTOMS
Nasal and sinus congestion
Itching of the nose or throat
Itchy, watery eyes
Sneezing
Running nose

4 FL. OZ.

4 Fl. Oz.

DIMETANE®
DECONGESTANT ELIXIR

A. H. Robins

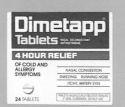

Dimetapp
Tablets

4 HOUR RELIEF

OF COLD AND
ALLERGY
SYMPTOMS

NASAL CONGESTION
SNEEZING   RUNNING NOSE
ITCHY, WATERY EYES

24 TABLETS

Available in consumer cartons of 24

DIMETAPP® TABLETS

A. H. Robins

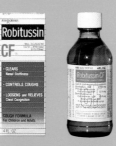

Robitussin
CF

- CLEARS
Nasal Stuffiness
- CONTROLS COUGHS
- LOOSENS and RELIEVES
Chest Congestion

COUGH FORMULA
For Children and Adults

Available in bottles of 4 Fl. Oz.,
8 Fl. Oz. and 16 Fl. Oz.

ROBITUSSIN-CF® SYRUP

A. H. Robins

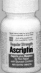
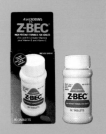

Z-BEC
HIGH POTENCY FORMULA FOR ADULTS
Zinc and B-Complex Vitamins
plus Vitamin E and Vitamin C

Available in bottles of 60 and 500

Z-BEC® TABLETS

A. H. Robins

Dimetane®
Decongestant

NASAL DECONGESTANT · ANTIHISTAMINE

ALLERGY & CONGESTION RELIEF

OF HAY FEVER SYMPTOMS
Nasal and sinus congestion
Itching of the nose or throat
Itchy, watery eyes · Sneezing · Running nose

24 CAPLETS

Available in consumer cartons of
24 and 48

DIMETANE® DECONGESTANT
CAPLETS

A. H. Robins

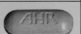

Dimetapp
PLUS

NASAL DECONGESTANT,
ANTIHISTAMINE, ANALGESIC

WITH NON-ASPIRIN PAIN RELIEVER

RELIEF OF
MAJOR
COLD & ALLERGY
SYMPTOMS

NASAL CONGESTION
SNEEZING   RUNNING NOSE
ITCHY, WATERY EYES
FEVER   ACHES & PAINS

24 CAPLETS

Available in consumer cartons
of 24 and bottles of 48

DIMETAPP® PLUS CAPLETS

A. H. Robins

Robitussin
DM

- CONTROLS COUGHS
(6 to 8 Hours)
- LOOSENS and RELIEVES
Chest Congestion

COUGH FORMULA
For Children and Adults

Available in bottles of 4 Fl. Oz.,
8 Fl. Oz., 16 Fl. Oz. and 128 Fl. Oz.

ROBITUSSIN-DM® SYRUP

Regular Strength
Ascriptin
Aspirin plus Maalox
for Pain Relief with Stomach Comfort
100 COATED TABLETS

bottles of 50, 100,
225 & 500 tablets

REGULAR STRENGTH
ASCRIPTIN®

(Aspirin [325 mg] and Maalox
[magnesium hydroxide 50 mg, dried
aluminum hydroxide gel 50 mg],
buffered with calcium carbonate)

A. H. Robins

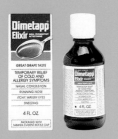

Dimetapp
Elixir

NASAL DECONGESTANT
ANTIHISTAMINE

GREAT GRAPE TASTE

TEMPORARY RELIEF
OF COLD AND
ALLERGY SYMPTOMS

NASAL CONGESTION

ITCHY, WATERY EYES
SNEEZING

4 FL. OZ.

Available in bottles of 4 Fl. Oz.,
8 Fl. Oz., 16 Fl. Oz. and 128 Fl. Oz.

DIMETAPP® ELIXIR

A. H. Robins

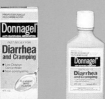

PROFESSIONALLY
RECOMMENDED

Donnagel®
ANTI-DIARRHEAL MEDICATION

FAST RELIEF FOR
Diarrhea
and Cramping

- Low Dosage
Concentration
- Non-constipating

PLEASANT
FLAVOR

Available in bottles of 4 Fl. Oz.,
8 Fl. Oz. and 16 Fl. Oz.

DONNAGEL®

A. H. Robins

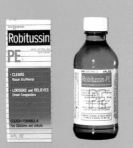

Robitussin
PE

- CLEARS
Nasal Stuffiness
- LOOSENS and RELIEVES
Chest Congestion

COUGH FORMULA
For Children and Adults

Available in bottles of 4 Fl. Oz.,
8 Fl. Oz. and 16 Fl. Oz.

ROBITUSSIN-PE® SYRUP

Rorer Consumer

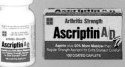
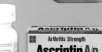

Arthritis Strength
Ascriptin A/D
Aspirin plus 50% More Maalox than
Regular Strength Ascriptin for Extra Stomach Comfort
100 COATED CAPLETS

bottles of 100,
225 & 500 caplets

FOR ARTHRITIS PAIN
ASCRIPTIN® A/D

(Aspirin [325 mg] and Maalox
[magnesium hydroxide 75 mg, dried
aluminum hydroxide gel 75 mg],
buffered with calcium carbonate)

Rorer Consumer

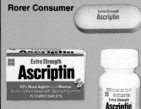
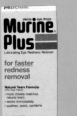

bottles of 36 & 75 caplets

EXTRA STRENGTH ASCRIPTIN®

(Aspirin [500 mg] and Maalox [magnesium hydroxide 80 mg, dried aluminum hydroxide gel 80 mg], buffered with calcium carbonate)

Rorer Consumer

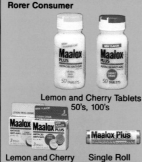

Lemon and Cherry Tablets 50's, 100's

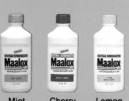

Lemon and Cherry   Single Roll
3 roll pack   Lemon only

MAALOX® PLUS

(magnesium hydroxide 200 mg, dried aluminum hydroxide gel 200 mg, and simethicone 25 mg)

Rorer Consumer

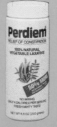

Granules
100 gm. and 250 gm.

PERDIEM®
100% Natural Vegetable Laxative
82 percent psyllium (Plantago Hydrocolloid)
18 percent senna (Cassia Pod Concentrate)

Ross

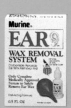

0.5 Fl. Oz.

MURINE® PLUS
Lubricating Eye Redness Reliever

Also available in 1.0 Fl. Oz.

Rorer Consumer

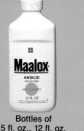

Bottles of 50 Tablets

Suspension
12 fl. oz.

CAMALOX®
(magnesium hydroxide 200 mg, dried aluminum hydroxide gel 225 mg and calcium carbonate 250 mg)

Rorer Consumer

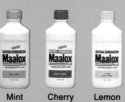

Mint   Cherry   Lemon
12 oz.
Suspension
Lemon
26 oz.

EXTRA STRENGTH MAALOX® PLUS
(magnesium hydroxide 450 mg, aluminum hydroxide gel 500 mg, and simethicone 40 mg)

Rorer Consumer

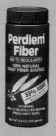

Granules
100 gm. and 250 gm.

PERDIEM® FIBER
100% Natural Daily Fiber Source
100% Psyllium (Plantago Hydrocolloid)

Ross

0.5 Fl. Oz.   0.5 Fl. Oz.

MURINE® EAR   **MURINE®**
WAX REMOVAL   **EAR DROPS**
SYSTEM

Rorer Consumer

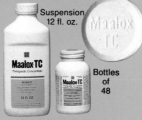

Bottles of 100 tablets

Bottles of 5 fl. oz., 12 fl. oz. & 26 fl. oz.

MAALOX®
Magnesia and Alumina Oral Suspension and Tablets, Rorer
(225 mg of aluminum hydroxide [200 mg tablets] and 200 mg of magnesium hydroxide)

Rorer Consumer

Suspension
12 fl. oz.

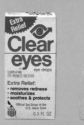

Bottles of 48

MAALOX® TC
(Therapeutic Concentrate)
Magnesium and Aluminum Hydroxides Oral Suspension and Tablets, Rorer

(300 mg of magnesium hydroxide and 600 mg of aluminum hydroxide per 5 ml/tablet)

0.5 Fl. Oz.

CLEAR EYES®
Lubricating Eye Redness Reliever

Also available in 1.0 Fl. Oz.

Ross   4 Fl. Oz.

For Oily   For Dry   For Normal   For All
Hair   Hair   Hair   Hair Types

SELSUN BLUE®
Dandruff Shampoo

Also available in 7 and 11 Fl. Oz.

Extra Medicated
For All Hair Types

Rorer Consumer

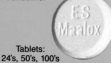

Tablets:
24's, 50's, 100's

EXTRA STRENGTH MAALOX®
(dried aluminum hydroxide gel 400 mg and magnesium hydroxide 400 mg)

Rorer Consumer

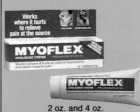

2 oz. and 4 oz.
Tube, 3 oz. Pump,
8 oz. and 16 oz. Jar

- Odorless   • Non-Burning
- Stainless   • Wrappable

MYOFLEX®
Analgesic Creme (trolamine salicylate)

Ross

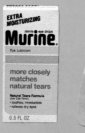

0.5 Fl. Oz.

MURINE® EYE LUBRICANT
More Closely Matches Natural Tears

Also available in 1.0 Fl. Oz.

Ross

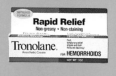

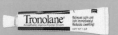

1 Oz. Tube With Applicator

TRONOLANE®
Anesthetic Cream for Hemorrhoids

Also available in a 2 oz. tube.

Ross

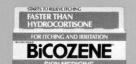
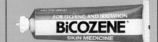

10 Suppositories

TRONOLANE®
Anesthetic Suppositories for
Hemorrhoids

Also available in size 20's.

RYDELLE

Regular   For Dry Skin
AVEENO® BATH

Normal to Oily Skin   Dry Skin

AVEENO®
For Acne   **BAR**

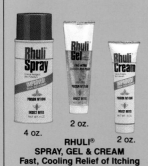

Shower and
Bath Oil   Lotion

AVEENO®
With Natural Colloidal Oatmeal
For the Relief of Dry, Itchy Skin

Rydelle

Rhuli
Spray   Rhuli
Gel   Rhuli
Cream

4 oz.   2 oz.   2 oz.

RHULI®
SPRAY, GEL & CREAM
Fast, Cooling Relief of Itching

SANDOZ
Consumer Division

STARTS TO RELIEVE ITCHING
FASTER THAN
HYDROCORTISONE

FOR ITCHING AND IRRITATION
BiCOZENE
SKIN MEDICINE

FOR ITCHING AND IRRITATION
BiCOZENE
SKIN MEDICINE

1 oz. (28.4 g.)

BICOZENE® CREME

Sandoz Consumer Division

4 oz., 8 oz.
DORCOL®
Children's Cough
Syrup

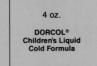

4 oz.
DORCOL®
Children's Liquid
Cold Formula

4 oz.
DORCOL®
Children's
Decongestant
Liquid

4 oz.
DORCOL®
Children's
Fever & Pain
Reducer

DORCOL®
PEDIATRIC FORMULAS

Sandoz Consumer Division

Gentle
Overnight Relief-
Guaranteed

EX·LAX
LAXATIVE PILLS

Pill

8's, 30's, 60's

Gentle Overnight Relief-
Guaranteed

EX·LAX
CHOCOLATED LAXATIVE

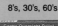

6's, 18's, 48's and 72's
Chocolated
Tablet
EX·LAX®

Sandoz Consumer Division

**EXTRA
GENTLE
EX·LAX®**

LAXATIVE PILLS
WITH SOFTENER

GENTLE
OVERNIGHT RELIEF-
GUARANTEED

24's
24 PILLS

EXTRA GENTLE EX·LAX®

Sandoz Consumer Division

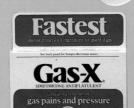
GAS·X

12's, 36's

Fastest
doctor prescribed ingredient for painful gas

Gas·X
SIMETHICONE-ANTIFLATULENT
for relieving symptoms of
gas pains and pressure

GAS·X®
(80 mg. simethicone)

Sandoz Consumer Division

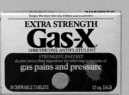
GAS·X

18 tablets

**EXTRA STRENGTH
Gas·X**
SIMETHICONE-ANTIFLATULENT
STRONGEST, FASTEST
doctor-prescribed ingredient for relieving symptoms of
gas pains and pressure

EXTRA-STRENGTH GAS·X®
(125 mg. simethicone)

Sandoz Consumer Division

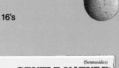

16's

GENTLE NATURE®
from *EX·LAX*

for natural-feeling relief overnight
Natural Vegetable Laxative

16 tablets

GENTLE NATURE®
(20 mg. sennosides)

Sandoz Consumer Division

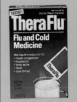

NEW!   NEW!
TheraFlu   **TheraFlu**
Flu and Cold   Flu, Cold &
Medicine   Cough
                Medicine

6 single dose packets

THERA FLU®   **THERA FLU®**
Flu and Cold   Flu, Cold &
Medicine   Cough Medicine

Sandoz Consumer Division

Triaminic-12
TWELVE HOUR RELIEF
Oral Nasal Decongestant/Antihistamine

TRIAMINIC-12®
Tablets
(Sustained Release)

10's, 20's

24's
TRIAMINIC®
Cold Tablets

Triaminic
COLD TABLETS

4 oz., 8 oz.
TRIAMINIC®
Cold Syrup   **TRIAMINIC®**

Sandoz Consumer Division

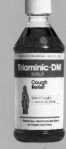

Triaminic-DM
SYRUP
Cough
Relief

4 oz., 8 oz.

TRIAMINIC-DM®
COUGH FORMULA

Sandoz Consumer Division

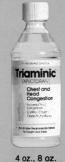
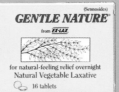

Triaminic
EXPECTORANT
Chest and
Head
Congestion

4 oz., 8 oz.

TRIAMINIC®
EXPECTORANT

Sandoz Consumer Division

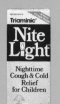
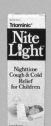

8 oz.   4 oz.

**TRIAMINIC®
NITE LIGHT™**
Nighttime Cough & Cold
Relief for Children

Schering

Safety Sealed

**AFRIN®
NASAL SPRAY
0.05%**

(oxymetazoline hydrochloride, USP)

Schering

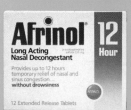

**AFRINOL®
EXTENDED RELEASE
TABLETS**

(pseudoephedrine sulfate)

Schering

009

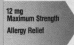

**CHLOR-TRIMETON®
MAXIMUM STRENGTH
TIMED RELEASE
ALLERGY TABLETS**

(12 mg chlorpheniramine maleate)

Sandoz Consumer Division

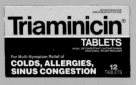

12's, 24's, 48's, 100's

**TRIAMINICIN®
TABLETS**

Schering

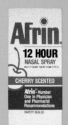

Safety Sealed

**AFRIN®
CHERRY SCENTED
NASAL SPRAY
0.05%**

**AFRIN®
MENTHOL
NASAL SPRAY
0.05%**

(oxymetazoline hydrochloride, USP)

Schering

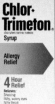

**CHLOR-TRIMETON®
ALLERGY SYRUP**

(2 mg chlorpheniramine maleate)

Schering

901

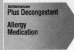

**CHLOR-TRIMETON®
DECONGESTANT TABLETS**

(4 mg chlorpheniramine maleate
and 60 mg pseudoephedrine sulfate)

Sandoz Consumer Division

4 oz., 8 oz.

**TRIAMINICOL®
MULTI-SYMPTOM
RELIEF**

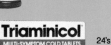

24's

**TRIAMINICOL®
MULTI-SYMPTOM COLD TABLETS**

Schering

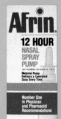

Safety Sealed

AFRIN® NASAL SPRAY PUMP

(oxymetazoline hydrochloride 0.05%)

Schering

TW

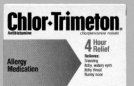

**CHLOR-TRIMETON®
ALLERGY TABLETS**

(4 mg chlorpheniramine maleate)

Schering

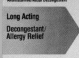

**LONG ACTING
CHLOR-TRIMETON®
DECONGESTANT REPETABS®**

(8 mg chlorpheniramine maleate and
120 mg pseudoephedrine sulfate)

SCHERING

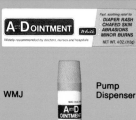

WMJ   Pump
Dispenser

A and D Reg. ™ Ointment

Schering

Safety Sealed

Nose Drops
0.05%

Children's Strength
Nose Drops
0.025%

AFRIN® NOSE DROPS

(oxymetazoline hydrochloride)

Schering

374

**CHLOR-TRIMETON®
LONG ACTING ALLERGY
REPETABS® TABLETS**

(8 mg chlorpheniramine maleate)

Schering

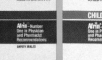

**CHLOR-TRIMETON®
SINUS CAPLETS**

(2 mg chlorpheniramine maleate, 12.5 mg
phenylpropanolamine HCl, and 500 mg
acetaminophen)

Schering

PKD
or
SN
or
171
or
522

AT THE FIRST SIGN OF
COLD & FLU
SYMPTOMS

ASPIRIN-FREE
SAFETY
SEALED
Coricidin
TABLETS
24 TABLETS

CORICIDIN® TABLETS
(2 mg chlorpheniramine maleate and
325 mg acetaminophen)

Schering

DRIXORAL
ANTIHISTAMINE/NASAL DECONGESTANT
12 hour relief

Temporarily relieves
nasal congestion due
to the common cold
and associated with
sinusitis. Alleviates
running nose and
sneezing due to hay fever.

20 SUSTAINED-ACTION TABLETS

**DRIXORAL®
SUSTAINED-ACTION TABLETS**
(6 mg dexbrompheniramine maleate and
120 mg pseudoephedrine sulfate)

Schering/Emko Product Line

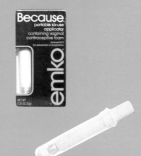

Because
portable six-use
applicator
containing vaginal
contraceptive foam
for prevention of pregnancy

Net wt .35 oz (10g)

emko

BECAUSE® CONTRACEPTOR®
(nonoxynol-9)

Schering

Tinactin
JOCK ITCH CREAM
KILLS JOCK ITCH FUNGI
■ Stops jock itch fungi
■ Soothes irritation, relieves itching
■ Odorless

Tinactin ANTIFUNGAL
JOCK ITCH
CREAM

Tinactin
ANTIFUNGAL
JOCK ITCH
Spray Powder
KILLS
JOCK ITCH
FUNGI
■ Stops jock itch fungi
■ Relieves itching

Net Wt 100g (3.5 ounce)

**TINACTIN® JOCK ITCH
CREAM AND SPRAY POWDER**
(tolnaftate 1%)

Schering

871
or
307

FOR CONGESTED
COLD, FLU &
SINUS SYMPTOMS

ASPIRIN-FREE
SAFETY
SEALED
Coricidin D.
DECONGESTANT TABLETS
24 TABLETS

**CORICIDIN 'D'®
DECONGESTANT TABLETS**
(2 mg chlorpheniramine maleate, 12.5 mg
phenylpropanolamine HCl, and 325 mg
acetaminophen)

Schering

DRIXORAL PLUS
ANTIHISTAMINE / NASAL DECONGESTANT
PAIN RELIEVER
FEVER REDUCER
12 hour relief

For temporary relief of:
■ Nasal & sinus congestion
■ Running nose
■ Sneezing due to hay fever
■ Runny watery eyes
■ Fever
■ Minor aches, pain & headache

24 EXTENDED-RELEASE
TABLETS

PACKAGE NOT CHILD-RESISTANT

**DRIXORAL® PLUS
EXTENDED-RELEASE TABLETS**
(60 mg pseudoephedrine sulfate, 3 mg
dexbrompheniramine maleate and 500 mg
acetaminophen)

Schering/Emko Product Line

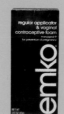

regular applicator
& vaginal
contraceptive foam
for prevention of pregnancy

Net wt .82 oz (40g)

emko

**EMKO®
CONTRACEPTIVE
FOAM**
(nonoxynol-9)

Schering

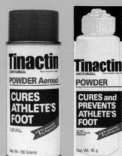

Tinactin
ANTIFUNGAL
POWDER Aerosol
CURES
ATHLETE'S
FOOT
1%

Net Wt. 100 Grams

Tinactin
ANTIFUNGAL
POWDER
CURES and
PREVENTS
ATHLETE'S
FOOT
1%

Net Wt. 45 g

**TINACTIN® POWDER AEROSOL
AND POWDER**
(tolnaftate 1%)

Schering

NDC 0085-0575-01

FOR
YOUR CHILD'S
CONGESTED
COLD,
FLU &
SINUS
SYMPTOMS

Coricidin
DEMILETS® TABLETS
ASPIRIN-FREE

Analgesic
antihistamine
decongestant
36 chewable tablets

CORICIDIN® DEMILETS® TABLETS
(1.0 mg chlorpheniramine maleate,
80 mg acetaminophen, 6.25 mg phenylpropanolamine HCl)

Schering

DRIXORAL NON-DROWSY
FORMULA

NEW LONG-ACTING
NASAL DECONGESTANT

Up to 12-Hour Relief

For up to 12 hours relief from
nasal congestion due to the
common cold, hay fever or other
upper respiratory allergies
without drowsiness.

WITHOUT DROWSINESS

10 EXTENDED-RELEASE TABLETS

**DRIXORAL®
NON-DROWSY FORMULA
EXTENDED-RELEASE TABLETS**
(120 mg pseudoephedrine sulfate)

Schering

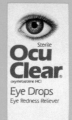

Sterile
**Ocu
Clear.**
oxymetazoline HCl
Eye Drops
Eye Redness Reliever

Safety Sealed
**OCUCLEAR®
EYE DROPS**
(oxymetazoline HCl 0.025%)

Schering

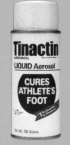

Tinactin
ANTIFUNGAL
LIQUID Aerosol
CURES
ATHLETE'S
FOOT
1%

Net Wt. 100 Grams

**TINACTIN®
LIQUID AEROSOL**
(tolnaftate 1%)

Schering

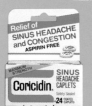

Coricidin.
SINUS

Relief of
SINUS HEADACHE
and CONGESTION
ASPIRIN FREE

MAXIMUM
STRENGTH
Coricidin
SINUS
HEADACHE
CAPLETS
Safety Sealed
24 COATED CAPLETS

**CORICIDIN® SINUS
HEADACHE CAPLETS**

(500 mg acetaminophen, 2 mg chlorpheniramine maleate, and 12.5 mg
phenylpropanolamine HCl)

Schering

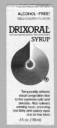

ALCOHOL-FREE!
WILD CHERRY FLAVOR

**DRIXORAL
SYRUP**
ANTIHISTAMINE/NASAL DECONGESTANT

Temporarily relieves
nasal congestion due
to the common cold and
sinusitis. Also relieves
running nose, sneezing,
and itchy and watery eyes
due to hay fever.

4 fl. oz. (118ml)

Safety Sealed
DRIXORAL® SYRUP
(2 mg brompheniramine maleate and
30 mg pseudoephedrine sulfate)

Schering

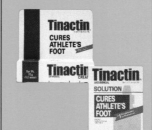

Tinactin
CURES
ATHLETE'S
FOOT

Tinactin
Tinactin
CREAM

Tinactin
SOLUTION
CURES
ATHLETE'S
FOOT
1%

**TINACTIN®
CREAM AND SOLUTION**
(tolnaftate 1%)

While every effort has
been made to reproduce
products faithfully, this
section is to be consid-
ered a Quick-Reference
identification aid.

SCHWARZ PHARMA

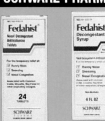

24 tablets   4 fl oz

Tablets also available in
bottles of 100

FEDAHIST®
Tablets and Decongestant
Syrup

Schwarz Pharma

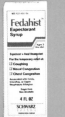

4 fl oz   1 fl oz

FEDAHIST®
Expectorant Syrup
and Expectorant Pediatric Drops

Schwarz Pharma

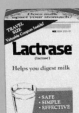

Available in
cartons of
10 and 30 and
bottles of 100

LACTRASE® Capsules
(lactase) 250 mg

SMITHKLINE BEECHAM

Consumer Brands

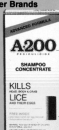

4 fl. oz.

A-200® PEDICULICIDE SHAMPOO

Also available:
A-200® Pediculicide Shampoo, 2 fl. oz.
A-200® Pediculicide Gel, 1 oz.

SmithKline Beecham Consumer Brands

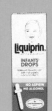

1.16 fl. oz.   4 fl. oz.
Fruit Flavored Drops and
Cherry Elixir
Alcohol Free
Child Resistant Safety Cap

LIQUIPRIN®
Acetaminophen

SmithKline Beecham Consumer Brands

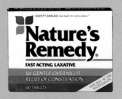

60 tablets

NATURE'S REMEDY®

Also available:
Box 12s and 30s

SmithKline Beecham Consumer Brands

OXY® 5
Vanishing

OXY® 5
Tinted

OXY® 10
Vanishing

OXY® 10
Tinted

SmithKline Beecham Consumer Brands

REGULAR   MAXIMUM
STRENGTH   STRENGTH

Regular   Maximum
Strength   Strength

Sensitive
Skin
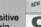

50 pads
Also available: 90 pads
OXY CLEAN®
MEDICATED PADS

SmithKline Beecham Consumer Brands

Medicated   Lathering
Cleanser   Facial
4 fl. oz.   Scrub
    2.65 oz.

Medicated Soap
3.25 oz.
OXY CLEAN®

SmithKline Beecham Consumer Brands

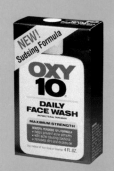

OXY 10® DAILY FACE WASH

SmithKline Beecham Consumer Brands

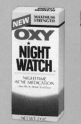

Maximum   Sensitive
Strength   Skin

OXY NIGHT WATCH™

SmithKline Beecham Consumer Brands

TUMS®
Peppermint

TUMS®
Assorted Flavors

SmithKline Beecham Consumer Brands

TUMS E-X®
Wintergreen

TUMS E-X®
Cherry

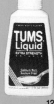

TUMS E-X®
Peppermint

TUMS E-X®
Assorted Flavors

SmithKline Beecham Consumer Brands

Available in Extra Strength and
Extra Strength with Simethicone

12 fl. oz.

TUMS® LIQUID
Extra Strength Antacid
(calcium carbonate)

SMITHKLINE

Consumer Products

1 oz. tube

ACNOMEL® ACNE CREAM
(resorcinol, sulfur, alcohol)

SmithKline Consumer Products

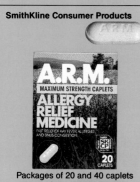

Packages of 20 and 40 caplets

A.R.M.® ALLERGY RELIEF MEDICINE

(chlorpheniramine maleate, phenylpropanolamine HCl)

SmithKline Consumer Products

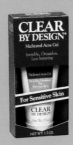

1.5 oz. tube

CLEAR BY DESIGN®
Medicated Acne Gel

(benzoyl peroxide 2.5%)

SmithKline Consumer Products

Packages of 10, 20 and 40 caplets

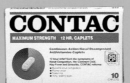

CONTAC®
CONTINUOUS ACTION
NASAL DECONGESTANT
ANTIHISTAMINE CAPLETS

SmithKline Consumer Products

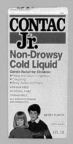

Includes dose-by-weight cup

CONTAC JR.®
COLD MEDICINE FOR CHILDREN

SmithKline Consumer Products

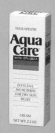

2.5 oz. tube

AQUA CARE® CREAM
with 10% Urea

SmithKline Consumer Products

60 Pads

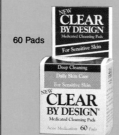

CLEAR BY DESIGN®
Medicated
Cleansing Pads

SmithKline Consumer Products

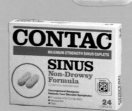

Packages of 24

CONTAC®
MAXIMUM STRENGTH
SINUS CAPLETS
NON-DROWSY FORMULA

SmithKline Consumer Products

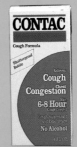

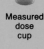

Measured dose cup

CONTAC®
COUGH FORMULA

SmithKline Consumer Products

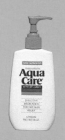

8 oz. and 16 oz. bottles

AQUA CARE® LOTION
with 10% Urea

SmithKline Consumer Products

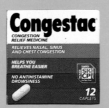

Packages of 12 and 24 caplets

CONGESTAC®
Congestion Relief Medicine
Decongestant/Expectorant

SmithKline Consumer Products

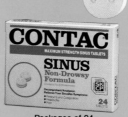

Packages of 24

CONTAC®
MAXIMUM STRENGTH
SINUS TABLETS
NON-DROWSY FORMULA

SmithKline Consumer Products

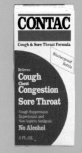

Measured dose cup

CONTAC®
COUGH & SORE THROAT FORMULA

SmithKline Consumer Products

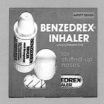

1 inhaler per package

BENZEDREX® INHALER

(propylhexedrine)

SmithKline Consumer Products

Packages of 10, 20 and 40 capsules

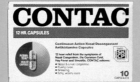

CONTAC®
CONTINUOUS ACTION
NASAL DECONGESTANT
ANTIHISTAMINE CAPSULES

SmithKline Consumer Products

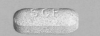

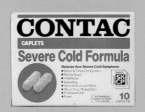

Packages of 10, 20 and 40 caplets

CONTAC®
SEVERE COLD FORMULA

SmithKline Consumer Products

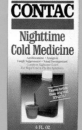

Measured dose cup

CONTAC®
NIGHTTIME
COLD MEDICINE

SmithKline Consumer Products	**SmithKline Consumer Products**	**SmithKline Consumer Products**	**SmithKline Consumer Products**

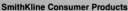
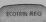
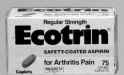

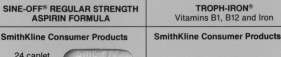

75 caplet bottle

**REGULAR STRENGTH
ECOTRIN® CAPLETS**
Duentric® coated 5 gr. aspirin

**16 oz. bottle
FEOSOL® ELIXIR**
(ferrous sulfate USP)

Packages of 24,
48, and 100 tablets

**SINE-OFF® REGULAR STRENGTH
ASPIRIN FORMULA**

4 oz. liquid

TROPH-IRON®
Vitamins B1, B12 and Iron

SmithKline Consumer Products	**SmithKline Consumer Products**	**SmithKline Consumer Products**	**SmithKline Consumer Products**

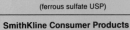
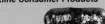
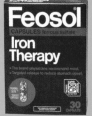
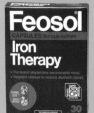

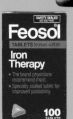

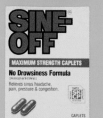
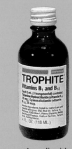

24 caplet
package

50 caplet bottle

**MAXIMUM STRENGTH
ECOTRIN® CAPLETS**
Duentric® coated 7.7 gr. aspirin

**Packages of 30 and
60 capsules and bottles of 500**

FEOSOL® CAPSULES
(ferrous sulfate USP)

**SINE-OFF®
MAXIMUM STRENGTH ALLERGY/
SINUS FORMULA CAPLETS**

4 oz. liquid

TROPHITE® LIQUID
Vitamins B1, B12

SmithKline Consumer Products	**SmithKline Consumer Products**	**SmithKline Consumer Products**

24 caplet
package

**In 100, 250 and 1000
tablet bottles**

**REGULAR STRENGTH
ECOTRIN® TABLETS**
Duentric® coated 5 gr. aspirin

In 100 and 1000 tablet bottles

FEOSOL® TABLETS
(ferrous sulfate USP)

**SINE-OFF®
MAXIMUM STRENGTH
NO DROWSINESS FORMULA CAPLETS**

While every effort has
been made to reproduce
products faithfully, this
section is to be consid-
ered a Quick-Reference
identification aid.

SmithKline Consumer Products	**SmithKline Consumer Products**	**SmithKline Consumer Products**

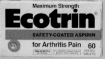

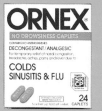

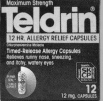

Packages of 12, 24   12 mg.
and 48 capsules

**In 60 and 150
tablet bottles**

**MAXIMUM STRENGTH
ECOTRIN® TABLETS**
Duentric® coated 7.7 gr. aspirin

**Packages of 24 and
48 caplets**

ORNEX® CAPLETS
Decongestant/Analgesic

**TELDRIN®
TIMED-RELEASE CAPSULES**
(chlorpheniramine maleate)

For more detailed in-
formation on products
illustrated in this sec-
tion, consult the Prod-
uct Information Section
or manufacturers may
be contacted directly.

SQUIBB	**STELLAR**	Stuart	Stuart

THERAGRAN® STRESS FORMULA
High Potency Multivitamin Formula
with Iron and Biotin

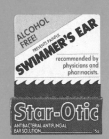

STAR-OTIC®
Prevent Swimmer's Ear
Antibacterial • Antifungal

Bottles
of
60 tablets

FERANCEE®-HP
High Potency Hematinic

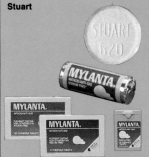

Available in boxes of 40 and 100,
bottles of 180, flip-top Convenience
Packs of 48 and 12 tablet rolls
MYLANTA® TABLETS
Antacid/Anti-Gas

E. R. Squibb & Sons

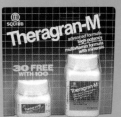

**ADVANCED FORMULA
THERAGRAN-M®**
High Potency Multivitamin
Formula with Minerals

STUART

12 oz

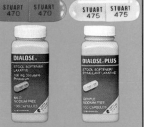

5 oz

ALternaGEL®
High Potency Aluminum Hydroxide
Antacid

Stuart

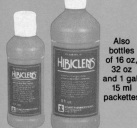

Also
bottles
of 16 oz,
32 oz
and 1 gal;
15 ml
packettes

4 oz   8 oz
HIBICLENS®
(chlorhexidine gluconate)
Antiseptic Antimicrobial
Skin Cleanser

Stuart

Also available:
24 oz and
5 oz

Packs of 24

Tablet Roll
Boxes of
60 tablets

MYLANTA®-II LIQUID and TABLETS
Double Strength Antacid/Anti-Gas

E. R. Squibb & Sons

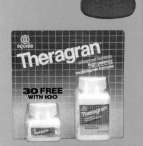

**ADVANCED FORMULA
THERAGRAN®**
High Potency Multivitamin
Formula

Stuart

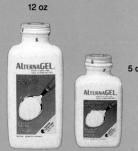

Bottles of 36
and 100 capsules
DIALOSE®
(docusate potassium,
100 mg)

Bottles of 36, 100
and 500 capsules
DIALOSE® PLUS
(docusate potassium,
100 mg and casan-
thranol, 30 mg)
Stool Softeners

Stuart

Bottles of 30 and 60 capsules

KASOF®
(docusate potassium, 240 mg)

High Strength Stool Softener

Stuart

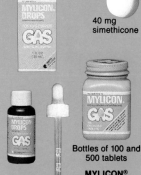

40 mg
simethicone

Bottles of 100 and
500 tablets

MYLICON®
Antiflatulent

1 fl oz

E. R. Squibb & Sons

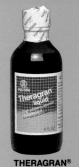

**THERAGRAN®
LIQUID**
High Potency Liquid
Vitamin Supplement

Stuart

Available in
9 oz and 16 oz
bottles

EFFER-SYLLIUM®

Packets in
cartons of
12s & 24s

EFFER-SYLLIUM®
Natural Fiber Bulking Agent

Stuart

Sodium Free

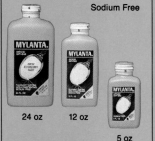

24 oz   12 oz

5 oz

MYLANTA® LIQUID
Antacid/Anti-Gas

(magnesium and alumi-
num hydroxides with
simethicone)

Stuart

80 mg
100 tablets simethicone

Convenience
Package
of 48s

Convenience
Package of 12s

MYLICON®-80
Antiflatulent

Stuart

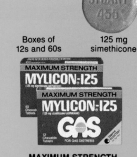

Boxes of 12s and 60s   125 mg simethicone

MAXIMUM STRENGTH
MYLICON®-125
Antiflatulent

Stuart

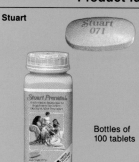

Bottles of 100 tablets

STUART PRENATAL® TABLETS
Multivitamin/Multimineral Supplement
for pregnant or lactating women

Thompson Medical Company, Inc.

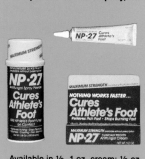

Available in ½, 1 oz. cream; ½ oz.
solution; 3.5 oz. spray powder

NP-27®
(tolnaftate 1%)

Upjohn

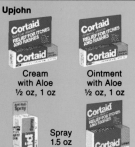

Cream with Aloe ½ oz, 1 oz

Ointment with Aloe ½ oz, 1 oz

Spray 1.5 oz

Lotion 1 oz

CORTAID®
Cream & Ointment with Aloe; Lotion
(hydrocortisone acetate)
Spray (hydrocortisone)

Stuart

Bottles of 100 tablets

OREXIN®
Therapeutic Vitamin Supplement

Stuart

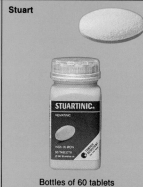

Bottles of 60 tablets

STUARTINIC®
Hematinic

Thompson Medical Company, Inc.

Fall Asleep Fast
MAXIMUM STRENGTH
Sleepinal

Available in 16, 32 capsule sizes

SLEEPINAL™
(diphenhydramine HCl 50 mg.)

Upjohn

HALTRAN®
Relieves Cramps Right From The Start   200 mg

HALTRAN
MENSTRUAL PAIN AND CRAMP RELIEVER

Available in Blister Packages of 12;
Bottles of 30

HALTRAN® Tablets
(ibuprofen tablets, USP)

Stuart

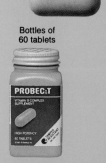

Bottles of 60 tablets

PROBEC®-T
High potency B complex supplement
with 600 mg of vitamin C

THOMPSON MEDICAL

Cortizone·5 CREME

RASH, ECZEMA, PSORIASIS†
Doctor Recommended
Itch & Rash Relief

MAXIMUM STRENGTH
Cortizone·5 CREME

Available in ½, 1, 2 oz. creme;
1 oz. ointment

CORTIZONE-5
(hydrocortisone 0.5%)

Thompson Medical Company, Inc.

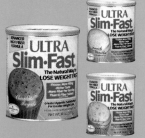

ULTRA Slim·Fast

Available in Chocolate Royale,
French Vanilla and Strawberry
Supreme; 14 oz. can

ULTRA SLIM-FAST®

Upjohn

Kaopectate   Kaopectate

Tablets   Chewable Tablets

Kaopectate   Kaopectate

Regular   Peppermint
Concentrated Anti-Diarrheal
KAOPECTATE®

Stuart

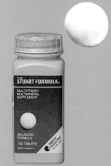

Bottles of 100 and 250 tablets

STUART FORMULA® TABLETS
Multivitamin/Multimineral Supplement

Thompson Medical Company, Inc.

LONG LASTING FORMULA
LOSE WEIGHT FAST
MAXIMUM STRENGTH
dexatrim

Available in 10, 20 and 40 capsule sizes

LONG LASTING FORMULA
LOSE WEIGHT FAST
MAXIMUM STRENGTH
dexatrim

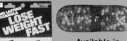

Available in 10, 20 and 40 caplet sizes

MAXIMUM STRENGTH DEXATRIM®
Capsules & Caplets
Plus Vitamin C

UPJOHN

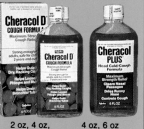

Cheracol D
COUGH FORMULA
Maximum Strength Cough Relief

Cheracol PLUS
Head Cold/Cough Formula

2 oz, 4 oz, 6 oz   4 oz, 6 oz

CHERACOL D®   CHERACOL PLUS®
Cough Formula   Head Cold/Cough
                              Formula

Upjohn

Motrin IB   Motrin IB

200 mg

Motrin IB   Motrin IB

Available in 24's and 50's

MOTRIN® IB
Caplets and Tablets

(ibuprofen, USP)

Upjohn

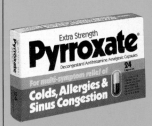

½ oz & 1 oz tubes
MYCITRACIN®
Triple Antibiotic Ointment

(bacitracin-polymyxin-neomycin
topical ointment)

WALKER, CORP

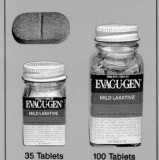

35 Tablets   100 Tablets

EVAC-U-GEN®
Mild Laxative

Wallace

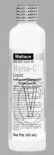

1 pint
(473 ml)

Also available: 4 fl oz (118 ml)
RYNA-C® LIQUID
(antitussive-antihistamine-decongestant)

Warner-Lambert Co.

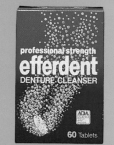

60 Tablets

**PROFESSIONAL STRENGTH
EFFERDENT®**

Denture Cleanser

Upjohn

Available in blister packs
of 24 and bottles of 500

Nasal Decongestant/Antihistamine/
Analgesic

PYRROXATE® Capsules

WALLACE

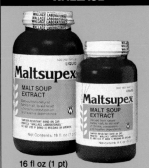

16 fl oz (1 pt)

MALTSUPEX® LIQUID
(malt soup extract)

Wallace

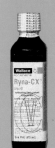

1 pint
(473 ml)

Also available: 4 fl oz (118 ml)
RYNA-CX® LIQUID
(antitussive-decongestant-expectorant)

Warner-Lambert Co.

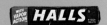
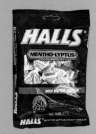

HALLS® Mentho-Lyptus®
Cough Tablets

Upjohn

UNICAP M® Tablets
Advanced formula
dietary supplement
Bottle of 120

UNICAP Sr.™
Tablets
Multivitamin
supplement
Bottle of 120

UNICAP T® Tablets
Stress Formula
Bottle of 60

Wallace

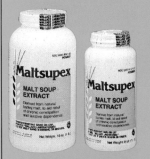

16 oz (1 lb)   8 oz (½ lb)

MALTSUPEX® POWDER
(malt soup extract)

Wallace

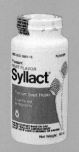

SYLLACT™
(powdered psyllium seed husks)

Warner-Lambert Co.

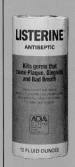

12 oz.

LISTERINE® ANTISEPTIC

WAKUNAGA

KYOLIC®
Aged Garlic Extract
with B₁, B₁₂

KYOLIC®
Aged Garlic Extract
Super Formula
101-Capsules

Wallace

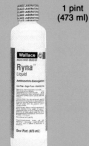

1 pint
(473 ml)

Also available: 4 fl oz (118 ml)
RYNA™ LIQUID
(antihistamine-decongestant)

WARNER-LAMBERT CO.

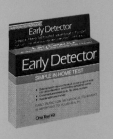

EARLY DETECTOR®
In-Home Test
for Fecal Occult Blood

Warner-Lambert Co.

24
Lozenges

LISTERINE®
Antiseptic Throat Lozenges

24
Lozenges

**MAXIMUM STRENGTH
LISTERINE®**
Antiseptic Throat Lozenges

Warner-Lambert Co.	Warner-Lambert Co.	**WESTWOOD**	Westwood

Warner-Lambert Co.

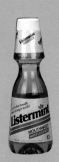

LISTERMINT™ with FLUORIDE
Anticavity Dental Rinse & Mouthwash

Warner-Lambert Co.

Spearmint

Wintergreen

Regular
ROLAIDS®

Fast, Safe, Lasting Relief from Heartburn, Sour Stomach or Acid Indigestion and Upset Stomach Associated with these Symptoms

WESTWOOD
Moisture Rich Body Oil

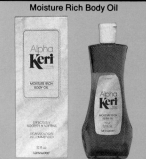

ALPHA KERI®
Shower and Bath Products

Westwood

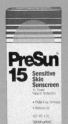

Sensitive Skin Sunscreen 15 / Sensitive Skin Sunscreen 29

PRESUN®
Creamy, Lotion, Facial, Sensitive Skin and Stick Formulas

Warner-Lambert Co.

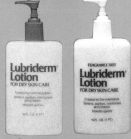

Scented / Unscented

**LUBRIDERM®
LOTION**

For Dry Skin Care

Warner-Lambert Co.

SODIUM FREE* ROLAIDS®

Sodium Free Relief from Heartburn, Sour Stomach or Acid Indigestion and Upset Stomach Associated with these Symptoms

Westwood

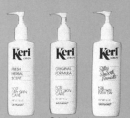

Fresh Herbal Scent / Original Formula / Silky Smooth Formula

KERI® LOTION
For Dry Skin Care

Advil / **Advil**

Coated Tablets in Bottles of 8, 24, 50, 100, 165 and 250. Coated Caplets in Bottles of 24, 50, 100 and 165.
ADVIL®
Ibuprofen Tablets and Caplets, USP

Warner-Lambert Co.

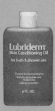

8 fl. oz.

**LUBRIDERM®
SKIN CONDITIONING OIL**

For Dry Skin Care

Warner-Lambert Co.

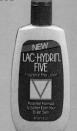

Cherry

Assorted Fruit

CALCIUM RICH ROLAIDS®

Calcium Rich, Sodium Free Relief from Heartburn, Sour Stomach or Acid Indigestion and Upset Stomach Associated with these Symptoms

Westwood

8 oz.

LAC-HYDRIN® FIVE
Fragrance Free Lotion

Patented Formula To Soften Your Driest Skin

Whitehall

CoAdvil

CoAdvil
advanced formula for cold & sinus relief™

Coated Caplets in Packages of 20 and Bottles of 48 and 100.

CoADVIL™
Ibuprofen/Pseudoephedrine Caplets

Warner-Lambert Co.

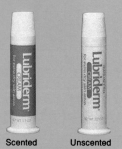

Scented / Unscented

LUBRIDERM® CREAM

For Extra Dry Skin Areas

Warner-Lambert Co.

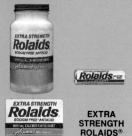

EXTRA STRENGTH ROLAIDS®

Extra Strength Calcium, Sodium Free Relief from Heartburn, Sour Stomach or Acid Indigestion and Upset Stomach Associated with these Symptoms

Westwood

Lotion / Cream / Cleanser

**Fragrance-Free
MOISTUREL®**

Whitehall

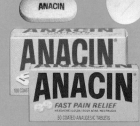

ANACIN

**ANACIN
FAST PAIN RELIEF**

Coated Tablets in Tins of 12 and Bottles of 30, 50, 100, 200 and 300. Coated Caplets in Bottles of 30, 50 and 100.
ANACIN®
Analgesic Tablets and Caplets

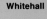

Whitehall

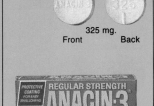

325 mg.
Front   Back

Coated Tablets: Bottles
of 24, 50 and 100.

REGULAR STRENGTH ANACIN-3®
Acetaminophen Tablets

Whitehall

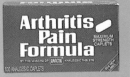

Available in Bottles of 40, 100 and
175 Caplets.

ARTHRITIS PAIN FORMULA
by the makers of ANACIN®
Analgesic Tablets

Whitehall

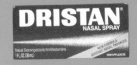

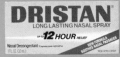

Both Available in Bottles of
15 ml. and 30 ml.
and Metered Dose Pumps of 15 ml.

DRISTAN®
Nasal Spray

Whitehall   Ointment
1 oz. and 2 oz. Tubes

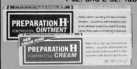

Cream
0.9 oz. and 1.8 oz. Tubes

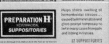

Suppositories
12s, 24s, 36s and 48s
PREPARATION H®
Hemorrhoidal Ointment, Cream
and Suppositories

Whitehall

Front   Back
500 mg.

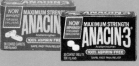

Coated Tablets: Tins of 12, Bottles
of 30, 60 and 100. Coated Caplets:
Bottles of 30, 60 and 100.

MAXIMUM STRENGTH ANACIN-3®
Acetaminophen Tablets and Caplets

Whitehall

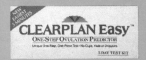

**CLEARPLAN™
OVULATION PREDICTOR**
One-Step Ovulation
Predictor Test

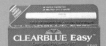

CLEARBLUE EASY™
One-Step Pregnancy Test

Whitehall

Front
Back
Front

Back

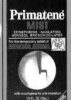

Coated Tablets: Tins of 12, Packages
of 24, 48 and Bottles of 100. Coated
Caplets: Packages of 20 and 40.
**DRISTAN®
COATED TABLETS AND CAPLETS**
Decongestant/Antihistamine/
Analgesic

Whitehall

Available in 15 cc.
Inhaler Unit and
15 cc. and 22.5 cc.
Refills.

PRIMATENE® MIST

Asthma Remedy

Whitehall

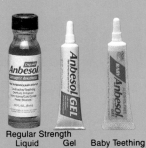

Regular Strength
Liquid
.31 oz.
and
.74 oz.

Gel
.25 oz.

Baby Teething
Gel
.25 oz.

ANBESOL®

Whitehall

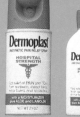

Regular   Mountain
Fresh
Herbal   Shampoo &
Conditioner

4 oz., 8 oz.
& 12 oz.
Bottles

Extra Strength

DENOREX®
Medicated Shampoo

Whitehall

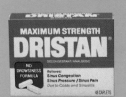

Coated Caplets: Packages of
24, 48 and Bottles of 100.

MAXIMUM STRENGTH DRISTAN®
(acetaminophen 500 mg., pseudoephedrine
HCl 30 mg.)

Whitehall
Regular

Front   Back

P Formula

Front   Back

M Formula

Front   Back

PRIMATENE® TABLETS
Asthma Remedy

Whitehall

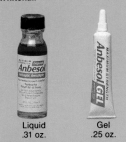

Liquid
.31 oz.

Gel
.25 oz.

**MAXIMUM STRENGTH
ANBESOL®**
Anesthetic for Oral Topical
Pain Relief

Whitehall

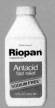

DERMOPLAST®
Anesthetic Pain Relief Spray
and Lotion

Available in 2¾ oz. Spray and
3 oz. Lotion

Whitehall

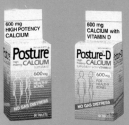

High Potency Calcium Supplement
and High Potency Calcium
Supplement with Vitamin D

Both available in Bottles of 60
POSTURE® and POSTURE®-D
(elemental calcium/Vitamin D)

Whitehall

RIOPAN®
Antacid
(magaldrate)

RIOPAN PLUS®
Antacid plus
Anti-Gas
(magaldrate and
simethicone)

Both products available in 12 fl. oz.
Suspension, Chew Tablets, 60's and 100's,
and Rollpacks. RIOPAN also available
in Swallow Tablets, 60's and 100's.

Whitehall

Available in 12 fl. oz. Suspension and Chew Tablets (60s)

RIOPAN PLUS® 2
High-Potency Antacid plus Anti-Gas
(magaldrate and simethicone)

Winthrop Consumer Products

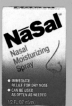

CAMPHO-PHENIQUE®
Cold Sore Gel
.23 oz and .5 oz

Winthrop Consumer Products

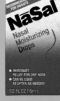

15 ml   15 ml

NāSal™
Nasal Moisturizer
Spray and Drops

WYETH-AYERST

Tamper-Resistant/Evident Packaging
Statements alerting consumers to the specific type of Tamper-Resistant/Evident Packaging appear on the bottle labels and cartons of all over-the-counter products of Wyeth-Ayerst. This includes plastic cap seals on bottles, individually wrapped tablets or suppositories, and sealed cartons. This packaging has been developed to better protect the consumer.

Whitehall

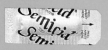

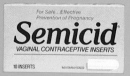

Available in Packages of 10 and 20.

SEMICID®
Vaginal Contraceptive
Inserts

Winthrop Consumer Products

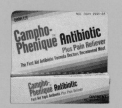

Available in ½ oz and 1 oz tubes

CAMPHO-PHENIQUE®
First Aid Triple Antibiotic plus
Pain Reliever Ointment

Winthrop Consumer Products

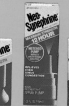

NEO-SYNEPHRINE®
Nasal Decongestant

Spray, Spray Pump or Drops

Wyeth-Ayerst

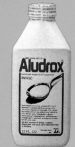

12 Fl. Oz.

ALUDROX® SUSPENSION
Antacid

Whitehall

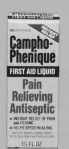

Available in Packages of 3, 6 and 12.

Contraceptive Sponge

TODAY®
Vaginal Contraceptive Sponge

Winthrop Consumer Products

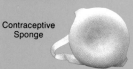

CAMPHO-PHENIQUE®
First Aid Liquid
.75 oz, 1.5 oz, 4 oz

Winthrop Consumer Products

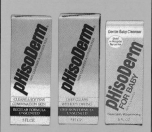

Unscented   Oily Skin   Baby
Regular   Formula   Cleanser
    Available in   5 oz
5 oz, 9 oz (regular), 16 oz
and Lightly Scented
pHisoDerm®

Wyeth-Ayerst

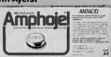

100 tablets

0.6 gram (10 gr.)

AMPHOJEL® TABLETS
and
SUSPENSION
Antacid

12 Fl. Oz.
Also available in 0.3 gram (5 gr.) tablets

WINTHROP

Consumer Products

Available in 15 cc Inhaler Units and 15 cc and 22.5 cc Refills.

Available in packages of 24 and 60 tablets.

BRONKAID®
Mist and Tablets
Asthma Remedy

Winthrop Consumer Products

Available in bottles of
100, 500 and 1,000

FERGON® (IRON)
Tablets

Winthrop Consumer Products

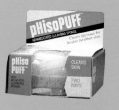

pHisoPUFF®
Exfoliating Sponge

Wyeth-Ayerst

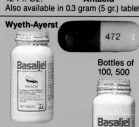

472

Bottles of
100, 500

Bottles
of 100

473

BASALJEL®
TABLETS and CAPSULES

Antacid

Wyeth-Ayerst

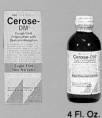

12 Fl. Oz.

**BASALJEL®
SUSPENSION**

Antacid

Wyeth-Ayerst

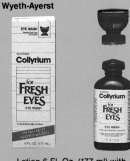

Lotion 6 Fl. Oz. (177 ml) with
separate eyecup bottle cap

**COLLYRIUM for FRESH EYES
Eye Wash**

Wyeth-Ayerst

Also available in
Ready-to-Feed
Liquid and Powder

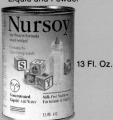

13 Fl. Oz.

Iron Fortified

**NURSOY®
SOY PROTEIN ISOLATE FORMULA
Concentrated Liquid**

Wyeth-Ayerst

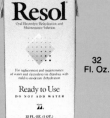

32
Fl. Oz.

**RESOL®
ORAL ELECTROLYTE REHYDRATION
AND MAINTENANCE SOLUTION**
Ready to Use

Wyeth-Ayerst

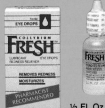

4 Fl. Oz.

CEROSE-DM®

Cough/Cold Preparation
with Dextromethorphan

Also available in 1-pint bottles

Wyeth-Ayerst

½ Fl. Oz. (15 ml)

COLLYRIUM FRESH™

Eye drops with tetrahydrozoline
HCl plus glycerin

Wyeth-Ayerst

12 Suppositories

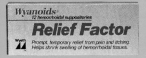

Also available in boxes of 24

**WYANOIDS®
RELIEF FACTOR**
Hemorrhoidal Suppositories

Wyeth-Ayerst

Also available in Ready-to-Feed
Liquid and Powder

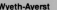

Lo-Iron   Iron
            Fortified

13 Fl. Oz.

S • M • A® INFANT FORMULA
Concentrated Liquid

ZILA

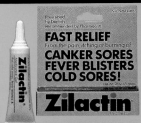

ZILACTIN®
Fast relief from canker sores,
fever blisters, and cold sores.

Also available from Zila
Pharmaceuticals: ZilaBrace for fast
relief from brace sores. ZilaDent for
fast relief from denture sores.

Conversion Tables

Metric Doses With Approximate Apothecary Equivalents

The approximate dose equivalents represent the quantities usually prescribed by physicians using, respectively, the metric and apothecary system of weights and measures. When prepared dosage forms such as tablets, capsules, etc. are prescribed in the metric system, the pharmacist may dispense the corresponding approximate equivalent in the apothecary system and vice versa. (Note: A milliliter [mL] is the approximate equivalent of a cubic centimeter [cc]). Exact equivalents, which appear in the United States Pharmacopeia and the National Formulary, must be used to calculate quantities in pharmaceutical formulas and prescription compounding:

LIQUID MEASURE Metric	Approximate Apothecary Equivalents	LIQUID MEASURE Metric	Approximate Apothecary Equivalents	LIQUID MEASURE Metric	Approximate Apothecary Equivalents	LIQUID MEASURE Metric	Approximate Apothecary Equivalents
1000 mL	1 quart	3 mL	45 minims	30 mL	1 fluid ounce	0.25 mL	4 minims
750 mL	1½ pints	2 mL	30 minims	15 mL	4 fluid drams	0.2 mL	3 minims
500 mL	1 pint	1 mL	15 minims	10 mL	2½ fluid drams	0.1 mL	1½ minims
250 mL	8 fluid ounces	0.75 mL	12 minims	8 mL	2 fluid drams	0.06 mL	1 minim
200 mL	7 fluid ounces	0.6 mL	10 minims	5 mL	1¼ fluid drams	0.05 mL	¾ minim
100 mL	3½ fluid ounces	0.5 mL	8 minims	4 mL	1 fluid dram	0.03 mL	½ minim
50 mL	1¾ fluid ounces	0.3 mL	5 minims				

WEIGHT Metric	Approximate Apothecary Equivalents	WEIGHT Metric	Approximate Apothecary Equivalents	WEIGHT Metric	Approximate Apothecary Equivalents	WEIGHT Metric	Approximate Apothecary Equivalents
30g	1 ounce	30mg	1/2 grain	500mg	7½ grains	1.2 mg	1/50 grain
15g	4 drams	25mg	3/8 grain	400mg	6 grains	1 mg	1/60 grain
10g	2½ drams	20mg	1/3 grain	300mg	5 grains	800 μg	1/80 grain
7.5g	2 drams	15mg	1/4 grain	250mg	4 grains	600 μg	1/100 grain
6g	90 grains	12mg	1/5 grain	200mg	3 grains	500 μg	1/120 grain
5g	75 grains	10mg	1/6 grain	150mg	2½ grains	400 μg	1/150 grain
4g	60 grains (1 dram)	8mg	1/8 grain	125mg	2 grains	300 μg	1/200 grain
3g	45 grains	6mg	1/10 grain	100mg	1½ grains	250 μg	1/250 grain
2g	30 grains (½ dram)	5mg	1/12 grain	75mg	1¼ grains	200 μg	1/300 grain
1.5g	22 grains	4mg	1/15 grain	60mg	1 grain	150 μg	1/400 grain
1g	15 grains	3mg	1/20 grain	50mg	¾ grain	120 μg	1/500 grain
750mg	12 grains	2mg	1/30 grain	40mg	⅔ grain	100 μg	1/600 grain
600mg	10 grains	1.5mg	1/40 grain				

Approximate Household Equivalents

For household purposes, an American Standard Teaspoon is defined by the American National Standards Institute as containing 4.93 ± 0.24 mL. The USP states that in view of the almost universal practice of employing teaspoons ordinarily available in the household for administration of medicine, the teaspoon may be regarded as representing 5 mL. Household units of measure often are used to inform patients of the size of a liquid dose. Because of difficulties involved in measuring liquids under normal conditions of use, household spoons are not appropriate when accurate measurement of a liquid dose is required. When accurate measurement of a liquid dose is required, the USP recommends that a calibrated oral syringe or dropper be used.

1 fluid dram = 1 teaspoonful = 5 mL
2 fluid drams = 1 dessertspoonful = 10 mL
4 fluid drams = 1 tablespoonful = 15 mL
2 fluid ounces = 1 wineglassful = 60 mL
4 fluid ounces = 1 teacupful = 120 mL
8 fluid ounces = 1 tumblerful = 240 mL

Temperature Conversion Table:

$$9 \times °C = (5 \times °F) - 160$$
$$\text{Centigrade to Fahrenheit} = (°C \times 9/5) + 32 = °F$$
$$\text{Fahrenheit to Centigrade} = (°F - 32) \times 5/9 = °C$$

Milliequivalents per Liter (mEq/L)

$$mEq/L = \frac{\text{weight of salt (g)} \times \text{valence of ion} \times 1000}{\text{molecular weight of salt}}$$

$$\text{weight of salt (g)} = \frac{mEq/L \times \text{molecular weight of salt}}{\text{valence of ion} \times 1000}$$

Pounds—Kilograms (kg) Conversion

1 pound = 0.453592 kg
1 kg = 2.2 pounds

SECTION 6
Product Information Section

This section is made possible through the courtesy of the manufacturers whose products appear on the following pages. The information concerning each product has been prepared, edited and approved by the manufacturer.

Products described in this edition comply with labeling regulations. Copy may include all the essential information necessary for informed usage such as active ingredients, indications, actions, warnings, drug interactions, precautions, symptoms and treatment of oral overdosage, dosage and administration, professional labeling, and how supplied. In some cases additional information has been supplied to complement the foregoing. The Publisher has emphasized to manufacturers the necessity of describing products comprehensively so that all information essential for intelligent and informed use is available. In organizing and presenting the material in this edition the Publisher is providing all the information made available by manufacturers.

In presenting the following material to the medical profession, the Publisher is not necessarily advocating the use of any product.

Abbott Laboratories
Pharmaceutical Products Division
NORTH CHICAGO, IL 60064

DAYALETS® Filmtab®
[dāy'a-lets]
Multivitamin Supplement for adults and children 4 or more years of age

DAYALETS® PLUS IRON Filmtab®
Multivitamin Supplement with Iron for adults and children 4 or more years of age

Description: Dayalets provide 100% of the recommended daily allowances of essential vitamins. Dayalets Plus Iron provides 100% of the recommended daily allowances of essential vitamins plus the mineral iron.

Daily dosage (one Dayalets tablet) provides:

VITAMINS			% U.S. RDA
Vitamin A.. (1.5 mg)..	5000	IU	100%
Vitamin D.. (10 mcg).	400	IU	100%
Vitamin E	30	IU	100%
Vitamin C	60	mg	100%
Folic Acid	0.4	mg	100%
Thiamine (Vitamin B_1)	1.5	mg	100%
Riboflavin (Vitamin B_2)	1.7	mg	100%
Niacin	20	mg	100%
Vitamin B_6	2	mg	100%
Vitamin B_{12}	6	mcg	100%

Ingredients: Ascorbic acid, cellulose, dl-alpha tocopheryl acetate, niacinamide, povidone, pyridoxine hydrochloride, riboflavin, thiamine hydrochloride, vitamin A acetate, vitamin A palmitate, folic acid, FD&C Yellow No. 6, cholecalciferol, and cyanocobalamin in a film-coated tablet with vanillin flavoring and artificial coloring added.
Each Dayalets Plus Iron Filmtab® represents all the vitamins in the Dayalets formula in the same concentrations, plus the mineral iron 18 mg (100% U.S. R.D.A.), as ferrous sulfate. Dayalets Plus Iron contain the same ingredients as Dayalets.
These products contain no sugar and essentially no calories.

Indications: Dietary supplement and supplement with iron for adults and children 4 or more years of age.

Administration and Dosage: One Filmtab tablet daily.

How Supplied: Dayalets® Filmtab® in bottles of 100 tablets (NDC 0074-3925-01).
Dayalets® Plus Iron Filmtab in bottles of 100 tablets (NDC 0074-6667-01).
® Filmtab—Film-sealed tablets, Abbott.
Abbott Laboratories
North Chicago, IL 60064
Ref. 02-6903-8/R9, Ref. 02-6906-7/R7

OPTILETS®–500
[op'te-lets]
High potency multivitamin for use in treatment of multivitamin deficiency.

OPTILETS–M–500®
High potency multivitamin for use in treatment of multivitamin deficiency.
Mineral supplementation added.

Description: A therapeutic formula of ten important vitamins, with and without minerals, in a small tablet with the Abbott Filmtab® coating. Each Optilets-500 tablet provides:
Vitamin C
(as sodium ascorbate) ....500 mg
Niacinamide ....100 mg
Calcium Pantothenate ....20 mg
Vitamin B_1
(thiamine mononitrate) ....15 mg
Vitamin B_2 (riboflavin) ....10 mg
Vitamin B_6
(pyridoxine hydrochloride) ....5 mg
Vitamin A (as palmitate
1.5 mg, as acetate 1.5 mg—
total 3 mg) ....10,000 IU
Vitamin B_{12}
(cyanocobalamin) ....12 mcg
Vitamin D
(cholecalciferol) ....(10 mcg) 400 IU
Vitamin E (as dl-alpha
tocopheryl acetate) ....30 IU

Inactive Ingredients: Cellulosic polymers, corn starch, D&C Yellow No. 10, FD&C Yellow No. 6, iron oxide, polyethylene glycol, povidone, stearic acid, talc, titanium dioxide and vanillin.
Each Optilets-M-500 Filmtab contains all the vitamins (vitamin C—ascorbic acid) in the same quantities provided in Optilets-500, plus the following minerals and inactive ingredients:
Magnesium (as oxide) ....80 mg
Iron (as dried ferrous sulfate) ......20 mg
Copper (as sulfate) ....2 mg
Zinc (as sulfate) ....1.5 mg
Manganese (as sulfate) ....1 mg
Iodine (as calcium iodate) ....0.15 mg

Inactive Ingredients: Cellulosic polymers, colloidal silicon dioxide, corn starch, D&C Red No. 7, FD&C Blue No. 1, iron oxide, magnesium stearate, microcrystalline cellulose, polyethylene glycol, povidone, propylene glycol, sorbic acid and titanium dioxide.

Dosage and Administration: Usual adult dosage is one Filmtab tablet daily, or as directed by physician.

How Supplied: Optilets-500 tablets are supplied in bottles of 100 (NDC 0074-4287-13). Optilets-M-500 tablets are supplied in bottles of 30 (NDC 0074-4286-30) and 100 (NDC 0074-4286-13).
®Filmtab—Film-sealed Tablets, Abbott.
Abbott Laboratories
North Chicago, IL 60064
Ref. 07-5628-7/R18, Ref. 07-5627-7/R17

SURBEX®
[sir'bex]
Vitamin B-complex

SURBEX® with C
Vitamin B-complex with vitamin C

Description: Each Surbex Filmtab tablet provides:
Niacinamide ....30 mg
Calcium Pantothenate ....10 mg
Vitamin B_1
(thiamine mononitrate) ....6 mg
Vitamin B_2 (riboflavin) ....6 mg
Vitamin B_6
(pyridoxine hydrochloride)........2.5 mg
Vitamin B_{12} (cyanocobalamin) .....5 mcg
Each Surbex with C Filmtab tablet provides the same ingredients as Surbex, plus 250 mg Vitamin C (as sodium ascorbate).

Inactive Ingredients
Surbex tablets: Cellulosic polymers, corn starch, D&C Yellow No. 10, dibasic calcium phosphate, FD&C Yellow No. 6, magnesium stearate, polyethylene glycol, povidone, propylene glycol, stearic acid, titanium dioxide, and vanillin.
Surbex with C Tablets: Cellulosic polymers, corn starch, D&C Yellow No. 10, FD&C Yellow No. 6, lactose, magnesium stearate, microcrystalline cellulose, polyethylene glycol, povidone, propylene glycol, titanium dioxide, and vanillin.

Indications: Surbex is indicated for treatment of Vitamin B-Complex deficiency.
Surbex with C is indicated for use in treatment of Vitamin B-Complex with Vitamin C deficiency.

Dosage and Administration: Usual adult dosage is one tablet twice daily or as directed by physician.

How Supplied: Surbex is supplied as bright orange-colored tablets in bottles of 100 (NDC 0074-4876-13).
Surbex with C is supplied as yellow-colored tablets in bottles of 100 (NDC 0074-4877-13).
Abbott Pharmaceuticals, Inc.
North Chicago, IL 60064
Ref. 03-1615-5/R11, 03-1616-5/R12

SURBEX–T®
High-potency vitamin B-complex with 500 mg of vitamin C

Description: Each Filmtab® tablet provides:
Vitamin C (ascorbic acid) ....500 mg
Niacinamide ....100 mg
Calcium Pantothenate ....20 mg
Vitamin B_1 (thiamine
mononitrate) ....15 mg
Vitamin B_2 (riboflavin) ....10 mg
Vitamin B_6 (pyridoxine
hydrochloride) ....5 mg
Vitamin B_{12} (cyanocobalamin) ...10 mcg

Inactive Ingredients: Cellulosic polymers, colloidal silicon dioxide, corn starch, D&C Yellow No. 10, FD&C Yellow No. 6, magnesium stearate, microcrystalline cellulose, polyethylene glycol, povidone, propylene glycol, titanium dioxide, and vanillin.

Indications: For use in treatment of Vitamin B-Complex with Vitamin C deficiency.

Dosage and Administration: Usual adult dosage is one Filmtab tablet daily, or as directed by physician.

How Supplied: Orange-colored tablets in bottle of 100 (**NDC** 0074-4878-13). Also supplied in Abbo-Pac® unit dose packages of 100 tablets in strips of 10 tablets per strip (**NDC** 0074-4878-11).
®Filmtab—Film-sealed Tablets, Abbott. Abbott Pharmaceuticals, Inc.
North Chicago, IL 60064
Ref. 03-1483-7/R12

SURBEX®–750 with IRON
High-potency B-complex with iron, vitamin E and 750 mg vitamin C

Description: Each Filmtab® tablet provides:
VITAMINS
Vitamin C (as sodium ascorbate) 750 mg
Niacinamide .... 100 mg
Vitamin B$_6$ (pyridoxine
  hydrochloride) .... 25 mg
Calcium Pantothenate .... 20 mg
Vitamin B$_1$ (thiamine
  mononitrate) .... 15 mg
Vitamin B$_2$ (riboflavin) .... 15 mg
Vitamin B$_{12}$ (cyanocobalamin) 12 mcg
Folic Acid .... 400 mcg
Vitamin E (as dl-alpha tocopheryl
  acetate) .... 30 IU
MINERAL
Elemental Iron (as dried
  ferrous sulfate) .... 27 mg
  equivalent to 135 mg ferrous sulfate

Inactive Ingredients: Cellulosic polymers, colloidal silicon dioxide, FD&C Red No. 3, corn starch, iron oxide, magnesium stearate, microcrystalline cellulose, polyethylene glycol, povidone, and vanillin.

Indications: For the treatment of vitamin C and B-complex deficiencies and to supplement the daily intake of iron and vitamin E.

Dosage and Administration: Usual adult dosage is one tablet daily or as directed by physician.

How Supplied: Bottles of 50 tablets (**NDC** 0074-8029-50).
Abbott Pharmaceuticals, Inc.
North Chicago, IL 60064
Ref. 03-1489-4/R8

SURBEX®–750 with ZINC
High-potency B-complex with zinc, vitamin E and 750 mg of vitamin C. For persons 12 years of age or older

Description: Daily dose (one Filmtab® tablet) provides:

VITAMINS		%U.S. R.D.A.*
Vitamin E	30 IU	100%
Vitamin C	750 mg	1250%
Folic Acid	0.4 mg	100%
Thiamine (B$_1$)	15 mg	1000%
Riboflavin (B$_2$)	15 mg	882%
Niacin	100 mg	500%
Vitamin B$_6$	20 mg	1000%
Vitamin B$_{12}$	12 mcg	200%
Pantothenic Acid	20 mg	200%
MINERAL		
Zinc**	22.5 mg	150%

* % U.S. Recommended Daily Allowance for Adults.
** Equivalent to 100 mg of zinc sulfate.

Ingredients: Ascorbic acid, niacinamide, cellulose, dl-alpha tocopheryl acetate, zinc sulfate, povidone, pyridoxine hydrochloride, calcium pantothenate, riboflavin, thiamine mononitrate, cyanocobalamin, magnesium stearate, colloidal silicon dioxide, folic acid, in a film-coated tablet with vanillin flavoring and artificial coloring added.

Usual Adult Dose: One tablet daily.

How Supplied: Bottles of 50 tablets (**NDC** 0074-8152-50).
Abbott Pharmaceuticals, Inc.
North Chicago, IL 60064
Ref. 03-1490-4/R9

If desired, additional information on any Abbott Product will be provided upon request to Abbott Laboratories.

Adria Laboratories
Division of Erbamont Inc.
7001 POST ROAD
DUBLIN, OH 43017

Professional Labeling
EMETROL®
(Phosphorated Carbohydrate Solution)
For the relief of nausea associated with upset stomach

Description: EMETROL is an oral solution containing balanced amounts of dextrose (glucose) and levulose (fructose) and phosphoric acid with controlled hydrogen ion concentration. Available in pleasant-tasting lemon-mint and cherry flavors.

Ingredients: Each 5 mL teaspoonful contains dextrose (glucose), 1.87 g; levulose (fructose), 1.87 g; and phosphoric acid, 21.5 mg; and the following inactive ingredients: D&C yellow No. 10 (lemon-mint only), natural color (cherry only), flavors, glycerin, methylparaben and purified water.

Action: EMETROL quickly relieves nausea by local action on the wall of the hyperactive G.I. tract. It reduces smooth-muscle contraction in direct proportion to the amount used. Unlike systemic antinauseants, EMETROL works almost immediately to control nausea.

Indications: For the relief of nausea associated with upset stomach. For other conditions, take only as directed by your physician.

Advantages:
1. **Fast Action**—works almost immediately by local action on contact with the hyperactive G.I. tract.
2. **Effectiveness**—reduces smooth-muscle contractions in direct proportion to the amount used—stops nausea.
3. **Safety**—non-toxic—won't mask symptoms of organic pathology.
4. **Convenience**—can be recommended over the phone for any member of the family, even the children—no ℞ required.
5. **Patient Acceptance**—a low cost that patients appreciate—a pleasant lemon-mint or cherry flavor that both children and adults like.

Usual Adult Dose: One or two tablespoonfuls. Repeat every 15 minutes until distress subsides.
For nausea and upset stomach associated with morning sickness: take one or two tablespoonfuls immediately on arising, repeated every three hours or when symptoms threaten.

Usual Children's Dose: One or two teaspoonfuls. Repeat dose every 15 minutes until distress subsides. See *Caution*.

Important: Never dilute EMETROL or drink fluids of any kind immediately before or after taking a dose.

Caution: Not to be taken for more than one hour (5 doses) without consulting a physician. If upset stomach continues or recurs frequently, consult a physician promptly as it may be a sign of a serious condition.
WARNING: KEEP THIS AND ALL MEDICATIONS OUT OF THE REACH OF CHILDREN. As with any drug, if you are pregnant or nursing a baby, seek the advice of a health professional before using this product.
This product contains fructose and should not be taken by persons with hereditary fructose intolerance (HFI).

> **This product contains sugar and should not be taken by diabetics except under the advice and supervision of a physician.**

In case of accidental overdose, contact a poison control center, emergency medical facility, or physician immediately for advice.

How Supplied: Each 5 mL teaspoonful of EMETROL contains dextrose (glucose), 1.87 g; levulose (fructose), 1.87 g; and phosphoric acid, 21.5 mg in a lemon-mint or cherry syrup.
Lemon-Mint
NDC 0013-2113-45—Bottle of 4 fluid ounces (118 mL)
NDC 0013-2113-65—Bottle of 8 fluid ounces (236 mL)
NDC 0013-2113-51—Bottle of 1 pint (473 mL)
Cherry
NDC 0013-2114-45—Bottle of 4 fluid ounces (118 mL)
NDC 0013-2114-65—Bottle of 8 fluid ounces (236 mL)
NDC 0013-2114-51—Bottle of 1 pint (473 mL)

Continued on next page

Adria—Cont.

Store at room temperature.
NOTICE: Each bottle is protected by a printed band around the cap. Do not use if band is damaged or missing.

ADRIA LABORATORIES
Division of Erbamont Inc.
COLUMBUS, OH 43215
Shown in Product Identification Section, page 403

Professional Labeling
MODANE
[mō'dāne]
(phenolphthalein)

Description: MODANE TABLETS (rust red)—Each tablet contains white phenolphthalein 130 mg. Inactive ingredients include acacia, calcium carbonate, calcium sulfate, cornstarch, dibasic calcium phosphate, FD&C Red No. 40 aluminum lake, lactose, magnesium stearate, povidone, shellac, sodium benzoate, sucrose, talc, titanium dioxide, water and carnauba wax.

Clinical Pharmacology: Phenolphthalein, a stimulant laxative, acts primarily on the large intestine to produce a semifluid stool usually in 4–8 hours. It is dissolved by bile salts and alkaline intestinal secretions and may impart a red color to alkaline feces and urine.

Indications: For temporary relief of constipation.

Contraindications: Sensitivity to phenolphthalein.

Warnings: Do not use any laxative preparations when abdominal pain, nausea, or vomiting are present. Frequent and continued use may cause dependence upon laxatives.
KEEP THIS PRODUCT OUT OF REACH OF CHILDREN.
As with any drug, if the patient is pregnant or nursing a baby, she should consult a health professional before using.

Precautions: Phenolphthalein may color alkaline feces and urine red. If skin rash appears, do not use this product or any other preparation containing phenolphthalein.

Adverse Reactions: Excessive bowel activity, usually diarrhea or abdominal discomfort, nausea, vomiting, cramps, weakness, dizziness, palpitations, sweating and fainting may follow the administration of a laxative. Diarrhea may lead to fluid and electrolyte deficits. Allergic reactions, skin rashes attributed to phenolphthalein, have been reported.

Overdosage: Phenolphthalein is relatively nontoxic. Overdosage may be expected to result in excessive bowel activity. Treatment is symptomatic if the duration of effects is prolonged. Fluid and electrolyte deficits might result from prolonged catharsis.

Dosage and Administration:
MODANE Tablet (rust red)—Adults: One tablet daily, or as directed by a doctor. This strength is not recommended for children.

How Supplied: Each MODANE tablet contains white phenolphthalein 130 mg in a rust red, round, sugar-coated tablet printed with A on one side and 513 on the other. Store at room temperature.
Package of 10 tablets
NDC 0013-5131-07
Package of 30 tablets
NDC 0013-5131-13
Bottle of 100 tablets
NDC 0013-5131-17
Shown in Product Identification Section, page 403

Professional Labeling
MODANE PLUS
[mō'dāne plŭs]
(phenolphthalein and docusate sodium)

Description: Each tablet contains white phenolphthalein 65mg and docusate sodium 100mg. Inactive ingredients include acacia, calcium carbonate, calcium sulfate, croscarmellose sodium, FD&C yellow No. 6 aluminum lake, magnesium stearate, microcrystalline cellulose, povidone, shellac, silica gel, sodium benzoate, sucrose, talc, titanium dioxide, water and carnauba wax.
Phenolphthalein is classified as a stimulant laxative. Chemically phenolphthalein is 3,3-bis(p-hydroxyphenyl)phthalide.
Chemically, docusate sodium is butanedioic acid, sulfo-1,4-bis(2-ethylhexyl) ester, sodium salt. It is an anionic surfactant.

Clinical Pharmacology: Phenolphthalein, a stimulant laxative, acts primarily on the large intestine to produce a semifluid stool usually in 4–8 hours. It is dissolved by bile salts and alkaline intestinal secretions and may impart a red color to alkaline feces and urine.
Docusate sodium is classified as a stool softener. It is used in conditions in which it is desirable that the feces be kept soft and straining at the stool be avoided.

Indications: For temporary relief of constipation in adults.

Contraindications: Sensitivity to phenolphthalein. Mineral oil administration.

Warnings: Do not use any laxative preparations when abdominal pain, nausea, or vomiting are present. Frequent and continued use may cause dependence upon laxatives.
KEEP THIS PRODUCT OUT OF REACH OF CHILDREN.
As with any drug, if the patient is pregnant or nursing a baby, she should consult a health professional before using.

Precautions: Phenolphthalein may color alkaline feces and urine red. If skin rash appears, do not use this product or any other preparation containing phenolphthalein.
Docusate sodium may increase the intestinal absorption of mineral oil and/or

hepatic uptake of other drugs administered concurrently.

Adverse Reactions: Excessive bowel activity, usually diarrhea or abdominal discomfort, nausea, vomiting, cramps, weakness, dizziness, palpitations, sweating and fainting may follow the administration of a laxative. Diarrhea may lead to fluid and electrolyte deficits. Allergic reactions, skin rashes attributed to phenolphthalein, have been reported.

Overdosage: Phenolphthalein is relatively nontoxic. Overdosage may be expected to result in excessive bowel activity. Treatment is symptomatic if the duration of effects is prolonged. Fluid and electrolyte deficits might result from prolonged catharsis.

Dosage and Administration:
Adults: One tablet daily, or as directed by a doctor. This strength is not recommended for children.

How Supplied: Each MODANE PLUS tablet contains white phenolphthalein 65 mg and docusate sodium 100 mg in an orange, round, sugar-coated tablet printed with A on one side and 514 on the other.
Package of 10 tablets
NDC 0013-5151-07
Package of 30 tablets
NDC 0013-5151-13
Bottle of 100 tablets
NDC 0013-5151-17
Store at room temperature.
Shown in Product Identification Section, page 403

**Allergan
  Pharmaceuticals**
A Division of Allergan, Inc.
**2525 DUPONT DRIVE
IRVINE, CA 92715**

CELLUVISC™
**(carboxymethylcellulose sodium) 1%
Lubricant Ophthalmic Solution**

Contains: Active: Carboxymethylcellulose sodium 1%. Inactives: calcium chloride, potassium chloride, purified water, sodium chloride, and sodium lactate.

FDA APPROVED USES

Indications: FOR USE AS A LUBRICANT TO PREVENT FURTHER IRRITATION OR TO RELIEVE DRYNESS OF THE EYE.

Warnings: Do not reuse. Once opened, discard. To avoid contamination, do not touch tip of container to any surface. If you experience eye pain, changes in vision, continued redness or irritation of the eye, or if the condition worsens or persists for more than 72 hours, discontinue use and consult a doctor. If solution changes color or becomes cloudy, do not use. Keep this and all drugs out of the reach of children. In case of accidental ingestion, seek professional assistance or contact a poison control center immediately.

Directions: Instill 1 or 2 drops in the affected eye(s) as needed.

How Supplied: Celluvisc™ (carboxymethylcellulose sodium) 1% Lubricant Ophthalmic Solution is supplied in sterile, preservative-free, disposable, single-use containers of 0.01 fluid ounce each, in the following size:
30 SINGLE-USE CONTAINERS—
NDC 0023-4554-30
Shown in Product Identification Section, page 403

LACRI–LUBE® S.O.P.®
(white petrolatum 56.8%, mineral oil 42.5%)
Lubricant Ophthalmic Ointment

Contains: Actives: white petrolatum 56.8%, mineral oil 42.5%. Inactives: chlorobutanol (chloral deriv.) 0.5% and lanolin alcohols.

FDA APPROVED USES

Indications: FOR USE AS A LUBRICANT TO PREVENT FURTHER IRRITATION OR TO RELIEVE DRYNESS OF THE EYE.

Warnings: To avoid contamination, do not touch tip of container to any surface. Replace cap after using. If you experience eye pain, changes in vision, continued redness or irritation of the eye, or if the condition worsens or persists for more than 72 hours, discontinue use and consult a doctor. Keep this and all drugs out of the reach of children. In case of accidental ingestion, seek professional assistance or contact a poison control center immediately.

Directions: Pull down the lower lid of the affected eye and apply a small amount (one-fourth inch) of ointment to the inside of the eyelid.

How Supplied: Lacri-Lube S.O.P. (white petrolatum 56.8%, mineral oil 42.5%) Lubricant Ophthalmic Ointment is supplied in sterile, disposable unit-dose containers of 0.7 g each and sterile, ophthalmic ointment tubes as follows:
24 UNIT-DOSE CONTAINERS—
NDC 0023-0312-01
3.5 g TUBE—NDC 0023-0312-04
7.0 g TUBE—NDC 0023-0312-07
Shown in Product Identification Section, page 403

LACRIL®
(hydroxypropyl methylcellulose 0.5%, gelatin A 0.01%)
Lubricant Ophthalmic Solution

Contains: Actives: Hydroxypropyl methylcellulose 0.5% and gelatin A 0.01%. Inactives: calcium chloride, chlorobutanol (chloral deriv.) 0.5%, dextrose, magnesium chloride, polysorbate 80, potassium chloride, purified water, sodium acetate, sodium borate, sodium chloride, and sodium citrate. May also contain acetic acid to adjust pH.

FDA APPROVED USES

Indications: FOR USE AS A LUBRICANT TO PREVENT FURTHER IRRITATION OR TO RELIEVE DRYNESS OF THE EYE.

Warnings: To avoid contamination, do not touch tip of container to any surface. Replace cap after using. If you experience eye pain, changes in vision, continued redness or irritation of the eye, or if the condition worsens or persists for more than 72 hours, discontinue use and consult a doctor. If solution changes color or becomes cloudy, do not use. Keep this and all drugs out of the reach of children. In case of accidental ingestion, seek professional assistance or contact a poison control center immediately.

Directions: Instill 1 or 2 drops in the affected eye(s) as needed.

How Supplied: Lacril (hydroxypropyl methylcellulose 0.5%, gelatin A 0.01%) Lubricant Ophthalmic Solution is supplied in sterile plastic dropper bottles in the following size:
½ fl oz—NDC 0023-0045-15

LIQUIFILM FORTE®
(polyvinyl alcohol) 3.0%
Lubricant Ophthalmic Solution

Contains: Active: Polyvinyl alcohol 3.0%. Inactives: edetate disodium, mono- and dibasic sodium phosphates, purified water, sodium chloride, and thimerosal 0.002%. May also contain hydrochloric acid or sodium hydroxide to adjust pH.

FDA APPROVED USES

Indications: FOR USE AS A LUBRICANT TO PREVENT FURTHER IRRITATION OR TO RELIEVE DRYNESS OF THE EYE.

Warnings: To avoid contamination, do not touch tip of container to any surface. Replace cap after using. If you experience eye pain, changes in vision, continued redness or irritation of the eye, or if the condition worsens or persists for more than 72 hours, discontinue use and consult a doctor. This product contains thimerosal 0.002% as a preservative. Do not use this product if you are sensitive to thimerosal or any other ingredient containing mercury. If solution changes color or becomes cloudy, do not use. Keep this and all drugs out of the reach of children. In case of accidental ingestion, seek professional assistance or contact a poison control center immediately.

Directions: Instill 1 or 2 drops in the affected eye(s) as needed.

How Supplied: Liquifilm Forte® (polyvinyl alcohol) 3.0% Lubricant Ophthalmic Solution is supplied in sterile plastic dropper bottles in the following sizes:
½ fl oz—NDC 11980-187-15
1 fl oz—NDC 11980-187-30

LIQUIFILM TEARS®
(polyvinyl alcohol) 1.4%
Lubricant Ophthalmic Solution

Contains: Active: Polyvinyl alcohol 1.4%. Inactives: chlorobutanol (chloral deriv.) 0.5%, purified water, and sodium chloride. May also contain hydrochloric acid or sodium hydroxide to adjust pH.

FDA APPROVED USES

Indications: FOR USE AS A LUBRICANT TO PREVENT FURTHER IRRITATION OR TO RELIEVE DRYNESS OF THE EYE.

Warnings: To avoid contamination, do not touch tip of container to any surface. Replace cap after using. If you experience eye pain, changes in vision, continued redness or irritation of the eye, or if the condition worsens or persists for more than 72 hours, discontinue use and consult a doctor. If solution changes color or becomes cloudy, do not use. Keep this and all drugs out of the reach of children. In case of accidental ingestion, seek professional assistance or contact a poison control center immediately.

Directions: Instill 1 or 2 drops in the affected eye(s) as needed.

How Supplied: Liquifilm Tears® (polyvinyl alcohol) 1.4% Lubricant Ophthalmic Solution is supplied in sterile plastic dropper bottles in the following sizes:
½ fl oz—NDC 11980-025-15
1 fl oz—NDC 11980-025-30
Shown in Product Identification Section, page 403

PREFRIN™ Liquifilm®
(phenylephrine HCl 0.12%, polyvinyl alcohol 1.4%)
Vasoconstrictor (Redness Reliever) and Lubricant Eye Drops

Contains: Actives: Phenylephrine HCl 0.12% and polyvinyl alcohol 1.4%. Inactives: benzalkonium chloride, edetate disodium, purified water, sodium acetate, mono- and dibasic sodium phosphates and sodium thiosulfate. May also contain hydrochloric acid or sodium hydroxide to adjust pH.

FDA APPROVED USES

Indications: RELIEVES REDNESS OF THE EYE DUE TO MINOR EYE IRRITATIONS. FOR USE AS A LUBRICANT TO PREVENT FURTHER IRRITATION OR TO RELIEVE DRYNESS OF THE EYE.

Warnings: To avoid contamination, do not touch tip of container to any surface. Replace cap after using. If you experience eye pain, changes in vision, continued redness or irritation of the eye, or if the condition worsens or persists for more than 72 hours, discontinue use and consult a doctor. If you have glaucoma, do not use this product except under the advice and supervision of a doctor. Overuse of this product may produce increased redness of the eye. Pupils may dilate in some individuals. If solution changes color or becomes cloudy, do not use. Keep this and all drugs out of the reach of children. In case of accidental ingestion, seek professional assistance or contact a poison control center immediately.

Note: Not for use while wearing soft contact lenses.

Continued on next page

Allergan—Cont.

Directions: Instill 1 or 2 drops in the affected eye(s) up to four times daily.

How Supplied: Prefrin™ Liquifilm® (phenylephrine HCl 0.12%, polyvinyl alcohol 1.4%) Vasoconstrictor (Redness Reliever) and Lubricant Eye Drops is supplied in sterile plastic dropper bottles in the following size:

0.7 fl oz—NDC 11980-036-07
Shown in Product Identification Section, page 403

REFRESH®
(polyvinyl alcohol 1.4%, povidone 0.6%)
Lubricant Ophthalmic Solution

Contains: Actives: Polyvinyl alcohol 1.4% and povidone 0.6%. Inactives: purified water and sodium chloride. May also contain hydrochloric acid or sodium hydroxide to adjust pH.

FDA APPROVED USES

Indications: FOR USE AS A LUBRICANT TO PREVENT FURTHER IRRITATION OR TO RELIEVE DRYNESS OF THE EYE.

Warnings: Do not reuse. Once opened, discard. To avoid contamination, do not touch tip of container to any surface. If you experience eye pain, changes in vision, continued redness or irritation of the eye, or if the condition worsens or persists for more than 72 hours, discontinue use and consult a doctor. If solution changes color or becomes cloudy, do not use. Keep this and all drugs out of the reach of children. In case of accidental ingestion, seek professional assistance or contact a poison control center immediately.

Directions: Instill 1 or 2 drops in the affected eye(s) as needed.

How Supplied: Refresh® (polyvinyl alcohol 1.4%, povidone 0.6%) Lubricant Ophthalmic Solution is supplied in sterile, preservative-free, disposable, single-use containers of 0.01 fluid ounce each, in the following sizes:

30 SINGLE-USE CONTAINERS—
NDC 0023-0506-01
50 SINGLE-USE CONTAINERS—
NDC 0023-0506-50
Shown in Product Identification Section, page 403

REFRESH® P.M.
(white petrolatum 56.8%, mineral oil 41.5%)
Lubricant Ophthalmic Ointment

Contains: Actives: white petrolatum 56.8%, mineral oil 41.5%. Inactives: lanolin alcohols, purified water and sodium chloride.

FDA APPROVED USES

Indications: FOR USE AS A LUBRICANT TO PREVENT FURTHER IRRITATION OR TO RELIEVE DRYNESS OF THE EYE.

Warnings: To avoid contamination, do not touch tip of container to any surface. Replace cap after using. If you experience eye pain, changes in vision, continued redness or irritation of the eye, or if the condition worsens or persists for more than 72 hours, discontinue use and consult a doctor. Keep this and all drugs out of the reach of children. In case of accidental ingestion, seek professional assistance or contact a poison control center immediately.

Directions: Pull down lower lid of the affected eye and apply a small amount (one-fourth inch) of the ointment to the inside of the eyelid.

How Supplied: Refresh P.M. (white petrolatum 56.8%, mineral oil 41.5%) Lubricant Ophthalmic Ointment is supplied in sterile, preservative-free, ophthalmic ointment tubes in the following size:

3.5 g—NDC 0023-0667-04
Shown in Product Identification Section, page 403

RELIEF®
(phenylephrine HCl 0.12%, polyvinyl alcohol 1.4%)
Vasoconstrictor (Redness Reliever) and Lubricant Eye Drops

Contains: Actives: Phenylephrine HCl 0.12% and polyvinyl alcohol 1.4%. Inactives: edetate disodium, purified water, sodium acetate, mono- and dibasic sodium phosphates and sodium thiosulfate. May also contain hydrochloric acid or sodium hydroxide to adjust pH.

FDA APPROVED USES

Indications: RELIEVES REDNESS OF THE EYE DUE TO MINOR EYE IRRITATIONS. FOR USE AS A LUBRICANT TO PREVENT FURTHER IRRITATION OR TO RELIEVE DRYNESS OF THE EYE.

Warnings: Do not reuse. Once opened, discard. To avoid contamination, do not touch tip of container to any surface. If you experience eye pain, changes in vision, continued redness or irritation of the eye, or if the condition worsens or persists for more than 72 hours, discontinue use and consult a doctor. If you have glaucoma, do not use this product except under the advice and supervision of a doctor. Overuse of this product may produce increased redness of the eye. Pupils may dilate in some individuals. If solution changes color or becomes cloudy, do not use. Keep this and all drugs out of the reach of children. In case of accidental ingestion, seek professional assistance or contact a poison control center immediately.

Note: Not for use while wearing soft contact lenses.

Directions: Instill 1 or 2 drops in the affected eyes(s) up to four times daily.

How Supplied: Relief® (phenylephrine HCl 0.12%, polyvinyl alcohol 1.4%) Vasoconstrictor (Redness Reliever) and Lubricant Eye Drops is supplied in sterile, preservative-free, disposable, single-use containers of 0.01 fluid ounce each, in the following sizes:

30 SINGLE-USE CONTAINERS—
NDC 0023-0507-01
Shown in Product Identification Section, page 403

TEARS PLUS®
(polyvinyl alcohol 1.4%, povidone 0.6%)
Lubricant Ophthalmic Solution

Contains: Actives: Polyvinyl alcohol 1.4% and povidone 0.6%. Inactives: chlorobutanol (chloral deriv.) 0.5%, purified water and sodium chloride. May also contain hydrochloric acid or sodium hydroxide to adjust pH.

FDA APPROVED USES

Indications: FOR USE AS A LUBRICANT TO PREVENT FURTHER IRRITATION OR TO RELIEVE DRYNESS OF THE EYE.

Warnings: To avoid contamination, do not touch tip of container to any surface. Replace cap after using. If you experience eye pain, changes in vision, continued redness or irritation of the eye, or if the condition worsens or persists for more than 72 hours, discontinue use and consult a doctor. If solution changes color or becomes cloudy, do not use. Keep this and all drugs out of the reach of children. In case of accidental ingestion, seek professional assistance or contact a poison control center immediately.

Directions: Instill 1 or 2 drops in the affected eye(s) as needed.

How Supplied: Tears Plus® (polyvinyl alcohol 1.4%, povidone 0.6%) Lubricant Ophthalmic Solution is supplied in sterile, plastic dropper bottles in the following sizes:

½ fl oz—NDC 11980-165-15
1 fl oz—NDC 11980-165-30
Shown in Product Identification Section, page 403

B.F. Ascher & Company, Inc.
**15501 WEST 109th STREET
LENEXA, KS 66219
Mailing address:
P.O. BOX 717
SHAWNEE MISSION, KS
66201-0717**

AYR® Saline Nasal Mist and Drops
[ār]

AYR Mist or Drops restores vital moisture to provide prompt relief for dry, crusted and inflamed nasal membranes due to chronic sinusitis, colds, low humidity, overuse of nasal decongestant drops and sprays, allergies, minor nose bleeds and other minor nasal irritations. AYR provides a soothing way to thin thick secretions and aid their removal from the nose and sinuses. AYR can be used as often as needed without the side effects associated with overuse of decongestant nose drops and sprays.

SAFE AND GENTLE ENOUGH FOR CHILDREN AND INFANTS

AYR Drops are particularly convenient for easy application with infants and children. AYR is formulated to prevent stinging, burning and irritation of delicate nasal tissue, even that of babies.

Directions For Use: SPRAY—Squeeze twice in each nostril as often as needed. DROPS—Two to four drops in each nostril every two hours as needed, or as directed by your physician.

AYR is a specially formulated, buffered, isotonic saline solution containing sodium chloride 0.65% adjusted to the proper tonicity and pH with monobasic potassium phosphate/sodium hydroxide buffer to prevent nasal irritation. AYR also contains the non-irritating antibacterial and antifungal preservatives thimerosal and benzalkonium chloride and is formulated with deionized water.

How Supplied: AYR Mist in 50 ml spray bottles, AYR Drops in 50 ml dropper bottles.

Shown in Product Identification Section, page 403

MOBIGESIC® Analgesic Tablets
[mō'bĭ-jē'zĭk]

Active Ingredients: Each tablet contains 325 mg of magnesium salicylate with 30 mg of phenyltoloxamine citrate.

Also Contains: Microcrystalline cellulose, magnesium stearate and colloidal silicon dioxide which aid in the formulation of the tablet and its dissolution in the gastrointestinal tract.

Indications: MOBIGESIC acts fast to provide relief from the pain and discomfort of simple headaches and colds; for temporary relief of the pain and tension accompanying muscle soreness and fatigue, neuralgia, minor menstrual cramps, T.M.J. and pain of tooth extraction. The unique formula provides relief of pain due to sinusitis and in the fever and inflammation of colds.

Caution: When used for the temporary symptomatic relief of colds, if relief does not occur within 7 days (3 days for fever), discontinue use and consult physician. This preparation may cause drowsiness. Do not drive or operate machinery while taking this medication. Do not administer to children under 6 years of age or exceed recommended dosage unless directed by physician.

Warnings: Keep this and all drugs out of the reach of children. In case of accidental overdose, call your doctor or poison control center immediately. As with any drug, if you are pregnant or nursing a baby, seek the advice of a health professional before using this product.

Usual Dosage: Adults—1 or 2 tablets every four hours, up to 10 tablets daily. Children (6 to 12 years)—1 tablet every 4 hours, up to 5 tablets daily. Do not use more than 10 days unless directed by physician.

Store at room temperature (59°–86°F).

How Supplied: Packages of 18's, 50's and 100's.

Shown in Product Identification Section, page 403

MOBISYL® Analgesic Creme
[mō'bĭ-sĭl]

Active Ingredient: Trolamine salicylate 10%. Also Contains: Glycerin, methylparaben, mineral oil, polysorbate 60, propylparaben, sorbitan stearate, sorbitol, stearic acid, and water.

Description: MOBISYL is a greaseless, odorless, penetrating, non-burning, non-irritating analgesic creme.

Indications: For adults and children, 12 years of age and older, MOBISYL is indicated for the temporary relief of minor aches and pains of muscles and joints, such as simple backache, lumbago, arthritis, neuralgia, strains, bruises and sprains.

Actions: MOBISYL penetrates fast into sore, tender joints and muscles where pain originates. It works to reduce inflammation. Helps soothe stiff joints and muscles and gets you going again.

Warnings: For external use only. Avoid contact with the eyes. Discontinue use if condition worsens or if symptoms persist for more than 7 days, and consult a physician. Do not use on children under 12 years of age except under the advice and supervision of a physician. In case of accidental ingestion, seek professional assistance or contact a Poison Control Center immediately. Close cap tightly. Keep this and all drugs out of the reach of children. Store at room temperature.

Dosage and Administration: Place a liberal amount of MOBISYL Creme in your palm and massage into the area of pain and soreness three or four times a day, especially before retiring. MOBISYL may be worn under clothing or bandages.

How Supplied: MOBISYL is available in 1.25 oz tubes, 3.5 oz tubes, 8 oz jars.

Shown in Product Identification Section, page 403

PEN•KERA® Creme with Keratin Binding Factor
A Therapeutic Creme for Chronic Dry Skin

Ingredients: Water, octyl palmitate, glycerin, mineral oil, polysorbate 60, sorbitan stearate, carbomer 940, triethanolamine, wheat germ glycerides, diazolidinyl urea, polyamino sugar condensate (and) urea, and dehydroacetic acid.

Indications: PEN•KERA Therapeutic Creme for Chronic Dry Skin contains Keratin Binding Factor, a polyamino sugar condensate and urea, which is synthesized to match the same biological components as those found in skin. The Keratin Binding Factor in PEN•KERA Creme replaces the missing elements of

dehydrated skin which absorb and retain moisture. The Keratin Binding Factor actually simulates the natural moisturizing mechanism of the skin, relieving itching, flaking, sensitive, dry skin symptoms.

PEN•KERA is fragrance-free, dye-free, paraben-free, lanolin-free and non-greasy for smooth, fast absorption.

Dosage and Administration: Apply in a thin layer. Because it penetrates quickly and is non-greasy, PEN•KERA may be used under make-up or sun screens. Regular use will reduce the frequency of application and quantity required to achieve moisturized skin.

Precautions: FOR EXTERNAL USE ONLY

How Supplied: PEN•KERA Therapeutic Creme is available in 8 oz. bottles (0225-0440-35).

Shown in Product Identification Section, page 403

UNILAX® Softgel Capsules

Active Ingredients: Docusate sodium, USP 230 mg and yellow phenolphthalein, USP 130 mg.

Inactive Ingredients: D&C Yellow No. 10, FD&C Blue No. 1, FD&C Yellow No. 6, gelatin, glycerin, polyethylene glycol 400, sorbitol and titanium dioxide.

Indications: Constipation (irregularity).

Actions: UNILAX® is a dual-acting stool softener and stimulant laxative.

Warnings: Do not use laxative products when abdominal pain, nausea, or vomiting are present. As with all laxatives, frequent or prolonged use may result in dependence. If skin rash appears, do not use this or any other preparation containing phenolphthalein. As with any drug, if you are pregnant or nursing a baby, seek the advice of a health professional before using this product. Keep this and all drugs out of the reach of children. In case of accidental overdose, seek professional assistance or contact a poison control center immediately.

Dosage and Administration: Adults and children 12 years of age and over: Oral dosage is 1 softgel capsule daily (preferably at bedtime) or as directed by a physician. Do not use in children under 12 years of age.

How Supplied: Bottles of 15 and 60 softgel capsules.

Shown in Product Identification Section, page 403

Products are cross-indexed by generic and chemical names in the
YELLOW SECTION

Astra Pharmaceutical Products, Inc.
50 OTIS ST.
WESTBORO, MA 01581-4428

XYLOCAINE® (lidocaine) 2.5%
[zī'lo-caine]
OINTMENT

For temporary relief of pain and itching due to minor burns, sunburn, minor cuts, abrasions, insect bites and minor skin irritations.

Composition: Diethylaminoacet-2, 6-xylidide 2.5% in a water miscible ointment vehicle consisting of polyethylene glycols and propylene glycol.

Action and Uses: A topical anesthetic ointment for fast, temporary relief of pain and itching due to minor burns, sunburn, minor cuts, abrasions, insect bites and minor skin irritations. The ointment can be easily removed with water. It is ineffective when applied to intact skin.

Administration and Dosage: Apply topically in liberal amounts for adequate control of symptoms. When the anesthetic effect wears off additional ointment may be applied as needed.

Important Warning: *In persistent, severe or extensive skin disorders, advise patient to use only as directed. In case of accidental ingestion advise patient to seek professional assistance or to contact a poison control center immediately. Keep out of the reach of children.*

Caution: *Do not use in the eyes. Not for prolonged use. If the condition for which this preparation is used persists or if a rash or irritation develops, advise patient to discontinue use and consult a physician.*

How Supplied: Available in tube of 35 grams (approximately 1.25 ounces).
Shown in Product Identification Section, page 403

Au Pharmaceuticals
P. O. BOX 811233
DALLAS, TX 75381-1000

AURUM THE GOLD LOTION
Topical Analgesic and Anti-inflammatory
Therapeutic Gold
Topical Analgesic and Anti-inflammatory
TheraGold
Topical Analgesic and Anti-inflammatory

Active Ingredients: The active ingredients are methyl salicylate 10%; menthol 3%; camphor 2.5%. These are combined in a rich, nonpetroleum base for easy and effective topical application.

Other Selected Ingredients: Special inactive ingredients include **24 KARAT GOLD,** Eucalyptus Oil, Jojoba Oil, Ginseng Extract, Urea and Aloe Vera.

Indications: These lotions give fast, deep-penetrating, effective relief from stiff, sore, aching muscles and joints associated with arthritis, bursitis, tendinitis and muscle disorders. These lotions are also effective in reducing inflammation in acute and chronic inflammatory problems within the joints and soft tissues.

Actions: Methyl salicylate, menthol and camphor are classified as counterirritants which combine to provide both heat and cold stimulation to the pain receptors over and around the affected area. The lotions replace the perception of pain with the feeling of heat and/or cold to provide temporary relief of minor aches and pains.

Directions: Apply a liberal amount of lotion to painful area and allow to remain on skin for 30 seconds before rubbing remainder into skin. Apply product 3 or 4 times a day or as needed until pain is relieved, then reduce the frequency to as needed.

Warnings: Use only as directed. For external use only. Avoid contact with eyes, mucous membranes, broken or irritated skin. If condition worsens or persists for more than 7 days without relief, discontinue use of this product and consult a physician. Do not use on children under 2 years of age without consulting a physician.

How Supplied: These products are available in 8 ounce, 2 ounce and 1 ounce bottles.
National Drug Code Registration # 057646-12567.

Ayerst Laboratories
Division of American Home Products Corporation
685 THIRD AVE.
NEW YORK, NY 10017-4071

For information for Ayerst's consumer products, see product listings under Whitehall Laboratories.
Please turn to Whitehall Laboratories, page 743.

Baker Cummins Dermatologicals, Inc.
8800 NORTHWEST 36TH STREET
MIAMI, FL 33178

ACNO® Cleanser

Description: Astringent cleanser for oily skin. ACNO® cleanser is an antiseptic astringent for treatment of acne and other oily skin conditions. It helps remove excess oil and grime and leaves skin feeling fresh and clean.

Ingredients: 60% Isopropyl Alcohol, Water, Laureth-23, Fragrance, Tetrasodium EDTA.

Warnings: FOR EXTERNAL USE ONLY. Keep out of reach of children. In case of accidental ingestion, seek professional assistance or contact a Poison Control Center immediately. Avoid contact with eyes or mucous membranes. FLAMMABLE.

Dosage and Administration: Saturate a cotton pad with ACNO® cleanser and stroke on affected areas. Repeat two to three times daily.

How Supplied: 8 fl. oz. bottle (0575-1009-08).

ACNO® Lotion

Description: ACNO® Lotion was formulated for the management and treatment of acne. It dries acne blemishes and allows skin to heal.

Ingredients: 3% Sulfur, 2% Salicylic Acid.

Warnings: FOR EXTERNAL USE ONLY. Other topical acne medication should not be used at the same time as this medication. Do not get into eyes. If excessive skin irritation develops or increases, discontinue use and consult a doctor or pharmacist. Keep out of reach of children. In case of accidental ingestion, seek professional assistance or contact a Poison Control Center immediately.

Dosage and Administration: Shake well before using. Cleanse the skin thoroughly before applying ACNO® Lotion. Cover the entire affected area with a thin layer one to three times daily. Because excessive drying of the skin may occur, start with one application daily, then gradually increase to two or three times daily if needed or as directed by physician.

How Supplied: 4 fl. oz. bottle (NDC 0575-1008-04).

AQUA–A® Cream

Description: Contains the vitamin A derivative, retinyl palmitate. Moisture-enriched smoothing concentrate. Clinically proven for all skin types.

Ingredients: Water, Caprylic/Capric Triglyceride, Methyl Gluceth-10, Glyceryl Stearate, Squalane, Mineral Oil, PPG-20 Methyl Glucose Ether Distearate, Dimethicone, Stearic Acid, PPG-50 Stearate, Retinyl Palmitate, Sodium Hyaluronate, Lecithin, Sodium Polyglutamate, Ascorbyl Palmitate, Carbomer 934, Dichlorobenzyl Alcohol, Cetyl Alcohol, BHT, Diazolidinyl Urea, Xanthan Gum, Menthol, Sodium Hydroxide, Tetrasodium EDTA.

Directions for Use: Use morning or night or both.

How Supplied: 2 oz. jars (0575-2003-02).
Shown in Product Identification Section, page 404

AQUADERM™ Cream

Description: Ultrarich moisturizing cream concentrate. Softens, smooths, protects, absorbs quickly.

Ingredients: Water, Caprylic/Capric Triglyceride, Methyl Gluceth-10, Glyceryl Stearate, Mineral Oil, Squalane, PPG-20 Methyl Glucose Ether Distearate, Dimethicone, Stearic Acid, PEG-50 Stearate, Sodium Hyaluronate, Lecithin, Sodium Polyglutamate, Magnesium Aluminum Silicate, Carbomer 934, Dichlorobenzyl Alcohol, Cetyl Alcohol, BHT, Diazolidinyl Urea, Xanthan Gum, Menthol, Sodium Hydroxide, Tetrasodium EDTA.

Directions for Use: Apply to face or other dry areas morning or night or both.

How Supplied: 4 oz. jar (0575-2002-04).

Shown in Product Identification Section, page 404

AQUADERM™ Lotion

Description: Ultrarich moisturizing lotion concentrate. Smooths, softens, protects, absorbs quickly. Clinically proven for all skin types.

Ingredients: Water, Caprylic/Capric Triglyceride, Methyl Gluceth-10, Glyceryl Stearate, Dimethicone, Petrolatum, Mineral Oil, PPG-20 Methyl Glucose Ether Distearate, Squalane, PEG-50 Stearate, Stearic Acid, Sodium Hyaluronate, Lecithin, Sodium Polyglutamate, Magnesium Aluminum Silicate, Carbomer 934, Dichlorobenzyl Alcohol, Cetyl Alcohol, BHT, Diazolidinyl Urea, Xanthan Gum, Menthol, Tetrasodium EDTA, Sodium Hydroxide.

Directions for Use: Apply to hands and body morning or night or both.

How Supplied: 7.5 fl. oz. bottle (0575-2001-75).

Shown in Product Identification Section, page 404

P&S® Liquid

Ingredients: Mineral Oil, Water, Fragrance, Glycerin, Phenol, Sodium Chloride, D&C Yellow #11, D&C Red #17, D&C Green #6.

Indications: P&S® Liquid, used regularly, helps loosen and remove crusts and scales on the scalp.

Warnings: FOR EXTERNAL USE ONLY. Do not apply to large portions of body surfaces. Discontinue use if excessive skin irritation develops. Avoid contact with eyes or mucous membranes. Keep out of the reach of children. In case of accidental ingestion, seek professional assistance or contact a Poison Control Center immediately.

Directions for Use: Apply liberally to scalp lesions each night before retiring. Massage gently to loosen scales and crusts. Leave on overnight and shampoo the next morning. Use daily as needed.

How Supplied: 8 fl. oz. bottle (0575-4001-08); 4 fl. oz. bottle (0575-4001-04).

Shown in Product Identification Section, page 404

P&S® PLUS Tar Gel

Active Ingredients: 8% Coal Tar Solution (1.6% Crude Coal Tar, 6.4% Ethyl Alcohol), 2% Salicylic Acid.

Indications: For psoriasis and other scaling conditions. P&S® PLUS relieves the itching, irritation and skin flaking associated with seborrheic dermatitis, psoriasis and dandruff.

Warnings: FOR EXTERNAL USE ONLY. Avoid contact with the eyes; flush with water if product gets into eyes. If irritation develops, discontinue use. If condition worsens or does not improve after regular use of this product as directed, consult a physician. Do not use on children under 2 years of age except as directed by a physician. Use caution in exposing skin to sunlight after applying this product; it may increase your tendency to sunburn for up to 24 hours after application. Do not use product in or around the rectum or in the genital area or groin except on the advice of a physician. Keep this and all drugs out of reach of children. In case of accidental ingestion, seek professional assistance or contact a Poison Control Center immediately.

Directions for Use: Apply to affected areas of skin and scalp daily or as directed by physician.

How Supplied: 3.5 oz. tube (NDC 0575-4009-35).

Shown in Product Identification Section, page 404

P&S® Shampoo

Active Ingredient: 2% Salicylic Acid.

Indications: P&S® Shampoo relieves the itching, irritation and skin flaking associated with seborrheic dermatitis of the scalp. It also relieves the itching, redness, and scaling associated with psoriasis of the scalp. P&S® Shampoo may be used alone as well as following treatment with P&S® Liquid. Its rich conditioning formula improves hair's manageability and helps prevent tangles.

Warnings: FOR EXTERNAL USE ONLY. Avoid contact with eyes or mucous membranes. If this occurs, rinse thoroughly with water. If condition worsens or does not improve after regular use of this product as directed, consult a physician. Do not use on children under 2 years of age except as directed by a physician. Keep this and all drugs out of reach of children. In case of accidental ingestion, seek professional assistance or contact a Poison Control Center immediately.

Directions for Use: For best results use twice weekly or as directed by a physician. Wet hair, apply to scalp and massage vigorously. Rinse and repeat.

How Supplied: 4 fl. oz. bottle (NDC 0575-4007-04).

Shown in Product Identification Section, page 404

PANSCOL® Medicated Lotion and Ointment

Active Ingredients: 3% Salicylic Acid, 0.5% Phenol.

Indications: For dry, scaling skin. PANSCOL® Medicated Lotion and Ointment relieve the itching, irritation and skin flaking associated with seborrheic dermatitis of the body and relieves the itching, redness and scaling associated with psoriasis of the body.

Warnings: FOR EXTERNAL USE ONLY. Avoid contact with the eyes or mucous membranes. If contact occurs, rinse thoroughly with water. Discontinue use if excessive irritation of the skin develops. If condition worsens, or if symptoms persist for more than 7 days, consult a physician before continuing use of this product. Do not use on children under 2 years of age except under the advice and supervision of a physician. Keep out of reach of children. In case of accidental ingestion, seek professional assistance or contact a Poison Control Center immediately.

Directions for Use: Apply a thin layer to the affected areas one to two times daily.

How Supplied: *Lotion:* 4 fl. oz. bottle (NDC 0575-4003-04); *Ointment:* 3 oz. jar (NDC 0575-4005-03).

PHACID™ Shampoo

Description: PHACID™ is a mild, pH-balanced shampoo with a special blend of cleansers and conditioners. This unique formula is especially beneficial for problem hair and scalp conditions.

Ingredients: Sodium Lauryl Sulfate, Disodium Cocamido MIPA-Sulfosuccinate, Isostearoamphopropionate, Water, Propylene Glycol, Phosphoric Acid, Fragrance, Tetrasodium EDTA.

Warnings: FOR EXTERNAL USE ONLY. Keep out of reach of children. Avoid contact with eyes. Flush any lather out of eyes with water.

Directions for Use: Apply to wet hair, work up a good lather, rinse well. Repeat as necessary or as directed by a physician.

How Supplied: 8 fl. oz. bottle (0575-1012-08).

ULTRA DERM® Bath Oil

Ingredients: Mineral Oil, Lanolin Oil, Octoxynol-3, Fragrance.

Indications: A moisture bath for dry, sensitive skin. Relieves the discomfort of dry, chafed or itchy skin by replacing the moisture wind, sun or lack of humidity has removed.

Continued on next page

Baker Cummins Derm.—Cont.

Warnings: FOR EXTERNAL USE ONLY. Take precautions against slipping when used in tub.

Directions for Use:
Bath: 1 to 2 tablespoons in tub of warm water.
Shower: Apply with damp washcloth after showering while body is still wet.

How Supplied: 8 fl. oz. bottle (0575-1002-08).

ULTRA DERM® Moisturizer

Ingredients: Water, Propylene Glycol, Mineral Oil, Lanolin Oil, Petrolatum, Glycerin, Glyceryl Stearate, PEG-50 Stearate, Propylene Glycol Stearate SE, Cetyl Alcohol, Sorbitan Laurate, Potassium Sorbate, Phosphoric Acid, Tetrasodium EDTA, Fragrance.

Indications: For dry, sensitive skin. ULTRA DERM® Lotion combines lubricants and moisturizers in a formula that soothes, smooths and softens dry, itchy skin.

Warnings: FOR EXTERNAL USE ONLY.

Directions for Use: Apply as often as needed or as directed by a physician. Smooths readily into skin.

How Supplied: 8 fl. oz. bottle (0575-1001-08).

ULTRA MIDE 25™ Extra Strength Moisturizer

Ingredients: Water, Urea, Mineral Oil, Glycerin, Propylene Glycol, PEG-50 Stearate, Butyrolactone, Hydrogenated Lanolin, Sorbitan Laurate, Glyceryl Stearate, Magnesium Aluminum Silicate, Propylene Glycol Stearate SE, Cetyl Alcohol, Fragrance, Diazolidinyl Urea, Tetrasodium EDTA.

Indications: Extra strength moisturizer. Helps relieve discomfort of extra dry skin.
Contains ingredients to soften and moisturize areas of very dry, rough, cracked or calloused skin. The unique formula contains a stabilized form of urea (25%) to help prevent the stinging and irritation often associated with moisturizers containing urea. ULTRA MIDE 25 Lotion contains no parabens.

Warnings: FOR EXTERNAL USE ONLY. Keep out of reach of children. Discontinue use if irritation occurs. Caution should be taken when used near the eyes. In case of accidental ingestion, seek professional assistance or contact a poison control center immediately.

Directions for Use: Apply four times daily, or as directed by a physician. Each application should be rubbed in completely.

How Supplied: 8 fl. oz. bottle (0575-4200-08).

X-SEB® Shampoo

Active Ingredient: 4% Salicylic Acid.

Indications: X-SEB® Shampoo relieves the itching and scalp flaking associated with dandruff. Its conditioning formula leaves hair more manageable, with more body.

Warnings: FOR EXTERNAL USE ONLY. Avoid contact with eyes or mucous membranes. If this occurs, rinse thoroughly with water. If condition worsens or does not improve after regular use of this product as directed, consult a physician. Do not use on children under 2 years of age except as directed by a physician. Keep this and all drugs out of the reach of children. In case of accidental ingestion, seek professional assistance or contact a Poison Control Center immediately.

Directions for Use: For best results use twice weekly or as directed by a physician. Wet hair, apply to scalp and massage vigorously. Rinse and repeat.

How Supplied: 4 fl. oz. bottle (NDC 0575-1006-04).
Shown in Product Identification Section, page 404

X-SEB® PLUS Conditioning Shampoo

Active Ingredients: 1% Pyrithione Zinc, 2% Salicylic Acid.

Indications: For dandruff and seborrheic dermatitis. X-SEB® PLUS Shampoo relieves the itching, irritation and skin flaking associated with dandruff and seborrheic dermatitis. X-SEB® PLUS contains the plus of conditioners to leave hair soft and manageable. Pleasant fragrance.

Warnings: FOR EXTERNAL USE ONLY. Avoid contact with the eyes; if this happens, rinse thoroughly with water. Keep this and all drugs out of the reach of children. In case of accidental ingestion, seek professional assistance or contact a Poison Control Center immediately.

Directions for Use: Wet hair, apply to scalp and massage vigorously. Rinse and repeat. If irritation develops, discontinue use. Use at least twice a week for best results or as directed by a physician.

How Supplied: 4 fl. oz. bottle (NDC 0575-1016-04)
Shown in Product Identification Section, page 404

X-SEB® T Shampoo

Active Ingredients: 10% Coal Tar Solution (2% Crude Coal Tar, 8% Ethyl Alcohol), 4% Salicylic Acid.

Indications: X-SEB® T Shampoo relieves the itching, irritation and skin flaking associated with seborrheic dermatitis, psoriasis and dandruff.

Warnings: FOR EXTERNAL USE ONLY. Avoid contact with the eyes; flush with water if product gets in eyes. If

irritation develops, discontinue use. If condition worsens or does not improve after regular use of this product as directed, consult a physician. Do not use on children under 2 years of age except as directed by a physician. Use caution in exposing skin to sunlight after applying this product; it may increase your tendency to sunburn for up to 24 hours after application. Keep out of reach of children. In case of accidental ingestion, seek professional assistance or contact a Poison Control Center immediately.

Directions for Use: Wet hair, apply to scalp and massage vigorously. Rinse and repeat or as directed by a physician.

How Supplied: 4 fl. oz. bottle (NDC 0575-1005-04).
Shown in Product Identification Section, page 404

X-SEB® T PLUS Conditioning Shampoo

Active Ingredients: 10% Coal Tar Solution (equivalent to 2% Crude Coal Tar), 3% Salicylic Acid, 1% Menthol.

Indications: For psoriasis, seborrheic dermatitis and dandruff. X-SEB® T PLUS Shampoo relieves the itching, irritation and skin flaking associated with psoriasis, seborrheic dermatitis, and dandruff. X-SEB® T PLUS contains the plus of conditioners to leave hair soft and manageable. Pleasant color and fragrance.

Warnings: FOR EXTERNAL USE ONLY. Avoid contact with the eyes; if this happens, rinse thoroughly with water. Keep this and all drugs out of the reach of children. In case of accidental ingestion, seek professional assistance or contact a Poison Control Center immediately.

Directions for Use: Wet hair, apply to scalp and massage vigorously. Rinse and repeat. If irritation develops, discontinue use. Use daily until control is achieved. To maintain control, use at least twice a week or as directed by a physician.

How Supplied: 4 fl. oz. bottle (NDC 0575-1015-04).
Shown in Product Identification Section, page 404

IDENTIFICATION PROBLEM?
Consult the
Product Identification Section
where you'll find
products pictured
in full color.

Baker Cummins Pharmaceuticals, Inc.
8800 NORTHWEST 36TH STREET
MIAMI, FL 33178

SNAPLETS-D™
**Taste-Free Granules
Children's Cold and Allergy Formula**

Active Ingredients: Each pre-measured pack contains phenylpropanolamine hydrochloride 6.25 mg and chlorpheniramine maleate 1 mg.

Indications: Provides temporary relief of nasal congestion, sneezing, and runny and stuffy nose due to the common cold and allergies. Temporarily relieves itching of the nose or throat, and itchy, watery eyes due to hay fever or other allergies. Helps drain nasal and sinus passages.

Warnings: Keep this and all drugs out of the reach of children. In case of accidental overdose, seek professional assistance or contact a poison control center immediately. DO NOT EXCEED RECOMMENDED DOSE because at higher doses nervousness, dizziness, or sleeplessness may occur. DO NOT give this product to children for more than seven days. If symptoms do not improve or are accompanied by a fever, consult a doctor. UNLESS DIRECTED BY A DOCTOR, DO NOT give this product to children who have heart disease, high blood pressure, thyroid disease, diabetes, asthma or glaucoma or to children who are taking a prescription drug for high blood pressure or depression. May cause excitability, nervousness and insomnia in some children. May cause drowsiness. DO NOT give this product to children who are taking sedatives or tranquilizers without first consulting the child's doctor.

Dosage and Administration: The suggested dose for pediatric patients is:
Under 2 years—consult physician
2 years to under 6—1 Snaplets pack every 4 hours
6 years to under 12—2 Snaplets packs every 4 hours
Do not exceed 6 doses in 24 hours unless directed by a doctor. To administer, select the proper number of packs based on the child's age. Partially fill a teaspoon with a soft food that the child likes (applesauce, ice cream, jam, etc.). Hold Snaplets pack upright and snap open by bending it back at neck. Sprinkle entire contents of pack(s) onto the soft food in the spoon. Administer entire dose to child immediately (do not give partial contents).

How Supplied: Snaplets-D™ is available in boxes of 30 pre-measured packs (NDC 0575-3030-30).
Shown in Product Identification Section, page 404

SNAPLETS-DM™
**Taste-Free Granules
Children's Cough Formula**

Active Ingredients: Each pre-measured pack contains phenylpropanolamine hydrochloride 6.25 mg and dextromethorphan hydrobromide 5 mg.

Indications: Temporarily relieves cough due to minor throat and bronchial irritation associated with the common cold or inhaled irritants. For temporary relief of nasal congestion due to the common cold and allergies. Helps drain nasal and sinus passages.

Warnings: Keep this and all drugs out of the reach of children. In case of accidental overdose, seek professional assistance or contact a poison control center immediately. DO NOT EXCEED RECOMMENDED DOSE because at higher doses nervousness, dizziness or sleeplessness may occur. DO NOT give this product for more than 7 days. UNLESS DIRECTED BY A DOCTOR, DO NOT give this product to children who have heart disease, high blood pressure, thyroid disease or diabetes, or to children who are taking a prescription drug for high blood pressure or depression. A persistent cough may be a sign of a serious condition. If cough persists for more than 1 week, tends to recur, or is accompanied by a fever, rash or persistent headache, consult a doctor. DO NOT give this product for persistent or chronic cough such as occurs with asthma or if cough is accompanied by excessive phlegm (mucus) unless directed by a doctor.

Dosage and Administration: The suggested dose for pediatric patients is:
Under 2 years—consult doctor
2 years to under 6—1 Snaplets pack every 4 hours
6 years to under 12—2 Snaplets packs every 4 hours
Do not exceed 6 doses in 24 hours. To administer, select the proper number of packs based on the child's age. Partially fill a teaspoon with a soft food that the child likes (applesauce, ice cream, jam, etc.). Hold Snaplets pack upright and snap open by bending it back at neck. Sprinkle entire contents of pack(s) onto the soft food in the spoon. Administer entire dose to child immediately (do not give partial contents).

How Supplied: Snaplets-DM™ is available in boxes of 30 pre-measured packs (NDC 0575-3050-30).
Shown in Product Identification Section, page 404

SNAPLETS-EX™
**Taste-Free Granules
Children's Expectorant**

Active Ingredients: Each pre-measured pack contains phenylpropanolamine hydrochloride 6.25 mg and guaifenesin 50 mg.

Indications: Helps loosen phlegm (sputum) and bronchial secretions and rid the bronchial passages of bothersome mucus. Relieves irritated membranes in the respiratory passageways by preventing dryness through increased mucus flow. For temporary relief of nasal congestion due to colds and allergies. Helps drain the nasal and sinus passages.

Warnings: Keep this and all drugs out of the reach of children. In case of accidental overdose, seek professional assistance or contact a poison control center immediately. DO NOT EXCEED RECOMMENDED DOSE because at higher doses nervousness, dizziness or sleeplessness may occur. DO NOT GIVE this product for more than 7 days. UNLESS DIRECTED BY A DOCTOR, DO NOT give this product to children who have heart disease, high blood pressure, thyroid disease or diabetes, or to children who are taking a prescription drug for high blood pressure or depression. DO NOT give this product to children under 2 years unless directed by a doctor. A persistent cough may be a sign of a serious condition. If cough persists for more than 1 week, tends to recur, or is accompanied by a fever, rash or persistent headache, consult a doctor. DO NOT give this product for persistent or chronic cough such as occurs with asthma or where cough is accompanied by excessive phlegm (sputum) unless directed by a doctor.

Dosage and Administration: The suggested dose for pediatric patients is:
Under 2 years—consult doctor
2 years to under 6—1 Snaplets pack every 4 hours
6 years to under 12—2 Snaplets packs every 4 hours
Do not exceed 6 doses in 24 hours or give to children under 2 years of age unless directed by a doctor. To administer, select the proper number of packs based on the child's age. Partially fill a teaspoon with a soft food that the child likes (applesauce, ice cream, jam, etc.). Hold Snaplets pack upright and snap open by bending it back at neck. Sprinkle entire contents of pack(s) onto the soft food in the spoon. Administer entire dose to child immediately (do not give partial contents).

How Supplied: Snaplets-EX™ is available in boxes of 30 pre-measured packs (NDC 0575-3040-30).
Shown in Product Identification Section, page 404

SNAPLETS-FR™
**Taste-Free Granules
Children's Fever Reducer**

Active Ingredient: Each pre-measured pack contains acetaminophen 80 mg.

Indications: Provides effective temporary relief of fever and minor aches and pains associated with the common cold, "flu," teething, and immunizations.

Warnings: Keep this and all drugs out of the reach of children. In case of accidental overdose, seek professional assistance or contact a poison control center immediately. Prompt medical attention is critical even if you do not notice any

Continued on next page

Baker Cummins Pharm.—Cont.

signs or symptoms. DO NOT give this product for pain for more than five days or for fever for more than three days unless directed by a doctor. If pain or fever persists or gets worse, if new symptoms occur, or if redness or swelling is present, consult a doctor because these could be signs of a serious condition.

Dosage and Administration: The suggested dose for pediatric patients is:
4 months to under 2 years—1 Snaplets pack
2 to under 4 years—2 Snaplets packs
4 to under 6 years—3 Snaplets packs
6 to under 9 years—4 Snaplets packs
9 to under 11 years—4 to 5 Snaplets packs
11 to under 12 years—4 to 6 Snaplets packs
All doses may be repeated every 4 hours while symptoms persist but not more than 5 times daily or as directed by a doctor. Consult your doctor if fever persists for more than 3 days or if pain continues for more than 5 days. To administer, select the proper number of packs based on the child's age. Partially fill a teaspoon with a soft food that the child likes (applesauce, ice cream, jam, etc.). Hold Snaplets pack upright and snap open by bending it back at neck. Sprinkle entire contents of pack(s) onto the soft food in the spoon. Administer entire dose to child immediately (do not give partial contents).

How Supplied: Snaplets-FR™ is available in boxes of 32 pre-measured packs (NDC 0575-3010-32).
Shown in Product Identification Section, page 404

SNAPLETS–Multi™
Taste-Free Granules
Children's Cold Formula

Active Ingredients: Each pre-measured pack contains phenylpropanolamine hydrochloride 6.25 mg, chlorpheniramine maleate 1 mg, and dextromethorphan hydrobromide 5 mg.

Indications: Temporarily relieves cough due to minor throat and bronchial irritation associated with the common cold or inhaled irritants. For temporary relief of nasal congestion, sneezing, runny and stuffy nose due to the common cold and allergies. Temporarily relieves itching of the nose or throat, and itchy, watery eyes due to hay fever or other allergies. Helps drain nasal and sinus passages.

Warnings: Keep this and all drugs out of the reach of children. In case of accidental overdose, seek professional assistance or contact a poison control center immediately. DO NOT EXCEED RECOMMENDED DOSE because at higher doses nervousness, dizziness, or sleeplessness may occur. DO NOT give this product for more than 7 days. UNLESS DIRECTED BY A DOCTOR, DO NOT give this product to children who have heart disease, high blood pressure, thyroid disease, diabetes, asthma or glau-

coma or to children who are taking a prescription drug for high blood pressure or depression. A persistent cough may be a sign of a serious condition. If cough persists for more than 1 week, tends to recur, or is accompanied by a fever, rash or persistent headache, consult a doctor. DO NOT give this product for persistent or chronic cough such as occurs with asthma or if cough is accompanied by excessive phlegm (mucus) unless directed by a doctor. May cause excitability, nervousness and insomnia in some children. May cause drowsiness. DO NOT give this product to children who are taking sedatives or tranquilizers without first consulting the child's doctor.

Dosage and Administration: The suggested dose for pediatric patients is:
Under 2 years—consult physician
2 years to under 6—1 Snaplets pack every 4 hours
6 years to under 12—2 Snaplets packs every 4 hours
Do not exceed 6 doses in 24 hours unless directed by a doctor. To administer, select the proper number of packs based on the child's age. Partially fill a teaspoon with a soft food that the child likes (applesauce, ice cream, jam, etc.). Hold Snaplets pack upright and snap open by bending it back at neck. Sprinkle entire contents of pack(s) onto the soft food in the spoon. Administer entire dose to child immediately (do not give partial contents).

How Supplied: Snaplets-Multi™ is available in boxes of 30 pre-measured packs (NDC 0575-3060-30).
Shown in Product Identification Section, page 404

Bausch & Lomb
PERSONAL PRODUCTS DIVISION
1400 N GOODMAN ST.
ROCHESTER, NY 14692-0450

ALLERGY DROPS
Lubricant/Redness Reliever Eye Drops

Description: BAUSCH & LOMB Allergy Drops is a sterile lubricating eye drop that relieves minor irritation caused by allergens—pollen, dust, animal hair, air pollutants, and other common eye irritants. It relieves redness and keeps on working to protect eyes against further irritation.
Unlike other eye drops, BAUSCH & LOMB Allergy Drops contains a special ingredient that provides longer lasting relief from itching, burning, dry, irritated eyes.

Ingredients: Polyethylene glycol 300 (0.2%), naphazoline hydrochloride (0.012%). Also contains: boric acid, disodium edetate, sodium borate, sodium chloride; preserved with benzalkonium chloride (0.01%).

Indications: Relieves redness of the eye due to minor eye irritations. For the temporary relief of burning and irrita-

tion due to dryness of the eye and for use as a protectant against further irritation, or to relieve dryness of the eye.

Warnings: To avoid contamination, do not touch tip of container to any surface. Replace cap after using. If solution changes color or becomes cloudy, do not use. If you experience eye pain, changes in vision, continued redness or irritation of the eye, or if the condition worsens or persists for more than 72 hours, discontinue use and consult a doctor. If you have glaucoma, do not use this product except under the advice and supervision of a doctor. Overuse of this product may produce increased redness of the eye. Keep this and all medication out of the reach of children.
REMOVE CONTACT LENSES BEFORE USING.

Directions: Instill 1 or 2 drops in the affected eye(s) up to four times daily. Store at room temperature.

How Supplied: In plastic bottles of 0.5 fl oz.
Shown in Product Identification Section, page 404

DUOLUBE
Sterile Lubricant Eye Ointment

Description: White petrolatum 80% and mineral oil 20%. Contains no preservatives.

Indications: For use as a lubricant to prevent further irritation or to relieve dryness of the eye.

Directions: Pull down the lower lid of the affected eye and apply a small amount (one-fourth inch) of Duolube ointment to the inside of the eyelid.

Warnings: To avoid contamination, do not touch tip of container to any surface. Replace cap after using. If you experience eye pain, changes in vision, continued redness, irritation of the eye, or if the condition worsens or persists for more than 72 hours, discontinue use and consult a doctor. KEEP OUT OF REACH OF CHILDREN. NOT FOR USE WITH CONTACT LENSES.
DO NOT USE IF BOTTOM RIDGE OF CAP IS EXPOSED PRIOR TO INITIAL USE.
Store at room temperature.

How Supplied: In ⅛-oz (NDC 10119-020-13) tube.
Shown in Product Identification Section, page 404

EYE WASH
Sterile Isotonic Buffered Solution

Description: A sterile, isotonic solution that contains boric acid, purified water, sodium borate and sodium chloride; preserved with disodium edetate 0.025% and sorbic acid 0.1%. CONTAINS NO THIMEROSAL (MERCURY).

Indications: For cleansing the eye to help relieve irritation, burning, stinging and itching by removing loose, foreign material, air pollutants (smog or pollen) or chlorinated water.

Warnings: To avoid contamination, do not touch tip of container to any surface. Replace cap after using. If you experience eye pain, changes in vision, continued redness or irritation of the eye, or if the condition worsens or persists, consult a doctor. Obtain immediate medical treatment for all open wounds in or near the eyes. If solution changes color or becomes cloudy, do not use.
Use only as directed. If you experience any chemical burns, consult a doctor immediately. KEEP OUT OF REACH OF CHILDREN.

Directions: With Eye Cup—Rinse cup with BAUSCH & LOMB® Eye Wash immediately before and after each use. Avoid contamination of rim and inside surfaces of cup. Fill cup one-half full with BAUSCH & LOMB Eye Wash. Apply cup tightly to the affected eye to prevent spillage and tilt head backward. Open eyelids wide and rotate eyeball to thoroughly wash the eye.
NOTE: Enclosed eye cup is sterile if packaging intact.

Directions: Without Eye Cup—Flush the affected eye as needed, controlling the rate of flow of solution by pressure on the bottle.

How Supplied: In plastic dropper bottles of 4 fl oz, packaged with sterile eye cup.
Shown in Product Identification Section, page 404

MOISTURE DROPS®
Artificial Tears

Description: BAUSCH & LOMB MOISTURE DROPS Artificial Tears quickly provides soothing relief to dry, itchy, burning, irritated eyes. Its unique triple-action formula keeps on working, so your eyes stay moist, healthy, protected against further irritation. And unlike some eye drops, MOISTURE DROPS can be used as often as needed.

Ingredients: Hydroxypropyl methylcellulose (0.5%), dextran 70 (0.1%) and glycerin (0.2%). Also contains: boric acid, disodium edetate, potassium chloride, sodium borate, sodium chloride; preserved with benzalkonium chloride (0.01%).

Indications: For the temporary relief of burning and irritation due to dryness of the eye and for use as a protectant against further irritation, or to relieve dryness of the eye.

Warnings: To avoid contamination, do not touch tip of container to any surface. Replace cap after using. If you experience eye pain, changes in vision, continued redness or irritation of the eye, or if the condition worsens or persists for more than 72 hours, discontinue use and consult a doctor. If solution changes color or becomes cloudy, do not use.
Keep this and all medication out of the reach of children.
REMOVE CONTACT LENSES BEFORE USING.

Directions: Instill 1 or 2 drops in the affected eye(s) as needed.
Store at room temperature.

How Supplied: In plastic bottles of 0.5 fl oz.
Shown in Product Identification Section, page 404

Beach Pharmaceuticals
Division of BEACH PRODUCTS, INC.
5220 SOUTH MANHATTAN AVE. TAMPA, FL 33611

BEELITH Tablets
[bē-lith]
Magnesium Oxide with Vitamin B₆

Description: Each tablet contains magnesium oxide 600 mg and pyridoxine hydrochloride (Vitamin B_6) 25 mg equivalent to B_6 20 mg.

Inactive Ingredients: Castor oil, hydroxypropyl methylcellulose, magnesium stearate, microcrystalline cellulose, pharmaceutical glaze, povidone and sodium starch glycolate. May contain hydroxypropyl cellulose, polyethylene glycol and propylene glycol. Also contains: FD&C Blue #2, D&C Yellow #10, FD&C Yellow #6 (Sunset Yellow), and titanium dioxide.

Warning: Keep this and all drugs out of the reach of children. In case of accidental overdose seek professional assistance or contact a Poison Control Center immediately. As with any drug, if you are pregnant or nursing a baby, seek the advice of a health professional before using this product.

Actions and Uses: BEELITH is a dietary supplement for patients deficient in magnesium and/or pyridoxine. Each tablet yields approximately 362 mg of elemental magnesium & supplies 1000% of the Adult U.S. Recommended Daily Allowance (RDA) for Vitamin B_6 and 90% of the Adult RDA for magnesium.

Dosage: The usual adult dose is one or two tablets daily.

Precaution: Excessive dosage might cause laxation.

Caution: Use only under the supervision of a physician. Use with caution in renal insufficiency.

Drug Interaction Precautions: Do not take this product if you are presently taking a prescription antibiotic drug containing any form of tetracycline.

How Supplied: Golden yellow film coated tablet with the name **BEACH** and the number **1132** printed on each tablet. Bottles of 100 (NDC 0486-1132-01) tablets.

Shown on page 405 in the 1990 PHYSICIANS' DESK REFERENCE

Becton Dickinson Consumer Products
ONE BECTON DRIVE FRANKLIN LAKES, NJ 07417-1883

B–D Glucose Tablets

Indications and Usage: For fast relief from hypoglycemia. B-D Glucose Tablets contain D-Glucose (Dextrose), the most readily absorbed sugar, and are recommended for treatment of hypoglycemia. The tablets are chewable and dissolve quickly in the mouth to facilitate ingestion. Each tablet is 19 calories. When all symptoms have been alleviated, a light meal consisting of a longer acting carbohydrate and protein should be consumed.

Adverse Reactions: No adverse reactions have been reported with appropriate use of glucose. Occasional reports of nausea may be due to the hypoglycemia itself.

Dosage and Administration: The recommended dosage is two (2) to three (3) tablets (10.0 to 15.0 grams of dextrose) at the first sign of hypoglycemia. Repeat dosage as needed to counter additional hypoglycemic episodes that may be caused by longer acting insulins. Dosage may be regulated by taking fewer or more tablets, depending on severity of the reaction, age and body weight. Notify your physician of hypoglycemic episodes. Do not administer to anyone who is unconscious.

How Supplied: Box containing six chewable tablets. Tablets are packaged in durable three tablet blister packs.

Ingredients: Each tablet contains 5.0 grams dextrose. Other ingredients are flavors and tabletting aids: croscarmellose sodium, Type A and magnesium stearate. Contains no preservatives.

EDUCATIONAL MATERIALS

A complete, comprehensive diabetes education teaching system is available to health care professionals. These teaching aids are designed to help the patient and family members understand and manage diabetes. Materials include a series of brochures, patient take-home kits and audio visual aids.

IDENTIFICATION PROBLEM?
Consult the
Product Identification Section
where you'll find
products pictured
in full color.

Beiersdorf Inc
P.O. BOX 5529
NORWALK, CT 06856-5529

AQUAPHOR®
Ointment
NDC Numbers-10356-020-01
            10356-020-02
            10356-020-03
            10356-020-06
            10356-020-07

Composition: Petrolatum, mineral oil, mineral wax, wool wax alcohol.

Actions and Uses: Aquaphor is a stable, neutral, odorless, anhydrous ointment base. Miscible with water or aqueous solutions. Aquaphor will absorb several times its own weight, forming smooth, creamy water-in-oil emulsions. In its pure form, Aquaphor is recommended for use as a topical preparation to help soothe, protect and heal minor cuts and burns. Helps heal and protect chapped, cracked and extremely dry skin and lips.

Administration and Dosages: Use Aquaphor alone or in compounding virtually any ointment using aqueous solutions alone or in combination with other oil-based substances, and all common topical medications. Apply Aquaphor liberally to affected area. In the case of wounds, clean area prior to application.

Precautions: For external use only. Avoid contact with eyes. Not to be applied over third-degree burns, deep or puncture wounds, infections or lacerations. If condition worsens or does not improve within 7 days, patient should consult a doctor.

How Supplied:
1.75 oz. tube—List No. 45583
3.25 oz. jar—List No. 45584
16 oz. jar—List No. 45585
5 lb. jar—List No. 45586
Shown in Product Identification Section, page 404

BASIS® Soap
Combination Skin

Active Ingredient: Basis contains Acetulated Lanolin Alcohol, a special lanolin-derived emollient with sebum-solving properties to help remove excess oil in areas of the skin requiring additional cleansing.

Composition: A special formulation designed to clean all areas of your patients' combination skin gently and thoroughly. Contains a light fragrance and is noncomedogenic.

Action and Uses: This Basis formula has more cleansing ingredients to remove excess oil from oily areas of the face. Basis Combination Skin also contains the unique Basis Emollient System, to leave dry and normal areas soft, fresh and glowing—never overly dry.

Administration and Dosage: To be used twice or three times daily by patients with combination skin, as a facial cleanser. Since it is equally effective on dry and oily areas of the skin, it may also be used in the bath or shower as a gentle allover cleanser.

How Supplied: 1-, 3- and 5-oz. bars.
Shown in Product Identification Section, page 404

BASIS® Soap
Extra Dry Skin

Active Ingredient: Methyl Gluceth-20, an extra emollient chosen for its extreme mildness to the skin, as well as for its excellent cleansing and moisturizing properties. This emollient helps Basis Extra Dry smooth and soften even chapped extra-dry skin.

Composition: A mild, gentle natural soap product, formulated specifically to help moisturize dry, parched or chapped skin as it cleans. Contains a light fragrance, and is noncomedogenic.

Action and Uses: Basis Extra Dry Skin softens roughened or chapped skin by helping it retain its natural oils, while cleaning gently and thoroughly. Because of its extreme gentleness, Basis Extra Dry is an ideal hand soap for those who must wash often, such as doctors or nurses. It is also a very good choice for elderly patients' dry skin.

Administration and Dosage: To be used twice daily by elderly patients or patients with dry skin, as a moisturizing cleanser—for the face or hands—or to be used all over in the bath or shower.

How Supplied: 1-, 3- and 5-oz. bars.
Shown in Product Identification Section, page 404

BASIS® Soap
Normal to Dry Skin

Composition: Contains the unique Basis Emollient System, including coconut oil, petrolatum, lanolin alcohol and glycerin. Basis is a natural soap product containing sodium salts of fatty acids. Contains a light fragrance and is noncomedogenic.

Action and Uses: A mild, gentle non-drying cleanser—gentle enough to use on facial skin, yet effective enough to use all over. Because it is a natural soap product, Basis leaves no potentially irritating synthetic detergent residues on the skin and has been shown not to increase skin roughness or markedly change the pH value of the skin.

Administration and Dosage: To be used twice or three times daily by patients with normal or slightly dry skin, as a facial cleanser. For additional benefits, Basis may also be used in the bath or shower for allover cleansing and moisturizing.

How Supplied: 1-, 3- and 5 oz. bars.
Shown in Product Identification Section, page 404

BASIS® Soap
Sensitive Skin

Active Ingredient: Bisabolol, a proven anti-inflammatory agent found in chamomile, which acts to soothe and calm skin ordinarily irritated by washing with harsh soaps or cleansers.

Composition: An unscented, natural soap product, with emollients and one active ingredient, formulated to be extremely mild, effective and nonirritating. Basis Soap is noncomedogenic.

Action and Uses: Specially formulated to clean, smooth and soothe the skin of patients who tend to sting, itch or blotch after using regular soaps or toiletries—contains bisabolol, a gentle anti-inflammatory agent, to calm sensitive skin. Also for patients whose skin tends to be irritated by fragrance; ideal for children's skin.

Administration and Dosage: To be used twice daily by patients with sensitive skin, or children, as a facial cleanser. For additional benefits, patients may also use it in the bath or shower for allover cleansing and moisturizing.

How Supplied: 1-, 3- and 5-oz. bars.
Shown in Product Identification Section, page 404

EUCERIN® Cleansing Bar
[ū 'sir-in]
Unscented Moisturizing Formula

Composition: Sodium Cocoylisethionate. Triple Pressed Stearic Acid, Hydrogenated Tallow Fatty Acids, Water, Cocoamide, Petrolatum, Glycerine, Sodium Thiosulfate, Titanium Dioxide, Sodium Chloride, Lanolin Alcohol, Beeswax.

Actions and Uses: Eucerin® Cleansing Bar has been specially formulated for use on sensitive skin. The formulation contains Eucerite®, a special blend of ingredients that closely resemble the natural oils of the skin, thus providing excellent moisturizing properties. This formulation is unscented and noncomedogenic. Additional, the pH value of Eucerin Cleansing Bar is maintained at 5.5 in order to match the skin's normal acid mantle.

Directions: Use during shower, bath, or regular cleansing, or as directed by physician.

How Supplied: 3 ounce bar—List number 3852
Shown in Product Identification Section, page 404

EUCERIN® Creme
[ū 'sir-in]
Unscented Moisturizing Formula
NDC Numbers-10356-090-01
            10356-090-05
            10356-090-04

Composition: Water, petrolatum, mineral oil, mineral wax, wool wax alcohol, methylchloroisothiazolinone-methylisothiazolinone.

Actions and Uses: A gentle, non-comedogenic, unscented water-in-oil emulsion, Eucerin helps alleviate excessively dry skin and may be helpful in conditions such as chapped or chafed skin, sunburn, windburn, and itching associated with dryness.

Directions: Apply freely to affected areas of the skin as often as necessary or as directed by physician.

Precautions: For external use only.

How Supplied:
16 oz. jar—List Number 0090
8 oz. jar—List Number 3774
4 oz. jar—List Number 3797
*Shown in Product Identification
Section, page 404*

EUCERIN® Lotion
[*ū'sir-in*]
Unscented Moisturizing Formula
NDC Numbers-10356-793-01
                10356-793-04
                10356-793-06

Composition: Water, Mineral Oil, Isopropyl Myristate, PEG-40 Sorbitan Peroleate, Lanolin Acid Glycerin Ester, Sorbitol, Propylene Glycol, Cetyl Palmitate, Magnesium Sulfate, Aluminum Stearate, Lanolin Alcohol, BHT, Methylchloroisothiazolinone-Methylisothiazolinone.

Actions and Uses: Eucerin Lotion is a noncomedogenic, unscented, unique water-in-oil formulation that will help to alleviate and soothe excessively dry skin, and provide long-lasting moisturization.

Directions: Apply Eucerin Lotion all over body—hands arms, legs and feet—to help moisturize, smooth and soothe rough, dry skin.

Precautions: For external use only.

How Supplied:
4 fluid oz. plastic bottle—List Number 3771
8 fluid oz. plastic bottle—List Number 3793
16 fluid oz. plastic bottle—List number 3794
*Shown in Product Identification
Section, page 404*

NIVEA® BATH SILK
Moisturizing Bath Oil

Special Ingredients: Contains four different types of emollient oils: mineral oil; isohexadecane; soybean oil and castor oil; and octyldodecanol.

Composition: Nivea Bath Silk Bath Oil was specially developed to replace four of the natural classes of skin oils lost through bathing. It is a fragrant bath oil additive, containing four types of emollient oils, plus Eucerite®, the unique Beiersdorf emollient, for extra moisturizing.

Action and Uses: Whereas other bath oils contain only one emollient—mineral oil—Nivea Bath Silk contains *four different types* of emollient oils, thereby replac-

ing four of the major classes of lipids found in human sebum.
With repeated application, Nivea Bath Silk has been shown to increase the skin's moisture level over 24 hours. It can be recommended as a convenient whole-body moisturizer in patients with xerosis, before or after radiation therapy, or in infants with skin disorders related to dryness (i.e., cradle cap, etc.).

Administration and Dosage: To be added to the bath according to package instructions, as often as desired, to moisturize skin dried by the effects of bathing. May also be applied directly to the skin when showering. Especially effective when followed by an application of the appropriate Nivea Moisturizer.

How Supplied: 8-oz. bottle.

NIVEA® BATH SILK
Moisturizing Foam Bath & Shower Gel
Extra-Dry Skin

Special Ingredients: Contains twice the amount of the skin-caring ingredients found in Nivea Bath Silk Gel for normal-to-dry skin, including: two lipid components, a hydrolyzed protein derivative, and aloe.

Composition: A lightly scented moisturizing gel, for use in the bath or shower.

Action and Uses: Designed to clean gently while helping to retain the skin's natural moisturization level during bathing or showering for extra-dry skin.

Administration and Dosage: To be added to the bath according to package instructions, as often as desired, to help moisturize extra-dry skin. In the shower, Nivea Bath Silk Gel should be applied directly to the skin as a cleanser, then rinsed. Moisturizing is especially effective when followed with an application of the appropriate Nivea moisturizer.

How Supplied: 8-oz. bottle.

NIVEA® BATH SILK
Moisturizing Foam Bath & Shower Gel
Normal-to-Dry Skin

Special Ingredients: Contains two lipid components: Eucerite®, very similar to the skin's natural sebum; and PEG-7-glyceryl-cocoate, a modified triglyceride with hydrophilic properties. Also contains a hydrolyzed protein derivative, to help neutralize the effect of any detergent left on the skin, and aloe.

Composition: A mild, lightly scented moisturizing gel, for use in the bath or shower.

Action and Uses: Designed to clean gently while helping to retain the skin's natural moisturization level during bathing or showering for normal or slightly dry skin.

Administration and Dosage: To be added to the bath according to package instructions, as often as desired, to help

keep the natural moisture level of normal or slightly dry skin. In the shower, Nivea Bath Silk Gel should be applied as a cleanser directly to the skin and then rinsed off. Moisturizing is especially effective when followed with an application of the appropriate Nivea moisturizer.

How Supplied: 8-oz. bottle.

NIVEA® Moisturizing Creme

Composition: An extremely mild water-in-oil moisturizing creme, proven to be virtually nonirritating and safe for most patients with dry skin. Contains the unique Eucerite®, an emollient which has been shown to be unlike other common emulsifiers essentially free from irritancy. Noncomedogenic, with a light fragrance.

Action and Uses: For deep conditioning of hard-to-moisturize dry skin—especially useful on knees, feet, elbows and hands. Regular use of Nivea Creme has been shown to significantly improve the barrier function of the skin, as shown by reduced stinging reactions to lactic acid; markedly reduced transepidermal water loss; and a significant lowering of the amount of water-extractable amino acids from the skin during washing. Furthermore, Nivea Creme has been demonstrated to increase significantly the moisture content of the skin. Noncomedogenic, so it is ideal for facial use. Especially effective as a winter moisturizer, for moderate dry skin conditions such as xerosis, and for aging skin.

Administration and Dosage: To be used twice a day, or as often as needed, on dry skin on the hands, body or face. Particularly effective when used after bathing.

How Supplied: 4- and 6-oz. jars, and 2-oz. tube.
*Shown in Product Identification
Section, page 404*

NIVEA® Moisturizing Lotion
Extra Enriched Formula

Composition: A nongreasy but highly effective water-in-oil moisturizing lotion, created specifically for the treatments of extra-dry skin. Contains the unique Beiersdorf emollient, Eucerite®, which has been shown to reduce significantly the skin's transepidermal water loss. Noncomedogenic, with a light fragrance.

Action and Uses: For effective and long-lasting moisturizing of very dry skin on the hands and body. Because it is rapidly absorbed and noncomedogenic, Nivea Extra Enriched Lotion is also a good choice for facial use. Efficacy is due to the unique water-in-oil emulsion rather than to any active ingredients which could cause sensitization or unwanted reactions. Moisturization effects last at least 12 hours per application with continued use—longer than with standard oil-in-water formulations. Es-

Continued on next page

Beiersdorf—Cont.

pecially effective as a winter moisturizer, for moderate dry skin conditions such as xerosis, and for aging skin.

Administration and Dosage: To be used twice a day, or as often as needed, on the hands, body or face. Particularly effective when used after bathing.

How Supplied: 4-, 8- and 12-oz. bottles.
Shown in Product Identification Section, page 404

NIVEA® Moisturizing Lotion
Original Formula

Composition: A mild, light moisturizing lotion with a cooling, nongreasy feeling—ideal for daily moisturizing of normal or slightly dry skin. Contains the highly effective and unique Beiersdorf emollient, Eucerite®, which has been shown to reduce significantly the skin's transepidermal water loss. Noncomedogenic, with a light scent.

Action and Uses: Formulated to maintain the moisture content of healthy or slightly dry skin on the hands and body. Suitable for facial use, because it is noncomedogenic. Excellent as a summer moisturizer, when a lighter lotion may be preferred.

Administration and Dosage: To be used twice a day, or as needed, to maintain the moisture content of healthy normal skin—or to moisturize slightly dry skin—on the hands, body or face. Particularly effective when used after bathing.

How Supplied: 4-, 8- and 12-oz. bottles.
Shown in Product Identification Section, page 404

NIVEA® Moisturizing Oil

Composition: An extra effective moisturizing treatment for severely dry skin. Recently reformulated as an emulsion, so it is rapidly absorbed and nongreasy. Contains the unique Beiersdorf emollient, Eucerite®, which has been shown to reduce significantly the skin's transepidermal water loss. Noncomedogenic, with a light fragrance.

Action and Uses: Developed as an ultraeffective water-in-oil moisturizing emulsion to replace moisture in severely dry skin. Also useful as a cosmetic for patients who desire a glossy look after moisturizing. An ideal preparation to use for massage, especially for bedridden patients.

Administration and Dosage: For maximum efficacy, Nivea Moisturizing Oil should be applied after the shower or bath to areas of dry skin, while skin is still slightly damp. Also recommended as an effective overnight treatment. May be applied to skin as a lubricant before and during massage treatments. Alternatively, Nivea Moisturizing Oil may be used twice daily as an allover moisturizer, or applied as desired to add a cosmetic gloss to the skin.

How Supplied: 4-, 8- and 12-oz. bottles.
Shown in Product Identification Section, page 404

NIVEA® SUN
Moisturizing After Sun Lotion

Composition: A soothing, refreshing, light moisturizing lotion which contains alcohol, aloe and Eucerite®, the unique Beiersdorf emollient, which has been shown to reduce significantly the skin's transepidermal water loss. Lightly scented, rapidly absorbed, and noncomedogenic.

Action and Uses: Has a cooling effect on sunburned or parched skin. Moisturizes sun-exposed skin. Particularly effective used after bathing or showering.

Administration and Dosage: Recommended for use after coming in from the sun on sun-exposed or sunburned skin. May be used as often as desired. May be used on the face.

How Supplied: 4-oz. bottle.

NIVEA® SUN
SPF 15

Active Ingredients: Octyl Methoxycinnamate. Oxybenzone. Padimate O. 2-Phenylbenzimidazole-5-sulfonic Acid.

Composition: Nivea Sun adds effective sunblocking agents to a rich, moisturizing Nivea base, provides full UVA/UVB protection and has an SPF of 15. Nivea Sun contains emollients and moisturizers, including Eucerite®, the unique Beiersdorf emollient, which has been shown to reduce significantly the skin's transepidermal water loss. Noncomedogenic and lightly scented.

Action and Uses: Liberal and regular use of this product may help reduce premature aging and wrinkling of the skin, and skin cancer, due to long-term overexposure to the sun. Nivea Sun SPF 15 is noncomedogenic, so it is ideal for year-round daily facial use, as a moisturizing base under makeup.

Administration and Dosage: To be applied liberally during and before exposure to the sun. Must be reapplied after swimming. May also be recommended for year-round use on all sun-exposed areas of the skin.

How Supplied: In 4-oz. bottles.

NIVEA® VISAGE
Facial Nourishing Creme

Active Ingredients: Octyl Methoxycinnamate (2.7%). Benzophenone-3 (0.5%). These sunscreens give Nivea Visage Creme an SPF of 5.

Other Special Ingredients: Also contains aloe extract, tocopheryl acetate (Vitamin E USP), and Eucerite®, the unique Beiersdorf emollient, which has been shown to reduce significantly the skin's transepidermal water loss.

Composition: A rapidly absorbed but rich and effective moisturizing creme for the face. Contains emollients, aloe and Vitamin E for extra nourishment. Also contains an SPF 5 sunscreen to guard against damage and aging caused by UVA and UVB rays. Contains no other active ingredients, which could cause sensitization or unwanted reactions. Noncomedogenic, so it will not cause adult-onset acne. Lightly scented.

Action and Uses: Nivea Visage Creme was specially developed to replenish moisture lost from dried and aging facial skin. The creme form is particularly appropriate for winter moisturizing or for the more dry and sensitive areas of the face. A good choice for patients who have experienced adult-onset acne from using other, heavier products. Also recommended for younger patients who want a rich facial moisturizer that provides UVA/UVB protection.

Administration and Dosage: To be used on aging or extra-dry facial skin twice daily after washing, morning and evening, as a nourishing, protective moisturizer.

How Supplied: 2-oz. jars.

NIVEA® VISAGE
Facial Nourishing Lotion

Active Ingredients: Octyl Methoxycinnamate (2.7%). Benzophenone-3 (0.5%). These sunscreens give Nivea Visage Lotion an SPF of 5.

Other Special Ingredients: Also contains aloe extract, tocopheryl acetate (Vitamin E USP), and Eucerite®, the unique Beiersdorf emollient, which has been shown to reduce significantly the skin's transepidermal water loss.

Composition: A light, rapidly absorbed moisturizing lotion for the face. Contains emollients, aloe and Vitamin E for extra moisturization and protection. Also contains an SPF 5 sunscreen to guard against damage and aging caused by UVA and UVB rays. Contains no other active ingredients, which could cause sensitization or unwanted reactions. Noncomedogenic, so it will not cause adult-onset acne. Lightly scented.

Action and Uses: Nivea Visage Lotion was specially developed to replenish moisture lost from dry or aging facial skin. The lotion form is particularly appropriate for light summer moisturizing or for normal or slightly dry areas of the face. An ideal replacement product for patients who have experienced adult-onset acne as a result of using heavier facial preparations. Also recommended for younger patients who need UVA/UVB protection.

Administration and Dosage: To be used on facial skin twice daily, morning and evening after washing, as a nourishing, protective moisturizer.

How Supplied: 4-oz. bottles.

How Supplied: 4-, 8- and 12-oz. bottles.
Shown in Product Identification Section, page 404

Benson Pharmacal Co.
Div. of American Victor Co., Inc.
431 HEMPSTEAD AVENUE
WEST HEMPSTEAD, NY 11552

ALTOCAPS–400 CAPSULES
Vitamin E

Active Ingredient: Each capsule contains 400 mg vitamin E (*dl*-alpha-tocopheryl acetate) equivalent to 400 IU.

Inactive Ingredients: Excipient—soybean oil. Shell Ingredients—gelatin, glycerin, water.

Indication: As a vitamin E supplement.

Action: A main characteristic of vitamin E is its action as an antioxidant, preserving the wall membrane of body cells against adverse oxidation reactions.

Precaution: Keep out of the reach of children.

Dosage: Adults—one capsule daily or as directed by a physician.

How Supplied: Bottles of 25 soft-gel capsules.

ROYGEL 100 MG CAPSULES
Royal Jelly Plus Vitamin B Complex

Description: Royal jelly "Queen Bee Food" is a natural source rich in vitamin B complex, proteins, amino acids, fatty acids, major and trace elements; hence it has a high nutritional value.

Active Ingredients: Each capsule contains royal jelly 100 mg, vitamin B_1 10 mg, vitamin B_2 5 mg, vitamin B_6 1 mg, vitamin C 50 mg, vitamin B_{12} 3 μg, niacinamide, 30 mg, pantothenic acid 2 mg.

Inactive Ingredients: Excipients—refined soybean oil, hydrogenated vegetable oil, lecithin, beeswax. Shell Ingredients—gelatin, glycerin, purified water, titanium dioxide, methylparaben, propylparaben, FD&C Yellow No. 5, FD&C Red No. 40.

Indication: As a dietary supplement.

Precaution: Keep out of the reach of children.

Dosage: Adults—one capsule daily in the morning hours or as directed by a physician.

How Supplied: Bottles of 30 soft-gel capsules.

ROYGEL ULTIMA CAPSULES
Royal Jelly, Ginseng, Wheat Germ Oil

Active Ingredients: Each capsule contains royal jelly 100 mg, Korean ginseng powder 250 mg, wheat germ oil 100 mg.

Inactive Ingredients: Excipients—refined soybean oil, hydrogenated vegetable oil, beeswax, lecithin. Shell Ingredients—gelatin, glycerin, purified water, titanium dioxide, FD&C Red No. 40, methylparaben, propylparaben.

Indication: As a dietary supplement.

Precaution: Keep out of the reach of children.

Dosage: Adults—one capsule daily or as directed by a physician.

How Supplied: Bottles of 30 soft-gel capsules.

Blaine Company, Inc.
2700 DIXIE HIGHWAY
FT. MITCHELL, KY 41017

MAG–OX 400

Description: Each tablet contains Magnesium Oxide 400 mg. U.S.P. (Heavy), or 241.3 mg. Elemental Magnesium (19.86 mEq.)

Indications and Usage: Hypomagnesemia, magnesium deficiencies and/or magnesium depletion resulting from malnutrition, restricted diet, alcoholism or magnesium depleting drugs. An antacid. For increasing urinary magnesium excretion.

Warnings: Do not use this product except under the advice and supervision of a physician if you have a kidney disease. May have laxative effect.

Dosage: Adult dose 1 or 2 tablets daily or as directed by a physician.

Professional Labeling: Mag-Ox 400 Tablets for recurring calcium oxalate urinary calculi.
MAGNESIUM OXIDE U.S.P. is indicated in the reduction of crystalluria and calcium oxalate excretion in patients with recurring calcium oxalate lithiasis and to reduce the incidence of calculus formation in idiopathic, recurrent stone formers.

How Supplied: Bottles of 100 and 1000.

URO–MAG

Description: Each capsule contains Magnesium Oxide 140 mg. U.S.P. (Heavy), or 84.5 mg. Elemental Magnesium (6.93 mEq.)

Indications and Usage: Hypomagnesemia, magnesium deficiencies and/or magnesium depletion resulting from malnutrition, restricted diet, alcoholism or magnesium depleting drugs. An antacid. For increasing urinary magnesium excretion.

Warnings: Do not use this product except under the advice and supervision of a physician if you have a kidney disease. May have laxative effect.

Dosage: Adult dose 3–4 capsules daily or as directed by a physician.

Professional Labeling: URO-MAG Capsules for recurring calcium oxalate urinary calculi.
MAGNESIUM OXIDE U.S.P. is indicated in the reduction of crystalluria and calcium oxalate excretion in patients with recurring calcium oxalate lithiasis and to reduce the incidence of calculus formation in idiopathic, recurrent stone formers.

Dosage: Adults—one capsule daily or as directed by a physician.

How Supplied: Bottles of 30 soft-gel capsules.

How Supplied: Bottles of 100 and 1000.

EDUCATIONAL MATERIAL

Samples and literature available to physicians upon request.

Blistex Inc.
1800 SWIFT DRIVE
OAK BROOK, IL 60521

DYPROTEX®DIAPER RASH PADS

Description: Dyprotex contains micronized Zinc Oxide (40%), Cod Liver Oil (high in Vitamins A and D), and Dimethicone in a Petrolatum-Lanolin-Aloe Extract base suitable for topical application. The soft applicator pad provides easy handling, no-mess diaper area coverage. Each disposable pad is packaged in a resealable tub containing enough ointment for three applications. Dyprotex has a preferred fresh baby powder fragrance.

Actions and Uses: Dyprotex can provide prompt relief of diaper rash, superficial wounds, and other minor skin irritations. With regular use, it promotes the healing of these skin conditions, helps prevent diaper rash and protects against irritants present in the urine and feces. The presence of Zinc Oxide, Petrolatum and Dimethicone creates a long-lasting barrier coating over the skin. This coating serves to block the effects of high pH, enzymes, and ammonia resulting from the bacterial breakdown of urine—all significant factors contributing to the development and exacerbation of diaper rash. Zinc Oxide and Propyl Paraben provide antiseptic properties to prevent secondary infection and ensure that the applicator pad remains sanitary between each use.
Aloe Extract, Cod Liver Oil and Zinc Oxide relieve irritation and reduce surface inflammation due to their astringent and moisturizing properties.
Laboratory studies for protection showed that the barrier against baby urine formed by Dyprotex lasts three times longer than other commercially available diaper rash products under the same experimental conditions.
In clinical studies, twenty-five (25) babies with medically diagnosed diaper rash were treated with Dyprotex. After the initial application of Dyprotex to the diaper area, the subjects were examined two times per day for a period of five days. The severity of diaper dermatitis was graded at each visit. Dyprotex provided significant reduction of diaper rash by the second evaluation on day two, and the treated area continued to improve over the course of the study. A corresponding questionnaire also demonstrated a high degree of user satisfaction.

Continued on next page

Blistex—Cont.

which could be translated into improved patient compliance.

Directions: To relieve diaper rash, apply Dyprotex with each diaper change when inflammation is present or at the first sign of redness. When used daily, Dyprotex also protects against diaper rash reoccurrence. For external use only.

How Supplied: Dyprotex Diaper Rash Pads are available nationally in a 24 application package (eight .16 ounce applicator pads) and a 42 application (fourteen .16 ounce applicator pads).

Shown in Product Identification Section, page 404

Block Drug Company, Inc.
257 CORNELISON AVENUE JERSEY CITY, NJ 07302

ARTHRITIS STRENGTH BC® POWDER

Active Ingredients: Aspirin 742 mg in combination with 222 mg Salicylamide and 36 mg Caffeine per powder.

Indications: Arthritis Strength BC Powder is specially formulated with more of the pain relieving ingredients to provide fast temporary relief of minor arthritis pain and inflammation, neuralgia, neuritis and sciatica; relief of muscular aches, discomfort and fever of colds; and pain of tooth extraction.

Warning: Children and teenagers should not use this medicine for chicken pox or flu symptoms before a doctor is consulted about Reye Syndrome, a rare but serious illness reported to be associated with aspirin. Do not exceed recommended dosage or administer to children, including teenagers, with chicken pox or flu, unless directed by a physician. Do not take this product if you are allergic to aspirin, have asthma, gastric ulcer, or are taking a medication that affects the clotting of blood, except under the advice and supervision of a physician. If pain persists for more than 10 days or redness is present, discontinue use of this product and consult a physician immediately. Keep this and all medication out of children's reach. As with any drug, if you are pregnant or nursing a baby, consult your physician before using this product. Discontinue use if ringing in the ears occurs.
In case of accidental overdosage, contact a physician or poison control center immediately.

Dosage and Administration: Place one powder on tongue and follow with liquid. If you prefer, stir powder into glass of water or other liquid. May be used every three to four hours, up to 4 powders each 24 hours. For children under 12, consult a physician.

How Supplied: Available in tamper resistant cellophane wrapped envelopes of 6 powders, and tamper resistant cellophane wrapped boxes of 24 and 50 powders.

BC COLD POWDER
**BC Cold Powder Multi-Symptom Formula
BC Cold Powder Multi-Symptom Non-Drowsy Formula**

Active Ingredients: *Multi-Symptom Formula*—Aspirin 650 mg, Phenylpropanolamine Hydrochloride 25 mg, and Chlorpheniramine Maleate 4 mg per powder. *Non-Drowsy Formula*—Aspirin 650 mg and Phenylpropanolamine Hydrochloride 25 mg per powder.

Indications: *BC Cold Powder Multi-Symptom Formula* is for relief of cold symptoms such as body aches, fever, nasal congestion, sneezing, running nose, and watery itchy eyes. *BC Cold Powder Multi-Symptom Non-Drowsy Formula* is for relief of such symptoms as body aches, fever, and nasal congestions.

Warnings: CHILDREN AND TEENAGERS SHOULD NOT USE THIS MEDICINE FOR CHICKEN POX OR FLU SYMPTOMS BEFORE A DOCTOR IS CONSULTED ABOUT REYE SYNDROME, A RARE BUT SERIOUS ILLNESS REPORTED TO BE ASSOCIATED WITH ASPIRIN. KEEP THIS AND ALL MEDICINES OUT OF CHILDREN'S REACH. IN CASE OF ACCIDENTAL OVERDOSE, CONTACT A PHYSICIAN IMMEDIATELY. As with any drug, if you are pregnant or nursing a baby, seek the advice of a health professional before using this product. Do not exceed recommended dosage. If symptoms do not improve within 7 days, or are accompanied by high fever, consult a physician before continuing use. Do not take this product if you have high blood pressure, heart disease, diabetes, or thyroid disease except under the advice and supervision of a physician. Do not take this product if you are presently taking a prescription antihypertensive or antidepressant drug containing a monoamine oxidase inhibitor except under the advice and supervision of a physician. This product contains aspirin and should not be taken by individuals who are sensitive to aspirin. BC Cold Powder Multi-Symptom with antihistamine may cause drowsiness. Avoid alcoholic beverages while taking this product. Use caution when driving a motor vehicle or operating machinery.

Dosage and Administration: *Adults* —one powder into a glass of water or other liquid, or place powder on tongue and follow with liquid. May be used every 4 hours up to 4 times a day. *For children under 12*—consult a physician.

How Supplied: Available in tamper-resistant cellophane-wrapped envelopes of 6 powders, as well as tamper-resistant boxes of 24 powders.

BC® POWDER

Active Ingredients: Aspirin 650 mg per powder, Salicylamide 195 mg per powder and Caffeine 32 mg per powder.

Indications: BC Powder is for relief of simple headache; for temporary relief of minor arthritic pain, neuralgia, neuritis and sciatica; for relief of muscular aches, discomfort and fever of colds; and for relief of normal menstrual pain and pain of tooth extraction.

Warning: Children and teenagers should not use this medicine for chicken pox or flu symptoms before a doctor is consulted about Reye Syndrome, a rare but serious illness reported to be associated with aspirin. Do not exceed recommended dosage or administer to children, including teenagers, with chicken pox or flu, unless directed by a physician. Do not take this product if you are allergic to aspirin, have asthma, gastric ulcer, or are taking a medication that affects the clotting of blood, except under the advice and supervision of a physician. If pain persists for more than 10 days or redness is present, discontinue use of this product and consult a physician immediately. Keep this and all medication out of children's reach. As with any drug, if you are pregnant or nursing a baby, consult your physician before using this product. Discontinue use if ringing in the ears occurs.
In case of accidental overdosage, contact a physician or poison control center immediately.

Dosage and Administration: Stir one powder into a glass of water or other liquid, or place powder on tongue and follow with liquid. May be used every 3 or 4 hours up to 4 times a day. For children under 12 consult a physician.

How Supplied: Available in tamper resistant cellophane wrapped envelopes of 2 or 6 powders, as well as tamper resistant boxes of 24 and 50 powders.

NYTOL® TABLETS

Active Ingredient: Diphenhydramine Hydrochloride, 25 mg per tablet.

Indications: Diphenhydramine Hydrochloride is an antihistamine with anticholinergic and sedative effects which induces drowsiness and helps in falling asleep.

Warnings: Do not give children under 12 years of age. If sleeplessness persists continuously for more than 2 weeks, consult your physician. Insomnia may be a symptom of serious underlying medical illness. If pregnant or nursing, consult your physician before taking this or any medicine. Do not take this product if you have asthma, glaucoma, or enlargement of the prostate gland except under the advice and supervision of a physician. Take this product with caution if alcohol is being consumed. Keep this and all drugs out of the reach of children. In case of accidental overdose, contact a physician immediately.

Drug Interaction: Alcohol and other drugs which cause CNS depression will heighten the depressant effect of this product. Monoamine oxidase (MAO) inhibitors will prolong and intensify the anticholinergic effects of antihistamines.

Symptoms and Treatment of Oral Overdosage: In adults overdose may cause CNS depression resulting in hypnosis and coma. In children CNS hyperexcitability may follow sedation; the stimulant phase may bring tremor, delirium and convulsions. Gastrointestinal reactions may include dry mouth, appetite loss, nausea and vomiting. Respiratory distress and cardiovascular complications (hypotension) may be evident. Treatment includes inducing emesis, and controlling symptoms.

Dosage and Administration: Take 2 tablets 20 minutes before bed or as directed by a physician.

How Supplied: Available in tamper resistant packages of 16, 32, 48, and 72 tablets.

PROMISE® TOOTHPASTE
Desensitizing Dentifrice

Active Ingredients: 5% Potassium Nitrate in a pleasantly mint-flavored dentifrice.

Promise contains Potassium Nitrate for relief of dentinal hypersensitivity resulting from the exposure of tooth dentin due to periodontal surgery, cervical (gumline) erosion, abrasion or recession which causes pain on contact with hot, cold, or tactile stimuli.

Actions: Promise significantly reduces tooth hypersensitivity, with response to therapy evident after two weeks of use. Controlled double-blind clinical studies provide substantial evidence of the safety and effectiveness of Promise. The current theory on mechanism of action is that the potassium nitrate in Promise has an effect on neural transmission, interrupting the signal which would result in the sensation of pain.

Warning: When used as directed, it is important to remember that you have to brush for at least two weeks before relief begins to occur. If no improvement is seen after three months of use, consult your dentist.

Dosage and Administration: Use twice a day in place of regular toothpaste or as directed by a dental professional.

How Supplied: Promise Toothpaste is supplied in 1.6 oz. and 3.0 oz. tubes.

ORIGINAL SENSODYNE®
TOOTHPASTE
Desensitizing Dentifrice

Description: Each tube contains strontium chloride hexahydrate (10%) in a pleasantly flavored cleansing/polishing dentifrice.

Actions/Indications: Tooth hypersensitivity is a condition in which individuals experience pain from exposure to hot, cold stimuli, from chewing fibrous foods, or from tactile stimuli (e.g. toothbrushing.) Hypersensitivity usually occurs when the protective enamel covering on teeth wears away (which happens most often at the gum line) or if gum tissue recedes and exposes the dentin underneath.

Running through the dentin are microscopic small "tubules" which, according to many authorities, carry the pain impulses to the nerve of the tooth.

Sensodyne provides a unique ingredient—strontium chloride which is believed to be deposited in the tubules where it blocks the pain. The longer Sensodyne is used, the more of a barrier it helps build against pain.

The effect of Sensodyne may not be manifested immediately and may require a few weeks or longer of use for relief to be obtained. A number of clinical studies in the U.S. and other countries have provided substantial evidence of Sensodyne's performance attributes. Complete relief of hypersensitivity has been reported in approximately 65% of users and measurable relief or reduction in hypersensitivity in approximately 90%. Sensodyne has been commercially available for over 25 years and has received wide dental endorsement.

Contraindications: Subjects with severe dental erosion should brush properly and lightly with any dentifrice to avoid further removal of tooth structure.

Dosage: Use regularly in place of ordinary toothpaste or as recommended by dental professional.
NOTE: Individuals should be instructed to use SENSODYNE frequently since relief from pain tends to be cumulative. If relief does not occur after 3 months, a dentist should be consulted.

How Supplied: SENSODYNE Toothpaste is supplied as a paste in tubes of 4 oz. and 2.1 oz.
(U.S. Patent No. 3,122,483)

MINT SENSODYNE®
MINT GEL SENSODYNE®
TOOTHPASTES
Desensitizing Dentifrice

Active Ingredients: 5% Potassium Nitrate in a pleasantly mint-flavored dentifrice.
Mint Sensodyne and Mint Gel Sensodyne contain Potassium Nitrate for relief of dentinal hypersensitivity resulting from the exposure of tooth dentin due to periodontal surgery, cervical (gum line) erosion, abrasion or recession which causes pain on contact with hot, cold, or tactile stimuli.

Actions: Mint Sensodyne and Mint Gel Sensodyne significantly reduce tooth hypersensitivity, with response to therapy evident after two weeks of use. Controlled double-blind clinical studies provide substantial evidence of the safety and effectiveness of Mint Sensodyne and Mint Gel Sensodyne. The current theory on mechanism of action is that the potassium nitrate has an effect on neural transmission, interrupting the signal which would result in the sensation of pain.

Warning: When used as directed, it is important to remember that you have to brush for at least two weeks before relief begins to occur. If no improvement is seen after three months of use, consult your dentist.

Dosage and Administration: Use twice a day in place of regular toothpaste or as directed by a dental professional.

How Supplied: Mint Sensodyne and Mint Gel Sensodyne Toothpastes are supplied in 2.1 and 4.0 oz. tubes.
(U.S. Patent No. 3,863,006)

TEGRIN® MEDICATED SHAMPOO
[tĕg´rĭn]

Highly effective shampoo for moderate-to-severe dandruff and the relief of flaking, itching, and scaling associated with eczema, seborrhea, and psoriasis. Two commercial product versions are available: a lotion shampoo, in three formulas; herbal, original, and extra conditioning, and a gel concentrate, available in herbal scent.

Description: Each tube of gel shampoo or bottle of lotion shampoo contains 5% coal tar solution in a pleasantly scented, high-foaming, cleansing shampoo base with emollients, conditioners and other formula components.

Actions/Indications: Coal Tar is obtained in the destructive distillation of bituminous coal and is a highly effective agent for the local therapy of a number of dermatological disorders. The action of coal tar extract is believed to be keratolytic, antiseptic, antipruritic and astringent. The coal tar solution used in the Tegrin products is prepared in such a way as to reduce the pitch and other irritant components found in crude coal tar without reduction in therapeutic potency.

Coal tar solution has been used clinically for many years as a remedy for dandruff and for scaling associated with scalp disorders such as eczema, seborrhea, and psoriasis. Its mechanism of action has not been fully established, but it is believed to retard the rate of turnover of epidermal cells with regular use. A number of clinical studies have demonstrated the performance attributes of Tegrin Shampoo against dandruff and seborrheic dermatitis. In addition to relieving the above symptoms, Tegrin shampoo, used regularly, maintains scalp and hair cleanliness and leaves the hair lustrous and manageable.

Contraindications: For External Use Only—Should irritation develop, discontinue use. Avoid contact with eyes. Keep out of reach of children.

Dosage: Use regularly as a shampoo. Wet hair thoroughly. Rub Tegrin liberally into hair and scalp. Rinse thor-

Continued on next page

Block—Cont.

oughly. Briskly massage a second application of the shampoo into a rich lather. Rinse thoroughly.

How Supplied: Tegrin Concentrated Gel Shampoo is supplied in 2.5 oz. collapsible tubes.
Tegrin Lotion Shampoo is supplied in 3.75 and 6.6 oz. plastic bottles.

TEGRIN® for Psoriasis Lotion, Cream and Soap
[tĕg'rĭn]

Description: Each tube of cream or bottle of lotion contains special crude coal tar solution (5%) and allantoin (1.7%) in a greaseless, stainless vehicle. Tegrin Medicated Soap contains 2.0% crude coal tar solution.

Actions/Indications: Coal tar is obtained in the destructive distillation of bituminous coal and is a highly effective agent for the local therapy of a number of dermatological disorders. The action of coal tar is believed to be keratolytic, antiseptic, antipruritic and astringent. The coal tar solution used in the Tegrin products is prepared in such a way as to reduce the pitch and other irritant components found in crude coal tar. Allantoin (5-Ureidohydantoin) is a debriding and dispersing agent for psoriatic scales and is believed to accelerate proliferation of normal skin cells. The combination of coal tar extract and allantoin used in Tegrin has been demonstrated in a number of controlled clinical studies to have a high level of efficacy in controlling the itching and scaling of psoriasis.

Contraindications: Discontinue medication should irritation or allergic reactions occur. Avoid contact with eyes and mucous membranes. Keep out of reach of children.

Dosage and Administration: Apply lotion or cream 2 to 4 times daily as needed, massaging thoroughly into affected areas. Lather with Tegrin Soap in a hot bath before application to help soften heavy scales. Once condition is under control, maintenance therapy should be individually adjusted. Occlusive dressings are not required.

How Supplied: Tegrin Lotion 6 fl. oz., Tegrin Cream 2 oz. and 4.4 oz. tubes, Tegrin Soap 4.5 oz. bars.

IDENTIFICATION PROBLEM?
Consult the
Product Identification Section
where you'll find
products pictured
in full color.

Boehringer Ingelheim Pharmaceuticals, Inc.
90 EAST RIDGE
POST OFFICE BOX 368
RIDGEFIELD, CT 06877

DULCOLAX®
[dul'co-lax]
brand of bisacodyl USP
Tablets of 5 mg.................BI-CODE 12
Suppositories of 10 mg..BI-CODE 52
Laxative

Description: Dulcolax is a contact laxative acting directly on the colonic mucosa to produce normal peristalsis throughout the large intestine. Its unique mode of action permits either oral or rectal administration, according to the requirements of the patient. Because of its gentleness and reliability of action, Dulcolax may be used whenever constipation is a problem. In preparation for surgery, proctoscopy, or radiologic examination, Dulcolax provides satisfactory cleansing of the bowel, obviating the need for an enema.
The active ingredient in Dulcolax, bisacodyl, is a colorless, tasteless compound that is practically insoluble in water and alkaline solution. It is designated chemically bis(p-acetoxyphenyl)-2-pyridylmethane.
Each tablet contains bisacodyl USP 5 mg. Also contains acacia, acetylated monoglyceride, carnauba wax, cellulose acetate phthalate, corn starch, D&C Red No. 30 aluminum lake, D&C Yellow No. 10 aluminum lake, dibutyl phthalate, docusate sodium, gelatin, glycerin, iron oxides, kaolin, lactose, magnesium stearate, methylparaben, pharmaceutical glaze, polyethylene glycol, povidone, propylparaben, sodium benzoate, sorbitan monooleate, sucrose, talc, titanium dioxide, white wax.
Each suppository contains bisacodyl USP 10 mg. Also contains hydrogenated vegetable oil.
Dulcolax tablets and suppositories contain less than 0.2 mg per dosage unit which is considered sodium free.

Actions: Dulcolax differs markedly from other laxatives in its mode of action: it is virtually nontoxic, and its laxative effect occurs on contact with the colonic mucosa, where it stimulates sensory nerve endings to produce parasympathetic reflexes resulting in increased peristaltic contractions of the colon. Administered orally, Dulcolax is absorbed to a variable degree from the small bowel but such absorption is not related to the mode of action of the compound. Dulcolax administered rectally in the form of suppositories is negligibly absorbed. The contact action of the drug is restricted to the colon, and motility of the small intestine is not appreciably influenced. Local axon reflexes, as well as segmental reflexes, are initiated in the region of contact and contribute to the widespread peristaltic activity producing evacuation. For this reason, Dulcolax may often be employed satisfactorily in patients with ganglionic

blockage or spinal cord damage (paraplegia, poliomyelitis, etc.).

Indications: *Acute Constipation:* Taken at bedtime, Dulcolax tablets are almost invariably effective the following morning. When taken before breakfast, they usually produce an effect within six hours. For a prompter response and to replace enemas, the suppositories, which are usually effective in 15 minutes to one hour, can be used.
Chronic Constipation and Bowel Retraining: Dulcolax is extremely effective in the management of chronic constipation, particularly in older patients. By gradually lengthening the interval between doses as colonic tone improves, the drug has been found to be effective in redeveloping proper bowel hygiene. There is no tendency to "rebound".
Preparation for Radiography: Dulcolax tablets are excellent in eliminating fecal and gas shadows from x-rays taken of the abdominal area. For barium enemas, no food should be given following the administration of the tablets, to prevent reaccumulation of material in the cecum, and a suppository should be given one to two hours prior to examination.
Preoperative Preparation: Dulcolax tablets have been shown to be an ideal laxative in emptying the G.I. tract prior to abdominal surgery or to other surgery under general anesthesia. They may be supplemented by suppositories to replace the usual enema preparation. Dulcolax will not replace the colonic irrigations usually given patients before intracolonic surgery, but is useful in the preliminary emptying of the colon prior to these procedures.
Postoperative Care: Suppositories can be used to replace enemas, or tablets given as an oral laxative, to restore normal bowel hygiene after surgery.
Antepartum Care: Either tablets or suppositories can be used for constipation in pregnancy without danger of stimulating the uterus.
Preparation for Delivery: Suppositories can be used to replace enemas in the first stage of labor provided that they are given at least two hours before the onset of the second stage.
Postpartum Care: The same indications apply as in postoperative care, with no contraindication in nursing mothers.
Preparation for Sigmoidoscopy or Proctoscopy: For unscheduled office examinations, adequate preparation is usually obtained with a single suppository. For sigmoidoscopy scheduled in advance, however, administration of tablets the night before in addition will result in adequate preparation almost invariably.
Colostomies: Tablets the night before or a suppository inserted into the colostomy opening in the morning will frequently make irrigations unnecessary, and in other cases will expedite the procedure.

Contraindication: There is no contraindication to the use of Dulcolax, other than an acute surgical abdomen.
Caution for Patients: Do not use laxative products when abdominal pain, nausea or vomiting are present unless di-

rected by a doctor. As with all medicines, keep these tablets/suppositories out of reach of children. Frequent or continued use of this preparation may result in dependence on laxatives.

Adverse Reactions: As with any laxative, abdominal cramps are occasionally noted, particularly in severely constipated individuals.

Dosage:
Tablets
Tablets must be swallowed whole, not chewed or crushed, and should not be taken within one hour of antacids or milk.
Adults: Two or three (usually two) tablets suffice when an ordinary laxative effect is desired. This usually results in one or two soft, formed stools. Tablets when taken before breakfast usually produce an effect within 6 hours, when taken at bedtime usually in 8–12 hours.
Up to six tablets may be safely given in preparation for special procedures when greater assurance of complete evacuation of the colon is desired. In producing such thorough emptying, these higher doses may result in several loose, unformed stools.
Children: One or two tablets, depending on age and severity of constipation, administered as above. Tablets should not be given to a child too young to swallow them whole.
Suppositories
Adults: One suppository at the time a bowel movement is required. Usually effective in 15 minutes to one hour.
Children: Half a suppository is generally effective for infants and children under two years of age. Above this age, a whole suppository is usually advisable.
Combined
In preparation for surgery, radiography and sigmoidoscopy, a combination of tablets the night before and a suppository in the morning is recommended (see Indications).

How Supplied: Dulcolax, brand of bisacodyl: Yellow, enteric-coated tablets of 5 mg in boxes of 10, 25, 50 and 100; suppositories of 10 mg in boxes of 4, 8, 16 and 50.

Note: Store Dulcolax suppositories and tablets at temperatures below 77°F (25°C). Avoid excessive humidity.

Also Available: Dulcolax® Bowel Prep Kit. Each kit contains:
1 Dulcolax suppository of 10 mg bisacodyl;
4 Dulcolax tablets of 5 mg bisacodyl;
Complete patient instructions.

Clinical Applications: Dulcolax can be used in virtually any patient in whom a laxative or enema is indicated. It has no effect on the blood picture, erythrocyte sedimentation rate, urinary findings, or hepatic or renal function. It may be safely given to infants and the aged, pregnant or nursing women, debilitated patients, and may be prescribed in the presence of such conditions as cardiovascular, renal, or hepatic diseases.

Shown in Product Identification Section, page 404

NOSTRIL® Nasal Decongestant
[nō 'stril]
phenylephrine HCl, USP

Active Ingredient: Contains phenylephrine HCl, USP, 0.25% (¼% Mild strength) or phenylephrine HCl, USP, 0.5% (½% Regular strength). Also contains benzalkonium chloride 0.004% as a preservative, boric acid, sodium borate, water.

Indications: For temporary relief of nasal congestion due to the common cold, sinusitis, hay fever or other upper respiratory allergies.

Actions: NOSTRIL, the first metered one-way pump spray for nasal decongestion delivers measured, uniform doses. The medication constricts the smaller arterioles of the nasal passages, producing a gentle, predictable, decongestant effect. Nostril penetrates and shrinks swollen membranes, restoring freer breathing and unclogs sinus passages, bringing the effective medication in contact with inflamed, swollen tissues. It will not hurt tender membranes since it is formulated to match the pH of normal nasal secretions. The first one-way pump spray helps prevent draw-back contamination of the medication.

Warnings: Do not exceed recommended dosage because symptoms such as burning, stinging, sneezing, or increased nasal discharge may occur. Do not use for more than 3 days. If symptoms persist, consult a physician. Do not give Nostril 0.25% to children under 6 or Nostril 0.5% to children under 12 except under the advice and supervision of a physician. Nostril 0.5% for adult use only. Use of the dispenser by more than one person may spread infection. Keep this and all drugs out of reach of children.

Symptoms and Treatment of Oral Overdosage: In case of accidental ingestion, seek professional assistance or consult a poison control center immediately.

Dosage and Administration:
0.25% for adults and children 6 years and over: 1 to 2 sprays in each nostril not more frequently than every four hours.
0.5% for adults: 1 to 2 sprays in each nostril not more frequently than every four hours.
Remove protective cap. With head upright, insert metered pump spray nozzle in nostril. Hold bottle with thumb at base, nozzle between first and second fingers. Depress pump once or twice, all the way down with a firm even stroke and sniff deeply.
Note: Before using for the first time, remove the protective cap from the tip and depress the round tab firmly several times to prime the metering pump.

How Supplied: Metered one-way nasal pump spray in white plastic bottles of ½ fl. oz. (15 ml) packaged in tamper-resistant outer cartons.
0.25% (¼% Mild strength): for children 6 years and over and adults who prefer a

milder decongestant. (NDC 0597-0083-85)
0.5% (½% Regular strength): for adults and children 12 years or older (NDC 0597-0084-85)

NOSTRILLA™ Long Acting Nasal
[nō-stril 'a]
Decongestant
oxymetazoline HCl, USP

Active Ingredient: Contains oxymetazoline HCl, USP, 0.05%. Also contains benzalkonium chloride 0.02% as a preservative, glycine, sorbitol solution, water. (Mercury preservatives are not used in this product.)

Indications: For up to 12 hour relief of nasal congestion due to the common cold, sinusitis, hay fever or other upper respiratory allergies.

Actions: NOSTRILLA, the first metered one-way pump spray for nasal decongestion delivers measured, uniform doses. The medication constricts the smaller arterioles of the nasal passages, producing a prolonged (up to 12 hours), gentle, predictable, decongestant effect. Nostrilla penetrates and shrinks swollen membranes, restoring freer breathing and unclogs sinus passages, bringing the effective medication in contact with inflamed, swollen tissues. It will not hurt tender membranes since it is formulated to match the pH of normal nasal secretions. Use at bedtime restores freer nasal breathing through the night. The first one-way pump spray helps prevent draw-back contamination of the medication.

Warnings: Do not exceed recommended dosage because symptoms such as burning, stinging, sneezing or increased nasal discharge may occur. Do not use for more than 3 days. If symptoms persist, consult a physician. Do not give this product to children under 6 except under advice and supervision of a physician. Use of the dispenser by more than one person may spread infection. Keep this and all drugs out of reach of children.

Symptoms and Treatment of Oral Overdosage: In case of accidental ingestion, seek professional assistance or contact a poison control center immediately.

Dosage and Administration: Adults and children 6 and over: 1 to 2 sprays in each nostril 2 times daily (in the morning and evening).
Remove protective cap. With head upright, insert metered pump spray nozzle in nostril. Hold bottle with thumb at base, nozzle between first and second fingers. Depress pump once or twice, all the way down with a firm even stroke and sniff deeply.
Note: Before using for the first time, remove the protective cap from the tip and depress the round tab firmly several times to prime the metering pump.

Continued on next page

Boehringer Ingelheim—Cont.

How Supplied: Metered one-way nasal pump spray in white plastic bottles of ½ fl. oz. (15 ml) packaged in tamper-resistant outer cartons. (NDC 0597-0085-85).

Boiron-Borneman, Inc.
**1208 AMOSLAND ROAD
NORWOOD, PA 19074**

OSCILLOCOCCINUM®
[ŏ-sĭl ′ŏ-kŏk-sē ′nŭm]

Active Ingredient: Anas Barbariae Hepatis et Cordis Extractum HPUS 200C

Indications: For the relief of flu-like symptoms such as fever, chills, body aches and pains.

Actions: Like most Homeopathic remedies, Oscillococcinum® acts gently by stimulating the patient's natural defense mechanisms.

Warnings: If symptoms persist for more than three days or worsen, consult your physician. Keep all medication out of reach of children. As with any drug if you are pregnant or nursing a baby, seek professional advice before using this product.

Dosage and Administration: (Adults and Children over 2 years)
At the onset of symptoms, place the entire contents of one tube in your mouth and allow to dissolve under your tongue. Repeat every 6 hours as necessary. For maximum results, Oscillococcinum® should be taken early, at the onset of symptoms, and at least 15 minutes before or 1 hour after meals.

How Supplied: boxes of 3 unit-doses of 0.04 oz. (1 Gram) each. (NDC 51979-9756-43) Tamper resistant package.
Manufactured by Boiron, France.
Distributor: Boiron-Borneman, Inc.
Shown in Product Identification Section, page 405

"What 's Homeopathy?"
Booklet free to physicians and pharmacists.
"An Introduction to Homeopathy for the Practicing Pharmacist"
A free continuing education booklet for pharmacists.

Bristol Laboratories
**A Bristol-Myers Company
2400 W. LLOYD EXPRESSWAY
EVANSVILLE, IN 47721**

NALDECON CX® ADULT LIQUID℗
[nal ′dĕ-côn CX]
**Nasal Decongestant/
Expectorant/Cough Suppressant**

Description: Each teaspoonful (5 mL) of Naldecon CX Adult Liquid contains:
Phenylpropanolamine
hydrochloride .... 12.5 mg
Guaifenesin (glyceryl
guaiacolate) .... 200 mg
Codeine phosphate .... 10 mg
(Warning: May be Habit-Forming)
This combination product is antihistamine-free, alcohol-free and sugar-free.

Inactive Ingredients: Citric acid, FD&C Blue No. 1, FD&C Red No. 40, hydrogenated glucose syrup, natural and artificial flavor, polyethylene glycol, purified water, sodium benzoate, sodium citrate, sodium saccharin.

Indications: For the temporary relief of nasal congestion due to the common cold (cold), hay fever or other respiratory allergies (allergic rhinitis), or associated with sinusitis. Helps loosen phlegm (sputum) and thin bronchial secretions to rid the bronchial passageways of bothersome mucus. Temporarily quiets cough due to minor throat and bronchial irritation as may occur with a cold or inhaled irritants.

Contraindications: Do not take if hypersensitive to guaifenesin, codeine or sympathomimetic amines.

Warnings: As with any drug, if you are pregnant or nursing a baby, seek the advice of a health professional before using this product. Do not give this product to children under 12 years of age unless directed by a physician. Do not exceed recommended dosage because at higher doses nervousness, dizziness, or sleeplessness may occur. Do not take this product for more than 7 days. If symptoms do not improve or are accompanied by fever, consult a physician. Do not take this product if you have heart disease, high blood pressure, thyroid disease, diabetes, or difficulty in urination due to enlargement of the prostate gland unless directed by a physician.

Drug Interaction Precaution: Do not take this product if you are presently taking a prescription drug for high blood pressure or depression, without first consulting your physician. A persistent cough may be a sign of a serious condition. If cough persists for more than 1 week, tends to recur, or is accompanied by fever, rash, or persistent headache, consult a physician. Do not take this product for persistent or chronic cough such as occurs with smoking, asthma, chronic bronchitis, or emphysema, or if cough is accompanied by excessive phlegm (sputum) unless directed by a physician. Do not take this product if you have a chronic pulmonary disease or shortness of breath unless directed by a physician. May cause or aggravate constipation. Keep this and all drugs out of the reach of children. In case of accidental overdose, seek professional assistance or contact a Poison Control Center immediately.

Directions: Adults and children 12 years of age and over: Oral dosage is 2 teaspoonfuls every 4 hours, not to exceed 6 doses in 24 hours, or as directed by a physician.

How Supplied: NALDECON CX Adult Liquid—4 ounce and pint bottles.
Store at room temperature. Avoid excessive heat.

NALDECON DX® ADULT LIQUID
[nal ′dĕ-côn DX]
**Nasal Decongestant/
Expectorant/Cough Suppressant**

Description: Each teaspoonful (5 mL) of Naldecon DX Adult Liquid contains:
Phenylpropanolamine
hydrochloride..............................12.5 mg
Guaifenesin (glyceryl
guaiacolate)..................................200 mg
Dextromethorphan
hydrobromide................................10 mg
This combination product is antihistamine-free, sugar-free and alcohol-free.

Inactive Ingredients: Citric acid, FD&C Yellow No. 6, natural and artificial flavor, polyethylene glycol, purified water, sodium benzoate, sodium citrate, sodium saccharin and sorbitol.

Indications: For the temporary relief of nasal congestion due to the common cold (cold), hay fever or other respiratory allergies (allergic rhinitis), or associated with sinusitis. Helps loosen phlegm (sputum) and thin bronchial secretions to rid the bronchial passageways of bothersome mucus. Temporarily quiets cough due to minor throat and bronchial irritation as may occur with a cold or inhaled irritants.

Contraindications: Do not take if hypersensitive to guaifenesin, dextromethorphan or sympathomimetic amines.

Warnings: As with any drug, if you are pregnant or nursing a baby, seek the advice of a health professional before using this product. Do not give this product to children under 12 years of age unless directed by a physician. Do not exceed recommended dosage because at higher doses nervousness, dizziness or sleeplessness may occur. Do not take this product for more than 7 days. If symptoms do not improve or are accompanied by fever, consult a physician. Do not take this product if you have heart disease, high blood pressure, thyroid disease, diabetes, or difficulty in urination due to enlargement of the prostate gland unless directed by a physician.

Drug Interaction Precaution: Do not take this product if you are presently taking a prescription drug for high blood pressure or depression, without first consulting your physician. A persistent cough may be a sign of a serious condition. If cough persists for more than one week, tends to recur, or is accompanied by fever, rash, or persistent headache, consult a physician. Do not take this product for persistent or chronic cough such as occurs with smoking, asthma, chronic bronchitis, or emphysema, or if cough is accompanied by excessive phlegm (sputum) unless directed by a physician. Keep this and all drugs out of the reach of children. In case of accidental overdose, seek professional assistance or contact a poison control center immediately.

Directions: Adults and children 12 years of age and over: Oral dosage is 2 teaspoonfuls every 4 hours, not to exceed 6 doses in 24 hours, or as directed by a physician.

How Supplied: NALDECON DX Adult Liquid—4 ounce and pint bottles.
Store at room temperature. Avoid excessive heat.

NALDECON DX®
[nal 'dĕ-côn DX]
CHILDREN'S SYRUP
Nasal Decongestant/
Expectorant/Cough Suppressant

Description: Each teaspoonful (5 mL) of Naldecon DX Children's Syrup contains:

Phenylpropanolamine
   hydrochloride ....6.25 mg
Guaifenesin (glyceryl
   guaiacolate) ....100 mg
Dextromethorphan
   hydrobromide ....5 mg
This combination product is antihistamine-free.

Inactive Ingredients: Alcohol (5% V/V), FD&C Yellow No. 6, fructose, glycerin, natural and artificial flavors, purified water, sodium benzoate, sucrose and tartaric acid.

Indications: For the temporary relief of nasal congestion due to the common cold (cold), hay fever or other respiratory allergies (allergic rhinitis), or associated with sinusitis. Helps loosen phlegm (sputum) and thin bronchial secretions to rid the bronchial passageways of bothersome mucus. Temporarily quiets cough due to minor throat and bronchial irritation as may occur with a cold or inhaled irritants.

Contraindications: Do not take if hypersensitive to guaifenesin, dextromethorphan, or sympathomimetic amines.

Warnings: Do not exceed recommended dosage because at higher doses nervousness, dizziness, or sleeplessness may occur. Do not give this product to children for more than 7 days. If symptoms do not

improve or are accompanied by fever, consult a physician. Do not give this product to children who have heart disease, high blood pressure, thyroid disease, or diabetes, unless directed by a physician.

Drug Interaction Precaution: Do not give this product to a child who is taking a prescription drug for high blood pressure or depression, without first consulting the child's physician. A persistent cough may be a sign of a serious condition. If cough persists for more than 1 week, tends to recur, or is accompanied by fever, rash, or persistent headache, consult a physician. Do not give this product for persistent or chronic cough such as occurs with smoking, asthma, chronic bronchitis, or emphysema, or if cough is accompanied by excessive phlegm (sputum) unless directed by a physician. Keep this and all drugs out of the reach of children. In case of accidental overdose, seek professional assistance or contact a poison control center immediately.

Directions: Children 6 to under 12 years of age: Oral dosage is 2 teaspoonfuls every 4 hours, not to exceed 6 doses in 24 hours, or as directed by a physician. Children 2 to under 6 years of age: Oral dosage is 1 teaspoonful every 4 hours, not to exceed 6 doses in 24 hours, or as directed by a physician. Children under 2 years of age: consult a physician.

How Supplied: NALDECON DX Children's Syrup—4 ounce and pint bottles. Store at room temprature. Protect from excessive heat and freezing.

NALDECON DX® PEDIATRIC DROPS
[nal 'dĕ-côn DX]
Nasal Decongestant/
Expectorant/Cough Suppressant

Description: Each 1 mL of Naldecon DX Pediatric Drops contains:
Phenylpropanolamine
   hydrochloride .... 6.25 mg
Guaifenesin (glyceryl
   guaiacolate) .... 30 mg
Dextromethorphan
   hydrobromide .... 5 mg
Alcohol.................................... 0.6% V/V
This combination product is antihistamine-free and sugar-free.

Inactive Ingredients: Alcohol (0.6% V/V), citric acid, FD&C Yellow No. 6, natural and artificial flavors, propylene glycol, purified water, sodium benzoate, sodium saccharin and sorbitol.

Indications: For the temporary relief of nasal congestion due to the common cold (cold), hay fever or other respiratory allergies (allergic rhinitis), or associated with sinusitis. Helps loosen phlegm (sputum) and thin bronchial secretions to rid the bronchial passageways of bothersome mucus. Temporarily quiets cough due to minor throat and bronchial irritation as may occur with a cold or inhaled irritants.

Contraindications: Do not take if hypersensitive to guaifenesin, dextromethorphan, or sympathomimetic amines.

Warnings: Take by mouth only. Do not exceed recommended dosage because at higher doses nervousness, dizziness or sleeplessness may occur. Do not give this product to children for more than 7 days. If symptoms do not improve or are accompanied by fever, consult a physician. Do not give this product to children who have heart disease, high blood pressure, thyroid disease, or diabetes, unless directed by a physician.

Drug Interaction Precaution: Do not give this product to a child who is taking a prescription drug for high blood pressure or depression, without first consulting the child's physician. A persistent cough may be a sign of a serious condition. If cough persists for more than 1 week, tends to recur, or is accompanied by fever, rash, or persistent headache, consult a physician. Do not give this product for persistent or chronic cough such as occurs with smoking, asthma, chronic bronchitis, or emphysema, or if cough is accompanied by excessive phlegm (sputum) unless directed by a physician. Keep this and all drugs out of the reach of children. In case of accidental overdose, seek professional assistance or contact a poison control center immediately.

Directions: Children 2 to under 6 years of age: Oral dosage is 1 mL every 4 hours, not to exceed 6 doses in 24 hours, or as directed by a physician. Children under 2 years of age: consult a physician.

Professional Labeling—Children under 2 years of age: Dosage should be adjusted to age or weight and be administered every 4 hours as shown in the dosage table, not to exceed 6 doses in 24 hours.

Age	Weight	Dosage
1–3 months	8–12 lb	¼ mL
4–6 months	13–17 lb	½ mL
7–9 months	18–20 lb	¾ mL
10–24 months	21+ lb	1.0 mL

Bottle label reads as follows: Children under 2 years of age: Use only as directed by a physician.

How Supplied: NALDECON DX Pediatric Drops—30 mL bottle with calibrated dropper.
Store at room temperature. Protect from freezing.

NALDECON EX® CHILDREN'S SYRUP
[nal 'dĕ-côn EX]
Nasal Decongestant/Expectorant

Description: Each teaspoonful (5 mL) of Naldecon EX Children's Syrup contains:
Phenylpropanolamine
   hydrochloride...........................6.25 mg
Guaifenesin (glyceryl
   guaiacolate).................................100 mg

Continued on next page

Bristol—Cont.

Alcohol..0.5% V/V
This combination product is antihistamine-free and sugar-free.

Inactive Ingredients: Alcohol (5% V/V), D&C Yellow No. 10, glycerin, natural and artificial flavors, propylene glycol, purified water, sodium benzoate, sodium saccharin, sorbitol and tartaric acid.

Indications: For the temporary relief of nasal congestion due to the common cold (cold), hay fever or other respiratory allergies (allergic rhinitis), or associated with sinusitis. Helps loosen phlegm (sputum) and thin bronchial secretions to rid the bronchial passageways of bothersome mucus.

Contraindications: Do not take if hypersensitive to guaifenesin or sympathomimetic amines.

Warnings: Do not exceed recommended dosage because at higher doses nervousness, dizziness or sleeplessness may occur. Do not give this product to children for more than 7 days. If symptoms do not improve or are accompanied by fever, consult a physician. Do not give this product to children who have heart disease, high blood pressure, thyroid disease, or diabetes, unless directed by a physician.

Drug Interaction Precaution: Do not give this product to a child who is taking a prescription drug for high blood pressure or depression, without first consulting the child's physician. A persistent cough may be a sign of a serious condition. If cough persists for more than 1 week, tends to recur, or is accompanied by fever, rash, or persistent headache, consult a physician. Do not give this product for persistent or chronic cough such as occurs with smoking, asthma, chronic bronchitis, or emphysema, or if cough is accompanied by excessive phlegm (sputum) unless directed by a physician. Keep this and all drugs out of the reach of children. In case of accidental overdose, seek professional assistance or contact a poison control center immediately. Your physician or pharmacist is the best source of information on this medication.

Directions: Children 6 to under 12 years of age: Oral dosage is 2 teaspoonfuls every 4 hours, not to exceed 6 doses in 24 hours, or as directed by a physician. Children 2 to under 6 years of age: Oral dosage is 1 teaspoonful every 4 hours, not to exceed 6 doses in 24 hours, or as directed by a physician. Children under 2 years of age: consult a physician.

How Supplied: NALDECON EX Children's Syrup—4 ounce and pint bottles. Store at room temperature. Protect from excessive heat and freezing.

NALDECON EX® PEDIATRIC DROPS

[nal 'dĕ-côn EX]
Nasal Decongestant/Expectorant

Description: Each 1 mL of Naldecon EX Pediatric Drops contains:
Phenylpropanolamine
  hydrochloride ....6.25 mg
Guaifenesin (glyceryl
  guaiacolate) ....30 mg
This combination product is antihistamine-free.

Inactive Ingredients: Alcohol (0.6% V/V), citric acid, D&C Yellow No. 10, natural and artificial flavors, propylene glycol, purified water, sodium benzoate, and sucrose.

Indications: For the temporary relief of nasal congestion due to the common cold (cold), hay fever or other respiratory allergies (allergic rhinitis), or associated with sinusitis. Helps loosen phlegm (sputum) and thin bronchial secretions to rid the bronchial passageways of bothersome mucus.

Contraindications: Do not take if hypersensitive to guaifenesin or sympathomimetic amines.

Warnings: Take by mouth only. Do not exceed recommended dosage because at higher doses nervousness, dizziness or sleeplessness may occur. Do not give this product to children for more than 7 days. If symptoms do not improve or are accompanied by fever, consult a physician. Do not give this product to children who have heart disease, high blood pressure, thyroid disease, or diabetes, unless directed by a physician.

Drug Interaction Precaution: Do not give this product to a child who is taking a prescription drug for high blood pressure or depression, without first consulting the child's physician. A persistent cough may be a sign of a serious condition. If cough persists for more than 1 week, tends to recur, or is accompanied by fever, rash, or persistent headache, consult a physician. Do not give this product for persistent or chronic cough such as occurs with smoking, asthma, chronic bronchitis, or emphysema, or if cough is accompanied by excessive phlegm (sputum) unless directed by a physician. Keep this and all drugs out of the reach of children. In case of accidental overdose, seek professional assistance or contact a poison control center immediately. Your physician or pharmacist is the best source of information on this medication.

Directions: Children 2 to under 6 years of age: Oral dosage is 1 mL every 4 hours, not to exceed 6 doses in 24 hours, or as directed by a physician. Children under 2 years of age: consult a physician.

Professional Labeling—Children under 2 years of age: Dosage should be adjusted to age or weight and be administered every 4 hours as shown in the dosage table, not to exceed 6 doses in 24 hours.

Age	Weight	Dosage
1–3 months	8–12 lb	¼ mL
4–6 months	13–17 lb	½ mL
7–9 months	18–20 lb	¾ mL
10–24 months	21+ lb	1.0 mL

Bottle label reads as follows: Children under 2 years of age: Use only as directed by a physician.

How Supplied: NALDECON EX Pediatric Drops—30 mL bottle with calibrated dropper.
Store at room temperature. Protect from excessive heat and freezing.

NALDECON SENIOR DX®
Expectorant/Cough Suppressant Cough/Cold Liquid for Adults 50 and Over

Description: Each teaspoonful (5 mL) of Naldecon Senior DX Cough/Cold Liquid contains:
Guaifenesin ....200 mg
Dextromethorphan
  hydrobromide ....15 mg

Inactive Ingredients: Citric acid, FD&C Blue No. 1, FD&C Red No. 40, natural and artificial flavorings, polyethylene glycol, purified water, sodium benzoate, sodium citrate, sodium saccharin, sorbitol.

Indications: Non-narcotic cough suppressant for the temporary relief of coughing. Helps loosen phlegm (sputum) and bronchial secretions and rid the bronchial passageways of bothersome mucus.

Contraindications: Do not take if hypersensitive to guaifenesin or dextromethorphan.

Warnings: A persistent cough may be a sign of a serious condition. If cough persists for more than 1 week, tends to recur, or is accompanied by fever, rash, or persistent headache, consult a physician. Do not take this product for persistent or chronic cough such as occurs with smoking, asthma, emphysema, or if cough is accompanied by excessive phlegm (mucus) unless directed by a physician. Do not exceed recommended dose or give this product to children under 12 years of age unless directed by a physician. As with any drug, if you are pregnant or nursing a baby, seek the advice of a health professional before using this product. Keep this and all drugs out of the reach of children. In case of accidental overdose, seek professional assistance or contact a Poison Control Center immediately.

Directions: Adults: Oral dosage is 2 teaspoonfuls every 6 to 8 hours, not to exceed 4 doses in 24 hours, or as directed by a physician. Children under 12 years of age: consult a physician.

How Supplied: Naldecon Senior DX Cough/Cold Liquid—4 ounce and pint bottles.
Store at room temperature.

NALDECON SENIOR EX®
(guaifenesin)
Expectorant
Cough/Cold Liquid
for Adults 50 and Over

Description: Each teaspoonful (5 mL) of Naldecon Senior EX Cough/Cold Liquid contains:
Guaifenesin.....................................200 mg

Inactive Ingredients: Citric acid, FD&C Blue No. 1, FD&C Red No. 40, natural and artificial flavorings, polyethylene glycol, purified water, sodium benzoate, sodium citrate, sodium saccharin, sorbitol.

Indications: Helps loosen phlegm (sputum) and bronchial secretions and rid the bronchial passageways of bothersome mucus.

Contraindications: Do not take if hypersensitive to guaifenesin.

Warnings: A persistent cough may be a sign of a serious condition. If cough persists for more than 1 week, tends to recur, or is accompanied by fever, rash, or persistent headache, consult a physician. Do not take this product for persistent or chronic cough such as occurs with smoking, asthma, emphysema, or if cough is accompanied by excessive phlegm (mucus) unless directed by a physician. Do not exceed recommended dose or give this product to children under 12 years of age unless directed by a physician. As with any drug, if you are pregnant or nursing a baby, seek the advice of a health professional before using this product. Keep this and all drugs out of the reach of children. In case of accidental overdose, seek professional assistance or contact a Poison Control Center immediately.

Directions: Adults: Oral dosage is 2 teaspoonfuls every 4 hours, not to exceed 6 doses in 24 hours, or as directed by a physician. Children under 12 years of age: consult a physician.

How Supplied: Naldecon Senior EX Cough/Cold Liquid—4 ounce and pint bottles.
Store at room temperature.

Bristol-Myers Products
(A Bristol-Myers Company)
345 PARK AVENUE
NEW YORK, NY 10154

Tri-Buffered BUFFERIN®
[bŭf'fĕr-ĭn]
Analgesic

Composition:
Active Ingredient: Each coated tablet or caplet contains Aspirin 325 mg in a formulation buffered with Calcium Carbonate, Magnesium Oxide and Magnesium Carbonate.
Other Ingredients: Benzoic Acid, Carnauba Wax, Citric Acid, Corn Starch, FD&C Blue No. 1, Hydroxypropyl Methylcellulose, Mineral Oil, Polysorbate 20, Povidone, Propylene Glycol, Simethicone Emulsion, Sodium Phosphate, Sorbitan Monolaurate, Titanium Dioxide. May also contain: Glyceryl Behenate, Magnesium Stearate, Sodium Lauryl Sulfate, Sodium Stearyl Fumarate, Stearic Acid, Zinc Stearate.

Action and Uses: For effective relief from headaches, pain and fever of colds and flu, muscle aches, temporary relief of minor arthritis pain and inflammation, menstrual pain and toothaches. Buffered formulation helps prevent the stomach upset that plain aspirin can cause. Coated tablets for easy swallowing.

Contraindications: Hypersensitivity to salicylates.

Caution: If pain persists for more than 10 days or redness is present, or in arthritic or rheumatic conditions affecting children under 12, consult a physician immediately. Do not take without consulting a physician if under medical care. Consult a dentist for toothache promptly.

Warning: Children and teenagers should not use this medicine for chicken pox or flu symptoms before a doctor is consulted about Reye syndrome, a rare but serious illness reported to be associated with aspirin. KEEP THIS AND ALL MEDICINES OUT OF CHILDREN'S REACH. IN CASE OF ACCIDENTAL OVERDOSE, CONTACT A PHYSICIAN OR POISON CONTROL CENTER IMMEDIATELY. If dizziness, impaired hearing or ringing in the ears occurs, discontinue use. As with any drug, if you are pregnant or nursing a baby, seek the advice of a health professional before using this product.

Administration and Dosage: Adults: 2 tablets or caplets with water every 4 hours as needed. Do not exceed 12 tablets or caplets in 24 hours, unless directed by physician. For children 6 to under 12, one-half adult dose. Under 6, consult physician.

Overdose: (Symptoms and treatment) Typical of aspirin.

How Supplied: Tri-Buffered BUFFERIN is supplied as:
Coated circular white tablet with letter "B" debossed on one surface.
NDC 19810-0073-2 Bottle of 12's
NDC 19810-0073-3 Bottle of 36's
NDC 19810-0073-4 Bottle of 60's
NDC 19810-0073-5 Bottle of 100's
NDC 19810-0073-6 Bottle of 200's
NDC 19810-0093-2 Bottle of 275's
NDC 19810-0073-7 Bottle of 1000's for hospital and clinical use.
NDC 19810-0073-9 Boxed 200 × 2 tablet foil pack for hospital and clinical use.
Coated scored white caplet with letter "B" debossed on each side of scoring.
NDC 19810-0072-1 Bottle of 36's
NDC 19810-0072-2 Bottle of 60's
NDC 19810-0072-3 Bottle of 100's
All consumer sizes have child resistant closures except 100's for tablets and 60's for caplets which are sizes recommended for households without young children.
Store at room temperature.

Professional samples available on request.
Also described in PDR for Nonprescription Drugs.

Professional Labeling

1. Tri-Buffered BUFFERIN® FOR RECURRENT TRANSIENT ISCHEMIC ATTACKS

Indication: For reducing the risk of recurrent transient ischemic attacks (TIA's) or stroke in men who have had transient ischemia of the brain due to fibrin platelet emboli. There is inadequate evidence that aspirin or buffered aspirin is effective in reducing TIA's in women at the recommended dosage. There is no evidence that aspirin or buffered aspirin is of benefit in the treatment of completed strokes in men or women.

Clinical Trials: The indication is supported by the results of a Canadian study (1) in which 585 patients with threatened stroke were followed in a randomized clinical trial for an average of 26 months to determine whether aspirin or sulfinpyrazone, singly or in combination, was superior to placebo in preventing transient ischemic attacks, stroke, or death. The study showed that, although sulfinpyrazone had no statistically significant effect, aspirin reduced the risk of continuing transient ischemic attacks, stroke, or death by 19 percent and reduced the risk of stroke or death by 31 percent. Another aspirin study carried out in the United States with 178 patients, showed a statistically significant number of "favorable outcomes," including reduced transient ischemic attacks, stroke, and death (2).

Precautions: Patients presenting with signs and symptoms of TIA's should have a complete medical and neurologic evaluation. Consideration should be given to other disorders that resemble TIA's. Attention should be given to risk factors: it is important to evaluate and treat, if appropriate, other diseases associated with TIA's and stroke, such as hypertension and diabetes.
Concurrent administration of absorbable antacids at therapeutic doses may increase the clearance of salicylates in some individuals. The concurrent administration of nonabsorbable antacids may alter the rate of absorption of aspirin, thereby resulting in a decreased acetylsalicylic acid/salicylate ratio in plasma. The clinical significance of these decreases in available aspirin is unknown. Aspirin at dosages of 1,000 milligrams per day has been associated with small increases in blood pressure, blood urea nitrogen, and serum uric acid levels. It is recommended that patients placed on long-term aspirin treatment be seen at regular intervals to assess changes in these measurements.

Adverse Reactions: At dosages of 1,000 milligrams or higher of aspirin per day, gastrointestinal side effects include stomach pain, heartburn, nausea and/or

Continued on next page

Bristol-Myers—Cont.

vomiting, as well as increased rates of gross gastrointestinal bleeding.

Dosage and Administration: Adult oral dosage for men is 1,300 milligrams a day, in divided doses of 650 milligrams twice a day or 325 milligrams four times a day.

References:
(1) The Canadian Cooperative Study Group. "A Randomized Trial of Aspirin and Sulfinpyrazone in Threatened Stroke," *New England Journal of Medicine*, 299:53–59, 1978.
(2) Fields, W.S., et al., "Controlled Trial of Aspirin in Cerebral Ischemia," *Stroke* 8:301–316, 1977.

2. Tri-Buffered BUFFERIN® FOR MYOCARDIAL INFARCTION

Indication: Aspirin is indicated to reduce the risk of death and/or nonfatal myocardial infarction in patients with a previous infarction or unstable angina pectoris.

Clinical Trials: The indication is supported by the results of six, large, randomized multicenter, placebo-controlled studies[1-7] involving 10,816, predominantly male, post-myocardial infarction (MI) patients and one randomized placebo-controlled study of 1,266 men with unstable angina. Therapy with aspirin was begun at intervals after the onset of acute MI varying from less than 3 days to more than 5 years and continued for periods of from less than one year to four years. In the unstable angina study, treatment was started within 1 month after the onset of unstable angina and continued for 12 weeks and complicating conditions such as congestive heart failure were not included in the study.

Aspirin therapy in MI patients was associated with about a 20 percent reduction in the risk of subsequent death and/or nonfatal reinfarction, a median absolute decrease of 3 percent from the 12 to 22 percent event rates in the placebo groups. In the aspirin-treated unstable angina patients the reduction in risk was about 50 percent, a reduction in the event rate of 5% from the 10% rate in the placebo group over the 12 weeks of the study.

Daily dosage of aspirin in the post-myocardial infarction studies was 300 mg. in one study and 900 and 1500 mg. in five studies. A dose of 325 mg. was used in the study of unstable angina.

Adverse Reactions: Gastrointestinal Reactions: Doses of 1000 mg. per day of aspirin caused gastrointestinal symptoms and bleeding that in some cases were clinically significant. In the largest post-infarction study (The Aspirin Myocardial Infarction Study (AMIS) with 4,500 people), the percentage incidences of gastrointestinal symptoms for the aspirin (1000 mg. of a standard, solid-tablet formulation) and placebo-treated subjects, respectively, were: stomach pain (14.5%; 4.4%); heartburn (11.9%; 4.8%); nausea and/or vomiting (7.6%; 2.1%);

hospitalization for gastrointestinal disorder (4.8%; 3.5%). In the AMIS and other trials, aspirin treated patients had increased rates of gross gastrointestinal bleeding. Symptoms and signs of gastrointestinal irritation were not significantly increased in subjects treated for unstable angina with buffered aspirin in solution.

Cardiovascular and Biochemical:
In the AMIS trial, the dosage of 1000 mg. per day of aspirin was associated with small increases in systolic blood pressure (BP) (average 1.5 to 2.1 mm) and diastolic BP (0.5 to 0.6 mm), depending upon whether maximal or last available readings were used. Blood urea nitrogen and uric acid levels were also increased, but by less than 1.0 mg%.

Subjects with marked hypertension or renal insufficiency had been excluded from the trial so that the clinical importance of these observations for such subjects or for any subjects treated over more prolonged periods is not known. It is recommended that patients placed on long-term aspirin treatment, even at doses of 300 mg. per day, be seen at regular intervals to assess changes in these measurements.

References: 1. Elwood P.C., et al., "A Randomized Controlled Trial of Acetylsalicylic Acid in the Secondary Prevention of Mortality from Myocardial Infarction," *British Medical Journal*, 1:436–440, 1974. 2. The Coronary Drug Project Research Group, "Aspirin in Coronary Heart Disease," *Journal of Chronic Disease*, 29:625–642, 1976. 3. Breddin K, et al., "Secondary Prevention of Myocardial Infarction; Comparison of Acetylsalicylic Acid Phenprocoumon and Placebo," *Thromb. Haemost.*, 41:225–236, 1979. 4. Aspirin Myocardial Infarction Study Research Group, "A Randomized, Controlled Trial of Aspirin in Persons Recovered from Myocardial Infarction," *Journal American Medical Association*, 243:661–669, 1980. 5. Elwood P.C., and Sweetnam, P.M., "Aspirin and Secondary Mortality after Myocardial Infarction," *Lancet*, pp. 1313–1315, December 22–29, 1979. 6. The Persantine-Aspirin Reinfarction Study Research Group, "Persantine and Aspirin in Coronary Heart Disease," *Circulation* 62;449–460, 1980. 7. Lewis H.D., et al., "Protective Effects of Aspirin Against Acute Myocardial Infarction and Death in Men with Unstable Angina, Results of a Veterans Administration Cooperative Study," *New England Journal of Medicine*, 309;396–403, 1983.

Administration and Dosage: Although most of the studies used dosages exceeding 300 mg., two trials used only 300 mg. and pharmacologic data indicate that this dose inhibits platelet function fully. Therefore, 300 mg. or a conventional 325 mg. aspirin dose is a reasonable, routine dose that would minimize gastrointestinal adverse reactions.

Shown in Product Identification Section, page 405

Arthritis Strength Tri-Buffered BUFFERIN®
[*bŭf´fẽr-ĭn*]
Analgesic

Composition:
Active Ingredients: Aspirin (500 mg) in a formulation buffered with Calcium Carbonate, Magnesium Oxide and Magnesium Carbonate.
Other Ingredients: Benzoic Acid, Carnauba Wax, Citric Acid, Corn Starch, FD&C Blue No. 1, Hydroxpropyl Methylcellulose, Mineral Oil, Polysorbate 20, Povidone, Propylene Glycol, Simethicone Emulsion, Sodium Phosphate, Sorbitan Monolaurate, Titanium Dioxide. May also contain: Glyceryl Behenate, Magnesium Stearate, Sodium Lauryl Sulfate. Sodium Stearyl Fumarate, Stearic Acid, Zinc Stearate.

Action and Uses: For temporary relief from the minor aches and pains, stiffness, swelling and inflammation of arthritis. Buffered formulation helps prevent the stomach upset that plain aspirin can cause. Coated caplets for easy swallowing.

Contraindications: Hypersensitivity to salicylates.

Caution: If pain persists for more than 10 days or redness is present or in arthritic or rheumatic conditions affecting children under 12 consult physician immediately. Do not take without consulting physician if under medical care.

Warning: Children and teenagers should not use this medicine for chicken pox or flu symptoms before a doctor is consulted about Reye syndrome, a rare but serious illness reported to be associated with aspirin. KEEP THIS AND ALL MEDICINES OUT OF CHILDREN'S REACH. IN CASE OF ACCIDENTAL OVERDOSE, CONTACT A PHYSICIAN OR POISON CONTROL CENTER IMMEDIATELY. If dizziness, impaired hearing or ringing in the ears occurs, discontinue use. As with any drug, if you are pregnant or nursing a baby, seek the advice of a health professional before using this product.

Administration and Dosage: Adults: Two caplets with water every 4 hours as needed. Do not exceed 8 caplets in 24 hours, or give to children under 12 unless directed by a physician.

Overdose: (Symptoms and treatment) Typical of aspirin.

How Supplied: Arthritis Strength Tri-Buffered BUFFERIN® is supplied as:
Plain white coated caplet "ABS" debossed on one side.
NDC 19810-0051-1 Bottle of 40's
NDC 19810-0051-2 Bottle of 100's
The 40 caplet size does not have a child resistant closure and is recommended for households without young children.
Store at room temperature.
Professional samples available upon request.

Shown in Product Identification Section, page 405

	COMTREX Per Tablet or Caplet	COMTREX Liquid-Gel per Liqui-Gel	COMTREX Liquid Per Fl. Ounce
Acetaminophen:	325 mg.	325 mg.	650 mg.
Pseudoephedrine HCl:	30 mg.	—	60 mg.
Phenylpropanolamine HCl:	—	12.5 mg.	—
Chlorpheniramine Maleate:	2 mg.	2 mg.	4 mg.
Dextromethorphan HBr:	10 mg.	10 mg.	20 mg.

Other Ingredients:

Tablet	Caplet	Liqui-Gels	Liquid
Corn Starch	Benzoic Acid	D&C Yellow No. 10	Alcohol (20% by volume)
D&C Yellow No. 10 Lake	Carnauba Wax	FD&C Red No. 40	Citric Acid
FD&C Red No. 40 Lake	Corn Starch	Gelatin	D&C Yellow No. 10
Magnesium Stearate	D&C Yellow No. 10 Lake	Glycerin	FD&C Red No. 40
Methylparaben	FD&C Red No. 40 Lake	Polyethylene Glycol	Flavors
Propylparaben	Hydroxypropyl Methylcellulose	Povidone	Polyethylene Glycol
Stearic Acid	Magnesium Stearate	Propylene Glycol	Povidone
	Methylparaben	Silicon Dioxide	Sodium Citrate
	Mineral Oil	Sorbitol	Sucrose
	Polysorbate 20	Titanium Dioxide	Water
	Povidone	Water	
	Propylene Glycol		
	Propylparaben		
	Simethicone Emulsion		
	Sorbitan Monolaurate		
	Stearic Acid		
	Titanium Dioxide		

Extra Strength Tri-Buffered BUFFERIN®

[buf'fer-in]
Analgesic

Composition:
Active Ingredients: Aspirin (500 mg) in a formulation buffered with Calcium Carbonate, Magnesium Oxide and Magnesium Carbonate.
Other Ingredients: Benzoic Acid, Carnauba Wax, Citric Acid, Corn Starch, FD&C Blue No. 1, Hydroxypropyl Methylcellulose, Mineral Oil, Polysorbate 20, Povidone, Propylene Glycol, Simethicone Emulsion, Sodium Phosphate, Sorbitan Monolaurate, Titanium Dioxide. May also contain: Glyceryl Behenate, Magnesium Stearate, Sodium Lauryl Sulfate, Sodium Stearyl Fumarate, Stearic Acid, Zinc Stearate.

Action and Uses: Contains aspirin for relief from headaches, pain and fever of colds and flu, muscle aches, temporary relief of minor arthritis pain and inflammation, menstrual pain and toothaches. Buffered formulation which helps prevent the stomach upset that plain aspirin can cause. Each tablet is coated for easy swallowing.

Contraindications: Hypersensitivity to salicylates.

Caution: If pain persists for more than 10 days, or redness is present, or in arthritic or rheumatic conditions affecting children under 12, consult a physician immediately. Do not take without consulting a physician if under medical care. Consult a dentist for toothache promptly.

Warning: Children and teenagers should not use this medicine for chicken pox or flu symptoms before a doctor is consulted about Reye syndrome, a rare but serious illness reported to be associated with aspirin. KEEP THIS AND ALL MEDICINES OUT OF CHILDREN'S REACH. IN CASE OF ACCIDENTAL OVERDOSE, CONTACT A PHYSICIAN OR POISON CONTROL CENTER IMMEDIATELY. If dizziness, impaired hearing or ringing in the ears occurs, discontinue use. As with any drug, if you are pregnant or nursing a baby, seek the advice of a health professional before using this product.

Administration and Dosage: Adults: Two tablets with water every 4 hours as needed. Do not exceed 8 tablets in 24 hours, or give to children under 12 unless directed by a physician.

Overdose: (Symptoms and treatment) Typical of aspirin.

How Supplied: Extra Strength Tri-Buffered BUFFERIN® is supplied as: White elongated coated tablet with "ESB" debossed on one side.
NDC 19810-0074-1 Bottle of 30's
NDC 19810-0074-2 Bottle of 60's
NDC 19810-0074-3 Bottle of 100's
All sizes have child resistant closures except 60's which is recommended for households without young children.
Store at room temperature.
Professional samples available upon request.
Shown in Product Identification Section, page 405

COMTREX®

[cŏm'trĕx]
Multi-Symptom Cold Reliever

Composition: Each tablet, caplet, liqui-gel and fluid ounce (30 ml.) contains:
[See table above]

Actions and Uses: COMTREX® tablets, caplets, liqui-gels, and liquid contain four important ingredients for safe and effective relief. A **decongestant**—pseudoephedrine HCl—(Phenylpropanolamine HCl in Liqui-Gels) to relieve nasal and sinus congestion. An **antihistamine**—chlorpheniramine maleate—to dry up runny nose. A **cough suppressant**—dextromethorphan HBr—to quiet cough. A **non-aspirin analgesic**—acetaminophen—to relieve body aches and pain.

Contraindications: Hypersensitivity to acetaminophen or antihistamines.

Warning: KEEP THIS AND ALL OTHER MEDICATIONS OUT OF THE REACH OF CHILDREN. IN CASE OF ACCIDENTAL OVERDOSE, SEEK PROFESSIONAL ASSISTANCE OR CONTACT A POISON CONTROL CENTER IMMEDIATELY. PROMPT MEDICAL ATTENTION IS CRITICAL FOR ADULTS AS WELL AS CHILDREN EVEN IF YOU DO NOT NOTICE ANY SYMPTOMS. As with any drug, if you are pregnant or nursing a baby, seek the advice of a health professional before using this product. Do not take this product for more than 7 days (for adults) or 5 days (for children), or for fever for more than 3 days unless directed by a doctor. Do not exceed recommended dosage because at higher doses nervousness, dizziness or sleeplessness may occur. May cause excitability especially in children. A persistent cough may be a sign of a serious condition. If cough persists for more than 7 days, tends to recur, or is accompanied by rash, persistent headache, fever that lasts for more than 3 days or if new symptoms occur, consult a doctor. Do not take this product for persistent or chronic cough such as occurs with smoking, asthma or emphysema, or if cough is accompanied by excessive phlegm (mucus) unless directed by a doctor. If sore throat is severe, persists for more than 2 days, is accompanied or followed by a fever, headache, rash, nausea or vomiting, consult a doctor promptly. This product should not be taken by persons who have asthma, glaucoma, emphysema, chronic pulmonary disease, high blood pressure, heart disease, thyroid disease, diabetes, shortness of breath, difficulty in breathing or diffi-

Continued on next page

Bristol-Myers—Cont.

culty in urination due to enlargement of the prostate gland unless directed by a doctor. May cause marked drowsiness. Use caution when driving a motor vehicle or operating machinery. Avoid alcoholic beverages and do not take this product if you are taking sedatives or tranquilizers without first consulting your doctor.

Drug Interaction Precaution: This product should not be taken by any adult or child who is taking a prescription medication for high blood pressure or depression without first consulting a doctor.

Administration and Dosage:
Tablets or Caplets: **Adults,** 2 tablets or caplets every 4 hours as needed not to exceed 8 tablets or caplets in 24 hours. **Children** 6 to under 12 years: one tablet every 4 hours as needed, not to exceed 4 tablets or caplets in 24 hours. Under 6, consult a doctor.
Liqui-Gel: **Adults,** two liqui-gels every 4 hours as needed, not to exceed 12 liqui-gels in 24 hours. **Children** 6 to under 12 years; 1 liqui-gel every 4 hours as needed, not to exceed 6 liqui-gels in 24 hours. Under 6 consult a doctor.
Liquid: **Adults,** 1 fluid ounce (30 ml.) every 4 hours as needed, not to exceed 4 fluid ounces (120 ml.) in 24 hours. **Children** 6–12 years: ½ the adult dose. Under 6, consult a physician.

Overdose: For overdose treatment information, consult a regional poison control center. (Also see Allergy-Sinus COMTREX®, Cough Formula COMTREX®.)

How Supplied:
COMTREX® is supplied as:
Yellow tablet with letter "C" debossed on one surface.
NDC 19810-0790-1 Blister packages of 24's
NDC 19810-0790-2 Bottles of 50's
Coated yellow caplet with "Comtrex" printed in red on one side.
NDC 19810-0792-3 Blister packages of 24's
NDC 19810-0792-4 Bottles of 50's
Yellow Liqui-gel with "Comtrex" printed in red on one side.
NDC 19810-0561-1 Blister packages of 24's
NDC 19810-0561-2 Blister packages of 50's
Clear orange liquid:
NDC 19810-0791-1 6 oz. plastic bottles
NDC 19810-0791-2 10 oz. plastic bottles
All sizes packaged in child resistant closures except for 24's for tablets, caplets and liqui-gels and 6 oz. liquid which are sizes recommended for households without young children. Store caplets, tablets and liquid at room temperature. Store liqui-gels below 86° F. (30° C.). Keep from freezing.
Shown in Product Identification Section, page 405

ALLERGY–SINUS COMTREX
[cŏm 'trĕx]
Multi-Symptom Allergy/Sinus Formula

Composition: Active Ingredients: Each coated tablet or caplet contains 500 mg acetaminophen, 30 mg pseudoephedrine HCl, 2 mg chlorpheniramine maleate.
Other Ingredients: Benzoic acid, carnauba wax, corn starch, D&C yellow No. 10 lake, FD&C blue No. 1 lake, FD&C Red No. 40 lake, hydroxypropyl methylcellulose, mineral oil, polysorbate 20, povidone, propylene glycol, simethicone emulsion, sodium citrate, sorbitan monolaurate, stearic acid, titanium dioxide. May also contain: crospovidone, D&C yellow No. 10, erythorbic acid, FD&C blue No. 1, magnesium stearate, methylparaben, microcrystalline cellulose, polysorbate 80, propylparaben, silicon dioxide, wood cellulose.

Indications: ALLERGY-SINUS COMTREX provides temporary relief of these upper respiratory allergy, hay fever, and sinusitis symptoms: sneezing, itchy, watery eyes, runny nose, headache, nasal and sinus pressure and congestion.

Product Information: ALLERGY-SINUS COMTREX tablets and caplets contain three important ingredients for safe and effective relief. A maximum dose of **non-aspirin analgesic—** acetaminophen—to relieve sinus headache pain. A **decongestant**—pseudoephedrine HCl—to relieve nasal and sinus congestion. An **antihistamine**—chlorpheniramine maleate—to relieve sneezing, runny nose, and itchy eyes.

Contraindications: Hypersensitivity to acetaminophen, pseudoephedrine or antihistamines.

Warnings: KEEP THIS AND ALL MEDICINE OUT OF CHILDREN'S REACH. In case of accidental overdose, contact a physician or Poison Control Center immediately. Do not give to children under 12 or exceed recommended dosage. Reduce dosage if nervousness, restlessness or sleeplessness occurs. Do not use for more than 10 days unless directed by a physician. Do not take without consulting a physician if under medical care. Individuals with high blood pressure, diabetes, heart or thyroid disease, asthma, glaucoma, or difficulty in urination due to enlargement of the prostate gland should not take this preparation unless directed by a physician. As with any drug, if you are pregnant or nursing a baby, seek the advice of a health professional before using this product. Do not drive or operate machinery while taking this medicine as it may cause drowsiness.

Administration and Dosage: Adults, two tablets or caplets every 6 hours, as needed, not to exceed 8 tablets or caplets in 24 hours.

Overdose: For overdose treatment information, consult a regional poison control center. (See also Comtrex Tablets, Caplets and Liquid, Cough Formula Comtrex).

How Supplied: Allergy-Sinus COMTREX® is supplied as:
Coated green tablets with "Comtrex A/S" printed in black on one side.
NDC 19810-0774-1 Blister packages of 24's
NDC 19810-0774-2 Bottles of 50's
Coated green caplets with "A/S" debossed on one surface.
NDC 19810-0081-4 Blister packages of 24's
NDC 19810-0081-5 Bottles of 50's
All sizes packaged in child resistant closures except 24's for tablets and caplets which are sizes recommended for households without young children.
Store at room temperature.
Shown in Product Identification Section, page 405

Cough Formula COMTREX®
[cŏm 'trĕx]
Multi-Symptom Cough Formula

Composition:
Active Ingredients:
Each 4 teaspoonfuls (⅔ fl. oz.) contains:
—EXPECTORANT—200 mg Guaifenesin
—COUGH SUPPRESSANT—30 mg Dextromethorphan HBr
—ANALGESIC—500 mg Acetaminophen
—DECONGESTANT—60 mg Pseudoephedrine HCl

Other Ingredients:
Alcohol (20% by volume), Citric Acid, FD&C Red No. 40, Flavor, Menthol, Povidone, Saccharin Sodium, Sodium Citrate, Sucrose, Water.

Indications and Uses: For temporary relief of coughs, nasal and upper chest congestion fever and pain due to a chest cold.

BENEFITS OF COUGH FORMULA COMTREX
—Relieves upper chest congestion by loosening phlegm and mucus.
—Relieves your cough for up to 8 hours.
—Relieves muscle pain due to excessive coughing.
—Soothes irritated sore throat.
—Helps clear nasal passages to relieve congestion.

Contraindications: Hypersensitivity to Acetaminophen or Pseudoephedrine

Warning: KEEP THIS AND ALL OTHER MEDICATIONS OUT OF THE REACH OF CHILDREN. IN CASE OF ACCIDENTAL OVERDOSE, SEEK PROFESSIONAL ASSISTANCE OR CONTACT A POISON CONTROL CENTER IMMEDIATELY. PROMPT MEDICAL ATTENTION IS CRITICAL FOR ADULTS AS WELL AS FOR CHILDREN EVEN IF YOU DO NOT NOTICE ANY SYMPTOMS. As with any drug, if you are pregnant or nursing a baby, seek the advice of a health professional before using this product. Do not take this product for more than 7 days (for adults) or 5 days (for children) or for fever for more than 3 days unless directed by a doctor. Do not exceed recommended dosage because at higher doses nervousness, dizziness or sleeplessness may occur. A persistent cough may be a sign of a serious condition. If cough persists for more than 7 days, tends to recur or is accompanied by rash, persistent headache, fever that lasts for more than 3 days, or if new symptoms occur, consult a doctor. Do not take this product for persistent or chronic cough such as occurs with smoking, asthma, chronic bronchitis or emphysema or if cough is accompanied by excessive phlegm (mucus) unless directed by a doctor. If sore throat is severe, persists for more than 2 days, is accompanied or followed by a fever, headache, rash, nausea or vomiting, consult a doctor promptly. This product should not be taken by persons who have asthma, glaucoma, emphysema, chronic pulmonary disease, high blood pressure, thyroid disease, diabetes, shortness of breath, difficulty in breathing or difficulty in urination due to enlargement of the prostate gland unless directed by a doctor.

Precaution: This product should not be taken by any adult or child who is taking a prescription medication for high blood pressure or depression without first consulting a doctor.

Administration and Dosage:
Adult Dose: (12 years and over):
Take ⅔ fl. oz. in dosage cup or four teaspoonfuls. Repeat every 6 hours as needed. No more than 4 doses in a 24-hour period.
Child Dose: (6 to under 12 years):
Take ⅓ fl. oz. in dosage cup or two teaspoonfuls. Repeat every 6 hours as needed. No more than 4 doses in a 24-hour period.
DO NOT ADMINISTER TO CHILDREN UNDER 6 YEARS OF AGE.

Overdose: For overdose treatment information consult a regional poison control center.

How Supplied: Cough Formula COMTREX® is supplied as a clear red raspberry flavored liquid:
NDC 19810-0781-1 4 oz. plastic bottle
NDC 19810-0781-3 8 oz. plastic bottle
The 4 oz. size is not child resistant and is recommended for households without young children.
Store at room temperature.

CONGESPIRIN® for Children
Aspirin Free
Chewable Cold Tablets
[cŏn "gĕs'pir-in]

Composition: Each tablet contains acetaminophen 81 mg. (1¼ grains), phenylephrine hydrochloride 1¼ mg. Also Contains: Calcium Stearate, D&C Red No. 30 Aluminum Lake, D&C Yellow No. 10 Aluminum Lake, Ethyl Cellulose, Flavor, Mannitol, Microcrystalline Cellulose, Polyethylene, Saccharin, Calcium, Sucrose.

Action and Uses: A non-aspirin analgesic/nasal decongestant that temporarily reduces fever and relieves aches, pains and nasal congestion associated with colds and "flu."

Warnings: KEEP THIS AND ALL MEDICINES OUT OF CHILDREN'S REACH. IN CASE OF ACCIDENTAL OVERDOSE, CONTACT A PHYSICIAN IMMEDIATELY.

Caution: If child is under medical care, do not administer without consulting physician. Do not exceed recommended dosage. Consult your physician if symptoms persist or if high blood pressure, heart disease, diabetes or thyroid disease is present. Do not administer for more than 10 days unless directed by physician.

Dosage and Administration:
Under 2, consult your physician.
2–3 years ....2 tablets
4–5 years ....3 tablets
6–8 years ....4 tablets
9–10 years ....5 tablets
11–12 years ....6 tablets
over 12 years ....8 tablets
Repeat dose in four hours if necessary. Do not give more than four doses per day unless prescribed by your physician.

Overdose: For overdose treatment information consult a regional poison control center. See also: Congespirin for Children Aspirin Free Liquid Cold Medicine and Congespirin for Children Cough Syrup.

How Supplied: CONGESPIRIN Aspirin Free Chewable Cold Tablets are supplied as scored orange tablets with "C" on one side.
NDC 19810-0748-1 Bottles of 24's.
Bottles are child resistant.
Store at room temperature.
Shown in Product Identification Section, page 405

Extra–Strength DATRIL®
[dā 'trĭl]
Analgesic

Composition: Each tablet or caplet contains acetaminophen, 500 mg. Other Ingredients: (Tablets) Corn Starch, Stearic Acid. Tablets may also contain: Croscarmellose Sodium, Crospovidone, Erythorbic Acid, Methylparaben, Povidone, Propylparaben, Silicon Dioxide, Sodium Lauryl Sulfate, Wood Cellulose. Caplets also contain: Carnauba Wax, Corn Starch, FD&C Blue No. 1, Hydroxypropyl Methylcellulose, Mineral Oil, Polysorbate 20, Povidone, Propylene Glycol, Simethicone Emulsion, Sorbitan Monolaurate, Stearic Acid, Titanium Dioxide. May also contain: Benzoic Acid, Croscarmellose Sodium, Crospovidone, Erythorbic Acid, Methylparaben, Propylparaben, Silicon Dioxide, Sodium Lauryl Sulfate, Wood Cellulose.

Actions and Uses: Extra-Strength DATRIL contains non-aspirin acetaminophen which is less likely to irritate the stomach than plain aspirin. Extra-Strength DATRIL is intended for the temporary relief of minor aches, pains, headaches and fever. For most persons with peptic ulcer Extra-Strength DATRIL may be used when taken as directed for recommended conditions.

Contraindications: There have been rare reports of skin rash or glossitis attributed to acetaminophen. Discontinue use if a sensitivity reaction occurs. However, acetaminophen is usually well tolerated by aspirin-sensitive patients.

Caution: Severe or recurrent pain, high or continued fever may be indicative of serious illness. Under these conditions consult a physician. **If pain persists for more than 10 days or redness is present, or in arthritic conditions affecting children under 12, consult a physician immediately.** Do not take without consulting a physician if under medical care.

Warnings: Keep this and all medicines out of the reach of children. In case of accidental overdose, contact a physician or Poison Control Center immediately. Do not give to children 12 and under or use for more than 10 days unless directed by a physician. As with any drug, if you are pregnant or nursing a baby, seek the advice of a health professional before using this product.

Dosage: Adults: Two tablets or caplets. May be repeated in 4 hours if needed. Do not exceed 8 tablets or caplets in any 24 hour period.

Overdose:
MUCOMYST (acetylcysteine) As An Antidote For Acetaminophen Overdose)
Acetaminophen is rapidly absorbed from the upper gastrointestinal tract with peak plasma levels occurring between 30 and 60 minutes after therapeutic doses and usually within 4 hours following an overdose. The parent compound, which is nontoxic, is extensively metabolized in the liver to form principally the sulfate and glucuronide conjugates which are also nontoxic and are rapidly excreted in the urine. A small fraction of an ingested dose is metabolized in the liver by the cytochrome P-450 mixed function oxidase enzyme system to form a reactive, potentially toxic, intermediate metabolite which preferentially conjugates with hepatic glutathione to form the nontoxic cysteine and mercapturic acid derivatives which are then excreted by the kidney. Therapeutic doses of acetaminophen do not saturate the glucuronide and sulfate conjugation pathways and do not result in the formation of sufficient reactive metabolite to deplete glutathione stores. However, following ingestion of a large overdose (150 mg/kg or greater) the glucuronide and sulfate conjugation pathways are saturated resulting in a larger fraction of the drug being metabolized via the P-450 pathway. The increased formation of reactive metabolite may deplete the hepatic stores of glutathione with subsequent binding of the metabolite to protein molecules within the hepatocyte resulting in cellular necrosis. Acetylcysteine has been shown to reduce the extent of liver injury following acetaminophen overdose.

Continued on next page

Bristol-Myers—Cont.

Early symptoms following a potentially hepatotoxic overdose may include: nausea, vomiting, diaphoresis and general malaise. Clinical and laboratory evidence of hepatic toxicity may not be apparent until 48 to 72 hours postingestion. In adults and adolescents, regardless of the quantity of acetaminophen reported to have been ingested, administer MUCOMYST® acetylcysteine immediately. MUCOMYST acetylcysteine therapy should be initiated and continued for a full course of therapy. Its effectiveness depends on early administration, with benefit seen principally in patients treated within 16 hours of the overdose. If acetaminophen plasma assay capability is not available, and the estimated acetaminophen ingestion exceeds 150 mg/kg, MUCOMYST acetylcysteine therapy should be initiated and continued for a full course of therapy.
For full prescribing information, refer to the MUCOMYST package insert. Do not await the results of assays for acetaminophen level before initiating treatment with MUCOMYST acetylcysteine. The following additional procedures are recommended: The stomach should be emptied promptly by lavage or by induction of emesis with syrup of ipecac. A serum acetaminophen assay should be obtained as early as possible, but no sooner than four hours following ingestion. Liver function studies should be obtained initially and repeated at 24-hour intervals.
For additional emergency information call your regional poison center or toll-free (1-800-525-6115) to the Rocky Mountain Poison Center for assistance in diagnosis and for directions in the use of MUCOMYST acetylcysteine as an antidote.

How Supplied: Extra Strength DATRIL® is supplied as:
White circular tablets with "DATRIL" debossed on one surface.
NDC 19810-0705-1 Bottles of 30's
NDC 19810-0705-2 Bottles of 60's
NDC 19810-0705-3 Bottles of 100's
Coated white caplet with "Datril" debossed on one side.
NDC 19810-0799-1 Bottles of 24's
NDC 19810-0799-2 Bottles of 50's
All sizes packaged in child resistant closures except 50's for caplets and 60's for tablets which are sizes recommended for households without young children.
Store at room temperature.
Shown in Product Identification Section, page 405

EXCEDRIN® Extra-Strength Analgesic
[ĕx "cĕd 'rĭn]

Composition: Each tablet or caplet contains Acetaminophen 250 mg.; Aspirin 250 mg.; and Caffeine 65 mg.
OTHER INGREDIENTS: **(Tablets)** Microcrystalline Cellulose, Stearic Acid. Tablets may also contain: Hydroxypropylcellulose. **(Caplets)** Carnauba Wax, FD&C Blue No. 1, Hydroxypropyl Methylcellulose, Microcrystalline Cellulose, Mineral Oil, Polysorbate 20, Povidone, Propylene Glycol, Simethicone Emulsion, Sorbitan Monolaurate, Stearic Acid, Titanium Dioxide. Caplets may also contain: Benzoic Acid, Hydroxypropylcellulose.

Action and Uses: Extra-Strength EXCEDRIN is intended for the relief of pain from: headache, sinusitis, colds or 'flu', muscular aches and menstrual discomfort. Also recommended for temporary relief of toothaches and minor arthritic pains.

Contraindications: Hypersensitivity to salicylates or acetaminophen.

Caution: If pain persists for more than 10 days, or redness is present, or in arthritic conditions affecting children under 12, consult physician immediately. Consult dentist for toothache promptly. Do not take without consulting physician if under medical care. Store at room temperature.

Warning: Children and teenagers should not use this medicine for chicken pox or flu symptoms before a doctor is consulted about Reye syndrome, a rare but serious illness reported to be associated with aspirin. Do not exceed 8 tablets or caplets in 24 hours or use for more than 10 days unless directed by physician, or give to children under 12. KEEP THIS AND ALL MEDICINES OUT OF CHILDREN'S REACH. IN CASE OF ACCIDENTAL OVERDOSE, CONTACT A PHYSICIAN IMMEDIATELY. As with any drug, if you are pregnant or nursing a baby, seek the advice of a health professional before using this product.

Administration and Dosage: Tablets or Caplets—Individuals 12 and over, take 2 tablets or caplets every 4 hours as needed.

Overdose: For overdose treatment information, consult a regional poison control center.

How Supplied: Extra Strength EXCEDRIN® is supplied as:
White circular tablet with letter "E" debossed on one side.
NDC 19810-0700-2 Bottles of 12's
NDC 19810-0772-9 Bottles of 30's
NDC 19810-0700-4 Bottles of 60's
NDC 19810-0700-5 Bottles of 100's
NDC 19810-0700-6 Bottles of 165's
NDC 19810-0700-7 Bottles of 225's
NDC 19810-0782-2 Bottles of 275's
NDC 19810-0700-1 A metal tin of 12's
Coated white caplets with "Excedrin" printed in red on one side.
NDC 19810-0002-1 Bottles of 24's
NDC 19810-0002-2 Bottles of 50's
NDC 19810-0002-3 Bottles of 80's
All sizes packaged in child resistant closures except 100's for tablets, 80's for caplets which are sizes recommended for households without young children.
Store at room temperature.
Shown in Product Identification Section, page 405

EXCEDRIN P.M.®
[ĕx "cĕd 'rĭn]
Analgesic Sleeping Aid

Composition: Each tablet or caplet contains Acetaminophen 500 mg. and Diphenhydramine citrate 38 mg. Tablets also Contain: Corn Starch Pregelatinized, D&C Yellow No. 10, D&C Yellow No. 10 Aluminum Lake, FD&C Blue No. 1, FD&C Blue No. 1 Aluminum Lake, Magnesium Stearate, Methylparaben, Propylparaben, Stearic Acid. May Also Contain: Microcrystalline Cellulose, Povidone.
Caplets also Contain: Benzoic Acid; Carnauba Wax; Corn Starch; D&C Yellow No. 10; D&C Yellow No. 10 Aluminum Lake; FD&C Blue No. 1; FD&C Blue No. 1 Aluminum Lake; Hydroxypropyl Methylcellulose; Methylparaben; Magnesium Stearate; Propylene Glycol; Propylparaben; Simethicone Emulsion; Stearic Acid; Titanium Dioxide.

Action and Uses: For the temporary relief of occasional headaches and minor aches and pains with accompanying sleeplessness.

Contraindications: Hypersensitivity to acetaminophen or antihistamines.

Caution: Do not drive a car or operate machinery while taking this medication. Do not take without consulting physician if under medical care.

Warnings: KEEP THIS AND ALL MEDICINES OUT OF CHILDREN'S REACH. IN CASE OF ACCIDENTAL OVERDOSE, CONTACT A PHYSICIAN IMMEDIATELY. Do not give to children under 12 years of age or use for more than 10 days unless directed by a physician. Consult your physician if symptoms persist or new ones occur or if fever persists more than 3 days (72 hours) or recurs, or if sleeplessness persists continuously for more than two weeks. Insomnia may be a symptom of serious underlying medical illness. Take this product with caution if alcohol is being consumed. DO NOT TAKE THIS PRODUCT IF YOU HAVE ASTHMA, GLAUCOMA OR ENLARGEMENT OF THE PROSTATE GLAND EXCEPT UNDER THE ADVICE AND SUPERVISION OF A PHYSICIAN. As with any drug, if you are pregnant or nursing a baby, seek the advice of a health professional before using this product.

Administration and Dosage: Adults take two tablets at bedtime or as directed by a physician. Do not exceed recommended dosage.

Overdose: For overdose treatment information, consult a regional poison control center.

How Supplied:
EXCEDRIN P.M.® is supplied as:
Light blue circular tablets with "PM" debossed on one side.

NDC 19810-0763-6 Bottles of 10's
NDC 19810-0763-3 Bottles of 30's
NDC 19810-0763-4 Bottles of 50's
NDC 19810-0763-5 Bottles of 80's
Light blue coated caplet with "Excedrin P.M." imprinted on one side.
NDC 19810-0032-2 Bottles of 30's
NDC 19810-0032-3 Bottles of 50's
All sizes packaged in child resistant closures except 50's which is recommended for households without young children.
Store at room temperature.
Shown in Product Identification Section, page 405

Sinus EXCEDRIN®
[ex "cĕd 'rĭn]
Analgesic, Decongestant

Composition: Each coated tablet or caplet contains 500 mg Acetaminophen and 30 mg Pseudoephedrine HCl.

Other Ingredients: Corn Starch, D&C Yellow No. 10 Lake, FD&C Red No. 40 Lake, Hydroxypropylcellulose, Hydroxypropyl Methylcellulose, Mineral Oil, Polysorbate 20, Povidone, Propylene Glycol, Simethicone Emulsion, Sorbitan Monolaurate, Stearic Acid, Titanium Dioxide. May also contain: Benzoic Acid, Carnauba Wax.

Action and Uses: Sinus EXCEDRIN is intended for the temporary relief of headache and sinus pain and for the relief of sinus pressure due to sinusitis or the common cold.

Contraindications: Hypersensitivity to acetaminophen or pseudoephedrine.

Warnings: KEEP THIS AND ALL MEDICINES OUT OF CHILDREN'S REACH. In case of accidental overdose, contact a physician or Poison Control Center immediately. Do not exceed recommended dosage. Reduce dosage if nervousness, dizziness or sleeplessness occurs. Do not take this product for more than 7 days. If symptoms do not improve or are accompanied by a fever, consult a doctor. If you have heart disease, diabetes, high blood pressure, thyroid disease or difficulty in urination due to enlargement of the prostrate gland, or are presently taking a prescription drug for high blood pressure or depression, do not take this medicine unless directed by a physician. As with any drug, if you are pregnant or nursing a baby, seek the advice of a health professional before using this product.

Administration and Dosage: Adults and Children over 12: two tablets or caplets every 6 hours as needed, not to exceed 8 tablets or caplets in 24 hours. Children 12 and under should use only as directed by a doctor.

How Supplied: Sinus EXCEDRIN® is supplied as:
Coated circular orange tablets with "Sinus Excedrin" imprinted in green on one side.
NDC 19810-0080-1 Blister packages of 24's

NDC 19810-0080-2 Bottles of 50's
Coated orange caplets with "Sinus Excedrin" imprinted in green on one side.
NDC 19810-0077-1 Blister packages of 24's
NDC 19810-0077-2 Bottles of 50's
All sizes have child resistant closures except 24's for tablets and caplets which are recommended for households without young children.
Store at room temperature.
Shown in Product Identification Section, page 405 and page 406

4-WAY® Cold Tablets

Composition: "New Aspirin-Free Formula"
Each tablet contains acetaminophen 325 mg., phenylpropanolamine HCl 12.5 mg., and chlorpheniramine maleate 2 mg. Other Ingredients: Corn Starch, Corn Starch Pregelatinized, Microcrystalline Cellulose, Sodium Starch Glycolate, Stearic Acid, Sucrose.

Actions and Uses: For temporary relief of 1) nasal congestion, 2) runny nose, 3) fever, and 4) minor aches and pains as may occur in the common cold.

Dosage and Administration:
Adults—2 tablets every 4 hours, as needed. Do not exceed 12 tablets in 24 hours. Children 6 to under 12 years—one half the adult dosage.

Caution: Do not drive or operate machinery while taking this medication as it may cause drowsiness.

Warning: Keep this and all medicines out of children's reach. In case of accidental overdose, contact a physician or poison control center immediately. Do not exceed the recommended dosage. Do not give to children under 6 or use for more than 10 days (for adults) or 5 days (for children) unless directed by a physician. If symptoms do not improve or are accompanied by fever that lasts for more than 3 days or if new symptoms occur, consult a doctor. Persons with high blood pressure, diabetes, heart or thyroid disease, asthma, glaucoma, or difficulty in urination due to enlargement of the prostate gland or persons under a doctor's care should not use this preparation unless directed by a physician. May cause excitablity in children. Reduce dosage if nervousness, restlessness, or sleeplessness occurs. As with any drug, if you are pregnant or nursing a baby, seek the advice of a health professional before using this product. Do not drive a car or operate machinery while taking this medicine as it may cause drowsiness.

Drug Interaction Precaution: Do not take this product if you are presently taking a prescription drug for high blood pressure or depression without first consulting your doctor.

How Supplied: 4-WAY Cold Tablets are supplied as a white tablet with the number "4" debossed on one surface.

NDC 19810-0040-1 Bottle of 36's
NDC 19810-0040-2 Bottle of 60's
All sizes packaged in child resistant bottle closures.
Store at room temperature.
Shown in Product Identification Section, page 406

4-WAY® Fast Acting Nasal Spray

Composition: Phenylephrine hydrochloride 0.5%, naphazoline hydrochloride 0.05%, pyrilamine maleate 0.2%, in a buffered isotonic aqueous solution with thimerosal 0.005% added as a preservative. Also Contains: Benzalkonium Chloride, Poloxamer 188, Potassium Phosphate, Sodium Chloride, Sodium Phosphate, Water. Also available in a mentholated formula containing Phenylephrine hydrochloride 0.5%, naphazoline hydrochloride 0.05%, pyrilamine maleate 0.2%, in a buffered isotonic aqueous solution with thimerosal 0.005% added as a preservative. Also Contains: Benzalkonium Chloride, Camphor, Eucalyptol, Menthol, Poloxamer 188, Polysorbate 80, Potassium Phosphate, Sodium Chloride, Sodium Phosphate, Water.

Action and Uses: For prompt, temporary relief of nasal congestion due to the common cold, sinusitis, hay fever or other upper respiratory allergies.

Dosage and Administration: DOSAGE: Adults: Spray twice into each nostril. Repeat every 6 hours if needed. Do not give to children under 12 years of age unless directed by physician. **DIRECTIONS:** Remove protective cap. Hold bottle with thumb at base and nozzle between first and second fingers. With head upright, insert metered pump spray nozzle into nostril. Depress pump twice, all the way down, with a firm even stroke. Do not tilt head backward while spraying. Wipe tip clean after each use.

Warning: Do not exceed recommended dosage because symptoms may occur such as burning, stinging, sneezing or increase of nasal discharge. Overdosage in young children may cause marked sedation. Follow directions carefully. Do not use this product for more than 3 days. If symptoms persist, consult a physician. The use of this dispenser by more than one person may spread infection. Store at room temperature. Keep this and all medicines out of children's reach. In case of accidental ingestion, contact a physician or Poison Control Center immediately.

Overdosage: For overdose treatment information, contact a regional poison control center.

How Supplied:
4-WAY® Fast Acting Nasal Spray is supplied as:
Regular formula:
NDC 19810-0001-1 Atomizer of ½ fluid ounce
NDC 19810-0001-2 Atomizer of 1 fluid ounce.

Continued on next page

Bristol-Myers—Cont.

NDC 19810-0001-3 Metered pump of ½ fluid ounce.

Mentholated formula:

NDC 19810-0003-1 Atomizer of ½ fluid ounce.

NDC 19810-0003-2 Atomizer of 1 fluid ounce.

Store at room temperature.

Shown in Product Identification Section, page 406

4-WAY® Long Lasting Nasal Spray

Composition: Oxymetazoline Hydrochloride 0.05% in a buffered isotonic aqueous solution. Phenylmercuric Acetate 0.002% added as a preservative. **Also Contains:** Benzalkonium Chloride, Glycine, Sorbitol, Water.

Action and Uses: Provides temporary relief of nasal congestion due to the common cold, sinusitis, hay fever or other upper respiratory allergies.

Dosage and Administration: DOSAGE: Adults—and children 6 years of age and older (with adult supervision): Spray 2 or 3 times into each nostril twice daily—once in the morning and once in the evening. Not recommended for children under 6. **DIRECTIONS:** Remove protective cap. Hold bottle with thumb at base and nozzle between first and second fingers. With head upright, insert metered pump spray nozzle into nostril. Depress pump 2 or 3 times, all the way down, with a firm even stroke and sniff deeply. Repeat in other nostril. Do not tilt head backward while spraying. Wipe tip clean after each use.

Warning: Do not give this product to children under 6 years of age except under the advice and supervision of a physician. Do not exceed recommended dosage because symptoms may occur such as burning, stinging, sneezing or increase of nasal discharge. Do not use this product for more than 3 days. If symptoms persist, consult a physician. The use of this dispenser by more than one person may spread infection. Store at room temperature. Keep this and all medicines out of children's reach. In case of accidental ingestion, contact a physician or Poison Control Center immediately.

Overdosage: For overdose treatment information, contact a regional poison control center.

How Supplied: 4-WAY Long Lasting Nasal Spray is supplied as:

Atomizers and a metered pump:

NDC 19810-0728-1 Atomizers of ½ fluid ounce.

NDC 19810-0728-3 Metered pump of ½ fluid ounce.

Store at room temperature.

Shown in Product Identification Section, page 406

NO DOZ® Tablets

[nō 'dōz]

Composition: Each tablet contains 100 mg. Caffeine. Other Ingredients: Cornstarch, Flavors, Mannitol, Microcrystalline Cellulose, Stearic Acid, Sucrose.

Indications: Helps restore mental alertness or wakefulness when experiencing fatigue or drowsiness.

Dosage and Administration: Adults and children 12 years of age and over: One or two tablets not more often than every 3 to 4 hours.

Caution: Do not take without consulting physician if under medical care. No stimulant should be substituted for normal sleep in activities requiring physical alertness.

Warning: For occasional use only. Not intended for use as a substitute for sleep. If fatigue or drowsiness persists or continues to recur, consult a doctor. The recommended dose of this product contains about as much caffeine as a cup of coffee. Limit the use of caffeine-containing medications, foods, or beverages while taking this product because too much caffeine may cause nervousness, irritability, sleeplessness and, occasionally, rapid heart beat. Do not give to children under 12 years of age. **KEEP THIS AND ALL MEDICINES OUT OF THE REACH OF CHILDREN. IN CASE OF ACCIDENTAL OVERDOSE, SEEK PROFESSIONAL ASSISTANCE OR CONTACT A POISON CONTROL CENTER IMMEDIATELY. As with any drug, if you are pregnant or nursing a baby, seek the advice of a health professional before using this product.**

Overdose: Typical of caffeine.

How Supplied: NO DOZ® is supplied as:

A circular white tablet with "NoDoz" debossed on one side.

NDC 19810-0063-2 Blister pack of 16's

NDC 19810-0063-3 Blister pack of 36's

NDC 19810-0062-5 Bottle of 60's

Store at room temperature.

Shown in Product Identification Section, page 406

NUPRIN®
(ibuprofen)
Analgesic

Warning: ASPIRIN SENSITIVE PATIENTS should not take this product if they have had a severe allergic reaction to aspirin, e.g.—asthma, swelling, shock or hives, because even though this product contains no aspirin or salicylates, cross-reactions may occur in patients allergic to aspirin.

Composition: Each tablet or caplet contains ibuprofen USP, 200 mg. **Other Ingredients:** Carnauba wax, cornstarch, D&C Yellow No. 10, FD&C Yellow No. 6, hydroxypropyl methylcellulose, propylene glycol, silicon dioxide, stearic acid, titanium dioxide.

Action and Uses: For the temporary relief of minor aches and pains associated with the common cold, headache, toothache, muscular aches, backache, for the minor pain of arthritis, for the pain of menstrual cramps and for reduction of fever.

Warnings: The following warnings are stated on the Nuprin label: Do not take for pain for more than 10 days or for fever for more than 3 days unless directed by a doctor. If pain or fever persists or gets worse, if new symptoms occur, or if the painful area is red or swollen, consult a doctor. These could be signs of serious illness. If you are under a doctor's care for any serious condition, consult a doctor before taking this product. As with aspirin and acetaminophen, if you have any condition which requires you to take prescription drugs or if you have had any problems or serious side effects from taking any non-prescription pain reliever, do not take NUPRIN without first discussing it with your doctor. If you experience any symptoms which are unusual or seem unrelated to the condition for which you took ibuprofen, consult a doctor before taking any more of it. Although ibuprofen is indicated for the same conditions as aspirin and acetaminophen, it should not be taken with them except under a doctor's direction. Do not combine this product with any other ibuprofen-containing product. As with any drug, if you are pregnant or nursing a baby, seek the advice of a health professional before using this product. IT IS ESPECIALLY IMPORTANT NOT TO USE IBUPROFEN DURING THE LAST 3 MONTHS OF PREGNANCY UNLESS SPECIFICALLY DIRECTED TO DO SO BY A DOCTOR BECAUSE IT MAY CAUSE PROBLEMS IN THE UNBORN CHILD OR COMPLICATIONS DURING DELIVERY. Keep this and all drugs out of the reach of children. In case of accidental overdose, seek professional assistance or contact a poison control center immediately.

Caution: Store at room temperature. Avoid excessive heat 40°C (104°F).

Administration and Dosage: Directions. Adults: Take 1 tablet or caplet every 4 to 6 hours while symptoms persist. If pain or fever does not respond to 1 tablet or caplet, 2 tablets or caplets may be used but do not exceed 6 tablets or caplets in 24 hours, unless directed by a doctor. The smallest effective dose should be used. Take with food or milk if occasional and mild heartburn, upset stomach, or stomach pain occurs with use. Consult a doctor if these symptoms are more than mild or if they persist. Children: Do not give this product to children under 12 except under the advice and supervision of a doctor.

Overdosage: For overdose treatment information, consult a regional poison control center.

How Supplied:

NUPRIN® is supplied as:

Golden yellow round tablets with "NUPRIN" printed in black on one side.

NDC 19810-0767-5 Blister card of 8's
NDC 19810-0767-2 Bottles of 24's
NDC 19810-0767-3 Bottles of 50's
NDC 19810-0767-4 Bottles of 100's
NDC 19810-0767-7 Bottles of 150's
NDC 19810-0767-8 Bottles of 225's
Golden yellow caplets with "NUPRIN"
printed in black on one side.
NDC 19810-0796-1 Bottles of 24's
NDC 19810-0796-2 Bottles of 50's
NDC 19810-0796-3 Bottles of 100's
All sizes packaged in child resistant closures except 24's for tablets and 24's for caplets, which are sizes recommended for households without young children.
Store at room temperature. Avoid excessive heat 40°C. (104°F.).
Distributed by Bristol-Myers Company
*Shown in Product Identification
Section, page 406*

PAZO® Hemorrhoid Ointment/Suppositories

Composition:
Ointment: Triolyte®, [Bristol-Myers brand of the combination of benzocaine (0.8%) and ephedrine sulphate (0.2%)]; zinc oxide (4.0%); camphor (2.18%). Also Contains: Lanolin, Petrolatum.
Suppositories (per suppository): Triolyte® [Bristol-Myers brand of the combination of benzocaine (15.44 mg) and ephedrine sulfate (3.86 mg)]; zinc oxide (77.2 mg); camphor (42.07 mg). Also Contains: Hydrogenated Vegetable Oil.

Action and Uses: Pazo helps shrink swelling of inflamed hemorrhoid tissue. Provides prompt, temporary relief of burning itch and pain in many cases.

Administration:
Ointment—Apply Pazo well up in rectum night and morning, and after each bowel movement. Repeat as often during the day as may be necessary to maintain comfort. Continue for one week after symptoms subside. When applicator is used, lubricate applicator first with Pazo. Insert slowly, then simply press tube.
Suppositories—Remove foil and insert one Pazo suppository night and morning, and after each bowel movement. Repeat as often during the day as may be necessary to maintain comfort. Continue for one week after symptoms subside.

Warning: If the underlying condition persists or recurs frequently, despite treatment, or if any bleeding or hard irreducible swelling is present, consult your physician.
Keep out of children's reach. Keep in a cool place.

How Supplied: PAZO® ointment is supplied with a plastic applicator as:
NDC 19810-0768-1 One ounce tubes
NDC 19810-0768-2 Two ounce tubes
PAZO® suppositories are silver foil wrapped and supplied as:
NDC 19810-0703-1 Box of 12's
NDC 19810-0703-2 Box of 24's
Keep in a cool place.
*Shown in Product Identification
Section, page 406*

THERAPEUTIC MINERAL ICE

Active Ingredient: Menthol.
The cool blue Therapeutic Mineral Ice gel base is specially formulated to dry quickly with no grease or lingering unpleasant odor.

Indications: An external pain relieving coolant gel for the temporary relief of minor aches and pains of muscles and joints associated with arthritis, simple backache, strains, bruises, sprains and sports injuries. **USE ONLY AS DIRECTED. Read all warnings before use.**

Warning: KEEP OUT OF THE REACH OF CHILDREN. For external use only. Not for internal use. Avoid contact with eyes and mucous membranes. Do not use with other ointments, creams, sprays, or liniments. **Do not use with Heating Pads or Heating Devices.** If condition worsens, or if symptoms persist for more than 7 days, or clear up and occur again within a few days, discontinue use of this product and consult your doctor. Do not apply to wounds or damaged skin. Do not bandage tightly. If you have sensitive skin, consult doctor **before** use. If skin irritation develops, discontinue use and consult your doctor. As with any drug, if you are pregnant or nursing a baby, seek the advice of a health professional **before** using this product. Store in a cool place. Keep lid tightly closed. Do not use, pour, spill or store near heat or open flame. **Note:** you can always use Mineral Ice as directed, but its use is never intended to replace your doctor's advice.

Directions: Adults and children 2 years of age and older: Clean skin of all other ointments, creams, sprays, or liniments. Apply to affected areas not more than 3 to 4 times daily. May be used with wet or dry bandages or with ice packs. Not greasy. No protective cover needed. Children: Do not use on children under 2 years of age, except under the advice and supervision of a doctor.

How Supplied: Available in 3.5 oz., 8 oz., and 16 oz. containers.
*Shown in Product Identification
Section, page 406*

Burroughs Wellcome Co.
**3030 CORNWALLIS ROAD
RESEARCH TRIANGLE PARK,
NC 27709**

ACTIDIL® Syrup
ACTIDIL® Tablets
[ăk 'tuh-dĭl]

Indications: For the temporary relief of running nose, sneezing, itching of the nose or throat and itchy and watery eyes as may occur in allergic rhinitis (such as hay fever).

Directions: Syrup: Adults and children 12 years of age and over, 2 teaspoonfuls every 4 to 6 hours. Children 6 to under 12 years of age, 1 teaspoonful every 4 to 6 hours. Children under 6 years of age,

consult a physician. Do not exceed 4 doses in 24 hours.
Tablets: Adults and children 12 years of age and over, 1 tablet every 4 to 6 hours. Children 6 to under 12 years of age, ½ tablet every 4 to 6 hours. Children under 6 years of age, consult a physician. Do not exceed 4 doses in 24 hours.

Warnings: May cause excitability especially in children. May cause drowsiness. Do not take this product if you have asthma, glaucoma or difficulty in urination due to enlargement of the prostate gland except under the advice and supervision of a physician. Do not give this product to children under 6 years except under the advice and supervision of a physician. As with any drug, if you are pregnant or nursing a baby, seek the advice of a health professional before using this product.

Caution: Avoid driving a motor vehicle or operating heavy machinery. Avoid alcoholic beverages while taking this product.

KEEP THIS AND ALL DRUGS OUT OF THE REACH OF CHILDREN. In case of accidental overdose, seek professional assistance or contact a Poison Control Center immediately.

Syrup
Active Ingredients: Each 5 ml (1 teaspoonful) contains triprolidine hydrochloride 1.25 mg.

Inactive Ingredients: alcohol 4%; methylparaben 0.1% and sodium benzoate 0.1% (added as preservatives), FD&C Yellow No. 6, flavor, glycerin, purified water, and sorbitol.

Store at 15°–30°C (59°–86°F) and protect from light.

Tablets
Active Ingredients: Each scored tablet contains triprolidine hydrochloride 2.5 mg.

Inactive Ingredients: Corn and potato starch, lactose, magnesium stearate.

Store at 15°–30°C (59°–86°F) in a dry place and protect from light.

How Supplied: Syrup, 1 pint; Tablets, bottle of 100.
*Tablets Shown in Product Identification
Section, page 406*

ACTIFED® Capsules
[ăk 'tuh-fĕd]

Indications: For temporary relief of nasal congestion due to the common cold, hay fever or other upper respiratory allergies. Helps decongest sinus openings, sinus passages. For temporary relief of running nose, sneezing, itching of the nose or throat and itchy and watery eyes as may occur in allergic rhinitis (such as hay fever).

Directions: Adults and children 12 years of age and over, 1 capsule every 4 to 6 hours. Do not exceed 4 capsules in a 24

Continued on next page

Burroughs Wellcome—Cont.

hour period. Children under 12 years of age, consult a physician.

Warnings: May cause excitability especially in children. Do not give this product to children under 12 years except under the advice and supervision of a physician. May cause drowsiness. Do not exceed recommended dosage because at higher doses nervousness, dizziness or sleeplessness may occur. If symptoms do not improve within 7 days or are accompanied by high fever, consult a physician before continuing use. Do not take this product if you have high blood pressure, heart disease, diabetes, thyroid disease, asthma, glaucoma or difficulty in urination due to enlargement of the prostate gland except under the advice and supervision of a physician. As with any drug, if you are pregnant or nursing a baby, seek the advice of a health professional before using this product.

Drug Interaction Precaution: Do not take this product if you are presently taking a prescription antihypertensive or antidepressant drug containing a monoamine oxidase inhibitor except under the advice and supervision of a physician.

Caution: Avoid driving a motor vehicle or operating heavy machinery. Avoid alcoholic beverages while taking this product.

KEEP THIS AND ALL DRUGS OUT OF THE REACH OF CHILDREN. In case of accidental overdose, seek professional assistance or contact a Poison Control Center immediately.

Active Ingredients: Each capsule contains pseudoephedrine hydrochloride 60 mg and triprolidine hydrochloride 2.5 mg.

Inactive Ingredients: Corn starch and magnesium stearate. The capsule shell consists of gelatin, D&C Yellow No. 10, FD&C Yellow No. 6 and titanium dioxide. May contain one or more parabens. Printed with edible black ink.

Store at 15° to 25°C (59° to 77°F) in a dry place and protect from light.

How Supplied: Boxes of 10, 20.
Shown in Product Identification Section, page 406

ACTIFED® PLUS Caplets
[ăk 'tuh-fĕd]

Product Benefits: Each ACTIFED PLUS Caplet contains three important ingredients for maximum strength relief from symptoms of the common cold, seasonal allergies (hay fever) and sinus congestion.

The **ANTIHISTAMINE** temporarily dries runny nose and relieves sneezing associated with the common cold, hay fever or other upper respiratory allergies. Also relieves itching of the nose or throat, and itchy, watery eyes due to hay fever.

The **DECONGESTANT** temporarily relieves nasal congestion due to the common cold, hay fever or other upper respiratory allergies, or associated with sinusitis. Temporarily relieves nasal stuffiness. Reduces the swelling of nasal passages; shrinks swollen membranes; and temporarily restores freer breathing through the nose. Also, helps to decongest sinus openings and passages; relieves sinus pressure.

The non-aspirin **ANALGESIC** temporarily relieves occasional minor aches, pains and headache, and reduces fever due to the common cold.

Each ACTIFED PLUS Caplet Contains: acetaminophen 500 mg, pseudoephedrine hydrochloride 30 mg and triprolidine hydrochloride 1.25 mg. Also contains: D&C Yellow No. 10 Lake, FD&C Blue No. 1 Lake, hydroxypropyl cellulose, magnesium stearate, microcrystalline cellulose and povidone.

Directions: Adults and children 12 years and over, 2 caplets every 6 hours, not to exceed 8 caplets in a 24-hour period. Not recommended for children under 12 years of age.

Warnings: May cause excitability, especially in children. May cause drowsiness. Do not exceed recommended dosage because at higher doses nervousness, dizziness, or sleeplessness may occur. If symptoms do not improve within 7 days or are accompanied by high fever, consult a physician before continuing use. Do not take this product for more than 10 days. Do not take this product if you have high blood pressure, heart disease, diabetes, thyroid disease, asthma, glaucoma, or difficulty in urination due to enlargement of the prostate gland except under the advice and supervision of a physician. As with any drug, if you are pregnant or nursing a baby, seek the advice of a health professional before using this product. **Drug Interaction Precaution:** Do not take this product if you are presently taking a prescription antihypertensive or antidepressant drug containing a monoamine oxidase inhibitor except under the advice and supervision of a physician.

Caution: Avoid driving a motor vehicle or operating heavy machinery. Avoid alcoholic beverages while taking this product. **KEEP THIS AND ALL DRUGS OUT OF THE REACH OF CHILDREN.** In case of accidental overdose, seek professional assistance or contact a Poison Control Center immediately.

Store at 15°–25°C (59°–77°F) in a dry place and protect from light.

How Supplied: Boxes of 20, 40.
Shown in Product Identification Section, page 407

ACTIFED® 12–Hour Capsules
[ăk 'tuh-fĕd]

Indications: For temporary relief of nasal congestion due to the common cold, hay fever or other upper respiratory allergies. Helps decongest sinus openings,

sinus passages. For temporary relief of running nose, sneezing, itching of the nose or throat and itchy and watery eyes as may occur in allergic rhinitis (such as hay fever).

Directions: Adults and children 12 years of age and over—One capsule every 12 hours. Do not exceed two capsules in a 24 hour period. Children under 12 years of age, consult a physician.

Warnings: May cause excitability especially in children. Do not give this product to children under 12 years except under the advice and supervision of a physician. May cause drowsiness. Do not exceed recommended dosage because at higher doses nervousness, dizziness or sleeplessness may occur. If symptoms do not improve within 7 days or are accompanied by high fever, consult a physician before continuing use. Do not take this product if you have high blood pressure, heart disease, diabetes, thyroid disease, asthma, glaucoma or difficulty in urination due to enlargement of the prostate gland except under the advice and supervision of a physician. As with any drug, if you are pregnant or nursing a baby, seek the advice of a health professional before using this product.

Drug Interaction Precaution: Do not take this product if you are presently taking a prescription antihypertensive or antidepressant drug containing a monoamine oxidase inhibitor except under the advice and supervision of a physician.

Caution: Avoid driving a motor vehicle or operating heavy machinery. Avoid alcoholic beverages while taking this product.

KEEP THIS AND ALL DRUGS OUT OF THE REACH OF CHILDREN. In case of accidental overdose, seek professional assistance or contact a Poison Control Center immediately.

Active Ingredients: Each capsule contains pseudoephedrine hydrochloride 120 mg and triprolidine hydrochloride 5 mg.

Inactive Ingredients: Corn starch, D&C Yellow No. 10, sucrose, and other ingredients. The capsule shell consists of gelatin, D&C Yellow No. 10, FD&C Yellow No. 6, and titanium dioxide. May contain one or more parabens. Printed with edible black ink.

Store at 15°–25°C (59°–77°F) in a dry place and protect from light.

How Supplied: Boxes of 10, 20.
Shown in Product Identification Section, page 406

ACTIFED® Syrup
[ăk 'tuh-fĕd]

Indications: For temporary relief of nasal congestion due to the common cold, hay fever or other upper respiratory allergies. Helps decongest sinus openings, sinus passages. For temporary relief of running nose, sneezing, itching of the nose or throat and itchy and watery eyes as may occur in allergic rhinitis (such as hay fever).

Directions: Adults and children 12 years of age and over, 2 teaspoonfuls every 4 to 6 hours. Children 6 to under 12 years of age, 1 teaspoonful every 4 to 6 hours. Children under 6 years of age, consult a physician. Do not exceed 4 doses in 24 hours.

Warnings: May cause excitability especially in children. Do not give this product to children under 6 years except under the advice and supervision of a physician. May cause drowsiness. Do not exceed recommended dosage because at higher doses nervousness, dizziness or sleeplessness may occur. If symptoms do not improve within 7 days or are accompanied by high fever, consult a physician before continuing use. Do not take this product if you have high blood pressure, heart disease, diabetes, thyroid disease, asthma, glaucoma or difficulty in urination due to enlargement of the prostate gland except under the advice and supervision of a physician. As with any drug, if you are pregnant or nursing a baby, seek the advice of a health professional before using this product.

Drug Interaction Precaution: Do not take this product if you are presently taking a prescription antihypertensive or antidepressant drug containing a monoamine oxidase inhibitor except under the advice and supervision of a physician.

Caution: Avoid driving a motor vehicle or operating heavy machinery. Avoid alcoholic beverages while taking this product.

KEEP THIS AND ALL DRUGS OUT OF THE REACH OF CHILDREN. In case of accidental overdose, seek professional assistance or contact a Poison Control Center immediately.

Active Ingredients: Each 5 ml (1 teaspoonful) contains pseudoephedrine hydrochloride 30 mg and triprolidine hydrochloride 1.25 mg.

Inactive Ingredients: sodium benzoate 0.1% and methylparaben 0.1% (added as preservatives), D&C Yellow No. 10, glycerin, purified water, and sorbitol.

Store at 15°–30°C (59°–86°F) and protect from light.

How Supplied: Bottles of 4 fl oz and 1 pint.

Shown in Product Identification Section, page 406

ACTIFED® Tablets
[ăk 'tuh-fĕd]

Indications: For temporary relief of nasal congestion due to the common cold, hay fever or other upper respiratory allergies. Helps decongest sinus openings, sinus passages. For temporary relief of running nose, sneezing, itching of the nose or throat and itchy and watery eyes as may occur in allergic rhinitis (such as hay fever).

Directions: Adults and children 12 years of age and over, 1 tablet every 4 to 6 hours. Children 6 to under 12 years of age, ½ tablet every 4 to 6 hours. Children under 6 years of age, consult a physician. Do not exceed 4 doses in 24 hours.

Warnings: May cause excitability especially in children. Do not give this product to children under 6 years except under the advice and supervision of a physician. May cause drowsiness. Do not exceed recommended dosage because at higher doses nervousness, dizziness or sleeplessness may occur. If symptoms do not improve within 7 days or are accompanied by high fever, consult a physician before continuing use. Do not take this product if you have high blood pressure, heart disease, diabetes, thyroid disease, asthma, glaucoma or difficulty in urination due to enlargement of the prostate gland except under the advice and supervision of a physician. As with any drug, if you are pregnant or nursing a baby, seek the advice of a health professional before using this product.

Drug Interaction Precaution: Do not take this product if you are presently taking a prescription antihypertensive or antidepressant drug containing a monoamine oxidase inhibitor except under the advice and supervision of a physician.

Caution: Avoid driving a motor vehicle or operating heavy machinery. Avoid alcoholic beverages while taking this product.

KEEP THIS AND ALL DRUGS OUT OF THE REACH OF CHILDREN. In case of accidental overdose, seek professional assistance or contact a Poison Control Center immediately.

Active Ingredients: Each scored tablet contains pseudoephedrine hydrochloride 60 mg and triprolidine hydrochloride 2.5 mg.

Inactive Ingredients: Flavor, hydroxypropyl methylcellulose, lactose, magnesium stearate, polyethylene glycol, potato starch, povidone, sucrose, and titanium dioxide.

Store at 15°–25°C (59°–77°F) in a dry place and protect from light.

How Supplied: Boxes of 12, 24, 48 and bottles of 100 and 1000; unit dose pack box of 100.

Shown in Product Identification Section, page 407

ACTIFED® PLUS Tablets
[ăk 'tuh-fĕd]

Product Benefits: Each ACTIFED PLUS Tablet contains three important ingredients for maximum strength relief from symptoms of the common cold, seasonal allergies (hay fever) and sinus congestion.

The **ANTIHISTAMINE** temporarily dries runny nose and relieves sneezing associated with the common cold, hay fever or other upper respiratory allergies. Also relieves itching of the nose or throat, and itchy, watery eyes due to hay fever.

The **DECONGESTANT** temporarily relieves nasal congestion due to the common cold, hay fever or other upper respiratory allergies, or associated with sinusitis. Temporarily relieves nasal stuffiness. Reduces the swelling of nasal passages; shrinks swollen membranes; and temporarily restores freer breathing through the nose. Also, helps to decongest sinus openings and passages; relieves sinus pressure.

The non-aspirin **ANALGESIC** temporarily relieves occasional minor aches, pains and headache, and reduces fever due to the common cold.

Each ACTIFED PLUS Tablet Contains: acetaminophen 500 mg, pseudoephedrine hydrochloride 30 mg and triprolidine hydrochloride 1.25 mg. Also contains: D&C Yellow No. 10 Lake, FD&C Blue No. 1 Lake, hydroxypropyl cellulose, magnesium stearate, microcrystalline cellulose and povidone.

Directions: Adults and children 12 years and over, 2 tablets every 6 hours, not to exceed 8 tablets in a 24-hour period. Not recommended for children under 12 years of age.

Warnings: May cause excitability, especially in children. May cause drowsiness. Do not exceed recommended dosage because at higher doses nervousness, dizziness, or sleeplessness may occur. If symptoms do not improve within 7 days or are accompanied by high fever, consult a physician before continuing use. Do not take this product for more than 10 days. Do not take this product if you have high blood pressure, heart disease, diabetes, thyroid disease, asthma, glaucoma, or difficulty in urination due to enlargement of the prostate gland except under the advice and supervision of a physician. As with any drug, if you are pregnant or nursing a baby, seek the advice of a health professional before using this product. **Drug Interaction Precaution:** Do not take this product if you are presently taking a prescription antihypertensive or antidepressant drug containing a monoamine oxidase inhibitor except under the advice and supervision of a physician.

Caution: Avoid driving a motor vehicle or operating heavy machinery. Avoid alcoholic beverages while taking this product. **KEEP THIS AND ALL DRUGS OUT OF THE REACH OF CHILDREN.** In case of accidental overdose, seek professional assistance or contact a Poison Control Center immediately.

Store at 15°–25°C (59°–77°F) in a dry place and protect from light.

How Supplied: Boxes of 20, 40.

Shown in Product Identification Section, page 407

Continued on next page

Burroughs Wellcome—Cont.

ALLERACT™ Tablets
['al-ər-'akt]

Indications: For the temporary relief of running nose, sneezing, itching of the nose or throat and itchy and watery eyes as may occur in allergic rhinitis (such as hay fever).

Directions: Adults and children 12 years of age and over, 1 tablet every 4 to 6 hours. Children 6 to under 12 years of age, ½ tablet every 4 to 6 hours. Children under 6 years of age, consult a physician. Do not exceed 4 doses in 24 hours.

Warnings: May cause excitability especially in children. May cause drowsiness. Do not take this product if you have asthma, glaucoma or difficulty in urination due to enlargement of the prostate gland except under the advice and supervision of a physician. Do not give this product to children under 6 years except under the advice and supervision of a physician. As with any drug, if you are pregnant or nursing a baby, seek the advice of a health professional before using this product.

Caution: Avoid driving a motor vehicle or operating heavy machinery. Avoid alcoholic beverages while taking this product. **KEEP THIS AND ALL DRUGS OUT OF THE REACH OF CHILDREN.** In case of accidental overdose, seek professional assistance or contact a Poison Control Center immediately.

Active Ingredients: Each scored tablet contains triprolidine hydrochloride 2.5 mg.

Also Contains: Corn and potato starch, hydroxypropyl methylcellulose, lactose, magnesium stearate, polyethylene glycol, and titanium dioxide.

Store at 15°–25°C (59°–77°F) in a dry place and protect from light.

How Supplied: Boxes of 24.
Shown in Product Identification Section, page 407

ALLERACT™ DECONGESTANT Caplets
['al-ər-'akt]

Indications: For temporary relief of running nose, sneezing, itching of the nose or throat and itchy and watery eyes as may occur in allergic rhinitis (such as hay fever). For temporary relief of nasal congestion due to hay fever or other upper respiratory allergies.

Directions: Adults and children 12 years of age and over, 1 caplet every 4 to 6 hours. Children 6 to under 12 years of age, ½ caplet every 4 to 6 hours. Children under 6 years of age, consult a physician. Do not exceed 4 doses in 24 hours.

Warnings: May cause excitability especially in children. Do not give this product to children under 6 years except under the advice and supervision of a physician. May cause drowsiness. Do not exceed recommended dosage because at higher doses nervousness, dizziness or sleeplessness may occur. If symptoms do not improve within 7 days or are accompanied by high fever, consult a physician before continuing use. Do not take this product if you have high blood pressure, heart disease, diabetes, thyroid disease, asthma, glaucoma or difficulty in urination due to enlargement of the prostate gland except under the advice and supervision of a physician. As with any drug, if you are pregnant or nursing a baby, seek the advice of a health professional before using this product.

Drug Interaction Precaution: Do not take this product if you are presently taking a prescription antihypertensive or antidepressant drug containing a monoamine oxidase inhibitor except under the advice and supervision of a physician.

Caution: Avoid driving a motor vehicle or operating heavy machinery. Avoid alcoholic beverages while taking this product.

KEEP THIS AND ALL DRUGS OUT OF THE REACH OF CHILDREN. In case of accidental overdose, seek professional assistance or contact a Poison Control Center immediately.

Active Ingredients: Each scored caplet contains pseudoephedrine hydrochloride 60 mg and triprolidine hydrochloride 2.5 mg. **Also Contains:** Carnauba wax, hydroxypropyl methylcellulose, lactose, magnesium stearate, polyethylene glycol, potato starch, povidone, and titanium dioxide.

Store at 15°–25°C (59°–77°F) in a dry place and protect from light.

How Supplied: Boxes of 24.
Shown in Product Identification Section, page 407

ALLERACT™ DECONGESTANT Tablets
['al-ər-'akt]

Indications: For temporary relief of running nose, sneezing, itching of the nose or throat and itchy and watery eyes as may occur in allergic rhinitis (such as hay fever). For temporary relief of nasal congestion due to hay fever or other upper respiratory allergies.

Directions: Adults and children 12 years of age and over, 1 tablet every 4 to 6 hours. Children 6 to under 12 years of age, ½ tablet every 4 to 6 hours. Children under 6 years of age, consult a physician. Do not exceed 4 doses in 24 hours.

Warnings: May cause excitability especially in children. Do not give this product to children under 6 years except under the advice and supervision of a physician. May cause drowsiness. Do not exceed recommended dosage because at higher doses nervousness, dizziness or sleeplessness may occur. If symptoms do not improve within 7 days or are accompanied by high fever, consult a physician before continuing use. Do not take this product if you have high blood pressure, heart disease, diabetes, thyroid disease, asthma, glaucoma or difficulty in urination due to enlargement of the prostate gland except under the advice and supervision of a physician. As with any drug, if you are pregnant or nursing a baby, seek the advice of a health professional before using this product.

Drug Interaction Precaution: Do not take this product if you are presently taking a prescription antihypertensive or antidepressant drug containing a monoamine oxidase inhibitor except under the advice and supervision of a physician.

Caution: Avoid driving a motor vehicle or operating heavy machinery. Avoid alcoholic beverages while taking this product.

KEEP THIS AND ALL DRUGS OUT OF THE REACH OF CHILDREN. In case of accidental overdose, seek professional assistance or contact a Poison Control Center immediately.

Active Ingredients: Each scored tablet contains pseudoephedrine hydrochloride 60 mg and triprolidine hydrochloride 2.5 mg.

Also Contains: Hydroxypropyl methylcellulose, lactose, magnesium stearate, polyethylene glycol, potato starch, povidone, and titanium dioxide.

Store at 15°–25°C (59°–77°F) in a dry place and protect from light.

How Supplied: Boxes of 24 and 48.
Shown in Product Identification Section, page 407

BOROFAX® Ointment
[bôr 'uh-fǎks]

Description: Contains boric acid 5% and lanolin.

Inactive Ingredients: fragrances, glycerin, mineral oil, purified water and sodium borate.

Indications: A soothing application for burns, abrasions, chafing, and for infants' tender skin.

Directions: Apply topically as required.

Keep this and all medicines out of children's reach.

Store at 15°–25°C (59°–77°F).

How Supplied: Tube, 1¾ oz.

EMPIRIN® ASPIRIN
[ĕm 'puh-rŭn]

For relief of headache, minor muscular aches and pains, toothache, discomfort and fever of colds and flu, pain of the premenstrual and menstrual periods, and temporary relief of minor arthritis pain (see CAUTION below).

Directions: **Adults:** 1 or 2 tablets with a full glass of water. Repeat every 4 hours as needed, up to 12 tablets a day. **Children:** Consult a physician (see WARNINGS).

Caution: In arthritic conditions, if pain persists for more than 10 days or redness is present, consult a physician immediately.

Warnings: Children and teenagers should not use this medicine for chicken pox or flu symptoms before a doctor is consulted about Reye syndrome, a rare but serious illness reported to be associated with aspirin. Keep this and all medicines out of children's reach. In case of accidental overdose, contact a physician immediately.

High or continued fever, severe or persistent sore throat especially when accompanied by high fever, headache, nausea or vomiting, may be serious. Consult your physician. Do not exceed dose unless directed by a physician. Do not take this product if you are allergic to aspirin, have asthma, a gastric ulcer or its symptoms, or are taking a medication that affects the clotting of blood, except under the advice of a physician. As with any drug, if you are pregnant or nursing a baby, seek the advice of a health professional before using this product.

Active Ingredients: Each tablet contains aspirin 325 mg (5 gr).

Inactive Ingredients: microcrystalline cellulose and potato starch.

Store at 15° to 25°C (59° to 77°F) in a dry place.

How Supplied: Bottles of 50, 100, 250.
Shown in Product Identification Section, page 407

MAREZINE® Tablets
[mâr 'uh-zēn]

FDA APPROVED USES

Indications: For the prevention and treatment of the nausea, vomiting or dizziness associated with motion sickness.

Directions: Adults and children 12 years of age and older: 1 tablet every 4 to 6 hours, not to exceed 4 tablets in 24 hours or as directed by a doctor. Children 6 to under 12 years of age: ½ tablet every 6 to 8 hours, not to exceed 1½ tablets in 24 hours or as directed by a doctor. For prevention, take the first dose one-half hour before departure.

Warnings: Do not take this product if you have asthma, glaucoma, emphysema, chronic pulmonary disease, shortness of breath, difficulty in breathing or difficulty in urination due to enlargement of the prostate gland unless directed by a doctor. Do not give to children under 6 years of age unless directed by a doctor. May cause drowsiness; alcohol, sedatives and tranquilizers may increase the drowsiness effect. Avoid alcoholic beverages while taking this product. Do not take this product if you are taking sedatives or tranquilizers without first consulting your doctor. Use caution when driving a motor vehicle or operating machinery. As with any drug, if you are pregnant or nursing a baby, seek the advice of a health professional before using this product. Keep this and all drugs

out of the reach of children. In case of accidental overdose, seek professional assistance or contact a Poison Control Center immediately.

Active Ingredients: Each scored tablet contains cyclizine hydrochloride 50 mg.

Inactive Ingredients: Corn and potato starch, dextrin, lactose, and magnesium stearate.

Store at 15°–25°C (59°–77°F) in a dry place and protect from light.

How Supplied: Box of 12, bottle of 100.
Shown in Product Identification Section, page 407

Maximum Strength NEOSPORIN® Ointment
[nē 'uh-spō 'rŭn]

Indications: First aid to help prevent infection in minor cuts, scrapes and burns.

Directions: Clean the affected area. Apply a small amount of this product (an amount equal to the surface area of the tip of a finger) on the area 1 to 3 times daily. May be covered with sterile bandage.

Warnings: For external use only. Do not use in the eyes or apply over large areas of the body. In case of deep or puncture wounds, animal bites, or serious burns, consult a physician. Stop use and consult a physician if the condition persists or gets worse. Do not use longer than 1 week unless directed by a physician. Keep this and all drugs out of the reach of children. In case of accidental ingestion, seek professional assistance or contact a Poison Control Center immediately.

Each Gram Contains: polymyxin B sulfate 10,000 units, bacitracin zinc 500 units and neomycin 3.5 mg in a special white petrolatum base.

Store at 15° to 25°C (59° to 77°F).

How Supplied: ½ oz tube.

Professional Labeling: Consult *1990 Physicians' Desk Reference®*.
Shown in Product Identification Section, page 407

NEOSPORIN® Cream
[nē 'uh-spō 'rŭn]

Indications: First aid to help prevent infection in minor cuts, scrapes, and burns.

Directions: Clean the affected area. Apply a small amount of this product (an amount equal to the surface area of the tip of a finger) on the area 1 to 3 times daily. May be covered with sterile bandage.

Warnings: For external use only. Do not use in the eyes or apply over large areas of the body. In case of deep or puncture wounds, animal bites, or serious burns, consult a physician. Stop use and consult a physician if the condition persists or gets worse. Do not use longer

than 1 week unless directed by a physician. Keep this and all drugs out of the reach of children. In case of accidental ingestion, seek professional assistance or contact a Poison Control Center immediately.

Each Gram Contains: Aerosporin® (polymyxin B sulfate) 10,000 units and neomycin 3.5 mg. Also contains: methylparaben 0.25% (added as a preservative), emulsifying wax, mineral oil, polyoxyethylene polyoxypropylene compound, propylene glycol, purified water and white petrolatum.

Store at 15° to 25°C (59° to 77°F).

How Supplied: ½ oz tube; 1/32 oz (approx.) foil packets packed 144 per carton.

Professional Labeling: Consult *1990 Physicians' Desk Reference®*.
Shown in Product Identification Section, page 407

NEOSPORIN® Ointment
[nē 'uh-spō 'rŭn]

Indications: First aid to help prevent infection in minor cuts, scrapes and burns.

Directions: Clean the affected area. Apply a small amount of this product (an amount equal to the surface area of the tip of a finger) on the area 1 to 3 times daily. May be covered with sterile bandage.

Warnings: For external use only. Do not use in the eyes or apply over large areas of the body. In case of deep or puncture wounds, animal bites, or serious burns, consult a physician. Stop use and consult a physician if the condition persists or gets worse. Do not use longer than 1 week unless directed by a physician. Keep this and all drugs out of the reach of children. In case of accidental ingestion, seek professional assistance or contact a Poison Control Center immediately.

Each Gram Contains: Aerosporin® (polymyxin B sulfate) 5,000 units, bacitracin zinc 400 units and neomycin 3.5 mg in a special white petrolatum base.

Store at 15° to 25°C (59° to 77°F).

How Supplied: Tubes, ½ oz (with applicator tip), 1 oz; 1/32 oz (approx.) foil packets packed 144 per carton.

Professional Labeling: Consult *1990 Physicians' Desk Reference®*.
Shown in Product Identification Section, page 407

POLYSPORIN® Ointment
[pŏl 'ē-spō 'rŭn]

Indications: First aid to help prevent infection in minor cuts, scrapes and burns.

Directions: Clean the affected area. Apply a small amount of this product (an amount equal to the surface area of the

Continued on next page

Burroughs Wellcome—Cont.

tip of a finger) on the area 1 to 3 times daily. May be covered with a sterile bandage.

Warnings: For external use only. Do not use in the eyes or apply over large areas of the body. In case of deep or puncture wounds, animal bites, or serious burns, consult a physician. Stop use and consult a physician if the condition persists or gets worse. Do not use longer than 1 week unless directed by a physician. Keep this and all drugs out of the reach of children. In case of accidental ingestion, seek professional assistance or contact a Poison Control Center immediately.

Each Gram Contains: Aerosporin® (Polymyxin B Sulfate) 10,000 units and bacitracin zinc 500 units in a special white petrolatum base.

Store at 15° to 25°C (59° to 77°F).

How Supplied: Tubes, ½ oz with applicator tip, 1 oz; $\frac{1}{32}$ oz (approx.) foil packets packed in cartons of 144.
Shown in Product Identification Section, page 407

POLYSPORIN® Powder
[pŏl ´ē-spō ´rŭn]

Indications: First aid to help prevent infection in minor cuts, scrapes and burns.

Directions: Clean the affected area. Apply a light dusting of the powder on the area 1 to 3 times daily. May be covered with a sterile bandage.

Warnings: For external use only. Do not use in the eyes or apply over large areas of the body. In case of deep or puncture wounds, animal bites, or serious burns, consult a physician. Stop use and consult a physician if the condition persists or gets worse.
Do not use longer than 1 week unless directed by a physician. Keep this and all drugs out of the reach of children. In case of accidental ingestion, seek professional assistance or contact a Poison Control Center immediately.

Each Gram Contains: Aerosporin® (polymyxin B sulfate) 10,000 units and bacitracin zinc 500 units in a lactose base.
Store at 15° to 30°C (59° to 86°F). Do not store under refrigeration.

How Supplied: 0.35 oz (10 g) shaker-vial.
Shown in Product Identification Section, page 407

POLYSPORIN® Spray
[pŏl ´ē-spō ´rŭn]

Description: Each 85 gram can contains: Aerosporin® (polymyxin B sulfate) 200,000 units and bacitracin zinc 10,000 units. Propellant—dichlorodifluoromethane and trichloromonofluoromethane.

Each 1 second spray delivers approximately 2300 units of polymyxin B sulfate and 115 units of bacitracin zinc.

Indications: First aid to help prevent infection in minor cuts, scrapes and burns. Decreases the number of bacteria on the treated area.

Directions: Clean the affected area. SHAKE WELL before each spraying. Remove cap and press button to spray affected area. Hold container upright when spraying. Use one-second intermittent sprays from a distance of about eight inches. Prolonged spraying is unnecessary and wastes medication. Apply a small amount of this product one to three times daily. May be covered with a sterile bandage.

Warnings: Avoid spraying in eyes. Contents under pressure. Do not puncture or incinerate. Do not store at temperatures above 120°F. For external use only. Do not use in the eyes or apply over large areas of the body. In case of deep or puncture wounds, animal bites, or serious burns, consult a doctor. Stop use and consult a doctor if the condition persists or gets worse. Do not use longer than 1 week unless directed by a doctor. Keep this and all drugs out of the reach of children. In case of accidental ingestion, seek professional assistance or contact a Poison Control Center immediately.
Store at 15°–30°C (59°–86°F).

How Supplied: 3 oz (85 g) spray can.
Shown in Product Identification Section, page 407

Children's
SUDAFED® Liquid
[sū ´duh-fĕd]

Each 5 mL (1 teaspoonful) contains pseudoephedrine hydrochloride 30 mg. Also contains: methylparaben 0.1% and sodium benzoate 0.1% (added as preservatives), citric acid, FD&C Red No. 40, flavor, glycerin, purified water, sorbitol and sucrose.

Indications: For temporary relief of nasal congestion due to the common cold, hay fever or other upper respiratory allergies, and nasal congestion associated with sinusitis; promotes nasal and/or sinus drainage.

Directions: To be given every 4 to 6 hours. Do not exceed 4 doses in 24 hours. Children 6 to under 12 years of age, 1 teaspoonful. Children 2 to under 6 years of age, ½ teaspoonful. For children under 2 years of age, consult a physician.

Warnings: Do not exceed recommended dosage because at higher doses nervousness, dizziness or sleeplessness may occur. Do not give this product to children for more than 7 days. If symptoms do not improve or are accompanied by high fever, consult a physician. Do not give this product to children who have heart disease, high blood pressure, thyroid disease or diabetes unless directed by a physician.

Drug Interaction Precaution: Do not give this product to a child who is taking

a prescription drug for high blood pressure or depression, without first consulting the child's physician.

KEEP THIS AND ALL MEDICINES OUT OF CHILDREN'S REACH. In case of accidental overdose, seek professional assistance or contact a Poison Control Center immediately.

Store at 15° to 25°C (59° to 77°F) and protect from light.

How Supplied: Bottles of 4 fl oz.
Shown in Product Identification Section, page 407

SUDAFED® Cough Syrup
[sū ´duh-fĕd]

Each 5 mL (1 teaspoonful) contains pseudoephedrine hydrochloride 15 mg, dextromethorphan hydrobromide 5 mg and guaifenesin 100 mg. Also contains: alcohol 2.4%, methylparaben 0.1% and sodium benzoate 0.1% (added as preservatives), citric acid, D&C Yellow No. 10, FD&C Blue No. 1, flavor, glycerin, purified water, saccharin sodium, sodium chloride and sucrose.

Indications: For temporary relief of cough due to minor throat and bronchial irritation as may occur with the common cold or inhaled irritants. For temporary relief of nasal congestion due to the common cold. Helps loosen phlegm (sputum) and thin bronchial secretions to rid the bronchial passageways of bothersome mucus.

Directions: To be given every 4 hours. Do not exceed 4 doses in 24 hours. Adults and children 12 years of age and over, 4 teaspoonfuls. Children 6 to under 12 years of age, 2 teaspoonfuls. Children 2 to under 6 years of age, 1 teaspoonful. For children under 2 years of age, consult a physician.

Warnings: Do not give this product to children under 2 years of age unless directed by a physician. Do not exceed recommended dosage because at higher doses, nervousness, dizziness or sleeplessness may occur. Do not take this product for persistent or chronic cough such as occurs with smoking, asthma, chronic bronchitis, or emphysema, or where cough is accompanied by excessive phlegm (sputum) unless directed by a physician. A persistent cough may be a sign of a serious condition. If cough persists for more than 1 week, tends to recur, or is accompanied by fever, rash, or persistent headache, consult a physician. Do not take this preparation if you have high blood pressure, heart disease, diabetes, thyroid disease, or difficulty in urination due to enlargement of the prostate gland, except under the advice and supervision of a physician. As with any drug, if you are pregnant or nursing a baby, seek the advice of a health professional before using this product.

Drug Interaction Precaution: Do not take this product if you are presently taking a prescription antihypertensive or antidepressant drug containing a monoamine oxidase inhibitor except under the advice and supervision of a physician.

KEEP THIS AND ALL DRUGS OUT OF THE REACH OF CHILDREN. In case of accidental overdose, seek professional assistance or contact a Poison Control Center immediately.

Store at 15° to 25°C (59° to 77°F). DO NOT REFRIGERATE.

How Supplied: Bottles of 4 fl oz and 8 fl oz.

Shown in Product Identification Section, page 407

SUDAFED® Tablets 30 mg
[sū 'duh-fĕd]

Each tablet contains pseudoephedrine hydrochloride 30 mg. Also contains: acacia, carnauba wax, dibasic calcium phosphate, FD&C Red No. 3 Lake and Yellow No. 6 Lake, magnesium stearate, polysorbate 60, potato starch, povidone, sodium benzoate, stearic acid, sucrose and titanium dioxide.

Indications: For temporary relief of nasal congestion due to the common cold, hay fever or other upper respiratory allergies, and nasal congestion associated with sinusitis; promotes nasal and/or sinus drainage.

Directions: To be given every 4 to 6 hours. Do not exceed 4 doses in 24 hours. Adults and children 12 years of age and over, 2 tablets. Children 6 to under 12 years of age, 1 tablet. Children 2 to under 6 years of age, use Children's Sudafed Liquid. For children under 2 years of age, consult a physician.

Warnings: Do not exceed recommended dosage because at higher doses nervousness, dizziness or sleeplessness may occur. If symptoms do not improve within 7 days, or are accompanied by a high fever, consult a physician before continuing use. Do not take this preparation if you have high blood pressure, heart disease, diabetes, thyroid disease, or difficulty in urination due to enlargement of the prostate gland, except under the advice and supervision of a physician. As with any drug, if you are pregnant or nursing a baby, seek the advice of a health professional before using this product.

Drug Interaction Precaution: Do not take this product if you are presently taking a prescription antihypertensive or antidepressant drug containing a monoamine oxidase inhibitor except under the advice and supervision of a physician.

KEEP THIS AND ALL MEDICINES OUT OF CHILDREN'S REACH. In case of accidental overdose, seek professional assistance or contact a Poison Control Center immediately.

Store at 15° to 25°C (59° to 77°F) in a dry place and protect from light.

How Supplied: Boxes of 24, 48. Bottles of 100.

Shown in Product Identification Section, page 407

SUDAFED® Tablets 60 mg (Adult Strength)
[sū 'duh-fĕd]

Each tablet contains pseudoephedrine hydrochloride 60 mg. Also contains: acacia, carnauba wax, corn starch, dibasic calcium phosphate, hydroxypropyl methylcellulose, magnesium stearate, polysorbate 60, sodium starch glycolate, stearic acid, sucrose, titanium dioxide, and white shellac. Printed with edible red ink.

Indications: For temporary relief of nasal congestion due to the common cold, hay fever or other upper respiratory allergies, and nasal congestion associated with sinusitis; promotes nasal and/or sinus drainage.

Directions: To be given every 4 to 6 hours. Do not exceed 4 doses in 24 hours. Adults and children 12 years of age and over, 1 tablet. Children 6 to under 12 years of age, use Sudafed 30 mg Tablets. Children 2 to under 6 years of age, use Children's Sudafed Liquid. For children under 2 years of age, consult a physician.

Warnings: Do not exceed recommended dosage because at higher doses nervousness, dizziness or sleeplessness may occur. If symptoms do not improve within 7 days, or are accompanied by a high fever, consult a physician before continuing use. Do not take this preparation if you have high blood pressure, heart disease, diabetes, thyroid disease, or difficulty in urination due to enlargement of the prostate gland, except under the advice and supervision of a physician. As with any drug, if you are pregnant or nursing a baby, seek the advice of a health professional before using this product.

Drug Interaction Precaution: Do not take this product if you are presently taking a prescription antihypertensive or antidepressant drug containing a monoamine oxidase inhibitor, except under the advice and supervision of a physician.

KEEP THIS AND ALL MEDICINES OUT OF CHILDREN'S REACH. In case of accidental overdose, seek professional assistance or contact a Poison Control Center immediately.

Store at 15° to 25°C (59° to 77°F) in a dry place and protect from light.

How Supplied: Bottles of 100.
Shown in Product Identification Section, page 407

SUDAFED® PLUS Liquid
[sū 'duh-fĕd]

Each 5 ml (1 teaspoonful) contains pseudoephedrine hydrochloride 30 mg and chlorpheniramine maleate 2 mg. Also contains: methylparaben 0.1% and sodium benzoate 0.1% (added as preservatives), citric acid, D&C Yellow No. 10, FD&C Yellow No. 6, flavor, glycerin, purified water and sucrose.

Indications: For the temporary relief of nasal/sinus congestion associated with the common cold; also sneezing; watery,

itchy eyes; runny nose and other hay fever/upper respiratory allergy symptoms.

Directions: To be given every 4 to 6 hours. Do not exceed 4 doses in 24 hours. Adults and children 12 years of age and over, 2 teaspoonfuls. Children 6 to under 12 years of age, 1 teaspoonful. Children under 6 years of age, consult a physician.

Warnings: May cause excitability, especially in children. Do not give to children under 6 years except as directed by a physician. May cause drowsiness. Do not exceed recommended dosage because at higher doses nervousness, dizziness or sleeplessness may occur. If symptoms do not improve within 7 days, or are accompanied by a high fever, consult a physician before continuing use. Do not take this product if you have high blood pressure, heart disease, diabetes, thyroid disease, asthma, glaucoma or difficulty in urination due to enlargement of the prostate gland except under the advice and supervision of a physician. As with any drug, if you are pregnant or nursing a baby, seek the advice of a health professional before using this product.

Drug Interaction Precaution: Do not take this product if you are presently taking a prescription antihypertensive or antidepressant drug containing a monoamine oxidase inhibitor except under the advice and supervision of a physician.

Caution: Avoid driving a motor vehicle or operating heavy machinery. Avoid alcoholic beverages while taking this product.

KEEP THIS AND ALL MEDICINES OUT OF CHILDREN'S REACH. In case of accidental overdose, seek professional assistance or contact a Poison Control Center immediately.

Store at 15°–30°C (59°–86°F) and protect from light.

How Supplied: Bottles of 4 fl oz.
Shown in Product Identification Section, page 407

SUDAFED® PLUS Tablets
[sū 'duh-fĕd]

Each scored tablet contains pseudoephedrine hydrochloride 60 mg and chlorpheniramine maleate 4 mg. Also contains: lactose, magnesium stearate, potato starch and povidone.

Indications: For the temporary relief of nasal/sinus congestion associated with the common cold; also sneezing; watery, itchy eyes; runny nose and other hay fever/upper respiratory allergy symptoms.

Directions: To be given every 4 to 6 hours. Do not exceed 4 doses in 24 hours. Adults and children 12 years of age and over, 1 tablet. Children 6 to under 12 years of age, ½ tablet. Children under 6 years of age, consult a physician.

Warnings: May cause excitability, especially in children. Do not give to chil-

Continued on next page

Burroughs Wellcome—Cont.

dren under 6 years except as directed by a physician. May cause drowsiness. Do not exceed recommended dosage because at higher doses nervousness, dizziness or sleeplessness may occur. If symptoms do not improve within 7 days, or are accompanied by a high fever, consult a physician before continuing use. Do not take this product if you have high blood pressure, heart disease, diabetes, thyroid disease, asthma, glaucoma or difficulty in urination due to enlargement of the prostate gland except under the advice and supervision of a physician. As with any drug, if you are pregnant or nursing a baby, seek the advice of a health professional before using this product.

Drug Interaction Precaution: Do not take this product if you are presently taking a prescription antihypertensive or antidepressant drug containing a monoamine oxidase inhibitor except under the advice and supervision of a physician.

Caution: Avoid driving a motor vehicle or operating heavy machinery. Avoid alcoholic beverages while taking this product.

KEEP THIS AND ALL MEDICINES OUT OF CHILDREN'S REACH. In case of accidental overdose, seek professional assistance or contact a Poison Control Center immediately.

Store at 15°–30°C (59°–86°F) in a dry place and protect from light.

How Supplied: Boxes of 24, 48.
Shown in Product Identification Section, page 407

SUDAFED® SINUS Caplets
[sū 'dah-fĕd " 'sī-nəs]

Product Benefits:
- Maximum allowable levels of non-aspirin pain reliever and nasal decongestant provide temporary relief of sinus headache pain, pressure and nasal congestion due to colds or hay fever and other allergies.
- Contains no ingredients which may cause drowsiness.

Directions: Adults and children 12 years and over, 2 caplets every 6 hours, not to exceed 8 caplets in a 24-hour period. Not recommended for children under 12 years of age.

Each Caplet Contains: acetaminophen 500 mg and pseudoephedrine hydrochloride 30 mg. Also contains FD&C Yellow No. 6 Lake, magnesium stearate, microcrystalline cellulose, povidone and sodium starch glycolate.

Warnings: Do not exceed recommended dosage because at higher doses nervousness, dizziness, or sleeplessness may occur. If symptoms do not improve within 7 days or are accompanied by high fever, consult a physician before continuing use. Do not take this product for more than 10 days. Do not take this product if you have high blood pressure, heart dis-

ease, diabetes, thyroid disease, or difficulty in urination due to enlargement of the prostate gland except under the advice and supervision of a physician. As with any drug, if you are pregnant or nursing a baby, seek the advice of a health professional before using this product.

Drug Interaction Precaution: Do not take this product if you are presently taking a prescription antihypertensive or antidepressant drug containing a monoamine oxidase inhibitor except under the advice and supervision of a physician.

KEEP THIS AND ALL DRUGS OUT OF THE REACH OF CHILDREN. In case of accidental overdose, seek professional assistance or contact a Poison Control Center immediately.

Store at 15°–25°C (59°–77°F) in a dry place and protect from light.

How Supplied: Boxes of 24 and 48.
Shown in Product Identification Section, page 407

SUDAFED® SINUS Tablets
[sū 'dah-fĕd " 'sī-nəs]

Product Benefits:
- Maximum allowable levels of non-aspirin pain reliever and nasal decongestant provide temporary relief of sinus headache pain, pressure and nasal congestion due to colds or hay fever and other allergies.
- Contains no ingredients which may cause drowsiness.

Directions: Adults and children 12 years and over, 2 tablets every 6 hours, not to exceed 8 tablets in a 24-hour period. Not recommended for children under 12 years of age.

Each Tablet Contains: Acetaminophen 500 mg and pseudoephedrine hydrochloride 30 mg. Also contains FD&C Yellow No. 6 Lake, magnesium stearate, microcrystalline cellulose, povidone and sodium starch glycolate.

Warnings: Do not exceed recommended dosage because at higher doses nervousness, dizziness, or sleeplessness may occur. If symptoms do not improve within 7 days or are accompanied by high fever, consult a physician before continuing use. Do not take this product for more than 10 days. Do not take this product if you have high blood pressure, heart disease, diabetes, thyroid disease, or difficulty in urination due to enlargement of the prostate gland except under the advice and supervision of a physician. As with any drug, if you are pregnant or nursing a baby, seek the advice of a health professional before using this product.

Drug Interaction Precaution: Do not take this product if you are presently taking a prescription antihypertensive or antidepressant drug containing a monoamine oxidase inhibitor except under the advice and supervision of a physician.

KEEP THIS AND ALL DRUGS OUT OF THE REACH OF CHILDREN. In case of accidental overdose, seek professional assistance or contact a Poison Control Center immediately.

Store at 15°–25°C (59°–77°F) in a dry place and protect from light.

How Supplied: Boxes of 24 and 48.
Shown in Product Identification Section, page 407

SUDAFED® 12 Hour Capsules
[sū 'duh-fĕd]

Each capsule contains pseudoephedrine hydrochloride 120 mg. Also contains: corn starch, sucrose and other ingredients. The capsule shell consists of gelatin, FD&C Blues No. 1 and 2, and Red No. 3. May contain one or more parabens. Printed with edible black ink.

Indications: For temporary relief of nasal congestion due to the common cold, hay fever, or other upper respiratory allergies, and nasal congestion associated with sinusitis; promotes nasal and/or sinus drainage.

Directions: Adults and children 12 years and over—One capsule every 12 hours, not to exceed two capsules in 24 hours. Sudafed 12 Hour is not recommended for children under 12 years of age.

Warnings: Do not exceed recommended dosage because at higher doses nervousness, dizziness, or sleeplessness may occur. If symptoms do not improve within 7 days, or are accompanied by a high fever, consult a physician before continuing use. Do not take this preparation if you have high blood pressure, heart disease, diabetes, thyroid disease, or difficulty in urination due to enlargement of the prostate gland, except under the advice and supervision of a physician. As with any drug, if you are pregnant or nursing a baby, seek the advice of a health professional before using this product.

Drug Interaction Precaution: Do not take this product if you are presently taking a prescription antihypertensive or antidepressant drug containing a monoamine oxidase inhibitor, except under the advice and supervision of a physician.

KEEP THIS AND ALL DRUGS OUT OF THE REACH OF CHILDREN. In case of accidental overdose, seek professional assistance or contact a Poison Control Center immediately.

Store at 15°–25°C (59°–77°F) in a dry place and protect from light.

How Supplied: Boxes of 10, 20, 40.
Shown in Product Identification Section, page 408

WELLCOME® LANOLINE
[lăn 'ō-lŭn]

Description: Lanolin with solid and liquid petrolatum, fragrances, and glycerin.

Indications: A soothing and softening application for dry, rough skin and a protective application against the effects of harsh weather.

Directions: Apply topically to the hands and face as required.

Keep this and all medicines out of children's reach.

Store at 15°–25°C (59°–77°F).

How Supplied: Tubes, 1¾ oz.

Campbell Laboratories Inc.
**300 EAST 51st STREET
P.O. BOX 812, F.D.R. STATION
NEW YORK, NY 10150**

HERPECIN–L® Cold Sore Lip Balm
[*her "puh-sin-el "*]

Composition: A soothing, emollient, cosmetically pleasant lip balm incorporating pyridoxine HCl; allantoin; the sunscreen, octyl p-(dimethylamino)-benzoate (Padimate O); and titanium dioxide in a balanced, acidic lipid system. (All ingredients appear on the package. Has no "caines", antibiotics, phenol or camphor.) (NDC 38083-777-31)

Actions and Uses: HERPECIN-L® relieves dryness and chapping by providing a lipid barrier to help restore normal moisture balance to labial tissues. The sunscreen is effective in 2900-3200 AU range while titanium dioxide helps to block, scatter and reflect the sun's rays.

Administration: (1) *Recurrent "cold sores, sun and fever blisters ":* Simply put, users report the sooner and more often applied, the better the results. Frequent sufferers report that with *prophylactic* use (B.I.D./P.R.N.), their attacks are fewer and less severe. Most recurrent *herpes labialis* patients are aware of the *prodromal* symptoms: tingling, itching, burning. At this stage, or if the lesion has already developed, HERPECIN-L should be applied liberally as often as convenient—at least *every hour* (qq. hor.). The prodrome will often persist and remind the patient to continue to reapply HERPECIN-L. (2) *Outdoor sun/winter protection:* Apply during and after exposure (and after swimming) and again at bedtime (h.s.). (3) *Dry, chapped lips:* Apply as needed.

Note: HERPECIN-L is for peri-oral use only; not for "canker sores" (aphthous stomatitis). Primary attacks, usually in children and young adults, are normally intra-oral and accompanied by foul breath, pain and fever. Lasting up to six weeks, they are resistant to most treatments. Adjunctive therapy for pain, fever and secondary infection may be indicated. Excessive chapping may be from mouth breathing.

Adverse Reactions: A few, rare instances of topical sensitivity to pyridoxine HCl (Vitamin B$_6$) and/or the sunscreen have been reported. Discontinue use if allergic reaction develops.

Contraindications: HERPECIN-L does not contain any steroids. (Corticosteroids are normally contraindicated in *herpes* infections.)

How Supplied: 2.8 gm. swivel tubes. O.T.C.

Samples Available: Yes. (Please request on your Professional letterhead.)

Carnation Nutritional Products
**5045 WILSHIRE BLVD.
LOS ANGELES, CA 90036**

GOOD START™
[*'gud 'stärt*]
Iron-fortified Infant Formula

Composition: Product contains whey protein processed to make the formula well tolerated. Composition is similar to breast milk, including the osmolality, the ratios of the fatty acids and some minerals, the amino acid profile, and the carbohydrate source, which is 70% lactose and 30% maltodextrin. The maltodextrin aids digestibility, keeps the osmolality low, and thus helps prevent osmotic diarrhea.

Ingredients: 42% enzymatically hydrolyzed reduced minerals whey and whey protein concentrate, vegetable oils (14% palm olein, 5% high-oleic safflower and 4% coconut), 17% maltodextrin, 14% lactose, 1% soy lecithin, and less than 1% of each of the following: calcium chloride, potassium chloride, potassium citrate, calcium phosphate, choline bitartrate, sodium ascorbate (vitamin C), salt, magnesium chloride, taurine, ferrous sulfate (iron), inositol, zinc sulfate, L-carnitine, alpha-tocopheryl acetate (vitamin E), niacinamide, calcium pantothenate, copper sulfate, riboflavin, vitamin A acetate, pyridoxine hydrochloride (vitamin B$_6$), thiamine mononitrate, folic acid, phylloquinone (vitamin K), potassium iodide, vitamin D$_3$, manganese sulfate, biotin, vitamin B$_{12}$.

Indications and Usage: When a well-tolerated formula is indicated because mother cannot/chooses not to breast-feed, or needs to supplement with formula. This product contains complete nutrition for routine or long-term feeding. The cow's milk whey protein source is specially processed to make the formula well tolerated even by infants at high risk for cow's-milk-protein or soy-protein intolerance. Pleasant taste and aroma. Comparable in price to standard milk- or soy-based formula.

Precautions: GOOD START™ contains cow's milk whey protein which, although it has been specially processed to reduce allergenic potential, should be used only under direct medical supervision in cases of suspected milk allergy. GOOD START™ contains lactose and should not be given to infants with galactosemia.

Preparation: Standard dilution (20 cal/fl oz) is one level, unpacked scoop of powder (7.8 g) for each 2 fl oz of warm water. Cap bottle and shake well. Feed immediately, or refrigerate up to 24 hours. Discard formula left in bottle after feeding. Cover opened can and store in cool, dry place (not refrigerator). Use within 1 month of opening. Store unopened cans at room temperature. Each can makes approximately 87.2 fl oz (2.7 qt) of formula.

How Supplied: Powder, 12-oz cans, measuring scoop enclosed; 6 cans per case; No. 12021.
[See table above]

Shown in Product Identification Section, page 408

GOOD START™

Nutrients	Per 100 cal (5 fl oz)*		Minerals	Per 100 cal (5 fl oz)*	
Protein	2.4	g	Calcium	64	mg
Fat	5.1	g	Phosphorus	36	mg
Carbohydrate	11	g	Magnesium	6.7	mg
Water	135	g	Iron	1.5	mg†
Vitamins			Zinc	0.75	mg
Vitamin A	300	IU	Manganese	7	mcg
Vitamin C	8	mg	Copper	80	mcg
Vitamin D	60	IU	Iodine	8	mcg
Vitamin E	1.2	IU	Sodium	24	mg
Vitamin K	8.2	mcg	Potassium	98	mg
Thiamine	60	mcg	Chloride	59	mg
Riboflavin	135	mcg			
Vitamin B$_6$	75	mcg	**OTHERS**		
Vitamin B$_{12}$	0.22	mcg	Linoleic acid	450	mg
Niacin	750	mcg	Choline	12	mg
Folic acid	9	mcg	Inositol	6.1	mg
Pantothenic acid	450	mcg	L-Carnitine	10	mg/qt
Biotin	2.2	mcg	Taurine	50	mg/qt

*5 fl oz standard dilution provides 100 cal.
†The addition of iron to this formula conforms to the recommendation of the Committee on Nutrition of the American Academy of Pediatrics.

Chattem Consumer Products
Division of Chattem, Inc.
1715 WEST 38TH STREET
CHATTANOOGA, TN 37409

FLEX–ALL 454™ PAIN RELIEVING GEL

Active Ingredient: Menthol 7%.

Inactive Ingredients: Alcohol, Allantoin, Aloe Vera Gel, Boric Acid Carbomer 940, Diazolidinyl Urea, Eucalyptus Oil, Glycerin, Iodine, Methylparaben, Methyl Salicylate, Peppermint Oil, Polysorbate 60, Potassium Iodide, Propylene Glycol, Propylparaben, Thyme Oil, Triethanolamine, Water, 97-116.

Indications: To relieve the pain of minor arthritis, simple backache, strains, sprains, bruises, and cramps.

Actions: Flex-all is classified as a counterirritant which provides relief of deep-seated pain through cutaneous stimulation rather than through a direct analgesic effect.

Warnings: For external use only. Keep out of reach of children. If swallowed, call a physician or contact a poison control center. Keep away from eyes and mucous membranes, broken or irritated skin. Do not bandage tightly or use heating pad. If skin redness or irritation develops, or pain lasts more than 10 days, discontinue use and call a physician.

Dosage and Administration: Apply generously to painful muscles and joints and gently massage until Flex-all 454 disappears. Use before and after exercise. Repeat as needed for temporary relief of minor arthritis pain, simple backache, strains, sprains, bruises, and cramps.

How Supplied: Available in 2 oz. and 4 oz. bottles.

NORWICH® EXTRA–STRENGTH ASPIRIN
Aspirin (acetylsalicylic acid) tablets

Active Ingredient: Each tablet contains 500 mg (7.7 grains) of pure aspirin.

Inactive Ingredients: Starch, Hydroxypropyl Methylcellulose, Polyethylene Glycol.

Actions: Analgesic and antipyretic.

Indications: For fast, effective relief of headache, minor aches and pains, and for reduction of fever. Norwich® Extra Strength Aspirin also provides temporary relief of minor aches and pains of arthritis, rheumatism, menstrual discomfort, and toothaches.

Warnings: Children and teenagers should not use this medicine for chicken pox or flu symptoms before a doctor is consulted about Reye syndrome, a rare but serious illness. As with any drug, if you are pregnant or nursing a baby, seek the advice of a health professional before using this product. Keep all medicines out of the reach of children.

Caution: If pain persists for more than 10 days or if redness is present, or in conditions affecting children under 12, consult physician immediately. If asthmatic or taking medicines for anticoagulation (thinning the blood), diabetes, gout, or arthritis, consult physician before use. Discontinue if ringing in the ears occurs.

Treatment of Oral Overdosage: IN CASE OF ACCIDENTAL OVERDOSE, SEEK PROFESSIONAL ASSISTANCE OR CONTACT A POISON CONTROL CENTER IMMEDIATELY.

Dosage and Administration: Adults: Initial dose 2 tablets followed by 1 tablet every 3 hours or 2 tablets every 6 hours, not to exceed 8 tablets in any 24-hour period, or as directed by a physician. NOT RECOMMENDED FOR CHILDREN UNDER 12.

Professional Labeling: Same as outlined under Indications.

How Supplied: In child-resistant bottles of 150 tablets.

NORWICH® REGULAR STRENGTH ASPIRIN
Aspirin (acetylsalicylic acid) tablets

Active Ingredient: Each tablet contains 325 mg (5 grains) of pure aspirin.

Inactive Ingredients: Starch, Hydroxypropyl Methylcellulose, Polyethylene Glycol.

Actions: Analgesic and antipyretic.

Indications: For fast, effective relief of headache, minor aches and pains, and for reduction of fever, as well as temporary relief of minor aches and pains of arthritis, rheumatism, menstrual discomfort, and toothaches.

Warnings: Children and teenagers should not use this medicine for chicken pox or flu symptoms before a doctor is consulted about Reye syndrome, a rare but serious illness. As with any drug, if you are pregnant or nursing a baby, seek the advice of a health professional before using this product. Keep all medicines out of the reach of children.

Caution: If pain persists for more than 10 days or if redness is present, or in conditions affecting children under 12, consult physician immediately. Do not take if you have ulcers, ulcer symptoms or bleeding problems. If asthmatic or taking medicines for anticoagulation (thinning the blood), diabetes, gout, or arthritis, consult physician before use. Discontinue if ringing in the ears occurs.

Treatment of Oral Overdosage: IN CASE OF ACCIDENTAL OVERDOSE, SEEK PROFESSIONAL ASSISTANCE OR CONTACT A POISON CONTROL CENTER IMMEDIATELY.

Dosage and Administration: Adults: 1 or 2 tablets every 3–4 hours up to 6 times a day. Children: under 3 years, consult physician; 3–6 years, ½–1 tablet; over 6 years, 1 tablet. May be taken every 3–4 hours up to 3 times a day.

Professional Labeling: Same as outlined under Indications.

How Supplied: In child-resistant bottles of 500 tablets and bottles of 250 tablets.

NULLO® Deodorant Tablets

Active Ingredient: Each tablet contains 33.3 mg. Chlorophyllin Copper Complex.

Indications: Taken orally to control body odors due to fecal and urinary incontinence and odor due to colostomy and ileostomy.

Warning: Keep this and all drugs out of the reach of children. In case of accidental overdose, seek professional assistance or contact a poison control center immediately.

Drug Interaction: None has ever been reported.

Toxicity: None has ever been reported.

Dosage and Administration: Adult 12 years and older: swallow one or two tablets three times a day, before meals, until odor is eliminated (from two to seven days). Then take one tablet three times a day or as needed to control odor. For children under 12 years of age, consult a physician.
Ostomates may also place one or two tablets in empty pouch each time it is reused or changed.

Side Effects: Few side effects have been reported following the administration of chlorophyllin copper complex in oral doses of up to 800 mg. (in divided doses) daily for varying durations, each exceeding one week. Temporary mild diarrhea has occurred with a few humans along with the expected green coloration of the stool. One case of abdominal cramps and one case of excessive gas were reported.

How Supplied: Tamper-resistant bottles containing 30, 60, and 135 tablets.

PRĒMSYN PMS®
[preem 'sin pms]
Premenstrual Syndrome
Capsules/Caplets

Active Ingredients: Each capsule and caplet contain Acetaminophen 500 mg., Pamabrom 25 mg., and Pyrilamine Maleate 15 mg.

Indications: PRĒMSYN PMS® has been clinically proven to safely and effectively relieve premenstrual tension, irritability, nervousness, edema, backaches, legaches, and headaches that often accompany premenstrual syndrome. The formula in PRĒMSYN PMS® has been approved by an FDA-appointed panel.

Warning: KEEP THIS AND ALL DRUGS OUT OF THE REACH OF CHILDREN. In case of accidental overdose, seek professional assistance or contact a poison control center immediately.

Precautions: If drowsiness occurs, do not drive or operate machinery. As with any drug, if pregnant or nursing a baby, seek the advice of a health professional before using this product.

Dosage and Administration: Two capsules or caplets at first sign of premenstrual discomfort and repeat every three or four hours as needed, not to exceed 8 capsules/caplets in a 24-hour period.

How Supplied: Tamper-resistant bottles of 20 and 40 capsules and caplets.

Product Identification Marks: White caplet with PREMSYN PMS debossed on one surface. Grey and red capsules, film sealed with PREMSYN PMS printed on capsule.

EDUCATIONAL MATERIAL

NULLO®
Odor Control Following Ostomy Surgery
An information leaflet for patients with a colostomy, ileostomy, or urostomy. It contains basic information on odor, odor control, diet, and deodorants. Free to physicians, pharmacists, and patients.
Incontinence. A Review for Health Professionals
This 16-page booklet is aimed at increasing the dialogue between incontinent persons and health care givers. An overview of types of incontinence, assessment and management strategies are included. Free to physicians, pharmacists, and health professionals.
Incontinence, Prevalence • Types • Causes • Treatment Options • Daily Management
An information leaflet for persons experiencing temporary or long-term bladder control problems. It contains facts about incontinence, types of urinary incontinence, treatment options, and support groups for incontinent people. Free to physicians, pharmacists, health professionals, and patients.
Nullo® Internal Deodorant Tablets
The 12-page booklet provides the results of clinical studies in odor control for fecal incontinence, urinary incontinence, colostomy, and ileostomy. Free to physicians, pharmacists, and health professionals.

PREMSYN PMS®
Pamabrom and Pyrilamine Maleate, Two of the Active Ingredients in PREMSYN PMS®
The 22-page booklet presents information about the ingredients in PREMSYN PMS®. The booklet includes results of basic pharmacology and clinical studies. Free to physicians and pharmacists.
PMS: Premenstrual Syndrome, A Review for Health Professionals
This 16-page booklet is directed to the health professional. It is a review of premenstrual syndrome, the mechanism, the varying symptoms, and modes of treatment, including dietary tips and a daily symptom diary. Free to physicians and pharmacists.

PMS: Premenstrual Syndrome (3-Month Symptom Diary)
Two-page symptom diary to determine if the patient does have PMS. The diary covers three months using various symbols for symptoms and instructions for use. Free to physicians, pharmacists, clinics, and patients.
PMS: Premenstrual Syndrome (Slide Lecture Kit)
PMS, You're Not Alone (30-Minute Videotape)
Both are used by health professionals as instructional tools for educating either individual patients or groups of patients, other health professionals, and community groups. These can be obtained by writing Chattem, Inc.

Church & Dwight Co., Inc.
469 N. HARRISON STREET PRINCETON, NJ 08540

ARM & HAMMER®
Pure Baking Soda

Active Ingredient: Sodium Bicarbonate U.S.P.

Indications: For alleviation of acid indigestion, also known as heartburn or sour stomach. Not a remedy for other types of stomach complaints such as nausea, stomachache, abdominal cramps, gas pains, or stomach distention caused by overeating and/or overdrinking. In the latter case, one should not ingest solids, liquids or antacid but rather refrain from all physical activity and—if uncomfortable—call a physician.

Actions: ARM & HAMMER® Pure Baking Soda provides fast-acting, effective neutralization of stomach acids. Each level ½ teaspoon dose will neutralize 20.9 mEq of acid.

Warnings: Except under the advice and supervision of a physician: (1) do not take more than eight level ½ teaspoons per person up to 60 years old or four level ½ teaspoons per person 60 years or older in a 24-hour period, (2) do not use this product if you are on a sodium restricted diet, (3) do not use the maximum dose for more than two weeks, (4) do not ingest food, liquid or any antacid when stomach is overly full to avoid possible injury to the stomach.

Dosage and Administration: Level ½ teaspoon in ½ glass (4 fl. oz.) of water every two hours up to maximum dosage or as directed by a physician. Accurately measure level ½ teaspoon. Each level ½ teaspoon contains 20.9 mEq (.476 gm) sodium.

How Supplied: Available in 8 oz., 16 oz., 32 oz., and 64 oz. boxes.

OTIX™ DROPS
EAR WAX REMOVAL AID

Description: OTIX™ DROPS with Cotton Ear Plugs is an external ear wax removal aid that contains the active ingredient carbamide peroxide, 6.5%. OTIX™ DROPS Complete Ear Wax Removal Kit includes cotton ear plugs and a soft rubber bulb ear irrigator. Application of carbamide peroxide drops followed by warm water irrigation is an effective, medically recommended way to loosen excessive ear wax. OTIX™ DROPS is the only ear wax removal brand that supplies cotton ear plugs, which are recommended for use as a means to keep each product application in the ear for several minutes.

Indication: For occasional use as an aid to gently soften, loosen and remove excessive ear wax.

Ingredients: Carbamide Peroxide 6.5% in a base of Anhydrous Glycerin and Glyceryl Succinate.

Actions: OTIX™ DROPS patent pending formulation provides the foaming action of hydrogen peroxide with the solvent action of glycerin. In the bottle the carbamide peroxide is stabilized with the unique stabilizer glyceryl succinate. When contact is made with natural enzymes in the ear, oxygen is released. This oxygen release results in a foaming action which together with the solvent action of glycerin helps loosen and remove impacted ear wax. It is usually necessary to remove the loosened wax by gently flushing the ear with warm water using a soft rubber bulb ear irrigator.

Directions: FOR USE IN THE EAR ONLY. Adults and children over 12 years of age: Tilt head sideways and place 5 to 10 drops into ear. Tip of applicator should not enter ear canal. Keep drops in ear for several minutes by keeping head tilted or placing cotton in the ear. Use twice daily for up to 4 days if needed, or as directed by a physician. Any wax remaining after treatment may be removed by gently flushing the ear with warm water, using a soft rubber bulb ear irrigator. Children under 12 years of age: Consult a physician.

Warnings: Do not use if you have ear drainage or discharge, ear pain, irritation, or rash in the ear or are dizzy; consult a physician. Do not use if you have an injury or perforation (hole) of the eardrum or after ear surgery, unless directed by a physician.
Do not use for more than 4 days; if excessive ear wax remains after use of this product, consult a physician. Avoid contact with the eyes. Keep this and all drugs out of the reach of children. In case of accidental ingestion, consult a physician.

Caution: Avoid exposing bottle to excessive heat and direct sunlight.

How Supplied:
For Patients
OTIX™ DROPS with Cotton Ear Plugs and OTIX™ DROPS Complete Ear Wax Removal Kit with Cotton Ear Plugs and Rubber Bulb Irrigator each contain a ½ fl. oz. bottle which will provide 30 to 60 applications. Both are available in the

Continued on next page

Church & Dwight—Cont.

eye/ear sections of leading food and drug stores.

For Physicians

OTIX™ DROPS is also available in a 0.03 fl. oz. unit dose application for professional use only.

Shown in Product Identification Section, page 408

CIBA Consumer Pharmaceuticals

Division of CIBA-GEIGY Corporation
RARITAN PLAZA III
EDISON, NJ 08837

ACUTRIM® 16 HOUR*
PRECISION RELEASE™
APPETITE SUPPRESSANT
TABLETS
Caffeine Free

ACUTRIM® II—MAXIMUM STRENGTH
PRECISION RELEASE™
APPETITE SUPPRESSANT
TABLETS
Caffeine Free

ACUTRIM LATE DAY®
PRECISION RELEASE™
APPETITE SUPPRESSANT
TABLETS
Caffeine Free

Description:

ACUTRIM® Precision Release™ tablets deliver their maximum strength dosage of appetite suppressant at a precisely controlled, even rate.

This steady release is scientifically targeted to effectively distribute the appetite suppressant all day.

ACUTRIM makes it easier to follow the kind of reduced calorie diet needed for best weight control results.

A diet plan developed by an expert dietitian is included in the package for your personal use as a further aid.

ACUTRIM 16 Hour* *Breakfast to Bedtime* **™*** **Appetite Suppressant Contains no caffeine.**

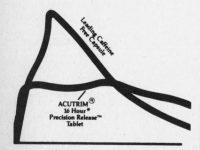

Hours　4　　8　　12　　16

Formula: Each Precision Release™ tablet contains: Active Ingredient—phenylpropanolamine HCl 75 mg. (appetite suppressant).

Inactive Ingredients—ACUTRIM® 16 HOUR*: Cellulose Acetate, Hydroxypropyl Methylcellulose, Stearic Acid—ACUTRIM® II MAXIMUM STRENGTH: Cellulose Acetate, D&C Yellow #10, FD&C Blue #1, FD&C Yellow #6, Hydroxypropyl Methylcellulose, Povidone, Propylene Glycol, Stearic Acid, Titanium Dioxide—ACUTRIM LATE DAY®: Cellulose Acetate, FD&C Yellow #6, Hydroxypropyl Methylcellulose, Isopropyl Alcohol, Propylene Glycol, Riboflavin, Stearic Acid, Titanium Dioxide.
*Extent of duration relates solely to blood levels.

Dosage: For best results, take one tablet daily directly after breakfast. Do not take more than one tablet every 24 hours. Recommended dosage may be used up to three months.

Caution: Do not give this product to children under 12. Do not exceed recommended dosage. If nervousness, dizziness, or sleeplessness occurs, stop taking this medication and consult your physician. If you are being treated for high blood pressure or depression, or have heart disease, diabetes, or thyroid disease, do not take this product, except under the supervision of a physician. If you are taking a cough/cold allergy medication containing any form of phenylpropanolamine, do not take this product.

Warning: As with any drug, if you are pregnant or nursing a baby, seek the advice of a health professional before using this product.
KEEP THIS AND ALL MEDICATION OUT OF THE REACH OF CHILDREN. In case of accidental overdose, seek professional assistance or contact a poison control center immediately.

Drug Interaction Precaution: If you are taking any prescription drugs, or any type of nasal decongestant, antihypertensive or antidepressant drug, do not take this product, except under the supervision of a physician.

How Supplied: Tamper-evident blister packages of 20 and 40 tablets. Do not use if individual seals are broken.
DO NOT STORE ABOVE 86°F
PROTECT FROM MOISTURE

12/86

Shown in Product Identification Section, page 408

EXTRA STRENGTH DOAN'S®
Analgesic Caplets

Indications: For temporary relief of minor backache.

Directions: Adults—Two caplets 3 or 4 times daily, not to exceed 8 caplets during a 24-hour period or as directed by a physician. Not intended for use by children or teenagers except under the advice of a physician. If pain persists for

more than 10 days, discontinue use and consult your physician.

Warning: Children and teenagers should not use this medicine for symptoms of chicken pox, flu or other viral illnesses before a doctor is consulted about Reye's syndrome, a rare but serious illness. As with any drug, if you are pregnant or nursing a baby, seek the advice of a health professional before using this product. Do not use this product if you are under medical care or are allergic to aspirin or salicylates, except under the advice and supervision of your physician.
Keep this and all medicines out of the reach of children. In case of accidental overdose, seek professional assistance or consult a Poison Control Center immediately.

Active Ingredient: Each caplet contains Magnesium Salicylate 500 mg.
Also Contains: Hydroxypropyl methylcellulose, magnesium stearate, microcrystalline cellulose, polyethylene glycol, polysorbate 80, propylene glycol, stearic acid and titanium dioxide.

How Supplied: Tamper-evident blister packages of 24 and 48 caplets. Do not use if individual seals are broken.
Store at 15°–30°C (59°–86°F). Protect from moisture.

Shown in Product Identification Section, page 408

REGULAR STRENGTH DOAN'S®
Analgesic Caplets

Indications: For temporary relief of minor backache.

Directions: Adults—Two caplets every 4 hours as needed, not to exceed 12 caplets during a 24-hour period or as directed by a physician. Not intended for use by children or teenagers except under the advice of a physician. If pain persists for more than 10 days, discontinue use and consult your physician.

Warning: Children and teenagers should not use this medicine for symptoms of chicken pox, flu or other viral illnesses before a doctor is consulted about Reye's syndrome, a rare but serious illness. As with any drug, if you are pregnant or nursing a baby, seek the advice of a health professional before using this product. Do not use this product if you are under medical care or are allergic to aspirin or salicylates, except under the advice and supervision of your physician. **Keep this and all medicines out of the reach of children.** In case of accidental overdose, seek professional assistance or consult a Poison Control Center immediately.

Active Ingredient: Each caplet contains Magnesium Salicylate 325 mg.
Also Contains: Magnesium Stearate, Microcrystalline Cellulose, Opadry Olive Green, Polyethylene Glycol, Purified Water, Stearic Acid.

How Supplied: Tamper-evident blister packages of 24 and 48 caplets. Do not use if individual seals are broken.

Store at 15°–30°C (59°–86°F). Protect from moisture.

Shown in Product Identification Section, page 408

FIBERALL® Chewable Tablets
[fi 'ber-all]
Lemon Creme Flavor

Description: Fiberall Chewable Tablets are a bulk-forming, nonirritant laxative which contains less than 1.5 grams of sugar per tablet. The active ingredient is polycarbophil, a bulk-forming man-made fiber. The smooth gelatinous bulk formed by Fiberall Chewable Tablets encourages peristaltic activity and a more normal elimination of the bowel contents.
The recommended dose of one tablet contains the equivalent to 1 gram of polycarbophil.
Inactive Ingredients: Crospovidone, dextrose, flavors, magnesium stearate and yellow No. 10 aluminum lake. Each dose contains less than 1 mg of sodium, 225 mg of calcium and less than 6 calories.

Indications: Fiberall Chewable Tablets are indicated for the management of chronic constipation, temporary constipation caused by illness or pregnancy, irritable bowel syndrome, and for constipation related to duodenal ulcer or diverticulosis. Fiberall Chewable Tablets are also indicated for stool softening in patients with hemorrhoids or after anorectal surgery.

Actions: After the tablet is chewed it readily disperses and acts without irritants or stimulants. Polycarbophil absorbs water in the gastrointestinal tract to form a gelatinous bulk which encourages a more normal bowel movement.

Dosage and Administration: *Adults and children 12 years and older:* chew and swallow 1 tablet, 1–4 times a day. *Children 6 to under 12 years:* chew and swallow one half tablet, 1–2 times a day. *Children under 6:* consult a physician. Drink a full glass (8 fl oz) of liquid with each dose. Additional liquid is helpful. Two to three days' usage may be required for optimal laxative benefits.

Contraindications: Fecal impaction or intestinal obstruction. Any disease state in which consumption of extra calcium is contraindicated.

Drug Interactions: This product contains calcium, which may interact with some forms of TETRACYCLINE if taken concomitantly. The tetracycline product should be taken 1 hour before or 2–3 hours after taking a Fiberall Chewable Tablet.

How Supplied: Boxes containing 18 tablets.

FIBERALL® Fiber Wafers
[fi 'ber-all]
Fruit & Nut

Description: Fiberall Fiber Wafers are a bulk-forming, nonirritant laxative. The active ingredient is psyllium hydrophilic mucilloid, a dietary fiber extracted from the seed husk of blond psyllium seed *(Plantago ovata)*. The smooth gelatinous bulk formed by Fiberall Wafers encourages peristaltic activity and a more normal elimination of the bowel contents.
One (1) Fiberall Fiber Wafer contains 3.4 g of psyllium hydrophilic mucilloid in a good-tasting wafer form, of which approximately 2.2 g is soluble fiber. One wafer is equivalent to one teaspoonful of Fiberall Powder.
Inactive Ingredients: Baking powder, brown sugar, butter flavor, cinnamon, corn syrup, crisp rice, dried ground apricots, flour, glycerin, granulated sugar, granulated walnuts, lecithin, margarine, molasses, oats, salt, vegetable oil shortening (soybean and cottonseed oil), water and wheat bran. Fiberall Fiber Wafers contain approximately 79 calories and 110 mg of sodium per serving.

Indications: Fiberall Fiber Wafers are indicated for the management of chronic constipation, temporary constipation caused by illness or pregnancy, irritable bowel syndrome, and for constipation related to duodenal ulcer or diverticulosis. Fiberall Wafers are also indicated for stool softening in patients with hemorrhoids or after anorectal surgery.

Actions: The homogenous high-fiber formula of Fiberall Fiber Wafers, eaten with 8 oz of a beverage of the patient's choice, acts without irritants or stimulants in the gastrointestinal tract.

Dosage and Administration: The recommended daily dosage for adults is one to two Fiberall Fiber Wafers with a full 8 oz glass of water or other liquid taken one to three times daily according to the individual response. The recommended daily dose for children 6 to 12 years old is one-half the usual adult dose (with liquid), or as recommended by a physician. For children under 6, consult a physician. Drinking additional liquid helps Fiberall work even more effectively. Two to three days' usage may be required for optimal laxative benefits.

Contraindications: Fecal impaction or intestinal obstruction.

How Supplied: Boxes containing 14 wafers.

Precaution: As with any grain product, inhaled or ingested psyllium powder may cause an allergic reaction in individuals sensitive to it.

Shown in Product Identification Section, page 408

FIBERALL® Fiber Wafers
[fi 'ber-all]
Oatmeal Raisin

Description: Fiberall Fiber Wafers are a bulk-forming, nonirritant laxative. The active ingredient is psyllium hydrophilic mucilloid, a dietary fiber extracted from the seed husk of blond psyllium seed *(Plantago ovata)*. The smooth gelatinous bulk formed by Fiberall Fiber Wa-

fers encourages peristaltic activity and a more normal elimination of the bowel contents.
One (1) Fiberall Fiber Wafer contains 3.4 g of psyllium hydrophilic mucilloid in a good-tasting wafer form, of which approximately 2.2 g is soluble fiber. One wafer is equivalent to one teaspoonful of Fiberall powder.
Inactive Ingredients: baking powder, cinnamon, cinnamon flavor, cloves, corn syrup, flour, glycerin, granulated sugar, lecithin, molasses, oats, raisins, vegetable oil shortening (soybean and cottonseed oil), water and wheat bran. Oatmeal Raisin Fiberall Fiber Wafers contain approximately 78 calories and 30 mg of sodium per serving.

Indications: Fiberall Fiber Wafers are indicated for the management of chronic constipation, temporary constipation caused by illness or pregnancy, irritable bowel syndrome, and for constipation related to duodenal ulcer or diverticulosis. Fiberall Wafers are also indicated for stool softening in patients with hemorrhoids or after anorectal surgery.

Actions: The homogenous high-fiber formula of Fiberall Fiber Wafers, eaten with 8 oz of a beverage of the patient's choice, acts without irritants or stimulants in the gastrointestinal tract.

Dosage and Administration: The recommended daily dosage for adults is one to two Fiberall Fiber Wafers with a full 8 oz glass of water or other liquid taken one to three times daily according to the individual response. The recommended daily dose for children 6 to 12 years old is one-half the usual adult dose (with liquid) or as recommended by a physician. For children under 6, consult a physician. Drinking additional liquid helps Fiberall work even more effectively. Two to three days' usage may be required for optimal laxative benefits.

Contraindications: Fecal impaction or intestinal obstruction.

How Supplied: Boxes containing 14 wafers.

Precaution: As with any grain product, inhaled or ingested psyllium powder may cause an allergic reaction in individuals sensitive to it.

Shown in Product Identification Section, page 408

FIBERALL® Powder, Natural Flavor
[fi 'ber-all]

Description: Fiberall is a bulk-forming, nonirritant laxative which contains no sugar. The active ingredient is psyllium hydrophilic mucilloid, a dietary fiber extracted from the seed husk of blond psyllium seed *(Plantago ovata)*. The

Continued on next page

The full prescribing information for each CIBA Consumer Pharmaceuticals product is contained herein and is that in effect as of December 1, 1989.

CIBA Consumer—Cont.

smooth gelatinous bulk formed by Fiberall encourages peristaltic activity and a more normal elimination of the bowel contents.

The recommended dose of one slightly rounded teaspoonful (5 g) contains 3.4 g psyllium hydrophilic mucilloid, of which approximately 2.2 g is soluble fiber.

Inactive Ingredients: Citric acid, flavor, polysorbate 60 and wheat bran. Each dose contains less than 10 mg of sodium, less than 60 mg of potassium, and provides less than 6 calories.

Indications: Fiberall is indicated for the management of chronic constipation, temporary constipation caused by illness or pregnancy, irritable bowel syndrome, and for constipation related to duodenal ulcer or diverticulosis. Fiberall is also indicated for stool softening in patients with hemorrhoids or after anorectal surgery.

Actions: The homogenous, high-fiber formula of Fiberall is readily dispersed in liquids and acts without irritants or stimulants in the gastrointestinal tract.

Dosage and Administration: The recommended daily dosage for adults is one slightly rounded teaspoonful (5 g) stirred into an 8 oz glass of cool water or other liquid and taken orally one to three times daily according to the individual response. The recommended daily dose for children 6 to 12 years old is one-half the usual adult dose (with liquid) or as recommended by a physician. For children under 6, consult a physician. Drinking additional liquid helps Fiberall work even more effectively. Two to three days' usage may be required for maximum laxative benefits.

Contraindications: Fecal impaction or intestinal obstruction.

How Supplied: Powder, in 10 or 15 oz containers.

Precaution: As with any grain product, inhaled or ingested psyllium powder may cause an allergic reaction in individuals sensitive to it.

Shown in Product Identification Section, page 408

FIBERALL® Powder, Orange Flavor
[fi 'ber-all]

Description: Fiberall is a bulk-forming, nonirritant laxative which contains no sugar. The active ingredient is psyllium hydrophilic mucilloid, a dietary fiber extracted from the seed husk of blond psyllium seed *(Plantago ovata).* The smooth gelatinous bulk formed by Fiberall encourages peristaltic activity and a more normal elimination of the lower bowel contents.

The recommended dose of one rounded teaspoonful (5.9 g) contains 3.4 g psyllium hydrophilic mucilloid, of which approximately 2.2 g is soluble fiber.

Inactive Ingredients: Beta-carotene, citric acid, flavors, polysorbate 60, saccharin, wheat bran and yellow No. 6

lake. Each dose contains less than 10 mg of sodium, less than 60 mg of potassium, and provides less than 10 calories.

Indications: Fiberall is indicated for the management of chronic constipation, temporary constipation caused by illness or pregnancy, irritable bowel syndrome, and for constipation related to duodenal ulcer or diverticulosis. Fiberall is also indicated for stool softening in patients with hemorrhoids or after anorectal surgery.

Actions: The homogenous, high-fiber formula of Fiberall is readily dispersed in liquids and acts without irritants or stimulants in the gastrointestinal tract.

Dosage and Administration: The recommended daily dosage for adults is one rounded teaspoonful (5.9 g) stirred into an 8 oz glass of cool water or other liquid and taken orally one to three times daily according to the individual response. The recommended daily dose for children 6 to 12 years old is one-half the usual adult dose (with liquid) or as recommended by a physician. For children under 6, consult a physician. Drinking additional liquid helps Fiberall work even more effectively. Two to three days' usage may be required for maximum laxative benefits.

Contraindications: Fecal impaction or intestinal obstruction.

How Supplied: Powder, in 10 and 15 oz containers.

Precaution: As with any grain product, inhaled or ingested psyllium powder may cause an allergic reaction in individuals sensitive to it.

Shown in Product Identification Section, page 408

NUPERCAINAL®
Hemorrhoidal and Anesthetic Ointment
Pain-Relief Cream

Caution:
Nupercainal products are not for prolonged or extensive use and should never be applied in or near the eyes. If the symptom being treated does not subside, or rash, irritation, swelling, pain, bleeding or other symptoms develop or increase, discontinue use and consult a physician.
Consult labels before using.
Keep this and all medications out of reach of children.
NUPERCAINAL SHOULD NOT BE SWALLOWED. IN CASE OF ACCIDENTAL INGESTION CONSULT A PHYSICIAN OR POISON CONTROL CENTER IMMEDIATELY.

Indications: Nupercainal Ointment and Cream are fast-acting, long-lasting pain relievers that you can use for a number of painful skin conditions. **Nupercainal Hemorrhoidal and Anesthetic Ointment** is for hemorrhoids as

well as for general use. **Nupercainal Pain-Relief Cream** is for general use only. The **Cream** is half as strong as the **Ointment.**

How to use Nupercainal Anesthetic Ointment (for general use). This soothing Ointment helps lubricate dry, inflamed skin and gives fast, temporary relief of pain, itching and burning. It is recommended for sunburn, nonpoisonous insect bites, minor burns, cuts and scratches. **DO NOT USE THIS PRODUCT IN OR NEAR YOUR EYES.**

Apply to affected areas gently. If necessary, cover with a light dressing for protection. Do not use more than 1 ounce of Ointment in a 24-hour period for an adult. Do not use more than one-quarter of an ounce in a 24-hour period for a child. If irritation develops, discontinue use and consult your doctor.

How to use Nupercainal Hemorrhoidal and Anesthetic Ointment for fast, temporary relief of pain and itching due to hemorrhoids (also known as piles).

Remove cap from tube and set it aside. Attach the white plastic applicator to the tube. Squeeze the tube until you see the Ointment begin to come through the little holes in the applicator. Using your finger, lubricate the applicator with the Ointment. Now insert the entire applicator gently into the rectum. Give the tube a good squeeze to get enough Ointment into the rectum for comfort and lubrication. Remove applicator from rectum and wipe it clean. Apply additional Ointment to anal tissues to help relieve pain, burning, and itching. For best results use Ointment morning and night and after each bowel movement. After each use detach applicator, and wash it off with soap and water. Put cap back on tube before storing. In case of rectal bleeding, discontinue use and consult your doctor.

Pain-Relief Cream for general use. This Cream is particularly effective for fast, temporary relief of pain and itching associated with sunburn, cuts, scrapes, scratches, minor burns and nonpoisonous insect bites. **DO NOT USE THIS PRODUCT IN OR NEAR YOUR EYES.** Apply liberally to affected area and rub in gently. This Cream is water-washable, so be sure to reapply after bathing, swimming or sweating. If irritation develops, discontinue use and consult your doctor.

Nupercainal Hemorrhoidal and Anesthetic Ointment contains 1% dibucaine USP. Also contains acetone sodium bisulfite, lanolin, light mineral oil, purified water, and white petrolatum. Available in tubes of 1 and 2 ounces. Store between 59°–86°F.

Nupercainal Pain-Relief Cream contains 0.5% dibucaine USP. Also contains acetone sodium bisulfite, fragrance, glycerin, potassium hydroxide, purified water, stearic acid, and trolamine. Available in 1½ ounce tubes.

Dibucaine USP is officially classified as a "topical anesthetic" and is one of the strongest and longest lasting of all topical pain relievers. It is not a narcotic.

C86-62 (Rev. 11/86)

Shown in Product Identification Section, page 408

NUPERCAINAL®
Suppositories

> **Caution:** Nupercainal suppositories are not for prolonged or extensive use. Contact with the eyes should be avoided.
> **Consult labels before using.**
> **Keep this and all medications out of reach of children.**
> NUPERCAINAL SUPPOSITORIES SHOULD NOT BE SWALLOWED. SWALLOWING CAN BE HAZARDOUS, PARTICULARLY TO CHILDREN. IN THE EVENT OF ACCIDENTAL SWALLOWING CONSULT A PHYSICIAN OR POISON CONTROL CENTER IMMEDIATELY.

Indications: Nupercainal Rectal Suppositories are for the temporary relief from itching, burning, and discomfort due to hemorrhoids or other anorectal disorders.

How to use Nupercainal Suppositories for hemorrhoids (also known as piles) or other anorectal disorders.
Tear off one suppository along the perforated line. Remove foil wrapper. Insert the suppository, rounded end first, well into the anus until you can feel it moving into your rectum. For best results, use one suppository after each bowel movement as needed, but not to exceed 6 in a 24-hour period. Each suppository is sealed in its own foil packet to reduce danger of leakage when carried in pocket or purse. **To prevent melting, do not store above 86°F (30°C).**
Each Nupercainal Suppository contains 2.4 gram cocoa butter, and .25 gram zinc oxide. Also contains acetone sodium bisulfite and bismuth subgallate.

C86-42 (Rev. 9/86)

Shown in Product Identification Section, page 408

OTRIVIN®
xylometazoline hydrochloride USP
Decongestant
Nasal Spray and Nasal Drops 0.1%
Pediatric Nasal Drops 0.05%

One application provides rapid and long-lasting relief of nasal congestion for up to 10 hours.
Quickly clears stuffy noses due to common cold, sinusitis, hay fever.
Nasal congestion can make life miserable—you can't breathe, smell, taste, or sleep comfortably. That is why Otrivin is so helpful. It clears away that stuffy feeling, usually within 5 to 10 minutes, and your head feels clear for hours.
Otrivin has been prescribed by doctors for many years. Here is how you use it:
Nasal Spray 0.1%—for adults and children 12 years and older. Spray 2 or 3 times into each nostril every 8–10 hours. With head upright, squeeze sharply and firmly while inhaling (sniffing) through the nose.
Nasal Drops 0.1%—for adults and children 12 years and older. Put 2 or 3 drops into each nostril every 8 to 10 hours. Tilt head as far back as possible. Immediately bend head forward toward knees, hold for a few seconds, then return to upright position.
Do not give Nasal Spray 0.1% or Nasal Drops 0.1% to children under 12 years except under the advice and supervision of a physician.
Pediatric Nasal Drops 0.05%—for children 2 to 12 years of age. Put 2 or 3 drops into each nostril every 8 to 10 hours. Tilt head as far back as possible. Immediately bend head forward toward knees, hold a few seconds, then return to upright position.
Do not give this product to children under 2 years except under the advice and supervision of a physician.
Otrivin Nasal Spray/Nasal Drops contain 0.1% xylometazoline hydrochloride, USP. Also contains benzalkonium chloride, potassium chloride, potassium phosphate monobasic, purified water, sodium chloride and sodium phosphate dibasic. They are available in an unbreakable plastic spray package of ½ fl oz (15 ml) and in a plastic dropper bottle of .66 fl oz (20 ml).
Otrivin Pediatric Nasal Drops contain 0.05% xylometazoline hydrochloride, USP. Also contains benzalkonium chloride, potassium chloride, potassium phosphate monobasic, purified water, sodium chloride and sodium phosphate dibasic. It is available in a plastic dropper bottle of .66 fl oz (20 ml).

Warnings: Do not exceed recommended dosage, because symptoms such as burning, stinging, sneezing, or increase of nasal discharge may occur. Do not use this product for more than 3 days. If symptoms persist, consult a physician. The use of this dispenser by more than one person may cause infection.
Keep this and all medicines out of the reach of children. Overdosage in young children may cause marked sedation. In case of accidental ingestion, seek professional assistance or contact a Poison Control Center immediately.
Store between 33°–86°F.

C86-44 (9/86)

Shown in Product Identification Section, page 408

PRIVINE®
naphazoline hydrochloride, USP
0.05% Nasal Solution
0.05% Nasal Spray

Caution: Do not use Privine if you have glaucoma. Privine is an effective nasal decongestant **when you use it in the recommended dosage.** If you use too much, too long, or too often, Privine may be harmful to your nasal mucous membranes and cause burning, stinging, sneezing or an increased runny nose. Do not use Privine by mouth.
Keep this and all medications out of the reach of children. Do not use Privine with children under 12 years of age, except with the advice and supervision of a doctor.
OVERDOSAGE IN YOUNG CHILDREN MAY CAUSE MARKED SEDATION AND IF SEVERE, EMERGENCY TREATMENT MAY BE NECESSARY. IF NASAL STUFFINESS PERSISTS AFTER 3 DAYS OF TREATMENT, DISCONTINUE USE AND CONSULT A DOCTOR.
Privine is a nasal decongestant that comes in two forms: Nasal Solution (in a bottle with a dropper) and Nasal Spray (in a plastic squeeze bottle). Both are for prompt, and prolonged relief of nasal congestion due to common colds, sinusitis, hay fever, etc.
How to use Nasal Solution. Squeeze rubber bulb to fill dropper with proper amount of medication. For best results, tilt head as far back as possible and put two drops of solution into your right nostril. Then lean head forward, inhaling and turning your head to the left. Refill dropper by squeezing bulb. Now tilt head as far back as possible and put two drops of solution into your left nostril. Then lean head forward, inhaling, and turning your head to the right.
Use only 2 drops in each nostril. Do not repeat this dosage more than every 3 hours.
The Privine dropper bottle is designed to make administration of the proper dosage easy and to prevent accidental overdosage. Privine will not cause sleeplessness, so you may use it before going to bed.
Important: After use, be sure to rinse the dropper with very hot water. This helps prevent contamination of the bottle with bacteria from nasal secretions. Use of the dispenser by more than one person may spread infection.
Note: Privine Nasal Solution may be used on contact with glass, plastic, stainless steel and specially treated metals used in atomizers. Do not let the solution come in contact with reactive metals, especially aluminum. If solution becomes discolored, it should be discarded.
How to use Nasal Spray. For best results do **not** shake the plastic squeeze bottle.
Remove cap. With head held upright, spray twice into each nostril. Squeeze the bottle sharply and firmly while sniffing through the nose.
For best results use every 4 to 6 hours. Do not use more often than every 3 hours. Avoid overdosage. Follow directions for use carefully.
Privine Nasal Solution contains 0.05% naphazoline hydrochloride USP. It also contains benzalkonium chloride, disodium edetate dihydrate, hydrochloric acid, purified water, sodium chloride, and trolamine. It is available in bottles of

Continued on next page

The full prescribing information for each CIBA Consumer Pharmaceuticals product is contained herein and is that in effect as of December 1, 1989.

CIBA Consumer—Cont.

.66 fl. oz. (20 ml) with dropper, and bottles of 16 fl. oz. (473 ml).
Privine Nasal Spray contains 0.05% naphazoline hydrochloride USP. It also contains benzalkonium chloride, disodium edetate dihydrate, hydrochloric acid, purified water, sodium chloride, and trolamine. It is available in plastic squeeze bottles of ½ fl. oz. (15 ml).
Store the nasal solution and nasal spray between 59°–86°F.

C86-43 (Rev. 9/86)
Shown in Product Identification Section, page 408

Q–VEL®
Muscle Relaxant Pain Reliever

Active Ingredient: Quinine Sulfate 1 gr. (64.8 mg).

Contains: Vitamin E (400 I.U. *dl*-alpha tocopheryl acetate) in a lecithin base.

Indications: For prevention and temporary relief of night leg cramps.

Warnings: Do not take if pregnant, nursing a baby or of childbearing potential, if sensitive to quinine, or under 12 years of age. Discontinue use and consult your physician if ringing in the ears, deafness, diarrhea, nausea, skin rash, bruising or visual disturbances occur. In case of accidental overdose, seek medical assistance or contact Poison Control Center at once. Keep this and all medicine out of reach of children.

Dosage: To prevent night leg cramps take 2 soft caplets after the evening meal plus 2 at bedtime. For relief in case of sudden attack, take 2 soft caplets at once plus 2 after ½ hour if needed. Do not exceed 4 soft caplets daily.

How Supplied: Bottles of 16, 30 and 50 softgels.
Shown in Product Identification Section, page 408

SLOW FE®
Slow Release Iron Tablets

Description: SLOW FE supplies ferrous sulfate for the treatment of iron deficiency and iron deficiency anemia with a significant reduction in the incidence of the common side effects of oral iron. The wax matrix delivery system of SLOW FE is designed to maximize the release of ferrous sulfate in the duodenum and the jejunum where it is best tolerated and absorbed. SLOW FE has been clinically shown to be associated with a lower incidence of constipation, diarrhea and abdominal discomfort when compared to regular iron tablets and the leading capsule.

Formula: Each tablet contains 160 mg. dried ferrous sulfate USP, equivalent to 50 mg. elemental iron. Also contains cetostearyl alcohol, colloidal silicon dioxide, hydroxypropyl methylcellulose, shellac, lactose, magnesium stearate, polyethylene glycol.

Dosage: ADULTS—one or two tablets daily or as recommended by a physician. A maximum of four tablets daily may be taken. CHILDREN—one tablet daily. Tablets must be swallowed whole.

Warning: The treatment of any anemic condition should be under the advice and supervision of a physician. As oral iron products interfere with absorption of oral tetracycline antibiotics, these products should not be taken within two hours of each other. As with any drug, if you are pregnant or nursing a baby, seek the advice of a health professional before using this product.
Keep this and all medicines out of reach of children. In case of accidental overdose, contact your physician or poison control center immediately.
Tamper-Resistant Packaging.

How Supplied: Blister packages of 30, 60 and bottles of 100.
Shown in Product Identification Section, page 409

SUNKIST CHILDREN'S CHEWABLE MULTIVITAMINS—REGULAR

Vitamin Ingredients: Each tablet contains:
[See table below].

Indication: Dietary supplementation.

Dosage and Administration: One chewable tablet daily for children two years and older.

Warning: Phenylketonurics: Contains Phenylalanine

How Supplied: SUNKIST Children's Multivitamins-Regular are supplied in bottles of 60 chewable tablets with child resistant caps.
Shown in Product Identification Section, page 409

SUNKIST CHILDREN'S CHEWABLE MULTIVITAMINS—PLUS EXTRA C

Vitamin Ingredients: Each tablet contains the ingredients of the Regular vitamin product plus extra Vitamin C (a total of 250 mg).

Indication: Dietary supplementation.

Dosage and Administration: One chewable tablet daily for adults and children two years and older.

Warning: Phenylketonurics: Contains Phenylalanine.

How Supplied: SUNKIST Children's Multivitamins Plus Extra C are supplied in bottles of 60 chewable tablets with child resistant caps.
Shown in Product Identification Section, page 409

SUNKIST CHILDREN'S CHEWABLE MULTIVITAMINS—PLUS IRON

Vitamin Ingredients: Each tablet contains the vitamins of the Regular product plus 15 mg of Iron.

Indication: Dietary supplementation.

Dosage and Administration: One chewable tablet daily for children two years and older.

Warning: Phenylketonurics: Contains Phenylalanine.

Precaution: Contains iron, which can be harmful in large doses. Close tightly and keep out of reach of children. In case of overdose, contact a physician or poison control center immediately.

How Supplied: SUNKIST Children's Multivitamins Plus Iron are supplied in bottles of 60 chewable tablets with child resistant caps.
Shown in Product Identification Section, page 409

SUNKIST CHILDREN'S CHEWABLE MULTIVITAMINS—COMPLETE

Vitamin Ingredients: Each tablet contains the following ingredients:
[See table on next page].

Indication: Dietary supplementation.

Dosage and Administration: Children ages 2 to 4 one-half chewable tablet daily; One chewable tablet daily for children four years and older.

Warning: Phenylketonurics: Contains Phenylalanine.

Precautions: Contains iron, which can be harmful in large doses. Close tightly and keep out of reach of children. In case

VITAMINS	QUANTITY PER TABLET	PERCENT U.S. RDA	
		FOR CHILD. 2 TO 4 YRS OF AGE (1 TABLET)	FOR ADULTS & CHILD. OVER 4 YRS OF AGE (1 TABLET)
Vitamin A (as Palmitate + Beta Carotene)	2500 IU	100	50
Vitamin D-3	400 IU	100	100
Vitamin E	15 IU	150	50
Vitamin C	60 mg	150	100
Folic Acid	0.3 mg	150	75
Niacinamide	13.5 mg	150	68
Vitamin B-6	1.05 mg	150	53
Vitamin B-12	4.5 mcg	150	75
Vitamin B-1	1.05 mg	150	70
Vitamin B-2	1.20 mg	150	71
Vitamin K-1	5 mcg	*	*

*Recognized as essential in human nutrition, but no U.S. RDA established.

of overdose, contact a physician or poison control center immediately.

How Supplied: SUNKIST Children's Multivitamins Complete are supplied in bottles of 60 chewable tablets with child resistant caps.
Shown in Product Identification Section, page 409

SUNKIST® VITAMIN C
Citrus Complex
Chewable Tablets
Easy to Swallow Caplets

Description: All Sunkist Vitamin C chewable tablets have a delicious orange flavor unlike any other Vitamin C tablet. Each 60 mg chewable tablet contains 100% of the U.S. RDA* of Vitamin C. Each 250 mg chewable tablet contains 417% of the U.S. RDA* of Vitamin C. Each 500 mg chewable tablet contains 833% of the U.S. RDA* of Vitamin C.

Each 500 mg easy to swallow caplet contains 833% of the U.S. RDA* of Vitamin C.

Sunkist Vitamin C chewable tablets and easy to swallow caplets do not contain artificial flavors, colors or preservatives.

*U.S. Recommended Daily Allowance for adults and children over 4 years of age.

Indication: Dietary supplement.

How Supplied: 60 mg Chewable Tablets—Rolls of 11.
250 mg and 500 mg Chewable Tablets—Bottles of 60.
500 mg Easy to Swallow Caplets—Bottles of 60.

Store in a cool dry place.

Sunkist® is a registered trademark of Sunkist Growers, Inc., Sherman Oaks, CA 91423.©
　　　　　　　　　　　　(12/86)
Shown in Product Identification Section, page 409

Colgate-Palmolive Company
A Delaware Corporation
300 PARK AVENUE
NEW YORK, NY 10022

COLGATE® JUNIOR FLUORIDE GEL TOOTHPASTE

Active Ingredient: Sodium Fluoride (NaF) 0.24% in a fruit-flavored toothpaste base.

Other Ingredients: Sorbitol, Glycerin, Hydrated Silica, Water, PEG-12, Sodium Lauryl Sulfate, Sodium Benzoate, Flavor, Cellulose Gum, Sodium Saccharin, Titanium Dioxide, FD&C Blue No. 1, D&C Yellow No. 10.

Indications: This toothpaste, with its anti-cavity ingredient Sodium Fluoride, provides clinically proven fluoride protection. It has been specially formulated to appeal to children 12 and under.

Actions: Clinical tests have shown Colgate® with Sodium Fluoride to be an effective aid in the reduction of the incidence of cavities. It is approved as a decay-preventive agent by the American Dental Association.

Contraindications: Sensitivity to any ingredient in the product.

Directions: Brush regularly as part of a dental health program.

How Supplied: 2.7 oz., 4.5 oz., 6.4 oz., and 8.2 oz. tubes. Also available in 4.5 oz. pump.
Shown in Product Identification Section, page 409

COLGATE Fluoride FLUORIDE GEL

Active Ingredient: Sodium Fluoride (NaF) 0.24% in a spearmint flavored gel toothpaste base.

Other Ingredients: Sorbitol, Glycerin, Hydrated Silica, Water, PEG-12, Sodium Lauryl Sulfate, Flavor, Sodium Benzoate, Cellulose Gum, Sodium Saccharin, Titanium Dioxide, FD&C Blue No. 1.

Indications: The gel toothpaste with the anti-cavity ingredient Sodium Fluoride providing maximum fluoride protection by a toothpaste and a fresh clean taste for the whole family.

Actions: Clinical tests have shown COLGATE® with Sodium Fluoride to be an effective aid in the reduction of the incidence of cavities. It is approved as a decay-preventive dentifrice by the American Dental Association.

Contraindications: Sensitivity to any ingredient in this product.

Directions: Brush regularly as part of a dental health program.

How Supplied: 1.4 oz., 2.6 oz., 4.6 oz., 6.4 oz., 8.2 oz. tubes. Also available in 4.5 and 6.4 oz. pumps.
Shown in Product Identification Section, page 409

COLGATE MFP® FLUORIDE TOOTHPASTE

Active Ingredient: Sodium Monofluorophosphate (MFP®) 0.76% in a doublemint flavored toothpaste base.

Other Ingredients: Dicalcium Phosphate Dihydrate, Water, Glycerin, Sodium Lauryl Sulfate, Cellulose Gum, Flavor, Sodium Benzoate, Tetrasodium Pyrophosphate, Sodium Saccharin.

Indications: The toothpaste with the anti-cavity ingredient MFP® Fluoride providing maximum fluoride protection by a toothpaste.

Actions: Clinical tests have shown COLGATE® with MFP® Fluoride to be an effective aid in the reduction of the incidence of cavities. It is approved as a decay-preventive dentifrice by the American Dental Association.

Contraindications: Sensitivity to any ingredient in this product.

Directions: Brush regularly as part of a dental health program.

How Supplied: 1.50 oz., 3.0 oz., 5.0 oz., 7.0 oz., 9.0 oz. tubes. Also available in 4.9 and 6.4 oz. pumps with Sodium Fluoride (NaF) 0.24%.
Shown in Product Identification Section, page 409

COLGATE® MOUTHWASH TARTAR CONTROL FORMULA

Ingredients: Water, SD Alcohol 38-B (15.3%), Glycerin, Tetrapotassium Pyrophosphate, Poloxamer 336, Poloxamer 407, Tetrasodium Pyrophosphate, Ben-

Continued on next page

VITAMINS	QUANTITY PER TABLET	PERCENT U.S. RDA FOR CHILD. 2 TO 4 YRS OF AGE (½ TABLET)	FOR ADULTS & CHILD. OVER 4 YRS OF AGE (1 TABLET)
Vitamin A (as Palmitate + Beta Carotene)	5000 IU	100	100
Vitamin D-3	400 IU	50	100
Vitamin E	30 IU	150	100
Vitamin C	60 mg	75	100
Folic Acid	0.4 mg	100	100
Biotin	40 mcg	13	13
Pantothenic Acid	10 mg	100	100
Niacinamide	20 mg	111	100
Vitamin B-6	2 mg	143	100
Vitamin B-12	6 mcg	100	100
Vitamin B-1	1.5 mg	107	100
Vitamin B-2	1.7 mg	106	100
Vitamin K-1	10 mcg	*	*
MINERALS			
Iron	18 mg	90	100
Magnesium	20 mg	5	5
Iodine	150 mcg	107	100
Zinc	10 mg	63	67
Manganese	1 mg	*	*
Calcium	100 mg	6	10
Phosphorus	78 mg	5	8
Copper	2 mg	100	100

*Recognized as essential in human nutrition, but no U.S. RDA established.

Colgate-Palmolive—Cont.

zoic Acid, PVM/MA Copolymer, Flavor, Sodium Saccharin, Sodium Fluoride, FD&C Blue #1, FD&C Yellow #5.

Indications: Highly effective in the inhibition of supragingival calculus, Colgate Mouthrinse Tartar Control Formula also provides effective breath odor control.

Actions: Clinical studies have shown that Colgate's exclusive combination of pyrophosphate and PVM/MA copolymer reduces calculus build-up by up to 37.7%.

Contraindications: Sensitivity to any ingredient in the product.

Directions: Adults and children 6 years of age and older. Use twice daily after brushing teeth with a toothpaste. Vigorously swish 10 ml. (2 teaspoons; or up to mark on cap) of rinse between teeth for 1 minute and then expectorate. Do not swallow rinse. Do not eat or drink for 30 minutes after rinsing. Children under 6 years of age: Consult a dentist or physician. Children under 12 years of age should be supervised in the use of this product.

How Supplied: 2 oz., 6 oz., 24 oz. and 32 oz. plastic bottles with dose-measure cap.
Shown in Product Identification Section, page 409

COLGATE® TARTAR CONTROL FORMULA

Active Ingredient: Sodium Fluoride 0.24% in a mint flavored toothpaste base.

Other Ingredients: Water, Hydrated Silica, Sorbitol, Glycerine, PEG-12, Tetrapotassium Pyrophosphate, Tetrasodium Pyrophosphate, Sodium Lauryl Sulfate, Flavor, PVM/MA Copolymer, Titanium Dioxide, Carrageenan, Sodium Saccharin. CONTAINS NO SUGAR.

Indications: This toothpaste with the anti-cavity ingredient sodium fluoride provides maximum fluoride protection by a toothpaste and is highly effective in inhibiting the formation of calculus. Repeated clinical studies have demonstrated an average 46% inhibition of calculus buildup.

Actions: Clinical tests have shown Colgate Tartar Control Formula to be effective in the reduction of calculus accumulation. It is also approved as a decay preventive dentifrice by the American Dental Association.

Contraindications: Sensitivity to any ingredient in the product.

Directions: Brush regularly as part of a dental health program.

How Supplied: 1.3 oz., 2.6 oz., 4.6 oz., 6.4 oz., and 8.2 oz. tubes. Also available in 4.5 oz. Pump.
Shown in Product Identification Section, page 409

COLGATE® TARTAR CONTROL GEL

Active Ingredient: Sodium Fluoride 0.24% in a mint flavored gel toothpaste base.

Other Ingredients: Water, Hydrated Silica, Sorbitol, Glycerine, PEG-12, Tetrapotassium Pyrophosphate, Tetrasodium Pyrophosphate, Sodium Lauryl Sulfate, Flavor, PVM/MA Copolymer, Carrageenan, Sodium Saccharin, FD&C Blue No. 1. CONTAINS NO SUGAR.

Indications: This gel toothpaste with the anti-cavity ingredient sodium fluoride provides maximum fluoride protection by a toothpaste and is highly effective in inhibiting the formation of calculus. Repeated clinical studies have demonstrated an average 46% inhibition of calculus buildup.

Actions: Clinical tests have shown Colgate Tartar Control Gel to be effective in the reduction of calculus accumulation. It is also approved as a decay preventive dentifrice by the American Dental Association.

Contraindications: Sensitivity to any ingredient in the product.

Directions: Brush regularly as part of a dental health program.

How Supplied: 1.3 oz., 2.6 oz., 4.6 oz., 6.4 oz., and 8.2 oz. tubes. Also available in 4.5 oz. Pump.
Shown in Product Identification Section, page 409

FLUORIGARD ANTI-CAVITY FLUORIDE RINSE
Fluorigard is accepted by the American Dental Association.

Active Ingredient: Sodium Fluoride (0.05%) in a neutral solution.

Other Ingredients: Water, Glycerin, SD Alcohol 38-B (6%), Poloxamer 338, Poloxamer 407, Sodium Benzoate, Sodium Saccharin, Benzoic Acid, Flavor, FD & C Blue No. 1, FD & C Yellow No. 5.

Indications: Good tasting Fluorigard Anti-Cavity Fluoride Rinse is fluoride in liquid form. It helps get cavity-fighting fluoride to back teeth, as well as front teeth; even floods those dangerous spaces between teeth where brushing might miss. 70% of all cavities happen in back teeth and between teeth.

Actions: Fluorigard Anti-Cavity Fluoride Rinse is a 0.05% Sodium Fluoride solution which has been proven effective in reducing cavities.

Contraindications: Sensitivity to any ingredient in this product.

Warnings: Do not swallow. For rinsing only. Not to be used by children under 6 years of age unless recommended by a dentist. Keep out of reach of young children. If an amount considerably larger than recommended for rinsing is swallowed, give as much milk as possible and contact a physician immediately.

Directions: Use once daily after thoroughly brushing teeth. For persons 6 years of age and over, fill measuring cap to 10 ml. level (2 teaspoons), rinse around and between teeth for one minute, then spit out. For maximum benefit, use every day and do not eat or drink for at least 30 minutes afterward. Rinsing may be most convenient at bedtime. This product may be used in addition to a fluoride toothpaste.

How Supplied: 6 oz., 12 oz., 18 oz. in shatterproof plastic bottles.
1 Gallon Professional Size for use in dentists' offices only.
Shown in Product Identification Section, page 409

Columbia Laboratories, Inc.
16400 N.W. 2ND AVENUE
MIAMI, FL 33169

REPLENS™
Replenishes vaginal moisture

Description: Replens vaginal gel relieves dryness and replenishes vaginal moisture. Replens is a greaseless lubricant that is nonstaining, fragrance free, unflavored and nonirritating.

Actions: When used as directed, Replens helps relieve vaginal dryness, discomfort and painful intercourse by providing continuous hydration to the vaginal cells.

Ingredients: Purified water, glycerin, mineral oil, polycarbophil, Carbomer 934P, hydrogenated palm oil glyceride, methylparaben, and sorbic acid.

Warnings: Keep out of the reach of children. Replens is not a contraceptive. Does not contain spermicide.

Dosage: Use 3 times a week.

How Supplied: Replens is available in boxes containing 12 prefilled disposable applicators. Each applicator contains 2.5 grams.
Shown in Product Identification Section, page 408

Commerce Drug Company, Inc.
Division Del Laboratories, Inc.
565 BROAD HOLLOW ROAD
FARMINGDALE, NY 11735

BOIL•EASE®

Active Ingredients: Benzocaine USP 5%, ichthammol USP 1.86%, precipitated sulfur USP 0.44%.

Inactive Ingredients: Anhydrous lanolin, camphor, eucalyptus oil, juniper tar, liquified phenol, menthol, paraffin, petrolatum, rosin, sexadecyl alcohol, thymol, yellow wax, zinc oxide.

Indications: Antiseptic, pain-relieving drawing salve for boils.

Actions: Benzocaine affords prompt, temporary relief of pain by creating surface anesthetic action on the affected area. Ichthammol NF is used topically and possesses a mild antiseptic, analgesic and *mild* local soothing effect. Sulfur is used for its mild keratolytic and antibacterial activity.

Warnings: For external use only. Avoid contact with the eyes. Do not use on boils on the lips, nose, cheeks, or forehead. Consult a doctor for treatment of boils in these areas. Do not use this product for more than 7 days. If condition worsens or does not improve, if fever occurs, or if redness around the boil develops, consult a doctor. Keep this and all drugs out of the reach of children.

Dosage and Administration: Apply Boil-Ease onto sterile gauze pad and then apply directly onto the affected area.

How Supplied: 1 oz plastic tube.

DERMAREST®

Active Ingredients: Diphenhydramine hydrochloride USP 2.0%, resorcinol USP 2.0%.

Inactive Ingredients: Aloe vera gel, benzalkonium chloride, edetate disodium, hydroxyethylcellulose, menthol, methylparaben, propylene glycol, purified water, sorbic acid.

Indications: This unique, medically proven, dual-action Dermarest formula provides fast, temporary relief of intense itching and pain associated with minor skin irritations, skin allergies, insect bites, hives, poison ivy and oak, rashes, sunburn, dry skin itch and bee stings.

Actions: Diphenhydramine hydrochloride is an antihistamine which depresses cutaneous sensory receptors. As an antihistamine, it relieves the discomfort of itching due to histamine release in allergic states when applied to the skin. The antihistamine competes with histamine at the H_1 receptors.

Resorcinol is primarily an antipruritic having some bactericidal and fungicidal activity.

Warnings: For external use only. Avoid contact with the eyes. Do not apply over large areas of the body. Do not apply to blistered, raw or oozing areas of the skin. If condition worsens, or if symptoms persist for more than 7 days, or clear up and occur again within a few days, discontinue use of this product and consult a physician. Keep this and all drugs out of the reach of children. In case of accidental ingestion, seek professional assistance or contact a poison control center immediately.

Dosage and Administration: For adults and children 2 years of age and older: Apply liberally to the affected area not more than three or four times daily, or as directed by your physician. For children under 2 years of age: Consult a physician.

How Supplied: Clear Gel in two sizes—1.25 oz and 0.65 oz tubes.

DIAPER GUARD®

Active Ingredients: Dimethicone NF 1.0%, white petrolatum USP 66%.

Inactive Ingredients: Benzalkonium chloride, cocoa butter, colloidal oatmeal, colloidal silicon dioxide, fragrance, magnesium silicate, methylparaben, paraffin, propylparaben, retinyl palmitate (vitamin A) with cholecalciferol (vitamin D_3), *dl* -alpha-tocopheryl acetate (vitamin E), zinc oxide.

Indications: The special wetness barrier in the Diaper Guard formula keeps baby drier, promotes healing of diaper rash, helps prevent and temporarily protect skin that is chafed, chapped, or windburned. It is freshly scented.

Actions: Dimethicone and petrolatum are both skin protectants, which form an occlusive barrier to water-soluble substances that can aggravate existing diaper rash. Dimethicone adheres to the skin and repels wetness, while petrolatum provides soothing emollient action. The combination helps prevent diaper rash.

Warning: For external use only. Avoid contact with the eyes. If condition worsens or does not improve within 7 days, consult a doctor. Not to be applied over deep or puncture wounds, infections, or lacerations. Keep this and all medications out of the reach of children. In case of accidental ingestion, seek professional assistance or contact a poison control center immediately.

Dosage and Administration: To help prevent diaper rash, apply Diaper Guard after each diaper change and at bedtime when exposure to wet diapers may be prolonged. If diaper rash is present, or at the first sign of redness, apply Diaper Guard to the diaper area three or more times daily as needed to promote healing. For best results apply to clean, dry skin.

How Supplied: 1.75 oz (49.69 g) tube.

OFF•EZY® WART REMOVAL KIT

Active Ingredients: Salicylic acid USP 17%.

Inactive Ingredients: Acetone, D&C Red No. 17, D&C Yellow No. 11, flexible collodion (containing 65% ether and 21% alcohol), methyl salicylate.

Indications: Off-Ezy Wart Removal Kit is a total regimen (liquid plus special skin buffer) for the effective removal of both common warts and plantar warts (on the bottom of the feet).

Actions: Warts are caused by specific DNA viruses which infect the epidermal cells, resulting in elevated epithelial growths. Salicylic acid is used in the treatment of warts due to its keratolytic effect on the epithelium. Collodion vehicles are often utilized to occlude the affected area, prevent migration and pro-

mote hydration of skin to receive the optimal effect of salicylic acid.

Warnings: Flammable. Keep away from fire or flame. For external use only. Do not use this product if you are a diabetic or have poor blood circulation except under a doctor's advice or supervision. Do not use on red, irritated, or infected skin. If discomfort persists, see a doctor. Do not use on moles, birthmarks, warts with hair growing from them, genital warts, or warts on the face or mucous membranes. Keep this and all medicines out of the reach of children. In case of accidental ingestion, seek professional assistance or contact a poison control center immediately.

Dosage and Administration: Wash affected area and dry thoroughly. Remove softened areas of the wart by *gently* rubbing with the enclosed skin buffer. Use the Accubrush® applicator to carefully apply Off-Ezy liquid, one drop at a time, directly to wart to sufficiently cover each wart. Avoid applying to surrounding skin. Let dry. For maximum effectiveness, reapply Off-Ezy liquid several hours later. Repeat entire treatment procedure once or twice daily for the next 6 to 7 days. Most warts should clear within this time period. However, if necessary, continue treatment for up to 12 weeks. Replace cap tightly after each use.

How Supplied: 0.45 fl oz bottle with: Double-textured skin buffer; Accubrush applicator.

BABY ORAJEL®
BABY ORAJEL® NIGHTTIME FORMULA

Active Ingredients: *Baby Orajel:* Benzocaine 7.5%. *Baby Orajel Nighttime Formula:* Benzocaine 10%.

Inactive Ingredients: *Baby Orajel:* FD&C Red No. 40, flavor, glycerin, polyethylene glycols, sodium saccharin, sorbic acid, sorbitol. *Baby Orajel Nighttime Formula:* FD&C Red No. 40, flavor, glycerin, polyethylene glycols, sodium saccharin, sorbic acid, sorbitol.

Indications: Baby Orajel is a soothing, cherry-flavored product which quickly relieves teething pain. In addition to the original alcohol-free formula (benzocaine 7.5%), Baby Orajel is also available in an alcohol-free Nighttime Formula (benzocaine 10%) which provides relief in intense nighttime teething discomfort.

Actions: Benzocaine is a topical, local anesthetic commonly used for pain, discomfort, or pruritis associated with wounds, mucous membranes and skin irritations. Local anesthetics inhibit conduction of nerve impulses from sensory nerves. This action results from an alteration of the cell membrane permeability to ions. These agents are poorly absorbed through the intact epidermis.

Warnings: Do not use if tube tip is out prior to opening. As with all products containing benzocaine, localized allergic

Continued on next page

Commerce—Cont.

reactions may occur after prolonged or repeated use. Keep this and all medications out of reach of children.

Precaution: For persistent or excessive teething pain, consult your physician.

Dosage and Administration: Wash hands. Cut open tip of tube on score mark. For infants 4 months of age and older, apply a *small* amount with fingertip or cotton applicator on affected area no more than four times daily.

How Supplied: Baby Orajel: Gel in ⅓ oz (9.45 g) tube.
Nighttime Formula Baby Orajel: ³⁄₁₆ oz (5.3 g) tube.

Maximum Strength ORAJEL®
[ōr 'ah-jel]

Active Ingredient: Benzocaine 20% in a special base.

Inactive Ingredients: Clove oil, flavors, polyethylene glycols, sodium saccharin, sorbic acid.

Indications: Maximum Strength Orajel is formulated to provide faster relief from toothache pain for hours.

Actions: Benzocaine is a topical, local anesthetic commonly used for pain, discomfort, or pruritis associated with wounds, mucous membranes and skin irritation. Local anesthetics inhibit conduction of nerve impulses from sensory nerves. This action results from an alteration of the cell membrane permeability to ions. These agents are poorly absorbed through the intact epidermis.

Warnings: Keep this and all drugs out of the reach of children. Do not use if tube tip is cut prior to opening.

Precaution: This preparation is intended for use in cases of toothache only as a temporary expedient until a dentist can be consulted. Do not use continuously.

Directions: Cut open tip of tube on score mark. Squeeze a small quantity of Maximum Strength Orajel directly into cavity and around gum surrounding the teeth.

How Supplied: Gel in two sizes—³⁄₁₆ oz (5.3 g) and ⅓ oz (9.45 g) tubes.

ORAJEL® Mouth-Aid
[ōr 'ah-jel]

Active Ingredients: Benzocaine 20%, benzalkonium chloride 0.12%, zinc chloride 0.1% in a special emollient base.

Inactive Ingredients: Allantoin, flavor, polyethylene glycols, propyl gallate, propylene glycol, purified water, sodium saccharin, sorbic acid, trisodium EDTA.

Indications: Orajel Mouth-Aid combines a fast-acting maximum strength pain reliever, soothing ingredients which aid healing, a germicide and an astringent to help provide relief of minor mouth and lip irritations.

Actions: Benzocaine is a topical, local anesthetic commonly used for pain, discomfort, or pruritis associated with wounds, mucous membranes and skin irritations. Local anesthetics inhibit conduction of nerve impulses from sensory nerves. This action results from an alteration of the cell membrane permeability to ions. These agents are poorly absorbed through the intact epidermis. Benzalkonium chloride is a rapidly acting surface disinfectant and detergent. Zinc chloride provides an astringent effect.

Warnings: Keep this and all medications out of reach of children. Do not use if tube tip is cut prior to opening.

Precaution: If condition persists, discontinue use and consult your physician or dentist. Not for prolonged use.

Directions: Cut open tip of tube on score mark. Apply directly to affected area as needed.

How Supplied: Gel in a ⅓ oz (9.45 g) tube.

PRONTO® Lice Killing Shampoo Kit

Active Ingredients: Pyrethrins 0.33%, piperonyl butoxide technical 4.00% [equivalent to 3.2% butylcarbityl (6-propylpiperonyl) ether and 0.80% related compounds].

Indications: One treatment pediculicide shampoo kills head, body and pubic lice on contact.

Actions: Pronto Lice Killing Shampoo contains the maximum strength of pyrethrins and piperonyl butoxide. Pyrethrins act directly on the nervous system of insects and piperonyl butoxide enhances the neurotoxic effect of pyrethrins by inhibiting the oxidative breakdown of the pyrethrins by the insect's detoxification system. This results in a longer amount of time which the pyrethrins may exert their toxic effect on the insect.

Warnings: May cause eye injury. Do not use near eyes or permit contact with eyes or nose. May cause skin irritation. Wash thoroughly with soap and water after handling. If product should get into eyes, immediately flush with water. Follow directions carefully.
Not to be used by persons allergic to ragweed. Harmful if swallowed. In case of infection or skin irritation, discontinue use and consult a physician. In order to prevent reinfestation with lice, all clothing and bedding must be sterilized or treated concurrent with the application of this preparation. Do not exceed two consecutive applications within 24 hours.

Precaution: If in eyes, flush with plenty of water and get medical attention.

Directions for Use: It is a violation of Federal Law to use this product in a manner inconsistent with its labeling.

Instruct child to close eyes and cover eyes with clean wet towel. Apply Pronto Shampoo Concentrate cautiously to dry hair, scalp or any affected areas. Add a generous amount of water to work Pronto Shampoo Concentrate into a rich lather. Allow the shampoo to remain on area for 10 minutes, but no longer. Rinse treated areas thoroughly with warm water. Rinse eyes out with water following use. A fine-toothed comb (included) may be used to help remove dead lice and their eggs (nits) from hair. Handy applicator gloves are provided for your convenience in applying the shampoo to avoid contact with lice.

Storage and Disposal: Do not reuse empty container. Rinse thoroughly. Securely wrap original container in several layers of newspaper and discard in waste container.

How Supplied: Shampoo in two sizes:
2 fl oz plastic bottle
4 fl oz plastic bottle

PRONTO® Fast Acting Lice Killing Spray
THIS PRODUCT IS NOT FOR USE ON HUMANS OR ANIMALS

Description:
Active Ingredients:
*3-Phenoxybenzyl *d-cis-* and *trans-**
2,2-dimethyl-3-(2-methylpropenyl)
cyclopropanecarboxylate   0.382%
Other isomers   0.018%
Petroleum distillates   4.256%
Inert Ingredients: 95.344%
                                     ‾‾‾‾‾‾‾‾‾‾
                                     100.000%

 d-(cis-trans-) phenothrin
 **cis/trans* isomer ratio: max. 25% (±) cis and min. 75% (±) *trans*.

Actions: Pronto Lice Killing Spray contains a synthetic pyrethroid which kills lice and their eggs on garments, bedding, furniture and other inanimate objects.

Warnings: Contents under pressure. Do not use or store near heat or open flame. Do not puncture or incinerate container. Exposure to temperatures above 130°F may cause bursting.

Precaution: Harmful if swallowed or absorbed through the skin. Avoid breathing vapors or spray mist. Avoid contact with skin and eyes. In case of contact, immediately flush eyes or skin with plenty of water. Obtain medical attention if irritation persists. If swallowed, do not induce vomiting. Call a physician immediately.
Do not apply directly to food. Cover or remove any food or food processing equipment during application. Do not apply while food processing is under way. After space spraying, wash all equipment with potable water (benches, shelving, etc, where exposed food will be handled.) All food processing surfaces and utensils should be covered during treatment or thoroughly washed before use. Remove pets and birds, and cover fish aquariums before spraying.
THIS PRODUCT IS NOT FOR USE ON HUMANS. If lice infestations should oc-

cur on humans, consult either your physician or pharmacist for a product for use on humans.

Directions for Use: It is a violation of Federal law to use this product in a manner inconsistent with its labeling. Shake well before each use. Remove protective cap. Aim spray opening away from person. Push button to spray. To kill lice and louse eggs: Spray in an inconspicuous area to test for possible staining or discoloration. Inspect again after drying, then proceed to spray entire area to be treated. Hold container upright with nozzle away from you. Depress valve and spray from a distance of 8 to 10 inches. Spray each square foot for 5 seconds or until damp. Spray only those garments, parts of bedding, including mattresses and furniture that cannot be either laundered or dry cleaned. Treat entire inner surface of all clothing to be worn next to the skin. Special attention should be given to seams and areas around the neck, armpits, waist, shirttails, and crotch of the pants. Allow all sprayed articles to dry thoroughly before use. Repeat treatment as necessary. Buyer assumes all risks of use, storage or handling of this material not in strict accordance with directions given herewith.

Storage and Disposal: Store in a cool area away from heat or open flame. Do not reuse empty container. Replace cap, securely wrap original container in several layers of newspaper and discard in trash.

How Supplied: 5 oz aerosol can.

PROPA pH® PERFECTLY CLEAR SKIN CLEANSER
For Normal/Combination Skin
For Sensitive Skin

Active Ingredients: Salicylic Acid USP 0.5%.

Inactive Ingredients: Aloe vera gel, benzophenone-4, edetate disodium, fragrance, menthol, purified water, SD alcohol 40 (25% by volume), sodium carbonate, sodium laureth-12 sulfate, triclosan.

Indications: Topical Skin Cleanser. Regular application is essential for persons who may develop acne since it removes dirt and excess oil which may clog pores. Helps clear up and prevent blackheads and acne blemishes.

Actions: Propa pH contains salicylic acid, a comedolytic and keratolytic agent, which penetrates and cleans oil-clogged pores.

Caution: For external use only. Use only as directed. If skin irritation develops, discontinue use and consult a physician. Keep away from eyes and mucous membranes. If contact occurs, flush thoroughly with water. Keep this and all drugs out of reach of children. Store at room temperature.

Dosage and Administration: Wash area to be treated. Saturate cotton ball or pad with Propa pH Skin Cleanser and stroke over face and neck. Repeat with fresh pads until no trace of dirt is visible.

Do not rinse. Use three times daily as part of cleansing routine.

How Supplied: 6 fl oz plastic bottle.

STYE™ OPHTHALMIC OINTMENT

Active Ingredients: Yellow mercuric oxide 1.0% in a sterile ophthalmic base.

Inactive Ingredients: Boric acid, light mineral oil, microcrystalline wax, wheat germ oil, white petrolatum.

Indications: Stye Ophthalmic Ointment is indicated for the relief of discomfort of styes and for the treatment of irritation and minor infections of eyelids.

Actions: Yellow mercuric oxide has antibacterial properties. These properties are useful in the treatment of blepharitis, stye, and conjunctivitis.

Warnings: Keep this and all drugs out of the reach of children. In case of accidental ingestion, seek professional assistance or contact a poison control center immediately.

Precaution: Do not use if rim of cap has been exposed prior to opening. In unopened tube, rim of cap is not exposed. Discontinue use if rash or irritation develops or if condition for which used persists. Use as indicated, but not for prolonged use.

Dosage and Administration: Apply night and morning directly from the tube to the affected lid. If irritation persists, consult your physician.

How Supplied: 0.125 oz (3.45 g) tube.

tANAC
LIQUID
ROLL-ON
STICK

Active Ingredients: *Liquid:* Benzocaine 10%, tannic acid 6%, and benzalkonium chloride 0.12%; *Roll-On:* Tannic acid 6%, benzocaine 5%, benzalkonium chloride 0.12%; *Stick:* benzocaine 7.5%, tannic acid 6%, benzalkonium chloride 0.12%.

Inactive Ingredients: *Liquid:* Flavor, polyethylene glycol 400, propylene glycol, sodium saccharin; *Roll-On:* flavor, glycerin, polyethylene glycol 400, sodium saccharin; *Stick:* allantoin, BHA, butylparaben, butyl stearate, candelilla wax, carnauba wax, castor oil, cetyl alcohol, citric acid, corn oil, flavor, glycerin, myristyl lactate, octyl dimethyl PABA, ozokerite, PEG-32, distearate, propylene glycol, sesame oil, stearic acid, titanium dioxide, white petrolatum, white wax, yellow wax.

Indications: Tanac Liquid is an effective first-aid treatment that helps relieve painful canker sores and gum irritations. Tanac Roll-On provides effective relief of painful cold sores, lip sores and chapped lips.
Tanac Stick promotes healing and relieves pain of cold sores, plus soothes and moisturizes even the most severely chapped or sunburned lips.

Actions: Benzocaine temporarily deadens sensations of nerve endings to provide relief of pain and discomfort. Benzalkonium Chloride is a rapidly acting surface antimicrobial. Tannic acid is an astringent which precipitates protein and furnishes a protective covering.

Warnings: Do not use if imprinted bottle-cap safety seal on Tanac Liquiud is broken or missing prior to opening. Do not use if carton-flap seals on Tanac Roll-On or Stick are broken or missing. Keep this and all drugs out of reach of children.

Precautions: If the condition for which this preparation is used persists, or if a rash or irritation develops, discontinue use and consult a physician. Use as indicated but not for more than 5 consecutive days. Not for prolonged use. Avoid getting into eyes.

Dosage and Administration: Apply directly to affected area(s) as required.

How Supplied: Tanac Liquid: 0.45 fl oz bottle; Tanac Roll-On: 0.30 fl oz bottle with applicator; Tanac Stick: 0.10 oz (2.84 g) plastic tube.

EDUCATIONAL MATERIAL

Teething Booklet From Baby Orajel®
Facts parents should know about tooth development and the teething process.
Fact & Fallacy Booklet From Pronto®
Answers questions about head lice control.

Cumberland-Swan, Inc.
ONE SWAN DRIVE
SMYRNA, TN 37167

SWAN CITROMA®, Laxative
Magnesium Citrate Oral Solution
Saline Laxative

Available in 3 Formulas:
1. REGULAR LEMON
2. LOW SODIUM SUGAR FREE LEMON
3. LOW SODIUM SUGAR FREE CHERRY

LOW SODIUM SUGAR FREE FORMULAS CONTAIN ONLY 2 mg. (0.085 mEq) OF SODIUM PER FL. OZ. AND ARE SUGAR FREE.

Description: Pleasant tasting, effervescent pasteurized liquid laxative. Also referred to as Citrate of Magnesia.

Active Ingredient: 1.745g Magnesium Citrate per fl. oz.

Indications: For the relief of constipation or irregularity. Bowel movement is generally produced in ½ to 6 hours. Also for use as part of a bowel cleansing regimen in preparing the patients for surgery, or the colon for x-ray or endoscopic examination.

Continued on next page

Cumberland-Swan—Cont.

Directions: Adults (12 yrs. and older) ½ to 1 full bottle. Children (6 to 12 yrs.) ⅓ to ½ bottle. Children under 6 consult a physician. Drink a full glass (8 oz) of liquid with each dose. The dose may be taken as a single daily dose or in divided doses. Do not exceed maximum daily dose. Discard unused product within 24 hours after opening bottle.

Warnings: Frequent and continued use may cause dependence upon laxatives. Do not use in excess of ten days. Do not use this product if you are on a low salt diet or have kidney disease unless directed by a physician. Do not use when abdominal pain, nausea or vomiting are present. Rectal blood or failure to have a bowel movement after use of a laxative may indicate a serious condition. Discontinue use and consult a physician. As with any drug, if you are pregnant or nursing a baby, seek the advice of a health professional before using this product.

Warning: KEEP THIS AND ALL DRUGS OUT OF THE REACH OF CHILDREN.
In case of accidental overdose, consult a physician or contact a Poison Control Center immediately.

Caution: (CHERRY FLAVOR ONLY) May cause a red color in the feces.

How Supplied: Bottles of 10 fluid ounces.
Shown in Product Identification Section, page 409

"Especially" Products Inc.
PO BOX 5477
PLAYA DEL REY, CA 90296

CRÈME de la FEMME

Description: The personal lubricant, CRÈME de la FEMME by "Especially", is a safe, fluid/film, natural-feeling, creme lubricant which forms a silky moistness instantly when applied to delicate tissues of the body.

Active Ingredients: Mineral oil and white petroleum.

Indications: CRÈME de la FEMME, especially formulated, is safe and enjoyed by women and men in eliminating friction and pain, as a sexual lubricant. Vaginal dryness is overcome instantly, and the product will not dry out. Not advised to be used with condoms or other latex devices. Also used for easy insertion of anal thermometer or enema nozzle.

Actions: Instantly overcomes dryness, forming a silky moistness which protects delicate tissue of female and significantly reduces postcoital urethritis due to long action. Its effectiveness enhances sexual pleasure. Is not a contraceptive.

Warnings: Do not get product into the eyes. Not to be swallowed internally.

Consult M.D. or pharmacist re possible allergies noted or suspected to petroleum products, before use.

Dosage and Administration: Apply small amount needed to coat vaginal orifice and clitoris. May also be applied to penis before insertion.

Professional Labeling: CRÈME de la FEMME® The Personal Lubricant.

How Supplied: 1 ounce tube—2 gram travel pak (foil).

Fisons
Consumer Health
Division
Fisons Pharmaceuticals
P.O. BOX 1212
ROCHESTER, NY 14603

AMERICAINE® HEMORRHOIDAL OINTMENT
[a-mer 'i-kān]

Active Ingredient: Benzocaine 20%.

Other Ingredients: Benzethonium Chloride; Polyethylene Glycol 300; Polyethylene Glycol 3350.

Indications: For the temporary relief of local pain, itching and soreness associated with hemorrhoids and anorectal inflammation.

Warnings: For external use only. If condition worsens, or does not improve within 7 days, consult a physician. Do not exceed the recommended daily dosage unless directed by a physician. In case of rectal bleeding, consult a physician promptly. Certain persons can develop allergic reactions to ingredients in this product. If the symptom being treated does not subside or if redness, irritation, swelling, pain, or other symptoms develop or increase, discontinue use and consult a physician. **Keep this and all drugs out of the reach of children.** In case of accidental ingestion, seek professional assistance or contact a Poison Control Center immediately.

Directions: *Adults:* When practical, cleanse the affected area with mild soap and warm water and rinse thoroughly. Gently dry by patting or blotting with toilet tissue or a soft cloth before application of this product. Apply externally to affected area up to 6 times daily. *Children under 12 years of age:* Consult a physician.

How Supplied: *Hemorrhoidal Ointment* —1 oz. tube.
Shown in Product Identification Section, page 409

AMERICAINE® TOPICAL ANESTHETIC SPRAY AND OINTMENT
[a-mer 'i-kān]

Active Ingredient: Benzocaine 20%.

Other Ingredients: *Spray* —Butane (propellant); Isobutane (propellant); Polyethylene Glycol 200; Propane (propel-

lant). *Ointment* —Benzethonium chloride; Polyethylene Glycol 300; Polyethylene Glycol 3350.

Indications: For the temporary relief of pain and itching associated with minor cuts, scrapes, burns, sunburn, insect bites, or minor skin irritations.

Warnings: For external use only. Avoid contact with the eyes. If condition worsens, or if symptoms persist for more than 7 days or clear up and occur again within a few days, discontinue use of this product and consult a physician. Keep this and all drugs out of the reach of children. In case of accidental ingestion, seek professional assistance or contact a Poison Control Center immediately. *For Spray only* —Contents under pressure. Do not puncture or incinerate. Flammable mixture; do not use near fire or flame. Do not store at temperature above 120°F. Use only as directed. Intentional misuse by deliberately concentrating and inhaling the contents can be harmful or fatal.

Directions: Adults and children 2 years of age and older: Apply liberally to affected area not more than 3 to 4 times daily. Children under 2 years of age: Consult a physician.

How Supplied: *Topical Anesthetic Spray* —⅔ oz., 2 oz. and 4 oz. aerosol containers. *Topical Anesthetic Ointment* —¾ oz. tube.
Shown in Product Identification Section, page 409

ALLEREST® TABLETS, CHILDREN'S CHEWABLE TABLETS, HEADACHE STRENGTH TABLETS, SINUS PAIN FORMULA TABLETS, 12 HOUR CAPLETS AND NO DROWSINESS ALLEREST™ TABLETS
[al 'e-rest]

Active Ingredients:
acetaminophen
  Headache Strength, 325 mg
  No Drowsiness, 325 mg
  Sinus Pain Formula, 500 mg
chlorpheniramine maleate
  Tablets, 2 mg
  Children's Chewables, 1 mg
  Sinus Pain Formula, 2 mg
  Headache Strength, 2 mg
  12 Hour Caplets, 2 mg
phenylpropanolamine HCl
  Tablets, 18.7 mg
  Children's Chewables, 9.4 mg
  Sinus Pain Formula, 18.7 mg
  Headache Strength, 18.7 mg
  12 Hour Caplets, 75 mg
pseudoephedrine HCl
  No Drowsiness, 30 mg

Other Ingredients:
Allerest Tablets — Blue 1; Dibasic Calcium Phosphate; Magnesium Stearate; Microcrystalline Cellulose; Povidone; Pregelatinized Starch; Sodium Starch Glycolate.
Children's Chewable Tablets —Blue 1; Calcium Stearate; Citric Acid; Flavor; Magnesium Trisilicate Mannitol; Red 3; Saccharin Sodium; Sorbitol.

Headache Strength and No Drowsiness Tablets —Magnesium Stearate; Microcrystalline Cellulose; Povidone; Pregelatinized Starch.

Sinus Pain Formula Tablets —Magnesium Stearate; Microcrystalline Cellulose; Povidone; Pregelatinized Starch; Sodium Starch Glycolate.

12 Hour Caplets —Carnauba Wax; Colloidal Silicon Dioxide; Lactose; Methylcellulose; Polyethylene Glycol; Povidone; Red 30; Stearic Acid; Titanium Dioxide; Yellow 6.

Indications: Allerest is indicated for symptomatic relief of hay fever, pollen allergies, upper respiratory allergies (perennial allergic rhinitis), allergic colds, sinusitis and nasal passage congestion. Those symptoms include headache pain, sneezing, runny nose, itchy/watery eyes, and itching nose and throat.

Actions: Allerest contains the antihistamine chlorpheniramine maleate which acts to suppress the symptoms of allergic rhinitis. In addition, it contains the decongestant phenylpropanolamine hydrochloride which acts to reduce swelling of the upper respiratory tract mucosa. Headache Strength and Sinus Pain Formula also contain acetaminophen to relieve headache pain.

No Drowsiness Allerest contains the decongestant pseudoephedrine hydrochloride and the analgesic acetaminophen to relieve headache pain and nasal congestion without causing drowsiness.

Contraindications: Known hypersensitivity to the ingredients in this drug.

Warnings: Allerest should be used with caution in patients with high blood pressure, heart disease, diabetes, thyroid disease, asthma, glaucoma, or difficulty in urination due to enlargement of the prostate gland. Since antihistamines may cause drowsiness, patients should be instructed not to operate a car or machinery. Products containing analgesics should not be taken for more than 10 days in adults and 5 days in children under 12. **Keep this and all drugs out of the reach of children.** In case of accidental ingestion, seek professional assistance or contact a Poison Control Center immediately.

Drug Interaction Precautions: Not to be taken by patients currently taking a prescription antihypertensive or antidepressant drug containing a monoamine oxidase inhibitor except under the advice and supervision of a physician.

Antihistamines and oral nasal decongestants have additive effects with alcohol and other CNS depressants.

Adverse Reactions: Drowsiness; excitability, especially in children; nervousness; and dizziness.

Overdosage: Acetaminophen in massive overdosage may cause hepatotoxicity.

Dosage and Administration:
Tablets and Headache Strength —Adults, 2 tablets every 4 hours. Not to exceed 8 tablets in 24 hours. Children (6–12)—half

the adult dose. Dosage for children under 6 should be individualized under the supervision of a physician. *Children's Chewable Tablets* —Children (6–12) 2 tablets every 4 hours. Not to exceed 8 tablets in 24 hours. Children under 6 consult a physician. Adults double the children's dose. *Sinus Pain Formula* —Adults, 2 tablets every 6 hours. Not to exceed 8 tablets in 24 hours. Not recommended for children 12 and under. *12 Hour Caplets* —Adults and children over 12 years of age, one caplet every 12 hours. Do not exceed 2 caplets in 24 hours.

How Supplied: *Tablets* —packaged on blister cards in 24, 48 and 72 count cartons. *Children's Chewable Tablets* —packaged on blister cards in 24 count cartons. *Headache Strength Tablets* —packaged on blister cards in 24 count cartons. *Sinus Pain Formula Tablets* —packaged on blister cards in 20 count cartons. *12 Hour Caplets* —packaged on blister cards in 10 count cartons. *No Drowsiness Tablets* —packaged on blister cards in 20 count cartons.

Shown in Product Identification Section, page 409

CaldeCORT® ANTI-ITCH CREAM AND SPRAY; CaldeCORT Light® CREAM
[kal 'de-kort]

Active Ingredient: *Cream, Light Cream* —Hydrocortisone Acetate (equivalent to Hydrocortisone 0.5%). *Spray* —Hydrocortisone 0.5%.

Other Ingredients: *Cream* —Glyceryl Monostearate; Lanolin Alcohol; Methylparaben; Mineral Oil; Polyoxyl 40 Stearate; Propylparaben; Sodium Metabisulfite; Sorbitol Solution; Stearyl Alcohol; Water; White Petrolatum; White Wax. *Light Cream* —Aloe Vera Gel; Isopropyl Myristate; Methylparaben; Polysorbate 60; Propylparaben; Sorbitan Monostearate; Sorbitol Solution; Stearic Acid; Water. *Spray* —Isobutane (propellant); Isopropyl Myristate; SD Alcohol 40-B 89.5% by volume.

Indications: For the temporary relief of itching associated with minor skin irritations, inflammation and rashes due to eczema, insect bites, poison ivy, poison oak, poison sumac, soaps, detergents, cosmetics and jewelry; and for external genital and anal itching.

Actions: Antidermatitis cream and spray for the temporary relief from itching and minor skin irritations.

Warnings: For external use only. Avoid contact with the eyes. If condition worsens, or if symptoms persist for more than 7 days or clear up and occur again within a few days, discontinue use and consult a doctor. Do not use if you have a vaginal discharge. Consult a doctor. Keep this and all drugs out of the reach of children. In case of accidental ingestion, seek professional assistance or contact a Poison Control Center immediately. *For Spray only* —Avoid spraying in eyes or on other mucous membranes. Contents under pressure. Do not puncture or incinerate. Flammable mixture, do not use near fire or flame. Do not store

at temperature above 120°F. Use only as directed. Intentional misuse by deliberately concentrating and inhaling the contents can be harmful or fatal.

Directions: Adults and children 2 years of age and older: Apply to affected area not more than 3 to 4 times daily. Children under 2 years of age: Consult a doctor.

How Supplied: *Anti-Itch Cream* —½ and 1 oz. tubes. *Anti-Itch Spray* —1½ oz. can. *Light Cream* —½ oz. tubes.

Shown in Product Identification Section, page 409

CALDESENE® MEDICATED POWDER AND OINTMENT
[kal 'de-sēn]

Active Ingredients: *Powder* —Calcium Undecylenate 10%. *Ointment* —Petrolatum 53.9%; Zinc Oxide 15%.

Other Ingredients: *Powder* — Fragrance; Talc. *Ointment* —Cod Liver Oil; Fragrance; Lanolin Oil; Methylparaben; Propylparaben; Talc.

Indications: Caldesene Medicated Powder is indicated to help heal, relieve and prevent diaper rash, prickly heat and chafing. Medicated Ointment helps prevent diaper rash and soothe minor skin irritations.

Actions: Antifungal and antibacterial Medicated Powder inhibits the growth of bacteria and fungi which cause diaper rash. Also, forms a protective coating to repel moisture, soothe and comfort minor skin irritations, helps heal and prevent chafing and prickly heat. Medicated Ointment forms a protective skin coating to repel moisture and promote healing of diaper rash, while its natural ingredients protect irritated skin against wetness. Soothes minor skin irritations, superficial wounds and burns.

Warnings: For external use only. Avoid contact with eyes. If condition worsens or does not improve within 7 days, consult a doctor. Do not apply ointment over deep or puncture wounds, infections and lacerations. Keep this and all drugs out of the reach of children. In case of accidental ingestion, seek professional assistance or contact a Poison Control Center immediately.

Directions: Cleanse and thoroughly dry affected area. Smooth on Caldesene 3–4 times daily, after every bath or diaper change, or as directed by a physician.

How Supplied: *Medicated Powder* —2.0 oz. and 4.0 oz. shaker containers. *Medicated Ointment* —1.25 oz. collapsible tubes.

Shown in Product Identification Section, page 409

CRUEX® ANTIFUNGAL POWDER, SPRAY POWDER AND CREAM
[kru 'ex]

Active Ingredients: *Powder* —Calcium Undecylenate 10%. *Spray Powder* —

Continued on next page

Fisons—Cont.

Total Undecylenate 19%, as Undecylenic Acid and Zinc Undecylenate.
Cream—Total Undecylenate 20%, as Undecylenic Acid and Zinc Undecylenate.

Other Ingredients: *Powder* —Colloidal Silicon Dioxide; Fragrance; Isopropyl Myristate; Talc. *Spray Powder* —Fragrance; Isobutane (propellant); Isopropyl Myristate; Menthol; Talc; Trolamine. *Cream* —Anhydrous Lanolin; Fragrance; Glycol Stearate SE; Methylparaben; PEG-6 Stearate; PEG-8 Laurate; Propylparaben; Sorbitol Solution; Stearic Acid; Trolamine; Water; White Petrolatum.

Indications: For the treatment of Jock Itch (tinea cruris) and relief of itching, chafing, burning rash and irritation in the groin area. Cruex powders also absorb perspiration.

Actions: Antifungal Powder, Spray Powder and Cream are proven clinically effective in the treatment of superficial fungus infections of the skin.

Warnings: Do not use on children under 2 years of age except under the advice and supervision of a doctor. For external use only. If irritation occurs, or if there is no improvement within 2 weeks, discontinue use and consult a doctor or pharmacist. Keep this and all drugs out of the reach of children. In case of accidental ingestion, seek professional assistance or contact a Poison Control Center immediately. *For Spray Powder only* —Avoid spraying in eyes or on other mucous membranes. Contents under pressure. Do not puncture or incinerate. Flammable mixture, do not use near a fire or flame. Do not store at temperature above 120° F. Use only as directed. Intentional misuse by deliberately concentrating and inhaling the contents can be harmful or fatal.

Directions: Cleanse skin with soap and water and dry thoroughly. Apply Cruex to affected area morning and night, before and after athletic activity, or as directed by a doctor. Best results are usually obtained with 2 weeks' use of this product. If satisfactory results have not occurred within this time, consult a doctor or pharmacist. Children under 12 years of age should be supervised in the use of this product. This product is not effective on the scalp or nails.

How Supplied: *Powder* —1.5 oz. plastic squeeze bottle. *Spray Powder* —1.8 oz., 3.5 oz. and 5.5 oz. aerosol containers. *Cream* —½ oz. tube.

Shown in Product Identification Section, page 409

DESENEX® ANTIFUNGAL POWDER, SPRAY POWDER, CREAM, OINTMENT, LIQUID AND PENETRATING FOAM; SOAP; FOOT & SNEAKER DEODORANT SPRAY
[dess'i-nex]

Active Ingredients: *Powder, Spray Powder* —Total Undecylenate 19%, as Undecylenic Acid and Zinc Undecylenate. *Cream* —Total Undecylenate 20%, as Undecylenic Acid and Zinc Undecylenate. *Ointment* —Total Undecylenate 22%, as Undecylenic Acid and Zinc Undecylenate. *Liquid, Penetrating Foam* —Undecylenic Acid 10%. *Foot & Sneaker Deodorant Spray* —Aluminum Chlorohydrex.

Other Ingredients: *Powder* — Fragrance; Talc. *Spray Powder* —Fragrance; Isobutane (propellant); Isopropyl Myristate; Menthol; Talc; Trolamine. *Cream, Ointment* —Anhydrous Lanolin; Fragrance; Glycol Stearate SE; Methylparaben; PEG-6 Stearate; PEG-8 Laurate; Propylparaben; Sorbitol Solution; Stearic Acid; Trolamine; Water; White Petrolatum. *Liquid* —Fragrance; Isopropyl Alcohol 47.1% by volume; Polysorbate 80; Propylene Glycol; Trolamine; Water. *Penetrating Foam* —Emulsifying Wax; Fragrance; Isobutane (propellant); Isopropyl Alcohol 35.2% by volume; Sodium Benzoate; Trolamine; Water. *Foot & Sneaker Deodorant Spray* —Colloidal Silicon Dioxide; Diisopropyl Adipate; Fragrance; Isobutane (propellant); Menthol; SD Alcohol 40-B 89.3% by volume; Talc; Tartaric Acid.

Indications: Desenex Antifungal Products cure athlete's foot (tinea pedis) and body ringworm (tinea corporis) exclusive of the nails and scalp. Relieves itching and burning. Desenex Foot & Sneaker Deodorant Spray helps stop odor and reduces wetness.

Actions: Desenex Antifungal Powders, Cream, Ointment, Liquid and Penetrating Foam are proven effective in the treatment of superficial fungus infections of the skin caused by the three major types of dermatophytic fungi (T. rubrum, T. mentagrophytes, E. floccosum). Penetrating Foam quickly dissolves into a highly concentrated liquid. Foot & Sneaker Deodorant Spray is specially formulated with a unique combination of ingredients including a deodorant, antiperspirant and a moisture-absorbing powder. So it cools, soothes your feet and helps keep them dry and comfortable.

Warnings: Do not use on children under 2 years of age except under the advice and supervision of a doctor. For external use only. If irritation occurs, or if there is no improvement within 4 weeks, discontinue use and consult a doctor or pharmacist. Keep this and all drugs out of the reach of children. In case of accidental ingestion, seek professional assistance or contact a Poison Control Center immediately. *For Spray Powder, Penetrating Foam and Foot & Sneaker Deodorant Spray only* —Avoid spraying in eyes or on other mucous membranes. Contents under pressure. Do not puncture or incinerate. Flammable mixture, do not use near fire or flame. Do not store at temperature above 120° F. Use only as directed. Intentional misuse by deliberately concentrating and inhaling the contents can be harmful or fatal.

Directions: *Powder, Spray Powder, Cream, Ointment, Liquid and Penetrating Foam* —Cleanse skin with soap and water and dry thoroughly. Apply over affected area morning and night or as directed by a doctor, paying special attention to the spaces between the toes. It is also helpful to wear well-fitting, ventilated shoes and to change shoes and socks at least once daily. Best results are usually obtained with 4 weeks' use of this product. If satisfactory results have not occurred within this time, consult a doctor or pharmacist. Children under 12 years of age should be supervised in the use of this product. This product is not effective on the scalp or nails. For persistent cases of athlete's foot, use Desenex Ointment or Cream at night and Desenex Powder or Spray Powder during the day. *Soap* —Use in conjunction with Desenex Antifungal Products. *Foot & Sneaker Deodorant Spray* —Spray on soles of feet and between toes daily. For maximum effectiveness, spray in your shoes or sneakers after wearing to keep them fresh and pleasantly scented.

How Supplied: *Powder* —1.5 oz. and 3.0 oz. shaker containers. *Spray Powder* —2.7 oz. and 5.5 oz. aerosol containers. *Cream* —½ oz. and 1 oz. tubes. *Ointment* —0.9 oz. and 1.8 oz. tubes. *Liquid* —1.5 oz. plastic squeeze bottle. *Penetrating Foam* —1.5 oz. aerosol container. *Soap* —3.25 oz. bar. *Foot & Sneaker Deodorant Spray* —3.0 oz. aerosol container.

Shown in Product Identification Section, page 409 and page 410

ISOCLOR® Timesule®
[ĭs'ŏ-klŏr]
Capsules

Description: Isoclor® Timesule® Capsules combine a nasal decongestant with an antihistamine in a special sustained release capsule to provide temporary relief of nasal congestion due to the common cold and associated with sinusitis. Also alleviates runny nose and sneezing as may occur in hay fever.
Each Isoclor Timesule Capsule contains 8 mg chlorpheniramine maleate, USP, and 120 mg pseudoephedrine hydrochloride, USP, in a special form designed to provide therapeutic effects up to 12 hours.

Indications: For temporary relief of nasal congestion due to the common cold, hay fever, or other upper respiratory allergies, or associated with sinusitis. Helps decongest sinus openings, sinus passages. Reduces swelling of nasal passages, shrinks swollen membranes, and temporarily restores freer breathing through the nose. Alleviates runny nose, sneezing, itching of the nose or throat, and itchy and watery eyes as may occur in allergic rhinitis (such as hay fever).

Directions: Adults and children 12 years and older—one capsule every 12 hours. Do not exceed two capsules in 24 hours.
FOR YOUR PROTECTION DO NOT USE IF IMPRINTED FOIL CAP SEAL OR IMPRINTED NECK SEAL IS BROKEN OR MISSING.

Drug Interaction Precaution: Do not take this product if you are currently taking a prescription drug for high blood pressure or depression without first consulting your physician.

Warnings: Do not exceed recommended dosage because at higher doses nervousness, dizziness, or sleeplessness may occur. Do not give this product to children under 12 years except under the advice and supervision of a physician. Do not take this product if you have asthma, glaucoma, emphysema, chronic pulmonary disease, shortness of breath, difficulty in breathing, difficulty in urination due to enlargement of the prostate gland, high blood pressure, heart disease, diabetes, or thyroid disease except under the advice and supervision of a physician. If symptoms do not improve within seven days or are accompanied by a high fever, consult a physician before continuing use. May cause drowsiness; alcohol may increase the drowsiness effect. May cause excitability especially in children. As with any drug, if you are pregnant or nursing a baby, seek the advice of a health professional before using this product.
Avoid driving a motor vehicle or operating heavy machinery. Avoid alcoholic beverages while taking this product.
Keep this and all drugs out of the reach of children. In case of accidental overdose, seek professional assistance or contact a Poison Control Center immediately.

Inactive Ingredients: Castor wax, ethylcellulose, gelatin capsule, mineral oil, silicone oil, sugar spheres, white petrolatum.

How Supplied: Bottles of 100 and 500. Store at room temperature (15°–30°C, 59°–86°F).
Protect from excessive moisture.
Isoclor® and Timesule® are registered trademarks of Fisons Corporation.
Distributed by:
FISONS
Consumer Health
Rochester, NY 14623 USA

SINAREST® TABLETS, EXTRA STRENGTH TABLETS AND NO DROWSINESS SINAREST™ TABLETS
[sĭn 'a-rest]

Active Ingredients:
acetaminophen:
  Tablets, 325 mg
  Extra Strength, 500 mg
  No Drowsiness, 500 mg
chlorpheniramine maleate
  Tablets 2 mg
  Extra Strength, 2 mg
phenylpropanolamine HCl
  Tablets, 18.7 mg
  Extra Strength, 18.7 mg
pseudoephedrine HCl
  No Drowsiness, 30 mg

Other Ingredients: *All Tablets —* Magnesium Stearate; Microcrystalline Cellulose; Povidone; Pregelatinized Starch. *Extra Strength Tablets and No*

*Drowsiness Tablets only —*Sodium Starch Glycolate. *Sinarest Tablets and Extra Strength Tablets only —*Yellow 10; Yellow 6.

Indications: Sinarest is indicated for symptomatic relief from the headache pain, pressure and congestion associated with sinusitis, allergic rhinitis or the common cold.

Actions: Sinarest Tablets and Extra Strength Sinarest contain an antihistamine (chlorpheniramine maleate) and a decongestant (phenylpropanolamine) for the relief of sinus and nasal passage congestion as well as an analgesic (acetaminophen) to relieve pain and discomfort. No Drowsiness Sinarest contains a decongestant (pseudoephedrine hydrochloride) and an analgesic (acetaminophen) for the relief of headache pain, sinus pressure and nasal congestion without causing drowsiness.

Contraindications: Known hypersensitivity to any of the ingredients in this compound.

Warnings: Sinarest should be used with caution in patients with high blood pressure, heart disease, diabetes, thyroid disease, asthma, glaucoma, or difficulty in urination due to enlargement of the prostate gland. Since antihistamines may cause drowsiness, patients should be instructed not to operate a car or machinery. Products containing analgesics should not be taken for more than 10 days in adults and 5 days in children under 12. **Keep this and all drugs out of the reach of children.** In case of accidental ingestion, seek professional assistance or contact a Poison Control Center immediately.

Drug Interaction Precautions: Not to be taken by patients currently taking a prescription drug for high blood pressure or depression except under the advice and supervision of a physician. Antihistamines and oral nasal decongestants may have additive effects with alcohol and other CNS depressants.

Adverse Reactions: Drowsiness; excitability, especially in children; nervousness; and dizziness.

Overdosage: Acetaminophen in massive overdosage may cause hepatotoxicity.

Dosage and Administration: *Tablets —*Adults—take 2 tablets every 4 hours. Not to exceed 8 tablets in 24 hours. Children (6–12 years)—One half of adult dosage. Dosage for children under 6 should be individualized under the supervision of a physician. *Extra Strength Tablets —*Adults and Children over 12—take 2 tablets every 6 hours. Not to exceed 8 tablets in 24 hours. Not recommended for children 12 and under. *No Drowsiness Tablets —*Adults and Children 12 years of age and over—take 2 tablets every 6 hours. Not to exceed 8 tablets in 24 hours. Not recommended for children under 12.

How Supplied: *Tablets —*Blister packages of 20, 40 and 80 tablets. *Extra*

*Strength tablets —*package of 24 tablets. *No Drowsiness tablets —*blister package of 20 tablets.

Fleming & Company
1600 FENPARK DR.
FENTON, MO 63026

CHLOR–3
Medicinal Condiment

Active Ingredients: A troika of sodium chloride (50% 24.3 mEq/half tsp. iodized); potassium chloride (30% 11.5 mEq/half tsp.); magnesium chloride (20% 5.6 mEq/half tsp.).

Indications: The first medicinal condiment to restore needed K^+ & Mg^{++} lost during diuresis, at the expense of Na^+. To restore electrolytes lost by overcooking foods, or to add to diets that lack green vegetables, bananas, etc. And to replace conventional salting of foods in culinary and gourmet arts.

Symptoms and Treatment of Oral Overdosage: Hyperkalemia and hypermagnesemia are not end-stage results of usage.

How Supplied: In 8-oz plastic shaker, tamper-evident bottles.

IMPREGON Concentrate

Active Ingredient: Tetrachlorosalicylanilide 2%

Indications: Diaper Rash Relief, 'Staph' control, Mold inhibitor.

Actions: This is a bacteriostatic/fungistatic agent for home usage and hospital usage.

Warnings: Impregon should not be exposed to direct sunlight for long periods after applications.

Precaution: Addition of bleach prior to diaper treatment negates application effects.

Dosage and Administration: One capful (5ml) per gallon of water to impregnate diapers in the diaper pail. Dilutions for many home areas accompany the full package.

Note: For disposable-type diapers, add one teaspoonful to 8 oz of water to a 'Windex-type' sprayer. Spray middle half area of diapers until damp, and allow to dry before using, to prevent rashes.

How Supplied: Four ounce amber plastic bottles.

MAGONATE TABLETS
MAGONATE LIQUID
Magnesium Gluconate (Dihydrate)

Active Ingredients: Each tablet contains magnesium gluconate (dihydrate) 500mg (27mg of Mg^{++}). Each 5cc of Magonate Liquid contains magnesium gluconate (dihydrate) 1000mg (54mg of Mg^{++}).

Continued on next page

Fleming—Cont.

Indications: Alcoholism; digitalis toxicity; cardiac arrhythmias; extrinsic asthma; dysmenorrhea; eclampsia; hypertension; insomnia; muscle twitching; tremors; anxiety; pancreatitis, and toxicity of chemotherapy.

Precaution: Excessive dosage may cause loose stools.

Dosage and Administration: Magonate is recommended during and for three weeks after a course in chemotherapy, then monitored regularly.
Adults and children over 12 yrs.—one or two tablets or ½ to 1 teaspoon of liquid t.i.d. Under 12 yrs.—one tablet or ½ teaspoon of liquid t.i.d. Dosage may be increased in severe cases.

How Supplied: Magonate Tablets are supplied in bottles of 100 and 1000 tablets. Magonate Liquid is supplied in pints and gallons.

MARBLEN Suspensions and Tablet

Composition: A modified 'Sippy Powder' antacid containing magnesium and calcium carbonates.

Action and Uses: The peach/apricot (pink) or unflavored (green) antacid suspensions are sugar-free and neutralize 18 mEq acid per teaspoonful with a low sodium content of 18mg per fl. oz. Each pink tablet consumes 18.0 mEq acid.

Administration and Dosage: One teaspoonful rather than a tablespoonful or one tablet to reduce patient cost by ⅔.

How Supplied: Plastic pints and bottles of 100 and 1000.

NEPHROX SUSPENSION
(aluminum hydroxide)
Antacid Suspension

Composition: A watermelon flavored aluminum hydroxide (320mg as gel)/mineral oil (10% by volume) antacid per teaspoonful.

Action and Uses: A sugar-free/saccharin-free pink suspension containing no magnesium and low sodium (19mg/oz). Extremely palatable and especially indicated in renal patients. Each teaspoon consumes 9 mEq acid.

Administration and Dosage: Two teaspoonfuls or as directed by a physician.

Caution: To be taken only at bedtime. Do not use at any other time or administer to infants, expectant women, and nursing mothers except upon the advice of a physician as this product contains mineral oil.

How Supplied: Plastic pints and gallons.

NICOTINEX Elixir
nicotinic acid

Composition: Contains niacin 50 mg./tsp. in a sherry wine base (amber color).

Action and Uses: Produces flushing when tablets fail. To increase micro-circulation of inner-ear in Meniere's, tinnitus and labyrinthine syndromes. For 'cold hands & feet', and as a vehicle for additives.

Administration and Dosage: One or two teaspoonsful on fasting stomach.

Side Effects: Patients should be warned of dermal flush. Ulcer and gout patients may be affected by 14% alcoholic content.

Contraindications: Severe hypotension and hemorrhage.

How Supplied: Plastic pints and gallons.

OCEAN MIST
(buffered saline)

Composition: Special isotonic saline, buffered with sodium bicarbonate to proper pH so as not to irritate the nose.

Action and Uses: Rhinitis medicamentosa, rhinitis sicca and atrophic rhinitis. For patients 'hooked on nose drops' and glaucoma patients on diuretics having dry nasal capillaries. OCEAN may be used as a mist or drop.

Administration and Dosage: One or two squeezes in each nostril.

Supplied: Plastic 45cc spray bottles and pints.

PURGE
(flavored castor oil)

Composition: Contains 95% castor oil (USP) in a sweetened lemon flavored base that completely masks the odor and taste of the oil.

Indications: Preparation of the bowel for x-ray, surgery and proctological procedures, IVPs, and constipation.

Dosage: Infants—1–2 teaspoonfuls. Children—adjust between infant and adult dose. Adult—2–4 tablespoonfuls.

Precaution: Not indicated when nausea, vomiting, abdominal pain or symptoms of appendicitis occur. Pregnancy, use only on advice of physician.

Supplied: Plastic 1 oz. & 2 oz. bottles.

Products are
indexed alphabetically
in the
PINK SECTION

Glenbrook Laboratories
Division of Sterling Drug Inc.
90 PARK AVENUE
NEW YORK, NY 10016

CHILDREN'S BAYER® CHEWABLE ASPIRIN
Aspirin (Acetylsalicylic Acid)

Active Ingredients: Children's Bayer Chewable Aspirin—Aspirin 1¼ grains (81 mg) per orange flavored chewable tablet.

Inactive Ingredients: Dextrose excipient, FD&C Yellow No. 6, flavor, saccharin sodium, starch.

Actions and Uses: Analgesic, antipyretic, anti-inflammatory, antiplatelet. For effective, gentle relief of painful discomforts, sore throat; fever of colds; headache; teething pain, toothache; and other minor aches and pains.

Warnings: Children and teenagers should not use this medicine for chicken pox or flu symptoms before a doctor is consulted about Reye syndrome, a rare but serious illness reported to be associated with aspirin. Keep this and all drugs out of the reach of children. In case of accidental overdose, seek professional assistance or contact a poison control center immediately. As with any drug, if you are pregnant or nursing a baby, seek the advice of a health professional before using this product.

Administration and Dosage: The following dosages are those provided in the packaging, as appropriate for self-medication.
Children's Dose: To be administered only under adult supervision. For children under 3 consult physician.

Age (Years)	Weight (lb)	Dosage
3 up to 4	32 to 35	2 tablets
4 up to 6	36 to 45	3 tablets
6 up to 9	46 to 65	4 tablets
9 up to 11	66 to 76	5 tablets
11 up to 12	77 to 83	6 tablets
12 and over	84 and over	8 tablets

Indicated dosage may be repeated every four hours up to but not more than five times a day. Larger dosage may be prescribed by a physician.
Ways to Administer: CHEW, then follow with a half glass of water, milk or fruit juice.
SWALLOW WHOLE with a half a glass of water, milk or fruit juice.
DISSOLVE ON TONGUE, follow with a half a glass of water, milk or fruit juice.
DISSOLVE TABLET in a little water, milk or fruit juice and drink the solution.
CRUSHED in a teaspoonful of water—followed with part of a glass of water.

How Supplied: Children's Bayer Chewable Aspirin 1¼ grains (81 mg)—
NDC 12843-131-05, bottle of 36 tablets with child-resistant safety closure.
Shown in Product Identification Section, page 410

BAYER® CHILDREN'S COLD TABLETS

Active Ingredients: Each tablet contains phenylpropanolamine HCl 3.125 mg, aspirin 1¼ gr (81 mg). The tablets are orange flavored and chewable.

Inactive Ingredients: Colloidal silicon dioxide, compressible sugar, ethylcellulose, FD&C Red No. 3, Red No. 40 and FD&C Yellow No. 6, flavor, mannitol, microcrystalline cellulose, povidone, saccharin sodium, starch, stearic acid.

Action and Uses: Bayer Children's Cold Tablets combine two effective ingredients: a gentle decongestant to relieve nasal congestion and ease breathing, and genuine Bayer Aspirin to reduce fever and relieve minor aches and pains of colds.

Administration and Dosage:
The following dosage is provided in the packaging:

Age (yr)	Weight (lb)	Dosage
3 up to 6	32–45	2 tabs
6 up to 12	46–83	4 tabs
12 and over	84 and over	8 tabs

Indicated dosage may be repeated every four hours up to but not more than five times a day. Larger dosage may be prescribed by your physician. For easy administration, tablets may be chewed, dissolved or swallowed whole. Follow with liquid.

Contraindications: Side effects at higher doses may include nervousness, dizziness, sleeplessness. To be used with caution in presence of high blood pressure, heart disease, diabetes, asthma, or thyroid disease.

Caution: Do not exceed recommended dosage. For larger or more frequent doses, or for children under 3, consult a physician. If symptoms persist or are accompanied by high fever or vomiting, consult your physician before continuing use.

Warnings: Children and teenagers should not use this medicine for chicken pox or flu symptoms before a doctor is consulted about Reye syndrome, a rare but serious illness reported to be associated with aspirin. Keep this and all drugs out of the reach of children. In case of accidental overdose, seek professional assistance or contact a poison control center immediately. As with any drug, if you are pregnant or nursing a baby, seek the advice of a health professional before using this product.

How Supplied:
NDC 12843-181-01, bottles of 30 tablets with child-resistant safety closure.
Shown in Product Identification Section, page 410

BAYER® CHILDREN'S COUGH SYRUP

Active Ingredients: Each 5 ml (1 tsp) contains phenylpropanolamine HCl 9 mg and dextromethorphan hydrobromide 7.5 mg.

Inactive Ingredients: Alcohol 5%, caramel, flavor, glycerin, liquid glucose, parabens, purified water, saccharin sodium, sorbitol solution. May also contain sodium chloride. Cherry flavored.

Action and Uses: Bayer Children's Cough Syrup combines two effective ingredients in a syrup with a very appealing cherry flavor: a gentle nasal decongestant and a cough suppressant. It is nonnarcotic, and contains no chloroform or red dyes.

Administration and Dosage: The following dosage is provided on the packaging. For children under 2 consult physician.

Age (yr)	Weight (lb)	Dosage
2 up to 6	27–45	1 tsp
6 up to 12	46–83	2 tsp
12 and over	84 and over	4 tsp

Dose may be repeated every 4 hours, not more than 4 times per day.

Contraindications and Precautions: To be used with caution in presence of high blood pressure, heart disease, diabetes, asthma, or thyroid disease.
Caution: Consult your physician if cough persists for more than 7 days or if cough is accompanied by high fever since either may be signs of a serious condition.

Warnings: Do not give this product to children under 2 years of age or exceed recommended dosage, unless directed by a physician. Keep this and all drugs out of the reach of children. In case of accidental overdose, seek professional assistance or contact a poison control center immediately. As with any drug, if you are pregnant or nursing a baby, seek the advice of a health professional before using this product.

How Supplied:
NDC 12843-401-02, 3.0 oz bottles.
Shown in Product Identification Section, page 410

GENUINE BAYER® ASPIRIN
Aspirin (Acetylsalicylic Acid) Tablets and Caplets

Active Ingredients: Each Bayer-Aspirin contains aspirin 5 grains (325 mg) in a thin, inert, hydroxypropyl methylcellulose coating for easier swallowing. This is not an enteric coating and does not alter the onset of action of Genuine Bayer Aspirin.

Inactive Ingredients: Starch and Triacetin.

Actions and Uses: Analgesic, antipyretic, anti-inflammatory, antiplatelet. For relief of headache; painful discomfort and fever of colds and flu; sore throats; muscular aches and pains; temporary relief of minor pains of arthritis, rheumatism, bursitis, lumbago, sciatica; toothache, teething pains, and pain following dental procedures; neuralgia and neuritic pain; functional menstrual pain; sleeplessness when caused by minor painful discomfort; painful discomfort and fever accompanying immunizations.

Caution: If pain persists for more than 10 days, or redness is present, or in conditions affecting children under 12 years of age, consult a physician immediately.

Warnings: Children and teenagers should not use this medicine for chicken pox or flu symptoms before a doctor is consulted about Reye syndrome, a rare but serious illness reported to be associated with aspirin. Keep this and all drugs out of the reach of children. In case of accidental overdose, seek professional assistance or contact a poison control center immediately. As with any drug, if you are pregnant or nursing a baby, seek the advice of a health professional before using this product.

Administration and Dosage: The following dosages are those provided in the packaging, as appropriate for self-medication. Larger or more frequent dosage may be necessary as appropriate to the condition or needs of the patient.
The hydroxypropyl methylcellulose coating makes Genuine Bayer Aspirin particularly appropriate for those who must take frequent doses of aspirin and for those who have difficulty in swallowing uncoated tablets and caplets.
Usual Adult Dose: One or two tablets/caplets with water. May be repeated every four hours as necessary up to 12 tablets/caplets a day.

FOR ANTIPLATELET USE: RECURRENT TIA
There is evidence that aspirin is safe and effective for reducing the risk of recurrent transient ischemic attacks or stroke in men who have had transient ischemia of the brain due to fibrin platelet emboli. There is no evidence that aspirin is effective in reducing TIAs in women, or that it is of benefit in the treatment of completed strokes in men or women. Patients presenting with signs and symptoms of TIAs should have a complete medical and neurologic evaluation. Consideration should be given to other disorders which resemble TIAs.
It is important to evaluate and treat, if appropriate, other diseases associated with TIAs and stroke, such as hypertension and diabetes.

Dosage: The recommended dosage for this new indication is 1,300 mg/day (650 mg twice a day or 325 mg four times a day).

Precautions: A complete medical and neurologic evaluation should be performed on the male patient with recurrent TIA prior to instituting antiplatelet therapy with aspirin. The differential diagnosis should include consideration of disorders that resemble TIAs. An assessment of the presence and need for treatment of other diseases associated with TIAs or stroke, such as diabetes and hypertension, should be made.

IN MI PROPHYLAXIS
Aspirin is indicated to reduce the risk of death and/or nonfatal myocardial infarction in patients with a previous infarction or unstable angina pectoris.

Continued on next page

Glenbrook—Cont.

Clinical Trials: The indication is supported by the results of six, large, randomized multicenter, placebo-controlled studies[1-6] by the word-studies involving 10,816, predominantly male, post–myocardial infarction (MI) patients and one randomized placebo-controlled study[7] by the word study of 1,266 men with unstable angina. Therapy with aspirin was begun at intervals after the onset of acute MI varying from less than 3 days to more than 5 years and continued for periods of from less than 1 year to 4 years. In the unstable angina study, treatment was started within 1 month after the onset of unstable angina and continued for 12 weeks and complicating conditions, such as congestive heart failure, were not included in the study.

Aspirin therapy in MI patients was associated with about a 20 percent reduction in the risk of subsequent death and/or nonfatal reinfarction, a median absolute decrease of 3 percent from the 12 to 22 percent event rates in the placebo groups. In aspirin-treated unstable angina patients the reduction in risk was about 50 percent, a reduction in event rate of 5 percent from the 10 percent rate in the placebo group over the 12 weeks of the study.

Daily dosage of aspirin in the post–myocardial infarction studies was 300 mg in one study and 900—1500 mg in five studies. A dose of 325 mg was used in the study of unstable angina.

Adverse Reactions: Gastrointestinal Reactions: Doses of 1000 mg per day of aspirin caused gastrointestinal symptoms and bleeding that in some cases were clinically significant. In the largest post–infarction study (the Aspirin Myocardial Infarction Study [AMIS] trial with 4,500 people), the percentage incidences of gastrointestinal symptoms for the aspirin (1000 mg of a standard, solid-tablet formulation) and placebo-treated subjects, respectively, were: stomach pain (14.5%; 4.4%); heartburn (11.9%; 4.8%); nausea and/or vomiting (7.6%; 2.1%) hospitalization for GI disorder (4.9%; 3.5%). In the AMIS and other trials, aspirin-treated patients had increased rates of gross gastrointestinal bleeding. Symptoms and signs of gastrointestinal irritation were not significantly increased in subjects treated for unstable angina with buffered aspirin in solution.

Cardiovascular and Biochemical: In the AMIS trial, the dosage of 1000 mg per day of aspirin was associated with small increases in systolic blood pressure (BP) (average 1.5 to 2.1 mm) and diastolic BP (0.5 to 0.6 mm), depending upon whether maximal or last available readings were used. Blood urea nitrogen and uric acid levels were also increased, but by less than 1.0 mg%. Subjects with marked hypertension or renal insufficiency had been excluded from the trial so that the clinical importance of these observations for such subjects or for any subjects treated over more prolonged periods is not known. It is recommended that patients placed on long-term aspirin treatment, even at doses of 300 mg per day, be seen at regular intervals to assess changes in these measurements.

Sodium in Buffered Aspirin for Solution Formulations: One tablet daily of buffered aspirin in solution adds 553 mg of sodium to that in the diet and may not be tolerated by patients with active sodium-retaining states such as congestive heart or renal failure. This amount of sodium adds about 30 percent to the 70 to 90 meq intake suggested as appropriate for dietary treatment of essential hypertension in the 1984 Report of the Joint National Committee on Detection, Evaluation, and Treatment of High Blood Pressure.[8]

Dosage and Administration: Although most of the studies used dosages exceeding 300 mg, two trials used only 300 mg, daily, and pharmacologic data indicate that this dose inhibits platelet function fully. Therefore, 300 mg or a conventional 325 mg aspirin dose daily, is a reasonable routine dose that would minimize gastrointestinal adverse reactions. This use of aspirin applies to both solid, oral dosage forms (buffered and plain aspirin) and buffered aspirin in solution.

REFERENCES
(1) Elwood, P.C., et al., A Randomized Controlled Trial of Acetylsalicylic Acid in the Secondary Prevention of Mortality from Myocardial Infarction, *British Medical Journal*, 1:436–440, 1974.
(2) The Coronary Drug Project Research Group, "Aspirin in Coronary Heart Disease," *Journal of Chronic Disease*, 29:625–642, 1976.
(3) Breddin, K., et al., "Secondary Prevention of Myocardial Infarction: A Comparison of Acetylsalicylic Acid, Phenprocoumon or Placebo," *Homeostasis*, 470:263–268, 1979.
(4) Aspirin Myocardial Infarction Study Research Group, "A Randomized, Controlled Trial of Aspirin in Persons Recovered from Myocardial Infarction," *Journal American Medical Association* 245:661–669, 1980.
(5) Elwood, P.C., and Sweetnam P.M., "Aspirin and Secondary Mortality after Myocardial Infarction," *Lancet*, pp. 1313–1315, December 22–29, 1979.
(6) The Persantine-Aspirin Reinfarction Study Research Group, "Persantine and Aspirin in Coronary Heart Disease," *Circulation*, 62: 449–460, 1980.
(7) Lewis, H.D., et al., "Protective Effects of Aspirin Against Acute Myocardial Infarction and Death in Men with Unstable Angina. Results of a Veterans Administration Cooperative Study," *New England Journal of Medicine* 309:396–403, 1983.
(8) "1984 Report of the Joint National Committee on Detection, Evaluation and Treatment of High Blood Pressure," U.S. Department of Health and Human Services and United States Public Health Service, National Institutes of Health.

How Supplied:
Genuine Bayer Aspirin 5 grains (325 mg)—
NDC 12843-101-10, packs of 12 tablets.
NDC 12843-101-11, bottles of 24 tablets.
NDC 12843-101-17, bottles of 50 tablets.
NDC 12843-101-12, bottles of 100 tablets.
NDC 12843-101-20, bottles of 200 tablets.
NDC 12843-101-13, bottles of 300 tablets.
NDC 12843-102-38, bottles of 50 caplets.
NDC 12843-102-39, bottles of 100 caplets.
NDC 12843-102-20, bottles of 200 caplets.
Child-resistant safety closures on 12's, 24's, 50's, 200's, 300's tablets and 50's and 200's caplets. Bottles of 100's tablets and caplets available without safety closure for households without small children.
Shown in Product Identification Section, page 410

MAXIMUM BAYER® ASPIRIN
Aspirin (Acetylsalicylic Acid)
Tablets and Caplets

Active Ingredients: Maximum Bayer Aspirin—Aspirin 500 mg (7.7 grains) contains a thin, inert, hydroxypropyl methylcellulose coating for easier swallowing. This is not an enteric coating and does not alter the onset of action of Bayer Aspirin.

Inactive Ingredients: Starch and triacetin.

Actions and Uses: Analgesic, antipyretic, anti-inflammatory. For relief of headache; painful discomfort and fever of colds and flu; sore throats; muscular aches and pains; temporary relief of minor pains of arthritis, rheumatism, bursitis, lumbago, sciatica; toothache, teething pains, and pain following dental procedures; neuralgia and neuritic pain; functional menstrual pain; sleeplessness when caused by minor painful discomforts; painful discomfort and fever accompanying immunizations.

Caution: If pain persists for more than 10 days or redness is present, or in conditions affecting children under 12 years of age, consult a physician immediately.

Warnings: Children and teenagers should not use this medicine for chicken pox or flu symptoms before a doctor is consulted about Reye syndrome, a rare but serious illness reported to be associated with aspirin. Keep this and all drugs out of the reach of children. In case of accidental overdose, seek professional assistance or contact a poison control center immediately. As with any drugs, if you are pregnant or nursing a baby, seek the advice of a health professional before using this product.

Administration and Dosage: The following dosages are those provided on the packaging, as appropriate for self-medication. Larger or more frequent dosage may be necessary as appropriate to the condition or needs of the patient.
The hydroxypropyl methylcellulose coating makes Maximum Bayer Aspirin particularly appropriate for those who must take frequent doses of aspirin and for those who have difficulty in swallowing uncoated tablets/caplets.
Maximum Bayer Aspirin—500 mg (7.7 grains) tablets/caplets.

Usual Adult Dose: One or two tablets/caplets with water. May be repeated every four hours as necessary up to 8 tablets/caplets a day.

How Supplied:
Maximum Bayer Aspirin 500 mg (7.7 grains)
NDC 12843-161-53, bottles of 30 tablets.
NDC 12843-161-56, bottles of 60 tablets.
NDC 12843-161-58, bottles of 100 tablets.
NDC 12843-202-30, bottles of 30 caplets.
NDC 12843-202-56, bottles of 60 caplets.
Child-resistant safety closures on 30's bottles of tablets and caplets, 60's, bottles of caplets, and 100's bottles of tablets. Bottle of 60's tablets available without safety closure for households without small children.
Shown in Product Identification Section, page 410

8-HOUR BAYER®
TIMED-RELEASE ASPIRIN
Aspirin (acetylsalicylic acid)

Active Ingredients: Each oblong white scored caplet contains 10 grains (650 mg) of aspirin in microencapsulated form.

Inactive Ingredients: Guar gum, microcrystalline cellulose, starch and other ingredients.

Indications: 8-Hour Bayer Timed-Release Aspirin is indicated for the temporary relief of low-grade pain amenable to relief with salicylates, such as in rheumatoid arthritis, osteoarthritis, spondylitis, bursitis and other forms of rheumatism, as well as in many common musculoskeletal disorders. It possesses the same advantages for other types of prolonged aches and pains, such as minor injuries, dental pain and dysmenorrhea. Its long-lasting effectiveness should also make it valuable as an analgesic in simple headache, colds, grippe, flu and other similar conditions in which aspirin is indicated for symptomatic relief, either by itself or as an adjunct to specific therapy.

Caution: If pain persists for more than 10 days, or redness is present, or in conditions affecting children under 12 years, consult a physician immediately.

Warnings: Children and teenagers should not use this medicine for chicken pox or flu symptoms before a doctor is consulted about Reye syndrome, a rare but serious illness reported to be associated with aspirin. Keep this and all drugs out of the reach of children. In case of accidental overdose, seek professional assistance or contact a poison control center immediately. As with any drug, if you are pregnant or nursing a baby, seek the advice of a health professional before using this product.

Administration and Dosage: Two 8-Hour Bayer Timed-Release Aspirin caplets q. 8 h. provide effective long-lasting pain relief. This two-caplet (20 grain or 1300 mg) dose of timed-release aspirin promptly produces salicylate blood levels greater than those achieved by a 10-grain (650 mg) dose of regular aspirin, and in the second 4-hour period produces

a salicylate blood level curve which approximates that of two successive 10-grain (650 mg) doses of regular aspirin at 4-hour intervals. The 10-grain (650 mg) scored 8-Hour Bayer Timed-Release Aspirin caplets permit administration of aspirin in multiples of 5 grains (325 mg) allowing individualization of dosage to meet the specific needs of the patient. For the convenience of patients on a regular aspirin dosage schedule, two 10-grain (650 mg) 8-Hour Bayer Timed-Release Aspirin caplets may be administered with water every 8 hours. Whenever necessary, two caplets (20 grains or 1300 mg) should be given before retiring to provide effective analgesic and anti-inflammatory action—for relief of pain throughout the night and lessening of stiffness upon arising. Do not exceed 6 caplets in 24 hours. 8-Hour Bayer Timed-Release Aspirin has been made in a special caplet to permit easy swallowing. However, for patients who do have difficulty, 8-Hour Bayer Timed-Release Aspirin caplets may be gently crumbled in the mouth and swallowed with water without loss of timed-release effect. There is no bitter "aspirin" taste. For children under 12, consult physician.

Side Effects: Side effects encountered with regular aspirin may be encountered with 8-Hour Bayer Timed-Release Aspirin. Tinnitus and dizziness are the ones most frequently encountered.

Contraindications and Precautions: 8-Hour Bayer Timed-Release Aspirin is contraindicated in patients with marked aspirin hypersensitivity, and should be given with extreme caution to any patient with a history of adverse reaction to salicylates. It may cautiously be tried in patients intolerant to aspirin because of gastric irritation, but the usual precautions for any form of aspirin should be observed in patients with gastric ulcers, bleeding tendencies, asthma, or hypoprothrombinemia.

How Supplied:
NDC 12843-191-72, Caplets in Bottle of 30's.
NDC 12843-191-74, Caplets in Bottle of 72's.
NDC 12843-191-76, Caplets in Bottle of 125's.
All sizes packaged in child-resistant safety closure except 72's, which is a size recommended for households without young children.
Shown in Product Identification Section, page 410

THERAPY BAYER® ASPIRIN
Delayed-Release Enteric Aspirin (Acetylsalicylic Acid) Caplets
Antiarthritic, Antiplatelet

Composition: Therapy BAYER is 325 mg enteric-coated aspirin available in caplet form. The enteric coating prevents disintegration in the stomach and promotes dissolution in the duodenum, where there is a more neutral-to-alkaline environment. This action aids in protecting the stomach against injuries that

may occur as a result of ingesting non-enteric-coated aspirin (see **Safety**).

Inactive Ingredients: D&C Yellow No. 10, FD&C Yellow No. 6, hydroxypropyl methylcellulose, methacrylic acid, copolymer, starch, titanium dioxide, triacetin, polysorbate 80, and sodium lauryl sulfate.

Indications: Therapy BAYER is an anti-inflammatory, analgesic, and antiplatelet agent indicated for the relief of painful discomfort and muscular aches and pains associated with conditions requiring long-term aspirin therapy, e.g., arthritis or rheumatism and for situations where compliance with aspirin is hindered by the gastrointestinal side effects of non-enteric-coated or buffered aspirin.

Dosage: For analgesic or anti-inflammatory indications, the OTC maximum dosage for aspirin is 4,000 mg per day in divided doses, i.e., two 325 mg caplets every 4 hours or three 325 mg caplets every six hours. For antiplatelet effect dosage, see the **Antiplatelet Effect** section.

Caution: If pain persists for more than 10 days or redness is present, or in conditions affecting children under 12 years of age, consult a physician immediately.

Consumer Warning: Children and teenagers should not use this medicine for chicken pox or flu symptoms before a doctor is consulted about Reye's syndrome, a rare but serious illness reported to be associated with aspirin. Keep this and all drugs out of the reach of children. In case of accidental overdose, seek professional assistance or contact a poison control center immediately. As with any drug, if you are pregnant or nursing a baby, seek the advice of a health professional before using this product.

Professional Warning: Occasional reports have documented individuals with impaired gastric emptying in whom there may be retention of one or more enteric-coated aspirin caplets over time. This phenomenon may occur as a result of outlet obstruction from ulcer disease alone or combined with hypotonic gastric peristalsis. Because of the integrity of the enteric coating in an acidic environment, these caplets may accumulate and form a bezoar in the stomach. Individuals with this condition may present with complaints of early satiety or of vague upper abdominal distress. Diagnosis may be made by endoscopy or by abdominal films, which show opacities suggestive of a mass of small caplets.[1] Management may vary according to the condition of the patient. Options include gastrotomy and alternating slightly basic and neutral lavage.[2] While there have been no clinical reports, it has been suggested that such individuals may also be treated with parenteral cimetidine (to reduce acid secretion) and then given sips of slightly basic liquids to effect gradual dissolution of the enteric coating. Progress may be followed with plasma salicyl-

Continued on next page

Glenbrook—Cont.

ate levels or via recognition of tinnitus by the patient.

It should be kept in mind that individuals with a history of partial or complete gastrectomy may produce reduced amounts of acid and therefore have less acidic gastric pH. Under these circumstances, the benefits offered by the acid-resistant enteric coating may not exist.

Safety: The safety of enteric-coated aspirin has been demonstrated in a number of endoscopic studies comparing enteric-coated aspirin and plain aspirin, as well as plain buffered and "arthritis-strength" preparations. In these studies, endoscopies were performed in healthy volunteers before and after either two-day or 14-day administration of aspirin doses of 3,900 or 4,000 mg/day. Compared to all the other preparations, the enteric-coated aspirin produced significantly less damage to the gastric mucosa. There was also statistically less duodenal damage when compared with the plain, i.e., non-enteric-coated, aspirin.

Bioavailability: The bioavailability of aspirin from Therapy BAYER has been confirmed. In a single-dose study[3] in which plasma acetylsalicylic acid and salicylic acid levels were measured, measurable plasma concentrations were achieved within 15 minutes after dosing. Maximum concentrations were achieved at approximately five hours postdosing. Therapy BAYER, when compared with plain aspirin, achieves maximum plasma salicylate levels not significantly different from plain, ie, not enteric-coated, aspirin. Dissolution of the enteric coating occurs at a neutral-to-basic pH and is therefore dependent on gastric emptying into the duodenum. With continued dosing, appropriate therapeutic plasma levels are maintained.

Antiplatelet Effect:
IN MI PROPHYLAXIS

Indication: Aspirin is indicated to reduce the risk of death and/or nonfatal myocardial infarction in patients with a previous infarction or unstable angina pectoris.

Clinical Trials: The indication is supported by the results of six large randomized, multicenter, placebo-controlled studies[4–10] involving 10,816, predominantly male, post–myocardial infarction (MI) patients and one randomized placebo-controlled study of 1,266 men with unstable angina. Therapy with aspirin was begun at intervals after the onset of acute MI varying from less than three days to more than five years and continuing for periods of from less than 1 year to 4 years. In the unstable angina study, treatment was started within 1 month after the onset of unstable angina and continued for 12 weeks, and complicating conditions, such as congestive heart failure, were not included in the study. Aspirin therapy in MI patients was associated with about a 20% reduction in the risk of subsequent death and/or nonfatal rein-

farction, a median absolute decrease of 3% from the 12% to 22% event rates in the placebo groups. In the aspirin-treated unstable angina patients the reduction in risk was about 50%, a reduction in event rate of 5% from the 10% rate in the placebo group over the 12 weeks of the study.

Daily dosage of aspirin in the post–myocardial infarction studies was 300 mg in one study and 900–1,500 mg in five studies. A dose of 325 mg was used in the study of unstable angina.

Adverse Reactions: Gastrointestinal reactions: Doses of 1,000 mg per day of aspirin caused gastrointestinal symptoms and bleeding that, in some cases were clinically significant. In the largest postinfarction study (the Aspirin Myocardial Infarction Study [AMIS] with 4,500 people), the percentage of incidences of gastrointestinal symptoms for the aspirin (1,000 mg of a standard, solid-tablet formulation) and placebo-treated subjects, respectively, were: stomach pain (14.5%; 4.4%); heartburn (11.9%; 4.8%); nausea and/or vomiting (7.6%; 2.1%); hospitalization for GI disorder (4.9%; 3.5%). In the AMIS and other trials, aspirin-treated patients had increased rates of gross gastrointestinal bleeding. Symptoms and signs of gastrointestinal irritation were not significantly increased in subjects treated for unstable angina with buffered aspirin in solution.

Cardiovascular and Biochemical: In the AMIS trial, the dosage of 1,000 mg per day of aspirin was associated with small increases in systolic blood pressure (BP) (average 1.5 to 2.1 mm) and diastolic BP (0.5 to 0.6 mm), depending upon whether maximal or last available readings were used. Blood urea nitrogen and uric acid levels were also increased but by less than 1.0 mg percent. Subjects with marked hypertension or renal insufficiency had been excluded from the trial so that the clinical importance of these observations for such subjects or for any subjects treated over more prolonged periods is not known. It is recommended that patients placed on long-term aspirin treatment, even at doses of 300 mg per day, be seen at regular intervals to assess changes in these measurements.

Sodium in Buffered Aspirin for Solution Formulations: One tablet daily of buffered aspirin in solution adds 553 mg of sodium to that in the diet and may not be tolerated by patients with active sodium-retaining states, such as congestive heart or renal failure. This amount of sodium adds about 30% to the 70 to 90 meq intake suggested as appropriate for dietary treatment of essential hypertension in the 1984 Report of the Joint National Committee on Detection, Evaluation, and Treatment of High Blood Pressure.[11]

Dosage and Administration: Although most of the studies used dosages exceeding 300 mg, two trials used only 300 mg daily, and pharmacologic data indicate

that this dose inhibits platelet function fully. Therefore, 300 mg or a conventional 325 mg aspirin dose daily, is a reasonable routine dose that would minimize gastrointestinal adverse reactions. This use of aspirin applies to both solid oral dosage forms (buffered and plain aspirin) and buffered aspirin in solution.

For Recurrent TIAs in Men: There is evidence that aspirin is safe and effective for reducing the risk of recurrent transient ischemic attacks (TIAs) or stroke in men who have had transient ischemia of the brain due to fibrin platelet emboli. There is no evidence that aspirin is effective in reducing TIAs in women or is of benefit in the treatment of completed strokes in men or women.

Patients presenting with signs and/or symptoms of TIAs should have a complete medical and neurologic evaluation. Consideration should be given to other disorders that may resemble TIAs. It is important to evaluate and treat, if appropriate, other diseases associated with TIAs and stroke, such as hypertension and diabetes.

Dosage: The recommended dosage for this new indication is 1300 mg/day (650 mg b.i.d. or 325 mg q.i.d.). Store at controlled room temperature (59°–86°F).

References: 1. Bogacz, K, Caldron, P: Enteric-coated aspirin bezoar: Elevation of serum salicylate level by barium study. *Am J Med* 1987;83:783–786. 2. Baum, J: Enteric-coated aspirin and the problem of gastric retention. *J Rheumatol* 1984; 11:250–251. 3. Data on file, Glenbrook Laboratories. 4. Elwood, PC, et al: A randomized controlled trial of acetylsalicylic acid in the secondary prevention of mortality from myocardial infarction. *Br Med J* 1974;1:436–440. 5. The Coronary Drug Project Research Group: Aspirin in coronary heart disease. *J Chronic Dis* 1976;29:625–642. 6. Breddin, K, et al: Secondary prevention of myocardial infarction: A comparison of acetylsalicylic acid, phenprocoumon or placebo. *Homeostasis* 1979; 470:263–268. 7. Aspirin Myocardial Infarction Study Research Group: A randomized, controlled trial of aspirin in persons recovered from myocardial infarction. *JAMA* 1980; 245:661–669. 8. Elwood, PC, Sweetnam, PM: Aspirin and secondary mortality after myocardial infarction. *Lancet,* December 22–29, 1979, pp 1313–1315. 9. The Persantine-Aspirin Reinfarction Study Research Group: Persantine and aspirin in coronary heart disease. *Circulation* 1980;62:449–460. 10. Lewis, HD, et al: Protective effects of aspirin against acute myocardial infarction and death in men with unstable angina: Results of a Veterans Administration Cooperative Study. *N Eng J Med* 1983;309:396–403. 11. *1984 Report of the Joint National Committee on Detection, Evaluation and Treatment of High Blood Pressure,* U.S. Dept of Health and Human Services and US Public Health Service, National Institutes of Health.

How Supplied: Therapy BAYER 325 mg caplets in bottles of 50, 100.

Shown in Product Identification Section, page 410

HALEY'S M-O®

Active Ingredients: A suspension of magnesium hydroxide in purified water plus mineral oil. Haley's M-O contains 304 mg per teaspoon (5 mL) of magnesium hydroxide and 1.25 mL of mineral oil.

Inactive Ingredients: Purified water. For flavored Haley's M-O only, D&C Red No. 28, flavor, purified water, saccharin sodium.

Indications: For the relief of occasional constipation or irregularity accompanied by hemorrhoids.

Action at Laxative Dosage: Haley's M-O is a mild saline laxative which acts by drawing water into the gut, increasing intraluminal pressure, and increasing intestinal motility. This product generally produces bowel movement in ½ to 6 hours.

Administration and Dosage: As a laxative, especially for hemorrhoid sufferers, adults 1–2 tbsp at bedtime and upon arising. For constipation relief, adults 2 tbsp at bedtime and upon arising; children 6–12, minimum single dose; 1 tsp, maximum daily dose; 1 tbsp. For adults and children, as bowel function improves reduce dose gradually.

Caution: Do not take this product if you are presently taking a stool softener laxative unless directed by a doctor. Do not take with meals.

Warnings: Do not use laxative products when abdominal pain, nausea or vomiting are present unless directed by a doctor. If you have noticed a sudden change in bowel habits that persists over a period of 2 weeks, consult a doctor before using a laxative. Laxative products should not be used for a period longer than 1 week unless directed by a doctor. Rectal bleeding, or failure to have a bowel movement after use of a laxative may indicate a serious condition; discontinue use and consult your doctor. Do not administer to children under 6 years of age, to pregnant women, to bedridden patients, or to persons with difficulty swallowing. As with any drug, if you are nursing a baby, seek the advice of a health professional before using this product. Keep this and all drugs out of the reach of children. In case of accidental overdose, seek professional assistance or contact a poison control center immediately.

How Supplied: Haley's M-O is available in regular and flavored liquids:
Regular
4 fl oz NDC 12843-350-45; 12 fl oz NDC 12843-350-46; 26 fl oz NDC 12843-350-47.
Flavored
4 fl oz NDC 12843-360-67; 12 fl oz NDC 12843-360-68; 26 fl oz NDC 12843-360-69.

Shown in Product Identification Section, page 411

REGULAR STRENGTH MIDOL® MULTI-SYMPTOM FORMULA

Active Ingredients: Each caplet contains: acetaminophen 325 mg and pyrilamine maleate 12.5 mg.

Inactive Ingredients: Croscarmellose sodium type A, hydroxypropyl methylcellulose, magnesium stearate, microcrystalline cellulose, pregelatinized starch and triacetin.

Action and Uses: For relief of multiple symptoms suffered during menstrual cycle: cramps, bloating, headache, tension, irritability, and backache caused by menstrual discomfort.
Unlike general pain relievers, which contain only analgesics, Regular Strength Midol Multi-Symptom Formula has a unique combination of ingredients (an analgesic, tension and water retention reliever) specially formulated to give:
1. Relief from cramps, headaches, backaches and muscle aches.
2. Relief of irritability, anxiety and tension.
3. Relief from the discomforts of fluid retention and bloating.

Caution: May cause drowsiness. Use caution when driving or operating machinery. Alcohol, sedatives or tranquilizers may increase drowsiness.

Warnings: Keep this and all drugs out of the reach of children. In case of accidental overdose, seek professional assistance or contact a poison control center immediately. As with any drug, if you are pregnant or nursing a baby, seek the advice of a health professional before using this product.

Dosage: Take 2 caplets with water. Repeat every four hours as needed up to a maximum of 12 caplets per day. Under age 12: Consult your physician.

How Supplied:
White, capsule-shaped caplets.
NDC 12843-156-16, professional dispenser, 250 2-caplet packets for sample use.
NDC 12843-156-17, bottle of 12 caplets.
NDC 12843-156-18, bottle of 30 caplets.
NDC 12843-156-19, bottles of 60 caplets.
Child-resistant safety closures on bottles of 12 and 60 Caplets.

Shown in Product Identification Section, page 410

MAXIMUM STRENGTH MIDOL® PMS
Premenstrual Syndrome Formula

Active Ingredients: Each caplet contains acetaminophen 500 mg, pamabrom 25 mg, pyrilamine maleate 15 mg.

Inactive Ingredients: Croscarmellose sodium, hydrogenated vegetable oil, hydroxypropyl methylcellulose, magnesium stearate, microcrystalline cellulose, pregelatinized starch, talc and triacetin.

Action and Uses: Relieves the symptoms of premenstrual syndrome (PMS). Contains maximum strength medication for all these premenstrual symptoms: tension, irritability, anxiety, bloating, water-weight gain, cramps, backache, and headache. Unlike general pain relievers, which contain only analgesics, Midol PMS contains a combination of ingredients (an analgesic, diuretic, and a tension reliever) for the physical and emotional symptoms associated with PMS.

Dosage: Take 2 caplets with water. Repeat every 4 hours as needed, up to a maximum of 8 caplets per day. Under age 12: Take under the advice of your physician.

Caution: May cause drowsiness. Use caution when driving or operating machinery. Alcohol, sedatives or tranquilizers may increase drowsiness.

Warnings: Keep this and *all* drugs out of the reach of children. In case of accidental overdose, seek professional assistance or contact a poison control center immediately. As with any drug, if you are pregnant or nursing a baby, seek the advice of a health professional before using this product.

How Supplied:
White capsule-shaped caplets.
NDC 12843-163-46, bottles of 16 caplets.
NDC 12843-163-47, bottles of 32 caplets.
Child-resistant safety closure on bottles of 32 caplets.

Shown in Product Identification Section, page 410

MIDOL® 200 ADVANCED CRAMP FORMULA
Ibuprofen Tablets, USP
Menstrual Pain/Cramp Reliever

Warning: Aspirin-Sensitive Patients —Do not take this product if you have had a severe allergic reaction to aspirin, eg, asthma, swelling, shock or hives, because even though this product contains no aspirin or salicylates, cross-reactions may occur in patients allergic to aspirin.

Indications: For the temporary relief of painful menstrual cramps (dysmenorrhea); also headaches, backaches and muscular aches and pains associated with premenstrual syndrome.

Directions:
Adults: Take 1 tablet every 4 to 6 hours at the onset of menstrual symptoms and while pain persists. If pain does not respond to 1 tablet, 2 tablets may be used but do not exceed 6 tablets in 24 hours, unless directed by a doctor. The smallest effective dose should be used. Take with food or milk if occasional and mild heartburn, upset stomach, or stomach pain occurs with use. Consult a doctor if these symptoms are more than mild or if they persist. *Children:* Do not give this product to children under 12 except under the advice and supervision of a doctor.

Continued on next page

Glenbrook—Cont.

Warnings: Do not take for pain for more than 10 days unless directed by a doctor. If pain persists or gets worse, or if new symptoms occur, consult a doctor. These could be signs of serious illness. If you are under a doctor's care for any serious condition, consult a doctor before taking this product. As with aspirin and acetaminophen, if you have any condition which requires you to take prescription drugs or if you have had any problems or serious side effects from taking any nonprescription pain reliever, do not take this product without first discussing it with your doctor. If you experience any symptoms which are unusual or seem unrelated to the condition for which you took ibuprofen, consult a doctor before taking any more of it. Although ibuprofen is indicated for the same conditions as aspirin and acetaminophen, it should not be taken with them except under a doctor's direction. Do not combine this product with any other ibuprofen-containing product. As with any drug, if you are pregnant or nursing a baby, seek the advice of a health professional before using this product. **IT IS ESPECIALLY IMPORTANT NOT TO USE IBUPROFEN DURING THE LAST 3 MONTHS OF PREGNANCY UNLESS SPECIFICALLY DIRECTED TO DO SO BY A DOCTOR BECAUSE IT MAY CAUSE PROBLEMS IN THE UNBORN CHILD OR COMPLICATIONS DURING DELIVERY.** Keep this and *all* drugs out of the reach of children. In case of accidental overdose, seek professional assistance or contact a poison control center immediately. Ibuprofen is used for the relief of painful menstrual cramps and the pain associated with premenstrual syndrome. Ibuprofen has been proven more effective in relieving menstrual pain and cramps than aspirin and is gentler on the stomach. Ibuprofen had been widely prescribed for years and is now available in nonprescription strength.

Active Ingredients: Each tablet contains ibuprofen USP 200 mg.

Inactive Ingredients: Calcium phosphate, cellulose, magnesium stearate, silicon dioxide, sodium lauryl sulfate, sodium starch glycolate, stearic acid, titanium dioxide.
Store at room temperature; avoid excessive heat 40°C (104°F).

How Supplied:
White tablets NDC 12843-154-50, bottles of 16 tablets.
NDC 12843-154-51, bottles of 32 tablets.
Child-resistant safety closure on bottles of 32 tablets.
Shown in Product Identification Section, page 410

MAXIMUM STRENGTH MIDOL® MULTI-SYMPTOM FORMULA

Active Ingredients: Each caplet contains acetaminophen 500 mg and pyrilamine maleate 15 mg.

Inactive Ingredients: Croscarmellose sodium type A, hydroxypropyl methylcellulose, magnesium stearate, microcrystalline cellulose, pregelatinized starch and triacetin.

Action and Uses: Maximum strength medication for the relief of multiple symptoms suffered during menstrual cycle: cramps, bloating, headache, tension, irritability and backache caused by menstrual discomfort.
Unlike general pain relievers, which contain only analgesics, Midol Maximum Strength Multi-Symptom Formula has a unique combination of ingredients (an analgesic, tension reliever and water retention reliever) specially formulated to give:
1. Maximum strength relief from cramps, plus relief of headaches, backaches and muscle aches.
2. Maximum relief of irritability, anxiety and tension.
3. Maximum relief from the discomforts of fluid retention, bloating and water-weight gain.

Caution: May cause drowsiness. Use caution when driving or operating machinery. Alcohol, sedatives or tranquilizers may increase drowsiness.

Warnings: Keep this and all drugs out of the reach of children. In case of accidental overdose, seek professional assistance or contact a poison control center immediately. As with any drug, if you are pregnant or nursing a baby, seek the advice of a health professional before using this product.

Dosage: Take 2 caplets with water. Repeat every 4 hours, as needed, up to a maximum of 8 caplets per day.
Under age 12: Consult your physician.

How Supplied: White capsule-shaped caplets.
NDC 12843-157-16, professional dispenser, 250 2-caplet packets for sample use.
NDC 12843-157-17, bottles of 8 caplets.
NDC 12843-157-18, bottles of 16 caplets.
NDC 12843-157-19, bottles of 32 caplets.
Child-resistant safety closures on bottles of 8 and 32 caplets.
Shown in Product Identification Section, page 410

CHILDREN'S PANADOL®
Acetaminophen Chewable Tablets, Liquid, Drops

Description: Each Children's PANADOL Chewable Tablet contains 80 mg acetaminophen in a fruit-flavored sugarfree tablet. Children's PANADOL Acetaminophen Liquid is fruit-flavored, red in color, and is alcohol-free, sugar-free and aspirin-free. Each ½ teaspoonful contains 80 mg of acetaminophen. Infant's PANADOL Drops are fruit-flavored, red in color, and are alcohol-free, sugar-free and aspirin-free. Each 0.8 mL (one calibrated dropperful) contains 80 mg acetaminophen.

Actions and Indications: Acetaminophen, the active ingredient in PANA-

DOL, is the analgesic/antipyretic most widely recommended by pediatricians for fast, effective relief of children's fevers. It also relieves the aches and pains of colds and flu, earaches, headaches, teething, immunizations, tonsillectomy, and childhood illnesses.
Children's PANADOL Tablets, Liquid, and Drops are aspirin-free and contain no alcohol or sugar. The pleasant-tasting formulations are not likely to upset or irritate children's stomachs.

Usual Dosage: Dosing is based on single doses in the range of 10–15 mg/kg body weight. Doses may be repeated every four hours up to 4 or 5 times daily, but not to exceed 5 doses in 24 hours. To be administered to children under 2 years only on advice of a physician.
Children's PANADOL Chewable Tablets: 2–3 yr, 24–35 lb, 2 tablets; 4–5 yr, 36–47 lb, 3 tablets; 6–8 yr, 48–59 lb, 4 tablets; 9–10 yr, 60–71 lb, 5 tablets; 11–12 yr, 72–95 lb, 6 tablets. May be repeated every 4 hours, up to 5 times in a 24-hour period.
Children's PANADOL Liquid: (a special 3 teaspoon cup for accurate measurement is provided). 0–4 mo, 6–11 lb, ¼ teaspoonful; 4–11 mo, 12–17 lb, ½ teaspoonful; 12–23 mo, 18–23 lb, ¾ teaspoonful; 2–3 yr, 24–35 lb, 1 teaspoonful; 4–5 yr, 36–47 lb, 1½ teaspoonful; 6–8 yr, 48–59 lb, 2 teaspoonfuls; 9–10 yr, 60–71 lb, 2½ teaspoonfuls; 11–12 yr, 72–95 lb, 3 teaspoonfuls. May be repeated every 4 hours up to 5 times in a 24-hour period. May be administered alone or mixed with formula, milk, juice, cereal, etc.
Infant's PANADOL Drops: 0–4 mo, 6–11 lb, ½ dropperful (0.4 mL); 4–11 mo, 12–17 lb, 1 dropperful (0.8 mL); 12–23 mo, 18–23 lb, 1½ dropperfuls (1.2 mL); 2–3 yr, 24–35 lb, 2 dropperfuls (1.6 mL); 4–5 yr, 36–47 lb, 3 dropperfuls (2.4 mL); 6–8 yr, 48–59 lb, 4 dropperfuls (3.2 mL). May be repeated every 4 hours, up to 5 times in a 24-hour period. May be administered alone or mixed with formula, milk, juice, cereal, etc.

Warnings: Since Children's PANADOL Acetaminophen Chewable Tablets, Liquid, and Drops are available without a prescription as an analgesic/antipyretic, the following appears on the package labels: "WARNINGS: Do not take this product for more than 5 days. If symptoms persist or new ones occur, consult a physician. If fever persists for more than 3 days, or recurs, consult a physician. Keep this and *all* drugs out of the reach of children. In case of accidental overdose, seek professional assistance or contact a poison control center immediately. High fever, severe or persistent sore throat, cough, headache, nausea or vomiting may be serious; consult a physician."
Tamper Resistant: Children's PANADOL Acetaminophen Chewable Tablets packaging provides tamper-resistant features on both the outer carton and bottle. The following copy appears on the end flaps of this carton—"Purchase only if carton end flaps are sealed." The follow-

ing copy appears on the bottle—"Use only if printed seal under cap is intact." Children's PANADOL Liquid and Drops provide tamper-resistant features on the carton. The following copy appears on the carton—"Purchase only if Red Tear Tape and Plastic Overwrap are intact," and bottle—"Use only if Carton Overwrap and Red Tear Tape Are Intact."

Composition:
Tablets: Active Ingredient: Acetaminophen. Inactive Ingredients: FD&C Red No. 3, flavor, mannitol, saccharin sodium, starch, stearic acid and other ingredients.
Liquid: Active Ingredient: Acetaminophen. Inactive Ingredients: Benzoic acid, FD&C Red No. 40, flavor, glycerin, polyethylene glycol, potassium sorbate, propylene glycol, purified water, saccharin sodium, sorbitol solution. May also contain sodium chloride or sodium hydroxide.
Drops: Active Ingredient: Acetaminophen. Inactive Ingredients: Citric acid, FD&C Red No. 40, flavors, glycerin, parabens, polyethylene glycol, propylene glycol, purified water, saccharin sodium, sodium chloride, sodium citrate.

How Supplied: Chewable Tablets (colored pink and scored)—bottles of 30. Liquid (colored red)—bottles of 2 fl. oz. and 4 fl. oz. Drops (colored red)—bottles of ½ oz. (15 mL).
All packages listed above have child-resistant safety caps and tamper-resistant features.
Shown in Product Identification Section, page 410

JUNIOR STRENGTH PANADOL®

Description: Each Junior Strength PANADOL® Caplet contains 160 mg of acetaminophen.

Actions and Indications: Acetaminophen, the active ingredient in Junior Strength PANADOL®, is the analgesic/antipyretic most widely recommended by pediatricians for fast, effective relief of children's fevers. It also relieves the aches and pains of colds and flu, earaches, headaches, teething, immunizations, tonsillectomy, menstrual discomfort, and childhood illness.
Junior Strength PANADOL® Caplets are aspirin-free, sugar-free.

Usual Dosage: Dosing is based on single doses in the range of 10–15 mg/kg body weight. Doses may be repeated every 4 hours up to 4 or 5 times daily, but not to exceed 5 doses in 24 hours. To be administered to children under 2 years only on the advice of a physician.
2–3 yr, 24–35 lb, 1 caplet; 4–5 yr, 36–47 lb, 1½ caplets; 6–8 yr, 48–59 lb, 2 caplets; 9–10 yr, 60–71 lb, 2½ caplets; 11–12 yr, 72–95 lb, 3 caplets. Over 12 yr, 96 lb and over, 4 caplets. Dosage may be repeated every 4 hours, up to 5 times in a 24-hour period.

Inactive Ingredients: Hydroxypropyl methylcellulose, potassium sorbate, povidone, pregelatinized starch, starch, stearic acid, talc, triacetin.

Warnings: If symptoms persist or new ones occur, consult physician. If fever persists for more than 3 days, or recurs, consult a physician. Do not take this product for more than 5 days. Keep this and all drugs out of the reach of children. In case of accidental overdose, seek professional assistance or contact a poison control center immediately. As with any drug, if you are pregnant, or nursing a baby, seek the advice of a health professional before using this product.

How Supplied: Swallowable caplets (white)—blister-pack of 30. Package has child-resistant and tamper-resistant features.
NDC 12843-216-14

MAXIMUM STRENGTH PANADOL®
Tablets and Caplets

Active Ingredients: Each Maximum Strength PANADOL micro-thin coated tablet and caplet contains acetaminophen 500 mg.

Inactive Ingredients: Hydroxypropyl methylcellulose, potassium sorbate, povidone, pregelatinized starch, starch, stearic acid, talc, triacetin.

Actions: PANADOL acetaminophen has been clinically proven as a fast, effective analgesic (pain reliever) and antipyretic (fever reducer). PANADOL acetaminophen is a nonaspirin product designed to provide relief without stomach upset. Its patented micro-thin coating makes each 500 mg tablet or caplet easy to swallow.

Indications: For the temporary relief from pain of headaches, colds or flu, sinusitis, backaches, muscle aches, and menstrual discomfort. Also to reduce fever and for temporary relief of minor arthritis pain and headache.

Precautions: If a rare sensitivity reaction occurs, the drug should be stopped. PANADOL acetaminophen has rarely been found to produce any side effects. It is usually well tolerated by aspirin-sensitive patients.
Severe recurrent pain or high continued fever may indicate a serious condition. Under these circumstances consult a physician.

Warnings: As with other products available without prescription, the following appears on the label of PANADOL acetaminophen: Do not give to children under 12 or use for more than 10 days unless directed by a physician. Keep this and all drugs out of the reach of children. In case of accidental overdose, seek professional assistance or contact a poison control center immediately. As with any drug, if you are pregnant or nursing a baby, seek the advice of a health professional before using this product.

Usual Dosage: *Adults:* Two tablets or caplets every 4 hours as needed. Do not exceed 8 tablets or caplets in 24 hours unless directed by a physician.

Overdosage: In massive overdosage acetaminophen may cause hepatic toxicity

in some patients. Clinical and laboratory evidence of overdosage may be delayed up to 7 days. Under circumstances of suspected overdose, contact your regional poison control center immediately.

How Supplied: Tablets and caplets (white, micro-thin coated, imprinted "PANADOL" and "500"). Tablets packaged in tamper-evident bottles of 30 and 60. Caplets packaged in tamper-evident bottles of 24, 50.
Shown in Product Identification Section, page 410

PHILLIPS'® LAXCAPS®

Active Ingredients: A combination of phenolphthalein (90 mg) and docusate sodium (83 mg) per gelatin capsule.

Inactive Ingredients: FD&C Blue No. 1, Red No. 3, Red No. 40 and Yellow No. 6, gelatin, glycerin, PEG 400 and 3350, propylene glycol and sorbitol.

Indications: For relief of occasional constipation (irregularity).

Action: Phenolphthalein is a stimulant laxative which increases the peristaltic activity of the intestine. Docusate sodium is a stool softener which allows easier passage of the stool. This product generally produces bowel movement in 6 to 12 hours.

Administration and Dosage: Adults and children 12 and over take one (1) or two (2) capsules daily with a full glass (8 oz) of liquid, or as directed by a physician. For children under 12, consult your physician.

Warnings: Do not take any laxative if abdominal pain, nausea, vomiting, change in bowel habits persisting for over 2 weeks, rectal bleeding or kidney disease is present. Laxative products should not be used for a period longer than one week, unless directed by a physician. If there is a failure to have a bowel movement after use, discontinue and consult your doctor. If a skin rash appears do not take this or any other preparation which contains phenolphthalein. Keep this and all drugs out of the reach of children. In case of accidental overdose, seek professional assistance or contact a Poison Control Center immediately. As with any drug, if you are pregnant or nursing a baby, seek the advice of a health professional before using this product.

How Supplied: Blister packs for safety:
8's NDC 12843-384-18
24's NDC 12843-384-19

PHILLIPS' ® MILK OF MAGNESIA

Active Ingredients: A suspension of magnesium hydroxide in purified water meeting all USP specifications. Phillips' Milk of Magnesia contains 405 mg per teaspoon (5 mL) of magnesium hydroxide.

Inactive Ingredients: Purified water, and for Mint Flavored Phillips' Milk of

Continued on next page

Glenbrook—Cont.

Magnesia only—flavor, mineral oil and saccharin sodium.

Indications: For relief of occasional constipation (irregularity), relief of acid indigestion, sour stomach and heartburn.

Action at Laxative Dosage: Phillips' Milk of Magnesia is a mild saline laxative which acts by drawing water into the gut, increasing intraluminal pressure, and increasing intestinal motility. This product generally produces bowel movement in ½ to 6 hours.

At Antacid Dosage: Phillips' Milk of Magnesia is an effective acid neutralizer.

Administration and Dosage: As a laxative, adults and children 12 years and older, 2–4 tbsp; children 6–11, 1–2 tbsp; children 2–5, 1–3 tsp followed by a full glass (8 oz) of liquid. Children under 2, consult a physician.

As an antacid, 1–3 tsp with a little water, up to four times a day, or as directed by your physician.

Cautions: Antacids may interact with certain prescription drugs. If you are taking a prescription drug do not take this product without checking with your physician.

Laxative Warnings: Do not take any laxative if abdominal pain, nausea, vomiting, change in bowel habits persisting for over 2 weeks, rectal bleeding, or kidney disease is present. Laxative products should not be used for a period longer than 1 week, unless directed by a doctor. If there is a failure to have a bowel movement after use, discontinue and consult your doctor.

Antacid Warnings: Do not take more than the maximum recommended daily dosage in a 24-hour period (see Directions), or use the maximum dosage of this product for more than two weeks, or use this product if you have kidney disease, except under the advice and supervision of a physician. May have laxative effect.

General Warnings: As with any drug, if you are pregnant or nursing a baby, seek the advice of a health professional before using this product. Keep this and all drugs out of reach of children. In case of accidental overdose, seek professional assistance or contact a poison control center immediately.

How Supplied: Phillips' Milk of Magnesia is available in regular and mint flavor in bottles of:
Regular
4 fl oz NDC 12843-353-01, 12 fl oz NDC 12843-353-02, 26 fl oz NDC 12843-353-03.
Mint
4 fl oz NDC 12843-363-04, 12 fl oz NDC 12843-363-05, 26 fl oz NDC 12843-363-06.
Also available in tablet form.

Shown in Product Identification Section, page 411

PHILLIPS'® MILK OF MAGNESIA TABLETS

Active Ingredients: Each Tablet contains 311 mg of magnesium hydroxide.

Inactive Ingredients: Flavor, starch, sucrose. Product description not USP.

Indications: For relief of acid indigestion, sour stomach, heartburn and occasional constipation (irregularity).

Actions: *At Laxative Dosage:* Phillips' Milk of Magnesia Tablets offer the same mild saline laxative ingredient as liquid Phillips' Milk of Magnesia in a convenient, chewable tablet form. It acts by drawing water into the gut, increasing intraluminal pressure, and increasing intestinal motility. This product generally produces bowel movement in ½ to 6 hours.

At Antacid Dosage: Phillips' Milk of Magnesia Tablets are effective acid neutralizers.

Administration and Dosage:
As an Antacid —Adults chew thoroughly 2 to 4 tablets up to 4 times a day. Children 7 to 14 years, 1 tablet up to 4 times a day or as directed by a physician.
As a Laxative —Adults and children 12 years of age and older chew thoroughly 6 to 8 tablets. Children 6 to 11, 3 to 4 tablets; children 2 to 5, 1 to 2 tablets, preferably before bedtime and follow with a full glass (8 oz) of liquid. Children under 2, consult a physician.

Laxative Warnings: Do not take any laxative if abdominal pain, nausea, vomiting, change in bowel habits (that persists for over 2 weeks), rectal bleeding, or kidney disease are present. Laxative products should not be used for a period longer than 1 week, unless directed by a doctor. If there is a failure to have a bowel movement after use, discontinue and consult your doctor.

Antacid Warnings: Do not take more than the maximum recommended daily dosage in a 24-hour period (see Directions), or use the maximum dosage of this product for more than two weeks, or use this product if you have kidney disease, except under the advice and supervision of a physician. May have laxative effect.

General Warnings: As with any drug, if you are pregnant or nursing a baby, seek the advice of a health professional before using this product. Keep this and *all* drugs out of reach of children. In case of accidental overdose, seek professional assistance or contact a poison control center immediately.

How Supplied: Phillips' Milk of Magnesia Tablets are available in a mint flavored chewable tablet in blister packs of: 24. NDC 12843-373-19, Bottle of 100. NDC 12843-373-12, Bottle of 200. NDC 12843-373-09.
Also available in liquid form.

Shown in Product Identification Section, page 411

STRI-DEX® REGULAR STRENGTH PADS and STRI-DEX® MAXIMUM STRENGTH PADS STRI-DEX® REGULAR STRENGTH BIG PADS STRI-DEX® MAXIMUM STRENGTH BIG PADS

Active Ingredients:
Stri-Dex® Regular Strength: Salicylic acid 0.5%, alcohol 28% by volume.
Stri-Dex® Maximum Strength: Salicylic acid 2.0%, SD alcohol 40 44% by volume.

Inactive Ingredients:
Stri-Dex® Regular Strength: Citric acid, fragrance, purified water, simethicone emulsion, sodium carbonate, sodium dodecylbenzenesulfonate, sodium xylenesulfonate.
Stri-Dex® Maximum Strength: Ammonium xylenesulfonate, citric acid, fragrance, purified water, simethicone emulsion, sodium carbonate, sodium dodecylbenzenesulfonate.

Indications: For the treatment of acne. Reduces the number of acne pimples and blackheads, and allows the skin to heal. Helps prevent new acne pimples from forming.

Directions: Cleanse the skin thoroughly before using medicated pad. Use the pad to wipe the entire affected area one to three times daily. Because excessive drying of the skin may occur, start with one application daily, then gradually increase to two or three times daily if needed or as directed by a doctor.

Warning: FOR EXTERNAL USE ONLY. Using other topical acne medications at the same time or immediately following use of this product may increase dryness or irritation of the skin. If this occurs, only one medication should be used unless directed by a doctor.
Persons with very sensitive skin or known allergy to salicylic acid should not use this medication. If irritation or excessive dryness and/or peeling occurs, reduce frequency of use or dosage. If excessive itching, dryness, redness, or swelling occurs, discontinue use. If these symptoms persist, consult a physician promptly.
Keep away from eyes, lips, and other mucous membranes. Keep this and all drugs out of reach of children. In the case of accidental ingestion, seek professional assistance or contact a Poison Control Center immediately.

Dosage and Administration: See Labeling instructions for use.

How Supplied:
Stri-Dex Regular Strength is available in NDC 12843-087-13—Porta-Pak Refillable Plastic container consisting of 12 pads, 2″ in diameter.
NDC 12843-087-07—Plastic jar consisting of 42 pads, 2″ in diameter.
NDC 12843-087-08—Plastic jar consisting of 75 pads, 2″ in diameter.
NDC 12843-087-04—Stri-Dex Big Pads in a plastic jar consisting of 42 pads, 2⅞″ in diameter.

Stri-Dex Maximum Strength is available in:
NDC 12843-097-12—Porta-Pak Refillable Plastic container consisting of 12 pads, 2″ in diameter.
NDC 12843-097-09—Plastic jar consisting of 42 pads, 2″ in diameter.
NDC 12843-097-11—Plastic jar consisting of 75 pads, 2″ in diameter.
NDC 12843-097-03—Stri-Dex Big Pads in a plastic jar consisting of 42 pads, 2⅞″ in diameter.
Shown in Product Identification Section, page 411

VANQUISH® Analgesic Caplets

Active Ingredients: Each caplet contains aspirin 227 mg, acetaminophen 194 mg, caffeine 33 mg, dried aluminum hydroxide gel 25 mg, magnesium hydroxide 50 mg.

Inactive Ingredients: Acacia, colloidal silicon dioxide, hydrogenated vegetable oil, microcrystalline cellulose, powdered cellulose, sodium lauryl sulfate, starch, talc.

Action and Uses: A buffered analgesic, antipyretic for relief of headache; muscular aches and pains; neuralgia and neuritic pain; toothache; pain following dental procedures; for painful discomforts and fever of colds and flu; sinusitis; functional menstrual pain, headache and pain due to cramps; temporary relief from minor pains of arthritis, rheumatism, bursitis, lumbago, sciatica.

Caution: If pain persists for more than 10 days, or redness is present or in conditions affecting children under 12 years of age, consult a physician immediately.

Warnings: Children and teenagers should not use this medicine for chicken pox or flu symptoms before a doctor is consulted about Reye syndrome, a rare but serious illness reported to be associated with aspirin. Keep this and all drugs out of the reach of children. In case of accidental overdose, seek professional assistance or contact a poison control center immediately. As with any drug, if you are pregnant or nursing a baby, seek the advice of a health professional before using this product.

Usual Adult Dosage: Two caplets with water. May be repeated every four hours if necessary up to 12 tablets per day. Larger or more frequent doses may be prescribed by physician if necessary.

Contraindications: Hypersensitivity to salicylates and acetaminophen. (To be used with caution during anticoagulant therapy or in asthmatic patients.)

How Supplied:
White, capsule-shaped caplets in bottles of:
  30 Caplets—NDC 12843-171-44
  60 Caplets—NDC 12843-171-46
100 Caplets—NDC 12843-171-48
Shown in Product Identification Section, page 411

Goldline Laboratories
The Wellspring Division
1900 W. COMMERCIAL BLVD.
FT. LAUDERDALE, FL
33309-3018

NOSE BETTER® Non-Greasy Aromatic Gel

Composition: A custom blend of allantoin 0.50%, camphor 0.75%, menthol 0.50%; also contains: eucalyptus oil, solubilized lanolin, Vitamin E, FD&C Blue #1, fragrance, excipients and stabilizers.

Actions: Dermatologist tested, this unique dual-action vanishing gel soothes and relieves discomfort and irritation under the nose and around and inside the nostrils. Its penetrating aromatic vapors are cooling, soothing and refreshing.

Indications: The gel soothes and relieves sore, tender nose—outside and in—due to head cold, allergy, sinus, chafed nose, chapped nose, dryness.

Directions For Use: Gently rub gel around and inside nostrils and under nose. Breathe in penetrating vapors. Use as often as needed. Note: an occasional momentary initial "smarting" may be overcome by an immediate liberal second application of the gel.

Warning: For external use only. Avoid contact with eyes. Do not use on children under three. If condition worsens or does not improve in 7 days, consult your physician. Keep this and all medicines out of the reach of children.

How Supplied: Available in 0.46 oz (13 g) tube.

NOSE BETTER® Natural Mist® Moisturizing Spray

Composition: A buffered isotonic aqueous saline solution of 1% glycerin/0.35% sodium chloride with benzalkonium chloride as preservative. Formulated with deionized water, this gentle Natural Mist nasal spray also contains: potassium phosphate, fragrance, disodium EDTA, hydroxypropyl methylcellulose, and sodium hydroxide.

Actions and Uses: The spray instantly moisturizes and soothes dry, irritated nasal passages and restores vital nasal moisture. Ends dry nose and helps make breathing more comfortable. Provides prompt relief from nasal dryness, discomfort and irritation due to: dry air (low humidity), dust, smoke, air pollution, air conditioning, winter home heat, high altitudes, travel, oxygen therapy and overuse of decongestant sprays.

Directions For Use: Spray 2 or 3 times in each nostril as often as needed.

How Supplied: Available in 1 Fl Oz (30 ml) plastic spray bottle.

Herald Pharmacal, Inc.
6503 WARWICK ROAD
RICHMOND, VA 23225

AQUA GLYCOLIC LOTION

Description: Aqua Glycolic lotion is a high-potency moisturizer containing 12 per cent partially neutralized Glycolic Acid in an unscented lanolin-free lotion base.

How Supplied: 8 oz. bottles.

AQUA GLYCOLIC SHAMPOO®

Description: Cosmetically elegant shampoo, non-irritating, containing Glycolic Acid, leaves hair soft, manageable, helps eliminate itching, leaves scalp free from scale.

How Supplied: 8 oz. bottles.

AQUA GLYDE CLEANSER®

Description: A cleanser for acne and other oily skin conditions. Contains special denatured alcohol #40, purified water, and Glycolic Acid.

How Supplied: 8 oz. plastic bottles.

AQUARAY® 20 SUNSCREEN

Description: AQUARAY Sunscreen is free of the sensitizing ingredients PABA, Padimate O, fragrance, lanolin and parabens. It offers a wide range of protection from both UVA and UVB sun rays.

How Supplied: 4 fl. oz. bottles.

CAM LOTION®

Description: Lipid-free, soap-free skin cleanser for atopic dermatitis and other diseases aggravated by oily, greasy substances of animal and vegetable origin.

How Supplied: 8 and 16 oz. bottles.

Herbert Laboratories
2525 DUPONT DRIVE
IRVINE, CA 92715

AQUATAR®
Therapeutic Tar Gel

Active Ingredient: BioTar™ (coal tar extract—biologically active) 2.5%. **Inactive Ingredients:** DEA-oleth-3 phosphate; glycerin; imidurea; methylparaben; mineral oil; oleth-3; oleth-10; oleth-20; poloxamer 407; polysorbate 80; propylparaben; and purified water.

How Supplied: 3 oz tube.

BLUBORO® Powder
Astringent Soaking Solution

Active Ingredients: Aluminum sulfate 53.9% and calcium acetate 43%. **Inactive Ingredients:** boric acid and FD&C Blue No. 1.

Continued on next page

Herbert—Cont.

How Supplied: 12-packet carton, 100-packet carton (0.06 oz/packet).

DANEX®
Protein-Enriched Dandruff Shampoo

Active Ingredient: Pyrithione zinc 1%.

How Supplied: 4 oz bottle.

PHOTOPLEX®
Broad Spectrum Sunscreen Lotion
● **Contains Parsol® 1789: Absorbs Throughout the UVA Spectrum**
● **SPF 15+ UVB Protection**

Active Ingredients:
Avobenzone (Parsol®* 1789) 3.0%
Padimate O 7.0%
(octyl dimethyl p -aminobenzoic acid)

Inactive Ingredients: Benzyl alcohol; carbomer 934P; cetyl esters wax; edetate disodium; glycerin; imidurea; mineral oil (light); oleth-3 phosphate; purified water; stearyl alcohol (and) cetareth-20 and white petrolatum. May contain sodium hydroxide or hydrochloric acid to adjust pH.
NOTE: Store at room temperature. Protect from freezing.

Indications: Photoplex® Broad Spectrum Sunscreen Lotion provides protection from acute and long-term risks associated with UVA and UVB light exposure. Photoplex screens out the sun's burning rays to prevent sunburn. Overexposure to the sun may lead to premature aging of the skin and skin cancer. The liberal and regular use over the years of this product may help reduce the chance of these harmful effects.

Warnings: Do not use if sensitive to benzocaine, sulfonamides, aniline dyes, aminobenzoic acid (PABA) or related compounds or any other ingredient to this product. Use on children under six months of age only with the advice of physician.
For external use only. Avoid contact with eyes, eyelids and mouth. If contact with eyes occur, rinse thoroughly with water. Should skin irritation or rash develop, discontinue use. If irritation or rash persists, consult physician. Keep out of the reach of children. In case of accidental ingestion, seek professional assistance or contact a Poison Control Center immediately.

Caution: Photoplex Sunscreen Lotion may stain some fabrics.

Directions: Shake well before using. Prior to sun exposure, apply liberally and evenly over areas to be protected. To maintain maximal protection, reapply after 40 minutes in the water or after excessive perspiration. There is no recommended dosage for children under six months of age except under the advice and supervision of a physician.

How Supplied: Bottles of 4 oz. and 6 oz.

*Parsol® is a registered trademark of the Givaudan Corp.

VANSEB® Cream and Lotion Dandruff Shampoos

Active Ingredients: Salicylic acid 1% and sulfur 2%. **Inactive Ingredients:** Cocamide DEA.

How Supplied: 3 oz tube, 4 oz bottle.

VANSEB–T® Cream and Lotion Tar Dandruff Shampoos

Active Ingredients: Coal tar solution USP 5%; salicylic acid 1%; sulfur 2%. **Inactive Ingredients:** cocamide DEA.

How Supplied: 3 oz tube, 4 oz bottle.

Hoechst-Roussel Pharmaceuticals Inc.
SOMERVILLE, NJ 08876-1258

DOXIDAN®
Stimulant/Stool Softener Laxative

Ingredients: Each Liquigel™ contains 65 mg yellow phenolphthalein USP, 60 mg docusate calcium USP, and the following inactive ingredients: alcohol USP up to 1.5% (w/w), corn oil NF, FD&C Blue #1 and Red #40, gelatin NF, glycerin USP, hydrogenated vegetable oil NF, lecithin NF, parabens NF, sorbitol NF, titanium dioxide USP, vegetable shortening, yellow wax NF, and other ingredients.

Indications: Doxidan is a safe, reliable laxative for the relief of occasional constipation. The combination of a stimulant/stool softener laxative allows positive laxative action on a softened stool for gentle evacuation without straining. Doxidan generally produces a bowel movement in 6 to 12 hours. Doxidan may be of particular benefit when stool softening alone is insufficient and as an adjunct to bowel retraining.
SURGICAL AFTERCARE: Doxidan is useful in both pre- and post-operative conditions that require gentle peristaltic stimulation.
OBSTETRICS: The gentle, effective laxative action of Doxidan is useful in prenatal and postpartum patients where straining at stool is to be avoided.
GERIATRICS: Dietary changes, decreased physical activity and the use of certain drugs often contribute to constipation in the elderly patient.
Doxidan promotes a gentle laxation and eliminates the need for harsh cathartics.
ANORECTAL CONDITIONS: Doxidan contains an effective stool softener laxative that facilitates the passage of softened stools and their elimination from the rectum in patients with proctologic problems.

Warnings: Do not use when abdominal pain, nausea, or vomiting is present unless directed by a doctor. If you have no-

ticed a sudden change in bowel habits that persists over a period of 2 weeks, consult a doctor before using a laxative. Do not use for a period longer than 1 week unless directed by a doctor. Rectal bleeding or failure to have a bowel movement after use may indicate a serious condition. Discontinue use and consult your doctor. Occasional cramping may occur. If skin rash appears, do not use this product or any other preparation containing phenolphthalein. As with any drug, if you are pregnant or nursing a baby, seek the advice of a health professional before using this product.
Keep this and all medication out of the reach of children. In case of accidental overdose, seek professional assistance or contact a poison control center immediately.

Usual Dosage: Adults and children 12 years of age and over, one or two Liquigels by mouth daily. For use in children under 12 consult a physician. Store at controlled room temperature (59°–86°F) in a dry place.

How Supplied: Packages of 10, 30, 100 and 1,000 maroon Liquigels, and Unit Dose 100s (10 × 10 strips).
Liquigel TM R. P. Scherer
Doxidan REG TM Hoechst-Roussel
Manufactured by R. P. Scherer, Clearwater, FL, expressly for Hoechst-Roussel Pharmaceuticals Inc.
Shown in Product Identification Section, page 411

FESTAL® II
Digestive Aid

Composition: Each film-coated tablet contains lipase 6,000 USP units, amylase 30,000 USP units, protease 20,000 USP units and the following inactive ingredients: colloidal silicon dioxide NF, methacrylic acid copolymer NF, microcrystalline cellulose NF, opaque black, pharmaceutical glaze, polyethylene glycol NF, povidone USP, sodium chloride USP, sodium hydroxide NF, talc USP and titanium dioxide USP.

Actions and Uses: Festal® II provides a high degree of protected digestive activity in a formula of standardized enzymes. Enteric coating of the tablet prevents release of ingredients in the stomach so that high enzymatic potency is delivered to the site in the intestinal tract where digestion normally takes place.
Festal® II is indicated in any condition where normal digestion is impaired by insufficiency of natural digestive enzymes, or when additional digestive enzymes may be beneficial. These conditions often manifest complaints of discomfort due to excess intestinal gas, such as bloating, cramps and flatulence. The following are conditions or situations where Festal® II may be helpful: pancreatic insufficiency, chronic pancreatitis, pancreatic necrosis, and removal of gas prior to x-ray examination.
Keep this and all medication out of the reach of children.

Dosage: Usual adult dose is one or two tablets with each meal, or as directed by a physician. Store at controlled room temperature (59°–86°F). Store in a well-closed container in a dry place.

Contraindications: Festal® II should not be given to patients sensitive to protein of porcine origin.

How Supplied: Bottles of 100 and 500 white, film-coated enteric-coated tablets for oral use.
Festal REG TM Hoechst AG
Shown in Product Identification Section, page 411

SURFAK®
Stool Softener

Ingredients: Each 240 mg Liquigel™ contains 240 mg docusate calcium USP, alcohol USP up to 3% (w/w) and the following inactive ingredients: corn oil NF, FD&C Blue #1 and Red #40 gelatin NF, glycerin USP, parabens NF, sorbitol NF and other ingredients.
Each 50 mg Liquigel™ contains 50 mg docusate calcium USP, alcohol USP up to 1.3% (w/w) and the following inactive ingredients: corn oil NF, FD&C Red #3, and Red #40, gelatin NF, glycerin USP, parabens NF, sorbitol NF, soybean oil USP and other ingredients.

Actions: Surfak provides homogenization and formation of soft, easily evacuated stools without disturbance of body physiology, discomfort of bowel distention or oily leakage. Surfak is non-habit forming.

Indications: Surfak is indicated for the prevention and treatment of constipation in conditions in which hard stools may cause discomfort. Surfak is useful in patients who require only stool softening without propulsive action to accomplish defecation. Surfak does not cause peristaltic stimulation, and because of its safety it may be effectively used in patients with heart conditions, anorectal conditions, obstetrical patients, following surgical procedures, ulcerative colitis, diverticulitis and bedridden patients.

Warnings: Surfak has no known side effects or disadvantages, except for the unusual occurrence of mild, transitory cramping pains. If cramping pain occurs, discontinue the medication. As with any drug, if you are pregnant or nursing a baby, seek the advice of a health professional before using this product. Keep this and all medication out of reach of children.

Overdosage: Overdosage does not lead to systemic toxicity.

Dosage and Administration: Adults —one red 240 mg Liquigel by mouth daily for several days or until bowel movements are normal. Children and adults with minimal needs—one to three orange 50 mg Liquigels daily. For use in children under 6, consult a physician.

How Supplied: 240 mg red Liquigels—packages of 7 and 30, bottles of 100 and 500, and Unit Dose 100s (10 × 10

strips); 50 mg orange Liquigels—bottles of 30 and 100.
Store at controlled room temperature (59°–86°F) in a dry place.
Liquigel REG TM R.P. Scherer
Manufactured by R.P. Scherer, Clearwater, FL, expressly for Hoechst-Roussel Pharmaceuticals Inc.
Shown in Product Identification Section, page 411

EDUCATIONAL MATERIAL

Changes, Cycles and Constipation
Pamphlet describing constipation and its causes, with instructions on prevention and self-treatment, and when to consult a physician (English and Spanish).
What You Should Know About Hemorrhoids and Fissures
Pamphlet describing these conditions, with instructions on self-care and when to consult a physician (English and Spanish).

ICN Pharmaceuticals, Inc.
**ICN PLAZA
3300 HYLAND AVENUE
COSTA MESA, CA 92626**

INSTA–GLUCOSE
[*n-sta glū-cose*]
Liquid Glucose

Active Ingredient: Liquid Glucose NF, 30 grams. Each 31 g tube contains 24 g carbohydrate.

Indications: For relief from insulin reaction and hypoglycemia, Insta-Glucose is readily absorbed into the bloodstream from the digestive tract. The liquid gel is pleasant tasting and easy to swallow.

Dosage and Administration: The recommended dosage is one entire 31 g unit dose tube of Insta-Glucose (24 g carbohydrate). One tube will usually treat a mild to moderate insulin reaction. Notify your physician of hypoglycemic episodes.

How Supplied: Three 31 g unit dose tubes in a Tri-Pak container. 5-year shelf life.
Shown in Product Identification Section, page 411

IDENTIFICATION PROBLEM?
Consult the
Product Identification Section
where you'll find
products pictured
in full color.

Inter-Cal Corporation
**421 MILLER VALLEY RD.
PRESCOTT, AZ 86301**

ESTER–C®
(Calcium Ascorbate)

Description: Each Ester-C tablet contains 500 mg Vitamin C in the form of Calcium Ascorbate 550 mg, vegetable-derived cellulose, stearic acid, and magnesium stearate. Ester-C contains no preservatives, sugars, artificial colorings, or flavorings.
As the calcium salt of L-ascorbic acid, Ester-C has an empirical formula of $CaC_{12}H_{14}O_{12}$ and a formula weight of 390.3.

Actions: Vitamin C has been found to be essential for the prevention of scurvy. In humans, an exogenous source of the vitamin is required for collagen formation and tissue repair. Ascorbate ion is reversibly oxidized to dehydroascorbate ion in the body. Both of these are active forms of the vitamin and are considered to play important roles in biochemical oxidation-reduction reactions. The vitamin is involved in tyrosine metabolism, carbohydrate metabolism, iron metabolism, folic acid-folinic acid conversion, synthesis of lipids and proteins, resistance to infections, and cellular respiration.

Indications and Usage: Vitamin C and its salts, such as Calcium Ascorbate, are recommended as nutritional supplements in the prevention of scurvy. In scurvy, collagenous structures are primarily affected, and lesions develop in blood vessels and bones. Symptoms of mild deficiency may include faulty development of teeth and bones, bleeding gums, gingivitis, and loose teeth. An increased need for the vitamin exists in febrile states, chronic illness and infection, e.g., rheumatic fever, pneumonia, tuberculosis, whooping cough, diphtheria, sinusitis, etc. Additional increases in the daily intake of ascorbate are indicated in burns, delayed healing of bone fractures and wounds, and hemovascular disorders. Immature and premature infants require relatively larger amounts of Vitamin C.

Contraindications: Because of its calcium content, Ester-C is contraindicated in hypercalcemic states, e.g., from dosing with parathyroid hormone or overdosage of Vitamin D.
Diabetics, persons prone to recurrent renal calculi, those undergoing stool occult blood tests, and those on anticoagulant therapy should not take excessive doses of Vitamin C over extended periods of time.

Precautions: Because of its calcium content, Ester-C should be used with caution by those undergoing treatment with digitalis or cardiotonic glycosides such as digitoxin and digoxin.
Laboratory Tests—Diabetics taking more than 500 mg of Vitamin C may gen-

Continued on next page

Inter-Cal—Cont.

erate false readings in their urinary glucose tests. To avoid false-negative results, forms of the vitamin should not be taken as supplements for 48 to 72 hours before amine-dependent stool occult blood tests are conducted.

Drug Interactions—There is limited evidence suggesting that Vitamin C may influence the intensity and duration of action of bishydroxycoumarin.

Usage in Pregnancy—Pregnancy Category C—Animal reproduction studies have not been carried out with Ester-C tablets. It is also not known whether Ester-C can cause fetal harm when administered to a pregnant woman or can affect reproductive capacity.

Nursing Mothers—Caution should be exercised when Ester-C tablets are recommended for nursing mothers.

Adverse Reactions: There are no known adverse reactions following ingestion of Ester-C tablets. The gastric disturbances characteristic of the large doses of ascorbic acid are absent or greatly diminished when the pH-neutral form of calcium ascorbate present in Ester-C tablets is utilized as the source of Vitamin C supplementation.

Dosage and Administration: The minimum U.S. Recommended Daily Allowance for Vitamin C for the prevention of diseases such as scurvy is 60 mg per day. Optimum daily allowances, e.g., for the maintenance of increased plasma and cellular reserves, are significantly greater. For adults, the recommended average preventative dose of the vitamin is 70 to 150 mg daily. The recommended average optimum dose of Ester-C is 550 to 1650 mg (1 to 3 tablets) daily.

For frank scurvy, doses of 300 mg to one gram of Vitamin C daily have been recommended. Normal adults, however, have received as much as six grams of the vitamin without evidence of toxicity.

For enhancement of wound healing, doses of the vitamin approximating two Ester-C tablets daily for a week or ten days both preoperatively and postoperatively are generally considered adequate, although considerably larger amounts may be recommended. In the treatment of burns, the daily number of Ester-C tablets recommended is governed by the extent of tissue injury. For severe burns, daily doses of 2 to 4 tablets (approximately one to two grams of Vitamin C) are recommended.

In other conditions in which the need for increased Vitamin C is recognized, three to five times the optimum allowance appears to be adequate.

How Supplied: 550 mg tablets of Ester-C in plastic bottles of 100, 250, 90, and 225's. 4 oz. and 8 oz. powders, 275 mg tablet also available.
Store at room temperature.
U.S. Patent granted April 18, 1989; No. 4,822,816.

Literature revised: December, 1989.
    Mfd. by Inter-Cal Corp.
      Prescott, AZ 86301

Jackson-Mitchell Pharmaceuticals, Inc.
P.O. BOX 5425
SANTA BARBARA, CA 93150

MEYENBERG GOAT MILK
[my'en-berg]
Concentrated liquid • powder

Composition: A natural, mammalian milk more closely related to the structure of human milk than cow milk. Does not contain alpha S_1 casein. More easily digested.
Standard dilution (adults and babies over 6 months) supplies 20 calories/fl oz). EVAPORATED supplemented with folic acid and Vitamin D. POWDER, folic acid only.
NOTE: *Not a complete formula.* Vitamin supplement recommended if sole source of nutrition.

Action and Uses: For cow milk and/or soy milk sensitive adults and children.

Preparation: Adults—20 calories/fl oz with concentrated liquid—1 part to 1 part water. Refrigerate. Baby Formula—should be refrigerated and used within 48 hours.

MEYENBERG Evaporated GOAT MILK Fortified with Folic Acid and Vitamin D

	Evap. Milk	Water	Calories Fl. Oz.*
First or transitional dilution	1 part	2 parts	14
Standard dilution	1 part	1 part	20

*Increase calorie value as desired by the addition of a carbohydrate.

MEYENBERG Powdered GOAT MILK Fortified with Folic Acid

RECOMMENDED FOR BABIES OVER 1 YEAR BECAUSE OF FLAVOR

	Pwdr. Milk	Water	Calories Fl. Oz.*
Standard dilution	1 Tbsp.	2 Fl. Oz.	20

EDUCATIONAL MATERIAL

Is It Really Milk Allergy?
Brochure.
Meyenberg Story
Brochure.

Products are cross-indexed by generic and chemical names in the
YELLOW SECTION

Johnson & Johnson
Consumer Products, Inc
GRANDVIEW ROAD
SKILLMAN, NJ 08558

JOHNSON'S BABY SUNBLOCK
Ultra Sunblock (SPF 15) Cream
Ultra Sunblock (SPF 15) Lotion
Ultra Sunblock (SPF 30+) Lotion

Active Ingredients: Octyl Methoxycinnamate, Octyl Salicylate, Oxybenzone, Titanium Dioxide.

Inactive Ingredients: CREAM—Barium Sulfate, Benzyl Alcohol, Carbomer, Cetyl Alcohol, Dimethicone, Dioctyl Maleate, Disodium EDTA, Fragrance, Glycerin, Isopropyl Isostearate, Methyl Glucose Sesquistearate, Methylparaben, Propylene Glycol, Propylparaben, PVP/Eicosene Copolymer, Quaternium-15, Stearic Acid, Triethanolamine, Water.
LOTIONS—BHT, C12 –15 Alcohols Benzoate, Carbomer, Cetyl Alcohol, DEA-Cetyl Phosphate, Dimethicone, Dioctyl Sodium Sulfosuccinate, Disodium EDTA, Fragrance, Glyceryl Dilaurate, Isopropyl Isostearate, Isopropyl PPG-2-Isodeceth-7-Carboxylate, Isostearic Acid, Propylene Glycol, Quaternium-15, Simethicone, Tocopheryl Acetate, Water and other ingredients.

Indications: JOHNSON'S BABY SUNBLOCK products provide gentle effective protection. The PABA-free lotions and cream formulas each provide 15 and 30 times a child's natural sunburn protection, respectively. All are waterproof, providing protection for at least 80 minutes in water, and resist removal by sweating. Liberal and regular use of a sunblock (at least SPF 15) until age 18 can reduce the risk of skin cancer by 78%.

Actions: Blocks out ultraviolet rays (UVA and UVB).

Warning: For external use only. AVOID CONTACT WITH EYES. Should temporary stinging and tearing occur through accidental contact, thoroughly rinse eyes with water. Discontinue use if signs of irritation or rash appear. Use on children under six months of age only with the advice of a physician. Keep out of reach of children.

Dosage and Administration: Shake well. Apply generously and evenly to all exposed areas 30 minutes before sun exposure. Reapply after prolonged swimming or excessive perspiration.

How Supplied: Lotions in 4 fl. oz. plastic bottles; Cream in 2 oz. tube.
Shown in Product Identification Section, page 411

PURPOSE™ Dual Treatment Moisturizer With Sunscreen (SPF 12)

Active Ingredients: Octyl Methoxycinnamate, Oxybenzone.

Inactive Ingredients: Water, Glycerin, Cetyl Phosphate, DEA-Cetyl Phosphate, Cetyl Palmitate, Dimethicone, Stearoxytrimethylsilane, Octyl Stearate, Mineral Oil, Stearyl Alcohol, Cetyl Alcohol, Glyceryl Cocoate, Hydrogenated Coconut Oil, Ceteareth-25, Carbomer, Benzyl Alcohol, Methylparaben, Propylparaben, Disodium EDTA, Fragrance, Quaternium 15, BHT.

Indications: PURPOSE Dual Treatment Moisturizer with Sunscreen is a light, greaseless facial moisturizer with the added benefit of PABA-free sunscreens. This formula was created to allow for everyday sun protection as a part of a morning facial moisturizing routine. To this end, the PURPOSE formula is exceptionally cosmetically elegant and is particularly acceptable for under makeup base.

Warnings: For external use only. Avoid contact with eyes. Keep out of reach of children. Discontinue use if signs of irritation or rash appear.

Administration and Dosage: Apply daily under makeup or by itself.

How Supplied: Lotion in a 4 fluid ounce glass bottle (fragrance-free and lightly scented).

PURPOSE® Gentle Cleansing Soap

Ingredients: Sodium tallowate, Sodium cocoate, Water, Glycerin, Fragrance, Sodium chloride, BHT, Trisodium HEDTA, D&C Yellow No. 10, D&C Orange No. 4.

Indications: Mild PURPOSE Soap was created to wash tender, sensitive skin. Formulated especially to meet the need for a mild soap that dermatologists can recommend. This translucent washing bar is nonmedicated and free of harsh detergents or other ingredients that might dry or irritate skin.

Administration and Dosage: Wash face with PURPOSE Soap two or three times a day or as directed by your physician. Rinse with warm water. For complete skin care, use it also for bath and shower.

How Supplied: 3.6 oz. and 6 oz. bars.

SUNDOWN® SUNSCREENS
**Maximal Protection (SPF 8) LOTION
Ultra Protection (SPF 15) LOTION,
CREAM, STICK, and COMBI PACK
Ultra Protection (SPF 20) LOTION
Ultra Protection (SPF 25) LOTION
Ultra Protection (SPF 30+) LOTION
and STICK**

LOTIONS AND CREAM
Active Ingredients:
SPF 8, 15, 20, 25 and 30+: Octyl Methoxycinnamate, Octyl Salicylate, Oxybenzone, Titanium Dioxide.
Inactive Ingredients:
SPF 8, 15, 20, 25 and 30+ Lotions: BHT C12–15 Alcohols Benzoate, Carbomer, Cetyl Alcohol, DEA-Cetyl Phosphate, Dimethicone, Dioctyl Sodium Sulfosuccinate, Disodium EDTA, Fragrance, Glyceryl Dilaurate, Isopropyl Isostearate, Isopropyl PPG-2-Isodeceth-7-Carboxylate, Isostearic Acid, Propylene Glycol, Qua-

ternium-15, Simethicone, Tocopheryl Acetate, Water and other ingredients.
SPF 15 Cream: BHT C12–15 Alcohols Benzoate, Carbomer, Cetyl Alcohol, DEA-Cetyl Phosphate, Dimethicone, Dioctyl Sodium Sulfosuccinate, Dioctyl Maleate, Disodium EDTA, Fragrance, Glycerin, Glyceryl Dilaurate, Isopropyl PPG-2-Isodeceth-7- Carboxylate, Propylene Glycol, Quaternium-15, Simethicone, Stearyl Alcohol, Triethanolamine, Tocopheryl Acetate, Water and other ingredients.

STICKS
Active Ingredients:
SPF 15 and 30+: Octyl Methoxycinnamate, Octyl Salicylate, Oxybenzone.
Inactive Ingredients:
C12–15 Alcohols Benzoate, C18–36 Acid Glycol Ester, C18–36 Triglyceride, Dioctyl Maleate, Hydrogenated Castor Oil, Petrolatum, Phenoxyethanol, Synthetic Beeswax.

Indications: Sunscreens help prevent harmful effects from the sun. The SPF values designate that the products provide 8, 15, 20, 25 and 30+, times your natural sunburn protection, respectively. SPF 8 permits minimal tanning and SPF 15, 20, 25 and 30+ permit no tanning. Liberal and regular use may help reduce the chance of premature skin aging, skin wrinkling and skin cancer due to overexposure to the sun.

Actions: Blocks out ultraviolet rays (UVA and UVB).

Warning: For external use only. AVOID CONTACT WITH EYES. Should temporary stinging and tearing occur through accidental contact, thoroughly rinse eyes with water. Discontinue use if signs of irritation or rash appear. Use on children under six months of age only with the advice of a physician. Keep out of reach of children.

Dosage and Administration:
CREAM and LOTIONS: Shake well. For all products, apply generously and evenly to all exposed areas 30 minutes before sun exposure. Reapply after prolonged swimming or excessive perspiration.

How Supplied: LOTIONS in 4 fl. oz. plastic bottles; STICKS in 0.35 oz. sticks; CREAM in 2.0 oz. tube; COMBI PACK: Stick 0.04 oz; cream 0.70 oz.

Shown in Product Identification Section, page 411

IDENTIFICATION PROBLEM?
Consult the
Product Identification Section
where you'll find
products pictured
in full color.

Kremers Urban Company

See SCHWARZ PHARMA.

Lactaid Inc.
P.O. BOX 111
PLEASANTVILLE, NJ
08232-0111

LACTAID®
[lăkt′ād]
Lactaid Drops
and
Lactaid Caplets
(lactase enzyme)

PRODUCT OVERVIEW

Key Facts: Lactaid® lactase enzyme hydrolyzes lactose into digestible sugars: glucose and galactose. Lactaid Drops are added to milk for *in vitro* treatment; Lactaid Caplets are taken orally for *in vivo* hydrolysis.

Major Uses: Lactaid lactase enzyme (liquid and caplets) have proven to be clinically effective for lactose-intolerant people when consuming milk and/or dairy foods, by permitting consumption of lactose-containing foods without gas, cramps, bloating and/or diarrhea.

Safety Information: Lactaid enzyme should be discontinued in anyone who develops hypersensitivity to the enzyme.

PRESCRIBING INFORMATION
LACTAID®
[lăkt′ād]
Lactaid Drops
and
Lactaid Caplets
(lactase enzyme)

Description:
Drops: Each 5 drop dosage contains not less than 1250 NLU (Neutral Lactase Units) of Beta-D-galactosidase derived from *Kluyveromyces lactis* yeast. The enzyme is in a liquid carrier of glycerol (50%), water (30%), and inert yeast dry matter (20%). 5 drops hydrolyze approximately 70% of the lactose in 1 quart of milk at refrigerator temperature, at 43°F (6°C) in 24 hours, or will do the same in 2 hours at 85°F (30°C). Additional time and/or enzyme required for 100% lactose conversion. 1 U.S. quart of milk will contain approximately 50 g lactose prior to lactose hydrolysis and will contain 15 g or less, after 70% conversion.

Action: Hydrolysis converts the lactose into its simple sugar components: glucose and galactose.

Indications: Lactase insufficiency in the patient, suspected from GI disturbances after consumption of milk or milk-content products: e.g., bloat, distension, flatulence, diarrhea; or identified by a lactose tolerance test.

Continued on next page

Lactaid—Cont.

Usage: Added to milk. 5–15 drops per quart of milk depending on level of lactose conversion desired.

Other Uses: *In vivo* activity has been demonstrated, indicating usage in tube feedings and other lactose-content solid and liquid foods, with addition at time of consumption.

How Supplied: Lactase enzyme in a stable liquid form, in sales units of 12, 30 and 75 one-quart dosages at 5 drops per dose.

Caplets: Each caplet contains not less than 3000 FCC lactase units of Beta-D-Galactosidase from *Aspergillus oryzae.* One to two caplets taken with a meal will normally handle a lactose challenge equal to 1 glass of milk. In severe cases, 3 caplets may be required.

Toxicity: None.

Drug Interactions: None. Both liquid and tablets are classified as food, not drugs.

Warnings: Should hypersensitivity occur, discontinue use.

Precautions: Diabetics should be aware that the milk sugar will now be metabolically available and must be taken into account (17.5 g glucose and 17.5 g galactose per quart at 70% hydrolysis). No reports received of any diabetics' reactions. Galactosemics may not have milk in any form, lactase enzyme modified or not.

Adverse Reactions: The most frequently reported adverse reactions to Lactaid lactase caplets are gastrointestinal in nature, sometimes mimicking the symptoms of lactose intolerance. No reactions of any kind observed from Lactaid liquid drops. Total reactions to caplets estimated at under 0.1 ($\frac{1}{10}$) % of users.

How Supplied: In bottles of 100, bottles of 12 and boxes of 25 2-caplet "take along" packets.

Other Lactose Reduced Products: In most areas of the U.S.: Fresh lactose reduced lowfat milk from dairies, ready to drink, sold in food markets. Lactose hydrolysis level: 70%. If desired, further conversion of the dairy-treated milk can be done at home or institution with the Lactaid liquid enzyme. Also in some areas: Lactaid lactose reduced cottage cheese and American process cheese.
Any person or institution unable to locate Lactaid enzyme locally can order direct from Lactaid Inc. retail or wholesale. Samples and full product information to doctors, institutions and nutritionists on request.
Call toll-free 1-800-257-8650.
Shown in Product Identification
Section, page 411

EDUCATIONAL MATERIAL

Brochures
Patient brochure—"Why Lactaid? The Problem with Milk and the Answer"

Professional brochure—"Lactaid Specially Digestible Milk and Dairy Products as Part of a Nutritional Program"

Samples
Dispensing samples of Lactaid Caplets and Lactaid Drops.

PATIENT STARTER KITS

Contains patient brochure, 12 Lactaid Caplets and Lactaid Drops for treating 4 quarts of milk.
All literature, samples and patient starter kits are available free to physicians and dietitians.

Lakeside Pharmaceuticals
Division of Merrell Dow Pharmaceuticals Inc.
CINCINNATI, OH 45242-9553

CĒPACOL®/CĒPACOL MINT
[*sē'pǝ-cŏl*]
Mouthwash/Gargle

Description: Cēpacol Mouthwash contains: Ceepryn® (cetylpyridinium chloride) 0.05%. Also contains: Alcohol 14%, Edetate Disodium, FD&C Yellow No. 5 (tartrazine) as a color additive, Flavors, Glycerin, Polysorbate 80, Saccharin, Sodium Biphosphate, Sodium Phosphate, and Water.
Cēpacol Mint Mouthwash contains: Ceepryn® (cetylpyridinium chloride) 0.05%. Also contains: Alcohol 14.5%, D&C Yellow No. 10, FD&C Green No. 3, Flavor, Glucono Delta-Lactone, Glycerin, Poloxamer 407, Saccharin Sodium, Sodium Gluconate, and Water.

Actions: Cēpacol/Cēpacol Mint is a soothing, pleasant-tasting mouthwash/gargle. It kills germs that cause bad breath for a fresher, cleaner mouth. Cēpacol/Cēpacol Mint has a low surface tension, approximately ½ that of water. This property is the basis of the spreading action in the oral cavity as well as its foaming action. Cēpacol/Cēpacol Mint leaves the mouth feeling fresh and clean and helps provide soothing, temporary relief of dryness and minor mouth irritations.

Uses: Recommended as a mouthwash and gargle for daily oral care; as an aromatic mouth freshener to provide a clean feeling in the mouth; as a soothing, foaming rinse to freshen the mouth.
Used routinely before dental procedures, helps give patient confidence of not offending with mouth odor. Often employed as a foaming and refreshing rinse before, during, and after instrumentation and dental prophylaxis. Convenient as a mouth-freshening agent after taking dental impressions. Helpful in reducing the unpleasant taste and odor in the mouth following gingivectomy.
Used in hospitals as a mouthwash and gargle for daily oral care. Also used to refresh and soothe the mouth following emesis, inhalation therapy, and intuba-

tions, and for swabbing the mouths of patients incapable of personal care.

Warning: Keep out of the reach of children.

Directions for Use: Rinse vigorously before or after brushing or any time to freshen the mouth. Particularly useful after meals or before social engagements. Cēpacol/Cēpacol Mint leaves the mouth feeling refreshingly clean.
Use full strength every two or three hours as a soothing, foaming gargle, or as directed by a physician or dentist. May also be mixed with warm water.
Product label directions are as follows: Use full strength. Rinse mouth thoroughly before or after brushing or whenever desired or use as directed by a physician or dentist.

How Supplied:
Cēpacol Mouthwash: 12 oz, 18 oz, 24 oz, and 32 oz.
4 oz Hospital Bedside Bottles (not for retail sale), 4 oz trial size.
Cēpacol Mint Mouthwash: 12 oz, 18 oz, 24 oz, and 32 oz, 4 oz trial size.
Shown in Product Identification
Section, page 412

CĒPACOL®
[*sē'pǝ-cŏl*]
Throat Lozenges

Description: Each lozenge contains Ceepryn® (cetylpyridinium chloride) 0.07%, Benzyl Alcohol 0.3%. Also contains: FD&C Yellow No. 5 (tartrazine) as a color additive, Flavor, Glucose, and Sucrose.

Actions: Cetylpyridinium chloride (Ceepryn) is a cationic quaternary ammonium compound, which is a surface-active agent. Aqueous solutions of cetylpyridinium chloride have a surface tension lower than that of water.
Cetylpyridinium chloride in the concentration used in Cēpacol is nonirritating to tissues.

Indications: Cēpacol Lozenges stimulate salivation to help provide soothing temporary relief of dryness and minor irritations of mouth and sore throat and resulting cough.

Warnings: Severe sore throat or sore throat accompanied by high fever, headache, nausea, or vomiting, or any sore throat or mouth irritations persisting more than 2 days may be serious. Consult a physician promptly. Persons with a high fever or persistent cough should not use this preparation unless directed by a physician. Do not administer to children under 6 years of age unless directed by a physician or dentist. If sensitive to any of the ingredients, do not use. Keep this and all drugs out of the reach of children. In case of accidental overdose, seek professional assistance or contact a Poison Control Center immediately. As with any drug, if you are pregnant or nursing a baby, seek the advice of a health professional before using this product.

Dosage and Administration: Adults and children 6 years and older, dissolve

1 lozenge in the mouth every 2 hours, if needed. For children under 6 years, consult a physician or dentist.

How Supplied:
Trade Package: 18 lozenges in 2 pocket packs of 9 each.
Professional Package: 648 lozenges in 72 blisters of 9 each.
Store at room temperature, 59°–86°F (15°–30°C). Protect contents from humidity.

Shown in Product Identification Section, page 412

CĒPACOL®
[sē ′pǝ-cŏl]
Anesthetic Lozenges (Troches)

Description: Each lozenge contains Benzocaine 10 mg, Ceepryn® (cetylpyridinium chloride) 0.07%. Also contains: FD&C Blue No. 1, FD&C Yellow No. 5 (tartrazine) as a color additive, Flavors, Glucose, and Sucrose.

Actions: Cetylpyridinium chloride (Ceepryn) is a cationic quaternary ammonium compound, which is a surface-active agent. Aqueous solutions of cetylpyridinium chloride have a surface tension lower than that of water.
Cetylpyridinium chloride in the concentration used in Cēpacol is nonirritating to tissues.
Cēpacol Anesthetic Lozenges stimulate salivation to relieve dryness of the mouth and provide a mild anesthetic effect for pain relief.

Indications: *Sore Throat:* For prompt, temporary relief of pain and discomfort due to minor sore throat. For temporary relief of minor pain and discomfort associated with tonsillitis and pharyngitis. *Mouth Irritations:* For prompt, temporary relief of pain and discomfort due to minor mouth irritations. For temporary relief of discomfort associated with stomatitis. For adjunctive, temporary relief of minor pain and discomfort following periodontal procedures and minor surgery of the mouth.

Warnings: Severe sore throat or sore throat accompanied by high fever, headache, nausea, or vomiting, or any sore throat or mouth irritation persisting more than 2 days may be serious. Consult a physician promptly. Persons with a high fever or persistent cough should not use this preparation unless directed by a physician. Do not administer to children under 6 years of age unless directed by physician or dentist. If sensitive to any of the ingredients, do not use. As with any drug, if you are pregnant or nursing a baby, seek the advice of a health professional before using this product. Keep this and all drugs out of the reach of children. In case of accidental overdose, seek professional assistance or contact a Poison Control Center immediately.

Dosage and Administration: Adults and children 6 years and older, dissolve 1 lozenge in the mouth every 2 hours, if needed. For children under 6 years, consult a physician or dentist.

How Supplied:
Trade Package: 18 troches in 2 pocket packs of 9 each.
Professional Package: 324 troches in 36 blisters of 9 each.
Store at room temperature, below 86°F (30°C). Protect contents from humidity.
Shown in Product Identification Section, page 412

CĒPASTAT®
[sē ′pǝ-stăt]
Sore Throat Lozenges

Description: Each cherry flavor lozenge contains: Phenol 14.5 mg, Menthol 2.4 mg. Also contains: Antifoam Emulsion, D&C Red No. 33, FD&C Yellow No. 6, Flavor, Gum Crystal, Mannitol, Saccharin Sodium, and Sorbitol.
Each regular flavor lozenge contains: Phenol 29 mg, Menthol 2.4 mg. Also contains: Antifoam Emulsion, Caramel, Eucalyptus Oil, Gum Crystal, Mannitol, Saccharin Sodium, and Sorbitol.

Indications:
1. Sore throat:
   For prompt temporary relief of minor sore throat or discomfort associated with pharyngitis or tonsillitis or following tonsillectomy.
2. Mouth or gum irritation:
   For prompt temporary relief of minor pain or discomfort associated with pericoronitis or periodontitis or with dental procedures such as extractions, gingivectomies, and other minor oral surgery.

Actions: Phenol is a recognized topical anesthetic. Menthol provides a cooling sensation to aid in symptomatic relief and adds to the lozenge effect in stimulating salivary flow. The sugar-free formula should not promote tooth decay as sugar-based lozenges can.

Warnings*: Do not exceed recommended dosage. If soreness is severe, persists for more than 2 days, or is accompanied by high fever, headache, nausea, or vomiting, consult your physician or dentist promptly. Do not give to children under 6 years of age unless directed by a physician or dentist. Do not use for more than 10 days at a time. As with any drug, if you are pregnant or nursing a baby, seek the advice of a health professional before using this product.
KEEP THIS AND ALL DRUGS OUT OF THE REACH OF CHILDREN.
In case of accidental overdose, seek professional assistance or contact a Poison Control Center immediately.
Note to Diabetics*: Each lozenge contributes approximately 8 calories from 2 grams of sorbitol.

Dosage and Administration:
Lozenges–cherry flavor
ADULTS AND CHILDREN 12 YEARS AND OLDER: Dissolve 1 lozenge in the mouth, followed by another if needed, every 2 hours. Do not use more than 2 lozenges in 2 hours or more than 18 daily. CHILDREN 6 to UNDER 12 YEARS: Dissolve 1 lozenge in the mouth, followed by another if needed, every 3 hours. Do

not exceed 2 lozenges in 3 hours or more than 10 daily. CHILDREN UNDER 6 YEARS: Consult a physician or dentist.
Lozenges–regular flavor
ADULTS AND CHILDREN 12 YEARS AND OLDER: Dissolve 1 lozenge in the mouth every 2 hours. CHILDREN 6 TO UNDER 12 YEARS: Dissolve 1 lozenge in the mouth every 3 hours. Do not exceed 4 lozenges per day. CHILDREN UNDER 6 YEARS: Consult a physician or dentist.

How Supplied:
Lozenges–cherry flavor
   Trade package: Boxes of 18 lozenges as 2 pocket packs of 9 lozenges each. Professional package: 648 lozenges in 72 blisters of 9 lozenges each.
Lozenges–regular flavor
   Trade package: Boxes of 18 lozenges as 2 pocket packs of 9 lozenges each. Professional package: 648 lozenges in 72 blisters of 9 lozenges each.
Store at room temperature, below 86°F (30°C). Protect contents from humidity.
Shown in Product Identification Section, page 412

*This section appears on the label for the consumer.

Regular Flavor
CITRUCEL®
[sĭt ′rǝ-sĕl]
(Methylcellulose)
Bulk-forming Fiber Laxative

Description: Each 5.50 g adult dose (approximately one level measuring tablespoonful) contains Methylcellulose 2 g. Each 2.75 g child's dose (approximately one rounded measuring teaspoonful) contains Methylcellulose 1 g. Also contains: Malic Acid, Maltodextrin, Natural Citrus Flavor, Potassium Citrate, Riboflavin, Sucrose, and Other Ingredients. Each 5.50 g dose contains approximately 3 mg of sodium, 80 mg of potassium, and contributes 12 calories (from Maltodextrin and Sucrose).

Actions: Promotes elimination by providing additional fiber (bulk) to the diet. This product generally produces bowel movement in 12 to 72 hours.

Indications: For relief of constipation (irregularity). May also be used for relief of constipation associated with other bowel disorders such as irritable bowel syndrome, diverticular disease, and hemorrhoids as well as for bowel management during postpartum, postsurgical, and convalescent periods.

Contraindications: Intestinal obstruction, fecal impaction, known hypersensitivity to formula ingredients.

Precautions: Patients should be instructed to consult their physician before using any laxative if they have noticed a sudden change in bowel habits which persists for two weeks. Unless directed by a physician, patients should be advised not to use laxative products when abdominal pain, nausea or vomiting is

Continued on next page

Lakeside—Cont.

present. Patients should also be advised to discontinue use and consult a physician if rectal bleeding or failure to have a bowel movement occurs after use of any laxative product.

Dosage and Administration: Adults and children 12 years and older: *one level measuring* tablespoonful *stirred immediately and briskly* into 8 ounces of cold water or fruit juice, one to three times a day and administered promptly. Children 6 to under 12 years: *one rounded measuring* teaspoonful *stirred immediately and briskly* into 4 ounces of cold water or fruit juice, one to three times a day and administered promptly. Children under 6 years: use only as directed by a physician.
Continued use for two or three days may be necessary for full benefit.
Administering additional water is helpful.

How Supplied:
7 oz and 10 oz containers.
Store below 86°F (30°C). Protect contents from humidity; keep tightly closed.
Shown in Product Identification Section, page 412

Orange Flavor
CITRUCEL®
[sĭt 'rə-sĕl]
(Methylcellulose)
Bulk-forming Fiber Laxative

Description: Each 19 g adult dose (approximately one heaping measuring tablespoonful) contains Methylcellulose 2 g. Each 9.5 g child's dose (approximately 1 level measuring tablespoonful) contains Methylcellulose 1 g. Also contains: Citric Acid, FD&C Yellow No. 6, Orange Flavors (Natural and Artificial), Potassium Citrate, Riboflavin, Sucrose, and Other Ingredients. Each adult dose contains approximately 3 mg of sodium, 105 mg of potassium, and contributes 60 calories from 15 g of Sucrose.

Actions: Promotes elimination by providing additional fiber (bulk) to the diet. This product generally produces bowel movement in 12 to 72 hours.

Indications: For relief of constipation (irregularity). May also be used for relief of constipation associated with other bowel disorders such as irritable bowel syndrome, diverticular disease, and hemorrhoids as well as for bowel management during postpartum, postsurgical, and convalescent periods.

Contraindications: Intestinal obstruction, fecal impaction, known hypersensitivity to formula ingredients.

Precautions: Patients should be instructed to consult their physician before using any laxative if they have noticed a sudden change in bowel habits which persists for two weeks. Unless directed by a physician, patients should be advised not to use laxative products when abdominal pain, nausea, or vomiting is present. Patients should also be advised

to discontinue use and consult a physician if rectal bleeding or failure to have a bowel movement occurs after use of any laxative product.

Dosage and Administration: Adults and children 12 years and older: *one heaping measuring* tablespoonful stirred briskly into 8 ounces of cold water or fruit juice, one to three times a day and administered promptly. Children 6 to under 12 years: *one level measuring* tablespoonful stirred briskly into 4 ounces of cold water, one to three times a day and administered promptly. Children under 6 years: use only as directed by a physician.
Continued use for two or three days may be necessary for full benefit.
Administering additional water is helpful.

How Supplied:
16 oz and 30 oz containers.
Boxes of 20 single-dose packets.
Store below 86°F (30°C). Protect contents from humidity; keep tightly closed.
Shown in Product Identification Section, page 412

NOVAHISTINE® DMX
[nō "vă-hĭs 'tēn]
Cough/Cold Formula &
Decongestant

Description: Each 5 ml teaspoonful of NOVAHISTINE DMX contains: Dextromethorphan Hydrobromide 10 mg, Guaifenesin 100 mg, Pseudoephedrine Hydrochloride 30 mg. Also contains: Alcohol 10%, FD&C Red No. 40, FD&C Yellow No. 6, Flavors, Glycerin, Hydrochloric Acid, Invert Sugar, Saccharin Sodium, Sodium Chloride, Sorbitol, and Water. Dextromethorphan hydrobromide, a synthetic nonnarcotic antitussive, is the dextrorotatory isomer of 3-methoxy-N-methylmorphinan. Guaifenesin is the glyceryl ether of guaiacol. Pseudoephedrine hydrochloride is the salt of a pharmacologically active stereoisomer of ephedrine (1-phenyl-2-methylamino-1-propanol).

Actions: Dextromethorphan hydrobromide suppresses the cough reflex by a direct effect on the cough center in the medulla of the brain. Although it is chemically related to morphine, it produces no analgesia or addiction. Its antitussive activity is about equal to that of codeine.
Pseudoephedrine hydrochloride is an orally effective nasal decongestant. It is a sympathomimetic amine with peripheral effects similar to epinephrine and central effects similar to, but less intense than, amphetamines. Therefore, it has the potential for excitatory side effects. Pseudoephedrine hydrochloride at the recommended oral dosage has little or no pressor effect in normotensive adults. Patients taking pseudoephedrine orally have not been reported to experience the rebound congestion sometimes experienced with frequent, repeated use of topical decongestants. Pseudoephedrine is not known to produce drowsiness.

Guaifenesin acts as an expectorant by increasing respiratory tract fluid which reduces the viscosity of tenacious secretions, thus making expectoration easier.

Indications: NOVAHISTINE DMX is indicated when exhausting, nonproductive cough accompanies respiratory tract congestion. It is useful in the symptomatic relief of upper respiratory congestion associated with the common cold, influenza, bronchitis, and sinusitis.

Contraindications: NOVAHISTINE DMX is contraindicated in patients with severe hypertension, severe coronary artery disease, and in patients on MAO inhibitor therapy. Patient idiosyncrasy to adrenergic agents may be manifested by insomnia, dizziness, weakness, tremor, or arrhythmias.
Nursing mothers: Pseudoephedrine is contraindicated in nursing mothers because of the higher than usual risk for infants from sympathomimetic amines.
Hypersensitivity: NOVAHISTINE DMX is contraindicated in patients with hypersensitivity or idiosyncrasy to sympathomimetic amines, dextromethorphan, or to other formula ingredients.

Warnings: At dosages higher than the recommended dose, nervousness, dizziness, sleeplessness, nausea, or headache may occur. Do not take for more than 7 days. If symptoms do not improve, recur, or are accompanied by fever, rash, or persistent headache, patients should be advised to consult their physician before continuing use. Sympathomimetic amines should be used judiciously and sparingly in patients with hypertension, diabetes mellitus, ischemic heart disease, increased intracranial pressure, hyperthyroidism, or prostatic hypertrophy. Sympathomimetics may produce central nervous system stimulation with convulsions or cardiovascular collapse with accompanying hypotension. See Contraindications.
Use in elderly: The elderly (60 years and older) are more likely to have adverse reactions to sympathomimetics. Overdosage of sympathomimetics in this age group may cause hallucinations, convulsions, CNS depression, and death.
Use in children: NOVAHISTINE DMX should not be used in children under 2 years except under the advice and supervision of a physician.
Use in pregnancy: Safety for use during pregnancy has not been established. As with any drug, if you are pregnant or nursing a baby, seek the advice of a health professional before using this product.
If sensitive to any of the ingredients, do not use.
Keep this and all drugs out of the reach of children. In case of accidental overdose, seek professional assistance or contact a Poison Control Center immediately.

Precautions: Drugs containing pseudoephedrine should be used with caution in patients with diabetes, hypertension, cardiovascular disease, and hyperreactivity to ephedrine. See Contraindications.

Adverse Reactions: Adverse reactions occur infrequently with usual oral doses of NOVAHISTINE DMX. When they occur, adverse reactions may include gastrointestinal upset and nausea. Because of the pseudoephedrine in NOVAHISTINE DMX, hyperreactive individuals may display ephedrine-like reactions such as tachycardia, palpitations, headache, dizziness or nausea. Sympathomimetic drugs have been associated with certain untoward reactions including fear, anxiety, tenseness, restlessness, tremor, weakness, pallor, respiratory difficulty, dysuria, insomnia, hallucinations, convulsions, CNS depression, arrhythmias, and cardiovascular collapse with hypotension.

Note: Guaifenesin interferes with the colorimetric determination of 5-hydroxyindoleacetic acid (5-HIAA) and vanillylmandelic acid (VMA).

Drug Interactions: NOVAHISTINE DMX should not be used in patients taking a prescription drug for hypertension or depression without the advice of a physician. MAO inhibitors and beta-adrenergic blockers increase the effects of pseudoephedrine (sympathomimetics). Sympathomimetics may reduce the antihypertensive effects of methyldopa, mecamylamine, reserpine, and veratrum alkaloids.

Dosage and Administration: Adults and children 12 years and older, 2 teaspoonfuls every 4 hours. Children 6 to under 12 years, 1 teaspoonful every 4 hours. Children 2 to under 6 years, ½ teaspoonful every 4 hours. Not more than 4 doses every 24 hours. For children under 2 years of age, give only as directed by a physician.

How Supplied: As a red syrup in 4 fluid ounce bottles.
Keep tightly closed. Protect from excessive heat and light. Avoid freezing.
Shown in Product Identification Section, page 412

NOVAHISTINE® Elixir
[nō "vă-hǐs 'tĕn]
Cold & Hay Fever Formula

Description: Each 5 ml teaspoonful of NOVAHISTINE Elixir contains: Chlorpheniramine Maleate 2 mg, Phenylephrine Hydrochloride 5 mg. Also contains: Alcohol 5%, D&C Yellow No. 10, FD&C Blue No. 1, Flavors, Glycerin, Sodium Chloride, Sorbitol, and Water. Although considered sugar-free, each 5 ml contributes approximately 7 calories from sorbitol.

Actions: Phenylephrine is a nasal decongestant. Its effects are similar to epinephrine, but it is less potent on a weight basis, and has a longer duration of action. Phenylephrine produces peripheral effects similar to epinephrine, but has little or no central nervous system stimulation. After oral administration, nasal decongestion may occur within 15 or 20 minutes and persist for 2 to 4 hours. Chlorpheniramine maleate, an antihistaminic effective for the symptomatic relief of allergic rhinitis, possesses anticholinergic and sedative effects. Chlorpheniramine antagonizes many of the pharmacologic actions of histamine. It prevents released histamine from dilating capillaries and causing edema of the respiratory mucosa.

Indications: For the temporary relief of nasal congestion and eustachian tube congestion associated with the common cold, sinusitis, and hay fever (allergic rhinitis). Also provides temporary relief of runny nose, sneezing, itching of nose or throat, and itchy, watery eyes due to the common cold, hay fever (allergic rhinitis) or other upper respiratory allergies. May be given concomitantly, when indicated, with analgesics and antibiotics.

Contraindications: NOVAHISTINE Elixir is contraindicated in patients with severe hypertension, severe coronary artery disease, and in patients on MAO inhibitor therapy. Patient idiosyncrasy to adrenergic agents may be manifested by insomnia, dizziness, weakness, tremor, or arrhythmias.
NOVAHISTINE Elixir is also contraindicated in patients with narrow-angle glaucoma, urinary retention, peptic ulcer, asthma, emphysema, chronic pulmonary disease, shortness of breath, or difficulty in breathing.
Nursing mothers: Phenylephrine is contraindicated in nursing mothers.
Hypersensitivity: NOVAHISTINE Elixir is also contraindicated in patients with hypersensitivity or idiosyncrasy to sympathomimetic amines, antihistamines or to other formula ingredients.

Warnings: At dosages higher than the recommended dose, nervousness, dizziness, sleeplessness, nausea, or headache may occur. If symptoms do not improve within 7 days or are accompanied by high fever, patients should be advised to consult their physician before continuing use. Sympathomimetic amines should be used judiciously and sparingly in patients with hypertension, diabetes mellitus, ischemic heart disease, increased intraocular pressure, hyperthyroidism, or prostatic hypertrophy. Sympathomimetics may produce central nervous system stimulation with convulsions or cardiovascular collapse with accompanying hypotension. See Contraindications.
Use in elderly: The elderly (60 years and older) are more likely to have adverse reactions to sympathomimetics. Overdosage of sympathomimetics in this age group may cause hallucinations, convulsions, CNS depression, and death.
Use in children: May cause excitability. NOVAHISTINE Elixir should not be used in children under 6 years except under the advice and supervision of a physician.
Use in pregnancy: Safety for use during pregnancy has not been established. As with any drug, if you are pregnant or nursing a baby, seek the advice of a health professional before using this product.

If sensitive to any of the ingredients, do not use.
Keep this and all drugs out of the reach of children. In case of accidental overdose, seek professional assistance or contact a Poison Control Center immediately.

Precautions: Caution should be exercised if used in patients with high blood pressure, heart disease, diabetes or thyroid disease. The antihistamine may cause drowsiness, and ambulatory patients who operate machinery or motor vehicles should be cautioned accordingly.

Adverse Reactions: Drugs containing sympathomimetic amines have been associated with certain untoward reactions, including fear, anxiety, tenseness, restlessness, tremor, weakness, pallor, respiratory difficulty, dysuria, insomnia, hallucinations, convulsions, CNS depression, arrhythmias, and cardiovascular collapse with hypotension. Individuals hyperreactive to phenylephrine may display ephedrine-like reactions such as tachycardia, palpitation, headache, dizziness, or nausea.
Phenylephrine is considered safe and relatively free of unpleasant side effects when taken at recommended dosage. Patients sensitive to antihistamine drugs may experience mild sedation. Other side effects from antihistamines may include dry mouth, dizziness, weakness, anorexia, nausea, vomiting, headache, nervousness, polyuria, heartburn, diplopia, dysuria, and, very rarely, dermatitis.

Drug Interactions: Novahistine Elixir should not be used in patients taking a prescription drug for hypertension or depression without the advice of a physician. MAO inhibitors and beta-adrenergic blockers increase the effects of sympathomimetics. Sympathomimetics may reduce the antihypertensive effects of methyldopa, mecamylamine, reserpine, and veratrum alkaloids. Antihistamines have been shown to enhance one or more of the effects of tricyclic antidepressants, barbiturates, alcohol, and other central nervous system depressants.

Dosage and Administration: Adults and children 12 years and older, 2 teaspoonfuls every 4 hours; children 6 to under 12 years, 1 teaspoonful every 4 hours; children 2 to under 6 years, ½ teaspoonful every 4 hours.
For children under 2 years, at the discretion of the physician.
Product label dosage is as follows: Adults and children 12 years and older, 2 teaspoonfuls every 4 hours. Children 6 to under 12 years, 1 teaspoonful every 4 hours. Not more than 6 doses every 24 hours. For children under 6 years, give only as directed by a physician.

How Supplied: NOVAHISTINE Elixir, as a green liquid in 4 fluid ounce bottles. Keep tightly closed. Protect from excessive heat and light. Avoid freezing.
Shown in Product Identification Section, page 412

Continued on next page

Lakeside—Cont.

SINGLET® For Adults
[sĭng-lət]
**Decongestant/Antihistamine/
Analgesic (pain reliever)/Antipyretic
(fever reducer)**

Description: Each pink Singlet tablet contains Pseudoephedrine Hydrochloride 60 mg, Chlorpheniramine Maleate 4 mg, and Acetaminophen 650 mg. Also contains: FD&C Red No. 3, Hydroxypropyl Cellulose, Hydroxypropyl Methylcellulose 2910, Magnesium Stearate, Microcrystalline Cellulose, Pregelatinized Corn Starch, Sodium Starch Glycolate, Talc and Titanium Dioxide. May also contain: Ethylcellulose, Glycerin, Polyethylene Glycol 8000, and Sucrose.

Indications: For the temporary relief of nasal congestion, runny nose, occasional sinus headache, fever, sneezing, watery eyes or itching of the nose, throat, and eyes due to colds, hay fever, or other upper respiratory allergies.

Warnings: Do not take this product for more than 7 days. Unless directed by a physician, do not take this product if you have asthma, glaucoma, emphysema, chronic pulmonary disease, heart disease, high blood pressure, thyroid disease, diabetes, shortness of breath, difficulty in breathing, difficulty in urination due to enlargement of the prostate gland, or if you are presently taking a prescription drug for high blood pressure or depression. Do not exceed recommended dosage because severe liver damage, nervousness, dizziness, or sleeplessness may occur. May cause excitability. Consult your physician if symptoms persist, if new symptoms occur, or if redness or swelling is present, because these could be signs of a serious condition. Consult your physician if fever persists for more than 3 days (72 hours) or recurs. May cause drowsiness; alcohol, sedatives, and tranquilizers may increase the drowsiness effect. Avoid alcoholic beverages while taking this product. Do not take this product if you are taking sedatives or tranquilizers without first consulting your physician. Use caution when driving a motor vehicle or operating machinery. If sensitive to any of the ingredients, do not use.
As with any drug, if you are pregnant or nursing a baby, seek the advice of a health professional before using this product. KEEP THIS AND ALL DRUGS OUT OF THE REACH OF CHILDREN. In case of accidental overdose, seek professional assistance or contact a Poison Control Center immediately. Prompt medical attention is critical for adults as well as for children even if you do not notice any signs or symptoms.

Dosage and Administration: Adults and children 12 years and older: one tablet 3 to 4 times a day, taken with water, while symptoms persist. Do not take more than 1 tablet within a 4-hour period. Do not exceed 4 tablets in 24 hours.

Children under 12 years of age: consult a physician.

Storage: Protect from excessive heat and moisture.

How Supplied: Bottles of 100.

Lavoptik Company, Inc.
**661 WESTERN AVENUE N.
ST. PAUL, MN 55103**

LAVOPTIK® Eye Wash

Description: Isotonic LAVOPTIK Eye Wash is a buffered solution designed to help physically remove contaminants from the surface of the eye and lids. Formulated to buffer contaminants toward the safe range and help restore normal salts and water ratios in the tears.

Contents: Each 100 ml
Sodium Chloride	0.49	gram
Sodium Biphosphate	0.40	gram
Sodium Phosphate	0.45	gram
Preservative Agent		
Benzalkonium Chloride	0.005	gram

Precautions: If you experience severe eye pain, headache, rapid change in vision (side or straight ahead); sudden appearance of floating objects, acute redness of the eyes, pain on exposure to light or double vision consult a physician at once. If symptoms persist or worsen after use of this product, consult a physician. If solution changes color or becomes cloudy do not use. Keep this and all medicines out of reach of children. Keep container tightly closed. Do not use if safety seal is broken at time of purchase.

Administration: 6 ounce size with Eye Cup.
Rinse cup with clean water immediately before and after each use, avoid contamination of rim and inside surfaces of cup. Apply cup, half-filled with LAVOPTIK Eye Wash tightly to the eye. Tilt head backward. Open eyelids wide, rotate eyeball and blink several times to insure thorough washing. Discard washings. Repeat other eye. Tightly cap bottle. 32 ounce size.
Break seal as you remove cap and pour directly on contaminated area.

How Supplied: 6 ounce bottle with eyecup, NDC 10651-01040.
32 ounce bottle, NDC 10651-01019.

IDENTIFICATION PROBLEM?
Consult the
Product Identification Section
where you'll find
products pictured
in full color.

Lederle Laboratories
**A Division of American
Cyanamid Co.
ONE CYANAMID PLAZA
WAYNE, NJ 07470**

LEDERMARK®
Product Identification Code

Many Lederle tablets and capsules bear an identification code. A current listing appears in the Product Information Section of the 1990 PDR for Prescription Drugs.

CALTRATE®, JR.
[căl-trāte]
**Calcium Supplement For Children
Chewable Orange Flavored**

- Nature's most concentrated form of calcium®
- Made with pure calcium carbonate
- No lactose, no salt, no starch
- Great orange taste. Nonchalky.
- Plus Vitamin D to help absorb calcium.
- Children 4–10 years old need 1000 mg of calcium (U.S. RDA) every day to help keep teeth and bones strong.

ONE TABLET DAILY CONTAINS:
	Children 4+ % U.S. RDA
750 mg Calcium Carbonate which provides 300 mg elemental calcium	30%
60 I.U. Vitamin D	15%

Inactive Ingredients: Dextrose, dl-Alpha Tocopheryl, Gelatin, Magnesium Stearate, Malto Dextrin, Mannitol, Orange Flavor, Silica Gel, Sorbitol, Stearic Acid, Sucrose, Yellow 6, and other ingredients.

Recommended Intake: One or two tablets daily or as directed by a physician.
Keep out of the reach of children.

How Supplied: Bottle of 60—
NDC 0005-5516-19
Store at Room Temperature. Rev. 12/87
22043
*Shown in Product Identification
Section, page 412*

CALTRATE® 600
[căl-trāte]
**Smaller Tablet
High Potency Calcium Supplement
Nature's Most Concentrated Form of
Calcium®
No Sugar, No Salt, No Lactose, No
Cholesterol, No Preservatives,
Film-Coated for easy swallowing**

Inactive Ingredients: Croscarmellose Sodium, Hydroxypropyl Methylcellulose, Magnesium Stearate, Microcrystalline Cellulose, PVPP, Sodium Lauryl Sulfate, Titanium Dioxide, and other ingredients.
TWO TABLETS DAILY PROVIDE:
3000 mg Calcium Carbonate which

provides 1200 mg elemental calcium

For Adults—
Percentage of U.S.
Recommended Daily
Allowance (U.S. RDA)

120%

Recommended Intake: One or two tablets daily or as directed by the physician.

Warnings: Keep this and all medications out of the reach of children.

How Supplied: Bottle of 60—
NDC 0005-5510-19
Store at Room Temperature. Rev. 3/89
24192

*Shown in Product Identification
Section, page 412*

CALTRATE® 600+Iron & Vitamin D
[căl-trāte]
**High Potency Calcium Supplement
Nature's Most Concentrated Form of Calcium®
No Sugar, No Salt, No Lactose, No Cholesterol, Film-Coated for Easy Swallowing**

ONE TABLET DAILY CONTAINS:

	Adults— % U.S. RDA
1500 mg Calcium Carbonate which provides 600 mg elemental calcium	60%
18 mg elemental Iron in the Exclusive Optisorb® Time-Release System. (as ferrous fumarate)	100%
125 I.U. Vitamin D	31%

Inactive Ingredients: Diethyl Phthalate, Ethylcellulose, Hydroxypropyl Cellulose, Magnesium Stearate, Microcrystalline Cellulose, Pharmaceutical Glaze, Povidone, Red 40, Silica Gel, Sodium Lauryl Sulfate, Sodium Starch Glycolate, Stearic Acid, Talc, Titanium Dioxide and other ingredients.
• CALTRATE + Iron contains pure calcium and time-release iron for diets deficient in both minerals.
• Plus Vitamin D to help absorb calcium.

Recommended Intake: One or two tablets daily or as directed by the physician.
Keep out of the reach of children.

How Supplied: Bottle of 60—
NDC 0005-5523-19
Store at Room Temperature. Rev. 3/89
24190

*Shown in Product Identification
Section, page 412*

CALTRATE® 600 + Vitamin D
[căl-trāte]
**Smaller Tablet
High Potency Calcium Supplement
Nature's Most Concentrated Form of Calcium®
No Sugar, No Salt, No Lactose, No Cholesterol, Film-Coated for easy swallowing**

Inactive Ingredients: Blue 2, Croscarmellose Sodium, Hydroxypropyl Methyl-

cellulose, Magnesium Stearate, Microcrystalline Cellulose, Povidone, PVPP, Red 40, Sodium Lauryl Sulfate, Titanium Dioxide and Yellow 6.
TWO TABLETS DAILY PROVIDE:

	Adults— % U.S. RDA
3000 mg Calcium Carbonate which provides 1200 mg elemental calcium	120%
Vitamin D 250 I.U.	62%

Recommended Intake: Minimum dosage one tablet daily; two or more if directed by the physician.

Keep out of the reach of children.

How Supplied: Bottle of 60—
NDC 0005-5509-19
Store at Room Temperature. Rev. 6/89
22841

*Shown in Product Identification
Section, page 412*

CENTRUM®
[sĕn-trŭm]
**High Potency
Multivitamin/Multimineral Formula,
Advanced Formula
From A to Zinc®**

Each tablet contains:

	For Adults Percentage of U.S. Recommended Daily Allowance (U.S. RDA)
Vitamin A (as Acetate and Beta Carotene)	5000 I.U. (100%)
Vitamin E (as dl-Alpha Tocopheryl Acetate)	30 I.U. (100%)
Vitamin C (as Ascorbic Acid)	60 mg (100%)
Folic Acid	400 mcg (100%)
Vitamin B$_1$ (as Thiamine Mononitrate)	1.5 mg (100%)
Vitamin B$_2$ (as Riboflavin)	1.7 mg (100%)
Niacinamide	20 mg (100%)
Vitamin B$_6$ (as Pyridoxine Hydrochloride)	2 mg (100%)
Vitamin B$_{12}$ (as Cyanocobalamin)	6 mcg (100%)
Vitamin D	400 I.U. (100%)
Biotin	30 mcg (10%)
Pantothenic Acid (as Calcium Pantothenate)	10 mg (100%)
Calcium (as Dibasic Calcium Phosphate)	162 mg (16%)
Phosphorus (as Dibasic Calcium Phosphate)	125 mg (13%)
Iodine (as Potassium Iodide)	150 mcg (100%)
Iron (as Ferrous Fumarate)	18 mg (100%)
Magnesium (as Magnesium Oxide)	100 mg (25%)
Copper (as Cupric Oxide)	2 mg (100%)
Zinc (as Zinc Oxide)	15 mg (100%)
Manganese (as Manganese Sulfate)	2.5 mg*
Potassium (as Potassium Chloride)	40 mg*
Chloride (as Potassium Chloride)	36.3 mg*
Chromium (as Chromium Chloride)	25 mcg*

Molybdenum (as Sodium Molybdate)	25 mcg*
Selenium (as Sodium Selenate)	25 mcg*
Vitamin K$_1$ (as Phytonadione)	25 mcg*
Nickel (as Nickelous Sulfate)	5 mcg*
Tin (as Stannous Chloride)	10 mcg*
Silicon (as Sodium Metasilicate)	10 mcg*
Vanadium (as Sodium Metavanadate)	10 mcg*

*No U.S. RDA established.

Inactive Ingredients: Acacia Gum, Dextrose, Hydroxypropyl Methylcellulose, Lactose, Magnesium Stearate, Microcrystalline Cellulose, Methylparaben, Modified Food Starch, Mono- and Di-glycerides, Potassium Sorbate, Propylparaben, PVPP, Silica Gel, Sodium Aluminum Silicate, Sodium Benzoate, Sorbic Acid, Stearic Acid, Sucrose, and Yellow 6.

Recommended Intake: Adults, 1 tablet daily.

How Supplied:
Light peach, engraved CENTRUM C1.
Bottle of 60—NDC 0005-4239-19
Combopack*—NDC 0005-4239-30
*Bottles of 100 plus 30
Store at Room Temperature. Rev. 11/88
23965

*Shown in Product Identification
Section, page 412*

CENTRUM, JR.®
[sĕn-trŭm]
**Children's Chewable
Vitamin/Mineral Formula+Extra C
Tablets
Nutritional Support From Head to Toe®**

[See table on next page]

Inactive Ingredients: Acacia, Artificial Flavorings, Blue 1, Blue 2, Colloidal Silicon Dioxide, Dextrins, Dextrose, Gelatin, Hydrogenated Vegetable Oil, Hydrolyzed Protein, Lactose, Magnesium Stearate, Methylparaben, Microcrystalline Cellulose, Modified Food Starch, Mono- and Di-glycerides, Potassium Sorbate, Povidone, Propylparaben, Red 40, Sodium Benzoate, Sorbic Acid, Stearic Acid, Sucrose, Yellow 6.

Warnings: CONTAINS IRON, WHICH CAN BE HARMFUL IN LARGE DOSES. CLOSE TIGHTLY AND KEEP OUT OF THE REACH OF CHILDREN. IN CASE OF ACCIDENTAL OVERDOSE, CONTACT A PHYSICIAN OR POISON CONTROL CENTER IMMEDIATELY.

How Supplied: Bottle of 60—
NDC 0005-4249-19
Store at Room Temperature. Rev. 12/87
21343

*Shown in Product Identification
Section, page 412*

Continued on next page

Lederle—Cont.

CENTRUM, JR.®
[sĕn-trŭm]
**Children's Chewable
Vitamin/Mineral Formula+Extra
Calcium
Nutritional Support From Head to
Toe®**

[See table on next page].
Inactive Ingredients:
Acacia, Artificial Flavorings, Colloidal
Silicon Dioxide, Dextrins, Dextrose, Gelatin, Hydrogenated Vegetable Oil, Hydrolyzed Protein, Lactose, Magnesium
Stearate, Methylparaben, Microcrystalline Cellulose, Modified Food Starch,
Mono- and Di-glycerides, Potassium Sorbate, Propylparaben, Red 40, Sodium
Benzoate, Sodium Starch Glycolate, Sorbic Acid, Stearic Acid, Sucrose.

Warnings: CONTAINS IRON, WHICH
CAN BE HARMFUL IN LARGE DOSES.
CLOSE TIGHTLY AND KEEP OUT OF
THE REACH OF CHILDREN. IN CASE
OF ACCIDENTAL OVERDOSE, CONTACT A PHYSICIAN OR POISON CONTROL CENTER IMMEDIATELY.

Recommended Intake: 2 to 4 years of
age: chew one-half tablet daily. Over 4
years of age: chew one tablet daily.

How Supplied: Bottle of 60—
NDC 0005-4222-19.
Store at Room Temperature. Rev. 12/87
21340
*Shown in Product Identification
Section, page 412*

CENTRUM, JR.®
[sĕn-trŭm]
**Children's Chewable
Vitamin/Mineral Formula + Iron
Tablets
Nutritional Support From Head to
Toe®**

[See table on page 580]

Inactive Ingredients: Acacia, Artificial Flavorings, Blue 1, Blue 2, Colloidal
Silicon Dioxide, Dextrins, Dextrose, Gelatin, Hydrogenated Vegetable Oil, Hydrolyzed Protein, Lactose, Magnesium
Stearate, Methylparaben, Microcrystalline Cellulose, Modified Food Starch,
Mono- and Di-glycerides, Potassium Sorbate, Propylparaben, Red 40, Sodium
Benzoate, Sodium Starch Glycolate, Sorbic Acid, Stearic Acid, Sucrose, Yellow 6.

Recommended Intake: 2 to 4 years of
age: Chew one-half tablet daily. Over
4 years of age: Chew one tablet daily.

Warnings: CONTAINS IRON, WHICH
CAN BE HARMFUL IN LARGE DOSES.
CLOSE TIGHTLY AND KEEP OUT OF
THE REACH OF CHILDREN. IN CASE
OF ACCIDENTAL OVERDOSE, CONTACT A PHYSICIAN OR POISON CONTROL CENTER IMMEDIATELY.

How Supplied: Assorted Flavors—
Uncoated Tablet—Partially Scored
—Engraved Lederle C2 and
CENTRUM, JR. Bottle of 60 NDC 0005-
4234-19

Store at room temperature. Rev. 1/88
22048
*Shown in Product Identification
Section, page 412*

Dual Action
FERRO–SEQUELS®
[fĕrrō-sēēquals]
**High Potency Iron Supplement
Time-Release Iron Plus
Clinically Proven Anticonstipant
Easy-to-Swallow Tablets
Low Sodium, No Sugar, No Lactose**

Active Ingredients: Each tablet contains 150 mg of ferrous fumarate equivalent to 50 mg of elemental iron and 100
mg of docusate sodium (DSS).

Inactive Ingredients: Blue 1, Colloidal Silicon Dioxide, Corn Starch, Diethyl
Phthalate, Ethylcellulose, Hydroxypropyl Cellulose, Magnesium Stearate, Microcrystalline Cellulose, Pharmaceutical
Glaze, Povidone, Sodium Benzoate, Talc,
Titanium Dioxide, Yellow 10 and other
ingredients.

Warning: As with any drug, if you are
pregnant or nursing a baby, seek the advice of a health professional before using
this product. Keep this and all medications out of the reach of children. In case
of accidental overdose, seek professional
assistance or contact a Poison Control
Center immediately.

Recommended Intake: One tablet,
once or twice daily or as prescribed by a
physician.

How Supplied: Boxes of 30—
NDC 0005-5267-68
Bottle of 30—NDC 0005-5267-13
Bottle of 100—NDC 0005-5267-23
Unit Dose Pack 10×10—
NDC 0005-5267-60
Green, Capsule-shaped, film-coated tablets
Engraved LL and F2
Store at Room Temperature. Rev. 9/87
21560
*Shown in Product Identification
Section, page 413*

FIBERCON®
[fī-bĕr-cŏn]
**Calcium Polycarbophil
Bulk-Forming Fiber Laxative**

**Safe and effective, Less than one calorie per tablet, Sodium free, No preservatives, Film coated for easy swallowing, Calcium rich, No chemical
stimulants.**

Active Ingredient: Each tablet contains 625 mg calcium polycarbophil
equivalent to 500 mg polycarbophil.

Inactive Ingredients: Magnesium Stearate, Microcrystalline Cellulose, Silica
Gel, and other ingredients.

Indications: Relief of constipation (irregularity).

Actions: Increases bulk volume and
water content of the stool.

Warnings: If you have noticed a sudden change in bowel habits that persists

CENTRUM, JR.®
**Children's Chewable
Vitamin/Mineral Formula+Extra C**

EACH TABLET CONTAINS: VITAMINS	Quantity per tablet	Percentage of U.S. Recommended Daily Allowance (U.S. RDA)	
		For Children 2 to 4 (½ tablet)	For Children Over 4 (1 tablet)
Vitamin A (as Acetate)	5,000 I.U.	(100%)	(100%)
Vitamin D	400 I.U.	(50%)	(100%)
Vitamin E (as Acetate)	30 I.U.	(150%)	(100%)
Vitamin C (as Ascorbic Acid and Sodium Ascorbate)	300 mg	(375%)	(500%)
Folic Acid	400 mcg	(100%)	(100%)
Biotin	45 mcg	(15%)	(15%)
Thiamine (as Thiamine Mononitrate)	1.5 mg	(107%)	(100%)
Pantothenic Acid (as Calcium Pantothenate)	10 mg	(100%)	(100%)
Riboflavin	1.7 mg	(107%)	(100%)
Niacinamide	20 mg	(111%)	(100%)
Vitamin B_6 (as Pyridoxine Hydrochloride)	2 mg	(143%)	(100%)
Vitamin B_{12} (as Cyanocobalamin)	6 mcg	(100%)	(100%)
Vitamin K_1 (as Phytonadione)	10 mcg*		
MINERALS			
Iron (as Ferrous Fumarate)	18 mg	(90%)	(100%)
Magnesium (as Magnesium Oxide)	40 mg	(10%)	(10%)
Iodine (as Potassium Iodide)	150 mcg	(107%)	(100%)
Copper (as Cupric Oxide)	2 mg	(100%)	(100%)
Phosphorous (as Tribasic Calcium Phosphate)	50 mg	(3.12%)	(5.0%)
Calcium (as Tribasic Calcium Phosphate)	108 mg	(6.75%)	(10.8%)
Zinc (as Zinc Oxide)	15 mg	(93%)	(100%)
Manganese (as Manganese Sulfate)	1 mg*		
Molybdenum (as Sodium Molybdate)	20 mcg*		
Chromium (as Chromium Chloride)	20 mcg*		

*Recognized as essential in human nutrition but no U.S. RDA established.

CENTRUM, JR.®
Children's Chewable
Vitamin/Mineral Formula + Extra Calcium

EACH TABLET CONTAINS:	Quantity per tablet	Percentage of U.S. Recommended Daily Allowance (U.S. RDA)	
VITAMINS		For Children 2 to 4 (½ tablet)	For Children Over 4 (1 tablet)
Vitamin A (as Acetate)	5,000 I.U.	(100%)	(100%)
Vitamin D	400 I.U.	(50%)	(100%)
Vitamin E (as Acetate)	30 I.U.	(150%)	(100%)
Vitamin C (as Ascorbic Acid)	60 mg	(75%)	(100%)
Folic Acid	400 mcg	(100%)	(100%)
Biotin	45 mcg	(15%)	(15%)
Thiamine (as Thiamine Mononitrate)	1.5 mg	(107%)	(100%)
Pantothenic Acid (as Calcium Pantothenate)	10 mg	(100%)	(100%)
Riboflavin	1.7 mg	(107%)	(100%)
Niacinamide	20 mg	(111%)	(100%)
Vitamin B_6 (as Pyridoxine Hydrochloride)	2 mg	(143%)	(100%)
Vitamin B_{12} (as Cyanocobalamin)	6 mcg	(100%)	(100%)
Vitamin K_1 (as Phytonadione)	10 mcg*		
MINERALS			
Iron (as Ferrous Fumarate)	18 mg	(90%)	(100%)
Magnesium (as Magnesium Oxide)	40 mg	(10%)	(10%)
Iodine (as Potassium Iodide)	150 mcg	(107%)	(100%)
Copper (as Cupric Oxide)	2 mg	(100%)	(100%)
Phosphorus (as Dibasic Calcium Phosphate)	50 mg	(3.12%)	(5.0%)
Calcium (as Dibasic Calcium Phosphate and Calcium Carbonate)	160 mg	(10%)	(16%)
Zinc (as Zinc Oxide)	15 mg	(93%)	(100%)
Manganese (as Manganese Sulfate)	1 mg*		
Molybdenum (as Sodium Molybdate)	20 mcg*		
Chromium (as Chromium Chloride)	20 mcg*		

*Recognized as essential in human nutrition but no U.S. RDA established.

over a period of 2 weeks, consult a physician before using a laxative. If the recommended use of this product for 1 week has no effect, discontinue use and consult a physician.

Do not use laxative products when abdominal pain, nausea or vomiting is present except under the direction of a physician. Discontinue use and consult a physician if rectal bleeding occurs after use of any laxative product.

For chronic or continued constipation consult your physician.

Interaction Precaution: Contains calcium. Take this product at least one hour before or two hours after taking an oral dose of a prescription antibiotic containing any form of tetracycline.
KEEP THIS AND ALL MEDICINES OUT OF THE REACH OF CHILDREN. STORE AT CONTROLLED ROOM TEMPERATURE 15–30°C (59–86°F). PROTECT CONTENTS FROM MOISTURE.

Recommended Intake: Adults and children 12 years and older: swallow 2 tablets one to four times a day. Children 6 to 12 years: swallow 1 tablet one to three times a day. Children under 6 years: consult a physician. See package insert for additional information.

A FULL GLASS (8 fl. oz.) OF LIQUID SHOULD BE TAKEN WITH EACH DOSE.

How Supplied:
Film coated tablets, scored, engraved LL and F66.
Package of 36 tablets, NDC 0005-2500-02
Package of 60 tablets, NDC 0005-2500-86
Package of 90 tablets, NDC 0005-2500-33
Bottle of 500 tablets, NDC 0005-2500-31

Unit Dose Pkg. NDC 0005-2500-28
Travel size package of 8 tablets
Rev. 11/88
23491

Shown in Product Identification Section, page 412

FILIBON®
[fĭ-lĭ-bōn]
prenatal tablets

Each tablet contains:

	For Pregnant or Lactating Women Percentage of U.S. Recommended Daily Allowance (U.S. RDA)
Vitamin A (as Acetate)	5000 I.U. (63%)
Vitamin D_2	400 I.U. (100%)
Vitamin E (as dl-Alpha Tocopheryl Acetate)	30 I.U. (100%)
Vitamin C (Ascorbic Acid)	60 mg (100%)
Folic Acid	0.4 mg (50%)
Vitamin B_1 (as Thiamine Mononitrate)	1.5 mg (88%)
Vitamin B_2 (as Riboflavin)	1.7 mg (85%)
Niacinamide	20 mg (100%)
Vitamin B_6 (as Pyridoxine Hydrochloride)	2 mg (80%)
Vitamin B_{12} (as Cyanocobalamin)	6 mcg (75%)
Calcium (as Calcium Carbonate)	125 mg (10%)
Iodine (as Potassium Iodide)	150 mcg (100%)
Iron (as Ferrous Fumarate)	18 mg (100%)
Magnesium (as Magnesium Oxide)	100 mg (22%)

Inactive Ingredients: BHA, BHT, Dextrose, Ethylcellulose, Gelatin, Hydrolyzed Protein, Hydroxypropyl Meth-

ylcellulose, Lactose, Magnesium Stearate, Methylparaben, Modified Food Starch, Mono- and Di-glycerides, Polacrilin, Polysorbate 60, Povidone, Propylparaben, Red 40, Silica Gel, Sodium Benzoate, Sodium Bisulfite, Sodium Lauryl Sulfate, Sorbic Acid, Stearic Acid, Sucrose, Titanium Dioxide, Tricalcium Phosphate, and other ingredients.

Recommended Intake: 1 daily, or as prescribed by the physician.

How Supplied: Capsule-shaped tablets (film-coated, pink) engraved LL F4—bottle of 100 NDC-0005-4294-23
Store at Room Temperature. Rev. 10/86
18321

GEVRABON®
[jĕv-ra băn]
vitamin-mineral supplement

Composition: Each fluid ounce (30 mL) contains:

	For Adults Percentage of U.S. Recommended Daily Allowance (U.S. RDA)
Vitamin B_1 (as Thiamine Hydrochloride)	5 mg (333%)
Vitamin B_2 (as Riboflavin-5-Phosphate Sodium)	2.5 mg (147%)
Niacinamide	50 mg (250%)
Vitamin B_6 (Pyridoxine Hydrochloride)	1 mg (50%)
Vitamin B_{12} (as Cyanocobalamin)	1 mcg (17%)
Pantothenic Acid (as D-Pantothenyl Alcohol)	10 mg (100%)
Iodine (as Potassium Iodide)	100 mcg (67%)
Iron (as Ferrous Gluconate)	15 mg (83%)

Continued on next page

Lederle—Cont.

Magnesium (as Magnesium Chloride)....................2 mg (0.5%)
Zinc (as Zinc Chloride)..........2 mg (13%)
Choline (as Tricholine Citrate).....................................100 mg.*
Manganese (as Manganese Chloride).............................2 mg.*
*Recognized as essential in human nutrition but no U.S. RDA established.
Alcohol 18%

Inactive Ingredients: Alcohol, citric acid, glycerin, sherry wine, sucrose.

Indications: For use as a nutritional supplement. Shake well.

Warning: As with any drug, if you are pregnant or nursing a baby, seek the advice of a health professional before using this product. Keep this preparation out of the reach of children.

Administration and Dosage: Adult: One ounce (30 mL) daily or as prescribed by the physician as a nutritional supplement.

Important Note: In time a slight natural deposit, characteristic of the sherry wine base, may occur. This does not indicate in any way a loss of quality.

How Supplied: Syrup (sherry flavor) decanters of 16 fl. oz. NDC 0005-5250-35
Keep Out of Direct Sunlight
Store at Room Temperature, 15°–30°C (59°–86°F).

DO NOT FREEZE   Rev. 6/85
16520

GEVRAL®
[jĕv-ral]
Multivitamin and Multimineral Supplement
TABLETS

Composition: Each tablet contains:
For Adults
Percentage of U.S.
Recommended Daily
Allowance (U.S. RDA)

Vitamin A (as Acetate)	5000 I.U.	(100%)
Vitamin E (as dl-Alpha Tocopheryl Acetate)...	30 I.U.	(100%)
Vitamin C (as Ascorbic Acid)	60 mg	(100%)
Folic Acid	0.4 mg	(100%)
Vitamin B$_1$ (as Thiamine Mononitrate)	1.5 mg	(100%)
Vitamin B$_2$ (as Riboflavin)	1.7 mg	(100%)
Niacinaminde	20 mg	(100%)
Vitamin B$_6$ (as Pyridoxine Hydrochloride)	2 mg	(100%)
Vitamin B$_{12}$ (as Cyanocobalamin)	6 mcg	(100%)
Calcium (as Dibasic Calcium Phosphate)...	162 mg	(16%)
Phosphorus (as Dibasic Calcium Phosphate)...	125 mg	(13%)
Iodine (as Potassium Iodide)	150 mcg	(100%)
Iron (as Ferrous Fumarate)	18 mg	(100%)
Magnesium (as Magnesium Oxide)	100 mg	(25%)

Inactive Ingredients: Blue 2, Ethylcellulose, Gelatin, Hydrolyzed Protein, Hydroxypropyl Methylcellulose, Lactose, Magnesium Stearate, Methylparaben, Microcrystalline Cellulose, Modified Food Starch, Mono- and Di-glycerides, Polacrilin, Potassium Sorbate, Propylparaben, PVPP, Red 30, Silica Gel, Sodium Benzoate, Sorbic Acid, Stearic Acid, Sucrose, Titanium Dioxide, and Yellow 6.

Indications: Supplementation of the diet.

Administration and Dosage: One tablet daily or as prescribed by the physician.
Keep this and all medications out of the reach of children.

How Supplied: Capsule-shaped tablets (film-coated, brown) engraved LL G1—bottle of 100 NDC 0005-4289-23
Store at Room Temperature.
A SPECTRUM® Product   Rev. 5/89
22788

GEVRAL® T
[jĕv-ral t]
High Potency
Multivitamin and Multimineral Supplement
TABLETS

Each tablet contains:
For Adults
Percentage of U.S.
Recommended Daily
Allowance (U.S. RDA)

Vitamin A (as Acetate)	5000 I.U.	(100%)
Vitamin E (as dl-Alpha Tocopheryl Acetate)...	45 I.U.	(150%)
Vitamin C (as Ascorbic Acid)	90 mg	(150%)
Folic Acid	0.4 mg	(100%)
Vitamin B$_1$ (as Thiamine Mononitrate)	2.25 mg	(150%)
Vitamin B$_2$ (as Riboflavin)	2.6 mg	(153%)

CENTRUM, JR.®
Children's Chewable
Vitamin/Mineral Formula + Iron

EACH TABLET CONTAINS:	Quantity per tablet	Percentage of U.S. Recommended Daily Allowance (U.S. RDA) For Children 2 to 4 (½ tablet)	For Children Over 4 (1 tablet)
VITAMINS			
Vitamin A (as Acetate)	5,000 I.U.	(100%)	(100%)
Vitamin D	400 I.U.	(50%)	(100%)
Vitamin E (as Acetate)	30 I.U.	(150%)	(100%)
Vitamin C (as Ascorbic Acid)	60 mg	(75%)	(100%)
Folic Acid	400 mcg	(100%)	(100%)
Biotin	45 mcg	(15%)	(15%)
Thiamine (as Thiamine Mononitrate)	1.5 mg	(107%)	(100%)
Pantothenic Acid (as Calcium Pantothenate)	10 mg	(100%)	(100%)
Riboflavin	1.7 mg	(107%)	(100%)
Niacinamide	20 mg	(111%)	(100%)
Vitamin B$_6$ (as Pyridoxine Hydrochloride)	2 mg	(143%)	(100%)
Vitamin B$_{12}$ (as Cyanocobalamin)	6 mcg	(100%)	(100%)
Vitamin K$_1$ (as Phytonadione)	10 mcg*		
MINERALS			
Iron (as Ferrous Fumarate)	18 mg	(90%)	(100%)
Magnesium (as Magnesium Oxide)	40 mg	(10%)	(10%)
Iodine (as Potassium Iodide)	150 mcg	(107%)	(100%)
Copper (as Cupric Oxide)	2 mg	(100%)	(100%)
Phosphorus (as Dibasic Calcium Phosphate)	50 mg	(3.12%)	(5.0%)
Calcium (as Dibasic Calcium Phosphate and Calcium Carbonate)	108 mg	(6.75%)	(10.8%)
Zinc (as Zinc Oxide)	15 mg	(93%)	(100%)
Manganese (as Manganese Sulfate)	1 mg*		
Molybdenum (as Sodium Molybdate)	20 mcg*		
Chromium (as Chromium Chloride)	20 mcg*		

*Recognized as essential in human nutrition but no U.S. RDA established.

Niacinamide..................... 30 mg (150%)

Vitamin B$_6$ (as Pyridoxine
Hydrochloride)............ 3 mg (150%)

Vitamin B$_{12}$ (as
Cyanocobalamin)........ 9 mcg (150%)

Vitamin D$_2$...................... 400 I.U. (100%)

Calcium (as Dibasic
Calcium Phosphate)... 162 mg (16%)

Phosphorus (as Dibasic
Calcium Phosphate)... 125 mg (13%)

Iodine (as Potassium
Iodide)...........................225 mcg (150%)

Iron (as Ferrous
Fumarate).................... 27 mg (150%)

Magnesium (as
Magnesium Oxide)..... 100 mg (25%)

Copper (as Cupric Oxide) 1.5 mg (75%)

Zinc (as Zinc Oxide)....... 22.5 mg (150%)

Inactive Ingredients: BHA, BHT, Blue 2, Gelatin, Hydrolyzed Protein, Hydroxypropyl Methylcellulose, Lactose, Magnesium Stearate, Methylparaben, Microcrystalline Cellulose, Modified Food Starch, Mono- and Di-glycerides, Polacrilin, Polysorbate 60, Potassium Sorbate, Propylparaben, PVPP, Red 40, Silica Gel, Sodium Benzoate, Sodium Lauryl Sulfate, Sorbic Acid, Stearic Acid, Sucrose, Titanium Dioxide, and other ingredients.

Indications: For the treatment of vitamin and mineral deficiencies.

Dosage: 1 tablet daily or as prescribed by physician.
Keep this and all medications out of the reach of children.
Store at Room Temperature.

How Supplied: Tablets (film coated, maroon). Printed LL G2—bottle of 100
NDC 0005-4286-23
A SPECTRUM® Product
Rev. 10/86
14170

INCREMIN®
[*ĭn-cre-mĭn*]
WITH IRON SYRUP
Vitamins + Iron

DIETARY SUPPLEMENT
(Cherry Flavored)

Composition: Each teaspoonful (5 mL) contains:
Elemental Iron
(as Ferric Pyrophosphate)..........30 mg
L-Lysine HCl....................................300 mg
Thiamine HCl (B$_1$)...........................10 mg
Pyridoxine HCl (B$_6$)...........................5 mg
Vitamin B$_{12}$
(Cyanocobalamin).......................25 mcg
Sorbitol ....3.50 gm
Alcohol...0.75%

Inactive Ingredients: Alcohol, Flavorings, Red 33, Sodium Benzoate, Sorbic Acid.

Each teaspoonful (5 mL) supplies the following Minimum Daily Requirements:

	Child under 6	Child over 6	Adults
Vitamin B$_1$	20 MDR	13⅓ MDR	10 MDR
Iron	4 MDR	3 MDR	3 MDR

Indications: For the prevention and treatment of iron deficiency anemia in children and adults.

Warning: As with any drug, if you are pregnant or nursing a baby, seek the advice of a health professional before using this product.
Keep this and all medications out of the reach of children.

Administration and Dosage: or as prescribed by a physician.
Children: One teaspoonful (5 mL) daily for the prevention of iron deficiency anemia.
Adults: One teaspoonful (5 mL) daily for the prevention of iron deficiency anemia.

Notice: To protect from light always dispense in this container or in an amber bottle.
Store at Room Temperature.

How Supplied: Syrup (cherry flavor)—bottles of 4 fl. oz—NDC 0005-5604-58 and 16 fl. oz—NDC 0005-5604-65
Rev. 9/85
16846

NEOLOID®
[*nē̄-o-loid*]
emulsified castor oil
Peppermint Flavored

Composition: Emulsified Castor Oil USP 36.4% (w/w) with 0.1% (w/w) Sodium Benzoate and 0.2% (w/w) Potassium Sorbate added as preservatives, emulsifying and flavoring agents in water. Also contains the following inactive ingredients: Citric Acid, Glyceryl Monostearate, Polysorbate 80, Propylene Glycol, Sodium Alginate, Sodium Saccharin, Stearic Acid, Tenox II. NEOLOID is an emulsion with an exceptionally bland, pleasant taste.

Indications: For the treatment of isolated bouts of constipation.
SHAKE WELL

Administration and Dosage:
Infants —½ to 1½ teaspoonfuls
Children —Adjust between infant and adult dose.
Adult —Average dose, 2 to 4 tablespoonfuls or as prescribed by a physician.

Precautions: Not to be used when abdominal pain, nausea, vomiting, or other symptoms of appendicitis are present. Frequent or continued use of this preparation may result in dependence on laxatives. Do not use during pregnancy except on a physician's advice. Keep this and all drugs out of the reach of children.

Warning: As with any drug, if you are pregnant or nursing a baby, seek the advice of a health professional before using this product. In case of accidental over-

dose, seek professional assistance or contact a Poison Control Center immediately.

How Supplied: Bottles of 4 fl. oz. (118 mL) (peppermint flavor)
NDC-0005-5442-58
Store at Room Temperature.
DO NOT FREEZE
Rev. 9/85
16838

PERITINIC®
[*perĭ-tĭn-ĭc*]
hematinic with vitamins and fecal softener
Tablets
Film-Coated

Each tablet contains:
Elemental Iron
(as Ferrous Fumarate)..............100 mg
Docusate Sodium U.S.P. (DSS)
(to counteract the
constipating effect of iron).......100 mg
Vitamin B$_1$
(as Thiamine Mononitrate).......7.5 mg
(7½ MDR)
Vitamin B$_2$ (Riboflavin).................7.5 mg
(6¼ MDR)
Vitamin B$_6$
(Pyridoxine Hydrochloride).......7.5 mg
Vitamin B$_{12}$
(Cyanocobalamin) ....50 mcg
Vitamin C (Ascorbic Acid)..........200 mg
(6⅔ MDR)
Niacinamide.....................................30 mg
(3 MDR)
Folic Acid ....0.05 mg
Pantothenic Acid
(as D-Pantothenyl Alcohol)........15 mg
MDR—Adult Minimum Daily Requirement

Inactive Ingredients: Alginic Acid, Amberlite Resin, Blue 2, Ethyl Cellulose, FD&C Yellow No. 6,* Hydroxypropyl Methylcellulose, Lactose, Magnesium Stearate, Modified Food Starch, Povidone, Red 40, Silica Gel, Titanium Dioxide, and other ingredients.
*Contains FD&C Yellow No. 6 (Sunset Yellow) as a color additive.

Warning: As with any drug, if you are pregnant or nursing a baby, seek the advice of a health professional before using this product. In case of accidental overdose, seek professional assistance or contact a Poison Control Center immediately. Keep out of the reach of children.

Action and Uses: In the prevention of nutritional anemias, certain vitamin deficiencies, and iron-deficiency anemias.

Administration and Dosage:
Adults: 1 or 2 tablets daily.

How Supplied: Tablets (maroon, capsule-shaped, film coated) P8—bottle of 60
NDC 0005-5124-19
Rev. 5/87
18649

Continued on next page

Lederle—Cont.

STRESSTABS® Advanced Formula
[strĕss-tăbs]
High Potency
Stress Formula Vitamins

Each tablet contains:

For Adults-
Percentage of U.S.
Recommended Daily
Allowance (U.S. RDA)

Vitamin E (as *dl*-Alpha
Tocopheryl Acetate) 30 I.U. (100%)
Vitamin C (as Ascorbic
Acid) .... 500 mg (833%)
B VITAMINS
Folic Acid .... 400 mcg (100%)
Vitamin B₁ (as Thiamine
Mononitrate) .... 15 mg (1000%)
Vitamin B₂ (as
Riboflavin) .... 10 mg (588%)
Niacinamide ....100 mg (500%)
Vitamin B₆ (as Pyridoxine
Hydrochloride) .... 5 mg (250%)
Vitamin B₁₂
(as Cyanocobalamin) 12 mcg (200%)
Biotin ....45 mcg (15%)
Pantothenic Acid (as Calcium
Pantothenate USP) ... 20 mg (200%)

Inactive Ingredients: Calcium Carbonate, Dextrose, Dibasic Calcium Phosphate, Lactose, Hydroxypropyl Methylcellulose, Lactose, Magnesium Stearate, Microcrystalline Cellulose, Modified Food Starch, Silica Gel, Sodium Benzoate, Sorbic Acid, Stearic Acid, Titanium Dioxide, and Yellow 6.

Store at Room Temperature.

Recommended Intake: Adults, 1 tablet daily or as directed by the physician.

How Supplied:
Bottle of 30—NDC 0005-4124-13
Bottle of 60—NDC 0005-4124-19
Unit Dose Pack 10 × 10s—NDC 0005-4124-60

Rev. 8/89
22896
*Shown in Product Identification
Section, page 413*

STRESSTABS® + IRON
Advanced Formula
[strĕss-tăbs]
High Potency
Stress Formula Vitamins

Each tablet contains:

For Adults-
Percentage of U.S.
Recommended Daily
Allowance (U.S. RDA)

Vitamin E (as *dl*-Alpha
Tocopheryl Acetate) 30 I.U. (100%)
Vitamin C (as Ascorbic
Acid) .... 500 mg (833%)
B VITAMINS
Folic Acid .... 400 mcg (100%)
Vitamin B₁ (as Thiamine
Mononitrate) .... 15 mg (1000%)
Vitamin B₂ (as
Riboflavin) .... 10 mg (588%)
Niacinamide ....100 mg (500%)

Vitamin B₆ (as Pyridoxine
Hydrochloride) .... 5 mg (250%)
Vitamin B₁₂
(as Cyanocobalamin) 12 mcg (200%)
Biotin ....45 mcg (15%)
Pantothenic Acid (as Calcium
Pantothenate USP) ... 20 mg (200%)
Iron (as Ferrous
Fumarate) .... 27 mg (150%)

Inactive Ingredients: Calcium Carbonate, Dextrose, Dibasic Calcium Phosphate, Lactose, Magnesium Stearate, Microcrystalline Cellulose, Modified Food Starch, Red 40, Silica Gel, Sodium Benzoate, Sorbic Acid, Stearic Acid, Titanium Dioxide, and Yellow 6.

Recommended Intake: Adults, 1 tablet daily or as directed by physician.

How Supplied: Capsule-shaped tablets (film-coated, orange-red, scored) Engraved LL S2—
Bottle of 30—NDC 0005-4126-13
Bottle of 60—NDC 0005-4126-19
Store at Room Temperature. Rev. 8/89
22898
*Shown in Product Identification
Section, page 413*

STRESSTABS® + ZINC
Advanced Formula
[strĕss-tăbs]
High Potency
Stress Formula Vitamins

Each tablet contains:

For Adults-
Percentage of U.S.
Recommended Daily
Allowance (U.S. RDA)

Vitamin E (as *dl*-Alpha
Tocopheryl Acetate) 30 IU (100%)
Vitamin C
(as Ascorbic Acid) ...500 mg (833%)
B VITAMINS
Folic Acid ....400 mcg (100%)
Vitamin B₁ (as Thiamine Mononitrate)....15 mg (1000%)
Vitamin B₂
(as Riboflavin)............10 mg (588%)
Niacinamide.................100 mg (500%)
Vitamin B₆ (as Pyridoxine Hydrochloride)......5 mg (250%)
Vitamin B₁₂ (as Cyanocobalamin)...................12 mcg (200%)
Biotin.............................45 mcg (15%)
Pantothenic Acid (as Calcium Pantothenate USP) 20 mg (200%)
Copper (as Cupric Oxide)............................3 mg (150%)
Zinc (as Zinc Sulfate)23.9 mg (159%)

Inactive Ingredients: Calcium Carbonate, Dextrose, Dibasic Calcium Phosphate, Magnesium Stearate, Microcrystalline Cellulose, Modified Food Starch, Silica Gel, Sodium Benzoate, Stearic Acid, and Yellow 6.

Recommended Intake: Adults, 1 tablet daily or as directed by the physician.

How Supplied: Capsule-shaped Tablet (film coated, peach color) Engraved LL S3—
Bottle of 30—NDC 0005-4125-13
Bottle of 60—NDC 0005-4125-19

Store at Room Temperature. Rev. 8/89
22897
*Shown in Product Identification
Section, page 413*

ZINCON®
[zinc-ŏn]
Dandruff Shampoo

Contains: Pyrithione zinc (1%), water, sodium methyl cocoyl taurate, cocamide MEA, sodium chloride, magnesium aluminum silicate, sodium cocoyl isethionate, fragrance, glutaraldehyde, D&C green #5, citric acid or sodium hydroxide to adjust pH if necessary.

Indications: Relieves the itching and scalp flaking associated with dandruff. Relieves the itching, irritation, and skin flaking associated with seborrheic dermatitis of the scalp.

Directions: For best results use twice a week. Wet hair, apply to scalp and massage vigorously. Rinse and repeat.
SHAKE WELL BEFORE USING.

Warnings: Keep this and all drugs out of the reach of children. For external use only. Avoid contact with the eyes—if this happens, rinse thoroughly with water. If condition worsens or does not improve after regular use of this product as directed, consult a doctor. Do not use on children under 2 years of age except as directed by a doctor.

How Supplied:
4 oz. Bottle—NDC 0005-5455-58
8 oz. Bottle—NDC 0005-5455-61
Rev. 9/83
13918
*Shown in Product Identification
Section, page 413*

If desired, additional information on any Lederle product will be provided by contacting Lederle Professional Services Dept.

EDUCATIONAL MATERIAL

Are Our Children Getting Enough Calcium?
4-page pamphlet describing why children need to get enough calcium in their diets.
Calcium Supplements: The Differences Are Real
8-page pamphlet describing why today's women need to supplement their diet with calcium.
Fiber Action—The Secret to Healthy Regularity
8-page pamphlet describing the role of fiber in maintaining good digestive health.
Write to: Lederle Promotional Center
2200 Bradley Hill Road
Blauvelt, NY 10913

Leeming Division
Pfizer, Inc.
100 JEFFERSON ROAD
PARSIPPANY, NJ 07054

BEN–GAY® External Analgesic Products

Description: Ben-Gay is a combination of methyl salicylate and menthol in a suitable base for topical application. In addition to the Original Ointment (methyl salicylate, 18.3%; menthol, 16%), Ben-Gay is offered as a Greaseless/Stainless Ointment (methyl salicylate, 15%; menthol, 10%), an Extra Strength Arthritis Rub (methyl salicylate, 30%; menthol, 8%), a Lotion and a Clear Gel (both of which contain methyl salicylate, 15%; menthol, 7%) and Ben Gay Warming Ice (2.5% menthol in an alcohol base gel). Ben-Gay Sports-Gel (methyl salicylate 15%; menthol 10%) and Extra Strength Ben-Gay Sports-Balm (methyl salicylate 28%; menthol 10%) are available for use before and after exercise.

Action and Uses: Methyl salicylate and menthol are external analgesics which stimulate sensory receptors of warmth and cold. This produces a counter-irritant response which provides temporary relief of minor aches and pains of muscles and joints associated with simple bachache, arthritis, strains, bruises and sprains.

Several double-blind clinical studies of Ben-Gay products have shown the effectiveness of the menthol-methyl salicylate combination in counteracting minor pain of skeletal muscle stress and arthritis.

Three studies involving a total of 102 normal subjects in which muscle soreness was experimentally induced showed statistically significant beneficial results from use of the active product vs. placebo for lowered Muscle Action Potential (spasms), greater rise in threshold of muscular pain and greater reduction in perceived muscular pain.

Six clinical studies of a total of 207 subjects suffering from minor pain and skeletal muscular spasms due to osteoarthritis and rheumatoid arthritis showed the active product to give statistically significant beneficial results vs. placebo for lowered Muscle Action Potential (spasm), greater relief of perceived pain, increased range of motion of the affected joints and increased digital dexterity.

In two studies designed to measure the effect of topically applied Ben-Gay vs. Placebo on muscular endurance, discomfort, onset of exercise pain and fatigue, and cardiovascular efficiency, 30 subjects performed a submaximal three-hour run and another 30 subjects performed a maximal treadmill run. Ben-Gay was found to significantly decrease the discomfort during the submaximal and maximal run, and increase the time before onset of fatigue during the maximal run. It did not improve cardiovascular function or affect recovery. Applied before workouts, Ben-Gay exercise rubs

relax tight muscles and increase circulation to make exercising more comfortable, longer.

To help reduce muscle ache and soreness after exercise, a Ben-Gay exercise rub can be applied and allowed to work before taking a shower.

Directions: Rub generously into painful area, then massage gently until Ben-Gay disappears. Repeat as necessary.

Warning: Use only as directed. Do not use with a heating pad. Keep away from children to avoid accidental poisoning. Do not swallow. If swallowed, induce vomiting, call a physician. Keep away from eyes, mucous membrane, broken or irritated skin. If skin irritation develops, pain lasts 10 days or more, redness is present, or with arthritis-like conditions in children under 12, call a physician.

BONINE®
(meclizine hydrochloride)
Chewable Tablets

Actions: BONINE is an antihistamine which shows marked protective activity against nebulized histamine and lethal doses of intravenously injected histamine in guinea pigs. It has a marked effect in blocking the vasodepressor response to histamine, but only a slight blocking action against acetylcholine. Its activity is relatively weak in inhibiting the spasmogenic action of histamine on isolated guinea pig ileum.

Indications: BONINE is effective in the management of nausea, vomiting and dizziness associated with motion sickness.

Contraindications: Asthma, glaucoma, emphysema, chronic pulmonary disease, shortness of breath, difficulty in breathing, or difficulty in urination due to enlargement of the prostate gland unless directed by a doctor.

Warnings: May cause drowsiness; alcohol, sedatives and tranquilizers may increase the drowsiness effect. Avoid alcoholic beverages while taking this product. Do not take this product if you are taking sedatives or tranquilizers without first consulting your doctor. Do not drive or operate dangerous machinery while taking this medication.

Usage in Children: Clinical studies establishing safety and effectiveness in children have not been done; therefore, usage is not recommended in children under 12 years of age.

Usage in Pregnancy: As with any drug, if you are pregnant or nursing a baby, seek advice of a health care professional before taking this product.

Adverse Reactions: Drowsiness, dry mouth, and on rare occasions, blurred vision have been reported.

Dosage and Administration: For motion sickness 1 or 2 tablets of BONINE should be taken one hour prior to embarkation. Thereafter, the dose may be repeated every 24 hours for the duration of the journey.

How Supplied: BONINE (meclizine HCl) is available in convenient packets of 8 chewable tablets of 25 mg. meclizine HCl.

Inactive Ingredients: Cornstarch, FD&C Red #40, Lactose, Magnesium Stearate, Purified Siliceous Earth, Raspberry Flavor, Sodium Saccharin, Talc.

DESITIN® OINTMENT

Description: Desitin Ointment combines Zinc Oxide (40%) with Cod Liver Oil (high in Vitamins A & D), and Talc in a petrolatum-lanolin base suitable for topical application.

Actions and Uses: Desitin Ointment is designed to provide relief of diaper rash, superficial wounds and burns, and other minor skin irritations. It helps prevent incidence of diaper rash, protects against urine and other irritants, soothes chafed skin and promotes healing.

Relief and protection is afforded by Zinc Oxide, Cod Liver Oil, Lanolin and Petrolatum. They provide a physical barrier by forming a protective coating over skin or mucous membrane which serves to reduce further effects of irritants on the affected area and relieves burning, pain or itch produced by them. In addition to its protective properties, Zinc Oxide acts as an astringent that helps heal local irritation and inflammation by lessening the flow of mucus and other secretions.

Several studies have shown the effectiveness of Desitin Ointment in the relief and prevention of diaper rash.

Two clinical studies involving 90 infants demonstrated the effectiveness of Desitin Ointment in curing diaper rash. The diaper rash area was treated with Desitin Ointment at each diaper change for a period of 24 hours, while the untreated site served as controls. A significant reduction was noted in the severity and area of diaper dermatitis on the treated area.

Ninety-seven (97) babies participated in a 12-week study to show that Desitin Ointment helps prevent diaper rash. Approximately half of the infants (49) were treated with Desitin Ointment on a regular daily basis. The other half (48) received the ointment as necessary to treat any diaper rash which occurred. The incidence as well as the severity of diaper rash was significantly less among the babies using the ointment on a regular daily basis.

In a comparative study of the efficacy of Desitin Ointment vs. a baby powder, forty-five babies were observed for a total of eight weeks. Results support the conclusion that Desitin Ointment is a better prophylactic against diaper rash than the baby powder.

In another study, Desitin was found to be dramatically more effective in reducing the severity of medically diagnosed diaper rash than a commercially available diaper rash product in which only anhydrous lanolin and petrolatum are listed as ingredients. Fifty infants participated

Continued on next page

Leeming—Cont.

in the study, half of whom were treated with Desitin and half with the other product. In the group (25) treated with Desitin, seventeen infants showed significant improvement within 10 hours which increased to twenty-three improved infants within 24 hours. Of the group (25) treated with the other product, only three showed improvement at ten hours with a total of four improved within twenty-four hours. These results are statistically valid to conclude that Desitin Ointment reduces severity of diaper rash within ten hours.

Several other studies show that Desitin Ointment helps relieve other skin disorders, such as contact dermatitis.

Directions: Prevention: To prevent diaper rash, apply Desitin Ointment to the diaper area—especially at bedtime when exposure to wet diapers may be prolonged.

Treatment: If diaper rash is present, or at the first sign of redness, minor skin irritation or chafing, simply apply Desitin Ointment three or four times daily as needed. In superficial noninfected surface wounds and minor burns, apply a thin layer of Desitin Ointment, using a gauze dressing, if necessary. For external use only.

How Supplied: Desitin Ointment is available in 1 ounce (28g), 2 ounce (57g), 4 ounce (113g), 8 ounce (226g) tubes, and 1 lb. (452g) jar.

Shown in Product Identification Section, page 413

RHEABAN® Maximum Strength TABLETS
[rē'ăban]
(attapulgite)

Description: Maximum Strength Rheaban is an anti-diarrheal medication containing activated attapulgite and is offered in tablet form.

Each white Rheaban tablet contains 750 mg. of colloidal activated attapulgite. Rheaban provides the maximum level of medication when taken as directed. Rheaban contains no narcotics, opiates or other habit-forming drugs.

Actions and Uses: Rheaban is indicated for relief of diarrhea and the cramps and pains associated with it. Attapulgite, which has been activated by thermal treatment, is a highly sorptive substance which absorbs nutrients as well as noxious gases, irritants, toxins and some bacteria and viruses that are common causes of diarrhea.

In clinical studies to show the effectiveness in relieving diarrhea and its symptoms, 100 subjects suffering from acute gastroenteritis with diarrhea participated in a double-blind comparison of Rheaban to a placebo. Patients treated with the attapulgite product showed significantly improved relief of diarrhea and its symptoms vs. the placebo.

Dosage and Administration:
TABLETS

Adults—2 tablets after initial bowel movement, 2 tablets after each subsequent bowel movement.

Children 6 to 12 years—1 tablet after initial bowel movement, 1 tablet after each subsequent bowel movement.

Warnings: Do not exceed 12 tablets in 24 hours. Swallow tablets with water, do not chew. Do not use for more than two days, or in the presence of high fever. Tablets should not be used for infants or children under 6 years of age unless directed by physician. If diarrhea persists consult a physician.

How Supplied:
Tablets—Boxes of 12 tablets.

Inactive Ingredients: Colloidal Silicon Dioxide, Croscarmellose Sodium, Ethylcellulose, Hydroxypropyl Methylcellulose 2910, Pectin, Pharmaceutical Glaze, Sucrose, Talc, Titanium Dioxide, Zinc Stearate.

RID® Spray
Lice Control Spray

THIS PRODUCT IS NOT FOR USE ON HUMANS OR ANIMALS

Active Ingredient:

(5-Benzyl-3-Furyl) methyl 2,2-dimethyl-3-(2-methylpropenyl) cyclopropanecarboxylate	0.500%
Related Compounds	0.068%
Aromatic petroleum hydrocarbons	0.664%
Inert Ingredients	98.768%
	100.000%

Actions: A highly active synthetic pyrethroid for the control of lice and louse eggs on garments, bedding, furniture and other inanimate objects.

Warnings: Avoid contamination of feed and foodstuffs. Cover or remove fishbowls. HARMFUL IF SWALLOWED. This product is not for use on humans or animals. If lice infestations should occur on humans, consult either your physician or pharmacist for a product for use on humans.

Physical and Chemical Hazards: Contents under pressure. Do not use or store near heat or open flame. Do not puncture or incinerate container. Exposure to temperatures above 130° F may cause bursting.

CAUTION: Avoid spraying in eyes. Avoid breathing spray mist. Use only in well ventilated areas. Avoid contact with skin. In case of contact wash immediately with soap and water. Vacate room after treatment and ventilate before reoccupying.

Statement of Practical Treatment: If inhaled: Remove affected person to fresh air. Apply artificial respiration if indicated.

If in eyes: Flush with plenty of water. Contact physician if irritation persists.

If on skin: Wash affected areas immediately with soap and water.

Direction For Use: It is a violation of Federal law to use this product in a manner inconsistent with its labeling.

Shake well before each use. Remove protective cap. Aim spray opening away from person. Push button to spray.

To kill lice and louse eggs: Spray in an inconspicuous area to test for possible staining or discoloration. Inspect again after drying, then proceed to spray entire area to be treated.

Hold container upright with nozzle away from you. Depress valve and spray from a distance of 8 to 10 inches.

Spray each square foot for 3 seconds. Spray only those garments, parts of bedding, including mattresses and furniture that cannot be either laundered or dry cleaned.

Allow all sprayed articles to dry thoroughly before use. Repeat treatment as necessary.

Buyer assumes all risks of use, storage or handling of this material not in strict accordance with direction given herewith.

DISPOSAL OF CONTAINER

Wrap container and dispose of in trash. Do not incinerate.

How Supplied: 5 oz. aerosol can.

Also available in combination with RID® Lice Treatment Kit as the RID® Lice Elimination System.

RID®
Lice Killing Shampoo

Description: Rid contains a liquid pediculicide whose active ingredients are: pyrethrins 0.3% and piperonyl butoxide, technical 3.00%, equivalent to 2.4% (butylcarbityl) (6-propylpiperonyl) ether and to 0.6% related compounds. Also contains petroleum distillate 1.20% and benzyl alcohol 2.4%. Inert ingredients 93.1%.

Actions: RID kills head lice (*Pediculus humanus capitis*), body lice (*Pediculus humanus humanus*), and pubic or crab lice (*Phthirus pubis*), and their eggs.

The pyrethrins act as a contact poison and affect the parasite's nervous system, resulting in paralysis and death. The efficacy of the pyrethrins is enhanced by the synergist, piperonyl butoxide. Rid rinses out completely after treatment and is not designed to leave long-acting residues.

The active ingredients in RID are poorly absorbed through the skin. Of the relatively minor amounts that are absorbed, they are rapidly metabolized to water-soluble compounds and eliminated from the body without ill effects.

Indications: RID is indicated for the treatment of infestations of head lice, body lice and pubic (crab) lice, and their eggs.

Warning: RID should be used with caution by ragweed sensitized persons.

Precautions: This product is for external use only. It is harmful if swallowed. It should not be inhaled. It should be kept out of the eyes and contact with mucous membranes should be avoided. If accidental contact with eyes occurs, flush immediately with water. In case of infection or skin irritation, discontinue use and consult a physician. Consult a physician if infestation of eyebrows or eyelashes occurs. Avoid contamination of feed or foodstuffs.

Storage and Disposal: Do not store below 32°F (0°C). Do not reuse empty container. Wrap in several layers of newspaper and discard in trash.

Dosage and Administration: (1) Shake well. Apply undiluted RID to dry hair and scalp or to any other infested area until entirely wet. Do not use on eyelashes or eyebrows. (2) Allow RID to remain on area for 10 minutes but no longer. (3) Wash thoroughly with warm water and soap or shampoo. (4) Dead lice and eggs should be removed with the special nit comb provided. (5) Repeat treatment in 7 to 10 days to kill any newly hatched lice. Do not exceed two consecutive applications within 24 hours.
Since lice infestations are spread by contact, each family member should be examined carefully. If infested, he or she should be treated promptly to avoid spread or reinfestation of previously treated individuals. Contaminated clothing and other articles, such as hats, etc. should be dry cleaned, boiled or otherwise treated until decontaminated to prevent reinfestation or spread.

How Supplied: In 2, 4 and 8 fl. oz. plastic bottles. Exclusive nit removal comb that removes all the nits and patient instruction booklet (English and Spanish) are included in each package of RID. Also available in combination with RID Lice Control Spray as the RID Lice Elimination System.

UNISOM DUAL RELIEF®
Nighttime Sleep Aid and Pain Reliever

Description: Unisom Dual Relief® is a pale blue, capsule-shaped, coated tablet.

Active ingredients: 650 mg. acetaminophen and 50 mg. diphenhydramine HCl per tablet.

Inactive Ingredients: Corn starch, FD&C Blue #1, FD&C Blue #2, hydroxypropyl methylcellulose, magnesium stearate, polyethylene glycol, polysorbate 80, polyvinylpyrrolidone, stearic acid, titanium dioxide.

Indications: Unisom Dual Relief (diphenhydramine sleep aid formula) is indicated to help reduce difficulty in falling asleep while relieving accompanying minor aches and pains such as headache, muscle ache or menstrual discomfort. If there is difficulty in falling asleep, but pain is not being experienced at the same time, regular Unisom sleep aid is indicated which contains doxylamine succinate as its active ingredient.

Administration and Dosage: One tablet 30 minutes before retiring. Take once daily or as directed by a physician.

Warnings: DO NOT TAKE THIS PRODUCT IF YOU HAVE ASTHMA, GLAUCOMA OR ENLARGEMENT OF THE PROSTATE GLAND EXCEPT UNDER THE ADVICE AND SUPERVISION OF A PHYSICIAN.
Do not take this product for treatment of arthritis except under the advice and supervision of a physician. Do not exceed recommended dosage because severe liver damage may occur. If symptoms persist continuously for more than ten days, consult your physician. Insomnia may be a symptom of serious underlying medical illness. Take this product with caution if alcohol is being consumed. Do not take this product if pregnant or nursing a baby. For adults only. Do not give to children under 12 years of age. Keep this and all medications out of reach of children. IN CASE OF ACCIDENTAL OVERDOSE SEEK PROFESSIONAL ADVICE OR CONTACT A POISON CONTROL CENTER IMMEDIATELY.

Caution: This product contains an antihistamine and will cause drowsiness. It should be used only at bedtime.

Drug Interaction: Monoamine oxidase (MAO) inhibitors prolong and intensify the anticholinergic effects of antihistamines. The CNS depressant effect is heightened by alcohol and other CNS depressant drugs.

Attention: Use only if tablet blister seals are unbroken. Child resistant packaging.

How Supplied: Boxes of 8 and 16 tablets in child resistant blisters.

UNISOM® NIGHTTIME SLEEP AID
[yu 'na-som]
(doxylamine succinate)

Description: Pale blue oval scored tablets containing 25 mg. of doxylamine succinate, 2-[α-(2-dimethylaminoethoxy)α-methylbenzyl] pyridine succinate.

Action and Uses: Doxylamine succinate is an antihistamine of the ethanolamine class, which characteristically shows a high incidence of sedation. In a comparative clinical study of over 20 antihistamines on more than 3000 subjects, doxylamine succinate 25 mg. was one of the three most sedating antihistamines, producing a significantly reduced latency to end of wakefulness and comparing favorably with established hypnotic drugs such as secobarbital and pentobarbital in sedation activity. It was chosen as the antihistamine, based on dosage, causing the earliest onset of sleep. In another clinical study, doxylamine succinate 25 mg. scored better than secobarbital 100 mg. as a nighttime hypnotic. Two additional, identical clinical studies involving a total of 121 subjects demonstrated that doxylamine succinate 25 mg. reduced the sleep latency period by a third, compared to placebo. Duration of sleep was 26.6% longer with doxylamine succinate, and the quality of sleep was rated higher with the drug than with placebo. An EEG study of 6 subjects confirmed

the results of these studies. In yet another study, no statistically significant difference was found between doxylamine succinate and flurazepam in the average time required for 200 patients with mild to moderate insomnia to fall asleep over 5 nights following a nightly dose of doxylamine succinate 25 mg. or flurazepam 30 mg., nor was any statistically significant difference found in the total time the 200 patients slept. Patients on doxylamine succinate awoke an average of 1.2 times per night while those on flurazepam awoke an average of 0.9 times per night. In either case the patients awoke rested the following morning. On a rating scale of 1 to 5, doxylamine succinate was given a 3.0, flurazepam a 3.4 by patients rating the degree of restfulness provided by their medication (5 represents "very well rested"). Although statistically significant, the difference between doxylamine succinate 25 mg. and flurazepam 30 mg. in the number of awakenings and degree of restfulness is clinically insignificant.

Administration and Dosage: One tablet 30 minutes before retiring. Not for children under 12 years of age.

Side Effects: Occasional anticholinergic effects may be seen.

Precautions: Unisom® should be taken only at bedtime.

Contraindications: This product should not be taken by pregnant women, or those who are nursing a baby. This product is also contraindicated for asthma, glaucoma, enlargement of the prostate gland.

Warnings: Should be taken with caution if alcohol is being consumed. Product should not be taken if patient is concurrently on any other drug, without prior consultation with physician. Should not be taken for longer than two weeks unless approved by physician.

How Supplied: Boxes of 8, 32 or 48 tablets in child resistant blisters, and in boxes of 16 with non–child resistant packaging.

Inactive Ingredients: Dibasic Calcium Phosphate, FD&C Blue #1 Aluminum Lake, Magnesium Stearate, Microcrystalline Cellulose, Sodium Starch Glycolate.

VISINE®
Tetrahydrozoline Hydrochloride
Redness Reliever Eye Drops

Description: Visine is a sterile, isotonic, buffered ophthalmic solution containing tetrahydrozoline hydrochloride 0.05%, boric acid, sodium borate, sodium chloride and water. It is preserved with benzalkonium chloride 0.01% and edetate disodium 0.1%. Visine is a decongestant ophthalmic solution designed to provide symptomatic relief of conjunctival edema and hyperemia secondary to minor irritations, due to conditions such as smoke, dust, other airborne pollutants,

Continued on next page

Leeming—Cont.

swimming etc. and so-called nonspecific or catarrhal conjunctivitis. Relief is afforded by tetrahydrozoline hydrochloride, a sympathomimetic agent, which brings about decongestion by vasoconstriction. Reddened eyes are rapidly whitened by this effective vasoconstrictor, which limits the local vascular response by constricting the small blood vessels. The onset of vasoconstriction becomes apparent within minutes.

The effectiveness of Visine in relieving conjunctival hyperemia has been demonstrated by numerous clinicals, including several double-blind studies, involving more than 2,000 subjects suffering from acute or chronic hyperemia induced by a variety of conditions. Visine was found to be efficacious in providing relief from conjunctival hyperemia.

Indications: Relieves redness of the eye due to minor eye irritations.

Directions: Place 1 to 2 drops in the affected eye(s) up to four times daily.

Warning: To avoid contamination, do not touch tip of container to any surface. Replace cap after using. If you experience eye pain, changes in vision, continued redness or irritation of the eye, or if the condition worsens or persists for more than 72 hours, discontinue use and consult a doctor. If you have glaucoma, do not use this product except under the advice and supervision of a doctor. Overuse of this product may produce increased redness of the eye. If solution changes color or becomes cloudy, do not use. Remove contact lenses before using.

How Supplied: In 0.5 fl. oz., 0.75 fl. oz., and 1.0 fl. oz. plastic dispenser bottle and 0.5 fl. oz. plastic bottle with dropper.
Shown in Product Identification Section, page 413

VISINE A.C.®
Astringent/Redness Reliever Eye Drops

Description: Visine A.C. is a sterile, isotonic, buffered ophthalmic solution containing tetrahydrozoline hydrochloride 0.05%, zinc sulfate 0.25%, boric acid, sodium chloride, sodium citrate and purified water. It is preserved with benzalkonium chloride 0.01% and edetate disodium 0.1%. Visine A.C. is an ophthalmic solution combining the effects of the vasoconstrictor tetrahydrozoline hydrochloride with the astringent effects of zinc sulfate. The vasoconstrictor provides symptomatic relief of conjunctival edema and hyperemia secondary to minor irritation due to conditions such as dust and airborne pollutants as well as so-called nonspecific or catarrhal conjunctivitis, while zinc sulfate provides relief from hay fever, allergies, etc. Beneficial effects include amelioration of burning, irritation, pruritis, and removal of mucus from the eye. Relief is afforded by both ingredients, tetrahydrozoline hydrochloride and zinc sulfate.

Tetrahydrozoline hydrochloride is a sympathomimetic agent, which brings about decongestion by vasoconstriction. Reddened eyes are rapidly whitened by this effective vasoconstrictor, which limits the local vascular response by constricting the small blood vessels. The onset of vasoconstriction becomes apparent within minutes. Zinc sulfate is an ocular astringent which, by precipitating protein, helps to clear mucus from the outer surface of the eye.

The effectiveness of Visine A.C. in relieving conjunctival hyperemia and associated symptoms induced by allergies has been clinically demonstrated. In one double-blind study allergy sufferers experienced acute episodes of minor eye irritation. Visine A.C. produced statistically significant beneficial results versus a placebo of normal saline solution in relieving irritation of bulbar conjunctiva, irritation of palpebral conjunctiva, and mucous build-up. Treatment with Visine A.C. containing zinc sulfate also significantly improved burning and itching symptoms.

Indications: For temporary relief of discomfort and redness due to minor eye irritations.

Directions: Place 1 to 2 drops in the affected eye(s) up to 4 times daily.

Warning: To avoid contamination, do not touch tip of container to any surface. Replace cap after using. If you experience eye pain, changes in vision, continued redness or irritation of the eye, or if the condition worsens or persists for more than 72 hours, discontinue use and consult a doctor. If you have glaucoma, do not use this product except under the advice and supervision of a doctor. Overuse of this product may produce increased redness of the eye. If solution changes color or becomes cloudy, do not use. Remove contact lenses before using.

How Supplied: In 0.5 fl. oz. and 1.0 fl. oz. plastic dispenser bottle.
Shown in Product Identification Section, page 413

VISINE EXTRA®
Redness Reliever/Lubricant Eye Drops

Description: Visine Extra is a sterile, isotonic, buffered ophthalmic solution containing tetrahydrozoline hydrochloride 0.05%, polyethylene glycol 400 1.0%, boric acid, sodium borate, sodium chloride and water. It is preserved with benzalkonium chloride 0.013% and edetate disodium 0.1%.

Visine Extra is an ophthalmic solution combining the effects of the decongestant tetrahydrozoline hydrochloride with the demulcent effects of polyethylene glycol. It provides symptomatic relief of conjunctival edema and hyperemia secondary to ocular allergies, minor irritations and so-called nonspecific or catarrhal conjunctivitis. Tetrahydrozoline hydrochloride is a sympathomimetic agent, which brings about decongestion by vasoconstriction. Reddened eyes are rapidly

whitened by this effective vasoconstrictor, which limits the local vascular response by constricting the small blood vessels. The onset of vasoconstriction becomes apparent within minutes. Additional effects include amelioration of burning, irritation, pruritus, soreness, and excessive lacrimation. Relief is afforded by polyethylene glycol.

Polyethylene glycol is an ophthalmic demulcent which has been shown to be effective for the temporary relief of discomfort of minor irritations of the eye due to exposure to wind or sun. It is effective as a protectant and lubricant against further irritation or to relieve dryness of the eye.

The effectiveness of tetrahydrozoline hydrochloride in relieving conjunctival hyperemia and associated symptoms has been demonstrated by numerous clinicals, including several double-blind studies, involving more than 2000 subjects suffering from acute or chronic hyperemia induced by a variety of conditions. Visine Extra is a product that combines the redness relieving effects of a vasoconstrictor and the soothing moisturizing and protective effects of a demulcent.

Indications: Relieves redness of the eye due to minor eye irritations. For use as a protectant against further irritation or to relieve dryness.

Directions: Place 1 to 2 drops in the affected eye(s) up to 4 times daily.

Warning: To avoid contamination, do not touch tip of container to any surface. Replace cap after using. If you experience eye pain, changes in vision, continued redness or irritation of the eye, or if the condition worsens or persists for more than 72 hours, discontinue use and consult a doctor. If you have glaucoma, do not use this product except under the advice and supervision of a doctor. Overuse of this product may produce increased redness of the eye. If solution changes color or becomes cloudy, do not use. Remove contact lenses before using.

How Supplied: In 0.5 fl. oz. and 1.0 fl. oz. plastic dispenser bottle.
Shown in Product Identification Section, page 413

VISINE L. R.™ EYE DROPS
(oxymetazoline hydrochloride)

Description: Visine L. R. is a sterile, isotonic, buffered ophthalmic solution containing oxymetazoline hydrochloride 0.025%, boric acid, sodium borate, sodium chloride and water. It is preserved with benzalkonium chloride 0.01% and edetate disodium 0.1%.

Visine L. R. is produced by a process that assures sterility.

Indications: Visine L. R. is a decongestant ophthalmic solution designed for the relief of redness of the eye due to minor eye irritations. Visine L. R. is specially formulated to relieve redness of the eye in minutes with effective relief that lasts up to 6 hours.

Directions: *Adults and children 6 years of age and older*—Place 1 or 2 drops in the affected eye(s). This may be repeated as needed every 6 hours or as directed by a physician.

Parents: Before using with children under 6 years of age, consult your physician. Keep this and all other medications out of the reach of children. In case of accidental ingestion, seek professional assistance or contact a poison control center immediately.

Warning: If you experience eye pain, changes in vision, continued redness or irritation of the eye, or if the condition worsens or persists for more than 72 hours, discontinue use and consult a physician. If you have glaucoma, do not use this product except under the advice and supervision of a physician. As with any medication, if you are pregnant seek the advice of a physician before using this product. Overuse of this product may produce increased redness of the eye. If solution changes color or becomes cloudy, do not use. To avoid contamination of this product, do not touch tip of container to any surface. Replace cap after using. Remove contact lenses before using this product.

Caution: Should not be used if Visine imprinted neckband on bottle is broken or missing.

Storage: Store between 2° and 30°C (36° and 86°F).

How Supplied: In 0.5 fl. oz. and 1 fl. oz. plastic dispenser bottle.
Shown in Product Identification Section, page 413

WART–OFF®
Liquid

Active Ingredient: Salicylic Acid, U.S.P., 17%.

Inactive Ingredients: Alcohol, 18.1%, Camphor, Castor Oil, Ether 47.7%, Lactic Acid, Pyroxylin.

Indications: Removal of Warts

Warnings: Keep this and all medications out of reach of children to avoid accidental poisoning.
Flammable—Do not use near fire or flame. For external use only. In case of accidental ingestion, contact a physician or a Poison Control Center immediately. Do not use near eyes or on mucous membranes. Diabetics or other people with impaired circulation should not use Wart-Off®. Do not use on moles, birthmarks or unusual warts with hair growing from them. If wart persists, see your physician. If pain should develop, consult your physician. **Do not apply to surrounding skin.**

Instructions For Use: Read warning and enclosed instructional brochure. Apply Wart-Off® to warts only. Do not apply to surrounding skin. Make sure that surrounding skin is protected from acci-

dental application. Before applying, soak affected area in hot water for several minutes. If any tissue has been loosened, remove by rubbing surface of wart gently with cleaning brush enclosed in Wart-Off® package. Dry thoroughly. Warts are contagious, so don't share your towel. Apply once or twice daily. Using pinpoint applicator attached to cap, apply one drop at a time until entire wart is covered. Lightly cover with small adhesive bandage. Replace cap tightly to avoid evaporation. This treatment may be used daily for three to four weeks if necessary.

How Supplied: 0.5 fluid ounce bottle with special pinpoint plastic applicator, cleaning brush and instructional brochure.

Lehn & Fink
Division of Sterling Drug Inc.
Personal Products Division
225 SUMMIT AVENUE
MONTVALE, NJ 07645

DIAPARENE® BABY POWDER

Description: Powder comprised of corn starch, magnesium carbonate, methylbenzethonium chloride 0.055% and fragrance.

Action and Uses: Diaparene Baby Powder has a corn starch base for high absorbency to help keep baby's skin dry and for soothing diaper rash, prickly heat and chafing.

Administration and Dosage: Apply liberally to baby's skin after bath and with each diaper change.

How Supplied: Available in 4 oz, 9 oz, 14 oz containers.
Shown in Product Identification Section, page 413

DIAPARENE
[See table on next page]
Shown in Product Identification Section, page 413

DIAPARENE® SUPERS BABY WASH CLOTHS

Description: Wash cloths are impregnated with a cleansing solution containing water, SD alcohol-40, propylene glycol, PEG/60, lanolin, sodium nonoxynol-9-phosphate, sorbic acid, citric acid, disodium phosphate, oleth-20, and fragrance.

Action and Uses: Diaparene Baby Wash Cloths contain lanolin and a mild cleansing solution to clean and condition baby's skin.

Administration and Dosage: Wipe baby's skin with solution-impregnated wash cloths as required.

How Supplied: Available in canisters of 70 and 150 wash cloths.

Loma Linda Foods Inc.
11503 PIERCE STREET
RIVERSIDE, CA 92505

SOYALAC®   K PAREVE

Description: Soyalac is a nutritionally balanced, milk-free, soy formula based on the extract of the whole soybean. Soyalac is the only formula in the United States manufactured using the whole soybean as the initial raw materail. All of the protein, 30% of the fat and 30% of all other nutrients are derived from the soybeans.

Usage: As a beverage for infants, children and adults with an allergy or sensitivity to cow's milk. Feeding Soyalac may be recommended under the following circumstances:
—Cow's milk allergy or a family history of cow's milk allergy
—Lactose intolerance (primary or secondary following diarrhea)
—Vegetarianism

Preparation: Standard dilution is—
Ready to Use—as canned
Concentrate—one part mixed with an equal part of water
Powder (can)—four scoops to one cup of water (scoop supplied in can)

Availability:
Soyalac Ready to Use liquid:
32 fl oz cans, 6 cans per case
Soyalac Double Strength Concentrate:
13 fl oz cans, 12 cans per case
Soyalac Powder—Cans:
14 oz cans, 6 cans per case

Ingredients: Water, soybean solids, corn syrup, sucrose, soy oil, calcium carbonate, soy lecithin, sodium citrate, calcium citrate, calcium phosphate, salt, potassium phosphate, vitamins (ascorbic acid, alpha-tocopheryl acetate, niacinamide, calcium pantothenate, vitamin A palmitate, thiamine hydrochloride, riboflavin, pyridoxine hydrochloride, biotin, phytonadione, folic acid, cholecalciferol, cyanocobalamin), calcium carrageenan, L-methionine, potassium chloride, ferrous sulfate, taurine, zinc sulfate, L-carnitine, calcium chloride, cupric sulfate, potassium iodide.

Typical Analysis: Standard Dilution

SOYALAC	Nutrients per 100 Calories	per Liter
Protein (g)	3.1	21
Fat (g)	5.5	37
Carbohydrate (g)	10	68
Calories		675
Calories Per Fluid Ounce	20	
Essential Fatty Acids (linoleate) (g)	2.8	19.0
Vitamins:		
A (IU)	312	2110
D (IU)	62	420

Continued on next page

	Diaparene® **Medicated Cream**	**Diaparene®** **Peri-Anal®** **Medicated Ointment**	**Diaparene®** **Cradol®**
Description:	Special lotion formula to soothe and protect baby's skin. Contains: Methylbenzethonium Chloride 0.1% (w/w) Also contains: Dibasic Sodium Phosphate, Fragrance, Glycerine, Mineral Oil, Parabens, Polysorbate 60, Purified Water, Sorbitan Monostearate, Stearyl Alcohol, White Petrolatum.	Ointment that soothes and helps heal diaper rash, helps protect against wetness and irritation. Contains: Cod Liver Oil (vitamins A & D), Zinc Oxide, Methylbenzethonium Chloride 0.1% (w/w) Also contains: Calcium Caseinate, Fragrance, Lanolin, Lanolin Alcohol, Mineral Oil, Starch, Paraffin, White Petrolatum, Yellow Wax.	Medicated lotion scalp treatment for "cradle cap" developed by babies. Contains: Methylbenzethonium Chloride 0.07%. Also contains: Anhydrous Lanolin, Fragrance, Glyceryl Stearate, Lanolin, Lanolin Alcohol, Light Mineral Oil, Mineral Oil, Parabens, Paraffin, PEG-6 Stearate, Purified Water, Stearamidoethyl Diethylamine, Yellow Wax.
Action and Uses:	Nonstaining cream formula soothes and protects diaper area, knees, elbows—anywhere baby's skin needs comfort.	The antibacterial action of methylbenzethonium chloride combats ammonia-forming bacteria that can cause diaper rash and odor. Provides a water repellent shield to keep out wetness, and to protect skin from irritating urine, stool and perspiration.	Gently softens and separates crust and scales from the scalp. Helps prevent and treat local infection.
Administration and Dosage:	Directions: Apply anywhere skin chafing or irritation may develop. Use liberally, taking care to include skin folds where moisture collects.	Directions: At the first sign of redness or diaper rash, apply liberally to diaper area three times daily as needed. To help prevent diaper rash, apply to diaper area after each diaper change. Especially important at bedtime, or anytime that exposure to wet diapers may be prolonged. For minor skin irritations, apply a thin layer, using a gauze dressing if necessary.	Directions for "cradle cap" and scalp infection: Massage into wet or dry scalp 3 times daily for 3 days. Do not wash off or shampoo between applications. After 3 days, shampoo with mild soap and use a fine comb or scalp brush to gently brush away crusts and scales from baby's scalp. To prevent reoccurrence: Massage into wet or dry scalp 3 times weekly.
How Supplied:	NDC 12843-246-21 1 ounce tube NDC 12843-246-22 2 ounce tube NDC 12843-246-24 4 ounce tube	NDC 12843-236-10 1 ounce tube NDC 12843-236-20 2 ounce tube NDC 12843-236-40 4 ounce tube	NDC 12843-070-21 3 ounce bottle

E (IU)	2.3	16	Choline (mg)	16	110
K (mcg)	7.8	53	Inositol (mg)	16	110
B$_1$ (Thiamine) (mcg)	78	525	Minerals:		
B$_2$ (Riboflavin) (mcg)	94	635	Calcium (mg)	94	635
B$_6$ (Pyridoxine)			Phosphorus (mg)	55	370
(mcg)	70	475	Magnesium (mg)	12	81
B$_{12}$ (mcg)	0.31	2.1	Iron (mg)	1.9	13
Niacin (mcg)	1250	8450	Zinc (mg)	0.78	5.3
Folic Acid (mcg)	15.6	105	Manganese (mcg)	156	1055
Pantothenic Acid			Copper (mcg)	78	525
(mcg)	469	3170	Iodine (mcg)	7.8	53
Biotin (mcg)	9.4	64	Sodium (mg)	44	295
C (Ascorbic Acid)			Potassium (mg)	117	790
(mg)	12	81	Chloride (mg)	65	440

I-SOYALAC®   **K PAREVE**

Description: I-Soyalac is a nutritionally balanced, soy isolate infant formula

Products are cross-indexed by generic and chemical names in the
YELLOW SECTION

which is milk free, corn free and free of any animal ingredients.

Usage: As a beverage for infants, children and adults with an allergy or sensitivity to cow's milk. Feeding I-Soyalac may be recommended under the following circumstances:

—Intolerance to corn

—Cow's milk allergy or a family history of cow's milk allergy

—Lactose intolerance (primary or secondary following diarrhea)

—Galactosemia

—Common feeding problems

—Vegetarianism

Action and Uses: Same as Soyalac, with the added advantage that it may be used with confidence by infants, children and adults who may be sensitive to corn and corn products.

Preparation: Standard dilution is—
Ready to Serve—as canned
Concentrate—one part mixed with an equal part water

Ingredients: Water, sucrose, soy oil, soy protein isolate, tapioca dextrin, calcium phosphate, potassium citrate, soy lecithin, calcium carbonate, potassium chloride, calcium carrageenan, L-methionine, magnesium phosphate, vitamins (ascorbic acid, alpha-tocopheryl acetate, niacinamide, calcium pantothenate, vitamin A palmitate, thiamine hydrochloride, riboflavin, pyridoxine hydrochloride, folic acid, biotin, phytonadione, cholecalciferol, cyanocobalamin), calcium citrate, magnesium chloride, salt, choline chloride, ferrous sulfate, inositol, taurine, zinc sulfate, L-carnitine, cupric sulfate, potassium iodide.

Availability:
I-Soyalac Read-to-Use liquid
32 fl oz cans, 6 cans per case
I-Soyalac Double Strength Concentrate
13 fl oz cans, 12 cans per case

Typical Analysis: Standard Dilution
I-SOYALAC

	Nutrients per 100 Calories	per Liter
Protein (g)	3.1	21
Fat (g)	5.5	37
Carbohydrate (g)	10.0	68
Calories		675
Calories Per Fluid Ounce	20	
Essential Fatty Acids (linoleate) (g)	2.8	19.0
Vitamins:		
A (IU)	312	2110
D (IU)	63	425
E (IU)	2.3	16
K (mcg)	7.8	53
B_1 (Thiamine) (mcg)	94	635
B_2 (Riboflavin) (mcg)	94	635
B_6 Pyridoxine (mcg)	86	580
B_{12} (mcg)	0.31	2.1
Niacin (mcg)	1250	8450
Folic Acid (mcg)	15.6	105
Pantothenic Acid (mcg)	469	3170
Biotin (mcg)	7.8	53
C (Ascorbic Acid) (mg)	12	81
Choline (mg)	20	135
Inositol (mg)	17	115
Minerals:		
Calcium (mg)	102	690
Phosphorus (mg)	70	475
Magnesium (mg)	11	74
Iron (mg)	1.9	13
Zinc (mg)	0.78	5.3
Manganese (mcg)	47	320
Copper (mcg)	117	790
Iodine (mcg)	7.8	53
Sodium (mg)	42	285
Potassium (mg)	117	790
Chloride (mg)	78	525

EDUCATIONAL MATERIAL

Compare the Facts
Four-color 4-page brochure giving a comparison chart of Ingredients and Nutrition per 100 calories on all the leading soy-based infant formulas.
Congratulations on Your New Baby
New, updated version of the booklet on infant feeding.
Milk Allergy and Milk Substitutes
Booklet on milk allergies—diagnosis, symptoms, defense and course of action.
Milk-Free Recipes
Booklet of milk-free recipes.

Luyties Pharmacal Company
P.O. BOX 8080
ST. LOUIS, MO 63156

YELLOLAX
[*yel 'o-laks*]

Description: YELLOLAX is a combination of time proven Yellow-phenolphthalein, and the Homeopathic ingredients, Bryonia and Hydrastis. Clinically YELLOLAX is an oral laxative. Each tablet contains two grains of yellow phenolphthalein and the Bryonia and Hydrastis approximately one fortieth grain each.

Action: Yellow-phenolphthalein is an effective and safe laxative, which is not contraindicated in pregnancy. Homeopathic Bryonia is used to treat constipation and the pain associated with constipation. Homeopathic Bryonia tends to increase mucous membrane moisture. Homeopathic Hydrastis is also included in the treatment of constipation because, the Homeopathic Hydrastis provides some relief of constipation and the associated pain and headaches by relaxing mucous membranes and encouraging their secretion. YELLOLAX has been safely used in pregnancy, children, and as conjunctive treatment with hemorrhoidal complications.

Indications: YELLOLAX is indicated in the management of simple constipation. YELLOLAX is also indicated in those conditions which require a gentle laxative.

Contraindications: YELLOLAX and all laxatives are contraindicated in appendicitis. All laxatives containing phenolphthalein are contraindicated in patients who have hypersensitivity to phenolphthalein.

Warnings: Do not use laxatives in cases of severe colic, nausea and other symptoms of appendicitis. Do not use laxatives habitually nor continually. If condition persists consult physician. Keep this and all medication out of the reach of children. DO NOT exceed the recommended dosage.

Caution: Frequent or prolonged use may result in laxative dependence. If skin rash appears, discontinue use.

Side Effects: The phenolphthalein may impart a red color to the urine, (phenolphthalein is also used as a pH indicator), this is normal.

Dosage: For adults one or two tablets chewed before retiring. For children over six a quarter tablet to half tablet before retiring. Tablets should be well chewed. For younger children consult physician.

Supplied: Compressed tablets packed in glass bottles of 36 (NDC 0618-0832-55) and 100 (NDC 0618-0832-12), and in repackers of 1000 tablets.

Homoeopathic
Luyties also manufactures a complete line of homoeopathic products. If more information is needed contact them direct.

EDUCATIONAL MATERIAL

Packets are available containing descriptive literature on products manufactured by Luyties Pharmacal Company, company history, and pricing information.

Macsil, Inc.
1326 FRANKFORD AVENUE
PHILADELPHIA, PA 19125

BALMEX® BABY POWDER

Composition: Contains: Active Ingredient—zinc oxide; Inactive Ingredients—corn starch, calcium carbonate, BALSAN®(especially purified balsam Peru).

Action and Uses: Absorbent, emollient, soothing—for diaper irritation, intertrigo, and other common dermatological conditions. In acute, simple miliaria, itching ceases in minutes and lesions dry promptly. For routine use after bathing and each diaper change.

How Supplied: 8 oz. shaker-top plastic containers.

BALMEX® EMOLLIENT LOTION

Gentle and effective scientifically compounded infant's skin conditioner.

Continued on next page

Macsil—Cont.

Composition: Contains a special lanolin oil (non-sensitizing, dewaxed, moisturizing fraction of lanolin), BALSAN® (specially purified balsam Peru) and silicone.

Action and Uses: The special Lanolin Oil aids nature lubricate baby's skin to keep it smooth and supple. Balmex Emollient Lotion is also highly effective as a physiologic conditioner on adult's skin.

How Supplied: Available in 6 oz. dispenser-top plastic bottles.

BALMEX® OINTMENT

Composition: Contains: Active Ingredients—Bismuth Subnitrate, Zinc Oxide; Inactive Ingredients—Balsan (Specially Purified Balsam Peru), Benzoic Acid, Beeswax, Mineral Oil, Silicone, Synthetic White Wax, Purified Water, and other ingredients.

Action and Uses: Emollient, protective, anti-inflammatory, promotes healing—for diaper rash, minor burns, sunburn, and other simple skin conditions; also decubitus ulcers, skin irritations associated with ileostomy and colostomy drainage. Nonstaining, readily washes out of diapers and clothing.

How Supplied: 1, 2, 4 oz. tubes; 1 lb. plastic jars (½ oz. tubes for Hospitals only). Balmex Ointment-All Commercial Sizes-Safety Sealed.

Marion Laboratories, Inc.
Pharmaceutical Products Division
MARION INDUSTRIAL PARK
MARION PARK DRIVE
KANSAS CITY, MO 64137

DEBROX® Drops
[dē′brŏx]

Description: Carbamide peroxide 6.5%. Also contains citric acid, glycerin, propylene glycol, sodium stannate, water, and other ingredients.

Actions: DEBROX®, used as directed, cleanses the ear with sustained microfoam. DEBROX Drops foam on contact with earwax due to the release of oxygen.

Indications: DEBROX Drops provide a safe, nonirritating method of softening and removing earwax.

Directions: FOR USE IN THE EAR ONLY. Adults and children over 12 years of age: tilt head sideways and place 5 to 10 drops into ear. Tip of applicator should not enter ear canal. Keep drops in ear for several minutes by keeping head tilted or placing cotton in the ear. Use twice daily for up to four days if needed, or as directed by a doctor. Any wax remaining after treatment may be removed by gently flushing the ear with warm water, using a soft rubber bulb ear syringe. Children under 12 years of age: consult a doctor.

Warnings: Do not use if you have ear drainage or discharge, ear pain, irritation or rash in the ear, or are dizzy, unless directed by a physician. Do not use if you have an injury or perforation (hole) of the eardrum or after ear surgery unless directed by a physician. Do not use for more than four consecutive days. If excessive earwax remains after use of this product, consult a physician. Consult a physician prior to use in children under 12.

Cautions: Avoid exposing bottle to excessive heat and direct sunlight. Keep color tip on bottle when not in use. Avoid contact with eyes. Keep this and all drugs out of the reach of children. In case of accidental ingestion, seek professional assistance or contact a poison control center immediately.

How Supplied: DEBROX Drops are available in ½- or 1-fl-oz plastic squeeze bottles with applicator spouts.

Issued 1/89
Shown in Product Identification Section, page 413

GAVISCON® Antacid Tablets
[găv′ĭs-kŏn]

Composition: Each chewable tablet contains the following active ingredients:
Aluminum hydroxide dried gel... 80 mg
Magnesium trisilicate .... 20 mg
and the following inactive ingredients: alginic acid, calcium stearate, flavor, sodium bicarbonate, starch (may contain cornstarch), and sucrose.

Actions: Unique formulation produces soothing foam which floats on stomach contents. Foam containing antacid precedes stomach contents into the esophagus when reflux occurs to help protect the sensitive mucosa from further irritation. GAVISCON® acts locally without neutralizing entire stomach contents to help maintain integrity of the digestive process. Endoscopic studies indicate that GAVISCON Antacid Tablets are equally as effective in the erect or supine patient.

Indications: GAVISCON is specifically formulated for the temporary relief of heartburn (acid indigestion) due to acid reflux. GAVISCON is not indicated for the treatment of peptic ulcers.

Directions: Chew two to four tablets four times a day or as directed by a physician. Tablets should be taken after meals and at bedtime or as needed. For best results follow by a half glass of water or other liquid. DO NOT SWALLOW WHOLE.

Warnings: Do not take more than 16 tablets in a 24-hour period or 16 tablets daily for more than 2 weeks, except under the advice and supervision of a physician. Do not use this product except under the advice and supervision of a physician if you are on a sodium-restricted diet. Each GAVISCON Tablet contains approximately 0.8 mEq sodium.

Drug Interaction Precautions: Do not take this product if you are presently taking a prescription antibiotic drug containing any form of tetracycline.

Store at a controlled room temperature in a dry place.

Keep this and all drugs out of the reach of children. In case of accidental overdose, seek professional assistance or contact a poison control center immediately.

How Supplied: Available in bottles of 100 tablets and in foil-wrapped 2s in boxes of 30 tablets.

Issued 2/87
Shown in Product Identification Section, page 413

GAVISCON® EXTRA STRENGTH RELIEF FORMULA Antacid Tablets
[găv′ĭs-kŏn]

Composition: Each chewable tablet contains the following active ingredients:
Aluminum hydroxide .... 160 mg
Magnesium carbonate .... 105 mg
and the following inactive ingredients: alginic acid, calcium stearate, flavor, mannitol, sodium bicarbonate, stearic acid, and sucrose.

Directions: Chew 2 to 4 tablets four times a day or as directed by a physician. Tablets should be taken after meals and at bedtime or as needed. For best results follow by a half glass of water or other liquid. DO NOT SWALLOW WHOLE.

> **FDA Approved Uses:** For the relief of heartburn, sour stomach, and/or acid indigestion, and upset stomach associated with heartburn, sour stomach, and/or acid indigestion.

Warnings: Do not take more than 16 tablets in a 24-hour period or 16 tablets daily for more than 2 weeks, except under the advice and supervision of a physician. Do not use this product except under the advice and supervision of a physician if you are on a sodium-restricted diet. Each tablet contains approximately 1.3 mEq sodium.

Drug Interaction Precautions: Do not take this product if you are presently taking a prescription antibiotic drug containing any form of tetracycline.

Store at a controlled room temperature in a dry place.

Keep this and all drugs out of the reach of children.

In case of accidental overdose, seek professional assistance or contact a poison control center immediately.

How Supplied: Available in bottles of 100 tablets.

Issued 4/87
Shown in Product Identification Section, page 413

GAVISCON® EXTRA STRENGTH RELIEF FORMULA
Liquid Antacid
[găv 'ĭs-kŏn]

Composition: Each 2 teaspoonfuls (10 mL) contains the following active ingredients:

Aluminum hydroxide....................508 mg
Magnesium carbonate...................475 mg

And the following inactive ingredients: butylparaben, edetate disodium, flavor, glycerin, propylparaben, saccharin sodium, simethicone emulsion, sodium alginate, sorbitol solution, water, and xanthan gum.

FDA Approved Uses: For the relief of heartburn, sour stomach and/or acid indigestion, and upset stomach associated with heartburn, sour stomach and/or acid indigestion.

Directions: SHAKE WELL BEFORE USING. Take 2 to 4 teaspoonfuls four times a day or as directed by a physician. GAVISCON Extra Strength Relief Formula Liquid should be taken after meals and at bedtime, followed by half a glass of water. Dispense product only by spoon or other measuring device.

Warnings: Except under the advice and supervision of a physician, do not take more than 16 teaspoonfuls in a 24-hour period or 16 teaspoonfuls daily for more than 2 weeks. May have laxative effect. Do not use this product if you have a kidney disease; do not use this product if you are on a sodium-restricted diet. Each teaspoonful contains approximately 0.9 mEq sodium.

Drug Interaction Precautions: Do not take this product if you are presently taking a prescription antibiotic drug containing any form of tetracycline. Keep tightly closed. Avoid freezing. Store at a controlled room temperature. Keep this and all drugs out of the reach of children. In case of accidental overdose, seek professional assistance or contact a poison control center immediately.

How Supplied: Available in 12 fl oz (355 mL) bottles.

Issued 2/89
Shown in Product Identification Section, page 413

GAVISCON® Liquid Antacid
[găv 'ĭs-kŏn]

Composition: Each tablespoonful (15 ml) contains the following active ingredients:

Aluminum hydroxide .... 95 mg
Magnesium carbonate .... 412 mg

And the following inactive ingredients: D&C Yellow #10, edetate disodium, FD&C Blue #1, flavor, glycerin, paraben preservatives, saccharin sodium, sodium alginate, sorbitol solution, water, and xanthan gum.

FDA Approved Uses: For the relief of heartburn, sour stomach and/or acid indigestion, and upset stomach associated with heartburn, sour stomach and/or acid indigestion.

Directions: SHAKE WELL BEFORE USING. Take 1 or 2 tablespoonfuls four times a day or as directed by a physician. GAVISCON Liquid should be taken after meals and at bedtime, followed by half a glass of water. Dispense product only by spoon or other measuring device.

Warnings: Except under the advice and supervision of a physician, do not take more than 8 tablespoonfuls in a 24-hour period or 8 tablespoonfuls daily for more than 2 weeks. May have laxative effect. Do not use this product if you have a kidney disease; do not use this product if you are on a sodium-restricted diet. Each tablespoonful of GAVISCON Liquid contains approximately 1.7 mEq sodium.

Drug Interaction Precautions: Do not take this product if you are presently taking a prescription antibiotic drug containing any form of tetracycline. Keep tightly closed. Avoid freezing. Store at a controlled room temperature. Keep this and all drugs out of the reach of children. In case of accidental overdose, seek professional assistance or contact a poison control center immediately.

How Supplied: Bottles of 12 fluid ounce (355 ml) and 6 fluid ounce (177 ml).

Issued 2/87
Shown in Product Identification Section, page 414

GAVISCON®-2 Antacid Tablets
[găv 'ĭs-kŏn]

Composition: Each chewable tablet contains the following active ingredients:

Aluminum hydroxide dried gel...160 mg
Magnesium trisilicate .... 40 mg

and the following inactive ingredients: alginic acid, calcium stearate, flavor, sodium bicarbonate, starch (may contain cornstarch), and sucrose.

Indications: GAVISCON® is specifically formulated for the temporary relief of heartburn (acid indigestion) due to acid reflux. GAVISCON is not indicated for the treatment of peptic ulcers.

Directions: Chew one to two tablets four times a day or as directed by a physician. Tablets should be taken after meals and at bedtime or as needed. For best results follow by a half glass of water or other liquid. DO NOT SWALLOW WHOLE.

Warnings: Do not take more than eight tablets in a 24-hour period or eight tablets daily for more than 2 weeks, except under the advice and supervision of a physician. Do not use this product except under the advice and supervision of a physician if you are on a sodium-restricted diet. Each GAVISCON-2 Tablet contains approximately 1.6 mEq sodium.

Drug Interaction Precautions: Do not take this product if you are presently taking a prescription antibiotic drug containing any form of tetracycline. Store at a controlled room temperature in a dry place. Keep this and all drugs out of the reach of children. In case of accidental overdose, seek professional assistance or contact a poison control center immediately.

How Supplied: Boxes of 48 foil-wrapped tablets.

Issued 2/87
Shown in Product Identification Section, page 414

GLY-OXIDE® Liquid
[glī-ok 'sīd]

Description: GLY-OXIDE® Liquid contains carbamide peroxide 10%. Also contains citric acid, flavor, glycerin, propylene glycol, sodium stannate, water, and other ingredients.

Actions: GLY-OXIDE® Liquid has an oxygen-rich formula that works to relieve the pain of canker sores by cleaning and debriding damaged tissue so natural healing can occur.

Administration: Do not dilute. Apply directly from bottle. Replace color tip on bottle when not in use.

Indications: For local treatment and hygienic prevention of minor oral inflammation such as canker sores, denture irritation, and postdental procedure irritation. Place several drops on affected area four times daily, after meals and at bedtime, or as directed by a dentist or physician; expectorate after two or three minutes. Or place 10 drops onto tongue, mix with saliva, swish for several minutes, and expectorate.
As an adjunct to oral hygiene (orthodontics, dental appliances) after regular brushing, swish 10 or more drops vigorously. Continue for two to three minutes; expectorate.
When normal oral hygiene is inadequate or impossible (total care geriatrics, etc), swish 10 or more drops vigorously after meals and expectorate.

Precautions: Severe or persistent oral inflammation, denture irritation, or gingivitis may be serious. If these conditions or unexpected side effects occur, consult a dentist or physician immediately. Avoid contact with eyes. Protect from heat and direct light. Keep this and all drugs out of the reach of children. In case of accidental overdose, seek professional assistance or contact a poison control center immediately.

How Supplied: GLY-OXIDE® Liquid is available in ½-fl-oz and 2-fl-oz nonspill, plastic squeeze bottles with applicator spouts.

Issued 2/89
Shown in Product Identification Section, page 414

Continued on next page

Marion—Cont.

OS-CAL® 500 Chewable Tablets
[ăhs 'kăl]
(calcium supplement)

Each Tablet Contains: 1,250 mg of calcium carbonate.
Elemental calcium........................ 500 mg
Ingredients: calcium carbonate, dextrose monohydrate, maltodextrin, microcrystalline cellulose, magnesium stearate, Bavarian cream flavor, sodium chloride, and coconut cream flavor.

Directions: One tablet two to three times a day with meals, or as recommended by your physician.

Two Tablets Provide: 1,000 mg calcium, 100% of U.S. RDA for adults and children 12 or more years of age.

Three Tablets Provide: 1,500 mg calcium, 115% of U.S. RDA for pregnant and lactating women.

Store at room temperature. Keep out of reach of children.

How Supplied: OS-CAL® 500 Chewable Tablets is available in bottles of 60 tablets.

Issued 10/87
Shown in Product Identification Section, page 414

OS-CAL® 500 Tablets
[ăhs 'kăl]
(calcium supplement)

Each Tablet Contains: 1,250 mg of calcium carbonate from oyster shell, an organic calcium source.
Elemental calcium .... 500 mg
Ingredients: oyster shell powder, corn syrup solids, talc, hydroxypropyl methylcellulose, cornstarch, sodium starch glycolate, calcium stearate, polysorbate 80, pharmaceutical glaze, titanium dioxide, methyl propyl paraben, polyethylene glycol, polyvinylpyrrolidone, carnauba wax, D&C Yellow #10, acetylated monoglyceride, edetate disodium, FD&C Blue #1, and simethicone emulsion.

Directions: One tablet two or three times a day with meals, or as recommended by your physician.

Two Tablets Provide: 1,000 mg calcium, 100% of U.S. RDA for adults and children 12 or more years of age.

Three Tablets Provide: 1,500 mg calcium, 115% of U.S. RDA for pregnant and lactating women.

Store at room temperature. Keep out of reach of children.

How Supplied: OS-CAL® 500 is available in bottles of 60 and 120 tablets.
Issued 10/87
Shown in Product Identification Section, page 414

OS-CAL® 250+D Tablets
[ăhs 'kăl]
(calcium supplement with vitamin D)

Each Tablet Contains: 625 mg of calcium carbonate from oyster shell, an organic calcium source.
Elemental calcium .... 250 mg
Vitamin D .... 125 USP Units

Ingredients: oyster shell powder, corn syrup solids, talc, cornstarch, hydroxypropyl methylcellulose, calcium stearate, polysorbate 80, titanium dioxide, methyl propyl paraben, polyethylene glycol, pharmaceutical glaze, vitamin D, polyvinylpyrrolidone, carnauba wax, D&C Yellow #10, acetylated monoglyceride, edetate disodium, FD&C Blue #1, simethicone emulsion, and edible gray ink.

Directions: One tablet three times a day with meals, or as recommended by your physician.

Three Tablets Provide:

		% U.S. RDA for Adults
Calcium	750 mg	.... 75%
Vitamin D	375 Units	.... 94%

Store at room temperature. Keep out of reach of children.

How Supplied: OS-CAL® 250+D is available in bottles of 100, 240, 500, and 1,000 tablets.
Issued 10/87
Shown in Product Identification Section, page 414

OS-CAL® 500+D Tablets
[ăhs 'kăl]
(calcium supplement with vitamin D)

Each Tablet Contains: 1,250 mg of calcium carbonate from oyster shell, an organic calcium source.
Elemental calcium .... 500 mg
Vitamin D .... 125 USP Units

Ingredients: oyster shell powder, corn syrup solids, talc, hydroxypropyl methylcellulose, cornstarch, sodium starch glycolate, calcium stearate, polysorbate 80, pharmaceutical glaze, titanium dioxide, methyl propyl paraben, polyethylene glycol, polyvinylpyrrolidone, vitamin D, carnauba wax, D&C Yellow #10, acetylated monoglyceride, edetate disodium, FD&C Blue #1, and simethicone emulsion.

Directions: One tablet two or three times a day with meals, or as recommended by your physician.

Two Tablets Provide: 1,000 mg calcium, 100% of U.S. RDA for adults and children 12 or more years of age and 64% of vitamin D.

Three Tablets Provide: 1,500 mg calcium, 115% of U.S. RDA for pregnant and lactating women and 94% of vitamin D.
Store at room temperature. Keep out of reach of children.

How Supplied: OS-CAL® 500+D is available in bottles of 60 and 120.

Issued 10/87
Shown in Product Identification Section, page 414

OS-CAL® FORTIFIED Tablets
[ăhs 'kăl]
(multivitamin and minerals supplement with added calcium)

Each Tablet Contains:
Vitamin A (palmitate) 1668 USP Units
Vitamin D .... 125 USP Units
Thiamine mononitrate
  (vitamin B$_1$)................................ 1.7 mg
Riboflavin (vitamin B$_2$)................ 1.7 mg
Pyridoxine hydrochloride
  (vitamin B$_6$)................................ 2.0 mg
Ascorbic acid (vitamin C).......... 50.0 mg
dl-alpha-tocopherol acetate
  (vitamin E) .... 0.8 IU
Niacinamide .... 15.0 mg
Calcium (from oyster shell) .... 250.0 mg
Iron (as ferrous fumarate)........... 5.0 mg
Magnesium (as oxide)................... 1.6 mg
Manganese (as sulfate)................ 0.3 mg
Zinc (as sulfate)............................. 0.5 mg

Ingredients: oyster shell powder, ascorbic acid, corn syrup solids, niacinamide, D&C Yellow #10 Aluminum Lake, ferrous fumarate, calcium stearate, FD&C Blue #1 Aluminum Lake, cornstarch, vitamin A palmitate, polysorbate 80, magnesium oxide, pyridoxine, thiamine, riboflavin, vitamin E, pharmaceutical glaze, methyl paraben, zinc sulfate, manganese sulfate, propylparaben, povidone, vitamin D, hydroxypropyl methylcellulose, carnauba wax, titanium dioxide, ethylcellulose, and acetylated monoglyceride.

Indication: Multivitamin and mineral supplement with added calcium.

Dosage: One tablet three times daily with meals or as directed by physician. In case of accidental overdose, seek professional assistance or contact a poison control center immediately.

Keep out of reach of children.
Store at room temperature.

How Supplied: Bottles of 100 tablets.
Issued 6/89
Shown in Product Identification Section, page 414

OS-CAL® PLUS Tablets
[ăhs 'kăl]
(multivitamin and multimineral supplement)

Each Tablet Contains:
Elemental calcium (from oyster shell).. 250 mg
Vitamin D .... 125 USP Units
Vitamin A (palmitate) 1666 USP Units
Vitamin C (ascorbic acid)...... 33.0   mg
Vitamin B$_2$ (riboflavin).......... 0.66   mg
Vitamin B$_1$ (thiamine
  mononitrate) .... 0.5   mg
Vitamin B$_6$ (pyridoxine HCl) 0.5   mg

Niacinamide..............................	3.33	mg
Iron (as ferrous fumarate).....	16.6	mg
Zinc (as the sulfate).................	0.75	mg
Manganese (as the sulfate)....	0.75	mg

Ingredients: oyster shell powder, corn syrup solids, ferrous fumarate, ascorbic acid, calcium stearate, cornstarch, hydroxypropyl methylcellulose, polysorbate 80, titanium dioxide, vitamin A palmitate, niacinamide, ethylcellulose, manganese sulfate, methyl propyl paraben, zinc sulfate, pharmaceutical glaze, acetylated monoglyceride, riboflavin, thiamine mononitrate, pyridoxine hydrochloride, povidone, vitamin D, carnauba wax, and D&C Red #33.

Indications: As a multivitamin and multimineral supplement.

Dosage: One (1) tablet three times a day before meals or as directed by a physician. For children under 4 years of age, consult a physician.
Store at room temperature.
Keep out of reach of children. In case of accidental overdose, seek professional assistance or contact a poison control center immediately.

How Supplied: Bottles of 100 tablets.
Issued 10/87
Shown in Product Identification Section, page 414

THROAT DISCS® Throat Lozenges
[*thrōt dĭsks*]

Description: Each lozenge contains sucrose, starch (may contain cornstarch), acacia, glycyrrhiza extract (licorice), gum tragacanth, anethole, linseed, cubeb oleoresin, anise oil, peppermint oil, capsicum, and mineral oil.

Indications: Effective for soothing, temporary relief of minor throat irritations from hoarseness and coughs due to colds.

Precautions: For severe or persistent cough or sore throat, or sore throat accompanied by high fever, headache, nausea, and vomiting, consult physician promptly. Not recommended for children under 3 years of age.

Directions: Allow lozenge to dissolve slowly in mouth. One or two should give the desired relief.

How Supplied: Boxes of 60 lozenges.
Issued 9/88
Shown in Product Identification Section, page 414

IDENTIFICATION PROBLEM?
Consult the
Product Identification Section
where you'll find
products pictured
in full color.

Marlyn Health Care
6324 FERRIS SQUARE
SAN DIEGO, CA 92121

MARLYN PMS®
[*mar-lĭn pms*]
Nutritional Supplement for Women
Multi-Vitamin Mineral Pak
Five tablets/capsules per pak

Each Pak Contains   *% USRDA
VITAMIN A, D, & E CAPSULE

Vitamin A (Fish Liver Oil)	5000	IU	100
Vitamin D (Fish Liver Oil)	400	IU	100
Vitamin E (d-Alpha-Tocopherol)	200	IU	333

In a base of safflower oil containing:

Linoleic Acid	113.07	mg
Linolenic Acid	0.754	mg

VITAMIN B COMPLEX, SUSTAINED RELEASE W/PANCREATIN

Vitamin B_1 (Thiamine)	25	mg	1666
Vitamin B_2 (Riboflavin)	25	mg	1470
Niacinamide	25	mg	80
Vitamin B_6 (Pyridoxine)	125	mg	6250
Vitamin B_{12} (Cobalamin Conc)	50	mcg	833
Biotin	25	mcg	8.3
Pantothenic Acid (d-Cal Panto)	25	mg	250
Folic Acid	200	mcg	50
Choline (Bitartrate)	50	mg	**
Inositol	50	mg	**
Para-aminobenzoic Acid	50	mg	**

In a base containing pancreatin

VITAMIN C COMPLEX, SUSTAINED RELEASE

Vitamin C (Ascorbic Acid)	500	mg	833
Lemon Bioflavonoids	100	mg	**
Hesperidin	100	mg	**

MULTI-MINERALS, AMINO ACID CHELATED

Iron (Chelated Gluconate)	9	mg	50
Calcium (Dicalcium Phosphate & Bone Meal)	400	mg	40
Phosphorus (Dicalcium Phosphate & Bone Meal)	155	mg	15
Iodine (Kelp)	75	mcg	50
Zinc (Chelated Gluconate)	7.5	mg	50
Copper (Chelated Gluconate)	1	mg	50
Manganese (Chelated Gluconate)	5	mg	**
Potassium (Amino Acid Complex)	25	mg	**
Chromium (Organically Bound Yeast)	1	mcg	**
Selenium (Organically Bound Yeast)	50	mcg	**

MAGNESIUM TABLET, AMINO ACID CHELATED

Magnesium	250	mg	62

*United States recommended daily allowance.
**USRDA not established.

McNeil Consumer Products Company
Division of McNeil-PPC, Inc.
Fort Washington, PA 19034

IMODIUM® A-D
(loperamide hydrochloride)

PRODUCT OVERVIEW

Key Facts: IMODIUM® A-D is an antidiarrheal containing 2mg loperamide per caplet and 1mg loperamide per teaspoon. IMODIUM® A-D acts by slowing intestinal motility and by affecting water and electrolyte movement through the bowel.

Major Uses: IMODIUM® A-D is indicated for the control and symptomatic relief of acute nonspecific diarrhea.

Safety Information: No known drug interactions. Do not use if diarrhea is accompanied by high fever (greater than 101°F), or if blood is present in the stool.

PRESCRIBING INFORMATION
IMODIUM® A-D
(loperamide hydrochloride)

Description: Each caplet of Imodium A-D contains 2 mg of loperamide hydrochloride. They are coloured green and scored. Each 5 ml (teaspoon) of Imodium A-D liquid contains loperamide hydrochloride 1 mg. Imodium A-D liquid is stable, cherry flavored, and clear in color.

Actions: Imodium A-D contains a clinically proven antidiarrheal medication. Loperamide HCl acts by slowing intestinal motility and by affecting water and electrolyte movement through the bowel.

Indication: Imodium A-D is indicated for the control and symptomatic relief of acute nonspecific diarrhea.

Usual Dosage:
Adults: Take two caplets or four teaspoonfuls after first loose bowel movement. If needed, take 1 caplet or two teaspoonfuls after each subsequent loose bowel movement. Do not exceed four caplets or eight teaspoonfuls in any 24-hour period, unless directed by a physician.
9–11 years old (60–95 lb.): One caplet or two teaspoonfuls after first loose bowel movement, followed by one-half caplet or one teaspoonful after each subsequent loose bowel movement. Do not exceed three caplets or six teaspoonfuls a day.
6–8 years old (48–59 lb.): One caplet or two teaspoonfuls after first loose bowel movement, followed by one-half caplet or one teaspoonful after each subsequent loose bowel movement. Do not exceed two caplets or four teaspoonfuls a day.
Professional Dosage Schedule for children 2–5 years old (24–27 lb): one teaspoon af-

Continued on next page

McNeil Consumer—Cont.

ter first loose bowel movement, followed by one after each subsequent loose bowel movement. Do not exceed three tea-spoonfuls a day.

Warnings: Since Imodium A-D is available without a prescription, the following information appears on the package label: "WARNINGS: DO NOT USE FOR MORE THAN TWO DAYS UNLESS DIRECTED BY A PHYSICIAN. Do not use if diarrhea is accompanied by high fever (greater than 101°F), or if blood is present in the stool, or if you have had a rash or other allergic reaction to loperamide HCl. If you are taking antibiotics or have a history of liver disease, consult a physician before using this product. As with any drug, if you are pregnant or nursing a baby, seek the advice of a physician before using this product. Keep this and all drugs out of the reach of children. In case of accidental overdose, seek professional assistance or contact a poison control center immediately. Store at room temperature."

Overdosage: Overdosage of loperamide HCl in man may result in constipation, CNS depression, and nausea. A slurry of activated charcoal administered promptly after ingestion of loperamide hydrochloride can reduce the amount of drug which is absorbed. If vomiting occurs spontaneously upon ingestion, a slurry of 100 grams of activated charcoal should be administered orally as soon as fluids can be retained. If vomiting has not occurred, and CNS depression is evident, gastric lavage should be performed followed by administration of 100 grams of the activated charcoal slurry through the gastric tube. In the event of overdosage, patients should be monitored for signs of CNS depression for at least 24 hours. Children may be more sensitive to central nervous system effects than adults. If CNS depression is observed, naloxone may be administered. If responsive to naloxone, vital signs must be monitored carefully for recurrence of symptoms of drug overdose for at least 24 hours after the last dose of naloxone.

Inactive Ingredients:
Caplets: Corn starch, lactose, magnesium stearate, microcrystalline cellulose, FD&C Blue No. 1, and D&C Yellow No. 10.
Liquid: Alcohol (5.25%), citric acid, flavors, glycerin, methylparaben, propylparaben and purified water.

How Supplied:
Green, scored caplets 6's and 12's in tamper-resistant child-resistant blister packages.
Cherry-flavored liquid (clear) 2 fl. oz., 3 fl. oz., and 4 fl. oz. tamper-resistant bottles with child-resistant safety caps and special dosage cups.
BK403
Shown in Product Identification Section, page 416

MEDIPREN®
Ibuprofen Caplets and Tablets
Pain Reliever/Fever Reducer

WARNING
ASPIRIN SENSITIVE PATIENTS: Do not take this product if you have had a severe allergic reaction to aspirin (e.g., asthma, swelling, shock or hives) because even though this product contains no aspirin or salicylates, cross-reactions may occur in patients allergic to aspirin.

Description: Each MEDIPREN Caplet or Tablet contains ibuprofen 200 mg.

Indications: For the temporary relief of minor aches and pains associated with the common cold, headache, toothaches, muscular aches, backache, for the minor pain of arthritis, for the pain of menstrual cramps, and for reduction of fever.

Usual Dosage: *Adults:* One Caplet or Tablet every 4 to 6 hours while symptoms persist. If pain or fever does not respond to 1 Caplet or Tablet, 2 Caplets or Tablets may be used but do not exceed 6 Caplets or Tablets in 24 hours, unless directed by a doctor. The smallest effective dose should be used. Take with food or milk if occasional and mild heartburn, upset stomach, or stomach pain occurs with use. Consult a doctor if these symptoms are more than mild or if they persist.
Children: Do not give this product to children under 12 except under the advice and supervision of a doctor.

Warnings: Do not take for pain for more than 10 days or for fever for more than 3 days unless directed by a doctor. If pain or fever persists or gets worse, if new symptoms occur, or if the painful area is red or swollen, consult a doctor. These could be signs of serious illness. If you are under a doctor's care for any serious condition, consult a doctor before taking this product. As with aspirin and acetaminophen, if you have any condition which requires you to take prescription drugs or if you have had any problems or serious side effects from taking any nonprescription pain reliever, do not take this product without first discussing it with your doctor. If you experience any symptoms which are unusual or seem unrelated to the condition for which you took ibuprofen, consult a doctor before taking any more of it. Although ibuprofen is indicated for the same conditions as aspirin and acetaminophen, it should not be taken with them except under a doctor's direction. Do not combine this product with any other ibuprofen containing product. As with any drug, if you are pregnant or nursing a baby, seek the advice of a health professional before using this product. IT IS ESPECIALLY IMPORTANT NOT TO USE IBUPROFEN DURING THE LAST 3 MONTHS OF PREGNANCY UNLESS SPECIFICALLY DIRECTED TO DO SO BY A DOCTOR BECAUSE IT MAY CAUSE PROBLEMS IN THE UNBORN CHILD OR COMPLICATIONS DURING DELIVERY. Keep this and all drugs out of the reach of children.

Overdosage: In case of accidental overdose, contact a physician or poison control center.

Storage: Store at room temperature; avoid excessive heat 40°C (104°F).

Inactive Ingredients: Colloidal silicon dioxide, glyceryl triacetate, hydroxypropyl methylcellulose, microcrystalline cellulose, pregelatinized starch, sodium lauryl sulfate, sodium starch glycolate, titanium dioxide, FD&C blue #1 and D&C yellow #10.

How Supplied: Coated Caplets (colored white, imprinted "MEDIPREN")—bottles of 24's, 50's, 100's. Coated Tablets (colored white, imprinted "MEDIPREN")—bottles of 24's, 50's, 100's.
Shown in Product Identification Section, page 414

PEDIACARE® Cold Formula Liquid
PEDIACARE® Cough-Cold Formula Liquid and Chewable Tablets
PEDIACARE® NightRest Cough-Cold Formula Liquid
PEDIACARE® Infants' Oral Decongestant Drops

PRODUCT OVERVIEW

Key Facts: PediaCare® Cold Relief Products are formulated specifically for relief of pediatric cold and cough symptoms. These products are formulated to allow accurate dosing by age and weight, especially when using the enclosed dropper or dosage cup.
Recommended dosage schedules for Pediacare Infants' Drops, Cold Formula, Cough-Cold Formula are the same as recommended dosage schedules for Children's TYLENOL Infants' Drops, Elixir and Chewable Tablets, respectively.

PRESCRIBING INFORMATION

PEDIACARE® Cold Formula Liquid
PEDIACARE® Cough-Cold Formula Liquid and Chewable Tablets
PEDIACARE® NightRest Cough-Cold Formula Liquid
PEDIACARE® Infants' Oral Decongestant Drops

Description: Each 5 ml of PEDIACARE Cold Formula Liquid contains pseudoephedrine hydrochloride 15 mg and chlorpheniramine maleate 1 mg. Each 5 ml of PEDIACARE Cough-Cold Formula Liquid contains pseudoephedrine hydrochloride 15 mg, chlorpheniramine maleate 1 mg and dextromethorphan hydrobromide 5 mg. Each PEDIACARE Cough-Cold Formula Chewable Tablet contains pseudoephedrine hydrochloride 7.5 mg, chlorpheniramine maleate 0.5 mg and dextromethorphan hydrobromide 2.5 mg. Each 0.8 ml oral dropper of PEDIACARE Infants' Oral Decongestant Drops contains pseudoephedrine hydrochloride 7.5 mg. PEDIACARE NightRest contains pseudoephedrine hydrochloride 15 mg, chlorpheniramine maleate 1 mg and dextromethorphan hydrobromide 7.5 mg per 5 ml. PEDIACARE Liquid Products and Infants' Drops are stable, cherry flavored and red in color. PEDIACARE Cough-

Age Group	0–3 mo	4–11 mo	12–23 mo	2–3 yr	4–5 yr	6–8 yr	9–10 yr	11 yr	Dosage
Weight (lb)	6–11 lb	12–17 lb	18–23 lb	24–35 lb	36–47 lb	48–59 lb	60–71 lb	72–95 lb	
PEDIACARE Infants' Drops*	½ dropper (0.4 ml)	1 dropper (0.8 ml)	1½ droppers (1.2 ml)	2 droppers (1.6 ml)					q4–6h
PEDIACARE Cold Formula Liquid**				1 tsp	1½ tsp	2 tsp	2½ tsp	3 tsp	q4–6h
PEDIACARE Cough-Cold Formula Liquid**				1 tsp	1½ tsp	2 tsp	2½ tsp	3 tsp	q4–6h
Chewable Tablets**				2 tabs	3 tabs	4 tabs	5 tabs	6 tabs	q4–6h
PEDIACARE NightRest Liquid**									

*Administer to children under 2 years only on the advice of a physician.
**Administer to children under 6 years only on the advice of a physician.

Cold Formula Chewable Tablets are fruit flavored and pink in color.

Actions: PEDIACARE Cold Products are available in four different formulas, allowing you to select the ideal cold product to temporarily relieve the patient's cold symptoms. PEDIACARE Cold Formula Liquid contains a decongestant, pseudoephedrine hydrochloride, and an antihistamine, chlorpheniramine maleate, to provide temporary relief of nasal congestion, runny nose and sneezing due to the common cold, hay fever or other upper respiratory allergies. PEDIACARE Cough-Cold Formula Liquid and Chewable Tablets contain both of the above ingredients plus a cough suppressant, dextromethorphan hydrobromide, to provide temporary relief of nasal congestion, runny nose, sneezing and coughing due to the common cold, hay fever or other upper respiratory allergies. PEDIACARE NightRest Cough-Cold Formula Liquid contains a decongestant, pseudoephedrine hydrochloride, an antihistamine, chlorpheniramine maleate, and a cough suppressant, dextromethorphan hydrobromide to provide temporary relief of coughs, nasal congestion, runny nose and sneezing due to the common cold. PEDIACARE NightRest may be used day or night to relieve cough and cold symptoms. PEDIACARE Infants' Oral Decongestant Drops contain a decongestant, pseudoephedrine hydrochloride, to provide temporary relief of nasal congestion due to the common cold, hay fever or other upper respiratory allergies.

Professional Dosage: A calibrated dosage cup is provided for accurate dosing of the PEDIACARE Liquid formulas. A calibrated oral dropper is provided for accurate dosing of PEDIACARE Infants' Drops. All doses of PEDIACARE Cold Formula Liquid, PEDIACARE Cough-Cold Formula Liquid and Chewable Tablets and PEDIACARE Infants' Drops may be repeated every 4–6 hours, not to exceed 4 doses in 24 hours. PEDIACARE NightRest Liquid may be repeated every 6–8 hours, not to exceed 4 doses in 24 hours.
[See table above].
Note: Since PEDIACARE cold products are available without prescription, the following information appears on the package labels: "WARNINGS: Do not use if carton is opened, or if printed plastic bottle wrap or foil inner seal is broken. Keep this and all medication out of the reach of children. In case of accidental overdosage, contact a physician or poison control center immediately."
The following information appears on the appropriate package labels:
PEDIACARE Cold Formula Liquid: "Do not exceed the recommended dosage because nervousness, dizziness or sleeplessness may occur. If symptoms do not improve within seven days or are accompanied by fever, consult a physician before continuing use. This preparation may cause drowsiness, or in some cases, excitability. Do not give this product to children who have heart disease, high blood pressure, thyroid disease, diabetes, glaucoma or asthma, or are taking a prescription drug for high blood pressure or depression, except under the advice and supervision of a physician."
"*Inactive Ingredients:* Benzoic acid, citric acid, flavors, glycerin, polyethylene glycol, propylene glycol, sodium benzoate, sorbitol, sucrose, purified water, Red #33, Blue #1 and Red #40."
PEDIACARE Cough-Cold Formula Liquid and Chewable Tablets: "Do not exceed the recommended dosage because nervousness, dizziness or sleeplessness may occur. A persistent cough may be a sign of a serious condition. If symptoms do not improve within seven days, tend to recur, or are accompanied by fever, rash, excessive mucus, persistent cough or headache, consult a physician before continuing use. This preparation may cause drowsiness or, in some cases, excitability. Do not give this product to children who have heart disease, high blood pressure, thyroid disease, diabetes, glaucoma or asthma, or are taking a prescription drug for high blood pressure or depression, except under the advice and supervision of a physician."
PEDIACARE Cough-Cold Formula Liquid: *Inactive Ingredients:* Benzoic acid, citric acid, flavors, glycerin, polyethylene glycol, propylene glycol, sodium benzoate, sorbitol, sucrose, purified water, Red #33, Blue #1 and Red #40.
PEDIACARE Cough-Cold Formula Chewable Tablets also contain the warning, "Phenylketonurics: contains phenylalanine 3 mg per tablet," and the inactive ingredient listing, "*Inactive Ingredients:* Aspartame, cellulose, citric acid, dextrose, flavors, magnesium stearate, magnesium trisilicate, mannitol, starch, sucrose and Red #3."
PEDIACARE NightRest Cough-Cold Formula Liquid: "Do not exceed the recommended dosage because nervousness, dizziness or sleeplessness may occur. A persistent cough may be a sign of a serious condition. If symptoms do not improve within seven days, tend to recur, or are accompanied by fever, rash, excessive mucus, persistent cough or headache, consult a physician before continuing use. This preparation may cause drowsiness or, in some cases, excitability. Do not give this product to children who have heart disease, high blood pressure, thyroid disease, diabetes, glaucoma or asthma, or are taking a prescription drug for high blood pressure or depression, except under the advice and supervision of a physician."
PEDIACARE NightRest Cough-Cold Formula Liquid: *Inactive ingredients:* Benzoic acid, citric acid, flavors, glycerin, polyethylene glycol, propylene glycol, sodium benzoate, sorbitol, sucrose, purified water, Red #33, Blue #1 and Red #40.
PEDIACARE Infants' Oral Decongestant Drops: "Do not exceed the recommended dosage because at higher doses nervousness, dizziness or sleeplessness may occur. Do not give this product to children who have heart disease, high blood pressure, thyroid disease or diabetes unless directed by a physician. Do not give this product to children for more than seven days. If symptoms do not improve or are accompanied by fever, consult a physician. Do not give this product to children who are taking a prescription drug for high blood pressure or depression without first consulting a physician. Take by mouth only. Not for nasal use."
"*Inactive Ingredients:* Benzoic acid, citric acid, flavors, glycerin, polyethylene glycol, propylene glycol, purified water, sodium benzoate, sorbitol, sucrose and Red #40."

Overdosage: Acute dextromethorphan overdose usually does not result in serious signs and symptoms unless massive amounts have been ingested. Signs and symptoms of a substantial overdose may include nausea and vomiting, visual disturbances, CNS disturbances, and urinary retention. Symptoms from pseudoephedrine overdose consist most often of mild anxiety, tachycardia and/or mild hypertension. Symptoms usually appear within 4 to 8 hours of ingestion and are transient, usually requiring no treatment. Chlorpheniramine toxicity should be treated as you would an antihistamine/anticholinergic overdose and is

Continued on next page

McNeil Consumer—Cont.

likely to be present within a few hours after acute ingestion.

How Supplied: PEDIACARE Liquid products (colored red)—bottles of 4 fl oz with child-resistant safety cap and calibrated dosage cup. PEDIACARE Cough-Cold Formula Chewable Tablets (pink, scored)—bottles of 24 with child-resistant safety cap. PEDIACARE NightRest Cough-Cold Formula (colored red)—bottles of 4 fl oz with child-resistant safety cap and convenient dosage cup. PEDIACARE Infants' Drops (colored red)—bottles of ½ fl oz with calibrated dropper.

Shown in Product Identification Section, page 415

MAXIMUM STRENGTH SINE-AID® Sinus Headache Caplets and Tablets

Description: Each MAXIMUM STRENGTH SINE-AID® Caplet or tablet contains acetaminophen 500 mg and pseudoephedrine hydrochloride 30 mg.

Actions: MAXIMUM STRENGTH SINE-AID® Caplets and tablets contain a clinically proven analgesic-antipyretic and a decongestant. Maximum allowable nonprescription levels of acetaminophen and pseudoephedrine provide temporary relief of sinus congestion and pain. Acetaminophen is equal to aspirin in analgesic and antipyretic effectiveness and it is unlikely to produce many of the side effects associated with aspirin and aspirin-containing products. Acetaminophen produces analgesia by elevation of the pain threshold and antipyresis through action on the hypothalamic heat-regulating center. Pseudoephedrine hydrochloride is a sympathomimetic amine that promotes sinus cavity drainage by reducing nasopharyngeal mucosal congestion.

Indications: MAXIMUM STRENGTH SINE-AID® Caplets and Tablets provide effective symptomatic relief from sinus headache pain and congestion. SINE-AID® is particularly well-suited in patients with aspirin allergy, hemostatic disturbances (including anticoagulant therapy), and bleeding diatheses (e.g., hemophilia) and upper gastrointestinal disease (e.g., ulcer, gastritis, hiatus hernia).

Precautions: If a rare sensitivity occurs, the drug should be discontinued. Although pseudoephedrine is virtually without pressor effect in normotensive patients, it should be used with caution in hypertensives.

Usual Dosage: Adult dosage: Two caplets or tablets every four to six hours. Do not exceed eight caplets or tablets in any 24 hour period. **Note:** Since MAXIMUM STRENGTH SINE-AID® Caplets and Tablets are available without a prescription, the following appears on the package labels: "**WARNING:** Do not exceed the recommended dosage because at higher doses nervousness, dizziness or sleeplessness may occur. Do not administer to children under 12. If you have high

blood pressure, heart disease, diabetes, thyroid disease, difficulty in urination due to enlargement of the prostate gland, or are presently taking a prescription drug for the treatment of high blood pressure or depression, do not take except under the advice and supervision of a physician. Do not take this product for more than 7 days. If symptoms do not improve or are accompanied by high fever, consult a physician. **Do not use if carton is opened, or if printed red neck wrap or printed foil inner seal is broken. Keep this and all medication out of the reach of children. As with any drug, if you are pregnant or nursing a baby, seek the advice of a health professional before using this product. In case of accidental overdosage, contact a physician or poison control center immediately."**

Overdosage: Acetaminophen in massive overdosage may cause hepatic toxicity in some patients. In adults and adolescents, hepatic toxicity has rarely been reported following ingestion of acute overdoses of less than 10 grams. Fatalities are infrequent (less than 3–4% of untreated cases) and have rarely been reported with overdoses of less than 15 grams. In children, an acute overdosage of less than 150 mg/kg has not been associated with hepatic toxicity.

Early symptoms following a potentially hepatotoxic overdose may include: nausea, vomiting, diaphoresis and general malaise. Clinical and laboratory evidence of hepatic toxicity may not be apparent until 48 to 72 hours postingestion. In adults and adolescents, regardless of the quantity of acetaminophen reported to have been ingested, administer MUCOMYST® acetylcysteine immediately if 24 hours or less have elapsed from the reported time of ingestion. For full prescribing information, refer to the MUCOMYST package insert. Do not await results of assays for acetaminophen level before initiating treatment with MUCOMYST acetylcysteine. The following additional procedures are recommended: The stomach should be emptied promptly by lavage or by induction of emesis with syrup of ipecac. A serum acetaminophen assay should be obtained as early as possible, but no sooner than four hours following ingestion. Liver function studies should be obtained initially and repeated at 24-hour intervals.

Serious toxicity or fatalities are extremely infrequent in children, possibly due to differences in the way they metabolize acetaminophen. In children, the maximum potential amount ingested can be more easily estimated. If more than 150 mg/kg or an unknown amount was ingested, obtain an acetaminophen plasma level. The acetaminophen plasma level should be obtained as soon as possible, but no sooner than 4 hours following the ingestion. Induce emesis using syrup of ipecac. If the plasma level is obtained and falls above the broken line on the acetaminophen overdose nomogram, the MUCOMYST acetylcysteine therapy should be initiated and con-

tinued for a full course of therapy. If acetaminophen plasma assay capability is not available, and the estimated acetaminophen ingestion exceeds 150 mg/kg, MUCOMYST acetylcysteine therapy should be initiated and continued for a full course of therapy.

For additional emergency information, call your regional poison center or call the Rocky Mountain Poison Center toll-free (1-800-525-6115).

Symptoms from pseudoephedrine overdose consist most often of mild anxiety, tachycardia and/or mild hypertension. Symptoms usually appear within 4 to 8 hours of ingestion and are transient, usually requiring no treatment.

Inactive Ingredients: Cellulose, hydroxypropyl methylcellulose, magnesium stearate, polyethylene glycol, sodium starch glycolate, starch, titanium dioxide, Blue #1 and Red #40.

How Supplied: Caplets (colored white imprinted "Maximum SINE-AID")—blister pack of 24 and tamper-resistant bottles of 50. Tablets (colored white embossed "Sine-Aid")—blister package of 24 and tamper resistant bottles of 50 and 100.

Shown in Product Identification Section, page 415

CHILDREN'S TYLENOL® acetaminophen Chewable Tablets, Elixir, Drops

Description: Each Children's TYLENOL *Chewable Tablet* contains 80 mg. acetaminophen in a fruit or grape flavored tablet. Children's TYLENOL acetaminophen *Elixir* is stable and alcohol free; cherry flavored is red in color, grape flavored purple in color. Infants' TYLENOL *Drops* are stable, fruit flavored, orange in color and are alcohol free. Children's TYLENOL *Elixir:* Each 5 ml. contains 160 mg. acetaminophen. Infant's TYLENOL *Drops:* Each 0.8 ml. (one calibrated dropperful) contains 80 mg. acetaminophen.

Actions: Acetaminophen is a clinically proven analgesic/antipyretic. Acetaminophen produces analgesia by elevation of the pain threshold and antipyresis through action on the hypothalamic heat-regulating center. Acetaminophen is equal to aspirin in analgesic and antipyretic effectiveness and it is unlikely to produce many of the side effects associated with aspirin and aspirin-containing products.

Indications: Children's TYLENOL Chewable Tablets, Elixir and Drops are designed for treatment of infants and children with conditions requiring temporary relief of fever and discomfort due to colds and "flu," and of simple pain and discomfort due to teething, immunizations and tonsillectomy.

Precautions: If a rare sensitivity reaction occurs, the drug should be stopped.

Usual Dosage: All dosages may be repeated every 4 hours, but not more than 5 times daily. Administer to children under 2 years only on the advice of a physician. Children's TYLENOL *Chewable Tablets:* 2–3 years: two tablets; 4–5 years: three tablets; 6–8 years: four tablets; 9–10 years: five tablets; 11–12 years: six tablets. Children's TYLENOL *Elixir:* (special cup for measuring dosage is provided) 4–11 months: one-half teaspoon; 12–23 months: three-quarters teaspoon; 2–3 years: one teaspoon; 4–5 years: one and one-half teaspoons; 6–8 years: 2 teaspoons; 9–10 years: two and one-half teaspoons; 11–12 years: three teaspoons. Infants' TYLENOL *Drops:* 0–3 months: 0.4 ml.; 4–11 months: 0.8 ml.; 12–23 months: 1.2 ml.; 2–3 years: 1.6 ml.; 4–5 years: 2.4 ml.

Warning: Keep this and all medication out of reach of children. In case of accidental overdose, contact a physician or poison control center immediately. Consult your physician if fever persists for more than 3 days or if pain continues for more than 5 days. Store at room temperature.

Note: In addition to the above:
Children's TYLENOL® *Drops* —Do not use if printed carton overwrap or printed plastic bottle wrap is broken or missing or if carton is opened. Children's TYLENOL *Elixir* —Do not use if printed carton overwrap is broken or missing or if carton is opened. Do not use if printed plastic bottle wrap or printed foil inner seal is broken. Not a USP elixir. Children's TYLENOL *Chewables* —Do not use if carton is opened or if printed plastic bottle wrap or printed foil inner seal is broken. Phenylketonurics: contains phenylalanine 3 mg per tablet.

Overdosage: Acetaminophen in massive overdosage may cause hepatic toxicity in some patients. In adults and adolescents, hepatic toxicity has rarely been reported following ingestion of acute overdoses of less than 10 grams. Fatalities are infrequent (less than 3–4% of untreated cases) and have rarely been reported with overdoses of less than 15 grams. In children, an acute overdosage of less than 150 mg./kg. has not been associated with hepatic toxicity.
Early symptoms following a potentially hepatotoxic overdose may include: nausea, vomiting, diaphoresis and general malaise. Clinical and laboratory evidence of hepatic toxicity may not be apparent until 48 to 72 hours postingestion. In adults and adolescents, regardless of the quantity of acetaminophen reported to have been ingested, administer MUCOMYST® acetylcysteine immediately if 24 hours or less have elapsed from the reported time of ingestion. For full prescribing information, refer to the MUCOMYST package insert. Do not await results of assays for acetaminophen level before initiating treatment with MUCOMYST acetylcysteine. The following additional procedures are recommended: The stomach should be emptied promptly by lavage or by induction of emesis with syrup of ipecac. A serum acetaminophen assay should be obtained as early as possible, but no sooner than four hours following ingestion. Liver function studies should be ob-

tained initially and repeated at 24-hour intervals.
Serious toxicity or fatalities are extremely infrequent in children, possibly due to differences in the way they metabolize acetaminophen. In children, the maximum potential amount ingested can be more easily estimated. If more than 150 mg./kg. or an unknown amount was ingested, obtain an acetaminophen plasma level. The acetaminophen plasma level should be obtained as soon as possible, but no sooner than 4 hours following the ingestion. Induce emesis using syrup of ipecac. If the plasma level is obtained and falls above the broken line on the acetaminophen overdose nomogram, the MUCOMYST acetylcysteine therapy should be initiated and continued for a full course of therapy. If acetaminophen plasma assay capability is not available, and the estimated acetaminophen ingestion exceeds 150 mg./kg., MUCOMYST acetylcysteine therapy should be initiated and continued for a full course of therapy.
For additional emergency information, call your regional poison center or call the Rocky Mountain Poison Center toll free (1-800-525-6115).

Inactive Ingredients: Children's TYLENOL *Chewable Tablets* —Aspartame, Cellulose, Citric Acid, Ethylcellulose, Flavors, Hydroxypropyl Methylcellulose, Mannitol, Starch, Magnesium Stearate, Red #7 and Blue #1 (Grape only). Children's TYLENOL *Elixir* —Benzoic Acid, Citric Acid, Flavors, Glycerin, Polyethylene Glycol, Propylene Glycol, Sodium Benzoate, Sorbitol, Sucrose, Purified Water, Red #40. In addition to the above ingredients cherry flavored elixir contains Red #33 and grape flavored elixir contains malic acid and Blue #1. Infant's TYLENOL *Drops* —Flavors, Propylene Glycol, Saccharin, Purified Water, Yellow #6.

How Supplied: *Chewable Tablets* (pink colored fruit, purple colored grape, scored, imprinted "TYLENOL")—Bottles of 30 and child resistant blister packs of 48 (fruit only). *Elixir* (cherry colored red and grape colored purple)—bottles of 2 and 4 fl. oz. *Drops* (colored orange)—bottles of ½ oz. (15 ml.) with calibrated plastic dropper.
All packages listed above have child-resistant safety caps.

Shown in Product Identification Section, pages 414 and 415

Junior Strength TYLENOL® acetaminophen Coated Caplets

Description: Each Junior Strength Caplet contains 160 mg acetaminophen in a small, coated, capsule-shaped tablet.

Actions: Acetaminophen is a clinically proven analgesic/antipyretic. Acetaminophen produces analgesia by elevation of the pain threshold and antipyresis through action on the hypothalamic heat-regulating center. Acetaminophen is equal to aspirin in analgesic and antipyretic effectiveness and it is unlikely to

produce many of the side effects associated with aspirin and aspirin-containing products.

Indications: Junior Strength TYLENOL Caplets are designed for easy swallowability in older children and young adults to provide fast, effective temporary relief of fever and discomfort due to colds and "flu," and pain and discomfort due to simple headaches, minor muscle aches, sprains and overexertion.

Precautions: If a rare sensitivity reaction occurs, the drug should be stopped.

Usual Dosage: All dosages shouold be taken with liquid and may be repeated every 4 hours, but not more than 5 times daily. For ages: 6–8 years: two Caplets; 9–10 years: two and one-half Caplets; 11 years: three Caplets; 12–14 years: four Caplets.

Note: Since Junior Strength TYLENOL acetaminophen Caplets are available without a prescription as an analgesic, the following appears on the package labels:
Warnings: Do not use if carton is opened or if a blister unit is broken. Keep this and all medications out of the reach of children. In case of accidental overdosage, contact a physician or poison control center immediately. Consult your physician if fever persists for more than three days or if pain continues for more than five days. As with any drugs, if you are pregnant or nursing a baby, seek the advice of a health professional before using this product. Not for children who have difficulty swallowing tablets.

Overdosage: Acetaminophen in massive overdosage may cause hepatic toxicity in some patients. In adults and adolescents, hepatic toxicity has rarely been reported following ingestion of acute overdoses of less than 10 grams. Fatalities are infrequent (less than 3–4% of untreated cases) and have rarely been reported with overdoses of less than 15 grams. In children, an acute overdosage of less than 150 mg/kg has not been associated with hepatic toxicity.
Early symptoms following a potentially hepatotoxic overdose may include: nausea, vomiting, diaphoresis and general malaise. Clinical and laboratory evidence of hepatic toxicity may not be apparent until 48 to 72 hours postingestion. In adults and adolescents, regardless of the quantity of acetaminophen reported to have been ingested, administer MUCOMYST® acetylcysteine immediately if 24 hours or less have elapsed from the reported time of ingestion. For full prescribing information, refer to the MUCOMYST package insert. Do not await the results of assays for acetaminophen level before initiating treatment with MUCOMYST acetylcysteine. The following additional procedures are recommended: The stomach should be emptied promptly by lavage or by induction of emesis with syrup of ipecac. A serum acetaminophen assay should be

Continued on next page

McNeil Consumer—Cont.

obtained as early as possible, but no sooner than four hours following ingestion. Liver function studies should be obtained initially and repeated at 24-hour intervals.

Serious toxicity or fatalities are extremely infrequent in children, possibly due to differences in the way they metabolize acetaminophen. In children, the maximum potential amount ingested can be more easily estimated. If more than 150 mg/kg or an unknown amount was ingested, obtain an acetaminophen plasma level. The acetaminophen plasma level should be obtained as soon as possible, but no sooner than 4 hours following the ingestion. Induce emesis using syrup of ipecac. If the plasma level is obtained and falls above the broken line on the acetaminophen overdose nomogram, the MUCOMYST acetylcysteine therapy should be initiated and continued for a full course of therapy. If acetaminophen plasma assay capability is not available, and the estimated acetaminophen ingestion exceeds 150 mg/kg, MUCOMYST acetylcysteine therapy should be initiated and continued for a full course of therapy.

For additional emergency information, call your regional poison center or call the Rocky Mountain Poison Center toll-free (1-800-525-6115).

Inactive Ingredients: Cellulose, Ethylcellulose, Magnesium Stearate, Sodium Lauryl Sulfate, Sodium Starch Glycolate, Starch.

How Supplied: Coated Caplets (colored white, coated, scored, imprinted "TYLENOL 160"). Package of 30. All packages are safety sealed and use child resistant blister packaging.

Shown in Product Identification Section, page 415

Regular Strength TYLENOL® acetaminophen Tablets and Caplets

Description: Each Regular Strength TYLENOL Tablet or Caplet contains acetaminophen 325 mg.

Actions: Acetaminophen is a clinically proven analgesic and antipyretic. Acetaminophen produces analgesia by elevation of the pain threshold and antipyresis through action on the hypothalamic heat-regulating center. Acetaminophen is equal to aspirin in analgesic and antipyretic effectiveness and it is unlikely to produce many of the side effects associated with aspirin and aspirin-containing products.

Indications: Acetaminophen acts safely and quickly to provide temporary relief from: simple headache; minor muscular aches; the minor aches and pains associated with bursitis, neuralgia, sprains, overexertion, menstrual cramps; and from the discomfort of fever due to colds and "flu." Also for temporary relief of minor aches and pains of arthritis and rheumatism. Acetaminophen is particu-

larly well suited as an analgesic-antipyretic in the presence of aspirin allergy, hemostatic disturbances (including anticoagulant therapy), and bleeding diatheses (e.g., hemophilia) and upper gastrointestinal disease (e.g., ulcer, gastritis, hiatus hernia).

Precautions: If a rare sensitivity reaction occurs, the drug should be discontinued.

Usual Dosage: *Adults:* One to two tablets or caplets three or four times daily. *Children* (6 to 12): One-half to one tablet 3 or 4 times daily. (Junior Strength TYLENOL acetaminophen Swallowable Tablets, Chewable Tablets, Elixir and Drops are available for greater convenience in younger patients.)

Note: Since TYLENOL acetaminophen tablets and caplets are available without prescription as an analgesic, the following appears on the package labels: **Warning:** Do not take for pain for more than 10 days (for adult) or 5 days (for children) and do not take for fever for more than 3 days unless directed by a doctor. **Do not use if printed red neck wrap or printed foil inner seal is broken. Keep this and all medications out of the reach of children. As with any drug, if you are pregnant or nursing a baby, seek the advice of a health professional before using this product. In case of accidental overdosage, contact a doctor or poison control center immediately."**

Overdosage: Acetaminophen in massive overdosage may cause hepatic toxicity in some patients. In adults and adolescents, hepatic toxicity has rarely been reported following ingestion of acute overdoses of less than 10 grams. Fatalities are infrequent (less than 3–4% of untreated cases) and have rarely been reported with overdoses of less than 15 grams. In children, an acute overdose of less than 150 mg/kg has not been associated with hepatic toxicity.

Early symptoms following a potentially hepatotoxic overdose may include: nausea, vomiting, diaphoresis and general malaise. Clinical and laboratory evidence of hepatic toxicity may not be apparent until 48 to 72 hours postingestion. In adults and adolescents, regardless of the quantity of acetaminophen reported to have been ingested, administer MUCOMYST® acetylcysteine immediately if 24 hours or less have elapsed from the reported time of ingestion. For full prescribing information, refer to the MUCOMYST package insert. Do not await results of assays for acetaminophen level before initiating treatment with MUCOMYST acetylcysteine. The following additional procedures are recommended: The stomach should be emptied promptly by lavage or by induction of emesis with syrup of ipecac. A serum acetaminophen assay should be obtained as early as possible, but no sooner than four hours following ingestion. Liver function studies should be obtained initially and repeated at 24-hour intervals.

Serious toxicity or fatalities are extremely infrequent in children, possibly due to differences in the way they metabolize acetaminophen. In children, the maximum potential amount ingested can be more easily estimated. If more than 150 mg/kg or an unknown amount was ingested, obtain an acetaminophen plasma level. The acetaminophen plasma level should be obtained as soon as possible, but no sooner than 4 hours following the ingestion. Induce emesis using syrup of ipecac. If the plasma level is obtained and falls above the broken line on the acetaminophen overdose nomogram, the MUCOMYST acetylcysteine therapy should be initiated and continued for a full course of therapy. If acetaminophen plasma assay capability is not available, and the estimated acetaminophen ingestion exceeds 150 mg/kg, MUCOMYST acetylcysteine therapy should be initiated and continued for a full course of therapy.

For additional emergency information, call your regional poison center or call the Rocky Mountain Poison Center toll-free (1-800-525-6115).

Inactive Ingredients: *Tablets*—Calcium Stearate or Magnesium Stearate, Cellulose, Docusate Sodium and Sodium Benzoate or Sodium Lauryl Sulfate, and Starch. *Caplets*—Cellulose, Hydroxpropyl Methylcellulose, Magnesium Stearate, Polyethylene Glycol, Sodium Starch Glycolate and Starch.

How Supplied: Tablets (colored white, scored, imprinted "TYLENOL")—tins and vials of 12, and tamper-resistant bottles of 24, 50, 100 and 200. Caplets (colored white, "TYLENOL")—tamper-resistant bottles of 24, 50, 100. For additional pain relief, Extra-Strength TYLENOL® Tablets and Caplets, 500 mg, and Extra-Strength TYLENOL® Adult Liquid Pain Reliever are available (colored green; 1 fl. oz. = 1000 mg.)

Shown in Product Identification Section, page 414

Extra-Strength TYLENOL® acetaminophen Caplets, Gelcaps, Tablets

Description: Each Extra-Strength TYLENOL Caplet, Gelcap or Tablet contains acetaminophen 500 mg.

Actions: Acetaminophen is a clinically proven analgesic and antipyretic. Acetaminophen produces analgesia by elevation of the pain threshold and antipyresis through action on the hypothalamic heat-regulating center. Acetaminophen is equal to aspirin in analgesic and antipyretic effectiveness and it is unlikely to produce many of the side effects associated with aspirin and aspirin-containing products.

Indications: For the temporary relief of minor aches, pains, headaches and fever.

Precautions: If a rare sensitivity reaction occurs, the drug should be discontinued.

Usual Dosage: *Adults:* Two Caplets, Gelcaps or Tablets 3 or 4 times daily. No more than a total of eight Caplets, Gelcaps or Tablets in any 24-hour period.

Note: Since Extra-Strength TYLENOL acetaminophen is available without a prescription, the following appears on the package labels: "**Warning:** Do not take for more than 10 days or for fever for more than 3 days unless directed by a doctor. Severe or recurrent pain or high or continued fever may be indicative of serious illness. Under these conditions, consult a doctor. **Do not use if printed red neck wrap or printed foil inner seal is broken. Keep this and all medication out of the reach of children. As with any drug, if you are pregnant or nursing a baby, seek the advice of a health professional before using this product. In case of accidental overdosage, contact a doctor or poison control center immediately.**"

Overdosage: Acetaminophen in massive overdosage may cause hepatic toxicity in some patients. In adults and adolescents, hepatic toxicity has rarely been reported following ingestion of acute overdosage of less than 10 grams. Fatalities are infrequent (less than 3–4% of untreated cases) and have rarely been reported with overdoses of less than 15 grams. In children, an acute overdosage of less than 150 mg/kg has not been associated with hepatic toxicity.

Early symptoms following a potentially hepatotoxic overdose may include: nausea, vomiting, diaphoresis and general malaise. Clinical and laboratory evidence of hepatic toxicity may not be apparent until 48 to 72 hours postingestion. In adults and adolescents, regardless of the quantity of acetaminophen reported to have been ingested, administer MUCOMYST® acetylcysteine immediately if 24 hours or less have elapsed from the reported time of ingestion. For full prescribing information, refer to the MUCOMYST package insert. Do not await the results of assays for acetaminophen level before initiating treatment with MUCOMYST acetylcysteine. The following additional procedures are recommended: The stomach should be emptied promptly by lavage or by induction of emesis with syrup of ipecac. A serum acetaminophen assay should be obtained as early as possible, but no sooner than four hours following ingestion. Liver function studies should be obtained initially and repeated at 24-hour intervals.

Serious toxicity or fatalities are extremely infrequent in children, possibly due to differences in the way they metabolize acetaminophen. In children, the maximum potential amount ingested can be more easily estimated. If more than 150 mg/kg or an unknown amount was ingested, obtain an acetaminophen plasma level. The acetaminophen plasma level should be obtained as soon as possible, but no sooner than 4 hours following the ingestion. Induce emesis using syrup of ipecac. If the plasma level is obtained and falls above the broken line on the acetaminophen overdose nomogram, the MUCOMYST acetylcysteine therapy should be initiated and continued for a full course of therapy. If acetaminophen plasma assay capability is not available, and the estimated acetaminophen ingestion exceeds 150 mg/kg, MUCOMYST acetylcysteine therapy should be initiated and continued for a full course of therapy.

For additional emergency information, call your regional poison center or call the Rocky Mountain Poison Center toll-free (1-800-525-6115).

Inactive Ingredients: *Tablets* —Calcium Stearate or Magnesium Stearate, Cellulose, Docusate Sodium and Sodium Benzoate or Sodium Lauryl Sulfate and Starch. *Caplets* —Cellulose, Hydroxypropyl Methylcellulose, Magnesium Stearate, Polyethylene Glycol, Sodium Starch Glycolate, Starch and Red #40. *Gelcaps* —Benzyl Alcohol, Butylparaben, Castor Oil, Cellulose, Edetate Calcium Disodium, Gelatin, Hydroxypropyl Methylcellulose, Magnesium Stearate, Methylparaben, Propylparaben, Sodium Lauryl Sulfate, Sodium Propionate, Sodium Starch Glycolate, Starch, Titanium Dioxide, Blue #1 and #2, Red #40 and Yellow #10.

How Supplied: *Tablets* (colored white, imprinted "TYLENOL" and "500")—vials of 10 and tamper-resistant bottles of 30, 60, 100, and 200. *Caplets* (colored white, imprinted "TYLENOL 500 mg")—vials of 10 and tamper-resistant bottles of 24, 50, 100, 175, and 250's. *Gelcaps* (colored yellow and red, imprinted "Tylenol 500") tamper-resistant bottles of 24, 50 and 100. For adults who prefer liquids or can't swallow solid medication, Extra-Strength TYLENOL® Adult Liquid Pain Reliever, Mint Flavored is also available (colored green; 1 fl. oz. = 1000 mg).

Shown in Product Identification Section, page 414

**Extra-Strength
TYLENOL® acetaminophen
Adult Liquid Pain Reliever**

Description: Each 15 ml. (½ fl. oz. or one tablespoonful) contains 500 mg acetaminophen (alcohol 7%).

Actions: TYLENOL acetaminophen is a clinically proven analgesic and antipyretic. Acetaminophen produces analgesia by elevation of the pain threshold and antipyresis through action on the hypothalamic heat-regulating center. Acetaminophen is equal to aspirin in analgesic and antipyretic effectiveness and it is unlikely to produce many of the side effects associated with aspirin and aspirin-containing products.

Indications: Acetaminophen provides temporary relief of minor aches, pains, headaches and fevers.

Precautions: If a rare sensitivity reaction occurs, the drug should be discontinued.

Usual Dosage: Extra-Strength TYLENOL Adult Liquid Pain Reliever is an adult preparation for those adults who prefer liquids or can't swallow solid medication. Not for use in children under 12. Measuring cup is marked for accurate dosage. Extra-Strength Dose—1 fl. oz. (30 ml or 2 tablespoonsful, 1000 mg), which is equivalent to two 500 mg Extra-Strength TYLENOL Tablets or Caplets. Take every 4–6 hours, no more than 4 doses in any 24-hour period.

Note: Since Extra-Strength TYLENOL Adult Liquid Pain Reliever is available without a prescription, the following appears on the package labels: "**Warning:** Do not take for pain for more than 10 days (for adults) or 5 days (for children) and do not take for fever for more than 3 days unless directed by a doctor. Severe or recurrent pain or high or continued fever may be indicative of serious illness. Under these conditions, consult a physician. **Do not use if printed plastic over-wrap or printed foil inner seal is broken. Keep this and all medication out of the reach of children. As with any drug, if you are pregnant or nursing a baby, seek the advice of a health professional before using this product. In case of accidental overdosage, contact a doctor or poison control center immediately.**"

Overdosage: Acetaminophen in massive overdosage may cause hepatic toxicity in some patients. In adults and adolescents, hepatic toxicity has rarely been reported following ingestion of acute overdosage of less than 10 grams. Fatalities are infrequent (less than 3–4% of untreated cases) and have rarely been reported with overdoses of less than 15 grams. In children, an acute overdosage of less than 150 mg/kg has not been associated with hepatic toxicity.

Early symptoms following a potentially hepatotoxic overdose may include: nausea, vomiting, diaphoresis and general malaise. Clinical and laboratory evidence of hepatic toxicity may not be apparent until 48 to 72 hours postingestion. In adults and adolescents, regardless of the quantity of acetaminophen reported to have been ingested, administer MUCOMYST® acetylcysteine immediately if 24 hours or less have elapsed from the reported time of ingestion. For full prescribing information, refer to the MUCOMYST package insert. Do not await the results of assays for acetaminophen level before initiating treatment with MUCOMYST acetylcysteine. The following additional procedures are recommended: The stomach should be emptied promptly by lavage or by induction of emesis with syrup of ipecac. A serum acetaminophen assay should be obtained as early as possible, but no sooner than four hours following ingestion. Liver function studies should be obtained initially and repeated at 24-hour intervals.

Serious toxicity or fatalities are extremely infrequent in children, possibly due to differences in the way they metabolize acetaminophen. In children, the

Continued on next page

McNeil Consumer—Cont.

maximum potential amount ingested can be more easily estimated. If more than 150 mg/kg or an unknown amount was ingested, obtain an acetaminophen plasma level. The acetaminophen plasma level should be obtained as soon as possible, but no sooner than 4 hours following the ingestion. Induce emesis using syrup of ipecac. If the plasma level is obtained and falls above the broken line on the acetaminophen overdose nomogram, the MUCOMYST acetylcysteine therapy should be initiated and continued for a full course of therapy. If acetaminophen plasma assay capability is not available, and the estimated acetaminophen ingestion exceeds 150 mg/kg, MUCOMYST acetylcysteine therapy should be initiated and continued for a full course of therapy.

For additional emergency information, call your regional poison center or call the Rocky Mountain Poison Center toll-free (1-800-525-6115).

Inactive Ingredients: Alcohol, Citric Acid, Flavors, Glycerin, Polyethylene Glycol, Purified Water, Sodium Benzoate, Sorbitol, Sucrose, Yellow #6 (Sunset Yellow), Yellow #10 and Blue #1.

How Supplied: Mint-flavored liquid (colored green), 8 fl. oz. tamper-resistant bottle with child resistent safety cap and special dosage cup.

CHILDREN'S TYLENOL COLD®
Chewable Cold Tablets and Liquid Cold Formula

PRODUCT OVERVIEW

Key Facts: Children's Tylenol Cold® Products are formulated to relieve a child's fever, aches and pains, congestion and runny nose. The products are aspirin free and formulated for accurate dosing by age and weight.

Major Uses: Children's Tylenol Cold Products contain the same amount of acetaminophen as comparable Children's Tylenol Cold Products (80 mg per tablet, 160 mg. per 5 ml) for relief of fever and pain resulting from a cold in children ages 11 and under. Additionally, Children's Tylenol Cold Products contain pseudoephedrine hydrochloride (7.5 mg per tablet, 15 mg per 5 ml) for treatment of nasal congestion and chlorpheniramine maleate (0.5 mg per tablet, 1 mg per 5 ml) for treatment of runny noses and sneezing.

PRESCRIBING INFORMATION
CHILDREN'S TYLENOL COLD®
Chewable Cold Tablets and Liquid Cold Formula

Description: Each Children's Tylenol Cold Chewable Grape-Flavored Tablet contains acetaminophen 80 mg, chlorpheniramine maleate 0.5 mg and pseudoephedrine hydrochloride 7.5 mg. Children's Tylenol Cold Liquid Formula is grape flavored, and contains no alcohol. Each teaspoon (5 ml) contains acetamino-

phen 160 mg, chlorpheniramine maleate 1 mg, and pseudoephedrine hydrochloride 15 mg.

Actions: Children's Tylenol Cold Chewable Tablets and Liquid combine the analgesic-antipyretic acetaminophen with the decongestant pseudoephedrine hydrochloride and the antihistamine chlorpheniramine maleate to help relieve nasal congestion, dry runny noses and prevent sneezing as well as to relieve the fever, aches, pains and general discomfort associated with colds and upper respiratory infections.

Acetaminophen is equal to aspirin in analgesic and antipyretic effectiveness and it is unlikely to produce the side effects often associated with aspirin or aspirin-containing products.

Indications: Provides fast, effective temporary relief of nasal congestion, runny nose, sneezing, minor aches and pains, headaches and fever due to the common cold, hay fever or other upper respiratory allergies.

Usual Dosage: Administer to children under 6 years only on the advice of a physician. Children's Tylenol Cold Chewable Tablets: 2–5 years—2 tablets, 6–11 years—4 tablets.
Children's Tylenol Cold Liquid Formula: 2–5 years—1 teaspoonful; 6–11 years—2 teaspoonsful. Measuring cup is provided and marked for accurate dosing.
Doses may be repeated every 4-6 hours as needed, not to exceed 4 doses in 24 hours.
Note: Since Children's Tylenol Cold Chewable Tablets and Liquid Formula are available without prescription, the following information appears on the package labels. The Warnings are identical for the two dosage forms except the Liquid Cold Formula does not contain the phenylketonurics statement since the product does not contain aspartame.
Warning: Do not use if carton is opened, or if printed plastic bottle wrap or printed foil inner seal is broken.
Keep this and all medication out of the reach of children. In case of accidental overdosage, contact a physician or poison control center immediately. Phenylketonurics: contains phenylalanine, 4 mg per tablet. Do not exceed the recommended dosage because nervousness, dizziness or sleeplessness may occur. If fever persists for more than three days, or if symptoms do not improve or new ones occur within five days or are accompanied by high fever, consult a physician before continuing use. This preparation may cause drowsiness, or in some cases, excitability. Do not give this product to children who have heart disease, high blood pressure, thyroid disease, diabetes, glaucoma or asthma or are taking a prescription drug for high blood pressure or depression, except under the advice and supervision of a physician.

Overdosage: Acetaminophen in massive overdosage may cause hepatic toxicity in some patients. In adults and adolescents, hepatic toxicity has rarely been reported following ingestion of acute

overdosage of less than 10 grams. Fatalities are infrequent (less than 3–4% of untreated cases) and have rarely been reported with overdoses of less than 15 grams. In children, an acute overdosage of less than 150 mg/kg has not been associated with hepatic toxicity.
Early symptoms following a potentially hepatotoxic overdose may include: nausea, vomiting, diaphoresis and general malaise. Clinical and laboratory evidence of hepatic toxicity may not be apparent until 48 to 72 hours postingestion.
In adults and adolescents, regardless of the quantity of acetaminophen reported to have been ingested, administer MUCOMYST® acetylcysteine immediately if 24 hours or less have elapsed from the reported time of ingestion. For full prescribing information, refer to the MUCOMYST package insert. Do not await the results of assays for acetaminophen level before initiating treatment with MUCOMYST acetylcysteine. The following additional procedures are recommended: The stomach should be emptied promptly by lavage or by induction of emesis with syrup of ipecac. A serum acetaminophen assay should be obtained as early as possible, but no sooner than four hours following ingestion. Liver function studies should be obtained initially and repeated at 24-hour intervals.
Serious toxicity or fatalities are extremely infrequent in children, possibly due to differences in the way they metabolize acetaminophen. In children, the maximum potential amount ingested can be more easily estimated. If more than 150 mg/kg or an unknown amount was ingested, obtain an acetaminophen plasma level. The acetaminophen plasma level should be obtained as soon as possible, but no sooner than 4 hours following the ingestion. Induce emesis using syrup of ipecac. If the plasma level is obtained and falls above the broken line on the acetaminophen overdose nomogram, the MUCOMYST acetylcysteine therapy should be initiated and continued for a full course of therapy. If acetaminophen plasma assay capability is not available, and the estimated acetaminophen ingestion exceeds 150 mg/kg, MUCOMYST acetylcysteine therapy should be initiated and continued for a full course of therapy.
For additional emergency information, call your regional poison center or call the Rocky Mountain Poison Center toll-free (1-800-525-6115).
Chlorpheniramine toxicity should be treated as you would an antihistamine/anticholinergic overdose and is likely to be present within a few hours after acute ingestion.
Pseudoephedrine may produce central nervous system stimulation and sympathomimetic effects on the cardiovascular system which are likely to be manifested within a few hours following ingestion.

Inactive Ingredients: *Chewable Tablets*—Aspartame, citric acid, ethylcellulose, flavors, magnesium stearate, mannitol, microcrystalline cellulose, pregelatinized starch, sucrose, Blue #1 and Red #7. *Liquid*—Benzoic acid, citric acid, flavors, glycerin, malic acid, polyethylene glycol, propylene glycol, sodium benzoate, sorbitol, sucrose, purified water, Blue #1 and Red #40.

How Supplied: *Chewable Tablets* (colored purple, scored, imprinted "Tylenol Cold") on one side and "TC" on opposite side—bottles of 24. *Cold Formula*—bottles (colored purple) of 4 fl. oz.
Shown in Product Identification Section, page 415

TYLENOL® Cold Medication Liquid

Description: Each 30 ml (1 fl. oz.) contains acetaminophen 650 mg., chlorpheniramine maleate 4 mg., pseudoephedrine hydrochloride 60 mg., and dextromethorphan hydrobromide 30 mg. (alcohol 7%).

Actions: TYLENOL Cold Medication Liquid contains a clinically proven analgesic-antipyretic, decongestant, cough suppressant and antihistamine. Acetaminophen produces analgesia by elevation of the pain threshold and antipyresis through action on the hypothalamic heat-regulating center. Acetaminophen component is equal to aspirin in analgesic and antipyretic effectiveness and it is unlikely to produce many of the side effects associated with aspirin and aspirin-containing products. Pseudoephedrine hydrochloride is a sympathomimetic amine which provides temporary relief of nasal congestion. Dextromethorphan is a cough suppressant which provides temporary relief of coughs due to minor throat irritations that may occur with the common cold. Chlorpheniramine is an antihistamine which helps provide temporary relief of runny nose, sneezing and watery and itchy eyes.

Indications: TYLENOL Cold Medication Liquid provides effective temporary relief of runny nose, sneezing, watery and itchy eyes, nasal congestion, coughing, and aches, pains and fevers due to a cold or "flu."

Precautions: If a rare sensitivity reaction occurs, the drug should be stopped. Although pseudoephedrine is virtually without pressor effect in normotensive patients, it should be used with caution in hypertensives.

Usual Dosage: Measuring cup is provided and marked for accurate dosing. *Adults:* 1 fluid ounce (2 tbsp.) every 6 hours as needed, not to exceed 4 doses in 24 hours. Children (6–12 yr): ½ the adult dose (1 tbsp.) as indicated on the measuring cup provided, not to exceed 4 doses in 24 hours for 5 days.
Note: Since TYLENOL Cold Medication Liquid is available without a prescription, the following appears on the package label: "**WARNING:** Do not administer to children under 6 or exceed the recommended dosage because nervousness, dizziness or sleeplessness may occur. May cause excitability especially in children. A persistent cough may be a sign of a serious condition. If fever per-

sists for more than three days, or if symptoms do not improve or new ones occur within five days or are accompanied by high fever, rash, excessive mucus, persistent cough or headache, consult a physician before continuing use. This preparation may cause drowsiness; alcohol may increase the drowsiness effect. Avoid alcoholic beverages when taking this product. Use caution when driving a motor vehicle or operating machinery. Do not take this product if you have heart disease, high blood pressure, thyroid disease, diabetes, asthma, glaucoma, emphysema, chronic pulmonary disease, shortness of breath, difficulty in breathing, or difficulty in urination due to enlargement of the prostate gland or are taking a prescription drug for high blood pressure or depression, unless directed by a doctor. **Do not use if carton is opened, or if printed plastic overwrap or printed foil inner seal is broken. Keep this and all medication out of the reach of children. As with any drug, if you are pregnant or nursing a baby, seek the advice of a health professional before using this product. In case of accidental overdosage, contact a physician or poison control center immediately."**

Overdosage: Acetaminophen in massive overdosage may cause hepatic toxicity in some patients. In adults and adolescents, hepatic toxicity has rarely been reported following ingestion of acute overdosage of less than 10 grams. Fatalities are infrequent (less than 3–4% of untreated cases) and have rarely been reported with overdoses of less than 15 grams. In children, an acute overdosage of less than 150 mg/kg has not been associated with hepatic toxicity.
Early symptoms following a potentially hepatotoxic overdose may include: nausea, vomiting, diaphoresis and general malaise. Clinical and laboratory evidence of hepatic toxicity may not be apparent until 48 to 72 hours postingestion. In adults and adolescents, regardless of the quantity of acetaminophen reported to have been ingested, administer MUCOMYST® acetylcysteine immediately if 24 hours or less have elapsed from the reported time of ingestion. For full prescribing information, refer to the MUCOMYST package insert. Do not await results of assays for acetaminophen level before initiating treatment with MUCOMYST acetylcysteine. The following additional procedures are recommended: The stomach should be emptied promptly by lavage or by induction of emesis with syrup of ipecac. A serum acetaminophen assay should be obtained as early as possible, but no sooner than four hours following ingestion. Liver function studies should be obtained initially and repeated at 24-hour intervals.
Serious toxicity or fatalities are extremely infrequent in children, possibly due to differences in the way they metabolize acetaminophen. In children, the maximum potential amount ingested can be more easily estimated. If more than 150 mg/kg or an unknown amount

was ingested, obtain an acetaminophen plasma level. The acetaminophen plasma level should be obtained as soon as possible, but no sooner than 4 hours following the ingestion. Induce emesis using syrup of ipecac. If the plasma level is obtained and falls above the broken line on the acetaminophen overdose nomogram, the MUCOMYST acetylcysteine therapy should be initiated and continued for a full course of therapy. If acetaminophen plasma assay capability is not available, and the estimated acetaminophen ingestion exceeds 150 mg/kg, MUCOMYST acetylcysteine therapy should be initiated and continued for a full course of therapy.
For additional emergency information, call your regional poison center or call the Rocky Mountain Poison Center toll-free (1-800-525-6115).
Chlorpheniramine toxicity should be treated as you would an antihistamine/anticholinergic overdose and is likely to be present within a few hours after acute ingestion.
Symptoms from pseudoephedrine overdose consist most often of mild anxiety, tachycardia and/or mild hypertension. Symptoms usually appear within 4 to 8 hours of ingestion and are transient, usually requiring no treatment.
Acute dextromethorphan overdose usually does not result in serious signs and symptoms unless massive amounts have been ingested. Signs and symptoms of a substantial overdose may include nausea and vomiting, visual disturbances, CNS disturbances, and urinary retention.

Inactive Ingredients: Alcohol (7%), Citric Acid, Flavors, Glycerin, Liquid Polyethylene Glycol, Saccharin, Sodium Benzoate, Sorbitol, Sucrose, Purified Water, Yellow #6 (sunset yellow) and Blue #1.
How Supplied: Cherry/mint mentholated flavored (colored amber) in 5 oz. bottles with child-resistant safety cap, special dosage cup graded in ounces and tablespoons, and tamper-resistant packaging.
Shown in Product Identification Section, page 415

TYLENOL® Cold Medication Tablets and Caplets

Description: Each TYLENOL Cold Tablet or Caplet contains acetaminophen 325 mg., chlorpheniramine maleate 2 mg., pseudoephedrine hydrochloride 30 mg. and dextromethorphan hydrobromide 15 mg.

Actions: TYLENOL Cold Medication Tablets and Caplets contain a clinically proven analgesic-antipyretic, decongestant, cough suppressant and antihistamine. Acetaminophen produces analgesia by elevation of the pain threshold and antipyresis through action on the hypothalamic heat-regulating center. Acetaminophen is equal to aspirin in analgesic and antipyretic effectiveness and it is unlikely to produce many of the side effects associated with aspirin and aspirin-

Continued on next page

McNeil Consumer—Cont.

containing products. Pseudoephedrine hydrochloride is a sympathomimetic amine which provides temporary relief of nasal congestion. Dextromethorphan is a cough suppressant which provides temporary relief of coughs due to minor throat irritations that may occur with the common cold. Chlorpheniramine is an antihistamine which helps provide temporary relief of runny nose, sneezing and watery and itchy eyes.

Indications: TYLENOL Cold Medication provides effective temporary relief of runny nose, sneezing, watery and itchy eyes, nasal congestion, coughing, and aches, pains and fever due to a cold or "flu."

Precautions: If a rare sensitivity reaction occurs, the drug should be stopped. Although pseudoephedrine is virtually without pressor effect in normotensive patients, it should be used with caution in hypertensives.

Usual Dosage: *Adults:* Two tablets or caplets every 6 hours, not to exceed 8 tablets or caplets in 24 hours. Children (6–12 years): One caplet or tablet every 6 hours, not to exceed 4 tablets or caplets in 24 hours for 5 days.
Note: Since TYLENOL Cold Medication Tablets and Caplets are available without prescription, the following appears on the package label: "**WARNING:** Do not administer to children under 6 or exceed the recommended dosage because nervousness, dizziness or sleeplessness may occur. May cause excitability especially in children. A persistent cough may be a sign of a serious condition. If fever persists for more than three days, or if symptoms do not improve or new ones occur within five days or are accompanied by high fever, rash, excessive mucus, persistent cough or headache, consult a physician before continuing use. This preparation may cause drowsiness; alcohol may increase the drowsiness effect. Avoid alcoholic beverages when taking this product. Use caution when driving a motor vehicle or operating machinery. Do not take this product if you have heart disease, high blood pressure, thyroid disease, diabetes, asthma, glaucoma, emphysema, chronic pulmonary disease, shortness of breath, difficulty in breathing, or difficulty in urination due to enlargement of the prostate gland or are taking a prescription drug for high blood pressure or depression, unless directed by a doctor. **Do not use if carton is opened, or if printed green neck wrap or printed foil inner seal is broken. Keep this and all medication out of the reach of children. As with any drug, if you are pregnant or nursing a baby, seek the advice of a health professional before using this product. In case of accidental overdosage, contact a physician or poison control center immediately.**"

Overdosage: Acetaminophen in massive overdosage may cause hepatic toxicity in some patients. In adults and adolescents, hepatic toxicity has rarely been reported following ingestion of acute overdosage of less than 10 grams. Fatalities are infrequent (less than 3–4% of untreated cases) and have rarely been reported with overdoses of less than 15 grams. In children, an acute overdosage of less than 150 mg/kg has not been associated with hepatic toxicity.
Early symptoms following a potentially hepatotoxic overdose may include: nausea, vomiting, diaphoresis and general malaise. Clinical and laboratory evidence of hepatic toxicity may not be apparent until 48 to 72 hours postingestion. In adults and adolescents, regardless of the quantity of acetaminophen reported to have been ingested, administer MUCOMYST® acetylcysteine immediately if 24 hours or less have elapsed from the reported time of ingestion. For full prescribing information, refer to the MUCOMYST package insert. Do not await results of assays for acetaminophen level before initiating treatment with MUCOMYST acetylcysteine. The following additional procedures are recommended: The stomach should be emptied promptly by lavage or by induction of emesis with syrup of ipecac. A serum acetaminophen assay should be obtained as early as possible, but no sooner than four hours following ingestion. Liver function studies should be obtained initially and repeated at 24-hour intervals.
Serious toxicity or fatalities are extremely infrequent in children, possibly due to differences in the way they metabolize acetaminophen. In children, the maximum potential amount ingested can be more easily estimated. If more than 150 mg/kg or an unknown amount was ingested, obtain an acetaminophen plasma level. The acetaminophen plasma level should be obtained as soon as possible, but no sooner than 4 hours following the ingestion. Induce emesis using syrup of ipecac. If the plasma level is obtained and falls above the broken line on the acetaminophen overdose nomogram, the MUCOMYST acetylcysteine therapy should be initiated and continued for a full course of therapy. If acetaminophen plasma assay capability is not available, and the estimated acetaminophen ingestion exceeds 150 mg/kg, MUCOMYST acetylcysteine therapy should be initiated and continued for a full course of therapy.
For additional emergency information, call your regional poison center or call the Rocky Mountain Poison Center toll-free (1-800-525-6115).
Chlorpheniramine toxicity should be treated as you would an antihistamine/anticholinergic overdose and is likely to be present within a few hours after acute ingestion.
Symptoms from pseudoephedrine overdose consist most often of mild anxiety, tachycardia and/or mild hypertension. Symptoms usually appear within 4 to 8 hours of ingestion and are transient, usually requiring no treatment.
Acute dextromethorphan overdose usually does not result in serious signs and symptoms unless massive amounts have been ingested. Signs and symptoms of a substantial overdose may include nausea and vomiting, visual disturbances, CNS disturbances, and urinary retention.

Inactive Ingredients: *Tablets:* Cellulose, Starch, Magnesium Stearate, Yellow #6 and Yellow #10. *Caplets:* Cellulose, Glyceryl, Triacetate, Hydroxypropyl Methylcellulose, Magnesium Stearate, Sodium Starch Glycolate, Starch, Titanium Dioxide, Blue #1 and Yellow #6 & #10.

How Supplied: *Tablets* (colored yellow, imprinted "TYLENOL Cold")—blister packs of 24 and tamper-resistant bottles of 50. *Caplets* (light yellow, imprinted "TYLENOL Cold")—blister packs of 24 and tamper-resistant bottles of 50.
Shown in Product Identification Section, page 415

TYLENOL® Cold Medication No Drowsiness Formula Caplets

Description: Each TYLENOL Cold Medication No Drowsiness Formula Caplet contains acetaminophen 325 mg., pseudoephedrine hydrochloride 30 mg. and dextromethorphan hydrobromide 15 mg.

Actions: TYLENOL Cold Medication No Drowsiness Formula Caplets contain a clinically proven analgesic-antipyretic, decongestant and cough suppressant. Acetaminophen produces analgesia by elevation of the pain threshold and antipyresis through action on the hypothalamic heat-regulating center. Acetaminophen is equal to aspirin in analgesic and antipyretic effectiveness and it is unlikely to produce many of the side effects associated with aspirin and aspirin-containing products. Pseudoephedrine hydrochloride is a sympathomimetic amine which provides temporary relief of nasal congestion. Dextromethorphan is a cough suppressant which provides temporary relief of coughs due to minor throat irritations that may occur with the common cold.

Indications: TYLENOL Cold Medication No Drowsiness Formula provides effective temporary relief of the nasal congestion, coughing, and aches, pains and fever due to a cold or "flu."

Precautions: If a rare sensitivity reaction occurs, the drug should be stopped. Although pseudoephedrine is virtually without pressor effect in normotensive patients, it should be used with caution in hypertensives.

Usual Dosage:
Adults: Two caplets every 6 hours, not to exceed 8 caplets in 24 hours. *Children* (6–12 years): One caplet every 6 hours, not to exceed 4 tablets or caplets in 24 hours for 5 days.
Note: Since TYLENOL Cold Medication No Drowsiness Formula Caplets are available without prescription, the following appears on the package label: "**WARNING:** Do not administer to children under 6 or exceed the recommended

dosage because nervousness, dizziness or sleeplessness may occur. May cause excitability especially in children. A persistent cough may be a sign of a serious condition. If fever persists for more than three days, or if symptoms do not improve or new ones occur within five days or are accompanied by fever, rash, excessive mucus, persistent cough or headache, consult a physician before continuing use. Avoid alcoholic beverages when taking this product. Use caution when driving a motor vehicle or operating machinery. Do not take this product if you have heart disease, high blood pressure, thyroid disease, diabetes, asthma, glaucoma, emphysema, chronic pulmonary disease, shortness of breath, difficulty in breathing, or difficulty in urination due to enlargement of the prostate gland or are taking a prescription drug for high blood pressure or depression, unless directed by a doctor. Do not use if carton is opened, or if printed green neck wrap or printed foil inner seal is broken. Keep this and all medication out of the reach of children. As with any drug, if you are pregnant or nursing a baby, seek the advice of a health professional before using this product. In case of accidental overdosage, contact a physician or poison control center immediately."

Overdosage: Acetaminophen in massive overdosage may cause hepatic toxicity in some patients. In adults and adolescents, hepatic toxicity has rarely been reported following ingestion of acute overdosage of less than 10 grams. Fatalities are infrequent (less than 3–4% of untreated cases) and have rarely been reported with overdosage of less than 15 grams. In children, an acute overdosage of less than 150 mg/kg has not been associated with hepatic toxicity.

Early symptoms following a potentially hepatotoxic overdose may include: nausea, vomiting, diaphoresis and general malaise. Clinical and laboratory evidence of hepatic toxicity may not be apparent until 48 to 72 hours postingestion. In adults and adolescents, regardless of the quantity of acetaminophen reported to have been ingested, administer MUCOMYST® acetylcysteine immediately if 24 hours or less have elapsed from the reported time of ingestion. For full prescribing information, refer to the MUCOMYST package insert. Do not await results of assays for acetaminophen level before initiating treatment with MUCOMYST acetylcysteine. The following additional procedures are recommended: The stomach should be emptied promptly by lavage or by induction of emesis with syrup of ipecac. A serum acetaminophen assay should be obtained as early as possible, but no sooner than four hours following ingestion. Liver function studies should be obtained initially and repeated at 24–hour intervals.

Serious toxicity or fatalities are extremely infrequent in children, possibly due to differences in the way they metabolize acetaminophen. In children, the maximum potential amount ingested can be more easily estimated. If more than 150 mg/kg or an unknown amount was ingested, obtain an acetaminophen plasma level. The acetaminophen plasma level should be obtained as soon as possible, but no sooner than 4 hours following the ingestion. Induce emesis using syrup of ipecac. If the plasma level is obtained and falls above the broken line on the acetaminophen overdose nomogram, the MUCOMYST acetylcysteine therapy should be initiated and continued for a full course of therapy. If acetaminophen plasma assay capability is not available, and the estimated acetaminophen ingestion exceeds 150 mg/kg, MUCOMYST acetylcysteine therapy should be initiated and continued for a full course of therapy.

For additional emergency information, call your regional poison center or call the Rocky Mountain Poison Center toll-free (1-800-525-6115).

Symptoms from pseudoephedrine overdose consist most often of mild anxiety, tachycardia and/or mild hypertension. Symptoms usually appear within 4 to 8 hours of ingestion and are transient, usually requiring no treatment.

Acute dextromethorphan overdose usually does not result in serious signs and symptoms unless massive amounts have been ingested. Signs and symptoms of a substantial overdose may include nausea and vomiting, visual disturbances, CNS disturbances, and urinary retention.

Inactive Ingredients: Cellulose, Glyceryl, Triacetate, Hydroxypropyl Methylcellulose, Magnesium Stearate, Sodium Starch Glycolate, Starch, Titanium Dioxide, Blue #1 and Yellow #10.

How Supplied: *Caplets* (colored white, imprinted TYLENOL "cold")—blister packs of 24 and tamper-resistant bottles of 50.

Shown in Product Identification Section, page 415

Maximum-Strength
TYLENOL® Allergy Sinus Medication Caplets

Description: Each TYLENOL® Allergy Sinus Caplet contains acetaminophen 500 mg, chlorpheniramine maleate 2 mg, and pseudoephedrine hydrochloride 30 mg.

Actions: TYLENOL® Allergy Sinus Caplets contain a clinically proven analgesic-antipyretic, decongestant, and antihistamine. Acetaminophen produces analgesia by elevation of the pain threshold and antipyresis through action on the hypothalamic heat-regulating center. Acetaminophen is equal to aspirin in analgesic and antipyretic effectiveness, and it is unlikely to produce many of the side effects associated with aspirin and aspirin-containing products. Pseudoephedrine hydrochloride is a sympathomimetic amine which provides temporary relief of nasal congestion. Chlorpheniramine is an antihistamine which helps provide temporary relief of runny nose, sneezing and watery and itchy eyes.

Indications: TYLENOL® Allergy Sinus provides effective temporary relief of these upper respiratory allergy, hay fever and sinusitis symptoms: sneezing, itchy, watery eyes, runny nose, itching of the nose or throat, nasal and sinus congestion and sinus pain and headaches.

Precautions: If a rare sensitivity reaction occurs, the drug should be stopped. Although pseudoephedrine is virtually without pressor effect in normotensive patients, it should be used with caution in hypertensives.

Usual Dosage: *Adults:* Two caplets every 6 hours, not to exceed 8 caplets in 24 hours.

Note: Since TYLENOL® Allergy Sinus Caplets are available without a prescription, the following appears on the package label: "**WARNING:** Do not administer to children under 12 or exceed the recommended dosage because nervousness, dizziness, or sleeplessness may occur. May cause excitability, especially in children. This preparation may cause drowsiness; alcohol may increase the drowsiness effect. Avoid alcoholic beverages when taking this product. Use caution when driving a motor vehicle or operating machinery. Do not take this product if you have heart disease, high blood pressure, thyroid disease, diabetes, asthma, glaucoma, emphysema, chronic pulmonary disease, shortness of breath, difficulty in breathing or difficulty in urination due to enlargement of prostate gland unless directed by a doctor. Do not take this product for more than 7 days. If symptoms do not improve or are accompanied by a high fever, consult a physician." **DO NOT USE IF CARTON IS OPEN OR IF A BLISTER UNIT IS BROKEN. KEEP THIS AND ALL MEDICATION OUT OF THE REACH OF CHILDREN. AS WITH ANY DRUG, IF YOU ARE PREGNANT OR NURSING A BABY, SEEK THE ADVICE OF A HEALTH PROFESSIONAL BEFORE USING THIS PRODUCT. IN THE CASE OF ACCIDENTAL OVERDOSE, CONTACT A PHYSICIAN OR POISON CONTROL CENTER IMMEDIATELY.**

Drug Interaction Precaution: Do not take this product if you are presently taking a prescription drug for high blood pressure or depression without first consulting your doctor.

Overdosage: Acetaminophen in massive overdosage may cause hepatic toxicity in some patients. In adults and adolescents, hepatic toxicity has rarely been reported following ingestion of acute overdosage of less than 10 grams. Fatalities are infrequent (less than 3–4% of untreated cases) and have rarely been reported with overdoses of less than 15 grams. In children, an acute overdosage of less than 150 mg/kg has not been associated with hepatic toxicity.

Early symptoms following a potentially hepatotoxic overdose may include: nausea, vomiting, diaphoresis and general

Continued on next page

McNeil Consumer—Cont.

malaise. Clinical and laboratory evidence of hepatic toxicity may not be apparent until 48 to 72 hours postingestion. In adults and adolescents, regardless of the quantity of acetaminophen reported to have been ingested, administer MUCOMYST® acetylcysteine immediately if 24 hours or less have elapsed from the reported time of ingestion. For full prescribing information, refer to the MUCOMYST package insert. Do not await results of assays for acetaminophen level before initiating treatment with MUCOMYST acetylcysteine. The following additional procedures are recommended: The stomach should be emptied promptly by lavage or by induction of emesis with syrup of ipecac. A serum acetaminophen assay should be obtained as early as possible, but no sooner than four hours following ingestion. Liver function studies should be obtained initially and repeated at 24-hour intervals.

Several toxicity or fatalities are extremely infrequent in children, possibly due to differences in the way they metabolize acetaminophen. In children, the maximum potential amount ingested can be easily estimated. If more than 150 mg/kg or an unknown amount was ingested, obtain an acetaminophen plasma level. The acetaminophen plasma level should be obtained as soon as possible, but no sooner than 4 hours following ingestion. Induce emesis using syrup of ipecac. If the plasma level is obtained and falls above the broken line on the acetaminophen overdose nomogram, the MUCOMYST acetylcysteine therapy should be initiated and continued for a full course of therapy. If acetaminophen plasma assay capability is not available, and the estimated acetaminophen ingestion exceeds 150 mg/kg, MUCOMYST acetylcysteine therapy should be initiated and continued for a full course of therapy.

For additional emergency information, call your regional poison center or call the Rocky Mountain Poison Control Center toll-free (1-800-525-6115).

Chlorpheniramine toxicity should be treated as you would an antihistamine/anticholinergic overdose and is likely to be present within a few hours after acute ingestion.

Symptoms from pseudophedrine overdose consist most often of mild anxiety, tachycardia and/or hypertension. Symptoms usually appear within 4 to 8 hours of ingestion and are transient, usually requiring no treatment.

Inactive Ingredients: Cellulose, hydroxypropyl cellulose, hydroxypropyl methylcellulose, magnesium stearate, polyethylene glycol, sodium starch glycolate, starch, titanium dioxide, blue #1, yellow #6, yellow #10.

How Supplied: *Caplets:* (dark yellow, imprinted "TYLENOL Allergy Si-

nus")—Blister packs of 24 and tamper-resistant bottles of 50.

Shown in Product Identification Section, page 415

Maximum-Strength TYLENOL® Sinus Medication Tablets and Caplets

Description: Each Maximum-Strength TYLENOL® Sinus Medication tablet or caplet contains acetaminophen 500 mg and pseudoephedrine hydrochloride 30 mg.

Actions: TYLENOL Sinus Medication contains a clinically proven analgesic-antipyretic and a decongestant. Maximum allowable nonprescription levels of acetaminophen and pseudoephedrine provide temporary relief of sinus headache and congestion. Acetaminophen is equal to aspirin in analgesic and antipyretic effectiveness and it is unlikely to produce many of the side effects associated with aspirin and aspirin-containing products.

Acetaminophen produces analgesia by elevation of the pain threshold and antipyresis through action on the hypothalamic heat-regulating center. Pseudoephedrine hydrochloride is a sympathomimetic amine which promotes sinus cavity drainage by reducing nasopharyngeal mucosal congestion.

Indications: Maximum-Strength TYLENOL Sinus Medication provides effective symptomatic relief from sinus headache pain and congestion. Maximum-Strength TYLENOL Sinus Medication is particularly well-suited in patients with aspirin allergy, hemostatic disturbances (including anticoagulant therapy), and bleeding diatheses (e.g., hemophilia) and upper gastrointestinal disease (e.g., ulcer, gastritis, hiatus hernia).

Precautions: If a rare sensitivity occurs, the drug should be discontinued. Although pseudoephedrine is virtually without pressor effect in normotensive patients, it should be used with caution in hypertensives.

Usual Dosage: *Adult dosage:* Two tablets or caplets every four to six hours. Do not exceed eight tablets or caplets in any 24-hour period. **Note:** Since TYLENOL Sinus Medication tablets and caplets are available without a prescription, the following appears on the package labels: "**WARNING:** Do not exceed the recommended dosage because at higher doses nervousness, dizziness, or sleeplessness may occur. Do not administer to children under 12. If you have high blood pressure, heart disease, diabetes, thyroid disease, difficulty in urination due to enlargement of the prostate gland, or are presently taking a prescription drug for the treatment of high blood pressure or depression, do not take except under the advice and supervision of a physician. Do not take this product for more than 7 days. If symptoms do not improve or are accompanied by high fever, consult a physician. **Do not use if carton is opened or if printed green neck wrap or printed foil inner seal is broken. Keep this and all medication out of**

the reach of children. As with any drug, if you are pregnant or nursing a baby, seek the advice of a health professional before using this product. In case of accidental overdosage, contact a physician or poison control center immediately.

Overdosage: Acetaminophen in massive overdosage may cause hepatic toxicity in some patients. In adults and adolescents, hepatic toxicity has rarely been reported following ingestion of acute overdosage of less than 10 grams. Fatalities are infrequent (less than 3–4% of untreated cases) and have rarely been reported with overdoses of less than 15 grams. In children, an acute overdosage of less than 150 mg/kg has not been associated with hepatic toxicity.

Early symptoms following a potentially hepatotoxic overdose may include: nausea, vomiting, diaphoresis and general malaise. Clinical and laboratory evidence of hepatic toxicity may not be apparent until 48 to 72 hours postingestion. In adults and adolescents, regardless of the quantity of acetaminophen reported to have been ingested, administer MUCOMYST® acetylcysteine immediately if 24 hours or less have elapsed from the reported time of ingestion. For full prescribing information, refer to the MUCOMYST package insert. Do not await the results of assays for acetaminophen level before initiating treatment with MUCOMYST acetylcysteine. The following additional procedures are recommended: The stomach should be emptied promptly by lavage or by induction of emesis with syrup of ipecac. A serum acetaminophen assay should be obtained as early as possible, but no sooner than four hours following ingestion. Liver function studies should be obtained initially and repeated at 24-hour intervals.

Serious toxicity or fatalities are extremely infrequent in children, possibly due to differences in the way they metabolize acetaminophen. In children, the maximum potential amount ingested can be more easily estimated. If more than 150 mg/kg or an unknown amount was ingested, obtain an acetaminophen plasma level. The acetaminophen plasma level should be obtained as soon as possible, but no sooner than 4 hours following the ingestion. Induce emesis using syrup of ipecac. If the plasma level is obtained and falls above the broken line on the acetaminophen overdose nomogram, the MUCOMYST acetylcysteine therapy should be initiated and continued for a full course of therapy. If acetaminophen plasma assay capability is not available, and the estimated acetaminophen ingestion exceeds 150 mg/kg, MUCOMYST acetylcysteine therapy should be initiated and continued for a full course of therapy.

For additional emergency information, call your regional poison center or call the Rocky Mountain Poison Center toll-free (1-800-525-6115).

Symptoms from pseudoephedrine overdose consist most often of mild anxiety, tachycardia and/or mild hypertension.

Symptoms usually appear within 4 to 8 hours of ingestion and are transient, usually requiring no treatment.

Inactive Ingredients: *Caplets* —Cellulose, Hydroxypropyl Methylcellulose, Magnesium Stearate, Polysorbate 80, Sodium Starch Glycolate, Starch, Titanium Dioxide, Blue #1, Red #40 and Yellow #10. *Tablets* —Cellulose, Magnesium Stearate, Sodium Lauryl Sulfate, Starch, Yellow #6 (Sunset Yellow), Yellow #10 and Blue #1.

How Supplied: *Tablets* (colored light green, imprinted "Maximum-Strength TYLENOL Sinus")—tamper-resistant bottles of 24 and 50. *Caplets* (light green coating, printed "TYLENOL Sinus" in dark green) tamper resistant bottles of 24 and 50.

Shown in Product Identification Section, page 415

Mead Johnson Nutritionals
A Bristol-Myers Company
2400 W. LLOYD EXPRESSWAY
EVANSVILLE, IN 47721

Full-Year Formulas
Enfamil® Full-Year Formula™ [1]
Enfamil® With Iron Full-Year Formula™ [1]
Enfamil® Full-Year Formula™ Nursette
ProSobee® Soy Isolate Formula[1]
ProSobee® Soy Isolate Formula Nursette
Nutramigen® Protein Hydrolysate Formula[1]

[1]Concentrated liquid, powder, and ready-to-use
Oral Electrolyte Solution
Lytren® Oral Electrolyte Solution
Special Metabolic Diets
Lofenalac®
Low Methionine Diet Powder (Product 3200 K)
Low PHE-TYR Diet Powder (Product 3200 AB)
Mono- and Disaccharide-Free Diet Powder (Product 3232 A)
MSUD Diet Powder
Phenyl-Free®
Pregestimil®
Special Metabolic Modules
HIST 1
HIST 2
HOM 1
HOM 2
LYS 1
LYS 2
Moducal®
MSUD 1
MSUD 2
OS 1
OS 2
PKU 1
PKU 2
PKU 3
Protein-Free Diet Powder (Product 80056)

TYR 1
TYR 2
UCD 1
UCD 2
Detailed information may be obtained by contacting Mead Johnson Nutritionals Medical Affairs Department at (812) 429-6437.

Mead Johnson Pharmaceuticals
A Bristol-Myers Company
2400 W. LLOYD EXPRESSWAY
EVANSVILLE, IN 47721-0001

COLACE®
[*kōlās*]
docusate sodium, Mead Johnson capsules • syrup • liquid (drops)

Description: Colace (docusate sodium) is a stool softener.
Colace Capsules, 50 mg, contain the following inactive ingredients: citric acid, D&C Red No. 33, FD&C Red No. 40, non-porcine gelatin, edible ink, polyethylene glycol, propylene glycol, and purified water.
Colace Capsules, 100 mg, contain the following inactive ingredients: citric acid, D&C Red No. 33, FD&C Red No. 40, FD&C Yellow No. 6, non-porcine gelatin, edible ink, polyethylene glycol, propylene glycol, titanium dioxide, and purified water.
Colace Liquid, 1%, contains the following inactive ingredients: citric acid, D&C Red No. 33, methylparaben, poloxamer, polyethylene glycol, propylene glycol, propylparaben, sodium citrate, vanillin, and purified water.
Colace Syrup, 20 mg/5 mL, contains the following inactive ingredients: alcohol, citric acid, D&C Red No. 33, FD&C Red No. 40, flavor (natural), menthol, methylparaben, peppermint oil, poloxamer, polyethylene glycol, propylparaben, sodium citrate, sucrose, and purified water.

Actions and Uses: Colace, a surface-active agent, helps to keep stools soft for easy, natural passage. Not a laxative, thus not habit-forming. Useful in constipation due to hard stools, in painful anorectal conditions, in cardiac and other conditions in which maximum ease of passage is desirable to avoid difficult or painful defecation, and when peristaltic stimulants are contraindicated. *Note:* When peristaltic stimulation is needed due to inadequate bowel motility, see Peri-Colace® (laxative and stool softener).

Contraindications: There are no known contraindications to Colace.

Side Effects: The incidence of side effects—none of a serious nature—is exceedingly small. Bitter taste, throat irritation, and nausea (primarily associated with the use of the syrup and liquid) are the main side effects reported. Rash has occurred.

Administration and Dosage: *Orally* —Suggested daily Dosage: *Adults and*

older children: 50 to 200 mg *Children 6 to 12:* 40 to 120 mg *Children 3 to 6:* 20 to 60 mg. *Infants and children under 3:* 10 to 40 mg. The higher doses are recommended for initial therapy. Dosage should be adjusted to individual response. The effect on stools is usually apparent one to three days after the first dose. Give Colace liquid in half a glass of milk or fruit juice or in infant formula, to mask bitter taste. *In enemas* —Add 50 to 100 mg Colace (5 to 10 mL Colace liquid) to a retention or flushing enema.

Warning: As with any drug, if you are pregnant or nursing a baby, seek the advice of a health professional before using this product.

How Supplied: Colace capsules, 50 mg
NDC 0087-0713-01 Bottles of 30
NDC 0087-0713-02 Bottles of 60
NDC 0087-0713-03 Bottles of 250
NDC 0087-0713-05 Bottles of 1000
NDC 0087-0713-07 Cartons of 100 single unit packs
Colace capsules, 100 mg
NDC 0087-0714-01 Bottles of 30
NDC 0087-0714-02 Bottles of 60
NDC 0087-0714-03 Bottles of 250
NDC 0087-0714-05 Bottles of 1000
NDC 0087-0714-07 Cartons of 100 single unit packs
Note: Colace capsules should be stored at controlled room temperature (59°–86°F or 15°–30°C)
Colace liquid, 1% solution; 10 mg/mL (with calibrated dropper)
NDC 0087-0717-04 Bottles of 16 fl oz
NDC 0087-0717-02 Bottles of 30 mL
6505-00-045-7786 (Bottle of 30 mL) Defense
Colace syrup, 20 mg/5-mL teaspoon; contains not more than 1% alcohol
NDC 0087-0720-01 Bottles of 8 fl oz
NDC 0087-0720-02 Bottles of 16 fl oz
Shown in Product Identification Section, page 416

PERI-COLACE® capsules • syrup
casanthranol and docusate sodium

Description: Peri-Colace is a combination of the mild stimulant laxative casanthranol, and the stool-softener Colace® (docusate sodium). Each capsule contains 30 mg of casanthranol and 100 mg of Colace; the syrup contains 30 mg of casanthranol and 60 mg of Colace per 15-mL tablespoon (10 mg of casanthranol and 20 mg of Colace per 5-mL teaspoon) and 10% alcohol.
Peri-Colace Capsules contain the following inactive ingredients: D&C Red No. 33, FD&C Red No. 40, non-porcine gelatin, edible ink, polyethylene glycol, propylene glycol, titanium dioxide, and purified water.
Peri-Colace Syrup contains the following inactive ingredients: alcohol, citric acid, flavors, methyl salicylate, methylparaben, poloxamer, polyethylene glycol, propylparaben, sodium citrate, sorbitol solution, sucrose, and purified water.

Action and Uses: Peri-Colace provides gentle peristaltic stimulation and helps

Continued on next page

Mead Johnson Pharm.—Cont.

to keep stools soft for easier passage. Bowel movement is induced gently—usually overnight or in 8 to 12 hours. Nausea, griping, abnormally loose stools, and constipation rebound are minimized. Useful in management of chronic or temporary constipation.

Note: To prevent hard stools when laxative stimulation is not needed or undesirable, see Colace (stool softener).

Side Effects: The incidence of side effects—none of a serious nature—is exceedingly small. Nausea, abdominal cramping or discomfort, diarrhea, and rash are the main side effects reported.

Administration and Dosage:
Adults —1 or 2 capsules, or 1 or 2 tablespoons syrup at bedtime, or as indicated. In severe cases, dosage may be increased to 2 capsules or 2 tablespoons twice daily, or 3 capsules at bedtime. *Children* —1 to 3 teaspoons of syrup at bedtime, or as indicated.

Warnings: Do not use when abdominal pain, nausea, or vomiting are present. Frequent or prolonged use of this preparation may result in dependence on laxatives. As with any drug, if you are pregnant or nursing a baby, seek the advice of a health professional before using this product.

Overdosage: In addition to symptomatic treatment, gastric lavage, if timely, is recommended in cases of large overdosage.

How Supplied: Peri-Colace® Capsules
    NDC 0087-0715-01 Bottles of 30
    NDC 0087-0715-02 Bottles of 60
    NDC 0087-0715-03 Bottles of 250
    NDC 0087-0715-05 Bottles of 1000
    NDC 0087-0715-07 Cartons of 100 single unit packs
Note: Peri-Colace capsules should be stored at controlled room temperatures (59°–86°F or 15°–30°C).
Peri-Colace® Syrup
    NDC 0087-0721-01 Bottles of 8 fl oz
    NDC 0087-0721-02 Bottles of 16 fl oz
    Shown in Product Identification Section, page 416

Medicone Company
225 VARICK ST.
NEW YORK, NY 10014

MEDICONE® DERMA Ointment

Composition: Each gram contains: Benzocaine 2%; 8-Hydroxyquinoline Sulfate 1.05%; Menthol .48%; Zinc Oxide 13.73%; Ichthammol 1%; Lavender Perfume .08%; Petrolatum—Lanolin Base 79.87%.

Action and Uses: For prompt, temporary relief of intolerable itching, burning and pain associated with minor skin irritations. A bland, well balanced formula in a non-drying base which will not disintegrate or liquefy at body temperature and is not washed away by urine, perspiration or exudate. Exerts a soothing, cooling influence on irritated skin surfaces by affording mild anesthesia to control the scratch reflex, promotes healing of the affected area and checks the spread of infection. Useful for symptomatic relief in a wide variety of pruritic skin irritations resulting from insect bites, prickly heat, eczema, chafed and raw skin surfaces, sunburn, fungus infections, plant poisoning, pruritus ani and pruritus vulvae—mouth sores, cracked lips, under dentures.

Administration and Dosage: Apply liberally directly to site of irritation and gently rub into affected area for better penetration and absorption. Cover area with gauze if necessary.

Precautions: Do not use in the eyes. If the condition for which this preparation is used persists, or if rash or irritation develops, discontinue use and consult physician.

How Supplied: 1½ ounce tubes.
    Shown in Product Identification Section, page 416

MEDICONE® DRESSING Cream

Composition: Each gram contains: Benzocaine .50%; 8-Hydroxyquinoline Sulfate .05%; Cod Liver Oil 12.50%; Zinc Oxide 12.50%; Menthol .18%; Talcum 2.99%; Paraffin 1.66%; Petrolatum-Lanolin Base 65.53%; Lavender Perfume .10%.

Action and Uses: Meets the first requisite in the treatment of minor burns, wounds and other denuded skin lesions by exerting mild, cooling anesthetic action for the prompt temporary relief of pain, burning and itching. A stable, anesthetic dressing which does not liquefy or wash off at body temperature, nor is it decomposed by exudate, urine or perspiration. Promotes granulation and aids epithelization of affected tissue. The anesthetic, antipruritic, antibacterial properties make Medicone Dressing ideal for the treatment of 1st and 2nd degree burns, minor wounds, abrasions, diaper rashes and a wide variety of pruritic skin irritations.

Administration and Dosage: The smooth, specially formulated consistency allows comfortable application directly to the painful, irritated affected area. It may be spread on gauze before application or covered with gauze as desired.

Precautions: Do not use in the eyes. If the condition for which this preparation is used persists or if a rash or irritation develops, discontinue use and consult physician.

How Supplied: Tubes of 1½ ounce.
    Shown in Product Identification Section, page 416

MEDICONE® RECTAL OINTMENT

Composition: Each gram contains: Benzocaine, 2.01%; 8-Hydroxyquinoline Sulfate .5%; Menthol .4%; Zinc Oxide 10.04%; Balsam Peru 1.26%; Castor Oil 1.26%; Petrolatum—Lanolin Base 83.61%; Certified Color Added.

Action and Uses: A soothing, effective formulation which affords prompt, temporary relief of pain, burning and itching by exerting surface anesthetic action on the affected area in minor internal-external hemorrhoids and anorectal disorders. The active ingredients promote healing and protect against irritation, aiding inflamed tissue to retrogress to normal. The emollient petrolatum-lanolin base provides lubrication making bowel movements easier and more comfortable. Accelerates the normal healing process. Medicone Rectal Ointment and Medicone Rectal Suppositories are excellent for concurrent management of internal-external irritations.

Administration and Dosage: For internal use—attach pliable applicator and lubricate tip with a small amount of Ointment to ease insertion. Apply liberally into affected area morning and night and after each stool or as directed. When used externally, cover area with gauze. When used with Medicone Rectal Suppositories, insert a small amount of Ointment into the rectum before inserting suppository.

Precautions: If a rash or irritation develops or rectal bleeding occurs, discontinue use and consult physician.

How Supplied: 1½ ounce tubes with pliable rectal applicator.
    Shown in Product Identification Section, page 416

MEDICONE® RECTAL SUPPOSITORIES

Composition: Each suppository contains:
Benzocaine .... 2 gr.
8-Hydroxyquinoline sulfate.............¼ gr.
Zinc oxide... 3 gr.
Menthol..⅟₇ gr.
Balsam Peru .... 1 gr.
Cocoa butter—vegetable & petroleum
    oil base; Certified color added ....q.s.

Action and Uses: A soothing, comprehensive formula carefully designed to meet the therapeutic requirements in adequately treating simple hemorrhoids and minor anorectal disorders. Performs the primary function of promptly alleviating pain, burning and itching temporarily by exerting satisfactory local anesthesia. The muscle spasm, present in many cases of painful anal and rectal conditions, is controlled and together with the emollients provided, helps the patient to evacuate the bowel comfortably and normally. The active ingredients reduce congestion and afford antisepsis, accelerating the normal healing process. Used pre- and post-surgically in hemorrhoidectomy, in prenatal and postpartum care and whenever surgery is contraindicated for the comfort and well-being of the patient during treatment of an underlying cause.

Administration and Dosage: One suppository in the morning and one at night and after each stool, or as directed. Use of the suppositories should be continued for 10 to 15 days after cessation of discomfort to help protect against recurrence of symptoms. See Medicone Rectal Ointment for concurrent internal-external use.

Precautions: If a rash or irritation develops, or bleeding from the rectum occurs, discontinue use and consult physician.

How Supplied: Boxes of 12 and 24 individually foil-wrapped green suppositories.

Shown in Product Identification Section, page 416

MEDICONET®
(medicated rectal wipes)

Composition: Each cloth wipe medicated with Benzalkonium chloride, 0.02%; Ethoxylated lanolin, 0.5%; Methylparaben, 0.15%; Hamamelis water, 50%; Glycerin, 10%; Alkylaryl Polyether, Purified water, USP and Perfume, q.s.

Action and Uses: Soft disposable cloth wipes which fulfill the important requisite in treating anal discomfort by providing the facility for gently and thoroughly cleansing the affected area. For the temporary relief of intolerable pain, itching and burning in minor external hemorrhoidal, anal and outer vaginal discomfort. Lanolized, delicately scented, durable and delightfully soft. Antiseptic, antipruritic, astringent. Useful as a substitute for harsh, dry toilet tissue. May also be used as a compress in the pre- and post-operative management of anorectal discomfort. The hygienic Mediconet pad is generally useful in relieving pain, burning and itching in diaper rash, sunburn, heat rash, minor burns and insect bites.

How Supplied: Boxes of 20 individually packaged, pre-moistened cleansing cloths.

Shown in Product Identification Section, page 416

EDUCATIONAL MATERIAL

Clinical Evaluation Fact Cards and Samples
Medical study in the usage of our rectal suppositories.
The Latest Approach in Early Detection and Evaluation of Rectal Bleeding
A 16-page symposium for physicians of a medical mediconference.
Medical Mediconference
A discussion by experts on the latest approaches in Early Detection and Evaluation of Rectal Bleeding.

Mericon Industries, Inc.
8819 N. PIONEER RD.
PEORIA, IL 61615

DELACORT
(hydrocortisone USP ½%)

Active Ingredient: Hydrocortisone USP ½%.

Indications: For the temporary relief of minor skin irritations, itching and rashes due to eczema, dermatitis, insect bites, poison ivy, poison oak, poison sumac, soaps; detergents, cosmetics, and jewelry, and for itchy genital and anal areas.

Warnings: For external use only. Avoid contact with the eyes. If condition worsens, or if symptoms persist for more than 7 days discontinue use (of this product) and consult a physician. Do not use on children 2 years of age except under the advice and supervision of a physician.

Precaution: KEEP OUT OF REACH OF CHILDREN.

Dosage and Administration: For adults and children 2 years of age and older: Apply to affected area 3 or 4 times daily.

How Supplied: 2 oz. and 4 oz. squeeze bottle.

ORAZINC®
(zinc sulfate)

Active Ingredient: Zinc Sulfate U.S.P. 220 mg. and 110 mg. Capsules.

Indications: A Dietary Supplement containing Zinc.

Warnings: Should be taken with milk or meals to alleviate possible gastric distress.

Symptoms and Treatment of Oral Overdosage: Nausea, mild diarrhea or rash—to control, reduce dosage or discontinue.

Dosage and Administration: One capsule daily or as recommended by physician.

How Supplied: Bottles of 100 and 1000 Capsules each.

ORAZINC® LOZENGES
(zinc gluconate)

Active Ingredient: Zinc (Zinc Gluconate) 10 mg. Contains no starch, no artificial colors, flavors or preservatives. Sweetened with sorbitol and fructose.

Directions: As a dietary supplement, slowly dissolve one or two lozenges in mouth. To alleviate possible gastric distress, do not take on empty stomach.

Warnings: Keep this and all medications out of the reach of children.

How Supplied: Bottles of 100 Lozenges (NDC 0394-0495-02).

Miles Inc.
P. O. BOX 340
ELKHART, IN 46515

ALKA–MINTS® Chewable Antacid Rich in Calcium

Active Ingredient: Each ALKA-MINTS Chewable Antacid tablet contains calcium carbonate 850 mg. (340 mg of elemental calcium). Each tablet contains less than .5 mg sodium per tablet, and is dietarily sodium free.

Inactive Ingredients: Dioctyl sodium sulfosuccinate, flavor, hydrolyzed cereal solids, polyethylene glycol, sugar (compressible), magnesium stearate, sorbitol.

Indications: ALKA-MINTS is an antacid for occasional use for relief of acid indigestion, heartburn and sour stomach.

Actions: ALKA-MINTS has a natural, clean, spearmint taste that leaves the mouth feeling refreshed. Measured by the in-vitro standard established by the Food and Drug Administration, one ALKA-MINTS tablet neutralizes 15.9 mEq of acid.

Warnings: Do not take more than 9 tablets in a 24 hour period, or use the maximum dosage of this product for more than 2 weeks, except under the advice and supervision of a physician. May cause constipation. As with any drug, if you are pregnant or nursing a baby, seek the advice of a health professional before using this product. Keep this and all drugs out of the reach of children.

Dosage and Administration: Chew 1 tablet every 2 hours or as directed by a physician.

How Supplied: Cartons of 30's. Each carton contains convenient pocket-sized packs with individually sealed tablets so ALKA-MINTS stay fresh wherever you go.

Product Identification Mark:
ALKA-MINTS embossed on each tablet.
Shown in Product Identification Section, page 416

ALKA–SELTZER® ADVANCED FORMULA

Active Ingredients: Each tablet contains: acetaminophen 325 mg, calcium carbonate 280 mg, citric acid 900 mg, potassium bicarbonate 300 mg, heat-treated sodium bicarbonate 465 mg. Alka-Seltzer Advanced Formula in water contains principally the antacid citrates of sodium, potassium and calcium.

Inactive Ingredients: Each tablet contains: Aminoacetic acid, aspartame, calcium saccharin, flavors, hydrolyzed cereal solids, hydroxypropyl methylcellulose, lactose, sorbitol, tableting aids. Contains 75% less sodium per tablet than Original Alka-Seltzer. PHENYLKETONURICS: Contains 4.2 mg Phenylalanine per tablet.

Continued on next page

Miles—Cont.

Indications: For speedy relief of ACID INDIGESTION, SOUR STOMACH or HEARTBURN with HEADACHE, or BODY ACHES AND PAINS. Also for fast relief of UPSET STOMACH with HEADACHE from overindulgence in food and drink—especially recommended for taking before bedtime and again on arising. EFFECTIVE FOR PAIN RELIEF ALONE: HEADACHE or BODY and MUSCULAR ACHES and PAINS.

Warnings: Do not take more than 8 tablets in a 24-hour period or use the maximum dosage of this product for more than 10 days, except under the advice and supervision of a physician. May cause constipation. If symptoms persist or recur frequently or if you are on a sodium-restricted diet, do not take this product except under the supervision of a physician. As with any drug, if you are pregnant or nursing a baby, seek the advice of a health professional before using this product. Keep this and all drugs out of the reach of children. In case of accidental overdose, contact a physician or poison control center immediately. Each tablet contains 141 mg sodium.

Directions: Adults: Take 2 tablets fully dissolved in 4 ounces of water every 4 hours or as directed by a physician.

How Supplied: Tablets: Foil sealed; box of 36 tablets in 18 twin packs; box of 24 in 12 foil twin packs.
Shown in Product Identification Section, page 416

ALKA–SELTZER® Effervescent Antacid & Pain Reliever With Specially Buffered Aspirin

Active Ingredients: Each tablet contains: aspirin 325 mg., heat treated sodium bicarbonate 1916 mg., citric acid 1000 mg. ALKA-SELTZER® in water contains principally the antacid sodium citrate and the analgesic sodium acetylsalicylate. Buffered pH is between 6 and 7.

Inactive Ingredients: None.

Indications: ALKA-SELTZER® Effervescent Antacid & Pain Reliever is an analgesic and an antacid and is indicated for relief of sour stomach, acid indigestion or heartburn with headache or body aches and pains. Also for fast relief of upset stomach with headache from overindulgence in food and drink—especially recommended for taking before bed and again on arising. Effective for pain relief alone: headache or body and muscular aches and pains.

Actions: When the ALKA-SELTZER® Effervescent Antacid & Pain Reliever tablet is dissolved in water, the acetylsalicylate ion differs from acetylsalicylic acid chemically, physically and pharmacologically. Being fat insoluble, it is not absorbed by the gastric mucosal cells. Studies and observations in animals and

man including radiochrome determinations of fecal blood loss, measurement of ion fluxes and direct visualization with gastrocamera, have shown that, as contrasted with acetylsalicylic acid, the acetylsalicylate ion delivered in the solution does not alter gastric mucosal permeability to permit back-diffusion of hydrogen ion, and gastric damage and acute gastric mucosal lesions are therefore not seen after administration of the product. ALKA-SELTZER® Effervescent Antacid & Pain Reliever has the capacity to neutralize gastric hydrochloric acid quickly and effectively. In-vitro, 154 ml. of 0.1 N hydrochloric acid are required to decrease the pH of one tablet of ALKA-SELTZER® Effervescent Antacid & Pain Reliever in solution to 4.0. Measured against the in vitro standard established by the Food and Drug Administration one tablet neutralizes 17.2 mEq of acid. In vivo, the antacid activity of two ALKA-SELTZER® Antacid & Pain Reliever tablets is comparable to that of 10 ml. of milk of magnesia. ALKA-SELTZER® Effervescent Antacid & Pain Reliever is able to resist pH changes caused by the continuing secretion of acid in the normal individual and to maintain an elevated pH until emptying occurs.

ALKA-SELTZER® Effervescent Antacid & Pain Reliever provides highly water soluble acetylsalicylate ions which are fat insoluble. Acetylsalicylate ions are not absorbed from the stomach. They empty from the stomach and thereby become available for absorption from the duodenum. Thus, fast drug absorption and high plasma acetylsalicylate levels are achieved. Plasma levels of salicylate following the administration of ALKA-SELTZER® Effervescent Antacid & Pain Reliever solution (acetylsalicylate ion equivalent to 648 mg. acetylsalicylic acid) can reach 29 mg./liter in 10 minutes and rise to peak levels as high as 55 mg./liter within 30 minutes.

Warnings: Children and teenagers should not use this medicine for chicken pox or flu symptoms before a doctor is consulted about Reye Syndrome, a rare but serious illness reported to be associated with aspirin. As with any drug, if you are pregnant or nursing a baby, seek the advice of a health professional before using this product. Except under the advice and supervision of a physician, do not take more than, Adults: 8 tablets in a 24 hour period. (60 years of age or older: 4 tablets in a 24 hour period), or use the maximum dosage for more than 10 days. Do not use if you are allergic to aspirin or have asthma, if you have a coagulation (bleeding) disease, or if you are on a sodium restricted diet. Each tablet contains 567 mg. of sodium.
Keep this and all drugs out of the reach of children.

Dosage and Administration:
ALKA-SELTZER® Effervescent Antacid & Pain Reliever is taken in solution, approximately three ounces of water per tablet is sufficient.

Adults: 2 tablets every 4 hours. CAUTION: If symptoms persist or recur frequently, or if you are under treatment for ulcer, consult your physician.

Professional Labeling:

ASPIRIN FOR MYOCARDIAL INFARCTION

Indication: The Aspirin contained in ALKA-SELTZER is indicated to reduce the risk of death and/or non-fatal myocardial infarction in patients with a previous infarction or unstable angina pectoris.

Clinical Trials: The indication is supported by the results of six, large, randomized multicenter, placebo-controlled studies[1-7] involving 10,816, predominantly male, post-myocardial infarction (MI) patients and one randomized placebo-controlled study of 1,266 men with unstable angina. Therapy with aspirin was begun at intervals after the onset of acute MI varying from less than 3 days to more than 5 years and continued for periods of from less than one year to four years. In the unstable angina study, treatment was started within 1 month after the onset of unstable angina and continued for 12 weeks and complicating conditions such as congestive heart failure were not included in the study.

Aspirin therapy in MI patients was associated with about a 20 percent reduction in the risk of subsequent death and/or non-fatal reinfarction, a median absolute decrease of 3 percent from the 12 to 22 percent event rates in the placebo groups. In aspirin-treated unstable angina patients the reduction in risk was about 50 percent, a reduction in event rate of 5 percent from the 10 percent rate in the placebo group over the 12 weeks of the study.

Daily dosage of aspirin in the post-myocardial infarction studies was 300 mg in one study and 900 to 1500 mg in five studies. A dose of 325 mg was used in the study of unstable angina.

Adverse Reactions: Gastrointestinal Reactions: Symptoms and signs of gastrointestinal irritation were not significantly increased in subjects treated for unstable angina with buffered aspirin in solution. (ALKA-SELZER®.) Doses of 1000 mg per day of aspirin tablets caused gastrointestinal symptoms and bleeding that in some cases were clinically significant. In the largest post-infarction study (the Aspirin Myocardial Infarction Study (AMIS) with 4,500 cases), the percentage incidences of gastrointestinal symptoms for the aspirin (1000 mg of a standard, solid-tablet formulation) and placebo-treated subjects, respectively, were: stomach pain (14.5%; 4.4%); heartburn (11.9%; 4.8%); nausea and/or vomiting (7.6%; 2.1%); hospitalization for gastrointestinal disorder (4.9%; 3.5%). In the AMIS and other trials, aspirin treated patients had increased rates of gross gastrointestinal bleeding. As with all aspirin products ALKA-SELTZER is contraindicated in patients with aspirin sensitivity, with asthma, or with coagulation disease.

Cardiovascular and Biochemical: In the AMIS trial, the dosage of 1000 mg per day of aspirin was associated with small increases in systolic blood pressure (BP) (average 1.5 to 2.1 mm) and diastolic BP (0.5 to 0.6 mm), depending upon whether maximal or last available readings were used. Blood urea nitrogen and uric acid levels were also increased, but by less than 1.0 mg%. Subjects with marked hypertension or renal insufficiency had been excluded from the trial so that the clinical importance of these observations for such subjects or for any subjects treated over more prolonged periods is not known. It is recommended that patients placed on long-term aspirin treatment, even at doses of 300 mg per day, be seen at regular intervals to assess changes in these measurements.

Sodium in Buffered Aspirin for Solution Formulations: One tablet daily of buffered aspirin in solution adds 567 mg of sodium to that in the diet and may not be tolerated by patients with active sodium-retaining states such as congestive heart or renal failure. This amount of sodium adds about 30 percent to the 70 to 90 meq intake suggested as appropriate for dietary treatment of essential hypertension in the 1984 Report of the Joint National Committee on Detection, Evaluation, and Treatment of High Blood Pressure[8].

Dosage and Administration: Although most of the studies used dosages exceeding 300 mg, daily, two trials used only 300 mg and pharmacologic data indicate that this dose inhibits platelet function fully. Therefore, 300 mg or a conventional 325 mg aspirin dose daily is a reasonable, routine dose that would minimize gastrointestinal adverse reactions. This use of aspirin applies to both solid, oral dosage forms (buffered and plain aspirin) and buffered aspirin in solution.

References:
(1) Elwood, P. C., et al., A Randomized Controlled Trial of Acetysalicylic Acid in the Secondary Prevention of Mortality from Myocardial Infarction," *British Medical Journal* 1:436–440, 1974.
(2) The Coronary Drug Project Research Group, "Aspirin in Coronary Heart Disease," *Journal of Chronic Diseases,* 29:625–642, 1976.
(3) Breddin K., et al., "Secondary Prevention of Myocardial Infarction: A Comparison of Acetylsalicylic Acid, Phenprocoumon or Placebo," *International Congress Series* 470:263–268, 1979.
(4) Aspirin Myocardial Infarction Study Research Group, "A Randomized, Controlled Trial of Aspirin in Persons Recovered from Myocardial Infarction," *Journal American Medical Association* 245:661–669, 1980.
(5) Elwood, P. C., and P. M. Sweetnam, "Aspirin and Secondary Mortality after Myocardial Infarction," *Lancet* pp. 1313–1315, December 22–29, 1979.
(6) The Persantine-Aspirin Reinfarction Study Research Group, "Persantine and Aspirin in Coronary Heart Disease," *Circulation,* 62: 449–460, 1980.
(7) Lewis, H. D., et al., "Protective Effects of Aspirin Against Acute Myocardial Infarction and Death in Men with Unstable Angina, Results of a Veterans Administration Cooperative Study," *New England Journal of Medicine* 309:396–403, 1983.
(8) "1984 Report of the Joint National Committee on Detection, Evaluation, Treatment of High Blood Pressure," U.S. Department of Health and Human Services and United States Public Health Service, National Institutes of Health.

How Supplied: Tablets: foil sealed; box of 12 in 6 foil twin packs; box of 24 in 12 foil twin packs; box of 36 tablets in 18 foil twin packs; 100 tablets in 50 foil twin packs; carton of 72 tablets in 36 foil twin 96's card packs. Product Identification Mark: "ALKA-SELTZER" embossed on each tablet.

Shown in Product Identification Section, page 416

Flavored ALKA-SELTZER®
Effervescent Antacid & Pain Reliever

Active Ingredients: Each tablet contains: Aspirin 325 mg, heat treated sodium bicarbonate 1710 mg, citric acid 1220 mg. Alka-Seltzer in water contains principally the antacid sodium citrate and the analgesic sodium acetylsalicylate.

Inactive Ingredients: Flavors, Saccharin Sodium.

Indications: SPARKLING FRESH TASTE!
Flavored Alka-Seltzer®
For speedy relief of ACID INDIGESTION, SOUR STOMACH or HEARTBURN with HEADACHE, or BODY ACHES AND PAINS. Also for fast relief of UPSET STOMACH with HEADACHE from overindulgence in food and drink —especially recommended for taking before bed and again on arising. EFFECTIVE FOR PAIN RELIEF ALONE: HEADACHE or BODY and MUSCULAR ACHES and PAINS.

Warnings: Children and teenagers should not use this medicine for chicken pox or flu symptoms before a doctor is consulted about Reye Syndrome, a rare but serious illness reported to be associated with aspirin.
As with any drug, if you are pregnant or nursing a baby, seek the advice of a health professional before using this product.
Except under the advice and supervision of a physician: Do not take more than, ADULTS: 6 tablets in a 24-hour period, (60 years of age or older: 4 tablets in a 24-hour period), or use the daily maximum dosage for more than 10 days. Do not use if you are allergic to aspirin or have asthma, if you have a coagulation (bleeding) disease, or if you are on a sodium restricted diet. Each tablet contains 506 mg of sodium.
Keep this and all drugs out of the reach of children.

Directions: Alka-Seltzer must be dissolved in water before taking. ADULTS: 2 tablets every 4 hours. CAUTION: If symptoms persist or recur frequently or if you are under treatment for ulcer, consult your physician.

Professional Labeling:
ASPIRIN FOR MYOCARDIAL INFARCTION

Indication: The Aspirin contained in Alka-Seltzer is indicated to reduce the risk of death and/or non-fatal myocardial infarction in patients with a previous infarction or unstable angina pectoris.

Clinical Trials: The indication is supported by the results of six, large, randomized multicenter, placebo-controlled studies[1–7] involving 10,816, predominantly male, post-myocardial infarction (MI) patients and one randomized placebo-controlled study of 1,266 men with unstable angina. Therapy with aspirin was begun at intervals after the onset of acute MI varying from less than 3 days to more than 5 years and continued for periods of from less than one year to four years. In the unstable angina study, treatment was started within 1 month after the onset of unstable angina and continued for 12 weeks and complicating conditions such as congestive heart failure were not included in the study.
Aspirin therapy in MI patients was associated with about a 20 percent reduction in the risk of subsequent death and/or non-fatal reinfarction, a median absolute decrease of 3 percent from the 12 to 22 percent event rates in the placebo groups. In aspirin-treated unstable angina patients the reduction in risk was about 50 percent, a reduction in event rate of 5 percent from the 10 percent rate in the placebo group over the 12 weeks of the study.
Daily dosage of aspirin in the post-myocardial infarction studies was 300 mg in one study and 900 to 1500 mg in five studies. A dose of 325 mg was used in the study of unstable angina.

Adverse Reactions: Gastrointestinal Reactions: Symptoms and signs of gastrointestinal irritation were not significantly increased in subjects treated for unstable angina with buffered aspirin in solution (ALKA-SELTZER®). Doses of 1000 mg per day of aspirin tablets caused gastrointestinal symptoms and bleeding that in some cases were clinically significant. In the largest post-infarction study (the Aspirin Myocardial Infarction Study (AMIS) with 4,500 people), the percentage incidences of gastrointestinal symptoms for the aspirin (1000 mg of a standard, solid-tablet formulation) and placebo-treated subjects, respectively, were: stomach pain (14.5%; 4.4%); heartburn (11.9%; 4.8%); nausea and/or vomiting (7.6%; 2.1%); hospitalization for gastro-

Continued on next page

Miles—Cont.

intestinal disorder (4.9%; 3.5%). In the AMIS and other trials, aspirin treated patients had increased rates of gross gastrointestinal bleeding. As with all aspirin products Alka-Seltzer is contraindicated in patients with aspirin sensitivity, with asthma, or with coagulation disease.

Cardiovascular and Biochemical: In the AMIS trial, the dosage of 1000 mg per day of aspirin was associated with small increases in systolic blood pressure (BP) (average 1.5 to 2.1 mm) and diastolic BP (0.5 to 0.6 mm), depending upon whether maximal or last available readings were used. Blood urea nitrogen and uric acid levels were also increased, but by less than 1.0 mg%. Subjects with marked hypertension or renal insufficiency had been excluded from the trial so that the clinical importance of these observations for such subjects or for any subjects treated over more prolonged periods is not known. It is recommended that patients placed on long-term aspirin treatment, even at doses of 300 mg per day, be seen at regular intervals to assess changes in these measurements.

Sodium in Buffered Aspirin for Solution Formulations: One tablet daily of flavored buffered aspirin in solution adds 506 mg of sodium to that in the diet and may not be tolerated by patients with active sodium-retaining states such as congestive heart or renal failure. This amount of sodium adds about 30 percent to the 70 to 90 meq intake suggested as appropriate for dietary treatment of essential hypertension in the 1984 Report of the Joint National Committee on Detection, Evaluation, and Treatment of High Blood Pressure[8].

Dosage and Administration: Although most of the studies used dosages exceeding 300 mg, daily, two trials used only 300 mg and pharmacologic data indicate that this dose inhibits platelet function fully. Therefore, 300 mg or a conventional 325 mg aspirin dose daily is a reasonable, routine dose that would minimize gastrointestinal adverse reactions. This use of aspirin applies to both solid, oral dosage forms (buffered and plain aspirin) and buffered aspirin in solution.

References:
(1) Elwood, P. C., et al., A Randomized Controlled Trial of Acetysalicylic Acid in the Secondary Prevention of Mortality from Myocardial Infarction," *British Medical Journal* 1:436–440, 1974.
(2) The Coronary Drug Project Research Group, "Aspirin in Coronary Heart Disease," *Journal of Chronic Diseases,* 29:625–642, 1976.
(3) Breddin K., et al., "Secondary Prevention of Myocardial Infarction: A Comparison of Acetylsalicylic Acid, Phenprocoumon or Placebo," *International Congress Series* 470:263–268, 1979.
(4) Aspirin Myocardial Infarction Study Research Group, "A Randomized, Controlled Trial of Aspirin in Persons Recovered from Myocardial Infarction," *Journal American Medical Association* 245:661–669, 1980.
(5) Elwood, P. C., and P. M. Sweetnam, "Aspirin and Secondary Mortality after Myocardial Infarction," *Lancet* pp. 1313–1315, December 22–29, 1979.
(6) The Persantine-Aspirin Reinfarction Study Research Group, "Persantine and Aspirin in Coronary Heart Disease," *Circulation,* 62: 449–460, 1980.
(7) Lewis, H. D., et al., "Protective Effects of Aspirin Against Acute Myocardial Infarction and Death in Men with Unstable Angina, Results of a Veterans Administration Cooperative Study," *New England Journal of Medicine* 309:396–403, 1983.
(8) "1984 Report of the Joint National Committee on Detection, Evaluation, Treatment of High Blood Pressure," U.S. Department of Health and Human Services and United States Public Health Service, National Institutes of Health.

How Supplied: Foil sealed effervescent tablets in cartons of 12's in 6 foil twin packs; 24's in 12 foil twin packs; 36's in 18 foil twin packs.
Shown in Product Identification Section, page 416

ALKA–SELTZER® Effervescent Antacid

Active Ingredients: Each tablet contains heat treated sodium bicarbonate 958 mg., citric acid 832 mg., potassium bicarbonate 312 mg. ALKA-SELTZER® Effervescent Antacid in water contains principally the antacids sodium citrate and potassium citrate.

Inactive Ingredients: A tableting aid.

Indications: ALKA-SELTZER® Effervescent Antacid is indicated for relief of acid indigestion, sour stomach or heartburn.

Actions: The ALKA-SELTZER® Effervescent Antacid solution provides quick and effective neutralization of gastric acid. Measured by the in vitro standard established by the Food and Drug Administration one tablet will neutralize 10.6 mEq of acid.

Warnings: Except under the advice and supervision of a physician, do not take more than: Adults: 8 tablets in a 24 hour period (60 years of age or older: 7 tablets in a 24 hour period), Children: 4 tablets in a 24 hour period; or use the maximum dosage of this product for more than 2 weeks.
Do not use this product if you are on a sodium restricted diet. Each tablet contains 311 mg. of sodium.
Keep this and all drugs out of the reach of children. As with any drug, if you are pregnant or nursing a baby, seek the advice of a health professional before using this product.

Dosage and Administration: ALKA-SELTZER® Effervescent Antacid is taken in solution; approximately 3 oz. of water per tablet is sufficient. Adults: one or two tablets every 4 hours as needed. Children: ½ the adult dosage.

How Supplied: Boxes of 20 tablets in 10 foil twin packs; 36 tablets in 18 foil twin packs.
Shown in Product Identification Section, page 416

ALKA–SELTZER® Extra Strength Antacid & Pain Reliever

Active Ingredients: Each tablet contains: Aspirin 500mg, heat treated sodium bicarbonate 1985mg, citric acid 1000mg. Alka-Seltzer in water contains principally the antacid sodium citrate and the analgesic sodium acetylsalicylate.

Inactive Ingredients: Flavors

Indications: For speedy relief of acid indigestion, sour stomach or heartburn with headache or body aches and pains. Also, for fast relief of upset stomach with headache from overindulgence in food and drink—especially recommended for taking before bed and again on arising. Effective for pain relief alone. Headache or body and muscular aches and pains.

Warnings: Children and teenagers should not use this medicine for chicken pox or flu symptoms before a doctor is consulted about Reye Syndrome, a rare but serious illness reported to be associated with aspirin. As with any drug, if you are pregnant or nursing a baby, seek the advice of a health professional before using this product. Except under the advice and supervision of a physician, do not take more than, Adults: 7 tablets in a 24-hour period (60 years of age or older, 4 tablets in a 24-hour period), or use the daily maximum dosage for more than 10 days. Do not use if you are allergic to aspirin or have asthma, if you have a coagulation (bleeding) disease, or if you are on a sodium restricted diet. Each tablet contains 588mg of sodium. Keep this and all drugs out of the reach of children.

Dosage and Administration: Extra Strength Alka-Seltzer must be dissolved in water before taking. Adults: 2 tablets every 4 hours. Caution: If symptoms persist, or recur frequently, or if you are under treatment for ulcer, consult your physician.

How Supplied: Foil sealed effervescent tablets in cartons of 12's in 6 foil twin packs; 24's in 12 foil twin packs.
Shown in Product Identification Section, page 416

ALKA-SELTZER PLUS® Cold Medicine

Active Ingredients:
Each dry ALKA-SELTZER PLUS® Cold Tablet contains the following active ingredients: Phenylpropanolamine bitartrate 24.08 mg., chlorpheniramine maleate 2 mg., aspirin 325 mg. The product is

dissolved in water prior to ingestion and the aspirin is converted into its soluble ionic form, sodium acetylsalicylate.

Inactive Ingredients: Citric acid, flavors, sodium bicarbonate.

Indications: For relief of the symptoms of head colds, common flu, sinus congestion and hay fever.

Actions: Each tablet contains: A decongestant which helps restore free breathing, shrink swollen nasal tissue and relieve sinus congestion due to head colds or hay fever. An antihistamine which helps relieve the runny nose, sneezing, sniffles, itchy watering eyes that accompany colds or hay fever. Specially buffered aspirin which relieves headache, scratchy sore throat, general body aches and the feverish feeling of a cold and common flu.

Warnings: Children and teenagers should not use this medicine for chicken pox or flu symptoms before a doctor is consulted about Reye Syndrome, a rare but serious illness reported to be associated with aspirin. Do not exceed recommended dosage because at higher doses nervousness, dizziness or sleeplessness may occur. May cause excitability in children. Do not take this product if you are allergic to aspirin or have asthma, glaucoma, bleeding problems, emphysema, chronic pulmonary disease, shortness of breath, difficulty in breathing, heart disease, high blood pressure, thyroid disease, diabetes or difficulty in urination due to enlargement of the prostate gland or on a sodium-restricted diet unless directed by a doctor. Each tablet contains 506 mg of sodium. May cause drowsiness; alcohol, sedatives and tranquilizers may increase drowsiness effect. Avoid alcoholic beverages while taking this product. Do not take this product if you are taking sedatives or tranquilizers without first consulting your doctor. Use caution when driving a motor vehicle or operating machinery. Do not take this product for more than 7 days. If symptoms do not improve or are accompanied by fever or if fever persists for more than 3 days, consult a doctor. As with any drug, if you are pregnant or nursing a baby, seek the advice of a health professional before using this product. Keep this and all drugs out of the reach of children.

Drug Interaction Precaution: Do not take this product if you are presently taking a prescription drug for anticoagulation (thinning the blood), high blood pressure or depression without first consulting your doctor.

Dosage and Administration: ALKA-SELTZER PLUS® is taken in solution; approximately 3 ounces of water per tablet is sufficient. Adults: two tablets every 4 hours up to 8 tablets in 24 hours.

How Supplied: Tablets: carton of 12 tablets in 6 foil twin packs; 20 tablets in 10 foil twin packs; carton of 36 tablets in 18 foil twin packs.

Product Identification Mark: "Alka-Seltzer Plus" embossed on each tablet.
Shown in Product Identification Section, page 416

ALKA–SELTZER PLUS®
Night-Time Cold Medicine

Active Ingredients: Each tablet contains phenylpropanolamine bitartrate 24.08 mg, diphenhydramine citrate 38.33 mg, acetylsalicylic acid (aspirin) 325 mg. In water the aspirin is converted into its soluble ionic form, sodium acetylsalicylate.

Inactive Ingredients: Citric acid, flavors, heat-treated sodium bicarbonate, tableting aids.

Indications: For relief of the symptoms of head colds, common flu, sinus congestion and hay fever so you can get the rest you need.

Actions: Temporarily restores freer breathing through the nose, relieves runny nose, itching of the nose or throat, itchy watery eyes, and headache and minor body aches and pain due to common colds, hay fever, or common flu.

Warnings: Children and teenagers should not use this medicine for chicken pox or flu symptoms before a doctor is consulted about Reye Syndrome, a rare but serious illness reported to be associated with aspirin. Do not exceed recommended dosage because at higher doses nervousness, dizziness or sleeplessness may occur. May cause excitability in children. Do not take this product if you are allergic to aspirin or have asthma, glaucoma, bleeding problems, emphysema, chronic pulmonary disease, shortness of breath, difficulty in breathing, heart disease, high blood pressure, thyroid disease, diabetes or difficulty in urination due to enlargement of the prostate gland or on a sodium-restricted diet unless directed by a doctor. Each tablet contains 506 mg of sodium. May cause marked drowsiness; alcohol, sedatives and tranquilizers may increase drowsiness effect. Avoid alcoholic beverages while taking this product. Do not take this product if you are taking sedatives or tranquilizers without first consulting your doctor. Use caution when driving a motor vehicle or operating machinery. Do not take this product for more than 7 days. If symptoms do not improve or are accompanied by fever or if fever persists for more than 3 days, consult a doctor. As with any drug, if you are pregnant or nursing a baby, seek the advice of a health professional before using this product. Keep this and all drugs out of the reach of children.

Drug Interaction Precaution: Do not take this product if you are presently taking a prescription drug for anticoagulation (thinning the blood), high blood pressure or depression without first consulting your doctor.

Dosage and Administration: Adults: Take 2 tablets dissolved in water every 4 to 6 hours, not to exceed 8 tablets daily.

How Supplied: Tablets: carton of 20 tablets in 10 child-resistant foil twin packs; carton of 36 tablets in 18 child-resistant foil twin packs.

Product Identification Mark: "A/S PLUS NIGHT-TIME" etched on each tablet
Shown in Product Identification Section, page 416

BACTINE® Antiseptic·Anesthetic First Aid Spray

Active Ingredients: Benzalkonium Chloride 0.13% w/w, Lidocaine HCl 2.5% w/w.
Aerosol ingredients are % w/w of concentrate.

Inactive Ingredients:
Liquid—Edetate Disodium, Fragrances, Octoxynol 9, Propylene Glycol, Purified Water, Alcohol 3.17% w/w.
Aerosol—Dimethyl Polysiloxane Fluid 1000, Edetic Acid, Fragrances, Isobutane, Malic Acid, Povidone, Propylene Glycol, Purified Water, Sorbitol, and Emulsifier System.

Indications: Antiseptic/anesthetic for helping prevent infection, cleanse wounds, and for the temporary relief of pain and itching due to insect bites, minor burns, sunburn, minor cuts and minor skin irritations.

Warnings: (Aerosol Spray and Liquid Spray)
For external use only. Do not use in large quantities, particularly over raw surfaces or blistered areas. Avoid spraying in eyes, mouth, ears or on sensitive areas of the body. This product is not for use on wild or domestic animal bites. If you have an animal bite or puncture wound, consult your physician immediately. If condition worsens or if symptoms persist for more than 7 days, discontinue use of this product and consult a physician. Do not bandage tightly. Keep this and all drugs out of reach of children. In case of accidental ingestion, seek professional assistance or contact a Poison Control Center immediately.
(Aerosol Only): Contents under pressure. Do not puncture or incinerate. Do not store at temperature above 120° F. Use only as directed. Intentional misuse by deliberately concentrating and inhaling the contents can be harmful or fatal.

Dosage and Administration: For adults and children 2 years of age or older. For superficial skin wounds, cuts, scratches, scrapes, cleanse affected area thoroughly.

Directions: (Liquid) First Aid Spray
To apply, hold bottle 2 to 3 inches from injured area and squeeze repeatedly. To aid in removing foreign particles, dab injured area with clean gauze saturated with product. For sunburn, minor burns, insect bites, and minor skin irritations,

Continued on next page

Miles—Cont.

apply to affected area of skin for temporary relief. Product can be applied to affected area with clean gauze saturated with product.
(Aerosol First Aid Spray)
Shake well. For adults and children 2 years of age and older. For superficial skin wounds, cuts, scratches, scrapes, cleanse affected area thoroughly. Hold can upright 2 to 3 inches from injured area and spray until wet. To aid in removing foreign particles, dab injured area with clean gauze saturated with product. For sunburn, minor burns, insect bites, and minor skin irritations, hold can upright 4 to 6 inches from injured area and spray until wet. Product can be applied to affected area with clean gauze saturated with product.

How Supplied: 2 oz., 4 oz. liquid spray, 16 oz. liquid, 3 oz. aerosol.
Shown in Product Identification Section, page 417

BACTINE® First Aid Antibiotic Plus Anesthetic Ointment

Active Ingredients: Each gram contains Polymyxin B Sulfate 5000 units; Bacitracin 500 units; Neomycin Sulfate 5 mg (equivalent to 3.5 mg Neomycin base); Diperodon HCl 10 mg (pain reliever).

Inactive Ingredients: Mineral Oil, White Petrolatum.

Indications: First aid to help prevent infection, guard against bacterial contamination, relieve pain and itching in minor cuts, scrapes and burns.

Warning: For external use only. Do not use in the eyes or apply over large areas of the body. In case of deep or puncture wounds, animal bites or serious burns, consult a physician. Stop use and consult a physician if the condition persists or gets worse. Do not use longer than one (1) week unless directed by a physician. Keep this and all medicines out of children's reach. In case of accidental ingestion, seek professional assistance or contact a Poison Control Center immediately.

Directions: Clean the affected area. Apply a small amount of this product (an amount equal to the surface area of the tip of a finger) one to three times daily. May be covered with a sterile bandage.

How Supplied: ½ oz. tube.
Shown in Product Identification Section, page 417

BACTINE® Brand Hydrocortisone Skin Care Cream Antipruritic (Anti-Itch)

Active Ingredient: Hydrocortisone 0.5%.

Inactive Ingredients: Butylated Hydroxyanisole, Butylated Hydroxytoluene, Butylparaben, Carbomer, Cetyl Alcohol, Colloidal Silicon Dioxide, Corn oil (and) Gylceryl Oleate (and) Propylene Glycol (and) (BHA) (and) BHT (and) Propyl Gallate (and) Citric Acid, DEA-Oleth-3 Phosphate, Diisopropyl Sebacate, Edetate Disodium, Glycerin, Hydroxypropyl Methylcellulose 2906, Lanolin Alcohol, Methylparaben, Mineral Oil (and) Lanolin Alcohol, Propylene Glycol Stearate SE, Propylparaben, Purified Water.

Indications: For the temporary relief of minor skin irritations, itching, and rashes due to eczema, dermatitis, insect bites, poison ivy, poison oak, poison sumac, soaps, detergents, cosmetics, and jewelry.

Warnings: For external use only. Avoid contact with the eyes. If condition worsens or if symptoms persist for more than seven days, discontinue use and consult a physician.
Do not use on children under 2 years of age except under the advice and supervision of a physician.
Keep this and all drugs out of the reach of children. In case of accidental ingestion, seek professional assistance or contact a Poison Control Center immediately.

Directions: For adults and children 2 years of age and older. Gently massage into affected skin area not more than 3 or 4 times daily.

How Supplied: ½ oz. plastic tube.
Shown in Product Identification Section, page 417

BIOCAL® 500 mg Tablets Calcium Supplement

Each Tablet Contains: 1250 mg of calcium carbonate, U.S.P. which provides elemental calcium 500 mg.

Indications: Calcium supplementation.

Description: BIOCAL 500 mg Tablets are white, capsule-shaped tablets containing pure calcium carbonate. No sugar, salt, preservatives, artificial colors or flavors added.

Directions: Two tablets daily provide:

Elemental Calcium	For Adults % U.S. RDA	For Pregnant or Lactating Women % U.S. RDA
1000 mg	100%	77%

Take one or two tablets daily or as recommended by a physician.
Keep out of reach of children.

How Supplied: Bottles of 60 tablets in tamper-resistant package.
Shown in Product Identification Section, page 417

BUGS BUNNY™ Children's Chewable Vitamins (Sugar Free)
BUGS BUNNY™ Children's Chewable Vitamins Plus Iron (Sugar Free)
FLINTSTONES® Children's Chewable Vitamins
FLINTSTONES® Children's Chewable Vitamins Plus Iron

Vitamin Ingredients: Each multi-vitamin supplement with iron contains the ingredients listed in the chart below: [See table below].
BUGS BUNNY™ Children's Chewable Vitamins and FLINTSTONES® Children's Chewable Vitamins provide the same quantities of vitamins, but do not provide iron.

Indication: Dietary supplementation.

Dosage and Administration: One chewable tablet daily. For adults and children two years and older; tablet must be chewed.

Warning For Bugs Bunny Only: Phenylketonurics: Contains Phenylalanine.

Precaution:
IRON SUPPLEMENTS ONLY.
Contains iron, which can be harmful in large doses. Close tightly and keep out of reach of children. In case of overdose contact a Poison Control Center immediately.

How Supplied: Flintstones are supplied in bottles of 60 and 100, Bugs Bunny in bottles of 60 with child-resistant caps.
Shown in Product Identification Section, page 417

BUGS BUNNY™ Children's Chewable Vitamins Plus Iron (Sugar Free)
FLINTSTONES® Children's Chewable Vitamins Plus Iron

Vitamins	One Tablet Provides Quantity	% of U.S. RDA For Children 2 to 4 Years of Age	% of U.S. RDA For Adults and Children over 4 Years of Age
Vitamin A	2500 I.U.	100	50
Vitamin D	400 I.U.	100	100
Vitamin E	15 I.U.	150	50
Vitamin C	60 mg.	150	100
Folic Acid	0.3 mg.	150	75
Thiamine	1.05 mg.	150	70
Riboflavin	1.20 mg.	150	70
Niacin	13.50 mg.	150	67
Vitamin B₆	1.05 mg.	150	52
Vitamin B₁₂	4.5 mcg.	150	75
Mineral:			
Iron (Elemental)	15 mg.	150	83

FLINTSTONES® With Extra C
   Children's Chewable Vitamins
BUGS BUNNY™ With Extra C
   Children's Chewable Vitamins
   (Sugar Free)

Vitamin Ingredients: Each multivitamin supplement contains the ingredients listed in the chart.
[See table right]

Indication: Dietary supplementation.

Dosage and Administration: One tablet daily for adults and children two years and older; tablet must be chewed.

Warning For Bugs Bunny Only: Phenylketonurics: Contains Phenylalanine.

How Supplied: Flintstones in bottles of 60's & 100's, Bugs Bunny in bottles of 60 with child-resistant caps.
   *Shown in Product Identification
   Section, page 417*

FLINTSTONES® COMPLETE
   With Iron, Calcium & Minerals
   Children's Chewable Vitamins
BUGS BUNNY™ Children's
   Chewable Vitamins + Minerals
   With Iron and Calcium
   (Sugar Free)

Ingredients: Each supplement provides the ingredients listed in the chart below:

Indication: Dietary Supplementation.

Dosage and Administration: 2–4 years of age: Chew one-half tablet daily. Over 4 years of age: Chew one tablet daily.

Warning: Phenylketonurics: Contains Phenylalanine.

BUGS BUNNY™ With Extra C
   Children's Chewable Vitamins
   (Sugar Free)
FLINTSTONES® With Extra C
   Children's Chewable Vitamins

One Tablet Provides		% of U.S. RDA	
		For Children 2 To 4 Years of Age	For Adults and Children Over 4 Years of Age
Vitamins	Quantity		
Vitamin A	2500 I.U.	100	50
Vitamin D	400 I.U.	100	100
Vitamin E	15 I.U.	150	50
Vitamin C	250 mg.	625	417
Folic Acid	0.3 mg.	150	75
Thiamine	1.05 mg.	150	70
Riboflavin	1.20 mg.	150	70
Niacin	13.50 mg.	150	67
Vitamin B$_6$	1.05 mg.	150	52
Vitamin B$_{12}$	4.5 mcg.	150	75

Precaution: Contains iron, which can be harmful in large doses. Close tightly and keep out of reach of children. In case of overdose, contact a physician or poison control center immediately.

How Supplied: Bottles of 60's with child-resistant caps.
   *Shown in Product Identification
   Section, page 417*

**MILES® Nervine
Nighttime Sleep–Aid**

Active Ingredient: Each capsule-shaped tablet contains diphenhydramine HCl 25 mg.

Inactive Ingredients: Calcium Phosphate Dibasic, Calcium Sulfate, Carboxymethylcellulose Sodium, Corn Starch, Magnesium Stearate, Microcrystalline Cellulose.

Indications: Miles® Nervine helps you fall asleep and relieves occasional sleeplessness.

Actions: Antihistamines act on the central nervous system and produce drowsiness.

Warnings: Do not give to children under 12 years of age. Avoid alcoholic beverages while taking this product. Do not take this product if you are taking sedatives or tranquilizers without first consulting your doctor. If sleeplessness persists continuously for more than 2 weeks, consult your doctor. Insomnia may be a symptom of serious underlying medical illness. Do not take this product if you have asthma, glaucoma, emphysema, chronic pulmonary disease, shortness of breath, difficulty in breathing or difficulty in urination due to enlargement of the prostate gland unless directed by a doctor. As with any drug, if you are pregnant or nursing a baby, seek the advice of a health professional before using this product. Keep this and all drugs out of the reach of children. In case of accidental overdose, seek professional assistance or contact a poison control center immediately.

Dosage and Administration: Two tablets once daily at bedtime or as directed by a physician.

How Supplied: Blister pack 12's, bottle of 30's with a child-resistant cap.
   *Shown in Product Identification
   Section, page 417*

**ONE–A–DAY® Essential Vitamins
11 Essential Vitamins**

Ingredients: One tablet daily of ONE-A-DAY® Essential provides:

Vitamins	Quantity	U.S. RDA
Vitamin A (as Acetate and Beta Carotene)	5000 I. U.	100
Vitamin C	60 mg.	100
Thiamine (B$_1$)	1.5 mg.	100
Riboflavin (B$_2$)	1.7 mg.	100
Niacin	20 mg.	100
Vitamin D	400 I.U.	100
Vitamin E	30 I.U.	100
Vitamin B$_6$	2 mg.	100

FLINTSTONES® COMPLETE
Children's Chewable Vitamins
BUGS BUNNY™
Children's Chewable
Vitamins + Minerals
(Sugar Free)

| Vitamins | Quantity Per Tablet | Percentage of U.S. Recommended Daily Allowance (U.S. RDA) | |
		For Children 2 to 4 Years of Age (½ tablet)	For Adults & Children Over 4 Years of Age (1 tablet)
Vitamin A	5000 I.U.	100	100
Vitamin D	400 I.U.	50	100
Vitamin E	30 I.U.	150	100
Vitamin C	60 mg.	75	100
Folic Acid	0.4 mg.	100	100
Vitamin B-1 (Thiamine)	1.5 mg.	107	100
Vitamin B-2 (Riboflavin)	1.7 mg.	106	100
Niacin	20 mg.	111	100
Vitamin B-6 (Pyridoxine)	2 mg.	143	100
Vitamin B-12 (Cyanocobalamin)	6 mcg.	100	100
Biotin	40 mcg.	13	13
Pantothenic Acid	10 mg.	100	100

Minerals	Quantity	Percent U.S. RDA	
Iron (elemental)	18 mg.	90	100
Calcium	100 mg.	6	10
Copper	2 mg.	100	100
Phosphorus	100 mg.	6	10
Iodine	150 mcg.	107	100
Magnesium	20 mg.	5	5
Zinc	15 mg.	94	100

Continued on next page

Miles—Cont.

Folic Acid	0.4 mg.	100
Vitamin B$_{12}$	6 mcg.	100
Pantothenic Acid	10 mg.	100

Indication: Dietary supplementation.

Dosage and Administration: One tablet daily for adults and teens.

How Supplied: ONE-A-DAY® Essential, bottles of 60 and 100.
Shown in Product Identification Section, page 417

ONE-A-DAY® Maximum Formula Vitamins and Minerals Supplement for adults
The most complete ONE-A-DAY® brand.

Ingredients:
One tablet daily of ONE-A-DAY® Maximum Formula provides:

Vitamins	Quantity	% of U.S. RDA
Vitamin A Beta Carotene)	5000 I.U.	100
Vitamin A (as Acetate)	1500 I.U.	30
Vitamin C	60 mg.	100
Thiamine (B$_1$)	1.5 mg.	100
Riboflavin (B$_2$)	1.7 mg.	100
Niacin	20 mg.	100
Vitamin D	400 I.U.	100
Vitamin E	30 I.U.	100
Vitamin B$_6$	2 mg.	100
Folic Acid	0.4 mg.	100
Vitamin B$_{12}$	6 mcg.	100
Biotin	30 mcg.	10
Pantothenic Acid	10 mg.	100

Minerals	Quantity	% of U.S. RDA
Iron (Elemental)	18 mg.	100
Calcium	130 mg.	13
Phosphorus	100 mg.	10
Iodine	150 mcg.	100
Magnesium	100 mg.	25
Copper	2 mg.	100
Zinc	15 mg.	100
Chromium	10 mcg.	*
Selenium	10 mcg.	*
Molybdenum	10 mcg.	*
Manganese	2.5 mg.	*
Potassium	37.5 mg.	*
Chloride	34 mg.	*

*No U.S. RDA established

Indication: Dietary supplementation.

Dosage and Administration: One tablet daily for adults.

Precaution: Contains iron, which can be harmful in large doses. Close tightly and keep out of reach of children. In case of overdose, contact a physician or Poison Control Center immediately.

How Supplied: Bottles of 30, 60, and 100 with child-resistant caps.
Shown in Product Identification Section, page 417

ONE-A-DAY® Plus Extra C
Vitamins. For adults and teens.

Vitamin ingredients: One tablet daily of ONE-A-DAY® Plus Extra C provides:

Vitamins	Quantity	% of U.S. RDA
Vitamin A (as Beta Carotene)	2500 I.U.	100
Vitamin A (as Acetate)	2500 I.U.	
Vitamin C	300 mg.	500
Thiamine (B$_1$)	1.5 mg.	100
Riboflavin (B$_2$)	1.7 mg.	100
Niacin	20 mg.	100
Vitamin D	400 I.U.	100
Vitamin E	30 I.U.	100
Vitamin B$_6$	2 mg.	100
Folic Acid	0.4 mg.	100
Vitamin B$_{12}$	6 mcg.	100
Pantothenic Acid	10 mg.	100

Indication: Dietary supplementation.

Dosage and Administration: One tablet daily.

How Supplied: Bottles of 60's with child resistant caps.
Shown in Product Identification Section, page 417

STRESSGARD®
High Potency B Complex and C plus A, D, E, Iron and Zinc
The most complete stress product.
Multivitamin/Multimineral Supplement For Adults

Ingredients:

Vitamins	Quantity	% of U.S. RDA
Vitamin A (as Beta Carotene)	2500 I.U.	100
Vitamin A (as Acetate)	2500 I.U.	
Vitamin C	600 mg.	1000
Thiamine (B$_1$)	15 mg.	1000
Riboflavin (B$_2$)	10 mg.	588
Niacin	100 mg.	500
Vitamin D	400 I.U.	100
Vitamin E	30 I.U.	100
Vitamin B$_6$	5 mg.	250
Folic Acid	400 mcg.	100
Vitamin B$_{12}$	12 mcg.	200
Pantothenic Acid	20 mg.	200

Minerals	Quantity	% of U.S. RDA
Iron (Elemental)	18 mg.	100
Zinc	15 mg.	100
Copper	2 mg.	100

Indication: Dietary supplementation.

Dosage and Administration: Adults —one tablet daily with food.

Precaution: Contains iron, which can be harmful in large doses. Close tightly and keep out of reach of children. In case of overdose, contact a physician or Poison Control Center immediately.

How Supplied: Bottles of 60 with child-resistant caps.
Shown in Product Identification Section, page 417

WITHIN® Advanced Multivitamin for Women with Calcium, Extra Iron, Zinc and Beta-Carotene.
Provides calcium and extra iron Plus the daily nutritional support of 11 essential vitamins.

Ingredients: One tablet daily of WITHIN® provides:

Vitamins	Quantity	% of U.S. RDA
Vitamin A (as Beta Carotene)	2500 I.U.	100
Vitamin A (as Acetate)	2500 I.U.	
Vitamin C	60 mg.	100
Thiamine (B$_1$)	1.5 mg.	100
Riboflavin (B$_2$)	1.7 mg.	100
Niacin	20 mg.	100
Vitamin D	400 I.U.	100
Vitamin E	30 I.U.	100
Vitamin B$_6$	2 mg.	100
Folic Acid	0.4 mg.	100
Vitamin B$_{12}$	6 mcg.	100
Pantothenic Acid	10 mg.	100

Mineral	Quantity	% of U.S. RDA
Iron (Elemental)	27 mg.	150
Calcium (Elemental)	450 mg.	45
Zinc	15 mg.	100

Indication: Dietary supplementation.

Dosage and Administration: One tablet daily.

Precaution: Contains iron, which can be harmful in large doses. Close tightly and keep out of reach of children. In case of overdose, contact a physician or Poison Control Center immediately.

How Supplied: Bottles of 60 and 100 with child-resistant caps.
Shown in Product Identification Section, page 417

More Direct Health Products
6351-E YARROW DRIVE
CARLSBAD, CA 92009

CigArrest™
Smoking Deterrent Tablets

Active Ingredient: Lobeline sulfate 2 mg.

Indications: A temporary aid to breaking the cigarette habit. The effectiveness of the tablet is directly related to the user's motivation to stop smoking.

Use: Lobeline sulfate resembles nicotine both chemically and pharmacologically which aids the smoker in developing a sense of satiety for smoking almost identical to that obtained from tobacco. Not habit forming.

Warnings: As with any drug, if you are pregnant or nursing a baby, seek the advice of a health professional before using CigArrest.™ Keep this and all drugs out of the reach of children.

Symptoms and Treatment of Overdosage: In case of accidental overdose, seek the advice of a physician immediately.

Dosage and Administration: Take 1 (one) tablet at or after each meal, 3 (three) tablets per day. Recommended usage not to exceed six weeks.

How Supplied: Consumer packages of 15 (fifteen) blister packed tablets.

Murdock Pharmaceuticals, Inc.
1400 MOUNTAIN SPRINGS PARK
SPRINGVILLE, UTAH 84663

LACTASE
Lactose Digesting Enzyme

Description: 3450 FCC units (230 mg) Lactase enzyme in a neutral maltodextrin base.

Action: Lactose-digesting enzyme (Lactase) is recommended for individuals with lactose intolerance. Lactase is essentially the enzyme needed to break down milk sugar into digestible nutrients. Our Lactase is totally natural (containing no preservatives) and is easy-to-use in convenient capsule form.

Overdosage: No danger of overdosage. Safe for children's use.

Dosage and Administration: Take one to three capsules as needed before ingesting milk or other dairy products.

How Supplied: Available in double safety-sealed bottles of 60 capsules, 460 mg each.
Shown in Product Identification Section, page 417

SINUSTAT™
Nasal Decongestant

Description: Active Ingredient: 60 mg pseudoephedrine HCl extracted from *Ephedra sinica* (Chinese *Ephedra*). **Other Ingredients:** Golden seal root, sage leaf, *Echinacea angustifolia* root extract, plantain leaf, astragalus root extract, ginger root extract, hops flower extract, licorice root, gentian root extract, Ma Huang herb.

Indications: Maximum strength sinus decongestant for the temporary relief of symptoms associated with sinusitis and the common cold. Relieves sinus pressure, nasal congestion, promotes sinus drainage, shrinks swollen sinus and nasal membranes.

Warnings: Do not exceed your physician's recommended dosage. If you are pregnant or nursing, have high blood pressure, heart disease, diabetes, thyroid disease, prostate problems, or if currently taking a prescription drug, antihypertensive or antidepressant drug, consult your health care practitioner before taking this product. Do not continue to use this product, but seek medical as-

sistance immediately if symptoms are not relieved within one hour or become worse. Some users of this product may experience nervousness, tremor, sleeplessness, nausea, and loss of appetite. If these symptoms persist or become worse, consult your doctor.

Dosage and Administration: *Adults and children 12 and older* —One capsule every four to six hours. Do not exceed four capsules in 24 hours.

How Supplied: Available in double safety-sealed bottles of 30 capsules, 500 mg each.
Shown in Product Identification Section, page 417

EDUCATIONAL MATERIAL

Educational Services
Customer Service representatives are available via toll-free 1-800-962-8873 Monday-Friday, 8 am to 5 pm (MST) to give educational support to our products.
Samples
Sample cards (containing two capsules/tablets) of all Murdock Pharmaceuticals' products are available through area distributors. Please contact our Customer Service Department at 1-800-962-8873 for a distributor referral.

Muro Pharmaceutical, Inc.
890 EAST STREET
TEWKSBURY, MA 01876-9987

BROMFED® SYRUP
Antihistamine-Decongestant
(alcohol free)
ORANGE-LEMON FLAVOR

Each 5 mL (1 teaspoonful) contains: 2 mg brompheniramine maleate and 30 mg pseudoephedrine hydrochloride; also contains citric acid, FD & C Yellow #6, flavor, glycerin, methyl paraben, sodium benzoate, sodium citrate, sodium saccharin, sorbitol, sucrose, purified water.

Indications: For temporary relief of nasal congestion, sneezing, itchy and watery eyes and running nose due to common cold, hay fever or other upper respiratory allergies.

Directions: Adults and children 12 years of age and over: 2 teaspoonfuls every 4–6 hours. Children 6 to 12 years of age: 1 teaspoonful every 4–6 hours. Do not exceed 4 doses in 24 hours. Children under 6 years of age, consult a physician.

Warnings: If symptoms do not improve within 7 days or are accompanied by high fever, consult a physician before continuing use. May cause drowsiness. May cause excitability especially in children. DO NOT exceed recommended daily dosage because at higher doses nervousness, dizziness, or sleeplessness may occur. **Except under the advice and supervision of a physician:** DO NOT give this prod-

uct to children under 6 years. DO NOT take this product if you have asthma, glaucoma, difficulty in urination due to enlargement of the prostate gland, high blood pressure, heart disease, diabetes, or thyroid disease. As with any drug, if you are pregnant or nursing a baby, seek the advice of a health professional before using this product.

Caution: Avoid operating a motor vehicle or heavy machinery and alcoholic beverages while taking this product. Keep this and all drugs out of the reach of children.

Drug Interaction Precaution: Do not take this product if you are presently taking a prescription antihypertensive or antidepressant drug containing a monoamine oxidase inhibitor except under the advice and supervision of a physician.

Overdosage: In case of accidental overdose, seek professional assistance or contact a Poison Control Center immediately.

Store between 15° and 30°C (59° and 86°F). Dispense in tight, light resistant containers as defined in USP.

How Supplied: NDC 0451-4201-16 —16 fl. oz. (480 mL), NDC 0451-4201-04—4 fl. oz. (120 mL).

SALINEX NASAL MIST AND DROPS
Buffered Isotonic Saline Solutions

Ingredients: Sodium Chloride 0.4%. Also contains disodium phosphate, edetate disodium, hydroxypropyl methylcellulose, monosodium phosphate, polyethylene glycol, propylene glycol and purified water. Preservative used is benzalkonium chloride 0.01%.

Indications: Rhinitis Medicamentosa and Rhinitis Sicca. For relief of nasal congestion associated with overuse of nasal sprays, drops and inhalers.
To alleviate crusting due to nose bleeds; to compensate for nasal stuffiness and dryness due to lack of humidity.

Directions: Squeeze twice in each nostril as needed.

How Supplied: SPRAY: 50 ml plastic spray bottle. DROPS: 15 ml plastic dropper bottle.

IDENTIFICATION PROBLEM?
Consult the
Product Identification Section
where you'll find
products pictured
in full color.

Natren Inc.
3105 WILLOW LANE
WESTLAKE VILLAGE, CA 91361

BIFIDO FACTOR™
(Bifidobacterium bifidum)

Prominent probiotic in healthy adult large intestines.

Ingredients: Active—*Bifidobacterium bifidum,* strain Malyoth. Inactive—Whey and milk solids.

How Supplied:
2.5 oz. Powder NDC 53983-200-25.
4.5 oz. Powder NDC 53983-200-45.

LIFE START®
(Bifidobacterium infantis)

Prominent intestinal probiotic in healthy, breast-fed infants and small children.

Ingredients: Active—*Bifidobacterium infantis,* NLS strain. Inactive—Whey and milk solids.

How Supplied:
2.5 oz. Powder—NDC 53983-500-70.
4.5 oz. Powder—NDC 53983-500-75.

M.F.A.™—Milk-Free Acidophilus
(Dairy-free *Lactobacillus acidophilus*)

SUPERDOPHILUS®
(Lactobacillus acidophilus)

Most prominent probiotic in healthy adult small intestines.

Ingredients: Active—*Lactobacillus acidophilus,* strain DDS-1. Inactive—Whey and milk solids.

How Supplied:
2.5 oz. Powder—NDC 53983-100-15.
4.5 oz. Powder—NDC 53983-100-25.

National (800) 992-3323
California (800) 992-9393

Nature's Bounty, Inc.
90 ORVILLE DRIVE
BOHEMIA, NY 11716

ENER–B®
Vitamin B-12 Nasal Gel
Dietary Supplement

Description: ENER-B™ is the first intra-nasal application for Vitamin B-12. Each delivery supplies 400 mcg. of Vitamin B-12. This method of delivery provides the highest Vitamin B-12 blood levels that can be obtained without a prescription. Clinical tests show that ENER-B produced 8.4 to 10 times more Vitamin B-12 in the blood than tablets.

[See illustration above]

Clinical Tests results are available by writing Nature's Bounty.

Potency and Administration: Each nasal applicator delivers $\frac{1}{10}$ cc of gel into the nose which adheres to the mu-

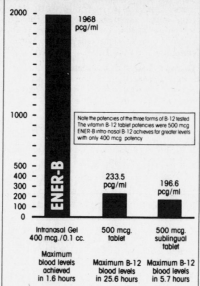

Measured Vitamin B-12 Increase in Blood Levels

Note the potencies of the three forms of B-12 tested The vitamin B-12 tablet potencies were 500 mcg ENER-B intra-nasal B-12 achieves for greater levels with only 400 mcg potency

1968 pcg/ml	233.5 pcg/ml	196.6 pcg/ml
Intranasal Gel 400 mcg./0.1 cc.	500 mcg. tablet	500 mcg. sublingual tablet
Maximum blood levels achieved in 1.6 hours	Maximum B-12 blood levels in 25.6 hours	Maximum B-12 blood levels in 5.7 hours

cous membranes providing 400 mcg. of Vitamin B-12. Odorless and non-irritating to the nose.

Directions: As a dietary supplement, one unit every two to three days.

How Supplied: Packages of 12 unit doses. Supplies 400 mcg. of B-12 each.
Shown in Product Identification Section, page 418

Neutrogena Corporation
5760 W. 96TH ST.
LOS ANGELES, CA 90045

NEUTROGENA® CLEANSING WASH

Inactive Ingredients: Purified water, glycerin, sodium oleate, sodium cocoate, lauroamphocarboxyl glycinate (and) sodium trideceth sulfate, cocamidopropyl betaine, lauramide DEA, triethanolamine, BHA, BHT, citric acid, trisodium HEDTA.

Indications: A mild-lather cleanser especially formulated for skin irritated by drying medications or for use in conjunction with dermabrasions, chemical peels or facial surgery.

Actions: Neutrogena Cleansing Wash is a gentle, glycerin-enriched formula designed to effectively cleanse skin, extremely sensitive skin or skin made hyperirritable by drying medications or facial procedures. It is residue-free so as not to interfere with skin treatments. It is fragrance-free, contains no color or parabens and is noncomedogenic.

Dosage and Administration: Use twice daily, or as directed by physician. Mix with water, work Neutrogena Cleansing Wash into a creamy lather and apply to face. Gently massage in a circular motion. Rinse completely.

How Supplied: Available in 6 oz pump dispenser bottle.
Shown in Product Identification Section, page 418

NEUTROGENA MOISTURE®

Active Ingredient: Octyl methoxycinnamate (SPF 5).

Inactive Ingredients: Purified water USP, glycerin, glyceryl stearate and PEG-100 stearate, petrolatum, isopropyl isostearate, octyl palmitate, soya sterol, cetyl alcohol NF, PEG-10 soya sterol, carbomer 954, methylparaben, imidazolidinyl urea, sodium hydroxide, tetrasodium EDTA, propylparaben, alpha-tocopherol.

Actions: Neutrogena Moisture is an extremely effective facial moisturizer for even the most fragile complexions. It is noncomedogenic, fragrance-free, and contains no color. Hypoallergenic. Provides an SPF 5 protection for the skin.

Dosage and Administration: Apply Neutrogena Moisture over face and throat morning and night, after thoroughly cleansing the skin.

How Supplied: 2 oz and 4 oz bottle.
Shown in Product Identification Section, page 418

NEUTROGENA MOISTURE® SPF 15 UNTINTED

Active Ingredients: Octyl methoxycinnamate and benzophenone-3.

Inactive Ingredients: Purified water, PPG-1 isoceteth-3 acetate, glycerin, emulsifying wax NF, glyceryl stearate, PEG-100 stearate, dimethicone, PEG-6000 monostearate, triethanolamine, methylparaben, imidazolidinyl urea, carbomer 954, propylparaben.

Actions: Effective 8 hours' moisturization with maximum sunblock protection (SPF 15) in a noncomedogenic facial moisturizer. Fragrance-free, hypoallergenic.

Dosage and Administration: Use daily after thorough cleansing of skin, alone or under makeup.

How Supplied: 4 oz bottle.
Shown in Product Identification Section, page 418

NEUTROGENA MOISTURE® SPF 15 WITH SHEER TINT

Active Ingredients: Octyl methoxycinnamate and benzophenone-3.

Inactive Ingredients: Purified water, PPG-1 Isoceteth-3 acetate, glycerin, emulsifying wax NF, glyceryl stearate, PEG-100 stearate, dimethicone, PEG-6000 monostearate, triethanolamine, methylparaben, imidazolidinyl urea, carbomer 954, propylparaben, iron oxide.

Actions: A PABA-free, noncomedogenic facial moisturizer that provides maximum sunblock protection (SPF 15). Fragrance-free, hypoallergenic. Moisturizes for 8 hours with just a hint of color.

Dosage and Administration: Use during the day with or without makeup.

How Supplied: 4 oz bottle.
Shown in Product Identification Section, page 418

NEUTROGENA® SUNBLOCK

Active Ingredients: Octyl methoxycinnamate and benzophenone-3.

Inactive Ingredients: Mineral oil, aluminum starch octenylsuccinate, silica, PVP/eicosene copolymer, glyceryl tribenate and calcium behenate, phenyltrimethicone, cyclomethicone and dimethiconol, titanium dioxide, C_{18}–C_{36} acid triglyceride, propylparaben.

Indications: Neutrogena Sunblock provides broad spectrum protection (UVA/UVB/IR) from the damaging rays of the sun.

Actions: Provides the highest level of SPF protection—SPF 15—recommended by the FDA. Liberal and regular use of Neutrogena Sunblock may help reduce the chance of premature aging of the skin and protects against the cancer-causing rays of the sun.

Waterproof: Stays on the skin even after long exposure in the water. Excellent for children above the age of 6 months. Remove with soap and water.

Rubproof/Sweatproof: Abrasion-resistant. Stays on even after rubbing or towel drying. Lower potential to run into eyes and cause stinging.

PABA-Free/Noncomedogenic: Suitable for those sensitive to PABA and its related compounds; won't clog pores. Fragrance-free. Hypoallergenic.

Warnings: For external use only, not to be swallowed. Avoid contact with eyes. Discontinue use if irritation or rash develops.

Dosage and Administration: For best results, apply to face and body 15 minutes before sun exposure. Reapply after rigorous swimming or exercise.

How Supplied: 2¼ oz tube.
Shown in Product Identification Section, page 418

New Life Health Products Corp.
P.O. BOX 9157
MORRIS PLAINS, NJ 07950-9157

NEW LIFE SMOKING DETERRENT LOZENGES™

Description: A temporary aid to those individuals who want to break the cigarette habit. Smoking Deterrent Lozenges contain silver acetate, the active ingredient which makes tobacco-based smoke taste bitterly unpleasant.

Active Ingredient: Each lozenge contains 2.5 mg silver acetate.

Indications and Usage: Use when necessary to deter smoking or to prevent relapse. It is recommended that usage be in conjunction with a formal stop-smoking plan, or with a physician-directed, hospital, clinical, or behavioral-modification program. Lozenges deter smoking best if partially or fully dissolved in the mouth prior to smoking. Deterrent action may last up to a few hours, depending on the smoker's genetic ability to taste the response, the condition of the smoker's taste receptors, and the concentration of the active ingredient in the mouth if flushed with food, drink, or toothpaste. About 85% of smokers will taste an aversive response.

Directions: Limit use to no more than six lozenges per day, one every four hours, for a maximum usage of three weeks.

Warnings: Frequent or prolonged use of this product is not recommended. This product contains a silver salt. While silver shows little evidence of systemic toxicity, chronic exposure to silver salts may cause argyrism, a harmless but otherwise permanent bluish discoloration of tissue.
Do not exceed 126 lozenges.
Keep this and all drugs out of the reach of children.
As with any drug, if you are pregnant or nursing a baby, seek professional assistance or contact a poison control center immediately.
STORE AT ROOM TEMPERATURE. AVOID EXCESSIVE HEAT, WHICH CAN MELT THE LOZENGE.

How Supplied: 168 lozenges/apothecary jar (Professionals Only; Display/-Sampler); 84 lozenges/package (two-week supply), 18 packages/case; 42 lozenges/package (one-week supply), 36 packages/case; 25 lozenges/package (sampler), net weight: 2.2 oz (62 g), 60 packages/case.
Shown in Product Identification Section, page 420

Order professional apothecary jar sampler with 168 lozenges (for professionals only) *direct* from manufacturer.

EDUCATIONAL MATERIAL

24-Page 4-Color Brochure
Free while supplies last:
Clearing the Air
How to quit smoking ... and quit for keeps
By US Department of Health and Human Services.

Products are cross-indexed by generic and chemical names in the
YELLOW SECTION

Noxell Corporation
11050 YORK ROAD
HUNT VALLEY, MARYLAND
21030-2098

NOXZEMA®
Antiseptic Skin Cleanser
Regular Formula

Active Ingredient: SD Alcohol 40 (63%)

Inactive Ingredients: Water, PPG-11 Stearyl Ether, Menthol, Camphor, Clove Oil, Eucalyptus Oil, Fragrance, FD&C Blue No. 1.

Indications: To deep clean oily, acne-prone skin without leaving skin dry and flaky.

Actions: Anti-bacterial skin cleanser specially formulated to remove dirt and oil without leaving skin dry.

Warnings: For external use only, avoid use around eyes and mucous membranes. Discontinue use if excessive irritation develops.

Precaution: Flammable until dry. Keep away from flame, fire and heat. Keep out of reach of children.

Dosage and Administration: Wash as you normally do. Moisten cotton pad. Scrub face and neck thoroughly. Repeat with fresh pads until no trace of dirt is visible. Don't rinse after use.

How Supplied: Noxzema Antiseptic Skin Cleanser Regular Formula is available in 4 oz. and 8 oz. bottles.
Shown in Product Identification Section, page 418

NOXZEMA®
Antiseptic Skin Cleanser
Extra Strength Formula

Active Ingredients: SD Alcohol 40 (36%), Isopropyl Alcohol (34%)

Inactive Ingredients: Water, Disodium Oleamido Peg-2 Sulfosuccinate, Menthol, Camphor, Clove Oil, Eucalyptus Oil, Fragrance, Yellow No. 5, Blue No. 1.

Indications: To deep clean oily, acne-prone skin.

Actions: Anti-bacterial skin cleanser specially formulated to deep clean and remove dirt and oil while leaving a refreshing feeling.

Warnings: For external use only. Avoid use around eyes and mucous membranes. Discontinue use if excessive irritation develops.

Precaution: Flammable until dry. Keep away from flame, fire and heat. Keep out of reach of children.

Dosage and Administration: Wash as you normally do. Moisten cotton pad. Scrub face and neck thoroughly. Repeat with fresh pads until no trace of dirt is visible. Don't rinse after use.

Continued on next page

Noxell—Cont.

How Supplied: Noxzema Antiseptic Skin Cleanser Extra Strength Formula is available in 4 oz. and 8 oz. bottles.

*Shown in Product Identification
Section, page 418*

NOXZEMA®
Antiseptic Skin Cleanser
Sensitive Skin Formula

Active Ingredient: Benzalkonium Chloride—0.13%

Inactive Ingredient: Water, SD Alcohol 40, Oleth 20, Phenoxyethanol, PPG-10 Methyl Glucose Ether, Menthol, Camphor, Clove Oil, Eucalyptus Oil, Fragrance, DMDM Hydantoin, Citric Acid, Sodium Citrate, Red No. 33, Red No. 4.

Indications: To gently deep clean oil and dirt from sensitive skin.

Actions: Anti-bacterial skin cleanser specially formulated to clean without being irritating. Leaves the skin fresh and soft.

Warnings: For external use only. Avoid use around eyes and mucous membranes. Discontinue use if excessive irritation develops.

Precaution: Flammable until dry. Keep away from flame, fire and heat. Keep out of reach of children.

Dosage and Administration: Wash as you normally do. Moisten cotton pad. Stroke over face and neck thoroughly. Repeat with fresh pads until no trace of dirt is visible. Don't rinse after use.

How Supplied: Noxzema Antiseptic Skin Cleanser Sensitive Skin Formula is available in 4 oz. and 8 oz. bottles.

*Shown in Product Identification
Section, page 418*

NOXZEMA CLEAR–UPS®
Anti-Acne Gel

Active Ingredient: Salicylic Acid 0.5%

Inactive Ingredients: Carbomer 940, DMDM Hydantoin, Glycerin, Methylparaben, Phenoxyethanol, Polyglycerylmethacrylate, Propylene Glycol, Tetrahydroxypropyl Ethylenediamine, Water.

Indications: Topical medication for treatment of acne vulgaris. Designed for effective treatment of pimples on sensitive or easily irritated skin.

Warnings: For external use only. Avoid use around eyes and mucous membranes. Discontinue use if excessive skin irritation develops.

How Supplied: Available in 0.50 ounce squeeze container.

*Shown in Product Identification
Section, page 418*

NOXZEMA CLEAR–UPS®
MAXIMUM STRENGTH LOTION
Vanishing
10% Benzoyl Peroxide

Active Ingredient: 10% Benzoyl Peroxide

Inactive Ingredients: DMDM Hydantoin, Glyceryl Stearate, Isopropyl Palmitate, Magnesium Aluminum Silicate, Methylparaben, Peg-20 Stearate, PPG-11 Stearyl Ether, Propylene Glycol, Propylparaben, Stearic Acid, Water, Xanthan Gum, Zinc Stearate.

Indications: Topical Medication for the treatment of acne vulgaris in vanishing base.

Actions: Noxzema Clear-Ups Maximum Strength Lotion contains benzoyl peroxide, which provides an anti-bacterial and keratolytic action. The product helps heal and prevent acne, helps eliminate blackheads and dries up excess oils.

Warnings: Persons with a known sensitivity to Benzoyl Peroxide should not use this medication. For external use only. Avoid contact with eyes, lips, mouth, or other sensitive areas. If swelling, itching, redness, or undue dryness occurs, discontinue use. Call physician if symptoms persist. Store at room temperature; avoid excess heat. Avoid contact with hair, fabrics and clothing since the oxidizing action of Benzoyl Peroxide may bleach colored or dyed fabrics.

Dosage and Administration: SHAKE WELL BEFORE USING. Wash skin thoroughly. For best results use Noxzema Skin Cream. Towel dry. Some people are sensitive to benzoyl peroxide so the first day of use, apply lotion lightly on a pimple or small affected area. If no discomfort occurs, apply Clear-Ups Maximum Strength Lotion directly on pimples and around affected areas twice daily. To help prevent pimples, apply lotion twice daily to areas where pimples and oily skin normally occur. Smooth in lotion with fingertips until it disappears. Re-cap tightly after use. See Caution.

How Supplied: Available in a 1 fluid ounce bottle.

*Shown in Product Identification
Section, page 418*

NOXZEMA CLEAR–UPS®
Medicated Pads
Regular Strength

Active Ingredient: Salicylic Acid 0.5%.

Other Ingredients: Camphor, clove oil, eucalyptus oil, fragrance, menthol, PPG-11 stearyl ether, SD Alcohol 40 63%, water.

Indications: Topical medication for the treatment of acne vulgaris. The abrasive pads provide astringency and deepdown cleaning. The salicylic acid works to clear acne and to prevent new pimples from forming. The product helps clear blackheads and absorbs excess oils.

Warnings: For external use only. Avoid use around eyes and mucous membranes. Discontinue use if excessive skin irritation develops.

How Supplied: In safety-sealed jars of 50 or 75 pads.

*Shown in Product Identification
Section, page 418*

NOXZEMA CLEAR–UPS®
Medicated Pads
Maximum Strength

Active Ingredient: Salicylic Acid 2.0%.

Other Ingredients: Camphor, clove oil, eucalyptus oil, fragrance, menthol, PEG 4, PPG-11 stearyl ether, SD Alcohol 40 64%, water.

Indications: Topical medication for the treatment of acne vulgaris. The abrasive pads provide astringency and deepdown cleaning. The salicylic acid works to clear acne and to prevent new pimples from forming. The product helps clear blackheads and absorbs excess oils.

Warnings: For external use only. Avoid use around eyes and mucous membranes. Discontinue use if excessive skin irritation develops.

How Supplied: In safety-sealed jars of 50 or 75 pads.

*Shown in Product Identification
Section, page 418*

NOXZEMA CLEAR–UPS®
ON-THE-SPOT TREATMENT
Tinted and Vanishing

Active Ingredient: 10% Benzoyl Peroxide

Inactive Ingredients: DMDM Hydantoin, Glyceryl Stearate, Iron Oxides (tinted only), Isopropyl Palmitate, Magnesium Aluminum Silicate, Methylparaben, Peg-20 Stearate, Peg-100 Stearate (tinted only), PPG-11 Stearyl Ether, Propylene Glycol, Propylparaben, Stearic Acid, Titanium Dioxide (tinted only), Water, Xanthan Gum, Zinc Stearate (vanishing only).

Indications: Topical medication for the treatment of acne vulgaris in one skin-toned shade to hide blemishes while they heal and 1 vanishing formulation to work invisibly. Comes in a unique, easy-to-use applicator to target problem areas.

Actions: Noxzema On-The-Spot contains benzoyl peroxide which provides an anti-bacterial and keratolytic action. The product helps heal and prevent acne and blackheads and comes in a unique, portable container with an easy-to-use applicator.

Warnings: Persons with a known sensitivity to Benzoyl Peroxide should not use this medication. For external use only. Avoid contact with eyes, lips, mouth or other sensitive areas. If swelling, itching, redness, or undue dryness occurs, discontinue use. Call physician if symptoms persist. Store at room temperature; avoid excess heat. Avoid contact with hair, fabrics and clothing since the oxidizing action of Benzoyl Peroxide may bleach colored or dyed fabrics.

Dosage and Administration:
1. SHAKE WELL BEFORE USING. Wash skin thoroughly. For best results use Noxzema Skin Cream. Towel dry.
2. Some people are sensitive to benzoyl peroxide, so for the first two days of use, apply lotion lightly on a pimple, or small affected area.
3. If no discomfort occurs, apply Clear-Ups On-The-Spot Treatment directly on pimples and around affected areas twice daily.
4. To help prevent pimples, smooth Clear-Ups On-The-Spot Treatment twice daily to areas where pimples and oily skin normally occur. Recap tightly after use. See caution.

How Supplied: Available in a .25 oz. unique container with an easy-to-use applicator. Clear-Ups On-The-Spot is available in one skin-tone, covering shade and one vanishing formulation.
Shown in Product Identification Section, page 418

NOXZEMA®
Medicated Skin Cream

Active Ingredients: Camphor, Phenol (less than 0.5%), Clove Oil, Eucalyptus Oil, Menthol.

Other Ingredients: Water, Stearic Acid, Linseed Oil, Soybean Oil, Fragrance, Propylene Glycol, Gelatin, Ammonium Hydroxide, Calcium Hydroxide.

Actions: Antipruritic, counterirritant and antiseptic.

Indications: This medicated skin product is an effective facial cleanser and has been demonstrated to be more effective than soap in an acne washing regimen. When used on sunburned skin, this medicated cream actually reduces the surface temperature of the skin to relieve pain almost instantly.

Additional Benefits: Noxzema is also an effective moisturizer. For an effective anti-acne program: instead of soap, wash with Noxzema and treat acne prone areas with Noxzema Acne 12.

Directions: (Wash) Morning and night wash your face with Noxzema Skin Cream. Scoop or pump out some Noxzema and spread over your face with a wet washcloth, gently work in using a circular motion. Rinse. (Sunburn) Apply Noxzema Skin Cream liberally to areas of burn or discomfort.

Contraindications: None.

Cautions: For persistent skin problems or serious burn, consult physician. Keep out of the reach of children.

How Supplied: Available on 2.5 oz., 4 oz., 6 oz., and 10 oz. jars. Also available in a 4.5 oz. tube and a 10.5 oz. pump container.
Shown in Product Identification Section, page 418

NuAge Laboratories, Ltd.
4200 LACLEDE AVENUE
ST. LOUIS, MO 63108

BIOCHEMIC TISSUE SALTS
[bīō"kem'ik tish'u sawlt]

Ingredients: Each tissue salt tablet provides Schuessler homoeopathic ingredients as the recommended triturated tablet in the required Lactose base per U.S.H.P.

Action: Biochemic Tissue Salts (or Cell Salts) work homoeopathically to help the body achieve relief and maintain health and fitness by stimulating the body's healing process.

History: The NuAge Biochemic Tissue Tablets were developed over one hundred years ago by Dr. Wm. Schuessler. Their use is explained in THE BIOCHEMIC HANDBOOK and many other publications. The Tissue Salts are "official" when made in accordance with the United States Homoeopathic Pharmacopoeia.

Contraindications: None

Warning: As with any drug, if nursing or pregnant seek the advice of a professional before using. Keep this and all medicine out of the reach of children. If symptoms persist or recur, consult a licensed medical practitioner.

Instructions: Use according to standard Homoeopathic indications.

EDUCATIONAL MATERIAL

The Biochemic Handbook
Published by Formur, Inc., a paperback pocket edition giving complete description of biochemic tissue salts and proper applications for noted symptoms. ($1.50)
Product Description Charts
Color sheet, 8½ × 11, describing each biochemic tissue salt and its proper application.

Numark Laboratories, Inc.
P.O. BOX 6321
EDISON, NJ 08818

CERTAIN DRI® ANTIPERSPIRANT

Active Ingredient: Aluminum Chloride

Actions: Antiperspirant protection—helps solve, control and lessen underarm perspiration.

Warnings: Do not apply after shaving, on broken skin, or immediately after bathing. If rash develops, discontinue use. Keep out of reach of children.

Directions: Must be applied sparingly on dry skin at bedtime only. Recommended for underarm use only.

How Supplied: 1.5 oz. unscented roll-on.

For more information contact NUMARK Laboratories, Inc., PO Box 6321, Edison, NJ 08818 for a free booklet, "Important Facts About Perspiration Problems." Call 1-800-331-0221.
Shown in Product Identification Section, page 418

O'Connor Pharmaceuticals
16400 N.W. 2ND AVENUE
MIAMI, FL 33169

DIASORB®
Nonfibrous Activated Attapulgite
Tablets and Liquid

Description: Diasorb relieves cramps and pains associated with diarrhea. It is available as easy-to-swallow tablets or as a liquid with a pleasant-tasting cola flavor. Diasorb is safe for children.

Active Ingredient: Each tablet or each liquid teaspoonful contains 750 mg nonfibrous activated attapulgite.

Inactive Ingredients: *Tablet*—D&C Red No. 30 aluminum lake, distilled acetylated monoglycerides, ethylcellulose, gelatin, hydroxypropyl methylcellulose, magnesium stearate, mannitol, titanium dioxide, and water. *Liquid*—Benzoic acid, citric acid, flavor, glycerin, magnesium aluminum silicate, methylparaben, polysorbate, propylene glycol, propylparaben, saccharin, sodium hypochlorite solution, sorbitol, xanthan gum, and water.

Directions for Use: Take the full recommended starting dose at the first sign of diarrhea, and repeat after each subsequent bowel movement. Do not exceed maximum recommended dose per day.
Swallow tablets with water. Do not chew. Shake liquid well before using.

Warning: Do not use for more than 2 days or in the presence of fever or in infants or children under 3, unless directed by a physician. In case of accidental overdose, seek professional assistance or contact a poison control center immediately.
Store at room temperature.
KEEP THIS AND ALL MEDICATIONS OUT OF THE REACH OF CHILDREN.

Dosage: See Table for recommended dosage for acute diarrhea.
[See table on next page].

How Supplied: *Tablets*—Packaged in blister packs of 6 in 24-count cartons. *Liquid*—In plastic bottles of 4 fl oz (120 mL).

Products are cross-indexed by generic and chemical names in the
YELLOW SECTION

Ohm Laboratories, Inc.
P. O. BOX 279
FRANKLIN PARK, NJ 08823

IBUPROHM®
Ibuprofen Tablets, USP
Ibuprofen Caplets, USP

Active Ingredient: Each tablet contains Ibuprofen USP, 200 mg.

Warning: ASPIRIN SENSITIVE PATIENTS: Do not take this product if you have had a severe allergic reaction to aspirin, e.g., asthma, swelling, shock or hives, because even though this product contains no aspirin or salicylates, cross-reactions may occur in patients allergic to aspirin.

Indications: For the temporary relief of minor aches and pains associated with the common cold, headache, toothache, muscular aches, backache, for the minor pain of arthritis, for the pain of menstrual cramps, and for reduction of fever.

Directions: *Adults:* Take 1 tablet every 4 to 6 hours while symptoms persist. If pain or fever does not respond to 1 tablet, 2 tablets may be used but do not exceed 6 tablets in 24 hours, unless directed by a doctor. The smallest effective dose should be used. Take with food or milk if occasional and mild heartburn, upset stomach, or stomach pain occurs with use. Consult a doctor if these symptoms are more than mild or if they persist. Children: Do not give this product to children under 12 except under the advice and supervision of a doctor.

Warnings: Do not take for pain for more than 10 days or for fever for more than 3 days unless directed by a doctor. If pain or fever persists or gets worse, if new symptoms occur, or if the painful area is red or swollen, consult a doctor. These could be signs of serious illness. If you are under a doctor's care for any serious condition, consult a doctor before taking this product. As with aspirin and acetaminophen, if you have any condition which requires you to take prescription drugs or if you have had any problems or serious side effects from taking any nonprescription pain reliever, do not take this product without first discussing it with your doctor. If you experience any symptoms which are unusual or seem unrelated to the condition for which you took ibuprofen, consult a doctor before taking any more of it. Although ibuprofen is indicated for the same conditions as aspirin and acetaminophen, it should not be taken with them except under a doctor's direction. Do not combine the product with any other ibuprofen-containing product. As with any drug, if you are pregnant or nursing a baby, seek the advice of a health professional before using this product. IT IS ESPECIALLY IMPORTANT NOT TO USE IBUPROFEN DURING THE LAST 3 MONTHS OF PREGNANCY UNLESS SPECIFICALLY DIRECTED TO DO SO BY A DOCTOR BECAUSE IT MAY CAUSE PROBLEMS IN THE UNBORN CHILD OR COMPLICATIONS DURING DELIVERY. Keep this and all drugs out of the reach of children. In case of accidental overdose, seek professional assistance or contact a poison control center immediately.

How Supplied: Coated tablets in bottles of 24, 50, 100, 165, 250, 500 and 1000. Coated caplets in bottles of 24, 50, 100 and 250.

Storage: Store at room temperature; avoid excessive heat 40° (104°F).
Shown in Product Identification Section, page 418

Ortho Pharmaceutical Corporation
Advanced Care Products
RARITAN, NJ 08869

CONCEPTROL®
Contraceptive Gel
Single Use Applicators

Description: An unscented, unflavored, colorless, greaseless and non-staining gel in convenient, easy-to-use disposable plastic applicators. Each applicator is filled with a single, pre-measured dose containing the active spermicide Nonoxynol-9—4.0%, (100 mg per application) at pH 4.5.

Indication: Contraception

Actions and Uses: A spermicidal gel for use whenever control of conception is desirable.

Warning: Occasional burning and/or irritation of the vagina or penis have been reported. If this occurs, discontinue use and consult a physician as necessary. Not effective if taken orally. Keep out of reach of children. When pregnancy is contraindicated, the contraceptive program should be discussed with a health care professional.

Dosage and Administration: One applicatorful of CONCEPTROL Contraceptive Gel should be inserted deeply into the vagina just before intercourse. An additional applicatorful is required each time intercourse is repeated. If intercourse has not occurred within one hour after the application of CONCEPTROL Contraceptive Gel, repeat the application of CONCEPTROL Contraceptive Gel before intercourse.
Douching is not recommended after using CONCEPTROL Gel. However, if desired for cleansing purposes, wait at least six hours following last intercourse to allow for full spermicidal activity of CONCEPTROL Gel.
While no method of contraception can provide an absolute guarantee against becoming pregnant, for maximum protection, CONCEPTROL Gel must be used according to directions.

Inactive Ingredients: Lactic Acid, Methylparaben, Povidone, Propylene Glycol, Purified Water, Sodium Carboxymethylcellulose, Sorbic Acid, Sorbitol Solution.

How Supplied: CONCEPTROL Gel is available in packages of 6 and 10 easy to use applicators, premeasured, prefilled, prewrapped.

Storage: Conceptrol Gel should be stored at room temperature.
Shown in Product Identification Section, page 418

CONCEPTROL CONTRACEPTIVE INSERTS

Description: A non-foaming, single dose vaginal contraceptive containing the active spermicide nonoxynol-9—8.34% (150 mg per insert). CONCEPTROL Inserts may be used with a condom or alone.

Indication: Contraception

Actions and Uses: A spermicidal insert for intravaginal contraception. For use with a condom or alone.

Warning: Occasional burning and/or irritation of the vagina or penis have been reported. Should sensitivity to the ingredients or irritation of the vagina or penis develop, discontinue use and consult a physician as necessary. Not effective if taken orally. Keep out of reach of children. When pregnancy is contraindicated, the contraceptive program should be discussed with a health care professional.

Dosage and Administration: CONCEPTROL should be inserted into the vagina at least ten minutes prior to male penetration to insure proper dispersion. CONCEPTROL provides protection from ten minutes to one hour after product insertion. Insert a new CONCEPTROL Contraceptive Insert each time intercourse is repeated. If a douche is desired for cleansing purposes, wait at least six hours following intercourse. CONCEPTROL is an effective method of contraception. While no method of birth

Age	Initial Dose	Maximum Dose per 24 hours
Adults and children over 12 years	4 Tablets or 4 tsp	12 Tablets or 12 tsp
Children 6–12 years	2 Tablets or 2 tsp	6 Tablets or 6 tsp
Children 3–6 years	1 Tablet or 1 tsp	3 Tablets or 3 tsp
Infants and children under 3 years	Only as directed by a physician	

control can provide an absolute guarantee against becoming pregnant, for maximum protection, CONCEPTROL must be used according to directions.

How Supplied: CONCEPTROL Contraceptive Inserts are available in packages containing 10 inserts.

Inactive Ingredients: Lauroamphodiacetate Sodium Trideceth Sulfate, Polyethylene Glycol 1000, Polyethylene Glycol 1450, Povidone.

Storage: Avoid excessive heat (over 86°F or 30°C).

Shown in Product Identification Section, page 418

DELFEN®
Contraceptive Foam

Description: A contraceptive foam in an aerosol dosage formulation containing 12.5% Nonoxynol-9 (100 mg. per application) and buffered to normal vaginal pH 4.5.

Indication: Contraception.

Action and Uses: A spermicidal foam for intravaginal contraception.

Warning: Occasional burning and/or irritation of the vagina or penis have been reported. In such cases, the medication should be discontinued and a physician consulted as necessary. Not effective if taken orally. Keep out of reach of children.
When pregnancy is contraindicated, the contraceptive program should be discussed with a health care professional.

Dosage and Administration: Insert DELFEN Contraceptive Foam just prior to each intercourse. You may have intercourse any time up to one hour after you have inserted the foam. If you repeat intercourse, insert another applicatorful of DELFEN Foam. After shaking the vial, place the measured-dose (5cc) applicator over the top of the vial, then press applicator down very gently. Fill to the top of the barrel threads. Remove applicator to stop flow of foam. Insert the filled applicator well into the vagina and depress the plunger. Remove the applicator with the plunger in depressed position. If a douche is desired for cleansing purposes, wait at least six hours after intercourse. Refer to directions and diagrams for detailed instructions. DELFEN Foam is a reliable method of birth control. While no method of birth control can provide an absolute guarantee against becoming pregnant, for maximum protection, DELFEN Foam must be used according to directions.

How Supplied: DELFEN Contraceptive Foam 0.70 oz. Starter vial with applicator. Also available in 0.70 oz. and 1.75 oz. Refill vials without applicator.

Inactive Ingredients: Benzoic Acid, Cetyl Alcohol, Diethylaminoethyl Stearamide, Glacial Acetic Acid, Methylparaben, Perfume, Phosphoric Acid, Polyvinyl Alcohol, Propellant 12, Propellant 114, Propylene Glycol, Purified Wa-

ter, Sodium Carboxymethylcellulose, Stearic Acid.

Storage: Contents under pressure. Do not puncture or incinerate container. Do not expose to heat or store at temperatures above 120°F.

Shown in Product Identification Section, page 419

GYNOL II® Original Formula
Contraceptive Jelly

Description: A colorless, unscented, unflavored, greaseless and non-staining contraceptive jelly containing the active spermicide Nonoxynol-9 (2%, 100 mg. per application) and having a pH of 4.5.

Indication: Contraception.

Actions and Uses: An aesthetically pleasing spermicidal jelly to be used in conjunction with a diaphragm whenever control of conception is desired.

Warning: Occasional burning and/or irritation of the vagina or penis have been reported. In such cases, the medication should be discontinued and a physician consulted as necessary. Not effective if taken orally. Keep out of reach of children. When pregnancy is contraindicated, the contraceptive program should be discussed with a health care professional.

Dosage and Administration: Used in conjunction with a vaginal diaphragm. Prior to insertion, put about a teaspoonful of GYNOL II Original Formula Contraceptive Jelly into the cup of the dome of the diaphragm and spread a small amount around the edge with your fingertip. This will aid in insertion and provide protection.
It is also important to remember that if intercourse occurs more than six hours after insertion, or if repeated intercourse takes place, an additional application of GYNOL II Original Formula is necessary. DO NOT REMOVE THE DIAPHRAGM—simply add more GYNOL II Original Formula with the applicator provided in the applicator package, being careful not to dislodge the diaphragm. Remember, another application of GYNOL II Original Formula is required each time intercourse is repeated, regardless of how little time has transpired since the diaphragm has been in place.
IMPORTANT—For contraceptive effectiveness, the diaphragm should remain in place for six hours after intercourse and should be removed as soon as possible thereafter. Continuous wearing of the diaphragm for more than 24 hours is not recommended. Retention of the diaphragm for prolonged periods may encourage the growth of certain bacteria in the vaginal tract. It has been suggested that under certain as yet unestablished conditions overgrowth of these bacteria may lead to symptoms of toxic shock syndrome (TSS). For further information, consult your physician.
If a douche is desired for cleansing purposes, wait at least six hours after intercourse. While no method of contraception can provide an absolute guarantee

against becoming pregnant, for maximum protection, GYNOL II Original Formula must be used according to directions.

Inactive Ingredients: Lactic Acid, Methylparaben, Povidone, Propylene Glycol, Purified Water, Sodium Carboxymethylcellulose, Sorbic Acid, Sorbitol Solution.

How Supplied: 2.5 oz Starter tube with measured dose applicator. Regular size 2.5 oz tube only. Large size 3.8 oz tube only.

Storage: Gynol II Original Formula should be stored at room temperature.

Shown in Product Identification Section, page 419

GYNOL II EXTRA STRENGTH
CONTRACEPTIVE JELLY

Description: GYNOL II Extra Strength Contraceptive Jelly is a clear, unscented, water-soluble, greaseless gel. It is mildly lubricating and non-staining. Each applicatorful contains 150 mg of nonoxynol-9 (3%), a potent spermicide which provides effective protection against pregnancy when used with a diaphragm or a condom or alone. A diaphragm alone is not effective protection against pregnancy.

Indication: Contraception.

Actions and Uses: An aesthetically pleasing spermicidal jelly for use alone, with a condom or a diaphragm whenever control of contraception is desired.

Warning: Occasional burning and/or irritation of the vagina or penis have been reported. In such cases, the medication should be discontinued and a physician consulted as necessary. Not effective if taken orally. Keep out of reach of children. When pregnancy is contraindicated, the contraceptive program should be discussed with a health care professional.

Dosage and Administration: When used in conjunction with a vaginal diaphragm. Prior to insertion, put about a teaspoonful of GYNOL II Extra Strength Contraceptive Jelly into the cup of the dome of the diaphragm and spread a small amount around the edge with your fingertip then insert.
It is also important to remember that if intercourse occurs more than six hours after insertion, or if repeated intercourse takes place, an additional application of GYNOL II Extra Strength is necessary. DO NOT REMOVE THE DIAPHRAGM, simply add more GYNOL II Extra Strength with the applicator provided in the applicator package, being careful not to dislodge the diaphragm. Remember, another application of GYNOL II Extra Strength is required each time intercourse is repeated, regardless of how little time has transpired since the diaphragm has been in place.
IMPORTANT—For contraceptive effectiveness, the diaphragm should remain

Continued on next page

Ortho Pharm.—Cont.

in place for six hours after intercourse and should be removed as soon as possible thereafter. Continuous wearing of the diaphragm for more than 24 hours is not recommended. Retention of the diaphragm for prolonged periods may encourage the growth of certain bacteria in the vaginal tract. It has been suggested that under certain as yet unestablished conditions overgrowth of these bacteria may lead to symptoms of toxic shock syndrome (TSS). For further information, consult your physician.

Dosage and Administration: For use with a condom or as a use-alone product. Insert an applicatorful of GYNOL II Extra Strength into the vagina as shown in the illustration. Intercourse should occur within one hour after GYNOL II Extra Strength has been inserted. An additional application must be used prior to each additional act of intercourse. This method of contraception must be used each and every time intercourse takes place, regardless of the time of the month.

Inactive Ingredients: Lactic Acid, Methylparaben, Povidone, Propylene Glycol, Purified Water, Sodium Carboxymethylcellulose, Sorbic Acid, Sorbitol Solution.

Shown in Product Identification Section, page 419

MASSÉ®
Breast Cream

Composition: MASSE Breast Cream.

Action and Uses: MASSE Breast Cream is especially designed for care of the nipples of pregnant and nursing women.

Administration and Dosage:
BEFORE BIRTH
During the last two or three months of pregnancy, it is often desirable to prepare the nipple and the nipple area of the breast for eventual nursing. In these cases, MASSE is used once or twice daily in the following manner: Carefully cleanse the breast with a soft, clean cloth and plain water and dry. Squeeze a ribbon of MASSE, approximately an inch long, and lightly massage into the nipple and immediate surrounding area. Do so until the cream has completely disappeared. The massage motion should be gentle and outward.
AFTER BABY IS BORN
During the nursing period MASSE is used as follows: BEFORE AND AFTER EACH NURSING cleanse the breasts with a clean cloth and water. After drying squeeze a ribbon of MASSE, approximately an inch long, and gently massage into the nipple and the immediate surrounding area.

Contraindications: MASSE should not be used in cases of acute mastitis or breast abscess.

Caution: In cases of excessive tenderness or irritation of any kind, consult your physician.

How Supplied: MASSE Breast Cream is available in a 2 oz. tube.

Inactive Ingredients: Purified Water, Glyceryl Stearate, Glycerin, Cetyl Alcohol, Peanut Oil, Sorbitan Stearate, Stearic Acid, Polysorbate 60, Sodium Benzoate, Propylparaben, Methylparaben, Potassium Hydroxide.

Storage: Massé should be stored at room temperature.
Shown in Product Identification Section, page 419

MICATIN®
['mī-kə-tin]
Antifungal For Athlete's Foot

Description: An antifungal containing the active ingredient miconazole nitrate 2%, clinically proven to cure athlete's foot, jock itch and ringworm.

Indications: Athlete's foot (tinea pedis), jock itch (tinea cruris), and ringworm (tinea corporis).

Actions and Uses: Proven clinically effective in the treatment of athlete's foot (tinea pedis), jock itch (tinea cruris), and ringworm (tinea corporis). For effective relief of the itching, scaling, burning and discomfort that can accompany these conditions.

Directions: Cleanse skin with soap and water and dry thoroughly. Apply a thin layer of MICATIN over affected area morning and night or as directed by a doctor. For athlete's foot, pay special attention to the spaces between the toes. It is also helpful to wear well-fitting, ventilated shoes and to change shoes and socks at least once daily. Best results in athlete's foot and ringworm are usually obtained with 4 weeks' use of this product and in jock itch with 2 weeks' use. If satisfactory results have not occurred within these times, consult a doctor or pharmacist. Children under 12 years of age should be supervised in the use of this product. This product is not effective on the scalp or nails.
Do not use on children under 2 years of age except under the advice and supervision of a doctor. For external use only. If irritation occurs, or if there is no improvement within 4 weeks (for athlete's foot or ringworm) or within 2 weeks (for jock itch), discontinue use and consult a doctor or pharmacist. Keep this and all drugs out of the reach of children. In case of accidental ingestion, seek professional assistance or contact a Poison Control Center immediately.

How Supplied:
MICATIN® Antifungal Cream is available in a 0.5 oz. tube and a 1.0 oz. tube.
MICATIN Antifungal Spray Powder is available in a 3.0 oz. aerosol can.
MICATIN Antifungal Deodorant Spray Powder is available in a 3.0 oz. aerosol can.
MICATIN Antifungal Powder is available in a 2.8 oz. plastic bottle.
MICATIN Antifungal Spray Liquid is available in a 3.5 oz. aerosol can.

Inactive Ingredients:
MICATIN Antifungal Cream: Benzoic Acid, BHA, Mineral Oil, Peglicol 5 Oleate, Pegoxol 7 Stearate, Purified Water.
MICATIN Antifungal Spray Powder: Alcohol, Propellant A-46, Sorbitan Sesquioleate, Stearalkonium Hectorite, Talc.
MICATIN Antifungal Deodorant Spray Powder: Alcohol, Propellant A-46, Talc, Stearalkonium Hectorite, Sorbitan Sesquioleate, Fragrance.
MICATIN Antifungal Powder: Talc.
MICATIN Antifungal Spray Liquid: Alcohol, Benzyl Alcohol, Cocamide DEA, Propellant A-46, Sorbitan Sesquioleate, Tocopherol.

Storage: Store at room temerature.
Shown in Product Identification Section, page 419

MICATIN®
['mī-kə-tin]
Antifungal For Jock Itch

Description: An antifungal containing the active ingredient miconazole nitrate 2%, clinically proven to cure jock itch.

Indications: Jock itch (tinea cruris).

Actions and Uses: Proven clinically effective in the treatment of jock itch (tinea cruris). For effective relief of the itching, scaling, burning and discomfort that can accompany this condition.

Directions: Cleanse skin with soap and water and dry thoroughly. Apply a thin layer of product over affected area morning and night or as directed by a doctor. Best results are usually obtained within 2 weeks' use of this product. If satisfactory results have not occurred within this time, consult a doctor or pharmacist. Children under 12 years of age should be supervised in the use of this product. This product is not effective on the scalp or nails.

Warnings: Do not use on children under 2 years of age except under the advice and supervision of a doctor. For external use only. If irritation occurs, or if there is no improvement of jock itch within 2 weeks, discontinue use and consult a doctor or pharmacist. Keep this and all drugs out of the reach of children. In case of accidental ingestion, seek professional assistance or contact a Poison Control Center immediately.

How Supplied:
MICATIN® Jock Itch Cream is available in a 0.5 oz. tube.
MICATIN Jock Itch Spray Powder is available in a 3.0 oz. aerosol can.

Inactive Ingredients:
MICATIN Jock Itch Cream: Benzoic Acid, BHA, Mineral Oil, Peglicol 5 Oleate, Pegoxol 7 Stearate, Purified Water.
MICATIN Jock Itch Spray Powder: Alcohol, Propellant A-46, Sorbitan Sesquioleate, Stearalkonium Hectorite, Talc.

Storage: Store at room temperature.

ORTHO–GYNOL®
Contraceptive Jelly

Description: ORTHO-GYNOL Contraceptive Jelly is a water dispersible spermicidal jelly having a pH of 4.5 and contains the active spermicide Octoxynol-9 (1%).

Indication: Contraception.

Action and Uses: An aesthetically pleasing spermicidal vaginal jelly for use with a vaginal diaphragm whenever the control of conception is desirable.

Warning: Occasional burning and/or irritation of the vagina or penis have been reported. In such cases, the medication should be discontinued and a physician consulted as necessary. Not effective if taken orally. Keep out of reach of children. When pregnancy is contraindicated, the contraceptive program should be discussed with a health care professional.

Dosage and Administration: Used in conjunction with a vaginal diaphragm. Prior to insertion, put about a teaspoonful of ORTHO-GYNOL Contraceptive Jelly into the cup of the dome of the diaphragm and spread a small amount around the edge with the fingertip. This will aid in insertion and provide protection.
It is also important to remember that if intercourse occurs more than six hours after insertion, or if repeated intercourse takes place, an additional application of ORTHO-GYNOL is necessary. DO NOT REMOVE THE DIAPHRAGM—simply add more ORTHO-GYNOL with the applicator provided in the applicator package, being careful not to dislodge the diaphragm.
Remember, another application of OR-THO-GYNOL is required each time intercourse is repeated, regardless of how little time has transpired since the diaphragm has been in place.
IMPORTANT—For contraceptive effectiveness, the diaphragm should remain in place for six hours after intercourse and should be removed as soon as possible thereafter. Continuous wearing of the diaphragm for more than 24 hours is not recommended. Retention of the diaphragm for prolonged periods may encourage the growth of certain bacteria in the vaginal tract. It has been suggested that under certain as yet unestablished conditions overgrowth of these bacteria may lead to symptoms of toxic shock syndrome (TSS). For further information, consult your physician.
If a douche is desired for cleansing purposes, wait at least 6 hours after intercourse. Refer to directions and diagrams for complete instructions. While no method of contraception can provide an absolute guarantee against becoming pregnant, for maximum protection OR-THO-GYNOL must be used according to directions.

How Supplied: 2.5 oz. and 3.8 oz. tube only packages.

Inactive Ingredients: Benzoic Acid, Castor Oil, Fragrance, Glacial Acetic Acid, Methylparaben, Potassium Hydroxide, Propylene Glycol, Purified Water, Sodium Carboxymethylcellulose, Sorbic Acid.

Storage: Ortho-Gynol should be stored at room temperature.
Shown in Product Identification Section, page 419

ORTHO® PERSONAL LUBRICANT

Description: ORTHO PERSONAL LUBRICANT is a non-staining, water soluble lubricating jelly that is safe for delicate tissues.

Indications: ORTHO PERSONAL LUBRICANT is especially formulated as a sexual lubricant that is designed to be gentle and non-irritating for both women and men. It may also be used for easy insertion of rectal thermometers, tampons, douche nozzles and enema nozzles.

Dosage and Administration: Apply a one (1″) to two (2″) inch ribbon of product, or desired amount, to external vaginal area and/or penis. Repeat applications may be used by one or both partners. If desired, this product may be used inside the vagina.

Precaution: ORTHO PERSONAL LUBRICANT does not contain spermicide. It is not a contraceptive.

How Supplied: ORTHO PERSONAL LUBRICANT is available in 2 oz. and 4 oz. tubes.

Inactive Ingredients: Glycerin, Methylparaben, Propylene Glycol, Purified Water, Sodium Alginate, Sodium Carboxymethylcellulose, Sorbic Acid.

Storage: Store at room temperature (59–86°F). Do not freeze.
Shown in Product Identification Section, page 419

P & S Laboratories
210 WEST 131st STREET
LOS ANGELES, CA 90061

See Standard Homeopathic Company

Paddock Laboratories, Inc.
3101 LOUISIANA AVE. NORTH
MINNEAPOLIS, MN 55427

ACTIDOSE–AQUA
(Highly Activated Charcoal Suspension)

Supplied in bottles containing 25 grams per 120ml and 50 grams per 240ml highly activated charcoal suspension. Each milliliter contains 208mg (0.208 grams) highly activated charcoal in aqueous suspension. Detailed blue color-coded attached package insert.

ACTIDOSE with SORBITOL
(Highly Activated Charcoal Suspension with Sorbitol)

Supplied in bottles containing 25 grams per 120ml and 50 grams per 240ml highly activated charcoal suspension. Each milliliter contains 208mg (0.208 grams) highly activated charcoal and 400mg (0.4 grams) sorbitol. Detailed red color-coded attached package insert.

EMULSOIL®
[*ē-muls-oil*]
Castor Oil

Emulsoil is a self-emulsifying, flavored castor oil formulated to instantly mix with any beverage.

Active Ingredient: Each 2-ounce bottle contains 95% w/w Castor Oil, USP with self-emulsifying and natural sugarless flavoring agents.

Indications: Emulsoil is used in the preparation of the small and large bowel for radiography, colonoscopy, surgery, proctologic procedures and exploratory IVP use. Can also be used for isolated bouts of constipation.

Warnings: Not to be used when abdominal pain, nausea, vomiting or other symptoms of appendicitis are present. Frequent or prolonged use may result in dependence on laxatives. Do not use during pregnancy except under competent advice.

Dosage and Administration: Adults: 1–4 tablespoonfuls. Children: 1–2 teaspoonfuls.

How Supplied: Available in 2-ounce bottles. Packaged 12 and 48 bottles per case.

GLUTOSE®
[*glū-tose*]
Dextrose Gel

Active Ingredient: Dextrose 40%, Each 80-gram bottle contains 32 grams dextrose in a dye free jel base.

Indications: Glutose is a concentrated glucose (40% Dextrose) used for insulin reactions and hypoglycemic states.

Dosage and Administration: Usual dose is ⅓ bottle Glutose (10 grams dextrose) orally, which can be repeated in 10 minutes if necessary. Response should be noticed in 10 minutes. The physician should then be notified when a hypoglycemic reaction occurs so that the insulin dose can be accurately adjusted. Glutose should not be given to children under 2 years of age unless otherwise directed by physician.

How Supplied: 80-gram squeeze bottle, 6 bottles/case. 25-gram unit-dose tube, 3 tubes/box.

IPECAC SYRUP
[*ip-ĕ-kak*]

Active Ingredients: Ipecac Syrup, USP contains in each 30 ml, not less than

Continued on next page

Paddock—Cont.

36.9 mg and not more than 47.1 mg of the total ether soluble alkaloids of ipecac. The content of emetine and cephaeline together is not less than 90.0% of the amount of the total ether-soluble alkaloids.

Indications: Ipecac Syrup is indicated for emergency use to cause vomiting in poisoning.

Warnings: Do not use in unconscious persons. Ordinarily, this drug should not be used if strychnine, corrosives such as alkalies, lye and strong acids, or petroleum distillates such as kerosene, gasoline, coal oil, fuel oil, paint thinners, or cleaning fluids have been ingested.

Dosage and Administration: Usual Dosage: One tablespoonful (15 ml) followed by one to two glasses of water, in persons over 1 year of age. Repeat dosage in 20 minutes if vomiting does not occur.

How Supplied: Available in 1-ounce bottles. Packaged 12 bottles per case.

Parke-Davis
Consumer Health Products Group
Division of Warner-Lambert
  Company
201 TABOR ROAD
MORRIS PLAINS, NJ 07950
(See also Warner-Lambert)

AGORAL® Plain
[ă'gō-răl"]
AGORAL® Raspberry
AGORAL® Marshmallow

Description: Each tablespoonful (15 mL) of Agoral Plain contains 4.2 grams mineral oil in a thoroughly homogenized emulsion.
Also contains acacia; agar; benzoic acid; egg albumin; flavors; glycerin; sodium benzoate; tragacanth; citric acid or sodium hydroxide to adjust pH; water.
Each tablespoonful (15 mL) of Agoral Raspberry (pink) or of Agoral Marshmallow (white) contains 4.2 grams mineral oil and 0.2 gram phenolphthalein in a thoroughly homogenized emulsion.
Also contains acacia; agar; benzoic acid; egg albumin; flavors; glycerin; saccharin sodium; sodium benzoate; tragacanth; citric acid or sodium hydroxide to adjust pH; water. Agoral Raspberry Flavor also contains D&C Red No. 30 Lake.

Actions: Agoral, containing mineral oil, facilitates defecation by lubricating the fecal mass and softening the stool. More effective than nonemulsified oil in penetrating the feces, Agoral thereby greatly reduces the possibility of oil leakage at the anal sphincter. Phenolphthalein gently stimulates motor activity of the lower intestinal tract. Agoral's combined lubricating-softening and peristaltic actions can help to restore a normal pattern of evacuation.

Indications: Relief of constipation. Agoral may be especially required when straining at stool is a hazard, as in hernia, cardiac, or hypertensive patients; during convalescence from surgery; before and after surgery for hemorrhoids or other painful anorectal disorders; for patients confined to bed.
The management of chronic constipation should also include attention to fluid intake, diet and bowel habits.

Contraindication: Sensitivity to phenolphthalein.

Warning: Do not use laxative products when abdominal pain, nausea, or vomiting are present unless directed by a physician. If you have noticed a sudden change in bowel habits that persists over a period of 2 weeks, consult a physician before using a laxative. Laxative products should not be used for a period longer than 1 week unless directed by a physician. Rectal bleeding or failure to have a bowel movement after use of a laxative may indicate a serious condition. Discontinue use and consult your physician. Do not administer to children under 6 years of age, to pregnant women, to bedridden patients or to persons with difficulty swallowing. As with any drug, if you are nursing a baby, seek the advice of a health professional before using this product. Do not take with meals. If skin rash appears, do not use this product or any other preparation containing phenolphthalein. Keep this and all drugs out of the reach of children. In case of accidental overdose, seek professional assistance or contact a Poison Control Center immediately. Drug interaction precaution: Do not take this product if you are presently taking a stool softener laxative.

Dosage: Agoral Plain—Adults—1 to 2 tablespoonfuls at bedtime only, unless other time is advised by physician. Children—Over 6 years, 2 to 4 teaspoonfuls at bedtime only, unless other time is advised by physician.
Agoral Raspberry and Marshmallow —Adults—½ to 1 tablespoonful at bedtime only, unless other time is advised by physician. Children—Over 6 years, ½ to ¾ teaspoonfuls at bedtime only, unless other time is advised by physician. This product generally produces bowel movement in 6 to 8 hours.

Supplied: Agoral Plain (without phenolphthalein), plastic bottles of 16 fl oz. Agoral (raspberry flavor), plastic bottles of 16 fl oz. Agoral (marshmallow flavor), plastic bottles of 8 fl oz and 16 fl oz.
Store between 15°–30° C (59°–86° F). Keep this and all drugs out of the reach of children.
In case of accidental overdose, seek professional assistance or contact a poison control center immediately.

ANUSOL®
[ă'nū-sōl"]
Suppositories/Ointment

Description:

	Anusol Suppositories each contains	Anusol Ointment each gram
Bismuth subgallate	2.25%	—
Bismuth Resorcin Compound	1.75%	—
Benzyl Benzoate	1.2 %	12 mg
Peruvian Balsam	1.8 %	18 mg
Zinc Oxide	11.0 %	110 mg
Analgine™ (pramoxine hydrochloride)	—	10 mg

Also contains the following inactive ingredients: calcium phosphate dibasic; coconut oil base, FD&C Blue No. 2 Lake and Red No. 40 Lake, hydrogenated fatty acid in a bland hydrogenated vegetable oil base.

Also contains the following inactive ingredients: calcium phosphate dibasic; cocoa butter; glyceryl monooleate; glyceryl monostearate; kaolin; mineral oil; polyethylene wax; Peruvian balsam.

Actions: Anusol Suppositories and Anusol Ointment help to relieve pain, itching and discomfort arising from irritated anorectal tissues. They have a soothing, lubricant action on mucous membranes. Analgine (pramoxine hydrochloride) in Anusol Ointment is a rapidly acting local anesthetic for the skin and mucous membranes of the anus and rectum. Analgine is also chemically distinct from procaine, cocaine, and dibucaine and can often be used in the patient previously sensitized to other surface anesthetics. Surface analgesia lasts for several hours.

Indications: For prompt, temporary symptomatic relief of minor pain, itching, burning and soreness of hemorrhoids and other simple anorectal irritation.

Contraindications: Anusol Suppositories and Anusol Ointment are contraindicated in those patients with a history of hypersensitivity to any of the components of the preparations.

Precautions: Symptomatic relief should not delay definitive diagnoses or treatment.
If irritation develops, these preparations should be discontinued. In case of rectal bleeding or persistence of the condition, consult your physician. Keep this and all drugs out of the reach of children. In case of accidental ingestion seek professional assistance or contact a Poison Control Center immediately. Do not use in the eyes or nose.

Adverse Reactions: Upon application of Anusol Ointment, which contains Analgine (pramoxine HCl), a patient may occasionally experience burning, especially if the anoderm is not intact. Sensitivity reactions have been rare; discontinue medication if suspected.

Dosage and Administration: Anusol Suppositories—Adults: Remove foil wrapper and insert suppository into the anus. Insert one suppository in the morning and one at bedtime, and one immediately following each evacuation.

Anusol Ointment—Adults: After gentle bathing and drying of the anal area, remove tube cap and apply freely to the exterior surface and gently rub in. Ointment should be applied every 3 or 4 hours.

NOTE: If staining from either of the above products occurs, the stain may be removed from fabric by hand or machine washing with household detergent.

How Supplied: Anusol Suppositories—boxes of 12, 24 and 48; in silver foil strips. Anusol Ointment—1-oz tubes and 2-oz tubes with plastic applicator. Store between 15° and 30°C (59° and 86°F).

Shown in Product Identification Section, page 419

BENADRYL Anti-Itch Cream

Active Ingredients: BENADRYL® (diphenhydramine hydrochloride USP) 1%.

Inactive Ingredients: Cetyl Alcohol, Methylparaben, Polyethylene Glycol Monostearate, Propylene Glycol and Water, Purified.

Indications: For the temporary relief of ITCHING and PAIN associated with minor skin irritations, allergic itches, rashes, insect bites and sunburn.

Actions: Benadryl, the most prescribed topical antihistamine, in a soothing, greaseless cream, is easily absorbed into the skin. It provides safe, effective, temporary relief from many different types of itching.

Warnings: For external use only. Do not use on chicken pox or measles unless supervised by a doctor. Do not use on extensive areas of the skin or for longer than 7 days except as directed by a doctor. Avoid contact with the eyes or other mucous membranes. If condition worsens, or if symptoms persist for more than 7 days, or clear up and occur again within a few days, discontinue use of this product and consult a physician. KEEP THIS AND ALL DRUGS OUT OF THE REACH OF CHILDREN. In case of accidental ingestion, seek professional assistance or contact a Poison Control Center immediately.

Dosage and Administration: For adults and children 6 years of age and older: Apply to the affected area not more than three to four times daily, or as directed by your physician. For children under 6 years of age: Consult a physician.

How Supplied: Benadryl Anti-Itch Cream is supplied in ½ oz. and 1 oz. tubes.

Shown in Product Identification Section, page 419

BENADRYL®
[bĕ'nă-drĭl]
Decongestant Elixir

Description: Each teaspoonful (5 mL) contains: Benadryl (diphenhydramine hydrochloride) 12.5 mg; pseudoephedrine hydrochloride 30 mg; alcohol 5%. Also contains: FD&C Yellow No. 6; glucose, liquid; glycerin, USP; flavors; menthol, USP; saccharin sodium, USP; sodium citrate, USP; sucrose, NF; water, purified, USP.

Indications: Temporarily relieves nasal congestion, runny nose, sneezing, itching of the nose or throat, itchy, watery eyes due to hay fever or other upper respiratory allergies, and runny nose, sneezing and nasal congestion of the common cold.

Warnings: Do not exceed recommended dosage because at higher doses nervousness, dizziness, or sleeplessness may occur. Do not take this product for more than 7 days. If symptoms do not improve or are accompanied by fever, consult a physician. Do not take this product if you have high blood pressure, heart disease, diabetes, thyroid disease, asthma, glaucoma, emphysema, chronic pulmonary disease, shortness of breath, difficulty in breathing or difficulty in urination due to enlargement of the prostate gland unless directed by a physician. May cause excitability, especially in children. May cause marked drowsiness; alcohol may increase the drowsiness effect. Avoid alcoholic beverages while taking this product. Use caution when driving a motor vehicle or operating machinery. As with any drug, if you are pregnant or nursing a baby seek the advice of a health professional before using this product. Keep this and all drugs out of the reach of children. In case of accidental overdose, seek professional assistance or contact a poison control center immediately.

Drug Interaction Precaution: Do not take this product if you are presently taking a prescription drug for high blood pressure or depression without first consulting your physician.

Directions: Children 6 to under 12 years oral dosage is one teaspoonful every 4 to 6 hours not to exceed 4 teaspoonfuls in 24 hours, or as directed by a physician. For children under 6 years of age, consult a physician. Adult oral dosage is two teaspoonfuls every 4 to 6 hours not to exceed 8 teaspoonfuls in 24 hours, or as directed by a physician.

How Supplied: Benadryl Decongestant Elixir is supplied in 4-oz bottles. Store below 30° C (86°F). Protect from freezing.

Shown in Product Identification Section, page 419

BENADRYL® Decongestant
[bĕ'nă-drĭl]
Decongestant Tablets and Kapseals®

Active Ingredients: Each tablet/Kapseal® contains: Benadryl® (diphenhydramine hydrochloride USP) 25 mg. and pseudoephedrine hydrochloride 60 mg.

Inactive Ingredients: Each tablet contains: Corn Starch, Croscarmelose Sodium, Dibasic Calcium Phosphate Dihydrate, FD&C Blue No. 1 Aluminum Lake, Hydroxypropyl Methylcellulose, Microcrystalline Cellulose, Polyethylene Glycol, Polysorbate 80, Stearic Acid, Titanium Dioxide and Zinc Stearate.
Each Kapseals® capsule contains: Calcium Stearate, Lactose (Hydrous), Syloid Silica Gel. The Kapseals® capsule shell contains: D&C Red No. 28, FD&C Blue No. 1 and Red No. 3, Gelatin, Glyceryl Monooleate, PEG-200 Ricinoleate and Titanium Dioxide.

Indications: Temporarily relieves nasal congestion, runny nose, sneezing, itching of the nose or throat, itchy, watery eyes due to hay fever or other upper respiratory allergies, and runny nose, sneezing and nasal congestion of the common cold.

Warning: Do not exceed recommended dosage because at higher doses nervousness, dizziness, or sleeplessness may occur. Do not take this product for more than 7 days. If symptoms do not improve or are accompanied by fever, consult a physician. Do not take this product if you have high blood pressure, heart disease, diabetes, thyroid disease, asthma, glaucoma, emphysema, chronic pulmonary disease, shortness of breath, difficulty in breathing or difficulty in urination due to enlargement of the prostate gland unless directed by a physician. May cause excitability, especially in children. May cause marked drowsiness: alcohol may increase the drowsiness effect. Avoid alcoholic beverages while taking this product. Use caution when driving a motor vehicle or operating machinery. Do not give this product to children under 12 years except under the advice and supervision of a physician. As with any drug, if you are pregnant or nursing a baby seek the advice of a health professional before using this product. Keep this and all drugs out of the reach of children. In case of accidental overdose, seek professional assistance or contact a poison control center immediately.

Drug Interaction Precaution: Do not take this product if you are presently taking a prescription drug for high blood

Continued on next page

This product information was prepared in November 1989. On these and other Parke-Davis Products, detailed information may be obtained by addressing PARKE-DAVIS, Consumer Health Products Group, Division of Warner-Lambert Company, Morris Plains, NJ 07950.

Parke-Davis—Cont.

pressure or depression without first consulting your physician.

Directions: Adults and children over 12 years of age: 1 tablet/Kapseal® every 4 to 6 hours not to exceed 4 tablets/Kapseals® in 24 hours. Benadryl Decongestant is not recommended for children under 12 years of age.

How Supplied: Benadryl Decongestant Tablets and Kapseals® are supplied in boxes of 24.
Store at room temperature 15°–30° C (59°–86° F).
Protect from moisture.
Shown in Product Identification Section, page 419

BENADRYL® Elixir

Active Ingredients: Each teaspoonful (5 mL) contains: Benadryl® (diphenhydramine hydrochloride USP) 12.5 mg. and Alcohol 14%.

Inactive Ingredients: Also contains: D&C Red No. 33, FD&C Red No. 40, Flavors, Sugar, and Water, Purified.

Indications: Temporarily relieves runny nose, sneezing, itching of the nose or throat and itchy, watery eyes due to hay fever or other upper respiratory allergies and runny nose and sneezing associated with the common cold.

Warnings: Do not take this product if you have asthma, glaucoma, emphysema, chronic pulmonary disease, shortness of breath, difficulty in breathing or difficulty in urination due to enlargement of the prostate gland unless directed by a physician. May cause excitability especially in children. May cause marked drowsiness; alcohol may increase the drowsiness effect. Avoid alcoholic beverages while taking this product. Use caution when driving a motor vehicle or operating machinery. As with any drug if you are pregnant or nursing a baby seek the advice of a healthy professional before using this product. Keep this and all drugs out of the reach of children. In case of accidental overdose, seek professional assistance or contact a Poison Control Center immediately.

Dosage and Administration: Children 6 to under 12 years of age oral dosage is 12.5 to 25 mg. (1 to 2 teaspoonfuls) every 4 to 6 hours not to exceed 12 teaspoonfuls in 24 hours, or as directed by a physician. For children under 6 years your physician should be contacted for the recommended dosage. Adult oral dosage is 25 mg. (2 teaspoonfuls) to 50 mg. (4 teaspoonfuls) every 4 to 6 hours not to exceed 24 teaspoonfuls in 24 hours, or as directed by a physician.

How Supplied: Benadryl Elixir is supplied in 4 oz. and 8 oz. bottles.
Shown in Product Identification Section, page 419

BENADRYL® 25
[bĕ′nă-drĭl]
Tablets and Kapseals®

Active Ingredient: Each tablet/Kapseal® contains: Benadryl® (diphenhydramine hydrochloride USP) 25 mg.

Inactive Ingredients: Each tablet contains: Corn Starch, Croscarmellose Sodium, Dibasic Calcium Phosphate Dihydrate, FD&C Red No. 3 Aluminum Lake, Hydroxypropyl Methylcellulose, Microcrystalline Cellulose, Polyethylene Glycol, Polysorbate 80, Stearic Acid, Titanium Dioxide and Zinc Stearate.
Each Kapseals® capsule contains: Lactose (Hydrous) and Magnesium Stearate. The Kapseals® capsule shell contains: D&C Red No. 28, FD&C Blue No. 1, Red No. 3 and Red No. 40, Gelatin, Glyceryl Monooleate, PEG-200 Ricinoleate and Titanium Dioxide.

Indications: Temporarily relieves runny nose, sneezing, itching of the nose or throat, itchy, watery eyes due to hay fever or other upper respiratory allergies and runny nose and sneezing of the common cold.

Warnings: Do not take this product if you have asthma, glaucoma, emphysema, chronic pulmonary disease, shortness of breath, difficulty in breathing or difficulty in urination due to enlargement of the prostate gland unless directed by physician. May cause excitability, especially in children. May cause marked drowsiness; alcohol may increase the drowsiness effect. Avoid alcoholic beverages while taking this product. Use caution when driving a motor vehicle or operating machinery. As with any drug if you are pregnant or nursing a baby seek the advice of a health professional before using this product. Keep this and all drugs out of the reach of children. In case of accidental overdose, seek professional assistance or contact a poison control center immediately.

Directions: Adult oral dosage is 25–50 mg (1 to 2 tablets/Kapseals®) every 4 to 6 hours not to exceed 12 tablets/Kapseals® in 24 hours, or as directed by a physician. Children 6 to under 12 years oral dosage is 12.5 mg to 25 mg (1 tablet/Kapseal®) every 4 to 6 hours, not to exceed 6 tablets/Kapseals® in 24 hours, or as directed by a physician. For children under 6 years your physician should be contacted for the recommended dosage.

How Supplied: Benadryl 25 Tablets and Kapseals® are supplied in boxes of 24 and 48.
Store at room temperature 15°–30° C (59°–86° F). Protect from moisture.
Shown in Product Identification Section, page 419

BENADRYL PLUS®
Tablets

Active Ingredients: Each tablet contains: Benadryl® (diphenhydramine hydrochloride USP) 12.5 mg., pseudoephedrine hydrochloride 30 mg., and acetaminophen 500 mg.

Inactive Ingredients: Each tablet contains: Carboxymethylcellulose, Croscarmellose Sodium, Hydroxypropyl Cellulose, Hydroxypropyl Methylcellulose, Magnesium Stearate, Microcrystalline Cellulose, Polyethylene Glycol, Propylene Glycol, Starch, Stearic Acid, Titanium Dioxide, and Zinc Stearate.

Indications: Temporarily relieves sneezing, running nose, nasal and sinus congestion, fever, minor sore throat pain, headache, sinus pressure, body aches and pain due to the common cold, and sneezing, runny nose, itching of the nose or throat, and itchy, watery eyes due to hay fever or other upper respiratory allergies.

Warnings: Do not exceed recommended dosage because at higher doses nervousness, dizziness, or sleeplessness may occur. Do not take this product if you have high blood pressure, heart disease, diabetes, thyroid disease, asthma, glaucoma, emphysema, chronic pulmonary disease, shortness of breath, difficulty in breathing, or difficulty in urination due to enlargement of the prostate gland unless directed by a physician. May cause excitability especially in children. May cause marked drowsiness; alcohol may increase the drowsiness effect. Avoid alcoholic beverages while taking this product. Use caution when driving a motor vehicle or operating machinery. If fever persists for more than 3 days (72 hours) or recurs, consult your physician. If sore throat persists for more than 2 days, is accompanied or followed by fever, headache, rash, nausea or vomiting, consult a physician promptly. As with any drug if you are pregnant or nursing a baby seek the advice of a health professional before using this product. Keep this and all drugs out of the reach of children. In case of accidental overdose, seek professional assistance or contact a Poison Control Center immediately. Do not give this product to children under 12 years except under the advice and supervision of a physician.

Drug Interaction Precaution: Do not take this product if you are presently taking a prescription drug for high blood pressure or depression without consulting your physician.

Directions: Adults (12 years and over): Two tablets every 6 hours, not to exceed 8 tablets in a 24-hour period. Benadryl Plus is not recommended for children under 12 years of age.

How Supplied: Benadryl Plus Tablets are supplied in boxes of 24 and 48.
Store at room temperature 15°–30°C (59°–86°F). Protect from moisture.
Shown in Product Identification Section, page 419

BENADRYL PLUS NIGHTTIME

Active Ingredients: Each fluid ounce or 2 tablespoons contains: Acetaminophen 1000 mg., diphenhydramine hydrochloride 50 mg., and pseudoephedrine hydrochloride 60 mg.

Inactive Ingredients: Alcohol 10%, citric acid, D&C Yellow No. 10, FD&C Red No. 40, FD&C Green No. 3, disodium edetate, flavoring, glycerin, polyethylene glycol, potassium sorbate, propyl gallate, propylene glycol, sodium benzoate, sodium citrate, sodium saccharin and purified water.

Indications: Benadryl Plus Nighttime provides temporary relief of nasal congestion, runny nose, sneezing, itching of the nose or throat, itchy watery eyes due to hay fever or other upper respiratory allergies and runny nose, sneezing and nasal congestion of the common cold, and fever, headache, sore throat pain, and body aches and pains associated with these conditions.

Warnings: Do not exceed recommended dosage because at higher doses nervousness, dizziness, or sleeplessness may occur. Do not take this product for more than 7 days. If symptoms do not improve or are accompanied by fever, consult a physician. Do not take this product if you have high blood pressure, heart disease, diabetes, thyroid disease, asthma, glaucoma, emphysema, chronic pulmonary disease, shortness of breath, difficulty in breathing, or difficulty in urination due to enlargement of the prostate gland unless directed by a physician. If fever persists for more than 3 days (72 hours) or recurs, consult your physician. If sore throat is severe, persists for more than 2 days, is accompanied or followed by fever, headache, rash, nausea or vomiting, consult a physician promptly. As with any drug if you are pregnant or nursing a baby seek the advice of a health professional before using this product. Keep this and all drugs out of the reach of children. In case of accidental ingestion, seek professional assistance or contact a Poison Control Center immediately. May cause marked drowsiness; alcohol may increase the drowsiness effect. Do not give this product to children under 12 years except under the advice of a physician.

Caution: Avoid alcoholic beverages while taking this product. Use caution when driving a motor vehicle or operating heavy machinery.

Drug Interaction Precaution: Do not take this product if you are presently taking a prescription drug for high blood pressure or depression without first consulting your physician.

Directions for Use: Adults take one fluid ounce using dosage cup or two (2) tablespoons at bedtime for nighttime relief. Dosage may be repeated every six (6) hours or as directed by a physician. Do not exceed 4 fluid ounces or eight (8) tablespoons in any 24-hour period. Children under 12 should use only as directed by a physician.

How Supplied: Benadryl Plus Nighttime is supplied in 6 ounce and 10 ounce bottles. Store at room temperature, 15°–30°C (59°–86°F).

Questions about Benadryl Plus® Nighttime?
Call us toll free 8 AM to 5 PM EST. Weekdays at 1-800-524-2624. In New Jersey call 1-800-338-0326.

Shown in Product Identification Section, page 419

BENADRYL® Spray

Active Ingredients: Benadryl® (diphenhydramine hydrochloride USP) 2% and Alcohol 90%.

Inactive Ingredients: Also contains: Acetylated Lanolin Alcohol, Povidone, Tris (Hydroxymethyl) Amino Methane, Water, Purified and Wheat Germ Glycerides.

Indications: For the temporary relief of ITCHING and PAIN associated with minor skin irritations, allergic itches, rashes, insect bites and sunburn.

Actions: Benadryl spray helps relieve itching. It forms an anti-itch "bandage" to protect and relieve affected areas. Its spray feature allows soothing relief without touching or rubbing the affected area. Benadryl spray is clear, won't stain clothing and won't rinse off (can be easily removed with soap and water).

Warnings: For external use only. Avoid contact with the eyes. Do not apply to blistered, raw or oozing areas of the skin. If condition worsens or if symptoms persist for more than 7 days, or clear up and occur again within a few days, discontinue use of this product and consult a physician. FLAMMABLE—Keep away from fire or flame. Keep this and all drugs out of the reach of children. In case of accidental ingestion, seek professional assistance or contact a Poison Control Center immediately.

Dosage and Administration: For adults and children over 2 years of age and older: Spray on affected area not more than three to four times daily, or as directed by your physician. For children under 2 years of age: Consult a physician.

How Supplied: Benadryl® Spray is available in a 2 oz. pump spray bottle.
Shown in Product Identification Section, page 419

BENYLIN® Cough Syrup

Description: Each teaspoonful (5 ml) contains:
Diphenhydramine
Hydrochloride   12.5 mg
Also contains: Alcohol 5%; Ammonium Chloride; Caramel; Citric Acid; D&C Red No. 33; FD&C Red No. 40; Flavor; Glucose Liquid; Glycerin; Menthol; Purified Water; Sodium Citrate; Sodium Saccharin; Sucrose.

Indications: For the temporary relief of cough due to minor throat and bronchial irritation as may occur with the common cold or with inhaled irritants.

Warnings: May cause marked drowsiness. Keep this and all drugs out of the reach of children. In case of accidental overdose, seek professional assistance or contact a poison control center immediately. Do not give to children under 6 years of age except under the advice and supervision of a physician. May cause excitability, especially in children. Do not take this product for persistent or chronic cough such as occurs with smoking, asthma, emphysema, or when cough is accompanied by excessive secretions, or if you have glaucoma, or difficulty in urination due to enlargement of the prostate gland except under the advice and supervision of a physician. As with any drug, if you are pregnant or nursing a baby, seek the advice of a health professional before using this product.

Caution: Avoid driving a motor vehicle or operating heavy machinery, or drinking alcoholic beverages. A persistent cough may be a sign of a serious condition. If cough persists for more than one week, tends to recur, or is accompanied by high fever, rash, or persistent headache, consult a physician.

Directions for Use:
Adults: (12 years and older): Take 2 teaspoonfuls every 4 hours. Do not exceed 12 teaspoonfuls in 24 hours.
Children (6–12 years): Take 1 teaspoonful every 4 hours. Do not exceed 6 teaspoonfuls in 24 hours.
Children (under 6 years): Consult physician for recommended dosage.

How Supplied: Benylin Cough Syrup is supplied in 4-oz and 8-oz bottles. Store at 59°–86°F.
Shown in Product Identification Section, page 420

BENYLIN DM®
dextromethorphan cough syrup

Description: Each teaspoonful (5 ml) contains:
Dextromethorphan
Hydrobromide   10 mg
Also contains: Alcohol 5%; Ammonium Chloride; Caramel; Citric Acid; D&C Red No. 33; Flavor; Glucose Liquid; Glycerin; Menthol; Purified Water; Sodium Citrate; Sucrose.

Indications: For temporary relief of coughs due to colds, bronchial irritation or upper respiratory allergies.

Warnings: Do not take this product for persistent or chronic cough such as occurs with smoking, asthma, emphysema, or when cough is accompanied by excessive secretions except under the advice

Continued on next page

This product information was prepared in November 1989. On these and other Parke-Davis Products, detailed information may be obtained by addressing PARKE-DAVIS, Consumer Health Products Group, Division of Warner-Lambert Company, Morris Plains, NJ 07950.

Parke-Davis—Cont.

and supervision of a physician. A persistent cough may be a sign of a serious condition. If cough persists for more than one week, tends to recur, or is accompanied by high fever, rash or persistent headache, consult a physician. Do not give to children under 2 years of age except under the advice and supervision of a physician. As with any drug, if you are pregnant or nursing a baby, seek the advice of a health professional before using this product. Keep this and all drugs out of the reach of children. In case of accidental overdose, seek professional assistance or contact a poison control center immediately.

Directions for Use:
Adults (12 years and older): Take 1 to 2 teaspoonfuls every 4 hours or 3 teaspoonfuls every 6 to 8 hours. Do not exceed 12 teaspoonfuls in 24 hours.
Children (6–12 years): Take ½–1 teaspoonful every 4 hours or 1½ teaspoonfuls every 6 to 8 hours. Do not exceed 6 teaspoonfuls in 24 hours.
Children (2–6 years): Take ¼ to ½ teaspoonful every 4 hours or ¾ teaspoonful every 6 to 8 hours. Do not exceed 3 teaspoonfuls in 24 hours.
Children (under 2 years): Consult physician for recommended dosage.

How Supplied: 4-oz bottles.
Store at 59°–86°F.
Shown in Product Identification Section, page 420

BENYLIN Decongestant

Description: Each teaspoonful (5 ml) contains:
Diphenhydramine
Hydrochloride   12.5 mg
Pseudoephedrine
Hydrochloride   30.0 mg
Also contains: Alcohol 5%; FD&C Yellow No. 6 (Sunset Yellow); Flavors; Glucose Liquid; Glycerin; Menthol; Purified Water; Saccharin Sodium; Sodium Citrate; Sucrose.

Indications: For the temporary relief of cough due to minor throat and bronchial irritations as may occur with the common cold or with inhaled irritants; and nasal congestion due to the common cold, hay fever, or other upper respiratory allergies.

Warnings: May cause marked drowsiness. Keep this and all drugs out of the reach of children. In case of accidental overdose, seek professional assistance or contact a poison control center immediately. Do not exceed recommended dosage because at higher doses nervousness, dizziness or sleeplessness may occur. Do not give to children under six years of age except under the advice and supervision of a physician. May cause excitability especially in children. Do not take this product for persistent or chronic cough such as occurs with smoking, asthma, emphysema or when cough is accompanied by excessive secretions, or if you have high blood pressure, heart

disease, diabetes, thyroid disease, glaucoma or difficulty in urination due to enlargement of the prostate gland except under the advice and supervision of a physician. If symptoms do not improve within seven days or are accompanied by high fever, consult a physician before continuing use. As with any drug, if you are pregnant or nursing a baby, seek the advice of a health professional before using this product.

Caution: Avoid driving a motor vehicle or operating heavy machinery, or drinking alcoholic beverages. A persistent cough may be a sign of a serious condition. If cough persists for more than one week, tends to recur or is accompanied by high fever, rash, or persistent headache, consult a physician.

Drug Interaction Precaution: Do not take this product if you are presently taking a prescription drug for high blood pressure or depression without consulting your doctor.

Directions for Use:
Adults (12 years and older): Take 2 teaspoonfuls every 4 hours. Do not exceed 8 teaspoonfuls in 24 hours.
Children (6–12 years): Take 1 teaspoonful every 4 hours. Do not exceed 4 teaspoonfuls in 24 hours.
Children (under 6 years): Consult physician for recommended dosage.

How Supplied: 4-oz. bottles. Store at 59°–86°F.
Shown in Product Identification Section, page 420

BENYLIN® Expectorant

Description: Each 4 teaspoonfuls (20 ml) contains:
Dextromethorphan
Hydrobromide   20.0 mg
Guaifenesin   400.0 mg
Also contains: Alcohol 5%; Citric Acid; FD&C Red No. 40; Flavors; Glycerin; Purified Water; Saccharin Sodium, Sodium Benzoate, Sodium Citrate; Sucrose.

Indications: For temporary relief of coughs plus accompanying upper chest congestion due to colds, bronchial irritation or upper respiratory allergies.

Warnings: Keep this and all drugs out of the reach of children. In case of accidental overdose, seek professional assistance or contact a poison control center immediately. Do not give to children under 2 years of age unless directed by a physician. Do not take this product for persistent or chronic cough such as occurs with smoking, asthma, emphysema, or when cough is accompanied by excessive secretions unless directed by a physician. A persistent cough may be a sign of a serious condition. If cough persists for more than one week, tends to recur, or is accompanied by high fever, rash, or persistent headache, consult a physician. As with any drug, if you are pregnant or nursing a baby, seek the advice of a health professional before using this product.

Directions for Use:
Adults (12 years and older): Take 2–4 teaspoonfuls every 4 hours (or fill dosage cup to the corresponding teaspoon level indicated). Do not exceed 24 teaspoonfuls in 24 hours.
Children (6–12 years): Take 1–2 teaspoonfuls every 4 hours (or fill dosage cup to the corresponding teaspoon level indicated). Do not exceed 12 teaspoonfuls in 24 hours.
Children (2–6 years): Take ½–1 teaspoonful every 4 hours (or fill dosage cup to the corresponding teaspoon level indicated). Do not exceed 6 teaspoonfuls in 24 hours.
Children (under 2 years): Consult your physician for recommended dosage.

How Supplied: Benylin Expectorant is supplied in 4-oz and 8-oz bottles. Store at 59°–86°F.
Shown in Product Identification Section, page 420

CALADRYL® Lotion
[că 'lă drĭl "]
CALADRYL Cream

Description: Caladryl Lotion—A drying, calamine-antihistamine lotion containing Calamine 8%, Benadryl® (diphenhydramine hydrochloride), 1%. Also contains: Alcohol 2%; Camphor; Fragrances; Glycerin; Sodium Carboxymethylcellulose; and Water, Purified.
Caladryl Cream—Calamine 8%, Benadryl (diphenhydramine hydrochloride) 1%. Also contains: Camphor; Cetyl Alcohol; Cresin White; Fragrance; Propylene Glycol; Proplyparaben; Polysorbate 60; Sorbitan Stearate; Water, Purified.

Indications: For relief of itching due to mild poison ivy or oak, insect bites, or other minor skin irritations, and soothing relief of mild sunburn

Warnings: For external use only. Do not apply to blistered, raw or oozing areas of the skin. Do not use on chicken pox or measles, unless supervised by a doctor. Do not use on extensive areas of the skin or for longer than 7 days except as directed by a doctor. Avoid contact with the eyes or other mucous membranes. Discontinue use if burning sensation or rash develops or condition persists. Remove by washing with soap and water.

KEEP THIS AND ALL DRUGS OUT OF THE REACH OF CHILDREN. In case of accidental ingestion seek professional assistance or contact a Poison Control Center immediately.

Directions: For adults and children 6 years or age and older: Apply sparingly to the affected area three to four times daily. Before each application cleanse skin with soap and water and dry affected area. Children under 6 years of age: Consult a doctor.

How Supplied: Caladryl Cream; 1½-oz tubes.

Caladryl Lotion—2½ fl.-oz. (75 ml) squeeze bottles and 6 fl.-oz. bottles.

Shown in Product Identification Section, page 420

GELUSIL®
[jĕl'ū-sĭl]
Antacid–Anti-gas
Liquid/Tablets
Sodium Free

Each teaspoonful (5 ml) or tablet contains:
200 mg aluminum hydroxide
200 mg magnesium hydroxide
25 mg simethicone
Also contains: Liquid: Citric Acid; Flavors; Hydroxypropyl Methylcellulose; Methylparaben; Propylparaben; Sodium Carboxymethyl Cellulose; Sodium Saccharin; Sorbitol Solution; Water; Xanthan Gum.
Tablets: Flavors; Magnesium Stearate; Mannitol; Sorbitol; Sugar.

Advantages:
● High acid-neutralizing capacity
● Sodium free
● Simethicone for antiflatulent activity
● Good taste for better patient compliance
● Fast dissolution of chewed tablets for prompt relief

Indications: For the relief of heartburn, sour stomach, acid indigestion and to relieve symptoms of gas.

Dosage and Administration: Two or more teaspoonfuls or tablets one hour after meals and at bedtime, or as directed by a physician.
Tablets should be chewed.

Warnings: Do not take more than 12 tablets or teaspoonfuls in a 24-hour period, or use this maximum dosage for more than two weeks, or use this product if you have kidney disease, except under the advice and supervision of a physician.
Keep this and all drugs out of the reach of children.

Drug Interaction Precaution: Do not take this product if you are presently taking a prescription antibiotic drug containing any form of tetracycline.

How Supplied:
Liquid—In plastic bottles of 12 fl oz.
Tablets—White, embossed Gelusil P-D 034—individual strips of 10 in boxes of 50 and 100.
Store at 59°–86°F (15°–30°C).
Shown in Product Identification Section, page 420

GELUSIL–II®
[jĕl'ū-sĭl]
Antacid–Anti-gas
Liquid/Tablets
High Potency
Sodium Free

Each teaspoonful (5 ml) or tablet contains:
400 mg aluminum hydroxide
400 mg magnesium hydroxide
  30 mg simethicone
Also contains: Liquid: Citric Acid; Flavors; Hydroxypropyl Methylcellulose; Sodium Saccharin; Sorbitol Solution; Water; Xanthan Gum
Tablets: Artificial Orange Flavor; Calcium Stearate; FD&C Yellow No. 6; Fumaric Acid; Mannitol; Povidone; Saccharin Sodium; Sorbitol; Sugar, Syloid 244.

Advantages:
● High acid-neutralizing capacity
● Sodium free
● Simethicone for antiflatulent activity
● Good taste for better patient compliance
● Fast dissolution of chewed tablets for prompt relief
● Double strength antacid

Indications: For the relief of heartburn, sour stomach, acid indigestion and to alleviate or relieve symptoms of gas.

Dosage and Administration: Two or more teaspoonfuls or tablets one hour after meals and at bedtime, or as directed by a physician. Tablets should be chewed.

Warnings: Do not take more than 8 tablets or teaspoonfuls in a 24-hour period, or use this maximum dosage for more than two weeks, or use this product if you have kidney disease, except under the advice and supervision of a physician. Keep this and all drugs out of the reach of children.

Drug Interaction Precaution: Do not take this product if you are presently taking a prescription antibiotic drug containing any form of tetracycline.

How Supplied:
Liquid—In plastic bottles of 12 fl oz.
Tablets—Double-layered white/orange, embossed P-D 043—individual strips of 10 in boxes of 80.
Store at 15°–30°C (59°–86°F).

GERIPLEX-FS® KAPSEALS®
[jĕ'rĭ-plĕx]

Composition: Each Kapseal represents:

Vitamin A ....(1.5 mg) 5,000 IU*	
(acetate)	
Vitamin C.. 50 mg	
(ascorbic acid)†	
Vitamin B₁ .... 5 mg	
(thiamine mononitrate)	
Vitamin B₂ .... 5 mg	
(riboflavin)	
Vitamin B₁₂, crystalline	
(cyanocobalamin) .... 2 mcg	
Choline dihydrogen	
citrate... 20 mg	
Nicotinamide .... 15 mg	
(niacinamide)	
Vitamin E (dl -alpha-tocopheryl acetate) .... (5 mg) 5 IU*.	
Iron‡ .... 6 mg	
Copper sulfate..................................... 4 mg	
Manganese sulfate	
(monohydrate).............................. 4 mg	

*International Units
†Supplied as sodium ascorbate
‡Supplied as dried ferrous sulfate equivalent to the labeled amount of elemental iron

Zinc sulfate .... 2 mg
Calcium phosphate, dibasic
  (anhydrous)................................ 200 mg
Taka-Diastase® (*Aspergillus oryzae* enzymes) ....2½ gr
Docusate sodium .... 100 mg
Also contains magnesium stearate, NF.

The capsule shell contains FD&C Blue No. 1, FD&C Red No. 3 and Gelatin.

Action and Uses: A preparation containing vitamins, minerals, and a fecal softener for middle-aged and older individuals. The fecal softening agent, docusate sodium, acts to soften stools and make bowel movements easier.

Administration and Dosage: USUAL DOSAGE —One capsule daily, with or immediately after a meal.

How Supplied: Bottles of 100.
Store at controlled room temperature 15°–30°C (59° to 86°F). Protect from light and moisture.

GERIPLEX-FS®
[jĕ'rĭ-plĕx]
LIQUID
Geriatric Vitamin Formula with Iron and a Fecal Softener

Composition: Each 30 ml represents vitamin B₁ (thiamine hydrochloride), 1.2 mg; vitamin B₂ (as riboflavin-5'-phosphate sodium), 1.7 mg; vitamin B₆ (pyridoxine hydrochloride), 1 mg; vitamin B₁₂ (cyanocobalamin) crystalline, 5 mcg; niacinamide, 15 mg; iron (as ferric ammonium citrate, green), 15 mg; Pluronic® F-68,* 200 mg; alcohol, 18%.
Also contains: Brandy, Caramel NF, Citric Acid Anhydrous NF, D&C Red No. 33, Flavors, FD&C Red No. 40, Glucono Delta Lactone, Glucose Liquid USP, Glycerin USP, Sodium Citrate USP, Sodium Saccharin NF, Sorbitol Solution USP, Sugar, Water Purified.

Administration and Dosage: USUAL ADULT DOSAGE—Two tablespoonfuls (30 ml) daily or as recommended by the physician.

How Supplied: 16-oz bottles.
Store below 30° (86°F). Protect from light and freezing.

*Pluronic is a registered trademark of BASF Wyandotte Corporation for polymers of ethylene oxide and propylene oxide.

This product information was prepared in November 1989. On these and other Parke-Davis Products, detailed information may be obtained by addressing PARKE-DAVIS, Consumer Health Products Group, Division of Warner-Lambert Company, Morris Plains, NJ 07950.

Parke-Davis—Cont.

MYADEC
High Potency Multivitamin Multimineral Formula

Each Tablet Represents:

		% of US Recommended Daily Allowances (US RDA)
Vitamins		
Vitamin A	9,000 IU*	180%
Vitamin D	400 IU	100%
Vitamin E	30 IU	100%
Vitamin C (ascorbic acid)	90 mg	150%
Folic Acid	0.4 mg	100%
Thiamine (vitamin B₁)	10 mg	667%
Riboflavin (vitamin B₂)	10 mg	588%
Niacin**	20 mg	100%
Vitamin B₆	5 mg	250%
Vitamin B₁₂	10 mcg	167%
Pantothenic Acid	20 mg	200%
Vitamin K	25 mcg	***
Biotin	45 mcg	15%
Minerals		
Iodine	150 mcg	100%
Iron	30 mg	167%
Magnesium	100 mg	25%
Copper	3 mg	150%
Zinc	15 mg	100%
Manganese	7.5 mg	***
Calcium	70 mg	7%
Phosphorus	54 mg	5%
Potassium	8 mg	***
Selenium	15 mcg	***
Molybdenum	15 mcg	***
Chromium	15 mcg	***

* International Units
** Supplied as niacinamide
*** No US Recommended Daily Allowance (US RDA) has been established for this nutrient.

Ingredients: Dicalcium phosphate, magnesium oxide, ferrous fumarate, niacinamide ascorbate, alcohol SD3A, dl-alpha tocopheryl acetate, microcrystalline cellulose, ascorbic acid, zinc sulfate, hydroxypropyl methylcellulose, calcium pantothenate, croscarmellose sodium, manganese sulfate, Vitamin A acetate, potassium chloride, purified water, povidone, FD&C Yellow No. 6 Al lake, thiamine mononitrate, riboflavin, silica gel, stearic acid, vitamin A and D crystalets, pyridoxine hydrochloride, titanium dioxide, FD&C Blue No. 2 Al lake, FD&C Red No. 40 Al lake, cupric sulfate, phytonadione, polyethylene glycol 3350, magnesium stearate, silicon dioxide, sterotex, citric acid, methyl paraben, folic acid, candelilla wax, hydroxypropyl cellulose, polysorbate 80, vanillin, potassium iodide, propyl paraben, chromium chloride, biotin, sodium molybdate, sodium selenate, cyanocobalamin.

Actions and Uses: High potency vitamin supplement with minerals for adults.

Dosage: One tablet daily with a full meal.

How Supplied: In bottles of 130. Store below 30°C (86°F). Protect from moisture.
Shown in Product Identification Section, page 420

NATABEC® KAPSEALS®

Each capsule represents:

Vitamins	
Vitamin A	4,000 IU*
Vitamin D	400 IU
Vitamin C	50 mg
Vitamin B₁	3 mg
Vitamin B₂	2.0 mg
Nicotinamide†	10 mg
Vitamin B₆	3 mg
Vitamin B₁₂	5 mcg
Minerals	
Precipitated Calcium carbonate	600 mg
Iron	30 mg

*IU = International Units
†Supplied as niacinamide

Action and Uses: A multivitamin and mineral supplement for use during pregnancy and lactation.

Dosage: One capsule daily, or as directed by physician.

How Supplied: In bottles of 100.
The color combination of the banded capsule is a Warner-Lambert trademark.

PROMEGA™
Natural Fish Oil Concentrate

Description: PROMEGA is a natural fish body oil concentrate which provides a rich dietary source of Omega-3 fatty acids, including eicosapentaenoic acid (EPA) and docosahexaenoic acid (DHA). Concentrated from certain oily cold water fish, not common in the American diet, these polyunsaturated fats can't be manufactured in the body. They must be obtained through the diet. If enough fish is not eaten, you may wish to include PROMEGA as part of a total dietary plan which includes reducing total fat and substituting polyunsaturated fats for some of the saturated animal fats in the diet to help lower the risk of heart disease. Other sensible steps such as regular exercise, smoking cessation, and weight control should be followed.
PROMEGA is cholesterol free (contains less than 1 mg cholesterol per softgel) and contains the highest percentage concentration of natural omega-3 available.

Recommended Adult Use: Take one to two softgels with each meal or together as a daily dietary supplement.
Each 1000 mg PROMEGA softgel supplies:

EPA (eicosapentaenoic acid)	280 mg
DHA (docosahexaenoic acid)	120 mg
Other Omega-3 fatty acids	100 mg
Vitamin E (d-alpha tocopherol)	1 IU

This and all dietary supplements should be kept out of reach of children.
MATERIALS IN THIS PRODUCT ARE DERIVED FROM ALL NATURAL SOURCES. PROMEGA contains no sugar, starch, wax, or artificial colors, flavors, preservatives. Excess saturated fats and environmental pollutants have been removed through the unique concentration process.

Ingredients: Fish oil concentrate, mixed tocopherols concentrate (antioxidant) in a softgel consisting of gelatin, glycerin and water.

Caution: If patients are taking anticoagulants or have bleeding problems a physician should be consulted before taking fish oil supplements.

How Supplied: Bottles of 30 or 60 softgels.

Storage: For maximum potency, store softgels at 59°F–86°F.
Shown in Product Identification Section, page 420

PROMEGA™ PEARLS
Natural Fish Oil Concentrate

Description: PROMEGA Pearls is a natural fish body oil concentrate which provides a rich dietary source of Omega-3 fatty acids, including eicosapentaenoic acid (EPA) and docosahexaenoic acid (DHA). Concentrated from certain oily cold water fish, not common in the American diet, these polyunsaturated fats can't be manufactured in the body. They must be obtained through the diet. If enough fish is not eaten, you may wish to include Promega as part of a total dietary plan which includes reducing total fat and substituting polyunsaturated fats for some of the saturated animal fats in the diet to help lower the risk of heart disease. Other sensible steps such as regular exercise, smoking cessation, and weight control should be followed.
PROMEGA is cholesterol free (contains less than 1 mg cholesterol per softgel) and contains the highest percentage concentration of natural omega-3 available.

Recommended Adult Use: Take one to two softgels with each meal or together as a daily dietary supplement.
Each 600 mg PROMEGA softgel pearl supplies:

EPA (eicosapentaenoic acid)	168 mg
DHA (docosahexaenoic acid)	72 mg
Other Omega-3 fatty acids	60 mg
Vitamin E (d-alpha tocopherol)	1 IU

This and all dietary supplements should be kept out of reach of children.
MATERIALS IN THIS PRODUCT ARE DERIVED FROM ALL NATURAL SOURCES. PROMEGA contains no sugar, starch, wax, or artificial colors, flavors, preservatives. Excess saturated fats and environmental pollutants have been removed through the unique concentration process.

Ingredients: Fish oil concentrate, mixed tocopherols concentrate (antioxidant) in a softgel consisting of gelatin, glycerin and water.

Caution: If patients are taking anticoagulants or have bleeding problems a physician should be consulted before taking fish oil supplements.

How Supplied: Bottles of 60 softgel Pearls

Storage: For maximum potency, store softgels at 59°F–86°F.

Shown in Product Identification Section, page 420

SINUTAB® Allergy Formula Sustained Action Tablets

Active Ingredients: Each sustained action tablet contains: Dexbrompheniramine maleate 6 mg., pseudoephedrine sulfate 120 mg.

Inactive Ingredients: Acacia, calcium carbonate, carnauba wax, confectioner's sugar, D&C yellow No. 10, FD&C blue No. 1, FD&C yellow No. 6, gelatin, hydrogenated castor oil, magnesium stearate, methylparaben, povidone, propylparaben, shellac, sodium benzoate, sucrose, talc, titanium dioxide.

Indications: For temporary relief of nasal congestion due to the common cold, hay fever or other upper respiratory allergies and associated with sinusitis. Combines a nasal decongestant with an antihistamine in a special continuous-acting, timed-release tablet to provide temporary relief from nasal congestion, running nose, and sneezing.

Actions: Sinutab Allergy Formula Sustained Action Tablets contain an antihistamine (dexbrompheniramine maleate) to help control upper respiratory allergic symptoms and a decongestant (pseudoephedrine sulfate) to reduce congestion of the nasopharyngeal mucosa. Half of the medication is released after the tablet is swallowed, and the remaining amount of medication is released hours later, providing continuous long-lasting relief for 12 hours.

Dexbrompheniramine maleate is an antihistamine incorporated to alleviate runny nose, sneezing, itching of the nose or throat, and itchy watery eyes as may occur in allergic rhinitis (such as hay fever). Pseudoephedrine sulfate, a sympathomimetic drug, provides vasoconstriction of the nasopharyngeal mucosa, resulting in a nasal decongestant effect (decongests sinus openings and passages, reduces swelling of nasal passages, shrinks swollen membranes, and temporarily restores free breathing through the nose).

Warnings: If symptoms do not improve within 7 days or are accompanied by high fever, consult a physician before continuing use. May cause drowsiness; alcohol may increase the drowsiness effect. May cause excitability, especially in children. Do not exceed recommended dosage because at higher doses nervousness, dizziness, or sleeplessness may occur. Do not give this product to children under 12 years except under the advice and supervision of a physician. Do not take this product if you have emphysema, chronic pulmonary disease, shortness of breath and difficulty in breathing, asthma, glaucoma, difficulty in urination due to en-largement of the prostate gland, high blood pressure, heart disease, diabetes, or thyroid disease except under the advice and supervision of a physician. As with any drug, if you are pregnant or nursing a baby, seek the advice of a health professional before using this product.

Caution: Avoid driving a motor vehicle or operating heavy machinery. Avoid alcoholic beverages while taking this product.

Drug Interaction: Do not take this product if you are presently taking a prescription antihypertensive or antidepressant drug containing a monoamine oxidase inhibitor except under the advice and supervision of a physician.

Precaution: Keep this and all drugs out of the reach of children.

Symptoms and Treatment of Oral Overdosage: In case of accidental overdose, seek professional assistance or contact a Poison Control Center immediately.

Dosage and Administration: Adults and children 12 years and over—1 tablet, every 12 hours. Do not exceed two tablets in 24 hours.

How Supplied: Sinutab Allergy Formula Sustained Action Tablets are green and coated. They are supplied in easy-to-open blister packs of 10 and 20 tablets.

Shown in Product Identification Section, page 420

SINUTAB® Regular Strength Without Drowsiness Formula Tablets

Active Ingredients: Each tablet contains: Acetaminophen 325 mg., pseudoephedrine hydrochloride 30 mg.

Inactive Ingredients: Cellulose microcrystalline, croscarmellose sodium, D&C red No. 33, FD&C red No. 40, hydroxypropyl cellulose, hydroxypropyl methylcellulose, magnesium stearate, propylene glycol, simethicone, starch pregelatinized, titanium dioxide, zinc stearate.

Indications: For temporary relief of sinus symptoms due to colds, flu, allergy and hay fever. Contains a nonaspirin analgesic to relieve headache pain and a decongestant to ease pressure and congestion.

Actions: Sinutab® Regular Strength Without Drowsiness Formula Tablets contain an analgesic (acetaminophen) to relieve pain and a decongestant (pseudoephedrine hydrochloride) to reduce congestion of the nasopharyngeal mucosa. Acetaminophen is both analgesic and antipyretic. Because acetaminophen is not a salicylate, Sinutab® Regular Strength Without Drowsiness Formula Tablets can be used by patients who are allergic to aspirin.

Pseudoephedrine hydrochloride, a sympathomimetic drug, provides vasoconstriction of the nasopharyngeal mucosa resulting in a nasal decongestant effect. The absence of antihistamine in the formula provides the added benefit of reduced likelihood of drowsiness side effects.

Warnings: Do not exceed recommended dosage. If symptoms persist, do not improve within 7 days, or are accompanied by high fever, or if new symptoms occur, see your doctor before continuing use. Do not take this product if you have high blood pressure, heart disease, diabetes, thyroid disease, or difficulty in urination due to an enlarged prostate except under doctor's supervision. Do not take this product for more than 10 days. As with any drug, if you are pregnant or nursing a baby, seek the advice of a health professional before using this product.

Drug Interaction: Do not take this product if you are presently taking a prescription drug for high blood pressure or depression without first consulting your doctor.

Precaution: Keep this and all drugs out of the reach of children.

Symptoms and Treatment of Oral Overdosage: In case of accidental overdose, seek professional help or contact a Poison Control Center immediately.

Dosage and Administration: Adults 2 tablets every 4 hours, not to exceed 8 tablets in 24 hours, or as directed by physician. Children under 12 should use only as directed by physician.

How Supplied: Sinutab® Regular Strength Without Drowsiness Formula Tablets are pink, uncoated and scored so that tablets may be split in half. They are supplied in child-resistant blister packs in boxes of 12 tablets and in easy-to-open (exempt) blister packs of 24 tablets, and in bottles of 100 tablets with child-resistant caps.

Shown in Product Identification Section, page 420

SINUTAB® Maximum Strength Formula Tablets and Caplets

Active Ingredients: Each tablet/caplet contains: Acetaminophen 500 mg., chlorpheniramine maleate 2 mg., pseudoephedrine hydrochloride 30 mg.

Inactive Ingredients:
Tablets contain: Carboxymethyl starch, cellulose, corn starch, croscarmellose sodium, hydroxypropyl cellulose, stearic acid, zinc stearate, D&C yellow No. 10 aluminum lake and FD&C yellow No. 6 aluminum lake.

Caplets contain: Cellulose, corn starch, croscarmellose sodium, hydroxypropyl cellulose, hydroxypropyl methylcellu-

Continued on next page

This product information was prepared in November 1989. On these and other Parke-Davis Products, detailed information may be obtained by addressing PARKE-DAVIS, Consumer Health Products Group, Division of Warner-Lambert Company, Morris Plains, NJ 07950.

Parke-Davis—Cont.

lose, magnesium stearate, polyethylene glycol, sodium starch glycolate, stearic acid, titanium dioxide, zinc stearate, D&C yellow No. 10 aluminum lake, and FD&C yellow No. 6 aluminum lake.

Indications: For temporary relief of sinus symptoms due to colds, flu, allergy and hay fever. Contains a nonaspirin analgesic to relieve headache pain, a decongestant to ease pressure and congestion and an antihistamine to dry up runny nose, watery eyes.

Actions: Sinutab® Maximum Strength Formula Tablets and Caplets contain an analgesic (acetaminophen) to relieve pain, a decongestant (pseudoephedrine hydrochloride) to reduce congestion of the nasopharyngeal mucosa, and an antihistamine (chlorpheniramine maleate) to help control allergic symptoms.
Acetaminophen is both analgesic and antipyretic. Because acetaminophen is not a salicylate, Sinutab® Maximum Strength Formula Tablets and Caplets can be used by patients who are allergic to aspirin.
Pseudoephedrine hydrochloride, a sympathomimetic drug, provides vasoconstriction of the nasopharyngeal mucosa resulting in a nasal decongestant effect. Chlorpheniramine maleate is an antihistamine incorporated to provide relief of running nose, sneezing, itching of the nose or throat, and itchy and watery eyes as may occur in allergic rhinitis.

Warnings: Do not exceed recommended dosage. If symptoms persist, do not improve within 7 days, or are accompanied by high fever, or if new symptoms occur, see your doctor before continuing use. Do not take this product if you have high blood pressure, heart disease, diabetes, thyroid disease, asthma, glaucoma, or difficulty in urination due to an enlarged prostate except under doctor's supervision. Do not take this product for more than 10 days. As with any drug, if you are pregnant or nursing a baby, seek the advice of a health professional before using this product. This product may cause drowsiness. Avoid driving a motor vehicle or operating heavy machinery and avoid alcoholic beverages while taking this product.

Drug Interaction: Do not take this product if you are presently taking a prescription drug for high blood pressure or depression without first consulting your doctor.

Precaution: Keep this and all drugs out of the reach of children.

Symptoms and Treatment of Oral Overdosage: In case of accidental overdose, seek professional help or contact a Poison Control Center immediately.

Dosage and Administration: Adults 2 tablets or caplets every 6 hours, not to exceed 8 tablets or caplets in 24 hours, or as directed by physician. Children under

12 should use only as directed by physician.

How Supplied: Sinutab® Maximum Strength Formula Caplets are yellow and coated. The Tablets are yellow and uncoated. They are supplied in child-resistant blister packs in boxes of 24 tablets or caplets.

Shown in Product Identification Section, page 420

SINUTAB® Maximum Strength Without Drowsiness Formula Tablets and Caplets

Active Ingredients: Each tablet/caplet contains: Acetaminophen 500 mg., pseudoephedrine hydrochloride 30 mg.

Inactive Ingredients:
Tablets contain: Carboxymethyl starch, cellulose, corn starch, croscarmellose sodium, hydroxypropyl cellulose, stearic acid, zinc stearate, D&C yellow No. 10 aluminum lake and FD&C yellow No. 6 aluminum lake.
Caplets contain: Cellulose, corn starch, croscarmellose sodium, hydroxypropyl cellulose, hydroxypropyl methylcellulose, magnesium stearate, polyethylene glycol, sodium starch glycolate, stearic acid, titanium dioxide, zinc stearate, D&C yellow No. 10 aluminum lake and FD&C yellow No. 6 aluminum lake.

Indications: For temporary relief of sinus symptoms due to colds, flu, allergy and hay fever. Contains a nonaspirin analgesic to relieve headache pain and a decongestant to ease pressure and congestion.

Actions: Sinutab® Maximum Strength Without Drowsiness Formula Tablets and Caplets contains an analgesic (acetaminophen) to relieve pain, and a decongestant (pseudoephedrine hydrochloride) to reduce congestion of the nasopharyngeal mucosa.
Acetaminophen is both analgesic and antipyretic. Because acetaminophen is not a salicylate, Sinutab® Maximum Strength Without Drowsiness Formula can be used by patients who are allergic to aspirin.
Pseudoephedrine hydrochloride, a sympathomimetic drug, provides vasoconstriction of the nasopharyngeal mucosa resulting in a nasal decongestant effect. The absence of antihistamine in the formula provides the added benefit of reduced likelihood of drowsiness side effects.

Warnings: Do not exceed recommended dosage. If symptoms persist, do not improve within seven days, or are accompanied by high fever, or if new symptoms occur, see your doctor before continuing use. Do not take this product if you have high blood pressure, heart disease, diabetes, thyroid disease, or difficulty in urination due to an enlarged prostate except under doctor's supervision. Do not take this product for more than 10 days. As with any drug, if you are pregnant or nursing a baby, seek the advice of a health professional before using this product.

Drug Interaction: Do not take this product if you are presently taking a prescription drug for high blood pressure or depression without first consulting your doctor.

Precaution: Keep this and all drugs out of the reach of children.

Symptoms and Treatment of Oral Overdosage: In case of accidental overdose, seek professional help or contact a Poison Control Center immediately.

Dosage and Administration: Adults 2 tablets every 6 hours, not to exceed 8 tablets in 24 hours or as directed by physician. Children under 12 should use only as directed by physician.

How Supplied: Sinutab® Maximum Strength Without Drowsiness Formula Caplets are orange and coated. The Tablets are orange and uncoated. They are supplied in child-resistant blister packs in boxes of 24 tablets or caplets and in bottles of 50 tablets with child-resistant caps.

Shown in Product Identification Section, page 420

THERA-COMBEX H-P®
High-Potency Vitamin B Complex with 500 mg Vitamin C

Composition: Each Kapseal contains:
Ascorbic acid
(vitamin C).................................. 500 mg
Thiamine (vitamin B_1)
mononitrate................................. 25 mg
Riboflavin
(vitamin B_2)............................. 15 mg
Pyridoxine hydrochloride
(vitamin B_6)............................. 10 mg
Vitamin B_{12}
(cyanocobalamin)....................... 5 mcg
Niacinamide.................................. 100 mg
dl-Panthenol .... 20 mg

Uses: For the prevention or treatment of vitamin B complex and vitamin C deficiencies.

Dosage: One or two capsules daily

How Supplied: Bottles of 100.

TUCKS®
Pre-moistened Hemorrhoidal/Vaginal Pads

Indications: For prompt, temporary relief of minor external itching, burning and irritation associated with hemorrhoids, rectal or vaginal surgical stitches and other minor rectal or vaginal irritation.
—Soothe, cool, and comfort itching, burning, and irritation of sensitive rectal and outer vaginal areas.
—As a compress, to help relieve discomfort from rectal/vaginal surgical stitches.
—Effective hygienic wipe to cleanse rectal area of irritation-causing residue.
—Solution buffered to help prevent further irritation.

Directions: For external use only. Use as a wipe following bowel movement, during menstruation, or after napkin or tampon change. Or, as a compress, apply to affected area 10 to 15 minutes as needed. Change compresses every 5 minutes.

Warnings: In case of rectal bleeding, consult physician promptly. In case of continued irritation, discontinue use and consult a physician. Keep this and all medication out of the reach of children. In case of accidental ingestion seek professional assistance or contact a Poison Control Center immediately.

Contains: Soft pads pre-moistened with a solution containing 50% Witch Hazel; 10% Glycerin USP; also contains: Benzalkonium Chloride NF 0.003%, Citric acid, USP; Methylparaben NF 0.1%; sodium citrate, USP; water, purified USP. Buffered to acid pH.

How Supplied: Jars of 40 and 100. Also available as Tucks Take-Alongs®, individual, foil-wrapped, nonwoven wipes, 12 per box
Shown in Product Identification Section, page 420

TUCKS® OINTMENT, CREAM

Composition: Tucks Ointment and Cream contain a specially formulated aqueous phase of 50% Witch Hazel (hamamelis water). Tucks Ointment also contains: alcohol 7%; arlacel; benzethonium chloride; lanolin anhydrous; sorbitol solution; and white petrolatum. Tucks Cream also contains: alcohol 7%; arlacel; benzethonium chloride; cetyl alcohol; lanolin anhydrous; polyethylene stearate; polysorbate; sorbitol solution; and white petrolatum.

Action and Uses: Both nonstaining Tucks Ointment and Tucks Cream exert a temporary soothing, cooling, mildly astringent effect on such superficial irritations as simple hemorrhoids, vaginal and rectal area itch, postepisiotomy discomfort and anorectal surgical wounds. Neither the Ointment nor the Cream contains steroids or skin-sensitizing "caine" type topical anesthetics.

Warning: If itching or irritation continues, discontinue use and consult your physician. In case of rectal bleeding, consult physician promptly. Keep this and all drugs out of the reach of children. In case of accidental ingestion seek professional assistance or contact a Poison Contol Center immediately.

Directions: Apply locally 3 or 4 times daily to temporarily soothe anal or outer vaginal irritation and itching, hemorrhoids, postepisiotomy and posthemorrhoidectomy discomfort.

How Supplied: Tucks Ointment and Tucks Cream (water-washable) in 40-g tubes with rectal applicators.

ZIRADRYL® Lotion
[zĭ'ră-drĭl]

Description: A zinc oxide-antihistaminic lotion of 1% Benadryl® (diphen-hydramine hydrochloride) and 2% zinc oxide; contains 2% alcohol. Also contains: camphor; chlorophylline sodium polysorbate; fragrances; glycerin; methocel; and water, purified.

Indications: For relief of itching due to mild poison ivy, poison oak or insect bites.

Directions: SHAKE WELL. For adults and children 6 years of age and older: Apply to the affected area not more than three to four times daily or as directed by your physician. Before each application, cleanse skin with soap and water and dry affected area. Temporary stinging sensation may follow application. Discontinue use if stinging persists. Removes easily with water. Children under 6 years of age: consult a physician.

Warnings: For external use only. Do not apply to blistered, raw or oozing areas of the skin. Do not use on chicken pox or measles unless supervised by a physician. Do not use on extensive areas of the skin or for longer than 7 days except as directed by a physician. Avoid contact with the eyes or other mucous membranes. If condition worsens or if symptoms persist for more than 7 days or clear up and occur again within a few days or if burning sensation or rash develops discontinue use of this product and consult a physician. KEEP THIS AND ALL DRUGS OUT OF REACH OF CHILDREN. In case of accidental ingestion, seek professional assistance or contact a Poison Control Center immediately.

How Supplied: 6-oz bottles. Protect from freezing.
Shown in Product Identification Section, page 420

Pharmafair, Inc.
**205-C KELSEY LANE
SILO BEND
TAMPA, FL 33619**

OPHTHALMICS

Eye Drops 15ml
NDC 24208-595-73
(Tetrahydrozoline HCl)

Eye Wash 4oz
NDC 24208-835-80

Lubrifair Ointment ⅛oz
NDC 24208-480-55
(White Petroleum, Mineral Oil, Lanolin Ocular Emolient)

Lubrifair Solution 15ml
NDC 24208-840-64
(Dextran 70, Hydroxypropyl Methylcellulose)

Ocugestrin Solution 15ml
NDC 24208-765-04
(Phenylephrine HCl 0.12%)

Dry Eyes Solution (Tearfair) 15ml
NDC 24208-755-04
(Polyvinyl Alcohol)

Tearfair Ointment
(White Petrolatum, Mineral Oil, Lanolin)
⅛oz tube: NDC 24208-760-02
0.7gm unit dose (24 per box) NDC 24208-760-07

EAR PREPARATIONS

Ear Drops 15ml
NDC 24208-531-73
(Carbamide Peroxide 6.5%)

DERMATOLOGICALS

Cortifair 0.5% Cream
(Hydrocortisone 0.5%)
15gm NDC 24208-510-82
30gm NDC 24208-510-84
425gm NDC 24208-510-90

Cortifair 0.5% Lotion
(Hydrocortisone 0.5%)
1oz NDC 24208-500-75

Tolnaftate 1% Cream 15gm
NDC 24208-985-52

Tolnaftate 1% Solution 10ml
NDC 24208-506-62

Topisporin Ointment
(Bacitracin Zinc, Neomycin Sulfate, Polymyxin B Sulfate)
15gm: NDC 24208-530-02
30gm: NDC 24208-530-04

TABLETS (ORAL PREPARATIONS)

Meclizine HCl Chewable Tablets 25mg
bottles of 100 NDC 24208-075-01
bottles of 1000 NDC 24208-075-10
unit dose 100's NDC 24208-075-11

Plough, Inc.
**3030 JACKSON AVENUE
MEMPHIS, TN 38151**

**AFTATE® Antifungal
Aerosol Liquid
Aerosol Powder
Gel
Powder**

Active Ingredient: Tolnaftate 1% (Also contains: Aerosol Spray Liquid-36% alcohol; Aerosol Spray Powder-14% alcohol.)

How Supplied:
AFTATE for Athlete's Foot
Sprinkle Powder—2.25 oz. bottle
Aerosol Spray Powder—3.5 oz can
Gel—.5 oz. tube.
Aerosol Spray Liquid—4 oz. can.

AFTATE for Jock Itch
Aerosol Spray Powder—3.5 oz. can
Sprinkle Powder—1.5 oz. bottle.
Gel—.5 oz. tube.
Shown in Product Identification Section, page 421

Continued on next page

Plough—Cont.

COPPERTONE® Waterproof Sunscreens

COPPERTONE® Sunscreen Lotion SPF 6
COPPERTONE® Sunscreen Lotion SPF 8
COPPERTONE® Sunblock Lotion SPF 15
COPPERTONE® Sunblock Lotion SPF 25
COPPERTONE® Sunblock Lotion SPF 30
COPPERTONE Sunblock Lotion SPF 45

New PABA-Free ingredients:
SPF 6–15: Ethylhexyl-p-methoxy-cinnamate, oxybenzone
SPF 25, 30: Ethylhexyl-p-methoxy-cinnamate, 2-ethylhexyl salicylate, homosalate, oxybenzone
SPF 45: Ethylhexyl-p-methoxy-cinnamate, 2-ethylhexyl salicylate, octocrylene, oxybenzone

How Supplied: 4 fl. oz. Plastic Bottles
Shown in Product Identification Section, page 421

COPPERTONE® Sun Spray Mist SPF 10

Active Ingredients: Ethylhexyl P-Methoxycinnamate, 2-Ethylhexyl Salicylate, Oxybenzone.

How Supplied: 7.25 oz. Plastic Bottle.

CORRECTOL®
Laxative
Tablets

Active Ingredients: Tablets—Yellow phenolphthalein, 65 mg. and docusate sodium, 100 mg. per tablet.

Inactive Ingredients: Butylparaben, calcium gluconate, calcium sulfate, carnauba wax, D&C No. 7 calcium lake, gelatin, magnesium stearate, sugar, talc, titanium dioxide, wheat flour, white wax, and other ingredients.

Indications: For relief of occasional constipation or irregularity. CORRECTOL generally produces bowel movement in 6 to 8 hours.

Actions: Yellow phenolphthalein—stimulant laxative; docusate sodium—fecal softener.

Warnings: Not to be taken in case of nausea, vomiting, abdominal pain, or signs of appendicitis. Take only as needed —as frequent or continued use of laxatives may result in dependence on them. If skin rash appears, do not use this or any other preparation containing phenolphthalein. As with any drug, if you are pregnant or nursing a baby, seek the advice of a health professional before using this product.

Dosage and Administration
Dosage: Adults—1 or 2 tablets daily as needed, at bedtime or on arising.
Children over 6 years—1 tablet daily as needed.

How Supplied: Tablets—Individual foil-backed safety sealed blister packaging in boxes of 15, 30, 60 and 90 tablets.
Shown in Product Identification Section, page 421

DI–GEL®
Antacid · Anti-Gas
Tablets/Liquid

DI-GEL Tablets: Active Ingredients: (Per Tablet)—Simethicone 20 mg., Calcium Carbonate 280 mg., Magnesium Hydroxide 128 mg. **Inactive Ingredients:** D & C yellow No. 10 aluminum lake, dextrin, FD&C yellow No. 6 aluminum lake, flavor, magnesium stearate, mannitol, polyvinyl-pyrrolidone, stearic acid, sucrose, talc.
Dietetically sodium free, calcium rich.

DI-GEL Liquid: Active Ingredients—per teaspoonful (5 ml): Simethicone 20 mg., aluminum hydroxide (equivalent to aluminum hydroxide dried gel USP) 200 mg., magnesium hydroxide 200 mg. **Also contains:** Flavor, methylcellulose, methylparaben, propylparaben, sodium saccharin, sorbitol, water.
Dietetically sodium free.

Indications: For fast, temporary relief of acid indigestion, heartburn, sour stomach and accompanying painful gas symptoms.

Actions: The antacid system in DI-GEL relieves and soothes acid indigestion, heartburn and sour stomach. At the same time, the simethicone "defoamers" eliminate gas.
When air becomes entrapped in the stomach, heartburn and acid indigestion can result, along with sensations of fullness, pressure and bloating.

Warnings: Do not take more than 20 teaspoonfuls or 24 tablets in a 24 hour period, or use the maximum dosage of this product for more than 2 weeks, except under the advice and supervision of a physician. If you have kidney disease do not use this product except under the advice and supervision of a physician. May cause constipation or have a laxative effect.

Drug Interaction: (Liquid Only) This product should not be taken if patient is presently taking a prescription antibiotic drug containing any form of tetracycline.

Dosage and Administration: Two teaspoonfuls or tablets every 2 hours, or after or between meals and at bedtime, not to exceed 20 teaspoonfuls or 24 tablets per day, or as directed by a physician.

How Supplied:
DI-GEL Liquid in Mint and Lemon/Orange Flavors - 6 and 12 fl. oz. bottles, safety sealed.
DI-GEL Tablets in Mint and Lemon/Orange Flavors - In boxes of 30 and 90 in handy portable safety sealed blister packaging. Also available in Mint 3-roll (36 tablets) and in Mint 60-tablet bottles.
Shown in Product Identification Section, page 421

DURATION®
Long Acting Nasal Decongestant Tablets

Active Ingredients: Pseudoephedrine Sulfate 120 mg.

Inactive Ingredients: Acacia, Butylparaben, Calcium Sulfate, Carnauba Wax, Corn Starch, Eiderdown Soap, FD&C Blue No. 1, FD&C Yellow No, 6, Gelatin, Lactose, Magnesium Stearate, Oleic Acid, Povidone, Rosin, Sugar, Talc, White Wax, Zein.

Indications: For temporary relief of nasal congestion due to cold, hay fever or other upper respiratory allergies, and nasal congestion associated with sinusitis; promotes nasal and/or sinus drainage. Relief lasts up to 12 hours without drowsiness.

Warnings: Do not exceed recommended dosage. Do not use if you have high blood pressure, heart disease, diabetes or thyroid disease except under the advice of a physician. If symptoms do not improve within 7 days or are accompanied by high fever, consult a physician before continuing use. If you are pregnant or nursing a baby, seek the advice of a health professional before using this product.

Drug Interaction: Do not take this product if you are presently taking a prescription antihypertensive or antidepressant drug containing a monoamine oxidase inhibitor, except under the advice and supervision of a physician.

Symptoms and Treatment of Oral Overdosage: In case of accidental overdose, seek professional assistance or contact a Poison Control Center immediately.

Dosage and Administration: Adults and children 12 years of age and over: One tablet every 12 hours. Not recommended for children under 12 years of age.

How Supplied: Available in packages of 10 and 20 individually sealed tablets.
Shown in Product Identification Section, page 421

DURATION®
12 Hour Nasal Spray
12 Hour Mentholated Nasal Spray
Topical Nasal Decongestant

Active Ingredient:
12 Hour Nasal Spray:
        Oxymetazoline HCl 0.05%

Other Ingredients:
12 Hour Nasal Spray: Preservative Phenylmercuric Acetate (Mentholated Nasal Spray also contains the following aromatics: menthol, camphor, eucalyptol).

Indications: Immediate relief for up to 12 hours of nasal congestion due to colds, hay fever and sinusitis.

Actions: The sympathomimetic action of DURATION constricts the smaller arterioles of the nasal passages, producing a gentle and predictable decongesting effect.

Warnings: Do not exceed recommended dosage because symptoms may occur such as burning, stinging, sneezing, or increase of nasal discharge. Do not use this product for more than 3 days. If symptoms persist, consult a physician. The use of dispenser by more than one person may spread infection.

Dosage and Administration:
DURATION 12 Hour Nasal Spray— With head upright, spray 2 or 3 times in each nostril twice daily—morning and evening. To spray, squeeze bottle quickly and firmly. Not recommended for children under 6.

How Supplied:
DURATION 12 Hour Nasal Spray—½ and 1 fl. oz. plastic squeeze bottle. DURATION 12 Hour Mentholated Nasal Spray—½ fl. oz. plastic squeeze bottle. All bottles in safety sealed cartons.
Shown in Product Identification Section, page 421

DURATION®
12 Hour Nasal Spray Pump

Active Ingredients: Oxymetazoline Hydrochloride 0.05%

Inactive Ingredients: Aminoacetic Acid, Benzalkonium Chloride, Phenylmercuric Acetate (Preservative), Sorbitol, Water.

Indications: Delivers a measured dosage every time. Immediate relief of nasal congestion for up to 12 hours due to common cold, hay fever and sinusitis.

Warnings: Do not exceed recommended dosage because symptoms may occur such as burning, stinging, sneezing, or increase of nasal discharge. Do not use this product for more than 3 days. If symptoms persist, consult a physician. The use of dispenser by more than one person may spread infection. Keep this and all medications out of the reach of children.

Symptoms and Treatment of Oral Overdosage: In case of accidental ingestion, seek professional assistance or contact a Poison Control Center immediately.

Dosage and Administration: Before using first time, remove protective cap. Prime the metered pump by depressing several times. Hold bottle with thumb at base and nozzle between first and second fingers. With head upright (do not tilt backward), insert metered pump-spray nozzle in nostril. Depress pump completely 2 or 3 times. Sniff deeply. Repeat in other nostril. Wipe tip clean after each use.

How Supplied: Available in ½ fl. oz. pump spray.
Shown in Product Identification Section, page 421

FEEN-A-MINT®
Laxative Gum/Pills

Active Ingredients: Gum—yellow phenolphthalein 97.2 mg. per tablet. Pills—yellow phenolphthalein, 65 mg., and docusate sodium 100 mg. per pill. Chocolated—yellow phenolphthalein, 65 mg.

Indications: For relief of occasional constipation or irregularity. FEEN-A-MINT generally produces bowel movement in 6 to 8 hours.

Inactive Ingredients: Gum—Acacia, butylated hydroxyanisole, gelatin, glycerin, glucose, gum base, peppermint oil, sodium benzoate, starch, sugar, talc, water.
Pills—Butylparaben, calcium gluconate, calcium slufate, carnauba wax, gelatin, magnesium stearate, sugar, talc, titanium dioxide, wheat flour, white wax and other ingredients.
Chocolated—Cocoa, partially hydrogenated cottonseed and palm kernel oils, peppermint oil (flavor), salt, soya lecithin, sugar, vanillin (flavor).

How Supplied: Gum—Individual foil-backed safety sealed blister packaging in boxes of 5, 16, and 40 tablets.
Pills—Safety sealed boxes of 15, 30, and 60 tablets.
Chocolated—Safety sealed boxes of 4, 18 and 36 tablets.
Shown in Product Identification Section, page 421

REGUTOL®
Stool Softener Tablets

Active Ingredient: Each tablet contains 100 mg. docusate sodium.

Inactive Ingredients: Acacia, butylparaben, calcium sulfate, carnauba wax, D&C yellow No. 10 aluminum lake, FD&C yellow No. 6 aluminum lake, gelatin, lactose, magnesium stearate, povidone, sugar, talc, titanium dioxide, white wax.

How Supplied: REGUTOL tablets in boxes of 30, 60 and 90 individually safety sealed blister packaging.
Shown in Product Identification Section, page 421

ST. JOSEPH®
ADULT CHEWABLE ASPIRIN
Low Strength Caplets (81 mg. each)

Active Ingredient: Each St. Joseph Adult Chewable Aspirin caplet contains 81 mg. (1.25 grains) aspirin in a chewable, pleasant citrus-flavored form.

Inactive Ingredients: D&C yellow No. 10 aluminum lake, FD&C yellow No. 6 aluminum lake, flavor, hydrogenated vegetable oil, maltodextrin, mannitol, saccharin, starch.

Indications: For safe, effective, temporary relief from: headache, muscular aches, minor aches and pain associated with overexertion, sprains, menstrual cramps, neuralgia, bursitis, and discomforts of fever due to colds.

Actions: Analgesic/Antipyretic.

Warnings: Children and teenagers should not use this medicine for chicken pox or flu symptoms before a doctor is consulted about Reye syndrome, a rare but serious illness reported to be associated with aspirin. As with any drug, if you are pregnant or nursing a baby, seek the advice of a health professional before using this product. Keep out of reach of children. In case of an accidental overdose, seek professional assistance or contact a poison control center immediately.

Dosage and Administration: Adult Dose—Analgesic/Antipyretic Indication: Take from 4 to 8 caplets (325 mg. to 650 mg.) every 4 hours as needed. Do not exceed 48 caplets in 24 hours. For professional dosage see below.
IN MYOCARDIAL INFARCTION PROPHYLAXIS

Indication: Aspirin is indicated to reduce the risk of death and/or nonfatal myocardial infarction in patients with a previous infarction or unstable angina pectoris.

Advantages of Product Form: Four St. Joseph Adult Chewable Aspirin caplets give patients the appropriate dosage (325 mg.) of aspirin to help prevent secondary MI. Because they're chewable, they can be taken anytime and anyplace. And they have a pleasant-tasting citrus flavor.

Clinical Trials: The indication is supported by the results of six, large, randomized, multicenter, placebo-controlled studies[1-7] involving 10,816, predominantly male, post–myocardial infarction (MI) patients and one randomized placebo-controlled study of 1,266 men with unstable angina. Therapy with aspirin was begun at intervals after the onset of acute MI varying from less than 3 days to more than 5 years and continued for periods of from less than 1 year to 4 years. In the unstable angina study, treatment was started within 1 month after the onset of unstable angina and continued for 12 weeks; complicating conditions, such as congestive heart failure were not included in the study.
Aspirin therapy in MI patients was associated with about a 20% reduction in the risk of subsequent death and/or nonfatal reinfarction, a median absolute decrease of 3% from the 12 to 22% event rates in the placebo groups. In aspirin-treated unstable angina patients the reduction in risk was about 50%, a reduction in event rate of 5% from the 10% rate in the placebo group over the 12 weeks of the study.
Daily dosage of aspirin in the post–myocardial infarction studies was 300 mg. in one study and 900 to 1500 mg. in five studies. A dose of 325 mg. was used in the study of unstable angina.

Adverse Reactions: Gastrointestinal Reactions—Doses of 1000 mg. per day of aspirin caused gastrointestinal symptoms and bleeding that in some cases were clinically significant. In the largest

Continued on next page

Plough—Cont.

postinfarction study, the Aspirin Myocardial Infarction Study (AMIS) trial with 4,500 people, the percentage incidences of gastrointestinal symptoms for the aspirin (1000 mg. of a standard, solid-tablet formulation) and placebo-treated subjects, respectively, were: stomach pain (14.3%; 4.4%); heartburn (11.9%; 4.3%); nausea and/or vomiting (7.3%; 2.1%); hospitalization for GI disorder (4.9%; 3.3%). In the AMIS and other trials, aspirin-treated patients had increased rates of gross gastrointestinal bleeding.

Cardiovascular and Biochemical: In the AMIS trial, the dosage of 1000 mg. per day of aspirin was associated with small increases in systolic blood pressure (BP) (average 1.5 to 2.1 mm) and diastolic BP (0.5 to 0.6 mm), depending upon whether maximal or last available readings were used. Blood urea nitrogen and uric acid levels were also increased, but by less than 1.0 mg.%. Subjects with marked hypertension or renal insufficiency had been excluded from the trial so that the clinical importance of these observations for such subjects or for any subjects treated over more prolonged periods is not known. It is recommended that patients placed on long-term aspirin treatment, even at doses of 300 mg. per day, be seen at regular intervals to assess changes in these measurements.

Dosage and Administration: Although most of the studies used dosages exceeding 300 mg., two trials used only 300 mg. daily, and pharmacologic data indicate that this dose inhibits platelet function fully. Therefore, 300 mg. or a conventional 325 mg. aspirin dose daily is a reasonable routine dose that would minimize gastrointestinal adverse reactions.

How Supplied: Chewable citrus-flavored caplets in plastic bottles of 36 caplets each.

References: (1) Elwood, P.C., et al.: A Randomized Controlled Trial of Acetylsalicylic Acid in the Secondary Prevention of Mortality from Myocardial Infarction, *British Medical Journal,* 1:436–440, 1974. (2) The Coronary Drug Project Research Group: "Aspirin in Coronary Heart Disease," *Journal of Chronic Disease,* 29:625–642, 1976. (3) Breddin, K., et al.: "Secondary Prevention of Myocardial Infarction: A Comparison of Acetylsalicylic Acid, Placebo and Phenprocoumon, *Homeostasis,* 9:325–344, 1980. (4) Aspirin Myocardial Infarction Study Research Group, "A Randomized, Controlled Trial of Aspirin in Persons Recovered from Myocardial Infarction," *Journal American Medical Association,* 245:661–669, 1980. (5) Elwood, P.C., and Sweetnam, P.M., "Aspirin and Secondary Mortality After Myocardial Infarction," *Lancet,* pp. 1313–1315, December 22–29, 1979. (6) The Persantine-Aspirin Reinfarction Study Research Group, "Persantine and Aspirin in Coronary Heart Disease," *Circulation,* 62: 449–460, 1980. (7) Lewis, H.D., et al., "Protective Effects of Aspirin Against Acute Myocardial Infarction and Death in Men with Unstable Angina. Results of a Veterans Administration Cooperative Study," *New England Journal of Medicine,* 309:396–403, 1983.

Shown in Product Identification Section, page 421

ST. JOSEPH® Aspirin–Free Fever Reducer for Children
Chewable Tablets, Liquid, Drops

Active Ingredient: Each Children's St. Joseph Aspirin-Free Chewable Tablet contains 80 mg. acetaminophen in a fruit-flavored tablet. Children's St. Joseph Aspirin-Free Liquid is stable, cherry flavored, red in color and alcohol-free and sugar-free. Each 5 ml. contains 160 mg. acetaminophen. Infant's St. Joseph Aspirin-Free Drops are stable, fruit flavored, orange in color and alcohol-free and sugar-free. Each 0.8 ml. (one calibrated dropperful) contains 80 mg. acetaminophen.

Inactive Ingredients: Tablets: Cellulose, D&C red No. 7 calcium lake, D&C red No. 30 aluminum lake, flavor, mannitol, silicon dioxide, sodium saccharin, zinc stearate.
Liquid: FD&C yellow No. 6, flavor, glycerin, maltol, polyethylene glycol, propylene glycol, saccharin, sodium benzoate, sodium chloride, sodium saccharin, water.
Drops: FD&C yellow No. 6, flavor, glycerin, maltol, polyethylene glycol, propylene glycol, saccharin, sodium benzoate, sodium chloride, sodium saccharin, water.

Indications: For temporary reduction of fever, relief of minor aches and pains of colds and flu.

Actions: Analgesic/Antipyretic

Warnings: Do not administer this product for more than 5 days. If symptoms persist or new ones occur, consult physician. If fever persists for more than three days, or recurs, consult physician. When using St. Joseph Aspirin-Free products do not give other medications containing acetaminophen unless directed by your physician. NOTE: SEVERE OR PERSISTENT SORE THROAT, HIGH FEVER, HEADACHES, NAUSEA OR VOMITING MAY BE SERIOUS. DISCONTINUE USE AND CONSULT PHYSICIAN IF NOT RELIEVED IN 24 HOURS. Do not exceed recommended dosage because severe liver damage may occur. As with any drug, if you are pregnant or nursing a baby, seek the advice of a health professional before using this product. [See table below].

Dosage and Administration: [See table below]
ST. JOSEPH Aspirin-Free Fever Reducer Tablets for Children may be given one of three ways. Always follow with ½ glass of water, milk or fruit juice.
1. Chewed, followed by liquid.
2. Crushed or dissolved in a teaspoon of liquid (for younger children).
3. Powdered for infant use, when so directed by physician.

How Supplied: Chewable fruit flavored tablets in plastic bottles of 30 tablets. Cherry tasting Liquid in 2 and 4 fl. oz. plastic bottles. Fruit flavored drops in ½ fl. oz. glass bottles, with calibrated plastic dropper.
All packages have child resistant safety caps and safety sealed packaging.

Shown in Product Identification Section, page 421

ST. JOSEPH CHILDREN'S DOSAGE CHART

Age	0–3 (months)	4–11 (months)	12–23 (months)	2–3 (years)	4–5 (years)	6–8 (years)	9–10 (years)	11 (years)	12+ (years)
Weight (lbs.)	7–12	13–21	22–26	27–35	36–45	46–65	66–76	77–83	84+
Dose of St. Joseph Acetaminophen Drops Dropperfuls	½	1	1½	2	3	4	5	—	—
Acetaminophen Liquid Teaspoonfuls	—	½	¾	1	1½	2	2½	3	4
Chewable Tablets Acetaminophen (80 mg. each)	—		1½	2	3	4	5	6	8

All dosages may be repeated every 4 hours, but do not exceed 5 dosages daily.
Note: Since St. Joseph pediatric products are available without prescription, parents are advised on the package label to consult a physician for use in children under two years.

ST. JOSEPH® Cold Tablets for Children

Active Ingredients: Per tablet: Acetaminophen 80 mg and phenylpropanolamine hydrochloride 3.125 mg.

Inactive Ingredients: Cellulose, FD&C Yellow No. 6 aluminum lake, flavor, mannitol, silica, sodium saccharin, zinc stearate.

How Supplied: In bottle with 30 fruit flavored chewable tablets.

ST. JOSEPH® Cough Suppressant for Children
Pediatric
Antitussive Suppressant

Active Ingredient: Dextromethorphan hydrobromide 7.5 mg. per 5 cc.

Inactive Ingredients: Caramel, citric acid, flavor, glycerin, methylparaben, propylparaben, sodium benzoate, sodium citrate, sucrose, water.

How Supplied: Alcohol-Free Cherry tasting suppressant in plastic bottle of 2 and 4 fl. ozs. In safety sealed packaging.
Shown in Product Identification Section, page 421

ST. JOSEPH® Measured Dose Nasal Decongestant

Active Ingredients: Phenylephrine Hydrochloride 0.125%

Inactive Ingredients: Cetyl pyridinium chloride, disodium phosphate, phenylmercuric acetate 0.002% (preservative), propylene glycol, sodium phosphate, sorbitol, water.

Indications: Gives temporary relief for up to 4 hours of nasal congestion due to colds, hay fever, sinusitis. The pump spray delivery system gives a measured dose every time (50 microliters).

Warnings: Do not exceed recommended dosage because symptoms may occur such as burning, stinging, sneezing, or increase of nasal discharge. Do not use this product for more than 3 days. If symptoms persist, consult a physician. Do not use in children under 2 years of age or who have heart disease, high blood pressure, thyroid disease or diabetes unless directed by a doctor. The use of the dispenser by more than one person may spread infection. Keep this and all medications out of the reach of children.

Symptoms and Treatment of Oral Overdosage: In case of accidental ingestion, seek professional assistance or contact a Poison Control Center immediately.

Dosage and Administration: For children 2 to under 6 years old. Before using first time, remove protective cap. Prime the metered pump by depressing several times. Hold bottle with thumb at base and nozzle between first and second fingers. With child's head upright (do not tilt child's head backward), insert metered pump spray nozzle in child's nos-

tril. Depress pump completely 1 or 2 times. Have child sniff deeply. Repeat in other nostil. Repeat application every 4 hours needed. Wipe tip clean after each use.

How Supplied: Available in ½ fl. oz. measured dose pump spray.
Shown in Product Identification Section, page 421

ST. JOSEPH® Nighttime Cold Medicine

Active Ingredients: Chlorpheniramine maleate, pseudoephedrine hydrochloride, acetaminophen, dextromethorphan hydrobromide

Inactive Ingredients: Citric acid, FD&C red No. 40, flavor, methylparaben, polyethylene glycol, propylene glycol, propylparaben, sodium benzoate, sodium citrate, sucrose, water

Indications: Temporary relief of major cold and flu symptoms

Actions: Antihistamine for relief of runny nose, sneezing, itchy watery eyes, scratchy throat and post-nasal drip; nasal decongestant for relief of nasal and sinus congestion; analgesic for aspirin-free relief to reduce fever of colds and flu and relieve body aches and pain; and cough suppressant to calm and quiet coughing.

Warning: For children under 6 years or 48 pounds, consult physician. Do not give this product to children for more than 5 days. If symptoms do not improve, or if new ones occur, or are accompanied by fever for over 3 days, consult physician. Do not exceed recommended dosage because at higher doses nervousness, dizziness, sleeplessness or severe liver damage may occur. May cause drowsiness or excitability. Keep this and all drugs out of reach of children.

Symptoms and Treatment of Oral Overdosage: In case of accidental overdose, seek professional assistance or contact a Poison Control Center immediately.

Dosage and Administration: One dose every 4 to 6 hours, not to exceed 3 times daily. Use the enclosed dosage cup to measure the right dose for your child.

Age/Weight Dosage Chart

AGE	WEIGHT	DOSE
Under 6 yrs.	Under 48 lbs.	Consult Physician
6–8 yrs.	48–65 lbs.	2 tsp.
9–10 yrs.	66–76 lbs.	2½ tsp.
11–12 yrs.	77–85 lbs.	3 tsp.

How Supplied: Alcohol-Free Cherry tasting syrup in plastic 4 oz. bottle. In safety sealed packaging.
Shown in Product Identification Section, page 421

SOLARCAINE®
Antiseptic·Topical Anesthetic
Lotion/Cream/Aerosol Spray Liquid

Active Ingredients:
SOLARCAINE Aloe Aerosol Spray—.5% lidocaine.
Also contains aloe vera and Vitamin E. Non-stinging and alcohol/fragrance free.

SOLARCAINE Aerosol Spray—to deliver benzocaine 20% (w/w), triclosan 0.13% (w/w). Also contains isopropyl alcohol 35% (w/w) in total contents.

SOLARCAINE Lotion—Benzocaine and triclosan.

SOLARCAINE Cream—Benzocaine and triclosan.

SOLARCAINE ALOE EXTRA™ Gel and Mist—Lidocaine HCl

SOLARCAINE Medicated Cream—Lidocaine

Indications: Medicated first aid to provide fast temporary relief of sunburn pain, minor burns, cuts, scrapes, chapping and skin injuries, poison ivy, detergent hands, insect bites (non-venomous). Aloe aerosol spray provides longer lasting/more cooling relief.

Actions: Lidocaine and benzocaine provide local anesthetic action to relieve itching and pain. Triclosan provides antimicrobial activity.

Caution: Not for use in eyes. Not for deep or puncture wounds or serious burns, nor for prolonged use. If condition persists, or infection, rash or irritation develops, discontinue use. Sunburns can be serious. In cases where skin is blistered or raw surfaces exist, do not use this product.

Warnings: For Aerosol Spray—Flammable—Do not spray while smoking or near fire. Do not spray into eyes or mouth. Avoid inhalation. Contents under pressure. For external use only.

Dosage and Administration: Lotion and Cream—Apply freely as needed. Sprays—Hold 3 to 5 inches from injured area. Spray until wet. To apply to face, spray on palm of hand. Use often for antiseptic protection.

How Supplied:
SOLARCAINE Aloe Aerosol Spray—4.5 oz. can.
SOLARCAINE Aerosol Spray—3- and 5-oz. cans.
SOLARCAINE Lotion—3- and 6-fl oz. bottles.
SOLARCAINE Cream—1-oz. tube.
SOLARCAINE Aloe Extra™ Gel—4- and 8-oz. bottles.
SOLARCAINE Aloe Extra™ Mist—3.75-fl.oz. bottle.
SOLARCAINE Cream—4 oz. jar.
Shown in Product Identification Section, page 421

Continued on next page

Plough—Cont.

SHADE® UVA/UVB Sunscreens

SHADE® Sunblock Lotion SPF 15
SHADE® Sunblock Lotion SPF 30
SHADE® Sunblock Lotion SPF 45
SHADE® Oil-Free Gel SPF 15
SHADE® Oil-Free Gel SPF 25
SHADE® Sunblock Stick SPF 30

Active Ingredients:
Lotions:
SPF 15—Ethylhexyl p-methoxycinnamate, oxybenzone
SPF 30—Ethylhexyl p-methoxycinnamate, oxybenzone, 2-ethylhexyl salicyylate
SPF 45—Ethylhexyl p-methoxycinnamate, oxybenzone, 2-ethylhexyl salicylate, octocrylene
Gels:
SPF 15, 25—Ethylhexyl p-methoxycinnamate, 2-ethylhexyl salicylate, oxybenzone
Shade Stick
SPF 30—Ethylhexyl p-methoxycinnamate, oxybenzone, 2-ethylhexyl salicylate, homosalate

Indications: Waterproof Paba-free sunscreens to help prevent harmful effects from the sun. SHADE screens both UVB and UVA rays. SHADE Protection Formulas provide 15, 25, 30, and 45 times your natural sunburn protection. Liberal and regular use may help reduce the chances of premature aging and wrinkling of skin, due to overexposure to the sun. All strengths are waterproof, maintaining sun protection for 80 minutes in water. Excellent for use on children.

Actions: Sunscreen

Warnings: For external use only. Avoid contact with eyes. Discontinue use if signs of irritation or rash appear.

Dosage and Administration: Apply evenly and liberally to all exposed skin. Reapply after prolonged swimming or excessive perspiration.

How Supplied: 4 fl. oz. Plastic Bottles
Shown in Product Identification Section, page 422

WATER BABIES® BY COPPERTONE

Water Babies® Sunblock Lotion SPF 15
Water Babies® Sunblock Cream SPF 25
Water Babies® Sunblock Lotion SPF 30
Water Babies® Sunblock Lotion SPF 45

Active Ingredients:
SPF 15: Ethylhexyl p-methoxycinnamate, oxybenzone
SPF 25: Ethylhexyl p-methoxycinnamate, oxybenzone, 2-ethylhexyl salicylate, homosalate
SPF 30: Ethylhexyl p-methoxycinnamate, 2-ethylhexyl salicylate, homosalate, oxybenzone
SPF 45: Ethylhexyl p-methoxycinnamate, 2-ethylhexyl salicylate, octocrylene, oxybenzone

How Supplied: SPF 15, SPF 30, SPF 45—In plastic bottles of 4.0 fl oz. SPF 25—In plastic tube (in carton) of 3.0 fl oz.
Shown in Product Identification Section, page 422

Procter & Gamble
P. O. BOX 599
CINCINNATI, OH 45201

DENQUEL® Sensitive Teeth Toothpaste
Desensitizing Dentifrice

Description: Each tube contains potassium nitrate (5%) in a low-abrasion, pleasant mint-flavored dentifrice.
Dentinal hypersensitivity is a condition in which pain or discomfort arises when various stimuli, such as hot, cold, sweet, sour or touch contact exposed dentin. Exposure of dentin often occurs as a result of either gingival recession or periodontal surgery.
Daily use of Denquel can provide, within the first 2 weeks of regular brushing, a significant decrease in hypersensitivity. See a dentist if tooth sensitivity is not reduced after 4 weeks of regular use, as this may indicate a dental condition other than hypersensitivity. The Council on Dental Therapeutics of the American Dental Association has given Denquel the ADA Seal of Acceptance as an effective desensitizing dentifrice for teeth sensitive to hot, cold or pressure (tactile) in otherwise normal teeth.

Dosage: Use twice a day or as directed by a dentist.

How Supplied: Denquel Sensitive Teeth Toothpaste is supplied in tubes containing 1.6, 3.0, or 4.5 ounces.

HEAD & SHOULDERS® SHAMPOO
Antidandruff Shampoo

Description: Head & Shoulders Shampoo offers effective dandruff control and beautiful hair in a formula that is pleasant to use. Independently conducted clinical testing (double-blind and dermatologist-graded) has proved that Head & Shoulders reduces dandruff flaking. Head & Shoulders is also gentle enough to use every day for clean, manageable hair.

Active Ingredient: 1.0% pyrithione zinc suspended in an anionic detergent system. Cosmetic ingredients are also included.

Indications: For effective control of dandruff and seborrheic dermatitis of the scalp.

Actions: Pyrithione zinc is substantive to the scalp and remains after rinsing. Its mechanism of action has not been fully established, but it is believed to control the microorganisms associated with dandruff flaking and itching.

Precautions: Not to be taken internally. Keep out of children's reach. Avoid getting shampoo in eyes—if this happens, rinse eyes with water.

Dosage and Administration: For best results in controlling dandruff, Head & Shoulders should be used regularly. It is gentle enough to use for every shampoo. In treating seborrheic dermatitis, a minimum of four shampooings are needed to achieve full effectiveness.

Composition: Lotion—Normal to Oily Formula: Pyrithione zinc in a shampoo base of water, ammonium laureth sulfate, ammonium lauryl sulfate, cocamide MEA, glycol distearate, ammonium xylenesulfonate, fragrance, citric acid, methylchloroisothiazolinone, methylisothiazolinone, and FD&C Blue No. 1. Lotion—Normal to Dry Formula: Pyrithione zinc in a shampoo base of water, ammonium laureth sulfate, ammonium lauryl sulfate, cocamide MEA, glycol distearate, ammonium xylenesulfonate, propylene glycol, fragrance, citric acid, methylchloroisothiazolinone, methylisothiazolinone, and FD&C Blue No. 1. Lotion—Dry Scalp Regular Formula: Pyrithione zinc in a shampoo base of water, ammonium laureth sulfate, ammonium lauryl sulfate, cocamide MEA, glycol distearate, dimethicone, ammonium xylenesulfonate, fragrance, tricetylmonium chloride, cetyl alcohol, stearyl alcohol, DMDM hydantoin, sodium chloride, FD&C Blue No. 1. Lotion—Dry Scalp Conditioning Formula: Pyrithione zinc in a shampoo base of water, ammonium laureth sulfate, ammonium lauryl sulfate, cocamide MEA, glycol distearate, dimethicone, ammonium xylenesulfonate, fragrance, tricetylmonium chloride, cetyl alcohol, stearyl alcohol, DMDM hydantoin, sodium chloride, FD&C Blue No. 1. Cream—Normal to Oily Formula: Pyrithione zinc in a shampoo base of water, sodium cocoglyceryl ether sulfonate, sodium chloride, sodium lauroyl sarcosinate, cocamide DEA, cocoyl sarcosine, fragrance, and FD&C Blue No. 1. Cream—Normal to Dry Formula: Pyrithione zinc in a shampoo base of water, sodium cocoglyceryl ether sulfonate, sodium chloride, sodium lauroyl sarcosinate, cocamide DEA, propylene glycol, cocoyl sarcosine, fragrance, and FD&C Blue No. 1.

How Supplied: Lotion available in 4.0, 7.0, 11.0, and 15.0 fl. oz. unbreakable plastic bottles. Dry scalp available in 7.0, 11.0, and 15.0 oz. Concentrate cream available in 5.5 oz. tube. Both lotion and concentrate are available in formulas for "Normal to Oily" and "Normal to Dry" hair. Dry scalp formula is available in "Regular" and "Conditioning."
Shown in Product Identification Section, page 422

Regular Flavor METAMUCIL® Powder
[met "uh-mū 'sil]
(psyllium hydrophilic mucilloid)

Description: Regular Flavor Metamucil is a bulk-forming natural therapeutic fiber for restoring and maintaining regularity. It contains hydrophilic mucilloid, a highly efficient dietary fiber derived from the husk of the psyllium seed (Plantago ovata). Metamucil contains no chemical stimulants and is nonaddictive. Each dose contains approximately 3.4 g of psyllium hydrophilic mucilloid. Inactive ingredients include dextrose (a carbohydrate). Each dose contains less than 10 mg of sodium, 31 mg of potassium, and 14 calories. Carbohydrate content is approximately 3.5 g.

Actions: Metamucil provides bulk that promotes normal elimination. The product is uniform, instantly miscible, palatable, and nonirritative in the gastrointestinal tract.

Indications: Metamucil is indicated in the management of chronic constipation, in irritable bowel syndrome, as adjunctive therapy in the constipation of diverticular disease, in the bowel management of patients with hemorrhoids, and for constipation during pregnancy, convalescence, and senility.

Contraindications: Intestinal obstruction, fecal impaction.

Precaution: May cause allergic reaction in people sensitive to inhaled or ingested psyllium powder.

Dosage and Administration: The usual adult dosage is one rounded teaspoonful (7 g) stirred into a standard 8-oz glass of cool water, fruit juice, milk or other beverage. It can be taken orally one to three times a day, depending on the need and response. It may require continued use for 2 or 3 days to provide optimal benefit. An additional glass of liquid after each dose is helpful. For children (6 to 12 years old), use ½ the adult dose in 8 oz of liquid, 1 to 3 times daily.

New Users: Medical research shows that high fiber intake is important for good digestive health. To help the body adjust and avoid the minor gas and bloating sometimes associated with high fiber intake, it may be necessary to increase fiber intake gradually. Initial dose: one teaspoonful of Metamucil per day. If minor gas or bloating occurs, reduce the amount for several days. Gradually increase to 3 teaspoonsful per day if needed.

How Supplied: Powder, containers of 7 oz, 14 oz, 21 oz and 32 oz (OTC); also available in cartons of 30 single-dose (7 g) packets and 100 single-dose (7 g) packets (Professional).

Shown in Product Identification Section, page 422

Sugar Free Regular Flavor METAMUCIL® Powder
[met "uh-mū 'sil]
(psyllium hydrophilic mucilloid)

Description: Sugar Free Regular Flavor Metamucil is a bulk-forming natural therapeutic fiber for restoring and maintaining regularity. It contains hydrophilic mucilloid, a highly efficient dietary fiber derived from the husk of the psyllium seed (Plantago ovata), which has been sweetened with NutraSweet®* brand sweetener (aspartame). It contains no chemical stimulants or sugar and is nonaddictive. Each dose contains approximately 3.4 g of psyllium hydrophilic mu-

cilloid. Inactive ingredients include aspartame and maltodextrin. Each dose contains about 1 calorie, less than 10 mg of sodium, 31 mg of potassium and 6 mg of phenylalanine. Carbohydrate content is 0.3 gram.

Actions: Metamucil provides bulk that promotes normal elimination. The product is uniform, instantly miscible, palatable, and nonirritative in the gastrointestinal tract.

Indications: Metamucil is indicated in the management of chronic constipation, in irritable bowel syndrome, as adjunctive therapy in the constipation of diverticular disease, in the bowel management of patients with hemorrhoids, and for constipation during pregnancy, convalescence, and senility.

Contraindications: Intestinal obstruction, fecal impaction.

Warning: Phenylketonurics should be aware that Sugar Free Metamucil contains phenylalanine.

Precaution: May cause allergic reaction in people sensitive to inhaled or ingested psyllium powder.

Dosage and Administration: The usual adult dosage is one rounded teaspoonful (3.7 g) stirred into a standard 8-oz glass of cool water, fruit juice, milk or other beverage. It can be taken orally one to three times a day, depending on the need and response. It may require continued use for 2 or 3 days to provide optimal benefit. An additional glass of liquid after each dose is helpful. For children (6–12 years old), use ½ the adult dose in 8 oz of liquid, 1 to 3 times daily.

New Users: Medical research shows that high fiber intake is important for good digestive health. To help the body adjust and avoid the minor gas and bloating sometimes associated with high fiber intake, it may be necessary to increase fiber intake gradually. Initial dose: one teaspoonful of Metamucil per day. If minor gas or bloating occurs, reduce the amount for several days. Gradually increase to 3 teaspoonsful per day if needed.

How Supplied: Powder, containers of 3.7 oz, 7.4 oz, 11.1 oz, and 16.9 oz (OTC); also available in cartons of 100 single-dose (3.7 g) packets (Professional).

Is This Product OTC?
Yes.

---

*NutraSweet is a registered trademark of the NutraSweet Company.
Shown in Product Identification Section, page 422

Orange Flavor METAMUCIL® Powder
[met "uh-mū 'sil]
(psyllium hydrophilic mucilloid)

Description: Orange Flavor Metamucil is a bulk-forming natural therapeutic fiber for restoring and maintaining regularity. It contains hydrophilic mucilloid, a highly efficient dietary fiber derived

from the husk of the psyllium seed (Plantago ovata). Metamucil contains no chemical stimulants and is nonaddictive. Each dose contains approximately 3.4 g of psyllium hydrophilic mucilloid. Inactive ingredients include citric acid, FD&C Yellow No. 6, flavoring, and sucrose (a carbohydrate). Each dose contains less than 10 mg of sodium, 31 mg of potassium, and 30 calories. Cabohydrate content is approximately 7.1 g.

Actions: Metamucil provides bulk that promotes normal elimination. The product is uniform, instantly miscible, palatable, and nonirritative in the gastrointestinal tract.

Indications: Metamucil is indicated in the management of chronic constipation, in irritable bowel syndrome, as adjunctive therapy in the constipation of diverticular disease, in the bowel management of patients with hemorrhoids, and for constipation during pregnancy, convalescence, and senility.

Contraindications: Intestinal obstruction, fecal impaction.

Precaution: May cause allergic reaction in people sensitive to inhaled or ingested psyllium powder.

Dosage and Administration: The usual adult dosage is one rounded tablespoonful (11 g) stirred into a standard 8-oz glass of cool water, fruit juice, milk or other beverage. It can be taken orally one to three times a day, depending on the need and response. It may require continued use for 2 or 3 days to provide optimal benefit. An additional glass of liquid after each dose is helpful. For children (6 to 12 years old), use ½ the adult dose in 8 oz of liquid, 1 to 3 times daily.

New Users: Medical research shows that high fiber intake is important for good digestive health. To help the body adjust and avoid the minor gas and bloating sometimes associated with high fiber intake, it may be necessary to increase fiber intake gradually. Initial dose: one tablespoonful of Metamucil per day. If minor gas or bloating occurs, reduce the amount for several days. Gradually increase to 3 tablespoonsful per day if needed.

How Supplied: Powder, containers of 7 oz, 14 oz, 21 oz, and 32 oz (OTC).
Shown in Product Identification Section, page 422

Strawberry Flavor METAMUCIL® Powder
[met "uh-mū 'sil]
(psyllium hydrophilic mucilloid)

Description: Strawberry Flavor Metamucil is a bulk-forming natural therapeutic fiber for restoring and maintaining regularity. It contains hydrophilic mucilloid, a highly efficient dietary fiber derived from the husk of the psyllium seed (Plantago ovata). Metamucil contains no chemical stimulants and is not addictive. Each dose contains approxi-

Continued on next page

Procter & Gamble—Cont.

mately 3.4 g of psyllium hydrophilic mucilloid. Inactive ingredients include citric acid, FD&C Red No. 40, flavoring, and sucrose (a carbohydrate). Each dose contains less than 10 mg of sodium, 31 mg of potassium, and 30 calories. Carbohydrate content is approximately 7.1 g.

Actions: Metamucil provides bulk that promotes normal elimination. The product is uniform, instantly miscible, palatable, and nonirritative in the gastrointestinal tract.

Indications: Metamucil is indicated in the management of chronic constipation, in irritable bowel syndrome, as adjunctive therapy in the constipation of diverticular disease, in the bowel management of patients with hemorrhoids, and for constipation during pregnancy, convalescence, and senility.

Contraindications: Intestinal obstruction, fecal impaction.

Precaution: May cause allergic reaction in people sensitive to inhaled or ingested psyllium powder.

Dosage and Administration: The usual adult dose is one rounded tablespoonful (11 g) stirred into a standard 8-oz glass of cool water, fruit juice, milk or other beverage. It can be taken orally one to three times a day, depending on the need and response. It may require continued use for 2 or 3 days to provide optimal benefit. An additional glass of liquid after each dose is helpful. For children (6–12 years old), use ½ tablespoonful in 8 oz of liquid, 1 to 3 times daily.

New Users: Medical research shows that high fiber intake is important for good digestive health. To help the body adjust and avoid the minor gas and bloating sometimes associated with high fiber intake, it may be necessary to increase fiber intake gradually. Initial dose: one tablespoonful of Metamucil per day. If minor gas or bloating occurs, reduce the amount for several days. Gradually increase to 3 tablespoonsful per day if needed.

How Supplied: Powder, containers of 7 oz, 14 oz, and 21 oz (OTC).
Shown in Product Identification Section, page 422

Sugar Free Orange Flavor EFFERVESCENT METAMUCIL®
[met "uh-mū 'sil]
(psyllium hydrophilic mucilloid)

Description: Sugar Free Orange Flavor Effervescent Metamucil is a bulk-forming natural therapeutic fiber for restoring and maintaining regularity. It contains hydrophilic mucilloid, a highly efficient dietary fiber derived from the husk of the psyllium seed (Plantago ovata), which has been sweetened with NutraSweet®* brand sweetener (aspartame). It contains no chemical stimulants or sugar and is nonaddictive. Each dose contains approximately 3.4 g of psyl-

---

lium hydrophilic mucilloid. Inactive ingredients include aspartame, citric acid, FD&C Yellow No. 6, flavoring, potassium bicarbonate, silicon dioxide, and sodium bicarbonate. Each packet provides less than 1 calorie, 310 mg of potassium, less than 10 mg of sodium, and 30 mg phenylalanine.

Actions: Effervescent Metamucil provides bulk that promotes normal elimination. It is effervescent and requires no stirring. The product is uniform, instantly miscible, palatable, and nonirritative in the gastrointestinal tract.

Indications: Effervescent Metamucil is indicated in the management of chronic constipation, in irritable bowel syndrome, as adjunctive therapy in the constipation of diverticular disease, in the bowel management of patients with hemorrhoids, and for constipation during pregnancy, convalescence, and senility.

Contraindications: Intestinal obstruction, fecal impaction.

Warning: Phenylketonurics should be aware that Sugar Free Effervescent Metamucil contains phenylalanine.

Precaution: May cause allergic reaction in people sensitive to inhaled or ingested psyllium powder.

Dosage and Administration: The usual adult dosage is the contents of one packet (0.18 oz) taken one to three times daily. The entire contents of a packet are poured into a standard 8-oz glass. The glass is slowly filled with cool water, fruit juice, milk or beverage. Drink promptly. An additional glass of liquid after each dose is helpful.

New Users: Medical research shows that high fiber intake is important for good digestive health. To help the body adjust and avoid the minor gas and bloating sometimes associated with high fiber intake, it may be necessary to increase fiber intake gradually. Initial dose: one packet of Metamucil per day. If minor gas or bloating occurs, reduce the amount for several days. Gradually increase to 3 packets per day if needed.

How Supplied: Cartons of 30 single-dose (0.18 oz) packets (OTC).

---

*NutraSweet is a registered trademark of the NutraSweet Company.
Shown in Product Identification Section, page 422

Sugar Free Lemon-Lime Flavor EFFERVESCENT METAMUCIL®
[met "uh-mū 'sil]
(psyllium hydrophilic mucilloid)

Description: Sugar Free Lemon-Lime Flavor Effervescent Metamucil is a bulk-forming natural therapeutic fiber for restoring and maintaining regularity. It contains hydrophilic mucilloid, a highly efficient dietary fiber derived from the husk of the psyllium seed (Plantago ovata), which has been sweetened with NutraSweet®* brand sweetener (aspar-

---

tame). It contains no chemical stimulants or sugar. Each dose contains approximately 3.4 g of psyllium hydrophilic mucilloid. Inactive ingredients include aspartame, calcium carbonate, citric acid, flavoring, potassium bicarbonate, silicon dioxide, and sodium bicarbonate. Each packet provides less than 1 calorie, 290 mg of potassium, less than 10 mg of sodium, and 30 mg phenylalanine.

Actions: Effervescent Metamucil provides bulk that promotes normal elimination. The product is effervescent and requires no stirring. It is uniform, instantly miscible, palatable, and nonirritative in the gastrointestinal tract.

Indications: Effervescent Metamucil is indicated in the management of chronic constipation, in irritable bowel syndrome, as adjunctive therapy in the constipation of diverticular disease, in the bowel management of patients with hemorrhoids, and for constipation during pregnancy, convalescence, and senility.

Contraindications: Intestinal obstruction, fecal impaction.

Warning: Phenylketonurics should be aware that Sugar Free Effervescent Metamucil contains phenylalanine.

Precaution: May cause allergic reaction in people sensitive to inhaled or ingested psyllium powder.

Dosage and Administration: The usual adult dosage is the contents of one packet (0.19 oz) taken one to three times daily. The entire contents of a packet are poured into a standard 8-oz glass. The glass is slowly filled with cool water, fruit juice, milk or beverage. Drink promptly. An additional glass of liquid after each dose is helpful.

New Users: Medical research shows that high fiber intake is important for good digestive health. To help the body adjust and avoid the minor gas and bloating sometimes associated with high fiber intake, it may be necessary to increase fiber intake gradually. Initial dose: one packet of Metamucil per day. If minor gas or bloating occurs, reduce the amount for several days. Gradually increase to 3 packets per day if needed.

How Supplied: Cartons of 30 single-dose (0.19 oz) packets (OTC) and 100 single-dose (0.19 oz) packets (Professional).

---

*NutraSweet is a registered trademark of the NutraSweet Company.
Shown in Product Identification Section, page 422

Sugar Free Orange Flavor METAMUCIL® Powder
[met "uh-mū 'sil]
(psyllium hydrophilic mucilloid)

Description: Sugar Free Orange Flavor Metamucil is a bulk-forming natural therapeutic fiber for restoring and maintaining regularity. It contains hydrophilic mucilloid, a highly efficient dietary fiber derived from the husk of the psyllium seed *(Plantago ovata),* which has been sweetened with NutraSweet®* brand sweetener (aspartame). It contains no chemical stimulants or sugar and is nonaddictive. Each dose contains approximately 3.4 g of psyllium hydrophilic mucilloid. Inactive ingredients include aspartame, citric acid, FD&C Yellow No. 6, flavoring, maltodextrin, and silicon dioxide. Each dose contains about 5 calories, less than 10 mg of sodium, 31 mg of potassium, and 30 mg of phenylalanine. Carbohydrate content is approximately 1.4 grams.

Actions: Metamucil provides bulk that promotes normal elimination. The product is uniform, instantly miscible, palatable, and nonirritative in the gastrointestinal tract.

Indications: Metamucil is indicated in the management of chronic constipation, in irritable bowel syndrome, as adjunctive therapy in the constipation of diverticular disease, in the bowel management of patients with hemorrhoids, and for constipation during pregnancy, convalescence, and senility.

Contraindications: Intestinal obstruction, fecal impaction.

Warning: Phenylketonurics should be aware that Sugar Free Metamucil contains phenylalanine.

Precautions: May cause allergic reaction in people sensitive to inhaled or ingested psyllium powder.

Dosage and Administration: The usual adult dosage is one rounded teaspoonful (5.2 g) stirred into a standard 8-oz glass of cool water, fruit juice, milk or other beverage. It can be taken orally one to three times a day, depending on the need and response. It may require continued use for 2 or 3 days to provide optimal benefit. An additional glass of liquid after each dose is helpful. For children (6–12 years old), use ½ the adult dose in 8 oz of liquid, 1 to 3 times daily.

New Users: Medical research shows that high fiber intake is important for good digestive health. To help the body adjust and avoid the minor gas and bloating sometimes associated with high fiber intake, it may be necessary to increase fiber intake gradually. Initial dose: one teaspoonful of Metamucil per day. If minor gas or bloating occurs, reduce the amount for several days. Gradually increase to 3 teaspoonsful per day if needed.

How Supplied: Powder, containers of 4.7 oz, 8.7 oz, 12.9 oz, and 20.7 oz (OTC).

---

*NutraSweet is a registered trademark of the NutraSweet Company.

Shown in Product Identification Section, page 422

PEPTO-BISMOL®
LIQUID AND TABLETS
For diarrhea, heartburn, indigestion, upset stomach and nausea.

Description: Each Pepto-Bismol Tablet contains 262 mg bismuth subsalicylate and each tablespoonful (15 ml) of Pepto-Bismol Liquid contains 262 mg bismuth subsalicylate. Each tablet contains 102 mg salicylate and each tablespoonful of liquid contains 130 mg salicylate. Liquid and tablets contain no sugar. Tablets are sodium-free (less than 2 mg/tablet) and Liquid is low in sodium (5 mg/tablespoonful). Inactive ingredients include (Tablets): calcium carbonate, FD&C Red. No. 27, flavor, magnesium stearate, mannitol, povidone, saccharin sodium and talc; (Liquid): FD&C Red No. 3, FD&C Red No 40, flavor, magnesium aluminum silicate, methylcellulose, saccharin sodium, salicylic acid, sodium salicylate and water.

Indications: Pepto-Bismol controls diarrhea within 24 hours, relieving associated abdominal cramps; soothes heartburn and indigestion without constipating; and relieves nausea and upset stomach.

Caution: This product contains salicylates. If taken with aspirin and ringing of the ears occurs, discontinue use. This product does not contain aspirin, but should not be administered to those patients who have a known allergy to aspirin or salicylates. Caution is advised in the administration to patients taking medication for anticoagulation, diabetes and gout.

Warning: Caution is advised in the administration to children, including teenagers, during or after recovery from chicken pox or flu. As with any drug, caution is advised in the administration to pregnant or nursing women.
Note: This medication may cause a temporary and harmless darkening of the tongue and/or stool. Stool darkening should not be confused with melena.

Dosage and Administration:
Tablets:
  Adults—Two tablets
  Children (according to age)—
    9–12 yr 1 tablet
    6–9 yr ⅔ tablet
    3–6 yr ⅓ tablet
Chew or dissolve in mouth. Repeat every ½ to 1 hour as needed, to a maximum of 8 doses in a 24-hour period.
Liquid: Shake well before using.
  Adults—2 tablespoonfuls
  Children (according to age)—
    9–12 yr 1 tablespoonful
    6–9 yr 2 teaspoonfuls
    3–6 yr 1 teaspoonful
Repeat dosage every ½ to 1 hour, if needed, to a maximum of 8 doses in a 24-hour period.
For children under 3 years, dose according to weight.

    28+ lb 1 teaspoonful
    14–18 lb ½ teaspoonful
Repeat every 4 hours, if needed, to a maximum of 6 doses in a 24-hour period.

How Supplied:
Pepto-Bismol Liquid is available in:
  NDC 37000-032-01 4 fl oz bottle
  NDC 37000-032-02 8 fl oz bottle
  NDC 37000-032-03 12 fl oz bottle
  NDC 37000-032-04 16 fl oz bottle
Pepto-Bismol Tablets are pink, triangular chewable, tablets imprinted with "Pepto-Bismol" on one side. Tablets are available in:
  NDC 37000-033-03 box of 24
  NDC 37000-033-04 box of 42
Shown in Product Identification Section, page 422

MAXIMUM STRENGTH
PEPTO-BISMOL®
LIQUID
For diarrhea, heartburn, indigestion, upset stomach and nausea.

Description: Each tablespoonful (15 mL) of Maximum Strength Pepto-Bismol Liquid contains 525 mg bismuth subsalicylate (230 mg salicylate). Maximum Strength Pepto-Bismol Liquid contains no sugar and is low in sodium (less than 5 mg/tablespoonful). Inactive ingredients include: FD&C Red No. 3, FD&C Red No. 40, flavor, magnesium aluminum silicate, methylcellulose, saccharin sodium, salicylic acid, sodium salicylate, and water.

Indications: Maximum Strength Pepto-Bismol controls diarrhea within 24 hours, relieving associated abdominal cramps; soothes heartburn and indigestion without constipating; and relieves nausea and upset stomach.

Caution: This product contains salicylates. If taken with aspirin and ringing of the ears occurs, discontinue use. This product does not contain aspirin, but should not be administered to those patients who have a known allergy to aspirin or salicylates. Caution is advised in the administration to patients taking medication for anticoagulation, diabetes, and gout.

Warning: Caution is advised in the administration to children, including teenagers, during or after recovery from chicken pox or flu. As with any drug, caution is advised in the administration to pregnant or nursing women.
Note: This medication may cause a temporary and harmless darkening of the tongue and/or stool. Stool darkening should not be confused with melena.

Dosage and Administration: Shake well before using.
Adults—2 tablespoonfuls
Children (according to age)—
  9–12 yr 1 tablespoonful
  6–9 yr 2 teaspoonfuls
  3–6 yr 1 teaspoonful
Repeat dosage every hour, if needed, to a maximum of 4 doses in a 24-hour period.

Continued on next page

Procter & Gamble—Cont.

How Supplied:
Maximum Strength Pepto-Bismol is available in:
NDC 37000-019-01   4 fl oz bottle
NDC 37000-019-02   8 fl oz bottle
NDC 37000-019-03   12 fl oz bottle
*Shown in Product Identification
Section, page 422*

EDUCATIONAL MATERIAL

Journal Reprints for Physicians
Reprints of published journal articles illustrating the effectiveness of bismuth subsalicylate (Pepto-Bismol) for the treatment of diarrhea.

Reed & Carnrick
**1 NEW ENGLAND AVENUE
PISCATAWAY, NJ 08855-9998**

**PHAZYME® and PHAZYME®-95
Tablets**

Description: A two-phase tablet. Contains specially-activated simethicone, both in the outer layer for release in the stomach and in the inner enteric-coated core for release in the small intestine.

Actions: PHAZYME is the only dual-approach to the problem of gastrointestinal gas. Simethicone minimizes gas formation and relieves gas entrapment in both the stomach and the lower G.I. tract. This action helps combat the painful sensation due to gastrointestinal gas. Also, for relief of gas distress associated with other functional or organic conditions such as: diverticulitis, spastic colitis, hyperacidity, postcholecystectomy syndrome and chronic cholecystitis.

Indications: PHAZYME is indicated for the relief of occasional or chronic discomfort caused by gas entrapped in the stomach or in the lower gastrointestinal tract—resulting from aerophagia, postoperative distention, dyspepsia and food intolerance.

Contraindications: A known sensitivity to any ingredient.

PHAZYME
Contains: Active ingredient: Specially-activated simethicone, both in the outer layer for release in the stomach and in the inner enteric-coated core for release in the small intestine, a total of 60 mg.
Inactive ingredients: Acacia, Calcium Sulfate, Carnauba Wax, Crospovidone, D&C Red No. 7 Lake, FD&C Blue No. 1 Lake, Gelatin, Lactose, Microcrystalline, Cellulose, Polyoxyl-40 Stearate, Polyvinyl Acetate Phthalate, Povidone, Pregelatinized Starch, Rice Starch, Sodium Benzoate, Sucrose, Titanium Dioxide.

Dosage: One or two tablets with each meal and at bedtime, or as directed by a physician.

How Supplied: Pink coated two-phase tablet in bottles of 50 and 100.

PHAZYME-95
Contains: Active ingredient: Specially-activated simethicone, both in the outer layer for release in the stomach and in the inner enteric-coated core for release in the small intestine, a total of 95 mg.
Inactive ingredients: Acacia, Calcium Sulfate, Carnauba Wax, Crospovidone, FD&C Yellow No. 6 Lake, FD&C Red No. 40 Lake, Gelatin, Lactose, Microcrystalline Cellulose, Polyoxyl-40 Stearate, Polyvinyl acetate Phthalate, Povidone, Pregelatinized Starch, Rice Starch, Sodium Benzoate, Sucrose, Titanium Dioxide.

Dosage: One tablet with each meal and at bedtime, or as directed by a physician.

How Supplied: Red coated two-phase tablet in 10 pack, bottles of 50 and 100.
*Shown in Product Identification
Section, page 422*

**Maximum Strength
PHAZYME®-125 Capsules**

Description: A red softgel containing the highest dose of simethicone available in a single capsule.
Active Ingredients: Simethicone 125 mg.
Inactive Ingredients: Soybean oil, gelatin, glycerin, vegetable shortening, polysorbate 80, purified water, hydrogenated soybean oil, yellow wax, lecithin, titanium dioxide, FD&C Red #40, methylparaben, propylparaben.

Actions: Simethicone minimizes gas formation and relieves gas entrapment in both the stomach and the lower G.I. tract. This action combats the painful sensation due to gastrointestinal gas. Also, for relief of gas distress associated with other functional or organic conditions such as diverticulitis, spastic colitis, hyperacidity, post-cholecystectomy syndrome and chronic cholecystitis.

Indications: PHAZYME-125 is indicated for the relief of acute severe lower intestinal discomfort due to gas—resulting from aerophagia, postoperative distention, dyspepsia and food intolerance.

Contraindications: A known sensitivity to any ingredient.

Dosage: One capsule with each meal and at bedtime, or as directed by a physician.

How Supplied: Red capsule in bottles of 50 and consumer 10 pack.
Rev. 8/87
*Shown in Product Identification
Section, page 422*

**proctoFoam®/non-steroid
(pramoxine HCl 1%)**

Description: proctoFoam is a foam for anal and perianal use.

Composition: Active ingredients: Pramoxine Hydrochloride 1%.

Inactive Ingredients: Butane, Cetyl Alcohol, Emulsifying Wax, Methylparaben, Mineral Oil, Polysorbate 60, Propane, Propylparaben, Sorbitan Seoquiolate, Trolamine, Water.

Actions: proctoFoam is an anesthetic mucoadhesive foam which medicates the anorectal mucosa, and provides prompt temporary relief from itching and pain. Its lubricating action helps make bowel evacuations more comfortable.

Indications: Prompt, temporary relief of anorectal inflammation, pruritus and pain associated with hemorrhoids, proctitis, cryptitis, fissures, postoperative pain and pruritus ani.

Contraindications: Contraindicated in persons hypersensitive to any of the ingredients.

Warning: Not for prolonged use. Do not use more than four consecutive weeks. If redness, pain, irritation or swelling persists or rectal bleeding occurs, discontinue use and consult a physician. Keep this and all medicines out of the reach of children.

Caution: Do not insert any part of the aerosol container into the anus. Contents of the container are under pressure, but not flammable. Do not burn or puncture the aerosol container. Store at room temperature. not over 120° F.

Dosage:
One applicatorful two or three times daily and after bowel evacuation.
1. To fill—Shake foam container vigorously before use. Hold container upright and insert into opening of applicator tip. With applicator drawn out all the way, press down on container cap. When the foam reaches fill line in the applicator, it is ready to use.
CAUTION: The aerosol container should never be inserted directly into the anus.
2. To administer—Separate applicator from container. Hold applicator by barrel and gently insert tip into the anus. With applicator in place, push plunger in order to expel foam, then withdraw applicator. (Applicator parts should be pulled apart for thorough cleaning with warm water.)
Note: To relieve itching place some foam on a tissue and apply externally.

How Supplied: Available in 15 g aerosol container, with special plastic applicator. The aerosol supplies approximately 18 applications.

Literature Available: Instruction pads with directions for use available upon request.
*Shown in Product Identification
Section, page 422*

R&C SHAMPOO®
Shampoo Pediculicide

Description: R&C SHAMPOO is a one-step pediculicide shampoo available without a prescription. Its active ingredients are: pyrethrins 0.30%, piperonyl butoxide technical 3.00%, equivalent to 2.40% (butylcarbityl) (6-propylpiperonyl) ether and 0.60% related compounds. Inert ingredients 96.70%.

Action: R&C SHAMPOO kills head lice (pediculus capitis), crab lice (phthirus pubis) and body lice (pediculus corporis) and their eggs.

Indications: R&C SHAMPOO is indicated for the treatment of infestations with head lice, crab lice and body lice.

Warning: R&C SHAMPOO should not be used by ragweed sensitized persons.

Caution: R&C SHAMPOO is for external use only. It can be harmful if swallowed or inhaled. It should be kept out of eyes and avoid contact with mucous membranes. If accidental contact with eyes occurs, flush immediately with water. In case of infection or skin irritation, discontinue use and consult a physician. Consult a physician if louse infestation of eyebrows and eyelashes occurs. Avoid contamination of feed or foodstuffs.

Storage and Disposal:
Storage: Store below 120°F.
Disposal: Do not reuse container. Rinse thoroughly before discarding in trash.

Dosage and Administration: (1) Apply a sufficient quantity of R&C SHAMPOO to thoroughly wet dry hair and skin, paying particular attention to the infested and adjacent hairy areas. (2) Allow R&C SHAMPOO to remain on the area for 10 minutes. (3) Add small quantities of water, working the shampoo into the hair and skin until a lather forms. (4) Rinse thoroughly. Dead lice and eggs will require removal with fine-tooth comb. If necessary, treatment may be repeated but do not exceed two consecutive applications within 24 hrs.
Since lice infestations are spread by contact, each family member should be examined carefully. If infested, he or she should be treated promptly to avoid spreading or reinfestation of previously treated individuals.
To eliminate infestation, it is important to wash all clothing, bedding, towels and combs and brushes, used by the infested person in hot water (130°). Dry clean nonwashable items.

How Supplied: In 2 and 4 fl oz. plastic bottles with pourable cap. Fine-tooth comb to aid in removal of dead lice and nits and patient booklet are included in each package of R&C SHAMPOO.

Literature Available: For free patient information brochures and filmstrips, please call 1-800-KIL-LICE. A Reed & Carnrick health consultant will be glad to assist you.
Shown in Product Identification Section, page 422

R&C SPRAY® III Lice Control Insecticide

Description: Active ingredients: 3-Phenoxybenzyl d-cis and trans 2,2-dimethyl-3-(2-methylpropenyl) cyclopropanecarboxylate 0.382%
Other Isomers 0.018%
Petroleum Distillates 4.255%
Inert Ingredients: 95.345%
100.000%

Actions: R&C SPRAY is specially formulated to kill lice and their nits on inanimate objects.

Indications: R&C SPRAY is recommended for use only on bedding, mattresses, furniture and other objects infested or possibly infested with lice which cannot be laundered or dry cleaned.

Warnings: Contents under pressure. Do not use or store near heat or open flame. Do not puncture or incinerate container. Exposure to temperatures above 130°F may cause bursting. It is a violation of Federal law to use this product in a manner inconsistent with its labeling. NOT FOR USE ON HUMANS OR ANIMALS.

Caution: Avoid spraying in eyes. Avoid breathing spray mist. Avoid contact with the skin. May be absorbed through the skin. In case of contact, wash immediately with soap and water. Harmful if swallowed. Vacate room after treatment and ventilate before reoccupying. Avoid contamination of feed and foodstuffs. Remove pets, birds and cover fish aquariums before spraying.

Directions: SHAKE WELL BEFORE AND OCCASIONALLY DURING USE. Spray on an inconspicuous area to test for possible staining or discoloration. Inspect after drying, then proceed to spray entire area to be treated.
Hold container upright with nozzle away from you. Depress valve and spray from a distance of 8 to 10 inches.
Spray each square foot for about three seconds. For mattresses, furniture, or similar objects (that cannot be laundered or dry cleaned): Spray thoroughly. Do not use article until spray is dry. Repeat treatment as necessary. Do not use in commercial food processing, preparation, storage or serving areas.

Storage and Disposal:
Storage: Store in a cool area away from heat or open flame.
Disposal: Wrap container and put in trash.

How Supplied: In 5 oz. and 10 oz. aerosol container.

Literature Available: For free patient information brochures and filmstrips, please call 1-800-KIL-LICE. A Reed & Carnrick health consultant will be glad to assist you.
Shown in Product Identification Section, page 422

EDUCATIONAL MATERIAL

Brochures
Questions and Answers About Head Lice
Available in English and Spanish to physicians, pharmacists and patients.

Questions and Answers About Treating Lice That Can Live Off the Body
Available to physicians, pharmacists and patients.
Gas Discomfort
A brochure about what gas discomfort is, why it hurts, and how to control it. Available to physicians, pharmacists and patients.

The Reese Chemical Co.
10617 FRANK AVENUE
CLEVELAND, OHIO 44106

REESE'S PINWORM MEDICINE
Pyrantel Pamoate

Active Ingredient: Pyrantel pamoate, 144 mg/cc (the equivalent of 50 mg pyrantel base per cc).

Indications: For the treatment of enterobiasis (pinworm infection) and ascariasis (common roundworm infection).

Warnings: Keep this and all drugs out of the reach of children. In case of accidental overdose, seek professional assistance or contact a poison control center immediately.

Precaution: If you are pregnant or have liver disease, do not take this product unless directed by a doctor.

Dosage and Administration: Adults and children 2 to 12 years of age—Oral dosage is a single dose of 5 mg of pyrantel pamoate per pound of body weight, not to exceed 1 gram.
Read package insert before taking this medicine. Do not administer to children under 2 years of age.

How Supplied: Reese's Pinworm Medicine is available in one-ounce bottles as a pleasant-tasting suspension which contains the equivalent of 50 mg pyrantel base per cc. It is supplied with English and Spanish label copy and directions.
Shown in Product Identification Section, page 423

Reid-Rowell
901 SAWYER ROAD
MARIETTA, GA 30062
AND
210 MAIN STREET W.
BAUDETTE, MN 56623

BALNEOL®
[băl 'nē-ŏl]
Perianal cleansing lotion

Composition: Contains water, mineral oil, propylene glycol, glyceryl stearate/PEG-100 stearate, PEG-40 stearate, laureth-4, PEG-4 dilaurate, lanolin oil, sodium acetate, carbomer-934, triethanolamine, methylparaben, dioctyl sodium sulfosuccinate, fragrance, acetic acid.

Action and Uses: BALNEOL is a soothing, emollient cleanser for hygienic

Continued on next page

Reid-Rowell—Cont.

cleansing of irritated perianal and external vaginal areas. It helps relieve itching and other discomforts. BALNEOL gently yet thoroughly cleanses and provides a soothing, protecting film.

Administration and Dosage: For cleansing without discomfort after each bowel movement, a small amount of BALNEOL is spread on tissue or cotton and used to wipe the perianal area. Also used between bowel movements and at bedtime for additional comfort. For cleansing and soothing the external vaginal area: to be used on clean tissue or cotton as often as necessary.

Caution: In all cases of rectal bleeding, consult physician promptly. If irritation persists or increases, discontinue use and consult physician.

How Supplied: 3 fl oz (89 mL) plastic bottle.
Shown in Product Identification Section, page 423

HYDROCIL® INSTANT
[hī'dro-sĭl]

Description: A concentrated hydrophilic mucilloid containing 95% psyllium. Inactive ingredients: polyethylene glycol and povidone. Hydrocil Instant mixes instantly, is sugar-free, low in potassium and contains less than 10 mg of sodium per dose.

Indications: Hydrocil Instant is a natural bulk-forming fiber useful in the treatment of constipation and other conditions as directed by a physician.

Directions: The usual adult dose is one packet or scoopful poured into an 8 oz glass. Add water, fruit juices or other liquid and stir. It mixes instantly. Drink immediately. Take in the morning and night or as directed by a physician. Follow each dose with another glass of liquid.

How Supplied: In unit-dose packets of 3.7 grams that are available in boxes of 30's or 500's. Also in 250 gram jars with a measuring scoop. Each packet or scoopful, 3.7 grams, contains one usual adult dose of psyllium hydrophilic mucilloid, 3.5 grams.

Rev. 8/88
Shown in Product Identification Section, page 423

Products are indexed alphabetically in the **PINK SECTION**

Requa, Inc.
BOX 4008
1 SENECA PLACE
GREENWICH, CT 06830

CHARCOAID
Poison Adsorbent, liquid has sweet, pleasant taste and feel; especially good for young patients.

Active Ingredient: Activated vegetable charcoal U.S.P., 30g per bottle, suspended in 70% sorbitol solution U.S.P., 110 g.

Indication: For the emergency treatment of acute poisoning.

Action: Adsorbent

Warnings: Before using call a poison control center, emergency room, or a physician for advice. If the patient has been given Ipecac Syrup, do not give activated charcoal until after patient has vomited. Do not use in a semi-conscious or unconscious person.

Precaution: May cause laxation. Careful attention to fluids and electrolytes is important, especially with young children and multiple dose therapy.

Dosage and Administration: Adults: Shake well and drink entire contents (add water if too sweet). To insure a full dose, rinse bottle with water and drink. For children, refer to Poison Control Center.

Professional Labeling: Some dilution may be necessary for administration via lavage tube. Add a small amount of water to bottle and shake.

How Supplied: 5 fl. oz. unit dose bottle, 30g activated charcoal U.S.P., suspended in 70% sorbitol solution U.S.P., 110 g.
U.S. Patent #4,122,169

CHARCOCAPS®
Activated Charcoal Capsules

Active Ingredient: Activated vegetable charcoal U.S.P., 260 mg per capsule.

Indications: Relief of intestinal gas, diarrhea, gastrointestinal distress associated with indigestion. Also to aid in the prevention of non-specific pruritus associated with kidney dialysis treatment.

Actions: Adsorbent, detoxicant, soothing agent. Reduces the volume of intestinal gas and allays related discomfort.

Warnings: As with all anti-diarrheals—not for children under 3 unless directed by physician. If diarrhea persists more than two days or is accompanied by high fever, consult physician.

Drug Interaction: Activated Charcoal USP can adsorb medication while they are in the digestive tract.

Precaution: General Guidelines—Take two hours before or one hour after medication including oral contraceptives.

Symptoms and Treatment of Oral Overdosage: Overdosage has not been

encountered. Medical evidence indicates that high dosage or prolonged use does not cause side effect or harm the nutritional state of the patient.

Dosage and Administration: Two capsules after meals or at first sign of discomfort. Repeat as needed up to eight doses (16 capsules) per day.

Professional Labeling: None.

How Supplied: Bottles of 8, 36, 100 capsules

EDUCATIONAL MATERIAL

Questions & Answers
Brochure with questions and answers about the use of activated charcoal.
Trial Size
Professional sample of Charcocaps, which includes coupon for regular size for the patient.

Richardson-Vicks Inc.
ONE FAR MILL CROSSING
SHELTON, CT 06484

CHILDREN'S CHLORASEPTIC® LOZENGES

Active Ingredients: Benzocaine 5 mg per lozenge.

Inactive Ingredients: Corn syrup, FD&C Blue No. 1, FD&C Red No. 40, flavor, sucrose.

Indications: For temporary relief of occasional minor sore throat pain and irritation. Also for temporary relief of pain associated with sore mouth, canker sores, tonsillitis, pharyngitis and throat infections.

Directions: Adults and children 2 years of age and older: Allow product to dissolve slowly in mouth. May be repeated every 2 hours as needed or as directed by a doctor or dentist. Children under 2 years of age: Consult a doctor or a dentist.

Warning: If sore throat is severe, persists for more than 2 days, is accompanied or followed by fever, headache, rash, nausea, or vomiting, consult a doctor promptly. If sore mouth symptoms do not improve in 7 days, see your doctor or dentist promptly. In case of accidental overdose, seek professional assistance or contact a poison control center immediately. As with any drug, if you are pregnant or nursing a baby, seek the advice of a health professional before using this product.
Store at room temperature.
KEEP THIS AND ALL MEDICINES OUT OF THE REACH OF CHILDREN.

How Supplied: Cartons of 18.
Shown in Product Identification Section, page 423

CHLORASEPTIC® LIQUID
(oral anesthetic, antiseptic)
Cherry, Menthol and Cool Mint
Flavors

Active Ingredients: Phenol 1.4%.

Inactive Ingredients:
Menthol Liquid: Alcohol (12.5%), citric acid, D&C Yellow No. 10, FD&C Green No. 3, flavor, glycerin, propylene glycol, sodium citrate, sodium saccharin, sorbitol and water.
Menthol Aerosol Spray: D&C Yellow No. 10, FD&C Green No. 3, flavor, glycerin, saccharin, sodium and water.
Cherry Liquid: Alcohol (12.5%), citric acid, FD&C Red No. 40, flavor, glycerin, propylene glycol, sodium citrate, sodium saccharin, sorbitol and water.
Cherry Aerosol Spray: FD&C Red No. 40, flavor, glycerin, saccharin sodium and water.
Cool Mint Liquid: Alcohol (12.5%), citric acid, FD&C Blue No. 1, flavor, glycerin, menthol, propylene glycol, sodium citrate, sodium saccharin, sorbitol and water.

Indications: For temporary relief of occasional minor irritations, pain, sore mouth, sore throat and pain associated with canker sores. Also for the temporary relief of pain associated with tonsillitis, pharyngitis and throat infections.

Administration and Dosage:
Chloraseptic Spray (Pump), Mouthwash and Gargle: Irritated throat: Spray 5 times (Children 2–12 years of age, 3 times) and swallow. May be used as a gargle. Repeat every 2 hours or as directed by dentist or doctor. Oral Hygiene: Dilute with equal parts of water and rinse thoroughly, or spray full strength, then expel remainder.
Chloraseptic Aerosol Spray: Irritated throat: Spray throat about 2 seconds (Children 2–12 years about 1 second) and swallow. Repeat every 2 hours or as directed by dentist or doctor.
Children under 12 years of age should be supervised in the use of these products.

Warning: If sore throat is severe, persists for more than 2 days, is accompanied or followed by fever, headache, rash, nausea, or vomiting, consult a doctor promptly. If sore mouth symptoms do not improve in 7 days, see your doctor or dentist promptly. In case of accidental overdose, seek professional assistance or contact a poison control center immediately. As with any drug, if you are pregnant or nursing a baby, seek the advice of a health professional before using this product. Do not administer to children under 2 years of age unless directed by a physician or dentist.
For 1.5 oz. Aerosol Spray—Avoid spraying in eyes. Contents under pressure. Do not puncture or incinerate. (Do not burn or throw in fire, as can will burst.) Do not store at temperature above 120°F. (Such high temperatures may cause bursting.) Store at room temperature.
KEEP THIS AND ALL MEDICINES OUT OF THE REACH OF CHILDREN.

How Supplied: Available in Menthol, Cherry, and Cool Mint flavors in 6 fl. oz. plastic bottles with sprayer. Menthol and Cherry Flavors also available in 12 fl. oz. gargle and 1.5 oz. nitrogen-propelled aerosol sprays.
Shown in Product Identification Section, page 423

CHLORASEPTIC® LOZENGES
Cherry, Menthol, and Cool Mint
Flavor

Active Ingredients:
Menthol and Cherry: Phenol (32.5 mg./lozenge)
Cool Mint: Benzocaine (6.0 mg./lozenge) and Menthol (10 mg./lozenge).

Inactive Ingredients:
Menthol: Corn syrup, D&C Yellow No. 10, FD&C Blue No. 1, FD&C Yellow No. 6, flavor and sucrose.
Cherry: Corn syrup, FD&C Blue No. 1, FD&C Red No. 40, flavor, and sucrose.
Cool Mint: Corn syrup, FD&C Blue No. 1, flavor and sucrose.

Indications: For temporary relief of occasional minor sore throat pain and irritation. Also, for temporary relief of pain associated with sore mouth, canker sores, tonsillitis, pharyngitis and throat infections.

Directions:
Cool Mint
Adults and children 2 years of age and older: Allow product to dissolve slowly in mouth. May be repeated every 2 hours as needed or as directed by a doctor or dentist. Children under 2 years of Age: Consult a doctor or a dentist.
Menthol and Cherry
Adults and children 12 years of age and older: May be repeated every two hours or as directed by dentist or doctor. Children 6 to under 12 years of age: Allow product to dissolve slowly in mouth. May be repeated every two hours, not to exceed 8 lozenges per day. Children under 6 years of age: Consult a dentist or a doctor.

Warning: If sore throat is severe, persists for more than 2 days, is accompanied or followed by fever, headache, rash, nausea, or vomiting, consult a doctor promptly. If sore mouth symptoms do not improve in 7 days, see your doctor or dentist promptly. In case of accidental overdose, seek professional assistance or contact a Poison Control Center immediately. As with any drug, if you are pregnant or nursing a baby, seek the advice of a health professional before using this product.
KEEP THIS AND ALL MEDICINES OUT OF THE REACH OF CHILDREN.

How Supplied: Available in Menthol and Cherry flavors in packages of 18 and 36. Also available in Cool Mint flavor in packages of 18.
Shown in Product Identification Section, page 423

CLEARASIL® Adult Care—
Medicated Blemish Cream

Active Ingredient: Sulfur, resorcinol (alcohol 10%) in a cream base which contains water, bentonite, glyceryl stearate SE, propylene glycol, isopropyl myristate, sodium bisulfite, dimethicone, methylparaben, propylparaben, fragrance, iron oxides.

Indications: For the topical treatment of acne vulgaris in adults or persons demonstrating sensitivity to benzoyl peroxide.

Actions: CLEARASIL Adult Care—Medicated Blemish Cream is a blemish medication specially suited for adult usage since it dries acne lesions without overdrying or irritating the skin the way many benzoyl peroxide-containing products do. The product contains sulfur and resorcinol to help heal acne pimples, and bentonite to absorb excess sebum.

Warnings: For external use only. Other topical acne medications should not be used at the same time as this medication. Apply to affected areas only. Do not use on broken skin or apply to large areas of the body. Do not get into eyes. Some people with sensitive skin may experience slight irritation after use of this product. If this occurs, discontinue use of this product. If condition persists, consult a doctor or pharmacist. Keep this and all medicine out of reach of children.

Symptoms and Treatment of Oral Overdosage: These symptoms are based upon medical judgement, not on actual experience. Theoretically, ingestion of very large amounts may cause nausea, vomiting, abdominal discomfort and diarrhea. Treatment is symptomatic, with bed rest and observation.

Dosage and Administration: Cleanse skin thoroughly before applying medication. To clear up the blemishes you have now, apply Clearasil Adult Care directly on and around the affected area two or three times daily. If excessive drying occurs, decrease usage to one or two applications per day.

How Supplied: Available in a .6 oz. tube.
Shown in Product Identification Section, page 424

CLEARASIL DOUBLECLEAR
REGULAR STRENGTH PADS AND
CLEARASIL DOUBLECLEAR
MAXIMUM STRENGTH PADS

Active Ingredients: *Regular Strength:* Salicylic Acid 1.25%, Alcohol 40% by volume. *Maximum Strength:* Salicylic Acid 2.00%, Alcohol 40% by volume.

Inactive Ingredients: Witch Hazel Distillate, Sodium Methyl Cocoyl Taurate, Purified Water, Quaternium-22, Aloe Vera Gel, Menthol, Fragrance.

Indications: Topical skin cleanser for the treatment of acne vulgaris.

Continued on next page

Richardson-Vicks—Cont.

Actions: Clearasil DoubleClear Pads contain a comedolytic agent that penetrates deep into the pores to clean out oil and dead skin cells that can clog pores and cause pimples.

Warnings: For external use only. If irritation or excessive dryness and/or peeling occurs, reduce frequency of use. If these symptoms persist, consult a physician promptly. May be irritating to eyes. If contact occurs, flush throughly with water. Keep away from extreme heat or open flame.

Drug Interactions: None known.

Symptoms and Treatment of Ingestion: Product contains Ethyl Alcohol and Salicylic Acid. If large amounts are ingested, nausea, vomiting, gastrointestinal irritation may develop. Bed rest and observation are indicated if ingested.

Directions for Use: After washing— 1. Wipe your face where pimples occur with the deep-cleaning side, to loosen embedded oil and dirt, and to treat existing pimples. 2. Use the superabsorbent side all over your face to absorb oil, remove dirt, and to help prevent new pimples from forming. 3. For maximum effectiveness do not rinse. 4. Use morning, evening, and whenever you wash your face.

How Supplied: Both Maximum and Regular Strength are supplied in 8 ounce jars containing 32 pads.
Shown in Product Identification Section, page 424

CLEARASIL® Maximum Strength Medicated Anti-Acne Cream Vanishing and Tinted

Active Ingredient: Benzoyl peroxide 10% in an odorless, greaseless cream base, containing water, propylene glycol, aluminum hydroxide, bentonite, glyceryl stearate SE, isopropyl myristate, dimethicone, PEG-12, potassium carbomer-940, methylparaben, and propylparaben. The tinted formula also contains titanium dioxide and iron oxides.

Indications: For the topical treatment of acne vulgaris.

Actions: CLEARASIL Maximum Strength Medicated Anti-Acne Cream contains benzoyl peroxide, an antibacterial and keratolytic agent as well as bentonite and aluminum hydroxide as oil absorbents. The product 1) helps heal and prevent acne pimples, 2) helps absorb excess skin oil often associated with acne blemishes, 3) helps your skin look fresh. The Vanishing formula works invisibly. The Tinted formula hides pimples while it works.

Warnings: Persons with a known sensitivity to benzoyl peroxide should not use this medication. Excessive dryness or peeling may occur especially in persons with unusually dry, sensitive, or maturing skin. If itching, redness, burning, swelling or undue dryness occurs, reduce

dosage or discontinue use. If symptoms persist, consult a physician promptly. For external use only. Keep from eyes, lips, mouth and sensitive areas of the neck. Avoid contact with hair, fabrics and clothing which may be bleached by the benzoyl peroxide in this product. Keep this and all medicine out of the reach of children.

Symptoms and Treatment of Ingestion: These symptoms are based upon medical judgement, not on actual experience. Theoretically, ingestion of very large amounts may cause nausea, vomiting, abdominal discomfort and diarrhea. Treatment is symptomatic, with bed rest and observation.

Directions For Use: 1. Wash thoroughly. (Clearasil® Antibacterial Soap and Clearasil® Medicated Astringent are excellent products to use in your cleansing regimen.) **2.** Try this sensitivity test. Apply cream sparingly with fingertips to one or two small affected areas during the first three days. If no discomfort or reaction occurs, apply up to two times daily, wherever pimples and oil are a problem. **3.** If bothersome dryness or peeling occurs, reduce dosage to one application per day or every other day.

How Supplied: Available in both Vanishing and Tinted formulas in 1 oz. and .65 oz. squeeze tubes.
Shown in Product Identification Section, page 424

**CLEARASIL®
10% Benzoyl Peroxide Medicated Anti-Acne Lotion**

Active Ingredient: Benzoyl Peroxide 10% in a colorless, greaseless lotion which contains water, aluminum hydroxide, isopropyl stearate, PEG-100 stearate, glyceryl stearate, cetyl alcohol, glycereth-26, isocetyl stearate, glycerin, dimethicone copolyol, sodium citrate, citric acid, methylparaben, propylparaben, fragrance.

Indications: For the topical treatment of acne vulgaris.

Actions: CLEARASIL 10% Benzoyl Peroxide Lotion contains benzoyl peroxide, an antibacterial and keratolytic agent. The product **1. Helps heal and prevent acne pimples.** Benzoyl peroxide dries up existing pimples and kills acne-causing bacteria to help prevent new ones.
2. Helps absorb excess skin oil often associated with acne blemishes. Contains aluminum hydroxide which is a special oil-absorbing ingredient that allows Clearasil Lotion to absorb **more** excess skin oil than 10% benzoyl peroxide alone.
3. Helps your skin look fresh. Extra oil absorption helps your skin look less oily, more natural.

Warnings: Persons with a known sensitivity to benzoyl peroxide should not use this medication. Excessive dryness or peeling may occur especially in persons with unusually dry, sensitive, or matur-

ing skin. If itching, redness, burning, swelling or undue dryness occurs, reduce dosage or discontinue use. If symptoms persist, consult a physician promptly. For external use only. Keep from eyes, lips, mouth and sensitive areas of the neck. Avoid contact with hair, fabrics and clothing which may be bleached by the benzoyl peroxide in this product. Keep this and all medicine out of the reach of children.

Symptoms and Treatment of Ingestion: These symptoms are based upon medical judgement, not on actual experience. Theoretically, ingestion of very large amounts may cause nausea, vomiting, abdominal discomfort and diarrhea. Treatment is symptomatic, with bed rest and observation.

**Directions For Use:
SHAKE WELL BEFORE USING.**
1. Wash thoroughly. (Clearasil® Antibacterial Soap and Clearasil® Medicated Astringent are excellent products to use in your cleansing regimen.) **2.** Try this sensitivity test. Apply lotion sparingly with fingertips to one or two small affected areas during the first three days. If no discomfort or reaction occurs, apply up to two times daily, wherever pimples and oil are a problem. **3.** If bothersome dryness or peeling occurs, reduce dosage to one application per day or every other day.

How Supplied: Available in a 1 fl. oz. squeeze bottle.

**CLEARASIL®
Medicated Astringent**

Active Ingredient: Salicylic Acid (0.5%), also contains ethyl alcohol (43%).

Indications: Topical Skin Cleanser for treatment of acne vulgaris.

Actions: Clearasil® Medicated Astringent contains a comedolytic agent that penetrates deep into pores to clean out oil and dead skin cells that can clog pores and cause pimples.

Warnings: For external use only. May be irritating to the eyes. If contact occurs, flush thoroughly with water. Keep away from extreme heat or open flame.

Drug Interaction: None known.

Symptoms and Treatment of Ingestion: Product contains ethyl alcohol. If large amounts are ingested, nausea, vomiting, gastrointestinal irritation may develop. Bed rest and observation are indicated if ingested.

Directions for Use: Use up to three times daily as part of your regular cleansing routine. Saturate cotton pad and clean face and neck thoroughly. Repeat with fresh cotton pads until no trace of dirt remains. Do not rinse after use.

How Supplied: 4 oz. plastic bottles.
Shown in Product Identification Section, page 424

DRAMAMINE® Liquid
[*dram 'uh-meen*]
(dimenhydrinate syrup USP)
DRAMAMINE® Tablets
(dimenhydrinate USP)
DRAMAMINE® Chewable Tablets
(dimenhydrinate USP)

Description: Dimenhydrinate is the chlorotheophylline salt of the antihistaminic agent diphenhydramine. Dimenhydrinate contains not less than 53% and not more than 56% of diphenhydramine, and not less than 44% and not more than 47% of 8-chlorotheophylline, calculated on the dried basis.

Inactive Ingredients:
Dramamine Tablets: Acacia, Carboxymethylcellulose Sodium, Corn Starch, Magnesium Stearate, and Sodium Sulfate.
Dramamine Liquid: Cherry Flavor, FD&C Red No. 40, Ethyl Alcohol 5%, Glycerin, Methylparaben, Sucrose, and Water.
Dramamine Chewable Tablets: Aspartame, Citric Acid, FD&C Yellow No. 6, Flavor, Magnesium Stearate, Methacrylic Acid Copolymer, Sorbitol.
Phenylketonurics: Contains Phenylalanine 1.5 mg per tablet.
Contains FD&C Yellow No. 5 (tartrazine) as a color additive.

Actions: While the precise mode of action of dimenhydrinate is not known, it has a depressant action on hyperstimulated labyrinthine function.

Indications: Dramamine is indicated for the prevention and treatment of the nausea, vomiting, dizziness or vertigo associated with motion sickness. Such an illness may arise from the motion of ships, planes, trains, automobiles, buses, swings, or even amusement park rides. Regardless of the cause of motion sickness, Dramamine has been found to be effective in its prevention or treatment.

Warnings: DRAMAMINE may cause marked drowsiness; alcohol, sedatives, and tranquilizers may increase the drowsiness effect. Avoid alcoholic beverages while taking this product. Do not take this product if you are taking sedatives or tranquilizers without first consulting your doctor. Use caution when driving a motor vehicle or operating machinery. Do not take this product if you have asthma, glaucoma, emphysema, chronic pulmonary disease, shortness of breath, difficulty in breathing, or difficulty in urination due to enlargement of the prostate gland unless directed by a doctor. Do not give to children under 2 years of age unless directed by a doctor. In case of accidental overdose, seek professional assistance or consult a poison control center immediately. As with any drug, if you are pregnant or nursing a baby, seek the advice of a health professional before using this product. Keep this and all medications out of the reach of children.

Dosage and Administration:
Dramamine Tablets: To prevent motion sickness, the first dose should be taken ½ to 1 hour before starting the activity.

Additional medication depends on travel conditions. *Adults:* 1 to 2 tablets every 4 to 6 hours, not to exceed 8 tablets in 24 hours. *Children 6 to 12 years:* ½ to 1 tablet every 6 to 8 hours, not to exceed 3 tablets in 24 hours. *Children 2 to 6 years:* Up to ½ tablet every 6 to 8 hours, not to exceed 1½ tablets in 24 hours. Children may also be given Dramamine cherry-flavored liquid in accordance with directions for use. Not for frequent or prolonged use except on advice of a physician. Do not exceed recommended dosage.
Dramamine Liquid: To prevent motion sickness, the first dose should be taken ½ to 1 hour before starting the activity. Additional medication depends on travel conditions. *Adults:* 4 to 8 teaspoonfuls (4 ml per teaspoonful) every 4 to 6 hours, not to exceed 32 teaspoonfuls in 24 hours. *Children 6 to 12 years:* 2 to 4 teaspoonfuls every 6 to 8 hours, not to exceed 12 teaspoonfuls in 24 hours. *Children 2 to 6 years:* 1 to 2 teaspoonfuls every 6 to 8 hours, not to exceed 6 teaspoonfuls in 24 hours. *Children under 2 years:* Only on advice of a physician.
Not for frequent or prolonged use except on advice of a physician. Do not exceed recommended dosage. Use of a measuring device is recommended for all liquid medication.
Dramamine Chewable Tablets: To prevent motion sickness, the first dose should be taken one-half to one hour before starting the activity. Additional medication depends on travel conditions. *Adults:* 1 to 2 tablets every 4 to 6 hours. *Children:* See directions for tablets above.

How Supplied: *Tablets* —scored, white tablets containing 50 mg of dimenhydrinate. Available in packets of 12 and 36 and bottles of 100 (OTC); *Liquid* —12.5 mg dimenhydrinate per 5 ml, ethyl alcohol 5%, bottles of 3 fl oz (OTC).
Shown in Product Identification Section, page 423

ICY HOT® Balm
[*ī 'see hot*]
(topical analgesic balm)
ICY HOT® Cream
(topical analgesic cream)
ICY HOT® Stick
(topical analgesic stick)

Active Ingredients: Icy Hot Balm contains methyl salicylate 29%, menthol 7.6%. Icy Hot Cream contains methyl salicylate 30%, menthol 10%. Icy Hot Stick contains methyl salicylate 30%, menthol 10%.
Inactive ingredients of Icy Hot Balm include paraffin and white petrolatum. Inactive ingredients of Icy Hot Cream include carbomer, cetyl esters wax, emulsifying wax, oleth-3 phosphate, stearic acid, trolamine, and water. Inactive ingredients of Icy Hot Stick include ceresin, cyclomethicone, hydrogenated castor oil, microcrystalline wax, paraffin, PEG-150 distearate, propylene glycol, stearic acid, and stearyl alcohol.

Description: Icy Hot Balm, Icy Hot Cream, and Icy Hot Stick are topically applied analgesics containing two active ingredients, methyl salicylate and menthol. It is the particular concentration of these ingredients, in combination with inert ingredients, that results in the distinct, combined heating/cooling sensation of Icy Hot.

Actions: Icy Hot is classified as a counterirritant which, when rubbed into the intact skin, provides relief of deep-seated pain through a counterirritant action rather than through a direct analgesic effect. In acting as a counterirritant, Icy Hot replaces the perception of pain with another sensation that blocks deep pain temporarily by its action on or near the skin surface.

Indications: Icy Hot helps bring temporary relief from minor arthritis pain and its stiffness, helps temporarily block minor pain from simple backache, and helps soothe sore muscles.

Warnings: For external use only as directed. Keep away from children to avoid accidental poisoning. If swallowed, induce vomiting and call a physician immediately. For children under 12, consult a physician before use. Avoid contact with eyes, mouth, genitalia, and mucous membranes. Do not apply to wounds or to damaged, irritated or very sensitive skin. Diabetics and people with impaired circulation should use Icy Hot only upon the advice of a physician. Do not wrap, bandage or apply external heat or hot water. If condition worsens, or if symptoms persist for more than 7 days or clear up and occur again within a few days, discontinue use of this product and consult a physician.

Adverse Reactions: The most common adverse reactions that may occur with Icy Hot use are skin irritation and blistering. The most serious adverse reaction is severe toxicity that occurs if the product is ingested.

Dosage and Administration: Apply Icy Hot to the painful area; massage until Icy Hot is completely absorbed. Repeat as necessary up to four times daily.

How Supplied: Icy Hot Balm is available in jars in two sizes, 3½ oz and 7 oz. Icy Hot Cream is available in tubes in two sizes, 1¼ oz and 3 oz. Icy Hot Stick is available as a 1¾ oz stick.
Shown in Product Identification Section, page 423

PERCOGESIC®
[*pĕr-kō-jē 'zĭk*]
Analgesic Tablets

Description: Each tablet contains:
Acetaminophen ....325 mg
Phenyltoloxamine citrate ....30 mg

Inactive Ingredients: Cellulose, Flavor, FD&C Yellow No. 6, Hydroxypropyl Methylcellulose, Magnesium Stearate, Polyethylene Glycol, Povidone, Silica Gel, Starch, Stearic Acid, Sucrose.

Continued on next page

Richardson-Vicks—Cont.

Indications: For temporary relief of minor aches and pains associated with colds, headaches, toothaches, muscular aches, backaches, premenstrual and menstrual periods, minor arthritis pain and to reduce fever.

Warning: May cause excitability especially in children. Don't take if you have asthma, glaucoma, emphysema, chronic pulmonary disease, shortness of breath, difficulty in breathing, or difficulty in urination due to enlargement of the prostate gland unless directed by a doctor. May cause drowsiness; alcohol, sedatives, and tranquilizers may increase drowsiness. Avoid alcoholic beverages while taking this product. Don't use if you're taking sedatives or tranquilizers without first consulting a doctor. Use caution when driving a motor vehicle or operating machinery. Don't take for pain for more then 10 days (adults) or 5 days (children), and don't take for fever for more than 3 days unless directed by a doctor. If pain or fever persists or worsens, new symptoms occur, or redness or swelling is present, consult a doctor as these could be signs of a serious condition. Don't give this product to children for arthritis pain unless directed by a doctor. If pregnant or nursing a baby, seek a health professional's advice before using this product. KEEP OUT OF REACH OF CHILDREN.

Overdosage: In case of overdosage, seek professional assistance or contact a poison control center immediately. Prompt medical attention is critical for adults and children, even if you don't notice signs or symptoms.

Dosage and Administration: *Adults* (12 years and over)—1 or 2 tablets every four hours. Maximum daily dose—8 tablets *Children* (6–12 years)—one tablet every 4 hours. Maximum daily dose—4 tablets.

How Supplied: Child-resistant bottles of 24 and 90 tablets, and bottles of 50 tablets.

Shown in Product Identification Section, page 423

VICKS® CHILDREN'S COUGH SYRUP
Expectorant, Antitussive Cough Syrup

Active Ingredients per tsp. (5 ml.): Dextromethorphan Hydrobromide 3.5 mg., Guaifenesin 50 mg., in a red, cherry-flavored, syrup base. This product contains no alcohol.

Inactive Ingredients: Citric Acid, FD&C Green No. 3, FD&C Red No. 40, Flavor, Methylparaben, Propylene Glycol, Purified Water, Sodium Citrate, Sodium Saccharin, Sucrose.

Indications: Provides temporary relief of coughs due to colds, helps loosen phlegm and mucus in the upper chest and promote drainage of bronchial tubes

so breathing is made easier. Coats and soothes a cough-irritated throat.

Actions: VICKS COUGH SYRUP is an antitussive and expectorant. It calms, quiets coughs of colds, flu and bronchitis; loosens phlegm, promotes drainage of bronchial tubes; and coats and soothes a cough irritated throat.

Warning: Do not take this product for persistent or chronic cough such as occurs with smoking, asthma, or emphysema, or if cough is accompanied by excessive phlegm (mucus) unless directed by a doctor. A persistent cough may be a sign of a serious condition. If cough persists for more than one week, tends to recur, or is accompanied by fever, rash, or persistent headache, consult a doctor. Do not give this product to children under two years of age unless directed by a doctor. As with any drug, if you are pregnant or nursing a baby, seek the advice of a health professional before using this product. **As with all medicines, keep out of children's reach.**

Overdosage: In case of accidental overdose seek professional assistance or contact a Poison Control Center immediately.

Dosage:
12 years and over:　4 teaspoonfuls
6–12 years:　2 teaspoonfuls
2–6 years:　1 teaspoonful
Repeat every 4 hours as needed.

How Supplied: Available in 4 fl. oz. bottles.

VICKS® COUGH SILENCERS
Cough Drops

Active Ingredients per drop: Dextromethorphan (expressed as Dextromethorphan Hydrobromide) 2.5 mg., Benzocaine 1 mg.

Inactive Ingredients: Corn Syrup, FD&C Blue No. 1, Silicon Dioxide, Sodium Chloride, Sucrose. Special Vicks Medication (menthol, anethole, peppermint oil) 0.35%.
Contains FD&C Yellow No. 5 (tartrazine).

Indications: Temporarily relieves cough and minor throat and bronchial irritation occurring with a cold.

Warning: A persistent cough may be a sign of a serious condition. If cough persists for more than one week, tends to recur, or is accompanied by fever, rash, or persistent headache, consult a doctor. Do not take this product for persistent chronic cough such as occurs with smoking, asthma, emphysema, or if cough is accompanied by excessive phlegm (mucus) unless directed by a doctor. As with any drug, if you are pregnant or nursing a baby, seek the advice of a health professional before using this product.

Overdosage: In case of accidental overdose, seek professional assistance or contact a poison control center immediately.

Directions for Use: Age 12 and over: 4 drops every four hours. Dissolve in mouth one at a time. Do not exceed 48 in 24 hours or as directed by doctor. Ages 6 to under 12: 2 to 4 drops every four hours. Dissolve in mouth one at a time. Do not exceed 24 in 24 hours or as directed by doctor. Ages 2 to under 6: 1 or 2 drops every four hours. Dissolve in mouth one at a time. Do not exceed 12 in 24 hours or as directed by doctor. Children under 2, consult doctor.

How Supplied: Available in boxes of 14's.

VICKS DAYCARE® LIQUID
VICKS DAYCARE® CAPLETS
Multi-Symptom Colds Medicine

Active Ingredients: LIQUID — per fluid ounce (2 Tbs.) or **CAPLET** — per **two** caplets, contains Acetaminophen 650 mg., Dextromethorphan Hydrobromide 20 mg., Pseudoephedrine Hydrochloride 60 mg., Guaifenesin 200 mg.

Inactive Ingredients:
Liquid: Citric Acid, FD&C Yellow No. 6, Flavor, Glycerin, Propylene Glycol, Purified Water, Saccharin, Sodium Benzoate, Sodium Citrate, Sucrose. Also contains Alcohol 10%.
Caplets: Cellulose, Croscarmellose Sodium, FD&C Yellow No. 6, Magnesium Stearate, Povidone, Starch, Stearic acid.

Indications: For temporary relief of major colds symptoms as follows:
Nasal and sinus congestion, coughing, aches and pains, fever, and cough-irritated throat of a cold or flu. Loosens upper chest congestion; restores freer breathing.

Actions: VICKS DAYCARE is a decongestant, antitussive, expectorant, analgesic and antipyretic. It helps clear stuffy nose, congested sinus openings. Calms, quiets coughing. Eases headache pain and the ache-all-over feeling. Reduces fever due to colds and flu. It relieves these symptoms without drowsiness. DAYCARE LIQUID also soothes a cough-irritated throat.

Warning: Do not exceed recommended dosage because at higher doses nervousness, dizziness, or sleeplessness may occur. Do not take this product for more than 7 days. If symptoms do not improve or are accompanied by fever, consult a doctor. Do not take this product if you have heart disease, diabetes, high blood pressure, thyroid disease, diabetes, or difficulty in urination due to enlargement of the prostate gland unless directed by a doctor. Do not take this product for persistent or chronic cough such as occurs with smoking, asthma, chronic bronchitis, or emphysema, or where cough is accompanied by excessive phlegm (mucus) unless directed by a doctor. A persistent cough may be a sign of a serious condition. If cough persists for more than 1 week, tends to recur, or is accompanied by fever, rash, or persistent headaches, consult a doctor. Do not take this product for pain for more than 10 days or for fever for more than 3 days unless directed by a doctor. If pain or fever persists or gets worse, if new symptoms occur, or if redness or swelling is present, consult a doctor because these could be signs of a serious condition. If sore throat is severe, persists for more than 2 days, is accompanied or followed by fever, headache, rash, nausea or vomiting, consult a doctor promptly. As with any drug, if you are pregnant or nursing a baby, seek the advice of a health professional before using this product.

Drug Interaction Precaution: Do not take this product if you are presently taking a prescription drug for high blood pressure or depression without first consulting your doctor. KEEP OUT OF REACH OF CHILDREN. TAKE ONLY AS DIRECTED.

Overdosage: In case of accidental overdose, seek professional assistance or contact a poison control center immediately. Prompt medical attention is critical for adults as well as for children even if you do not notice any signs or symptoms.

Dosage:
Adults: one fluid ounce (2 Tbs.) LIQUID, or 2 CAPLETS.
Children (6 to 12 years): One-half ounce (1 Tbs.) LIQUID, or 1 CAPLET.
Children (2 to 6 years): 1½ tsp LIQUID. May be repeated every 4 hours as needed. Maximum 4 doses per day.

How Supplied: Available in: **LIQUID** with child-resistant, tamper-evident cap—6 and 10 fl. oz. plastic bottles.
CAPLET in child-resistant packages—20.
Shown in Product Identification Section, page 423

VICKS FORMULA 44® COUGH CONTROL DISCS

Active Ingredients per disc: Dextromethorphan (expressed as Dextromethorphan Hydrobromide) 5 mg., Benzocaine 1.25 mg, Menthol 4.3 mg.

Inactive Ingredients: Anethole, Caramel, Corn Syrup, Flavor, Peppermint Oil, Silicon Dioxide, Sodium Chloride, Sucrose.

Indications: Provides temporary relief from coughs and relieves minor throat and bronchial irritation caused by colds, or inhaled irritants.

Actions: VICKS FORMULA 44 COUGH CONTROL DISCS are antitussive and local-anesthetic cough drops. They calm, quiet coughs and help coat and soothe irritated throats.

Warnings: A persistent cough may be a sign of a serious condition. If cough persists for more than 1 week, tends to recur, or is accompanied by fever, rash, or persistent headache, consult a doctor. Do not take this product for persistent or chronic cough such as occurs with smoking, asthma, emphysema, or if cough is accompanied by excessive phlegm (mucus) unless directed by a doctor. As with any drug, if you are pregnant or nursing

a baby, seek the advice of a health professional before using this product.
KEEP OUT OF THE REACH OF CHILDREN.

Overdosage: In case of accidental overdose, seek professional assistance or contact a poison control center immediately.

Dosage:
Adults 12 years and over:
 Dissolve two discs in mouth, one at a time. Repeat every 4 hours not to exceed 12 discs in 24 hours or as directed by doctor.
Children 2 to under 12 years:
 Dissolve one disc in mouth. Repeat every 4 hours not to exceed 6 discs in 24 hours or as directed by doctor.
Under 2 years, consult a doctor.

How Supplied: Available as individual foil-wrapped portable packets in boxes of 24.

VICKS FORMULA 44® COUGH MEDICINE

Active Ingredients per 2 tsp. (10 mL.): Dextromethorphan Hydrobromide 30 mg., Chlorpheniramine Maleate 4 mg. in a pleasant-tasting, dark brown syrup base. Also contains Alcohol 10%.

Inactive Ingredients: Caramel, Flavor, Propylene Glycol, Purified Water, Sodium Benzoate, Sodium Citrate, Invert Sugar.

Indications: For the temporary relief of coughs and runny nose due to colds, minor throat and bronchial irritation.

Actions: VICKS FORMULA 44 COUGH MIXTURE is a cough suppressant, antihistamine and demulcent. Calms and quiets coughs. Reduces sneezing and sniffling. Coats, soothes irritated throat.

Warning: May cause excitability especially in children. Do not take this product if you have asthma, glaucoma, emphysema, chronic pulmonary disease, shortness of breath, difficulty in breathing, or difficulty in urination due to enlargement of the prostate gland unless directed by a doctor. May cause drowsiness; alcohol may increase the drowsiness effect. Avoid alcoholic beverages while taking this product. Do not take this product if you are taking sedatives or tranquilizers without first consulting your doctor. Use caution when driving a motor vehicle or operating machinery. Do not take this product for persistent or chronic cough such as occurs with smoking, asthma, or emphysema, or if cough is accompanied by excessive phlegm (mucus) unless directed by a doctor. A persistent cough may be a sign of a serious condition. If cough persists for more than one week, tends to recur, or is accompanied by high fever, rash, or persistent headaches, consult a doctor.
As with any drug, if you are pregnant or nursing a baby, seek the advice of a health professional before using this preparation.

Overdosage: In case of accidental overdose, seek professional assistance or contact a Poison Control Center immediately.

Dosage:
Adults: 12 years and over—2 teaspoonfuls
Children: 6 to 12 years: 1 teaspoonful
Children under 6 consult a doctor.
Repeat every 6 hours as needed.
No more than 4 doses per day.

How Supplied: Available in 4 fl. oz. and 8 fl. oz. bottles.
Shown in Product Identification Section, page 423

VICKS FORMULA 44D® DECONGESTANT COUGH MEDICINE

Active Ingredients per 3 tsp. (15 ml.): Dextromethorphan Hydrobromide 30 mg., Pseudoephedrine Hydrochloride 60 mg., Guaifenesin (Glyceryl Guaiacolate) 200 mg. in a red, cherry-flavored, cooling syrup. Also contains alcohol 10%.

Inactive Ingredients: Citric Acid, FD&C Red No. 40, Flavor, Propylene Glycol, Purified Water, Sodium Benzoate, Sodium Citrate, Sodium Saccharin, Sucrose.

Indications: Relieves coughs, decongests nasal passages and loosens upper chest congestion due to colds, minor throat and bronchial irritation.

Actions: VICKS FORMULA 44D is an antitussive, nasal decongestant, expectorant. It calms, quiets coughs; relieves nasal congestion; loosens phlegm, mucus; and coats, soothes an irritated throat.

Warning: Do not exceed recommended dosage because at higher doses nervousness, dizziness, or sleeplessness may occur. Do not take this product for more than 7 days. If symptoms do not improve or are accompanied by fever, consult a doctor. Do not take this product if you have heart disease, high blood pressure, thyroid disease, diabetes, or difficulty in urination due to enlargement of the prostate gland unless directed by a doctor. Do not take this product for persistent or chronic cough such as occurs with smoking, asthma, or emphysema, or if cough is accompanied by excessive phlegm (mucus) unless directed by a doctor. A persistent cough may be a sign of a serious condition. If cough persists for more than 1 week, tends to recur, or is accompanied by high fever, rash, or persistent headaches, consult a doctor. Do not give this product to children under 2 years of age unless directed by a doctor. As with any drug, if you are pregnant, or nursing a baby, seek the advice of a health professional before using this product.

Drug Interaction Precaution: Do not take this product if you are presently taking a prescription drug for high blood pressure or depression without first consulting your doctor.

Continued on next page

Richardson-Vicks—Cont.

Overdosage: In case of accidental overdose, seek professional assistance or contact a Poison Control Center immediately.

Dosage:
ADULT DOSE 12 years and over— 3 teaspoonfuls
CHILD DOSE 6–12 years—
1½ teaspoonfuls
2–6 years—
¾ teaspoonful.
Repeat ever 6 hours as needed, no more than 4 doses per day.

How Supplied: Available in 4 fl. oz. and 8 fl. oz. bottles.
Shown in Product Identification Section, page 423

VICKS FORMULA 44M®
MULTI-SYMPTOM COUGH MEDICINE

Active Ingredients per 4 tsp. (20 ml.): Dextromethorphan Hydrobromide 30 mg., Pseudoephedrine Hydrochloride 60 mg., Guaifenesin 200 mg., Acetaminophen 500 mg. in a bluish-red fruit-flavored syrup. Also contains alcohol 20%.

Inactive Ingredients: Citric Acid, FD&C Blue No. 1, FD&C Red No. 40, Flavor, Glycerin, Purified Water, Sodium Benzoate, Sodium Citrate, Sodium Saccharin, Sucrose.

Indications: Relieves coughs, decongests nasal passages, loosens upper chest congestion, relieves headache, fever and muscular aches due to colds, minor throat and bronchial irritation due to cold, bronchitis, or flulike conditions.

Actions: VICKS FORMULA 44M is a cough suppressant, nasal decongestant, expectorant demulcent and analgesic. It calms, quiets coughs; relieves nasal congestion; loosens phlegm, mucus; and coats, soothes and eases the pain of an irritated throat.

Warning: Do not exceed recommended dosage because at higher doses nervousness, dizziness, or sleeplessness may occur. Do not take this product for more than 7 days. If symptoms do not improve or are accompanied by fever, consult a doctor. Do not take this product if you have heart disease, high blood pressure, thyroid disease, diabetes, or difficulty in urination due to enlargement of the prostate gland unless directed by a doctor. Do not take this product for persistent or chronic cough such as occurs with smoking, asthma, or emphysema, or if cough is accompanied by excessive phlegm (mucus) unless directed by a doctor. A persistent cough may be a sign of a serious condition. If cough persists for more than 1 week, tends to recur, or is accompanied by fever, rash, or persistent headache, consult a doctor. Do not give this product to children under 2 years of age unless directed by a doctor. Do not take this product for more than 10 days (adults), 5 days (children), and do not take for fever

for more than 3 days unless directed by a doctor. If pain or fever persists or gets worse, if new symptoms occur, or if redness or swelling is present, consult a doctor because these could be signs of a serious condition. Do not give this product to children for the pain of arthritis unless directed by a doctor. As with any drug, if you are pregnant or nursing a baby, seek the advice of a health professional before using this product.

Drug Interaction Precaution: Do not take this product if you are presently taking a prescription drug for high blood pressure or depression, without first consulting your doctor.

Overdosage: In case of accidental overdose, seek professional assistance or contact a Poison Control Center immediately.

Dosage: 12 years and over—4 teaspoonfuls
6–12 years—2 teaspoonfuls
Repeat every 6 hours as needed. No more than 4 doses per day.

How Supplied: Available in 4 fl. oz. and 8 fl. oz. bottles.
Shown in Product Identification Section, page 423

VICKS® PEDIATRIC FORMULA 44®
COUGH MEDICINE

Active Ingredients per 1 Tbs. (15 ml.): Dextromethorphan Hydrobromide USP 15 mg.

Inactive Ingredients: Carboxymethylcellulose Sodium, Cellulose, Citric Acid, FD&C Red No. 40, Flavor, Glycerin, Polysorbate 80, Potassium Sorbate, Propylene Glycol, Purified Water, Sodium Citrate, Sorbitol, Sucrose.

Indications: For the temporary relief of coughs due to the common cold or minor throat and bronchial irritation.

Administration and Dosage:
Directions for Use: SHAKE WELL BEFORE USING
Squeeze bottle to accurately dispense medicine into   (CUP INSIDE)
dosage cup provided.

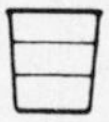

1 Tbs.
½ Tbs.

Dosage—Choose by weight (if weight is not known, choose by age):

Age, yr.	Weight, lb.	Dose
Under 2	Under 24	Consult physician*
2–5	24–47	Fill cup to ½ Tbs.
6–11	48–95	Fill cup to 1 Tbs.
12 and over	96 and over	2 Tbs. or Try one of the Adult Formula 44® Medicines

Repeat every 6–8 hours as needed, not to exceed 4 doses in 24 hours.
*Suggested doses for children 0–2 are:

Age, mo.	Weight, lb.	Dose
0–3	6–11	¼ tsp.
4–11	12–17	⅖ tsp.
12–23	18–23	½ tsp.

Warning: Do not exceed recommended dosage. Do not take this product for persistent or chronic cough such as occurs with smoking, asthma, or emphysema, or if cough is accompanied by excessive phlegm (mucus) unless directed by a doctor. A persistent cough may be a sign of a serious condition. If cough persists for more than 1 week, tends to recur, or is accompanied by fever, rash, or persistent headache, consult a doctor. In case of accidental overdose, seek professional assistance or contact a poison control center immediately. As with any drug, if you are pregnant or nursing a baby, seek the advice of a health professional before using this product.
KEEP OUT OF CHILDREN'S REACH. STORE AT ROOM TEMPERATURE. AVOID EXCESSIVE HEAT.

How Supplied: 4 fl. oz. squeeze bottles with VicksAccuTip™ Dispenser for clean, easy, accurate dosing. Calibrated dose cup accompanies each bottle.
Shown in Product Identification Section, page 423

VICKS® PEDIATRIC FORMULA 44®
COUGH & COLD MEDICINE

Active Ingredients: Per 1 Tbs. (15 ml.): Dextromethorphan Hydrobromide USP 15 mg., Pseudoephedrine Hydrochloride USP 30 mg., Chlorpheniramine Maleate USP 2 mg.

Inactive Ingredients: Carboxymethylcellulose Sodium, Cellulose, Citric Acid, FD&C Red No. 40, Flavor, Glycerin, Polysorbate 80, Potassium Sorbate, Propylene Glycol, Purified Water, Sodium Citrate, Sorbitol, Sucrose.

Indications: For the temporary relief of coughs, nasal congestion, runny nose and sneezing due to the common cold or upper respiratory allergies.

Administration and Dosage:
DIRECTIONS FOR USE: SHAKE WELL BEFORE USING
Squeeze bottle to accurately dispense medicine into   (CUP INSIDE)
dosage cup provided

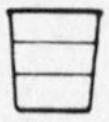

1 Tbs.
½ Tbs.

Dosage—Choose by weight (if weight is not known, choose by age):

Age, yr.	Weight, lb.	Dose
Under 6	Under 48	Consult physician*
6–11	48–95	Fill cup to 1 Tbs.
12 and over	96 and over	2 Tbs. or try one of the Adult Formula 44® Medicines

*Suggested dose for children 2–6 years (24–47 lb) ½Tbs.

Repeat every 6–8 hours as needed, not to exceed 4 doses in 24 hours.

Warning: Do not exceed recommended dosage because at higher doses nervousness, dizziness, or sleeplessness may occur. Do not take this product for more than 7 days. If symptoms do not improve or are accompanied by fever, consult a doctor. Do not take this product if you have heart disease, thyroid disease, diabetes, or difficulty in urination due to enlargement of the prostate gland unless directed by a doctor. Do not take this product for persistent or chronic cough such as occurs with smoking, asthma, or emphysema, or if cough is accompanied by excessive phlegm (mucus) unless directed by a doctor. A persistent cough may be a sign of a serious condition. If cough persists for more than 1 week, tends to recur, or is accompanied by fever, rash, or persistent headache, consult a doctor. May cause excitability especially in children. Do not take this product if you have asthma, glaucoma, emphysema, chronic pulmonary disease, shortness of breath or difficulty in breathing unless directed by a doctor. May cause drowsiness; alcohol, sedatives, and tranquilizers may increase the drowsiness effect. Avoid alcoholic beverages while taking this product. Do not take this product if you are taking sedatives or tranquilizers without first consulting your doctor. Use caution when driving a motor vehicle or operating machinery. In case of accidental overdose, seek professional assistance or contact a poison control center immediately. If pregnant or nursing a baby, consult a health professional before using this product.

Drug Interaction Precaution: Do not take this product if you are presently taking a prescription drug for high blood pressure or depression, without first consulting your doctor.

KEEP OUT OF CHILDREN'S REACH. STORE AT ROOM TEMPERATURE. AVOID EXCESSIVE HEAT.

How Supplied: 4 fl. oz. squeeze bottles with VicksAccuTip™ Dispenser for clean, easy, accurate dosing. Calibrated dose cup accompanies each bottle.
Shown in Product Identification Section, page 423

VICKS® PEDIATRIC FORMULA 44® COUGH & CONGESTION MEDICINE

Active Ingredients: Per 1 Tbs. (15 ml.): Dextromethorphan Hydrobromide USP 15 mg., Pseudoephedrine Hydrochloride USP 30 mg.

Inactive Ingredients: Carboxymethylcellulose Sodium, Cellulose, Citric Acid, FD&C Red No. 40, Flavor, Glycerin, Polysorbate 80, Potassium Sorbate, Propylene Glycol, Purified Water, Sodium Citrate, Sorbitol, Sucrose.

Indications: For the temporary relief of coughs and nasal congestion due to the common cold or upper respiratory allergies.

Administration and Dosage:
DIRECTIONS FOR USE: SHAKE WELL BEFORE USING
Squeeze bottle to accurately dispense medicine into (CUP INSIDE) dosage cup provided

1 Tbs.
½ Tbs.

Dosage—Choose by weight (if weight is not known, choose by age):

Age, yr.	Weight, lb.	Dose
Under 2	Under 24	Consult physician
2–5	24–47	Fill cup to ½ Tbs.
6–11	48–95	Fill cup to 1 Tbs.
12 and over	96 and over	2 Tbs. or Try one of the Adult Formula 44® Medicines

Repeat every 6–8 hours as needed, not to exceed 4 doses in 24 hours.

Warning:
Do not exceed recommended dosage because at higher doses nervousness, dizziness, or sleeplessness may occur. Do not take this product for more than 7 days. If symptoms do not improve or are accompanied by fever, consult a doctor. Do not take this product if you have heart disease, diabetes, or difficulty in urination due to enlargement of the prostate gland unless directed by a doctor. Do not take this product for persistent or chronic cough such as occurs with smoking, asthma, or emphysema, or if cough is accompanied by excessive phlegm (mucus) unless directed by a doctor. A persistent cough may be a sign of a serious condition. If cough persists for more than 1 week, tends to recur, or is accompanied by fever, rash, or persistent headache, consult a doctor. In case of accidental overdose, seek professional assistance or contact a poison control center immediately. If pregnant or nursing a baby, consult a health professional before using this product.

Drug Interaction Precaution: Do not take this product if you are presently taking a prescription drug for high blood pressure or depression, without first consulting your doctor.

KEEP OUT OF CHILDREN'S REACH. STORE AT ROOM TEMPERATURE. AVOID EXCESSIVE HEAT.

How Supplied: 4 fl. oz. squeeze bottles with VicksAccuTip™ Dispenser for clean, easy, accurate dosing. Calibrated dose cup accompanies each bottle.
Shown in Product Identification Section, page 423

VICKS® INHALER with decongestant action

Active Ingredients per inhaler: l-Desoxyephedrine 50 mg., Special Vicks Medication (menthol, camphor, bornyl acetate) 150 mg.

Inactive Ingredient: Fragrance.

Indications: Provides prompt, temporary relief of nasal congestion of colds and hay fever, allergies and sinusitis.

Actions: VICKS INHALER contains a volatile decongestant which, when inhaled, shrinks swollen membranes and provides fast relief from a stuffy nose.

Warning: Do not exceed recommended dosage because burning, stinging, sneezing, or increase of nasal discharge may occur. The use of this container by more than one person may spread infection. Do not use this product for more than 7 days. If symptoms persist, consult a doctor.

Overdosage: In case of accidental overdose, seek professional assistance or contact a Poison Control Center immediately.

Directions for Use: Adults (over 12 years): Inhale medicated vapors twice through each nostril while blocking off other nostril. Use every 2 hours as needed. Children (6–12): (With adult supervision) inhale once through each nostril every two hours as needed. Children (under 6): Consult a physician. VICKS INHALER is medically effective for 3 months after first use.

How Supplied: Available as a cylindrical plastic nasal inhaler (net weight: 0.007 oz.).

VICKS CHILDREN'S NYQUIL®

Children's NyQuil was specially formulated with the maximum allowable nonprescription levels of three effective ingredients to relieve nighttime cough, nasal congestion, and runny nose so children can rest. Children's NyQuil is alcohol free and analgesic free and has a pleasant cherry flavor.

Active Ingredients: Each ½ oz dose (1 tbs) Chlorpheniramine Maleate 2 mg, Pseudoephedrine HCl 30 mg, Dextromethorphan Hydrobromide 15 mg.

Inactive Ingredients: Citric Acid, Flavor, FD&C Red No. 40, Potassium Sorbate, Propylene Glycol, Purified Water, Sodium Citrate, Sucrose.

Indications: Specifically formulated for nighttime relief of nasal congestion, runny nose, sneezing and cough to help children rest.

Administration and Dosage:
[See table on next page].
Note: Since Children's NyQuil is available without a prescription, the following information appears on the label.

Warning: Do not exceed recommended dosage because at higher doses nervousness, dizziness or sleeplessness may occur. Do not give this product to children for more than 7 days. If symptoms do not improve or are accompanied by fever, consult a physician. Do not give this product to children who have heart disease, high blood pressure, diabetes or

Continued on next page

Richardson-Vicks—Cont.

thyroid disease, unless directed by a physician. May cause excitability especially in children. Do not give this product to children who have asthma or glaucoma unless directed by a physician. May cause drowsiness. Do not give this product to children under 6 years except on advice and supervision of a physician. Do not give this product for persistent or chronic cough such as occurs with asthma or if cough is accompanied by excessive mucus unless directed by a physician. A persistent cough may be a sign of a serious condition. If cough persists for more than 1 week, tends to recur, or is accompanied by fever, rash, or persistent headache, consult a physician. In case of accidental overdose, seek professional assistance or contact a poison control center immediately.

Drug Interaction Precaution: Do not give this product to a child who is taking a prescription drug for high blood pressure or depression, without first consulting the child's physician. TAKE ONLY AS DIRECTED. KEEP OUT OF REACH OF CHILDREN. Store at room temperature.

How Supplied: 4 fl. oz. and 8 fl. oz. bottles with child-resistant, tamper-evident cap, and a dosage cup.
Shown in Product Identification Section, page 423

VICKS NYQUIL®
[nī'quil]
**Nighttime Colds Medicine
in oral liquid form.
Original and Cherry Flavor**

Active Ingredients per fluid oz. (2 Tbs.): Acetaminophen 1000 mg., Doxylamine Succinate 7.5 mg., Pseudoephedrine HCl 60 mg, and Dextromethorphan Hydrobromide 30 mg. Also contains Alcohol 25%.

Inactive Ingredients: Original Flavor: Citric Acid, FD&C Blue No. 1, Flavor, Glycerin, Purified Water, Sodium Benzoate, Sodium Citrate, Sucrose. Contains FD&C Yellow No. 5 (tartrazine) as a color additive. Cherry Flavor: Citric Acid, FD&C Blue No. 1, FD&C Red No. 40, Flavor, Glyc-

erin, Purified Water, Sodium Citrate, Sodium Saccharin, Sucrose.

Indications: For the temporary relief of major cold and flu symptoms, as follows: nasal and sinus congestion, coughing, sneezing, minor sore throat pain, aches and pains, runny nose, headache, fever.

Actions: Decongestant, antipyretic, antihistaminic, antitussive, analgesic. Helps decongest nasal passages and sinus openings, relieves sniffles and sneezing, eases aches and pains, reduces fever, soothes headache, minor sore throat pain, and quiets coughing due to a cold. By relieving these symptoms, also helps patient to sleep and get the rest he needs.

Warning: Do not exceed recommended dosage because at higher doses nervousness, dizziness or sleeplessness may occur. Do not take this product for more than 7 days. If symptoms do not improve or are accompanied by fever, consult a doctor. Do not take this product if you have heart disease, high blood pressure, thyroid disease, diabetes, or difficulty in urination due to enlargment of the prostate gland unless directed by a doctor. Do not take this product for persistent or chronic cough such as occurs with smoking, asthma, or emphysema, or if cough is accompanied by excessive phlegm (mucus) unless directed by a doctor. A persistent cough may be a sign of a serious condition. If cough persists for more than 1 week, tends to recur, or is accompanied by high fever, rash, or persistent headaches, consult a doctor. May cause marked drowsiness. May cause excitability especially in children. Do not take this product if you have asthma or glaucoma, except under the advice and supervision of a physician. Avoid driving a motor vehicle or operating heavy machinery. If fever persists for more than 3 days, or recurs, consult your physician. Avoid alcoholic beverages while taking this product. As with any drug, if you are pregnant or nursing a baby, seek the advice of a health professional before using this product.

Drug Interaction Precaution: Do not take this product if you are presently taking a prescription drug for high blood pressure or depression without first consulting your doctor.

KEEP OUT OF REACH OF CHILDREN.
TAKE ONLY AS DIRECTED.

Overdosage: In case of accidental overdose, seek professional assistance or contact a Poison Control Center immediately.

Dosage and Dosage Form: A plastic measuring cup with 2 tablespoonful gradation is supplied.
ADULTS (12 and over): One fluid ounce in medicine cup (2 tablespoonfuls) at bedtime.
Not recommended for children.
If confined to bed or at home, a total of 4 doses may be taken per day, each 6 hours apart.

How Supplied: Available in 6, 10, and 14 fl. oz. plastic bottles with child-resistant, tamper-evident cap.
Shown in Product Identification Section, page 423

VICKS SINEX™
[sī'něx]
Decongestant Nasal Spray and Ultra Fine Mist

Active Ingredients: Phenylephrine Hydrochloride 0.5%.

Inactive Ingredients: Aromatic Vapors (Camphor, Eucalyptol, Menthol), Potassium Phosphate, Purified Water, Sodium Chloride, Sodium Phosphate, Tyloxapol. Cetylpyridinium Chloride 0.04%. Preservative: Thimerosal 0.001%.

Indications: For temporary relief of nasal congestion due to colds, hay fever, upper respiratory allergies or sinusitis.

Actions: *Provides fast decongestant relief*—Sinex gives fast relief of nasal stuffiness that often accompanies colds and hay fever. A strong decongestant shrinks swollen nasal membranes and relieves sinus pressure so your can breathe more freely.

Warning: Do not exceed recommended dosage because burning, stinging, sneezing or increase of nasal discharge may occur. Do not use this product for more than 3 days. If symptoms persist, consult a physician. Do not take this product if you have heart disease, high blood pressure, thyroid disease, diabetes, or difficulty in urination due to enlargement of the prostate gland unless directed by a doctor. The use of this dispenser by more than one person may spread infection. KEEP THIS AND ALL MEDICINES OUT OF THE REACH OF CHILDREN.

Accidental Ingestion: In case of accidental ingestion, seek professional assistance or contact a Poison Control Center immediately.

Dosage and Administration: Keep head and dispenser upright. May be used every 4 hours as needed.
Ultra Fine Mist: Remove protective cap. Hold atomizer with thumb at base and nozzle between first and second fingers. Without tilting head, insert nozzle into nostril. Fully depress rim with a

---

Dosage Instructions   Take at bedtime as directed. Use medicine cup provided.

Age, yrs.	Weight, lb.	Dose
Under 2	Under 24	Physician's Discretion.
2–5	24–47	¼ oz. (½ Tbs.)*
6–11	48–95	½ oz. (1 Tbs.)
12 and over	Over 95	Use NyQuil Nighttime Cold Medicine Adult Formula as directed.

If cold symptoms keep child confined to bed or at home, a total of 4 doses may be taken per day, each 6–8 hours apart.
*Administer to children under 6 only on the advice of a physician.

firm even stroke and sniff deeply. *Adults:* 2 or 3 sprays in each nostril not more often than every 4 hours. Not for use by children under 12 years of age unless directed by a doctor.

Squeeze Bottle: *Adults:* 2 or 3 sprays in each nostril not more often than every 4 hours. Not for use by children under 12 years of age unless directed by a doctor.

How Supplied: Available in ½ fl. oz. and 1 fl. oz. plastic squeeze bottles and ½ fl. oz. measured dose atomizer.

Shown in Product Identification Section, page 423

VICKS SINEX™ LONG-ACTING

[sī 'nĕx]

12-hour Formula Decongestant Nasal Spray and Ultra Fine Mist

Active Ingredient: Oxymetazoline Hydrochloride 0.05%.

Inactive Ingredients: Aromatic Vapors (Camphor, Eucalyptol, Menthol), Potassium Phosphate, Purified Water, Sodium Chloride, Sodium Phosphate, Tyloxapol. Preservative: Thimerosal 0.001%.

Indications: For temporary relief of nasal congestion due to colds, hay fever, upper respiratory allergies or sinusitis.

Actions: Oxymetazoline constricts the arterioles of the nasal passages—resulting in a nasal decongestant effect which lasts up to 12 hours, restoring freer breathing through the nose. SINEX LONG-ACTING helps decongest sinus openings and sinus passages, thus promoting sinus drainage.
- *Quickly helps you breathe more freely:* Shrinks swollen nasal membranes and opens up nasal passages.
- *Works effectively up to 12 hours:* Contains the strongest topical decongestant available to provide longer-lasting relief.
- *Provides special extra feeling of relief:* Unique Vicks vapors provide a cool, soothing feeling of relief.

Warning: Do not exceed recommended dosage because burning, stinging, sneezing or increase of nasal discharge may occur. Do not use this product for more than 3 days. If symptoms persist, consult a physician. Do not take this product if you have heart disease, high blood pressure, thyroid disease, diabetes, or difficulty in urination due to enlargement of the prostate gland unless directed by a doctor. The use of this dispenser by more than one person may spread infection. KEEP THIS AND ALL MEDICINES OUT OF THE REACH OF CHILDREN.

Accidental Ingestion: In case of accidental ingestion, seek professional assistance or contact a Poison Control Center immediately.

Dosage and Administration: Keep head and dispenser upright. May be used twice daily (morning and evening) or as directed by a physician.
Ultra Fine Mist: Remove protective cap. Hold atomizer with thumb at base and nozzle between first and second fin-

gers. Without tilting head, insert nozzle into nostril. Fully depress rim with a firm even stroke and sniff deeply. *Adults, and children 6 to under 12 years of age (with adult supervision):* 2 or 3 sprays in each nostril not more often than every 10 to 12 hours. Do not exceed 2 applications in any 24-hour period. Children under 6 years of age: consult a doctor.

Squeeze Bottle: *Adults, and children 6 to under 12 years of age (with adult supervision):* 2 or 3 sprays in each nostril not more often than every 10 to 12 hours. Do not exceed 2 applications in any 24-hour period. Children under 6 years of age: consult a doctor.

How Supplied: Available in ½ fl. oz. and 1 fl. oz. plastic squeeze bottles and ½ fl. oz. measured-dose atomizer.

Shown in Product Identification Section, page 424

VICKS® THROAT LOZENGES

Active Ingredients per lozenge: Benzocaine 5 mg.

Inactive Ingedients: Cetylpyridinium chloride, D&C Red No. 27, D&C Red No. 30, Flavor, Polyethylene Glycol, Sodium Citrate, Sucrose, Talc. Special blend of Vicks aromatics (menthol, camphor, eucalyptus oil).

Indications: For temporary relief of occasional minor irritation, pain, sore mouth, sore throat, and pain associated with canker sores.

Actions: VICKS THROAT LOZENGES are local anesthetic throat drops. They temporarily soothe minor sore throat irritations—ease pain—and relieve irritation and dryness of mouth and throat.

Warning: If sore throat is severe, persists for more than 2 days, is accompanied or followed by fever, headache, rash, nausea, or vomiting, consult a doctor promptly. If sore mouth symptoms do not improve in 7 days, see your dentist or doctor promptly. In case of accidental overdose, seek professional assistance or contact a poison control center immediately. As with any drug, if you are pregnant or nursing a baby, seek the advice of a health professional before using this product. Keep this and all medication out of the reach of children. Take only as directed.

Dosage: *Adults and Children 2 years and over:* allow one lozenge to dissolve slowly in mouth. Repeat every 2 hours as needed or as directed by a doctor. Children under 2 years of age: Consult a doctor.

How Supplied: Box of 12's.

VICKS® VAPORUB®

[vā 'pō-rub]

Decongestant Vaporizing Ointment For use as a rub

Active Ingredients: Special Vicks Medication (menthol 2.6%, camphor 4.73%, eucalyptus oil 1.2%) in a petrolatum base.

Inactive Ingredients: Cedarleaf Oil, Mineral Oil, Nutmeg Oil, Petrolatum, Thymol, Spirits of Turpentine.

Indications: For the temporary relief of nasal congestion and coughing associated with a cold to help you rest.

Actions: The inhaled vapors of VICKS VAPORUB have a decongestant and antitussive effect.

Warning: For external use only. Do not swallow or place in nostrils. A persistent cough may be a sign of a serious condition. If cough persists for more than a week, tends to recur, or is accompanied by fever, rash or persistent headache, consult a doctor. Do not take this product for persistent or chronic cough such as occurs with smoking, asthma, or emphysema, or if cough is accompanied by excessive phlegm (mucus) unless directed by a doctor. Never expose VAPORUB to flame or place in boiling water. **KEEP OUT OF CHILDREN'S REACH.**

Accidental Ingestion: In case of accidental ingestion, seek professional assistance or contact a Poison Control Center immediately.

Directions: *For adults and children (2 years and older)*—Direct Application: Rub a thick layer of Vicks VapoRub on chest and throat. If desired, cover with a dry, warm cloth, but keep clothing loose to let the vapors rise to nose and mouth. Repeat up to three times daily, especially at bedtime, or as directed by a doctor. Children under 2 years of age, consult a doctor.

How Supplied: Available in 1.5 oz., 3.0 oz. and 6.0 oz. plastic jars and 2.0 oz. tubes.

Shown in Product Identification Section, page 424

VICKS VAPOSTEAM®

[vā 'pō "stēm]

Liquid Medication for Hot Steam Vaporizers.

Active Ingredients: Menthol 3.2%, Camphor 6.2%, Eucalyptus Oil 1.5%.

Inactive Ingredients: Cedarleaf Oil, Nutmeg Oil, Poloxamer 124, Polyoxyethylene Dodecanol, Silicone, Alcohol 74%.

Indications: For temporary relief of nasal congestion due to a cold, hay fever or other respiratory allergies. Temporarily relieves cough occurring with a cold.

Actions: VAPOSTEAM increases the action of steam to help relieve colds symptoms in the following ways: relieves coughs of colds, eases nasal congestion, and moistens dry, irritated breathing passages.

Warning: For hot steam medication only. Do not use in cold steam vaporizers/humidifiers. Not to be taken by mouth. Keep away from open flame or extreme heat. Do not direct steam from vaporizer towards face. A persistent cough may be a sign of a serious condi-

Continued on next page

Richardson-Vicks—Cont.

tion. If cough persists for more than a week, tends to recur or is accompanied by fever, rash or persistent headache, consult a doctor. Do not use this product for persistent or chronic cough such as occurs with smoking, asthma, or emphysema, or if cough is accompanied by excessive phlegm (mucus) unless directed by a doctor.

KEEP OUT OF REACH OF CHILDREN.

Accidental Ingestion: In case of accidental ingestion, seek professional assistance or contact a Poison Control Center immediately.

Directions: In Hot Steam Vaporizers: VAPOSTEAM is formulated for use in HOT STEAM VAPORIZERS. Follow directions for use carefully.
Adults and children 2 years and older: Add 1 tablespoon of VAPOSTEAM for each quart of water directly to the water in a hot steam vaporizer, bowl or wash basin, or add 1½ teaspoonfuls of solution for each pint of water to an open container of boiling water. Breathe in medicated vapors. May be repeated up to three times daily or as directed by a doctor.
Children under 2 years of age: consult a doctor.

Consumer Information: For best performance, vaporizer should be thoroughly cleaned after each use according to manufacturer's instructions. In soft water areas, it may be necessary to add salt or other steaming aid to promote boiling. Follow directions of vaporizer manufacturer for best results.

How Supplied: Available in 4 fl. oz. and 6 fl. oz. bottles.

VICKS VATRONOL®
[*vătrōnŏl*]
Nose Drops

Active Ingredients: Ephedrine Sulfate 0.5% in an aqueous base.

Inactive Ingredients: Camphor, Cedarleaf Oil, Eucalyptol, Menthol, Nutmeg Oil, Potassium Phosphate, Purified Water, Sodium Chloride, Sodium Phosphate, Tyloxapol.
Preservative: Thimerosal 0.001%.

Indications: For temporary relief of nasal congestion due to a cold, hay fever or other respiratory allergies.

Actions: VICKS VATRONOL helps restore freer breathing by relieving nasal stuffiness. Relieves sinus pressure.

Warning: Do not exceed recommended dosage because burning, stinging, sneezing, or increase of nasal discharge may occur. The use of this container by more than one person may spread infection. Do not use this product for more than 3 days. If symptoms persist, consult a doctor. Do not use this product if you have heart disease, high blood pressure, thyroid disease, diabetes, or difficulty in urination due to enlargement of the pros-

tate gland unless directed by a doctor.
KEEP OUT OF REACH OF CHILDREN.

Overdosage: In case of accidental overdose, seek professional assistance or contact a Poison Control Center immediately.

Dosage: *Adults:* Fill dropper to upper mark. *Children (6–12 years):* Fill dropper to lower mark. *Children under 6 years of age:* consult a doctor.
Apply up one nostril, repeat in other nostril.
Repeat not more than every 4 hours as needed.

How Supplied: Available in ½ fl. oz. and 1 fl. oz. dropper bottles.

A. H. Robins Company, Inc.
CONSUMER PRODUCTS DIVISION
3800 CUTSHAW AVENUE
RICHMOND, VIRGINIA 23230

ALLBEE® C–800 TABLETS
[*all-be'*]
ALLBEE® C–800
plus IRON TABLETS

Allbee C-800

One tablet daily provides:	Percentage of U.S. Recommended Daily Allowances (U.S. RDA)	
Vitamin E	150	45 I.U.
Vitamin C	1333	800 mg
Thiamine (Vitamin B₁)	1000	15 mg
Riboflavin (Vitamin B₂)	1000	17 mg
Niacin	500	100 mg
Vitamin B₆	1250	25 mg
Vitamin B₁₂	200	12 mcg
Pantothenic Acid	250	25 mg

Ingredients: Ascorbic Acid, Niacinamide Ascorbate, Modified Starch, Vitamin E Acetate, Hydrolyzed Protein, Calcium Pantothenate, Hydroxypropyl Methylcellulose, Pyridoxine Hydrochloride, Riboflavin, Stearic Acid, Thiamine Mononitrate, Artificial Color, Silicon Dioxide, Lactose, Magnesium Stearate, Povidone, Polyethylene Glycol 400 or 4000, Vanillin, Gelatin, Polysorbate 20 or 80, Sorbic Acid, Sodium Benzoate, Cyanocobalamin. May also contain: Hydroxypropylcellulose and Propylene Glycol.

Allbee C-800 plus Iron

One tablet daily provides: Vitamin Composition	Percentage of U.S. Recommended Daily Allowances (U.S. RDA)	
Vitamin E	150	45.0 I.U.
Vitamin C	1333	800.0 mg
Folic Acid	100	0.4 mg
Thiamine (Vitamin B₁)	1000	15.0 mg
Riboflavin (Vitamin B₂)	1000	17.0 mg
Niacin	500	100.0 mg
Vitamin B₆	1250	25.0 mg
Vitamin B₁₂	200	12.0 mcg
Pantothenic Acid	250	25.0 mg

Mineral Composition

Iron	150	27.0 mg

Ingredients: Ascorbic Acid, Niacinamide Ascorbate, Ferrous Fumarate, Modified Starch, Vitamin E Acetate, Hydrolyzed Protein, Calcium Pantothenate, Hydroxypropyl Methylcellulose, Pyridoxine Hydrochloride, Riboflavin, Stearic Acid, Thiamine Mononitrate, Povidone, Silicon Dioxide, Artificial Color, Lactose, Magnesium Stearate, Polyethylene Glycol 400 or 4000, Vanillin, Gelatin, Folic Acid, Polysorbate 20 or 80, Sorbic Acid, Sodium Benzoate, Cyanocobalamin. May also contain: Hydroxypropylcellulose and Propylene Glycol.

Actions and Uses: The components of Allbee C-800 have important roles in general nutrition, healing of wounds, and prevention of hemorrhage. Allbee C-800 is recommended for nutritional supplementation of these components in conditions such as febrile diseases, chronic or acute infections, burns, fractures, surgery, physiologic stress, alcoholism, prolonged exposure to high temperature, geriatrics, gastritis, peptic ulcer, and colitis; and in weight-reduction and other special diets.
In dentistry, Allbee C-800 is recommended for nutritional supplementation of its components in conditions such as herpetic stomatitis, aphthous stomatitis, cheilosis, herpangina and gingivitis.
In addition, Allbee C-800 Plus Iron is recommended as a nutritional source of iron. The iron is present as ferrous fumarate, a well-tolerated salt. The ascorbic acid in the formulation enhances the absorption of iron.

Precautions: Do not take Allbee C-800 Plus Iron within two hours of oral tetracycline antibiotics, since oral iron products interfere with absorption of tetracycline. Not intended for treatment of iron-deficiency anemia.

Adverse Reactions: Iron-containing medications may occasionally cause gastrointestinal discomfort, nausea, constipation or diarrhea.

Dosage: The recommended OTC dosage for adults and children twelve or more years of age is one tablet daily. Under the direction and supervision of a physician, the dose and frequency of administration may be increased in accordance with the patient's requirements.

How Supplied: Allbee C-800—orange, film-coated, elliptically-shaped tablets in bottles of 60 (NDC 0031-0677-62). Allbee C-800 Plus Iron—red, film-coated, elliptically-shaped tablets in bottles of 60 (NDC 0031-0678-62).
Shown in Product Identification Section, page 424

ALLBEE® WITH C CAPLETS
[*all-be'*]

One caplet daily provides:	Percentage of U.S. Recommended Daily Allowance (U.S. RDA)	
Vitamin C	500	300.0 mg
Thiamine (Vitamin B₁)	1000	15.0 mg

Riboflavin		
(Vitamin B$_2$)	600	10.2 mg
Niacin	250	50.0 mg
Vitamin B$_6$	250	5.0 mg
Pantothenic Acid	100	10.0 mg

Ingredients: Niacinamide Ascorbate; Ascorbic Acid; Microcrystalline Cellulose; Corn Starch; Thiamine Mononitrate; Calcium Pantothenate; Riboflavin; Hydroxypropyl Methylcellulose; Pyridoxine Hydrochloride; Magnesium Stearate; Silicon Dioxide; Propylene Glycol; Lactose; Methacrylic Acid Copolymer; Triethyl Citrate; Titanium Dioxide; Polysorbate 20; Artificial Flavor; Saccharin Sodium; Sodium Sorbate.

Action and Uses: Allbee with C is a high-potency formulation of B and C vitamins. Its components have important roles in general nutrition, healing of wounds, and prevention of hemorrhage. It is recommended for deficiencies of B-vitamins and ascorbic acid in conditions such as febrile diseases, chronic or acute infections, burns, fractures, surgery, toxic conditions, physiologic stress, alcoholism, prolonged exposure to high temperature, geriatrics, gastritis, peptic ulcer, and colitis; and in conditions involving special diets and weight-reduction diets.

In dentistry, Allbee with C is recommended for deficiencies of B-vitamins and ascorbic acid in conditions such as herpetic stomatitis, aphthous stomatitis, cheilosis, herpangina, gingivitis.

Dosage: The recommended OTC dosage for adults and children twelve or more years of age, is one caplet daily. Under the direction and supervision of a physician, the dose and frequency of administration may be increased in accordance with the patient's requirements.

How Supplied: Yellow caplets, monogrammed AHR and Allbee C in bottles of 130 (NDC 0031-0673-66), 1,000 caplets (NDC 0031-0673-74), and in Dis-Co® Unit Dose Packs of 100 (NDC 0031-0673-64).

Shown in Product Identification Section, page 424

CHAP STICK® Lip Balm

Active Ingredients: 44% Petrolatums, 1.5% Padimate O (2-ethyl-hexyl *p*-dimethylaminobenzoate, 1% Lanolin, 1% Isopropyl Myristate, 0.5% Cetyl Alcohol.

Inactive Ingredients:
Regular: Arachadyl Propionate, Camphor, Carnauba Wax, D&C Red 6 Barium Lake, FD&C Yellow 5 Aluminum Lake, Fragrance, Isopropyl Lanolate, Methylparaben, Mineral Oil, 2-Octyl Dodecanol, Oleyl Alcohol, Polyphenylmethylsiloxane 556, Propylparaben, Titanium Dioxide, Wax Paraffin, White Wax.
Cherry: Arachadyl Propionate, Camphor, Carnauba Wax, D&C Red 6 Barium Lake, Flavors, Isopropyl Lanolate, Methylparaben, Mineral Oil, 2-Octyl Dodecanol, Polyphenylmethylsiloxane 556, Pro-

pylparaben, Saccharin, Wax Paraffin, White Wax.
Mint: Arachadyl Propionate, Carnauba Wax, FD&C Blue 1 Aluminum Lake, FD&C Yellow 5 Lake, Flavors, Isopropyl Lanolate, Methylparaben, Mineral Oil, 2-Octyl Dodecanol, Polyphenylmethylsiloxane 556, Propylparaben, Saccharin, Wax Paraffin, White Wax.
Orange: Arachadyl Propionate, Carnauba Wax, FD&C Yellow 6 Aluminum Lake, Flavors, Isopropyl Lanolate, Methylparaben, Mineral Oil, 2-Octyl Dodecanol, Polyphenylmethylsiloxane 556, Propylparaben, Saccharin, Wax Paraffin, White Wax.
Strawberry: Arachadyl Propionate, Camphor, Carnauba Wax, D&C Red 6 Barium Lake, Flavors, Isopropyl Lanolate, Methylparaben, Mineral Oil, 2-Octyl Dodecanol, Polyphenylmethylsiloxane 556, Propylparaben, Saccharin, Wax Paraffin, White Wax.

Indications: Helps prevention and healing of dry, chapped, sun and wind-burned lips.

Actions: A specially designed lipid complex hydrophobic base containing Padimate O which forms a barrier to prevent moisture loss and protect lips from the drying effects of cold weather, wind and sun which cause chapping. The special emollients soften the skin by forming an occlusive film thus inducing hydration, restoring suppleness to the lips, and preventing drying from evaporation of water that diffuses to the surface from the underlying layers of tissue. Chap Stick also protects the skin from the external environment and its sunscreen offers protection from exposure to the sun.

Warning: Discontinue use if signs of irritation appear.

Symptoms and Treatment of Oral Ingestion: The oral LD$_{50}$ in rats is greater than 5 gm/kg. There have been no reported overdoses in humans. There are no known symptoms of overdosage.

Dosage and Treatment: For dry, chapped lips apply as needed. To help prevent dry, chapped sun or windburned lips, apply to lips as needed before, during and following exposure to sun, wind, water and cold weather.
Professional Labeling: None.

How Supplied: Available in 4.25 gm tubes in Regular, Mint, Cherry, Orange, and Strawberry flavors.
Shown in Product Identification Section, page 424

CHAP STICK® SUNBLOCK 15 Lip Balm

Active Ingredients: 44% Petrolatums, 7% Padimate O, 3% Oxybenzone, 0.5% Lanolin, 0.5% Isopropyl Myristate, 0.5% Cetyl Alcohol.

Inactive Ingredients: Camphor, Carnauba Wax, D&C Red 6 Barium Lake, FD&C Yellow 5 Aluminum Lake, Fragrance, Isopropyl Lanolate, Methylparaben, Mineral Oil, Propylparaben, Tita-

nium Dioxide, Wax Paraffin, White Wax.

Indications: Ultra Sunscreen Protection (SPF-15). Helps prevention and healing of dry, chapped, sun and windburned lips. Overexposure to sun may lead to premature aging of skin and lip cancer. Liberal and regular use may help reduce the sun's harmful effects.

Actions: Ultra sunscreen protection for the lips, plus the attributes of Chap Stick® Lip Balm. The emollients in the specially designed lipid complex hydrophobic base soften the lips by forming an occlusive film while the two sunscreens have specific ultraviolet absorption ranges which overlap to offer ultra sunscreen protection (SPF-15).

Warning: Discontinue use if signs of irritation appear.

Symptoms and Treatment of Oral Ingestion: Toxicity studies indicate this product to be extremely safe. The oral LD$_{50}$ in rats is greater than 5 gm./kg. There are no known symptoms of overdosage.

Dosage and Treatment: For ultra sunscreen protection, apply evenly and liberally to lips before exposure to sun. Reapply as needed. For dry, chapped lips, apply as needed. To help prevent dry, chapped, sun, and windburned lips, apply to lips as needed before, during, and following exposure to sun, wind, water, and cold weather.

How Supplied: 4.25 gm. tube.
Shown in Product Identification Section, page 424

CHAP STICK® PETROLEUM JELLY PLUS

REGULAR:
Active Ingredients: 99% White Petrolatum, USP

Other Ingredients: Aloe, Butylated Hydroxytoluene, Flavor, Lanolin, Phenonip.

CHERRY:
Active Ingredients: 98.85% White Petrolatum, USP.

Other Ingredients: Aloe, Butylated Hydroxytoluene, D&C Red 6 Barium Lake, Flavors, Lanolin, Phenonip, and Saccharin.

Indications: Helps prevent and protect against dry, chapped, sun and windburned lips.

Actions: White Petrolatum, USP forms a barrier to prevent moisture loss and protect lips from the drying effects of cold weather, wind and sun which cause

Continued on next page

Prescribing information on A.H. Robins products listed here is based on official labeling in effect November 1, 1989 with Indications, Contraindications, Warnings, Precautions, Adverse Reactions, and Dosage stated in full.

Robins—Cont.

chapping. White Petrolatum, USP helps soften the skin by forming an occlusive film for inducing hydration and restoring suppleness to the lips and preventing drying from evaporation of water that diffuses to the surface from the underlying layers of tissue.

Warning: If condition worsens or does not improve within 7 days, consult a doctor.

Dosage and Treatment: To help prevent dry, chapped, sun or wind-burned lips, apply to lips as needed before, during and following exposure to sun, wind, water and cold weather.

How Supplied: Regular and Cherry flavored available in 0.35 oz. (10 grams) polyethylene tube.
Shown in Product Identification Section page 424

CHAP STICK® PETROLEUM JELLY PLUS WITH SUNBLOCK 15

Active Ingredients: 89% White Petrolatum, USP, 7% Padimate O, 3% Oxybenzone.

Other Ingredients: Aloe, Butylated Hydroxytoluene, Flavor, Lanolin, Phenonip.

Indications: Ultra Sunscreen Protection (SPF-15). Helps prevent and protect against dry, chapped, sun and windburned lips. Overexposure to sun may lead to premature aging of skin and skin cancer. Liberal and regular use may help reduce the sun's harmful effects.

Actions: Ultra sunscreen protection for the lips, plus the attributes of Chap Stick® Petroleum Jelly Plus. White Petrolatum, USP forms a barrier to prevent moisture loss and protect lips from the drying effects of wind and sun while two sunscreens, which have specific ultra violet absorption ranges, overlap to provide ultra sunscreen protection (SPF-15).

Warning: For external use only. Avoid contact with eyes. Discontinue use if signs of irritation or rash occur.

Dosage and Treatment: For ultra sunscreen protection, apply evenly and liberally to lips before exposure to sun. Reapply as needed. For dry chapped lips, apply as needed. To help prevent dry, chapped, sun and windburned lips, apply to lips as needed before, during and following exposure to sun, wind, water and cold weather.

How Supplied: Available in 0.35 oz (10 grams) polyethylene tube.
Shown in Product Identification Section, page 424

DIMACOL® Caplets
[di 'mă-col]

Description: Each caplet contains:
Guaifenesin, USP ....100 mg
Pseudoephedrine
　Hydrochloride, USP ....30 mg
Dextromethorphan
　Hydrobromide, USP ....10 mg

Inactive Ingredients: D&C Yellow 10 Aluminum Lake, FD&C Yellow 6 Aluminum Lake, Flavor, Hydroxypropyl Methylcellulose, Magnesium Stearate, Methacrylic Acid Copolymer, Methylparaben, Microcrystalline Cellulose, Polysorbate 20, Potassium Sorbate, Povidone, Propylene Glycol, Propylparaben, Saccharin Sodium, Silicon Dioxide, Titanium Dioxide, Triethyl Citrate, Xanthan Gum.

Indications: Temporarily relieves cough due to minor throat and bronchial irritation and nasal congestion as may occur with a cold. Expectorant action to help loosen phlegm and thin bronchial secretions to make coughs more productive.

Warnings: A persistent cough may be a sign of a serious condition. If cough persists for more than 1 week, tends to recur, or is accompanied by fever, rash, or persistent headache, patients should consult a doctor. Patients are advised not to take this product for persistent or chronic cough such as occurs with smoking, asthma, chronic bronchitis, emphysema, or if cough is accompanied by excessive phlegm (mucus) unless directed by a doctor. Likewise, persons with high blood pressure, heart disease, diabetes, thyroid disease or difficulty in urination due to enlargement of the prostate gland, are advised to use this product only as directed by a doctor. The recommended dosage should not be exceeded because at higher doses nervousness, dizziness, or sleeplessness may occur. As with any drug, women who are pregnant or nursing a baby should seek the advice of a health professional before using this product.

Contraindications: Hypersensitivity to any of the ingredients; marked hypertension, hyperthyroidism or in patients who are receiving monoamine oxidase inhibitors (MAOIs).

Adverse Reactions: The following adverse reactions may possibly occur: nausea, vomiting, dry mouth, nervousness, insomnia and rash (including urticaria).

NOTE: Guaifenesin has been shown to produce a color interference with certain clinical laboratory determinations of 5-hydroxyindoleacetic acid (5-HIAA) and vanillylmandelic acid (VMA).

Drug Interaction Precautions: Concomitant administration of pseudoephedrine with other sympathomimetic agents may produce additive effects and increased toxicity; with MAOIs may produce a hypertensive crisis; with certain antihypertensive agents may diminish their antihypertensive effect. Serious toxicity may result if dextromethorphan is used with MAOIs.

Directions: Adults and children 12 years and over, 2 caplets every 4 hours; children 6 to under 12 years of age, 1 caplet every 4 hours; children under 6 years—consult a doctor. DO NOT EXCEED 4 DOSES IN A 24-HOUR PERIOD.

How Supplied: Orange caplets in bottles of 100 (NDC 0031-1653-63), and 500 (NDC 0031-1653-70) and consumer packages of 12 (NDC 0031-1653-46), and 24 (NDC 0031-1653-54) (individually packaged).
Store at Controlled Room Temperature, Between 15°C and 30°C (59°F and 86°F).
Shown in Product Identification Section, page 424

DIMETANE®
[di 'mĕ-tāne]
brand of Brompheniramine Maleate, USP
Tablets—4 mg
Elixir—2 mg/5 mL (Alcohol, 3%)
Extentabs®—8 mg and 12 mg

Family Description: Dimetane® is Robins brand name for Brompheniramine Maleate, USP, an antihistamine. It comes in several oral dosage forms (tablets, elixir and Extentabs®) and can be used when an antihistamine is indicated.

Inactive Ingredients:
Tablets: Corn Starch, D&C Yellow 10 Aluminum Lake, Dibasic Calcium Phosphate, FD&C Yellow 6 Aluminum Lake, Lactose, Magnesium Stearate, Polyethylene Glycol.
Elixir: Citric Acid, FD&C Yellow 6, Flavors, Glucose, Saccharin Sodium, Sodium Benzoate, Water.
Extentabs® 8 mg: Acacia, Acetylated Monoglycerides, Calcium Carbonate, Calcium Sulfate, Carnauba Wax, Cellulose Acetate Phthalate, Corn Starch, Diethyl Phthalate, Edible Ink, FD&C Blue 2 Aluminum Lake, FD&C Red 3, Gelatin, Guar Gum, Magnesium Stearate, Pharmaceutical Glaze, Polysorbates, Stearic Acid, Sucrose, Titanium Dioxide, Wheat Flour, White Wax and other ingredients, one of which is a corn derivative. May contain FD&C Red 40 and FD&C Yellow 6 Aluminum Lakes.
Extentabs® 12 mg: Acacia, Acetylated Monoglycerides, Calcium Carbonate, Calcium Sulfate, Carnauba Wax, Cellulose Acetate Phthalate, Corn Starch, Diethyl Phthalate, Edible Ink, FD&C Blue 2 Aluminum Lake, FD&C Red 3, FD&C Yellow 6, Gelatin, Guar Gum, Magnesium Stearate, Pharmaceutical Glaze, Polysorbates, Stearic Acid, Sucrose, Titanium Dioxide, Wheat Flour, White Wax and other ingredients, one of which is a corn derivative. May contain FD&C Red 40 and FD&C Yellow 6 Aluminum Lakes.

Indications: For temporary relief of running nose, sneezing, itching of the nose or throat; and itchy, watery eyes as may occur in allergic rhinitis (such as hay fever).

Warnings: May cause drowsiness. May cause excitability, especially in children. This product should not be taken by patients who have asthma, glaucoma or difficulty in urination due to enlargement of the prostate gland. The tablets and liquid should not be given to children under six years, except under the advice and supervision of a physician. The Ex-

Product Name	Form	Strength	Package Size	Package Type	NDC 0031-
Dimetane Tablets	Peach-colored, compressed scored tablet	4 mg tablet	24	Blister Unit	1857-54
			100	Bottles	1857-63
Dimetane Elixir	Peach-colored liquid	2 mg/ 5 mL	4 fl. oz.	Bottles	1807-12
			1 Pint	Bottles	1807-25
Dimetane Extentabs 8 mg	Persian rose-colored, tablets	8 mg tablet	12	Blister Unit	1868-46
			100	Bottles	1868-63
Dimetane Extentabs 12 mg	Peach-colored, coated tablets	12 mg tablet	12	Blister Unit	1843-46
			100	Bottles	1843-63

tentabs should not be given to children under 12 years, except under the advice and supervision of a physician. Should not be taken if hypersensitivity to any of the ingredients exists. As with any drug, women who are pregnant or nursing a baby should seek the advice of a health professional before using these products.

Cautions: Patients should be warned to avoid driving a motor vehicle, operating heavy machinery, or consuming alcoholic beverages while taking this product.

Directions: Tablets and Liquid—The recommended OTC dosage is: Adults and children 12 years of age and over: 1 tablet or 2 teaspoonfuls every four to six hours, not to exceed 6 tablets or 12 teaspoonfuls in 24 hours. Children 6 to under 12 years: ½ tablet or 1 teaspoonful every four to six hours, not to exceed 3 whole tablets or 6 teaspoonfuls in 24 hours.

Professional Labeling: Children under 6 years: Use only as directed by a physician. The suggested dosage for children age 2 to under 6 years, only when the child is under the care of a physician, is ½ teaspoonful every 4 to 6 hours, not to exceed 6 doses in a 24-hour period. The dosage for a child under 2 years should be determined by the physician on the basis of the patient's weight, physical condition, or other appropriate consideration. Dimetane Elixir is contraindicated in neonates (children under the age of one month).

Extentabs®—The recommended OTC dosage is: Adults and children 12 years of age and over:
8 mg Extentab: One tablet every eight to twelve hours, NOT TO EXCEED 1 TABLET EVERY 8 HOURS OR 3 TABLETS IN A 24-HOUR PERIOD.
12 mg Extentab: One tablet every twelve hours, NOT TO EXCEED 1 TABLET EVERY 12 HOURS OR 2 TABLETS IN A 24-HOUR PERIOD.
Children under 12 years of age should use only as directed by a physician.

How Supplied: [See table above].
Store at Controlled Room Temperature, Between 15°C and 30°C (59°F and 86°F).
Shown in Product Identification Section, page 424 and 425

DIMETANE® DECONGESTANT ELIXIR
[di 'mĕ-tāne]
DIMETANE® DECONGESTANT CAPLETS

Elixir:
Each 5 mL (1 teaspoonful) contains:
Phenylephrine
  Hydrochloride, USP ....5 mg
Brompheniramine
  Maleate, USP ....2 mg
Alcohol 2.3%

Inactive Ingredients: Citric Acid, FD&C Blue 1, FD&C Red 40, Flavors, Sodium Benzoate, Sorbitol, Water.
Caplets:
Each caplet contains:
Phenylephrine
  Hydrochloride, USP ....10 mg
Brompheniramine
  Maleate, USP ....4 mg

Inactive Ingredients: Corn Starch, FD&C Blue 1 Aluminum Lake, Magnesium Stearate, Microcrystalline Cellulose.

Indications: For temporary relief of nasal congestion due to the common cold, sinusitis, hay fever or other upper respiratory allergies; runny nose, sneezing, itching of the nose or throat and itchy and watery eyes as may occur in allergic rhinitis (such as hay fever). Temporarily restores freer breathing through the nose.

Warnings: These products may cause excitability, especially in children. These products should not be taken by patients with asthma, glaucoma, difficulty in urination due to enlargement of the prostate gland, high blood pressure, heart disease, diabetes or thyroid disease except under the advice and supervision of a physician. Should not be taken by persons hypersensitive to any of the ingredients. May cause drowsiness. Doses in excess of the recommended dosage may cause nervousness, dizziness or sleeplessness. If symptoms do not improve within 7 days or are accompanied by fever, a physician should be consulted before continuing use. As with any drug, women who are pregnant or nursing a baby should seek the advice of a health professional before using this product.

Drug Interaction Precautions: Concomitant administration of phenylephrine with other sympathomimetic agents may produce additive effects and increased toxicity: with monoamine oxidase inhibitors (MAOIs) may produce a hypertensive crisis; with certain antihypertensive agents may diminish their antihypertensive effect.

Cautions: Patients should be warned about driving a motor vehicle, operating heavy machinery, or consuming alcoholic beverages while taking this product.

Directions: *Caplets:* Adults and children 12 years of age and over: 1 caplet every 4 hours, not to exceed 6 caplets in a 24-hour period; children 6 to under 12 years: ½ caplet every 4 hours, not to exceed 3 caplets in a 24-hour period; children under 6 years: use only as directed by a physician.
Elixir: Adults and children 12 years of age and over: 2 teaspoonfuls every 4 hours, not to exceed 12 teaspoonfuls in a 24-hour period; children 6 to under 12 years: 1 teaspoonful every 4 hours, not to exceed 6 teaspoonfuls in a 24-hour period. Children under 6 years: use only as directed by a physician.
Professional Labeling: The suggested dosage for children age 2 to under 6 years, only when the child is under the care of a physician, is ½ teaspoonful every 4 hours, not to exceed 6 doses in a 24-hour period. The dosage for a child under 2 years should be determined by the physician on the basis of the patient's weight, physical condition, or other appropriate consideration. Dimetane Decongestant is contraindicated in neonates (children under the age of one month).

How Supplied: *Caplets*—light blue, capsule-shaped caplets in cartons of 24 (NDC 0031-2117-54) and 48 (NDC 0031-2117-59) individually packaged blister units.
Elixir—red-colored, grape-flavored liquid in 4 fl oz bottle (NDC 0031-2127-12). Store at Controlled Room Temperature, Between 15°C and 30°C (59°F and 86°F).
Shown in Product Identification Section, page 425

Continued on next page

Prescribing information on A.H. Robins products listed here is based on official labeling in effect November 1, 1989 with Indications, Contraindications, Warnings, Precautions, Adverse Reactions, and Dosage stated in full.

Robins—Cont.

DIMETAPP® Elixir
[di 'mĕ-tap]

Description: Each 5 mL (1 teaspoonful) contains:
Brompheniramine
     Maleate, USP ....2 mg
Phenylpropanolamine
     Hydrochloride, USP ....12.5 mg
Alcohol 2.3%

Inactive Ingredients: Citric Acid, FD&C Blue 1, FD&C Red 40, Flavor, Saccharin Sodium, Sodium Benzoate, Sorbitol, Water.

Indications: For temporary relief of nasal congestion due to the common cold, hay fever or other upper respiratory allergies and associated with sinusitis; temporarily relieves running nose, sneezing, and itchy and watery eyes as may occur in allergic rhinitis (such as hay fever). Temporarily restores freer breathing through the nose.

Warnings: This product may cause excitability, especially in children. This product should not be taken by patients with high blood pressure, heart disease, diabetes, thyroid disease, asthma, glaucoma or difficulty in urination due to enlargement of the prostate gland, except under the advice and supervision of a physician. May cause drowsiness. Doses in excess of the recommended dosage may cause nervousness, dizziness, or sleeplessness. If symptoms do not improve within 7 days or are accompanied by high fever, a physician should be consulted before continuing use. Should not be taken by persons hypersensitive to any of the ingredients. As with any drug, women who are pregnant or nursing a baby should seek the advice of a health professional before using this product.

Caution: Patients should be warned to avoid driving a motor vehicle, operating heavy machinery or consuming alcoholic beverages while taking this product.

Drug Interaction Precaution: Do not take this product if you are presently taking a prescription antihypertensive or antidepressant drug containing a monoamine oxidase inhibitor, except under the advice and supervision of a physician.

Directions: Adults and children 12 years of age and over: 2 teaspoonfuls every 4 hours, children 6 to under 12 years: 1 teaspoonful every 4 hours; DO NOT EXCEED 6 DOSES IN A 24-HOUR PERIOD. Children under 6 years: use only as directed by a physician.
Professional Labeling: The suggested dosage for children age 2 to under 6 years, only when the child is under the care of a physician, is ½ teaspoonful every 4 hours, not to exceed 6 doses in a 24-hour period. The dosage for children under 2 years should be determined by the physician on the basis of the patients' weight, physical condition, or other appropriate consideration. Dimetapp Elixir

is contraindicated in neonates (children under the age of one month).

How Supplied: Purple, grape-flavored liquid in bottles of 4 fl. oz. (NDC 0031-2230-12), 8 fl. oz. (NDC 0031-2230-18), 12 fl. oz. (NDC 0031-2230-22), pints (NDC 0031-2230-25), gallons (NDC 0031-2230-29), and 5 mL Dis-Co® Unit Dose Packs (10 × 10s) (NDC 0031-2230-23).
Store at Controlled Room Temperature, Between 15°C and 30°C (59°F and 86°F).
Shown in Product Identification Section, page 425

DIMETAPP® Extentabs®
[di 'mĕ-tap]

Description: Each **Dimetapp Extentabs®** Tablet contains:
Brompheniramine Maleate,
     USP..12 mg
Phenylpropanolamine
     Hydrochloride, USP ....75 mg

Inactive Ingredients: Acacia, Acetylated Monoglycerides, Calcium Sulfate, Carnauba Wax, Castor Wax or Oil, Citric Acid, Edible Ink, FD&C Blue 1 and FD&C Blue 2 Aluminum Lake, Gelatin, Magnesium Stearate, Magnesium Trisilicate, Pharmaceutical Glaze, Polysorbates, Povidone, Silicon Dioxide, Stearyl Alcohol, Sucrose, Titanium Dioxide, Wheat Flour, White Wax. May contain FD&C Red 40 and FD&C Yellow 6 Aluminum Lakes.

Indications: For temporary relief of nasal congestion due to the common cold, hay fever or other upper respiratory allergies and associated with sinusitis; temporarily relieves running nose, sneezing, and itchy and watery eyes as may occur in allergic rhinitis (such as hay fever). Temporarily restores freer breathing through the nose.

Warnings: This product may cause excitability, especially in children. This product should not be taken by patients with high blood pressure, heart disease, diabetes, thyroid disease, asthma, glaucoma or difficulty in urination due to enlargement of the prostate gland, except under the advice and supervision of a physician. This product should not be given to children under 12 years except under the advice and supervision of a physician. May cause drowsiness. Doses in excess of the recommended dosage may cause nervousness, dizziness, or sleeplessness. If symptoms do not improve within 7 days or are accompanied by high fever, a physician should be consulted before continuing use. Should not be taken by persons hypersensitive to any of the ingredients. As with any drug, women who are pregnant or nursing a baby should seek the advice of a health professional before using this product.

Caution: Patients should be warned to avoid driving a motor vehicle, operating heavy machinery or consuming alcoholic beverages while taking this product.

Drug Interaction Precaution: Concomitant administration of phenylpropanolamine with other sympathomimetic

agents may produce additive effects and increased toxicity; with monoamine oxidase inhibitors (MAOIs) may produce a hypertensive crisis; with certain antihypertensive agents may diminish their antihypertensive effect.

Directions: Adults and children 12 years of age and over: one tablet every 12 hours. DO NOT EXCEED 1 TABLET EVERY 12 HOURS OR 2 TABLETS IN A 24-HOUR PERIOD.

How Supplied: Pale blue sugar-coated tablets monogrammed DIMETAPP AHR in bottles of 100 (NDC 0031-2277-63), 500 (NDC 0031-2277-70); Dis-Co® Unit Dose Packs of 100 (NDC 0031-2277-64); and consumer packages of 12 tablets (NDC 0031-2277-46), and 24 tablets (NDC 0031-2277-54) and 48 tablets (NDC 0031-2277-59) (individually packaged).
Store at Controlled Room Temperature, Between 15°C and 30°C (59°F and 86°F).
Dimetapp Extentabs® Tablets are the A. H. Robins Company's uniquely constructed extended action tablets.
Shown in Product Identification Section, page 425

DIMETAPP® Tablets
[di 'mĕ-tap]

Description: Each **Dimetapp** Tablet contains:
Brompheniramine
     Maleate, USP....................................4 mg
Phenylpropanolamine
     Hydrochloride, USP ....25 mg

Inactive Ingredients: Corn starch, FD&C Blue 1 Aluminum Lake, Magnesium Stearate, Microcrystalline Cellulose.

Indications: For temporary relief of nasal congestion due to the common cold, hay fever or other upper respiratory allergies and associated with sinusitis; temporarily relieves running nose, sneezing, and itchy and watery eyes as may occur in allergic rhinitis (such as hay fever). Temporarily restores freer breathing through the nose.

Warnings: This product may cause excitability, especially in children. This product should not be taken by patients with high blood pressure, heart disease, diabetes, thyroid disease, asthma, glaucoma or difficulty in urination due to enlargement of the prostate gland, except under the advice and supervision of a physician. May cause drowsiness. Doses in excess of the recommended dosage may cause nervousness, dizziness, or sleeplessness. If symptoms do not improve within 7 days or are accompanied by high fever, a physician should be consulted before continuing use. Should not be taken by persons hypersensitive to any of the ingredients. As with any drug, women who are pregnant or nursing a baby should seek the advice of a health professional before using this product.

Caution: Patients should be warned to avoid driving a motor vehicle, operating heavy machinery or consuming alcoholic beverages while taking this product.

	Initial	Every 3 Hours
Adults	2 tablespoonfuls (1 fl. oz.)	1 tablespoonful
Children:		
Over 12 Years:	2 tablespoonfuls	1 tablespoonful
6–12 Years:	2 teaspoonfuls	1–2 teaspoonfuls

Drug Interaction Precaution: Concomitant administration of phenylpropanolamine with other sympathomimetic agents may produce additive effects and increased toxicity; with monoamine oxidase inhibitors (MAOIs) may produce a hypertensive crisis; with certain antihypertensive agents may diminish their antihypertensive effect.

Directions: Adults and children 12 years of age and over: one tablet every 4 hours. Children 6 to under 12 years: one-half tablet every 4 hours. DO NOT EXCEED 6 DOSES IN A 24-HOUR PERIOD. Children under 6 years: Use only as directed by a physician.

How Supplied: Blue, scored compressed tablets engraved AHR and 2254 in consumer packages of 24 (NDC 0031-2254-54).
Store at Controlled Room Temperature, Between 15°C and 30°C (59°F and 86°F).
Shown in Product Identification Section, page 425

DIMETAPP PLUS® CAPLETS
[di 'me-tap]

Description: Each **Dimetapp PLUS®** **Caplet** contains:
Acetaminophen, USP.....................500 mg
Phenylpropanolamine
   Hydrochloride, USP ....12.5 mg
Brompheniramine Maleate, USP ...2 mg

Inactive Ingredients: Corn starch, FD&C Blue 2 Aluminum Lake, Hydroxypropyl Methylcellulose, Magnesium Stearate, Microcrystalline Cellulose, Polysorbate 20, Povidone, Propylene Glycol, Stearic Acid, Titanium Dioxide. May also contain Calcium Phosphate, Hydroxypropyl Cellulose, Methylparaben, Propylparaben.

Indications: For the temporary relief of minor aches, pains, and headache; for the reduction of fever; for the relief of nasal congestion due to the common cold or associated with sinusitis; and for the relief of runny nose, sneezing, itching of the nose or throat and itchy and watery eyes as may occur in allergic rhinitis (such as hay fever). Temporarily restores freer breathing through the nose.

Warnings: May cause drowsiness. May cause excitability, especially in children. If symptoms do not improve within 7 days or are accompanied by high fever, a physician should be consulted before continuing use. Patients who have asthma, glaucoma, heart disease, high blood pressure, thyroid disease, diabetes, emphysema, chronic pulmonary disease, shortness of breath, difficulty in urination due to enlargement of the prostate gland should not take this product unless directed by a physician. Recommended dosage should not be exceeded because at higher dosages severe liver damage, nervousness, dizziness, or sleeplessness may occur. As with any drug, women who are pregnant or nursing a baby should seek the advice of a health professional before using this product.

Caution: Patients should be warned to avoid driving a motor vehicle, operating heavy machinery or consuming alcoholic beverages while taking this product.

Drug Interaction Precaution: Concomitant administration of phenylpropanolamine with other sympathomimetic agents may produce additive effects and increased toxicity; with monoamine oxidase inhibitors (MAOIs) may produce a hypertensive crisis; with certain antihypertensive agents may diminish their antihypertensive effect.

Directions: Adults and children (12 years and over): Two caplets every 6 hours. DO NOT EXCEED 8 CAPLETS IN A 24-HOUR PERIOD.
Not recommended for children under 12 years of age.

How Supplied: Dimetapp Plus® Caplets are supplied as blue capsule-shaped film-coated tablets engraved AHR on one side and 2278 on the other in consumer packages of 24 (NDC 0031-2278-54), and 48 (NDC 0031-2278-59) (individually packaged).
Store at Controlled Room Temperature, Between 15°C and 30°C (59°F and 86°F).
Shown in Product Identification Section, page 425

DONNAGEL®
[don 'nă-jel]

Each 30 mL (1 fl. oz.) contains:
Kaolin, USP (90 gr) ....6.0 g
Pectin, USP (2 gr).......................142.8 mg
Hyoscyamine Sulfate, USP.....0.1037 mg
Atropine Sulfate, USP.............0.0194 mg
Scopolamine Hydrobromide,
   USP ....0.0065 mg
Sodium Benzoate, NF
   (preservative) ....60 mg
Alcohol...3.8%

Inactive Ingredients: Citric Acid, D&C Yellow 10, FD&C Blue 1, Flavors, Sodium Carboxymethylcellulose, Sodium Chloride, Sorbitol, Water.

Indications: Donnagel is indicated in the treatment of diarrhea and associated cramping.

Description: Donnagel combines the adsorbent and detoxifying effects of kaolin and pectin with the antispasmodic efficacy of the natural belladonna alkaloids. The latter, present in a specific, fixed ratio, help control hypermotility and hypersecretion in the gastrointestinal tract.

Warnings: As with any drug, women who are pregnant or nursing a baby should seek the advice of a health professional before taking this product.

Contraindications: Glaucoma or increased ocular pressure, advanced renal or hepatic disease or hypersensitivity to any of the ingredients.

Precautions: As with all preparations containing belladonna alkaloids, Donnagel must be administered cautiously to patients with incipient glaucoma or urinary bladder neck obstruction as in prostatic hypertrophy. Use with caution in elderly patients (where undiagnosed glaucoma or excessive pressure occurs most frequently).

Adverse Reactions: Blurred vision, dry mouth, difficult urination, flushing and dryness of the skin, dizziness or tachycardia may occur at higher dosage levels, rarely at the usual dose.

Dosage and Administration:
[See table above].
Do not take more than 4 doses in any 24-hour period.

How Supplied: Donnagel (light green, aromatic suspension) in 4 fl. oz. (NDC 0031-3016-12), 8 fl. oz. (NDC 0031-3016-18), and pint (NDC 0031-3016-25).
Store at Controlled Room Temperature, Between 15°C and 30°C (59°F and 86°F).
Shown in Product Identification Section, page 425

ROBITUSSIN®
(Guaifenesin Syrup, USP)
[ro "bĭ-tuss 'ĭn]

Active Ingredients per teaspoonful (5 mL)—Guaifenesin, USP 100 mg in pleasant tasting syrup with alcohol 3.5%.

Inactive Ingredients: Caramel, Citric Acid, FD&C Red 40, Flavors, Glucose, Glycerin, High Fructose Corn Syrup, Saccharin Sodium, Sodium Benzoate, Water.

Indications: Expectorant action to help loosen phlegm and thin bronchial secretions to make coughs more productive.

Warnings: A persistent cough may be a sign of a serious condition. If cough persists for more than 1 week, tends to recur, or is accompanied by fever, rash, or persistent headache, patients should consult a doctor. Patients are advised not to take this product for persistent or chronic cough such as occurs with smoking, asthma, chronic bronchitis, emphysema, or if cough is accompanied by excessive phlegm (mucus) unless directed

Continued on next page

Prescribing information on A.H. Robins products listed here is based on official labeling in effect November 1, 1989 with Indications, Contraindications, Warnings, Precautions, Adverse Reactions, and Dosage stated in full.

Robins—Cont.

by a doctor. As with any drug, women who are pregnant or nursing a baby should seek the advice of a health professional before using this product.

Contraindications: Hypersensitivity to any of the ingredients.

Adverse Reactions: Guaifenesin is well tolerated and has a wide margin of safety. Nausea and vomiting are the side effects that occur most commonly, and other reported adverse reactions have included dizziness, headache, and rash (including urticaria).
Note: Guaifenesin has been shown to produce a color interference with certain clinical laboratory determinations of 5-hydroxyindoleacetic acid (5-HIAA) and vanillylmandelic acid (VMA).

Directions: Adults and children 12 years and over: 2–4 teaspoonfuls every 4 hours; children 6 years to under 12 years: 1–2 teaspoonfuls every 4 hours. Children 2 years to under 6 years: ½–1 teaspoonful every 4 hours; children under 2 years—consult your doctor. DO NOT EXCEED RECOMMENDED DOSAGE.
Professional Labeling: Helps loosen phlegm and thin bronchial secretions in patients with stable chronic bronchitis.

How Supplied: Robitussin (wine-colored) in bottles of 4 fl. oz. (NDC 0031-8624-12), 8 fl. oz. (NDC 0031-8624-18), pint (NDC 0031-8624-25) and gallon (NDC 0031-8624-29).
Robitussin also available in 1 fl. oz. bottles (4 × 25's NDC 0031-8624-02) and Dis-Co® Unit Dose Packs of 10 × 10's in 5 mL (NDC 0031-8624-23), 10 mL (NDC 0031-8624-26 and 15 mL (NDC 0031-8624-28).
Store at Controlled Room Temperature, Between 15°C and 30°C (59°F and 86°F).
Shown in Product Identification Section, page 425

ROBITUSSIN–CF®
[*ro "bĭ-tuss 'ĭn*]

Active Ingredients per teaspoonful (5 mL)—Guaifenesin, USP 100 mg and Phenylpropanolamine Hydrochloride, USP 12.5 mg and Dextromethorphan Hydrobromide, USP 10 mg in pleasant-tasting syrup with alcohol 4.75%.

Inactive Ingredients: Citric Acid, FD&C Red 40, Flavors, Glycerin, Propylene Glycol, Saccharin Sodium, Sodium Benzoate, Sorbitol, Water.

Indications: Temporarily relieves coughs due to minor throat and bronchial irritation and nasal congestion as may occur with a cold. Expectorant action to help loosen phlegm and thin bronchial secretions to make cough more productive.

Warnings: A persistent cough may be a sign of a serious condition. If cough persists for more than 1 week, tends to recur, or is accompanied by fever, rash, or persistent headache, patients should consult a doctor. Patients are advised not to take this product for persistent or chronic cough such as occurs with smoking, asthma, chronic bronchitis, emphysema, or if cough is accompanied by excessive phlegm (mucus) unless directed by a doctor. Likewise, persons with high blood pressure, heart disease, diabetes, thyroid disease or difficulty in urination due to enlargement of the prostate gland are advised to use this product only as directed by a doctor. The recommended dosage should not be exceeded because at higher doses nervousness, dizziness, or sleeplessness may occur. As with any drug, women who are pregnant or nursing a baby should seek the advice of a health professional before using this product.

Contraindications: Hypersensitivity to any of the ingredients; marked hypertension; hyperthyroidism; patients who are receiving monoamine oxidase inhibitors (MAOIs).

Adverse Reactions: The following adverse reactions may occur: nausea, vomiting, dizziness, dry mouth, nervousness, insomnia, restlessness, headache, or rash (including urticaria).
Note: Guaifenesin has been shown to produce a color interference with certain clinical laboratory determinations of 5-hydroxyindoleacetic acid (5-HIAA) and vanillylmandelic acid (VMA).

Drug Interaction Precautions: Concomitant administration of phenylpropanolamine with other sympathomimetic agents may produce additive effects and increased toxicity; with MAOIs may produce a hypertensive crisis; with certain antihypertensive agents may diminish their antihypertensive effect. Serious toxicity may result if dextromethorphan is used with MAOIs.

Directions: Adults and children 12 years and over, 2 teaspoonfuls every 4 hours; children 6 years to under 12 years, 1 teaspoonful every 4 hours; children 2 years to under 6 years, ½ teaspoonful every 4 hours; children under 2 years —as directed by a physician. DO NOT EXCEED 6 DOSES IN A 24-HOUR PERIOD.

How Supplied: Robitussin-CF (red-colored) in bottles of 4 fl. oz. (NDC 0031-8677-12), 8 fl. oz. (NDC 0031-8677-18), and one pint (NDC 0031-8677-25).
Store at Controlled Room Temperature, Between 15°C and 30°C (59°F and 86°F).
Shown in Product Identification Section, page 425

ROBITUSSIN–DM®
[*ro "bĭ-tuss 'ĭn*]

Active Ingredients per teaspoonful (5 mL)—Guaifenesin, USP 100 mg and Dextromethorphan Hydrobromide, USP 15 mg in pleasant-tasting syrup with alcohol 1.4%.

Inactive Ingredients: Citric Acid, FD&C Red 40, Flavors, Glucose, Glycerin, High Fructose Corn Syrup, Saccharin Sodium, Sodium Benzoate, Water.

Indications: Temporarily relieves coughs due to minor throat and bronchial irritation as may occur with a cold. Expectorant action to help loosen phlegm and bronchial secretions to make coughs more productive.

Warnings: A persistent cough may be a sign of a serious condition. If cough persists for more than 1 week, tends to recur, or is accompanied by fever, rash, or persistent headache, patients should consult a doctor. Patients are advised not to take this product for persistent or chronic cough such as occurs with smoking, asthma, chronic bronchitis, emphysema, or if cough is accompanied by excessive phlegm (mucus), unless directed by a doctor. As with any drug, women who are pregnant or nursing a baby should seek the advice of a health professional before using this product.

Contraindications: Hypersensitivity to any of the ingredients, or in patients who are receiving monoamine oxidase inhibitors (MAOIs).

Adverse Reactions: The incidence of side effects is low. Reported side effects include nausea and vomiting, as well as diarrhea, drowsiness, and rash (including urticaria).
Overdose Symptoms may include ataxia, respiratory depression and convulsions in children, whereas adults may exhibit altered sensory perception, ataxia, slurred speech and dysphoria.
Note: Guaifenesin has been shown to produce a color interference with certain clinical laboratory determinations of 5-hydroxyindoleacetic acid (5- HIAA) and vanillylmandelic acid (VMA).

Drug Interaction Precaution: Serious toxicity may result if dextromethorphan is used with MAOIs.

Directions: Adults and children 12 years and over, 2 teaspoonfuls every 6 to 8 hours; children 6 years to under 12 years, 1 teaspoonful every 6 to 8 hours; children 2 years to under 6 years, ½ teaspoonful every 6 to 8 hours; children under 2 years—consult your doctor. DO NOT EXCEED 4 DOSES IN A 24-HOUR PERIOD.

How Supplied: Robitussin-DM (cherry-colored) in bottles of 4 fl. oz. (NDC 0031-8684-12), 8 fl. oz. (NDC 0031-8684-18), 12 fl. oz. (NDC 0031-8684-22), single doses: 6 premeasured doses—⅓ fl. oz. each (NDC 0031-8686-06), pint (NDC 0031-8684-25), and gallon (NDC 0031-8684-29).
Robitussin-DM also available in Dis-Co® Unit Dose Packs of 10 × 10's in 5 mL (NDC 0031-8684-23) and 10 mL (NDC 0031-8684-26).
Store at Controlled Room Temperature, Between 15°C and 30°C (59°F and 86°F).
Shown in Product Identification Section, page 425

ROBITUSSIN–PE®
[*ro "bĭ-tuss 'ĭn*]

Active Ingredients per teaspoonful (5 mL)— Guaifenesin, USP 100 mg and

Pseudoephedrine Hydrochloride, USP 30 mg in pleasant tasting syrup with alcohol 1.4%.

Inactive Ingredients: Citric Acid, FD&C Red 40, Flavors, Glucose, Glycerin, High Fructose Corn Syrup, Saccharin Sodium, Sodium Benzoate, Water.

Indications: Temporarily relieves nasal congestion as may occur with a cold. Expectorant action to help loosen phlegm and thin bronchial secretions to make coughs more productive.

Warnings: A persistent cough may be a sign of a serious condition. If cough persists for more than 1 week, tends to recur, or is accompanied by fever, rash, or persistent headache, patients should consult a doctor. Patients are advised not to take this product for persistent or chronic cough such as occurs with smoking, asthma, chronic bronchitis, emphysema, or if cough is accompanied by excessive phlegm (mucus) unless directed by a doctor. Likewise, persons with high blood pressure, heart disease, diabetes, thyroid disease or difficulty in urination due to enlargement of the prostate gland are advised to use this product only as directed by a doctor. The recommended dosage should not be exceeded because at higher doses nervousness, dizziness, or sleeplessness may occur. As with any drug, women who are pregnant or nursing a baby should seek the advice of a health professional before using this product.

Contraindications: Hypersensitivity to any of the ingredients; marked hypertension; hyperthyroidism; or in patients who are receiving monoamine oxidase inhibitors (MAOIs).

Adverse Reactions: Possible side effects include nausea, vomiting, nervousness, restlessness, rash (including urticaria), headache, or dry mouth.

Note: Guaifenesin has been shown to produce a color interference with certain clinical laboratory determinations of 5-hydroxyindoleacetic acid (5-HIAA) and vanillylmandelic acid (VMA).

Drug Interaction Precautions: Concomitant administration of pseudoephedrine with other sympathomimetic agents may produce additive effects and increased toxicity; with MAOIs may produce a hypertensive crisis; with certain antihypertensive agents may diminish their antihypertensive effect.

Directions: Adults and children 12 years and over, 2 teaspoonfuls every 4 hours; children 6 years to under 12 years, 1 teaspoonful every 4 hours; children 2 years to under 6 years, ½ teaspoonful every 4 hours; children under 2 years —as directed by physician. DO NOT EXCEED 4 DOSES IN A 24-HOUR PERIOD.

How Supplied: Robitussin-PE (orange-red) in bottles of 4 fl. oz. (NDC 0031-8695-12), 8 fl. oz. (NDC 0031-8695-18) and pint (NDC 0031-8695-25).

Store at Controlled Room Temperature, Between 15°C and 30°C (59°F and 86°F).

Shown in Product Identification Section, page 425

ROBITUSSIN NIGHT RELIEF®
[ro ″bĭ-tuss ′ĭn]
COLDS FORMULA
Composition:
Each fluid ounce contains:
Acetaminophen, USP ....650 mg
Phenylephrine HCl, USP ....10 mg
Pyrilamine Maleate, USP ....50 mg
Dextromethorphan
  Hydrobromide, USP ....30 mg

Inactive Ingredients: Citric Acid, FD&C Blue 1, FD&C Red 40, Flavors, Glycerin, Propylene Glycol, Saccharin Sodium, Sodium Benzoate, Sorbitol, Water.

Indications: Temporarily relieves cough, runny nose, sneezing and nasal congestion as may occur with a cold. Also relieves fever, headache, minor sore throat pain, and body aches and pains as may occur with a cold.

Warnings: This preparation may cause drowsiness. Patients should be warned not to drive or operate machinery or consume alcoholic beverages while taking this medication. This product should not be given to children under 6 years of age, except under the advice and supervision of a physician. Patients are cautioned not to use the product for more than 10 days. Persons with asthma, glaucoma, high blood pressure, diabetes, heart or thyroid disease or difficulty in urination due to enlargement of the prostate gland should use only as directed by a doctor. Dosage should be reduced if nervousness, restlessness or sleeplessness occurs. Since a persistent cough may be a sign of a serious condition, patients are advised to consult a physician if cough persists for more than 1 week, tends to recur, or is accompanied by high fever, rash or persistent headache. Likewise, patients are warned not to take this product for persistent or chronic cough such as occurs with smoking, asthma, chronic bronchitis, emphysema, or if cough is accompanied by excessive phlegm (mucus) unless directed by a doctor. As with any drug, women who are pregnant or nursing a baby should seek the advice of a health professional before using this product.

Contraindications: Hypersensitivity to any of the ingredients; marked hypertension; hyperthyroidism; patients who are receiving monoamine oxidase inhibitors (MAOIs).

Adverse Effects: The following adverse reactions may possibly occur: nausea, vomiting, dizziness, diarrhea, nervousness, insomnia and drowsiness.

Drug Interaction Precautions: Concomitant administration of phenylephrine with other sympathomimetic agents may produce additive effects and increased toxicity; with MAOIs may produce a hypertensive crisis; with certain antihypertensive agents may diminish their antihypertensive effect. Serious

toxicity may result if dextromethorphan is used with MAOIs.

Dosage: If your cold keeps you confined to bed or at home, take one dose every 6 hours, not to exceed 4 doses in a 24-hour period.
Adults (and children 12 years and over): one fluid ounce in medicine cup at bedtime (2 tablespoons). Children (6 years to under 12 years): ½ fluid ounce in medicine cup at bedtime (1 tablespoon). Under 6 years—consult your doctor.

How Supplied: Bottles of 4 fl. oz. (NDC 0031-8641-12) and 8 fl. oz. (NDC 0031-8641-18).
Store at Controlled Room Temperature, Between 15°C and 30°C (59°F and 86°F).
Shown in Product Identification Section, page 425

Z-BEC® Tablets
[zē ′běk]

One tablet daily provides:

Vitamin Composition		Percentage of U.S. Recommended Daily Allowance (U.S. RDA)
Vitamin E	150	45.0 I.U.
Vitamin C	1000	600.0 mg
Thiamine (Vitamin B$_1$)	1000	15.0 mg
Riboflavin (Vitamin B$_2$)	600	10.2 mg
Niacin	500	100.0 mg
Vitamin B$_6$	500	10.0 mg
Vitamin B$_{12}$	100	6.0 mcg
Pantothenic Acid	250	25.0 mg

Mineral Composition		
Zinc	150	22.5 mg*

*22.5 mg zinc (equivalent to zinc content in 100 mg zinc sulfate, USP)

Ingredients: Niacinamide Ascorbate; Ascorbic Acid; Microcrystalline Cellulose; Zinc Sulfate; Vitamin E Acetate; Hydrolyzed Protein; Calcium Pantothenate; Modified Starch; Hydroxypropyl Methylcellulose; Thiamine Mononitrate; Stearic Acid; Pyridoxine Hydrochloride; Riboflavin; Silicon Dioxide; Polysorbate 20; Magnesium Stearate; Lactose; Povidone; Propylene Glycol; Artificial Color; Vanillin; Hydroxypropyl Cellulose; Gelatin; Sorbic Acid; Sodium Benzoate; Cyanocobalamin.

Actions and Uses: Z-BEC is a high potency formulation. Its components have important roles in general nutrition, healing of wounds, and prevention of hemorrhage. It is recommended for deficiencies of these components in conditions such as febrile diseases, chronic or acute infections, burns, fractures, surgery, leg ulcers, toxic conditions, physiologic stress, alcoholism, prolonged expo-

Continued on next page

Prescribing information on A.H. Robins products listed here is based on official labeling in effect November 1, 1989 with Indications, Contraindications, Warnings, Precautions, Adverse Reactions, and Dosage stated in full.

Robins—Cont.

sure to high temperature, geriatrics, gastritis, peptic ulcer, and colitis; and in conditions involving special diets and weight-reduction diets.

In dentistry, Z-BEC is recommended for deficiencies of its components in conditions such as herpetic stomatitis, aphthous stomatitis, cheilosis, herpangina and gingivitis.

Precaution: Not intended for the treatment of pernicious anemia.

Dosage: The recommended OTC dosage for adults and children 12 or more years of age is one tablet daily with food or after meals. Under the direction and supervision of a physician, the dose and frequency of administration may be increased in accordance with the patient's requirements.

How Supplied: Green film-coated, capsule-shaped tablets in bottles of 60 (NDC 0031-0689-62), 500 (NDC 0031-0689-70), and Dis-Co® Unit Dose Packs of 100 (NDC 0031-0689-64).
Shown in Product Identification Section, page 425

Rorer Consumer Pharmaceuticals
a division of
Rorer Pharmaceutical Corporation
500 VIRGINIA DRIVE
FORT WASHINGTON, PA 19034

Regular Strength
ASCRIPTIN®
[ă"skrĭp'tin]
Analgesic
Aspirin plus Maalox®

Active Ingredients: Each coated tablet contains Aspirin (325 mg) and Maalox (Magnesium Hydroxide 50 mg, Dried Aluminum Hydroxide Gel 50 mg), buffered with Calcium Carbonate.

Inactive Ingredients: Hydroxypropyl Methylcellulose, Magnesium Stearate, Microcrystalline Cellulose, Starch, Talc, Titanium Dioxide, and other ingredients.

Description: Ascriptin is an excellent analgesic, antipyretic, and anti-inflammatory agent for general use, particularly where there is concern over aspirin-induced gastric distress. When large doses are used, as in arthritis and rheumatic disorders, gastric discomfort is rare. Coated tablets make swallowing easy.

Indications: As an analgesic for the relief of pain in such conditions as headache, neuralgia, minor injuries, and dysmenorrhea. As an analgesic and antipyretic in colds and influenza. As an analgesic and anti-inflammatory agent in arthritis and other rheumatic diseases. As an inhibitor of platelet aggregation, see MI's and TIA's indications.

Usual Adult Dose: Two or three tablets, four times daily. Do not exceed 12

tablets in a 24-hour period. For children under twelve, consult a doctor.

WARNINGS: Children and teenagers should not use this medicine for chicken pox or flu symptoms before a doctor is consulted about Reye syndrome, a rare but serious illness reported to be associated with aspirin. Keep this and all medicines out of children's reach. If pain persists more than 10 days, redness or swelling is present, fever persists more than 3 days, or symptoms worsen, consult a doctor immediately. If you are under medical care or have a history of stomach, kidney, or bleeding disorders or asthma, consult a doctor before using. Do not use if allergic to aspirin. As with any drug, if you are pregnant or nursing a baby, consult a doctor before using. **IMPORTANT:** Do not take this product during the last three months of pregnancy unless directed by a doctor. Aspirin taken near the time of delivery may cause bleeding problems in both mother and child. If ringing in the ears or loss of hearing occurs, consult a doctor before taking any more of this product. In case of accidental overdose, contact a doctor immediately. *Drug interaction precaution:* Do not use if taking a prescription drug for anticoagulation (blood thinning), diabetes, gout or arthritis, or a tetracycline antibiotic unless directed by a doctor.

Professional Labeling:
Aspirin for Myocardial Infarction

Indication: Aspirin is indicated to reduce the risk of death and/or non-fatal myocardial infarction in patients with a previous infarction or unstable angina pectoris.

Dosage and Administration: Although most of the studies used dosages exceeding 300 mg, two trials used only 300 mg, and pharmacologic data indicate that this dose inhibits platelet function fully. Therefore, 300 mg or a conventional 325-mg aspirin dose is a reasonable, routine dose that would minimize gastrointestinal adverse reactions. This use of aspirin applies to both solid, oral dosage forms (buffered and plain aspirin), and buffered aspirin in solution. *Note:* Complete information and references available.

RECURRENT TIA's IN MEN

Indications: For reducing the risk of recurrent transient ischemic attacks (TIA's) or stroke in men who have had transient ischemia of the brain due to fibrin platelet emboli. There is inadequate evidence that aspirin or buffered aspirin is effective in reducing TIA's in women at the recommended dosage. There is no evidence that aspirin or buffered aspirin is of benefit in the treatment of completed strokes in men or women.

Precautions: (1) Patients presenting with signs and symptoms of TIA's should have a complete medical and neurologic evaluation. Consideration should be given to other disorders which resemble TIA's. **(2)** Attention should be given to risk factors; it is important to evaluate and treat, if appropriate, other diseases

associated with TIA's and stroke such as hypertension and diabetes. **(3)** Concurrent administration of absorbable antacids at therapeutic doses may increase the clearance of salicylates in some individuals. The concurrent administration of nonabsorbable antacids may alter the rate of absorption of aspirin, thereby resulting in a decreased acetylsalicylic acid/salicylate ratio in plasma. The clinical significance on TIA's of these decreases in available aspirin is unknown.

Dosage: 1300 mg a day, in divided doses of 650 mg twice a day or 325 mg four times a day.

How Supplied: Bottles of 50 tablets (NDC 0067-0145-50), 100 tablets (NDC 0067-0145-68), and 225 tablets (NDC 0067-0145-77) with child-resistant caps. Bottles of 500 tablets (NDC 0067-0145-74) without child-resistant closures (for arthritic patients). Military Stock #NSN 6505-00-135-2783 V.A. Stock #6505-00-890-1979 (bottles of 500).
Shown in Product Identification Section, page 425

ASCRIPTIN® A/D for arthritis pain
Analgesic
Aspirin plus 50% more Maalox®
than Regular Strength Ascriptin for extra stomach comfort

Aspirin for arthritis pain relief plus contains 50% more Maalox than does Regular Strength Ascriptin.

Active Ingredients: Each coated caplet contains Aspirin (325 mg) and Maalox (Magnesium Hydroxide 75 mg, Dried Aluminum Hydroxide Gel 75 mg), buffered with Calcium Carbonate.

Inactive Ingredients: Hydroxypropyl Methylcellulose, Magnesium Stearate, Microcrystalline Cellulose, Starch, Talc, Titanium Dioxide, and other ingredients.

Description: Ascriptin A/D is a highly buffered analgesic, anti-inflammatory, and antipyretic agent for use in the treatment of rheumatoid arthritis, osteoarthritis, and other arthritic conditions. It is formulated with 50% more Maalox than Regular Strength Ascriptin to provide increased neutralization of gastric acid thus improving the likelihood of GI tolerance when large antiarthritic doses of aspirin are used. Coated caplets make swallowing easy.

Indications: As an analgesic, anti-inflammatory, and antipyretic agent in rheumatoid arthritis, osteoarthritis, and other arthritic conditions.

Usual Adult Dose: Two or three caplets, four times daily, or as directed by the physician for arthritis therapy. For children under twelve, at the discretion of the physician.

WARNINGS: Children and teenagers should not use this medicine for chicken pox or flu symptoms before a doctor is consulted about Reye syndrome, a rare but serious illness reported to be associated with aspirin. Keep this and all medicines out of children's reach. If pain persists more

than 10 days, redness or swelling is present, fever persists more than 3 days, or symptoms worsen, consult a doctor immediately. If you are under medical care or have a history of stomach, kidney, or bleeding disorders or asthma, consult a doctor before using. Do not use if allergic to aspirin. As with any drug, if you are pregnant or nursing a baby, consult a doctor before using. **IMPORTANT:** Do not take this product during the last three months of pregnancy unless directed by a doctor. Aspirin taken near the time of delivery may cause bleeding problems in both mother and child. If ringing in the ears or loss of hearing occurs, consult a doctor before taking any more of this product. **In case of accidental overdose, contact a doctor immediately.** *Drug interaction precaution:* Do not use if taking a prescription drug for anticoagulation (blood thinning), diabetes, gout or arthritis, or a tetracycline antibiotic unless directed by a doctor.

How Supplied: Available in bottles of 100 caplets (NDC 0067-0147-68), and 225 caplets (NDC 0067-0147-77) with child-resistant caps and in special bottles of 500 caplets (without child-resistant closures) for arthritic patients (NDC 0067-0147-74).

Shown in Product Identification Section, page 425

**Extra Strength
ASCRIPTIN®**
Analgesic
50% more Aspirin plus Maalox®
Extra pain relief with 50% more Aspirin than Regular Strength Ascriptin

Active Ingredients: Each coated caplet contains Aspirin (500 mg) and Maalox (Magnesium Hydroxide 80 mg, Dried Aluminum Hydroxide Gel 80 mg), buffered with Calcium Carbonate.

Inactive Ingredients: Hydroxypropyl Methylcellulose, Magnesium Stearate, Microcrystalline Cellulose, Starch, Talc, Titanium Dioxide, and other ingredients.

Description: Extra Strength Ascriptin contains 50% more aspirin than Regular Strength Ascriptin for fast, effective pain relief and Maalox for protection against aspirin-induced gastric distress. Coated caplets make swallowing easy.

Indications: For maximum relief of pain in headache, neuralgia, minor injuries, dysmenorrhea, discomfort and fever of ordinary colds. As an analgesic and anti-inflammatory agent in arthritis and other rheumatic diseases.

Usual Adult Dose: 2 caplets, three or four times daily. Not to exceed a total of 8 tablets in a 24-hour period, or as directed by a physician. For children under 12 at the discretion of physician.
WARNINGS: Children and teenagers should not use this medicine for chicken pox or flu symptoms before a doctor is consulted about Reye syndrome, a rare but serious illness reported to be associated with aspirin.

Keep this and all medicines out of children's reach. If pain persists more than 10 days, redness or swelling is present, fever persists more than 3 days, or symptoms worsen, consult a doctor immediately. If you are under medical care or have a history of stomach, kidney, or bleeding disorders or asthma, consult a doctor before using. Do not use if allergic to aspirin. As with any drug, if you are pregnant or nursing a baby, consult a doctor before using. **IMPORTANT:** Do not take this product during the last three months of pregnancy unless directed by a doctor. Aspirin taken near the time of delivery may cause bleeding problems in both mother and child. If ringing in the ears or loss of hearing occurs, consult a doctor before taking any more of this product. **In case of accidental overdose, contact a doctor immediately.** *Drug interaction precaution:* Do not use if taking a prescription drug for anticoagulation (blood thinning), diabetes, gout or arthritis, or a tetracycline antibiotic unless directed by a doctor.

How Supplied: Bottles of 36 caplets (NDC 0067-0146-63) without child-resistant closure and 75 caplets (NDC 0067-0146-75) with child-resistant caps.

Shown in Product Identification Section, page 426

CAMALOX®
[kăm 'ă-lŏx "]
Magnesium and Aluminum Hydroxides with Calcium Carbonate Oral Suspension and Tablets, Rorer High-potency antacid

Description: Camalox® Suspension is a carefully balanced formulation of 200 mg magnesium hydroxide, 225 mg dried aluminum hydroxide gel equivalent and 250 mg calcium carbonate per teaspoonful (5 mL). This combination of ingredients produces an antacid capability that exceeds that of other leading ethical products in terms of quantity of acid neutralized as well as the speed and duration of antacid activity as measured by laboratory tests. The formulation also minimizes the possibilities of both constipation and diarrhea. Camalox is prepared by a process which enhances its texture and vanilla-mint flavor, making it especially palatable even for patients who must take antacids for extended periods.

Inactive Ingredients: Citric acid, flavors, guar gum, methylparaben, propylparaben, silica, saccharin sodium, sorbitol solution, purified water.

Camalox® Tablets contain 200 mg magnesium hydroxide, 225 mg dried aluminum hydroxide gel equivalent and 250 mg calcium carbonate per tablet and have a delicate vanilla-mint flavor. They compare favorably with Camalox Suspension in terms of potency, as well as speed and duration of antacid activity; thus, Camalox Tablets overcome the usual deficiencies of antacid tablets. As measured by the *in vitro* test for acid neutralizing capacity, Camalox Tablets ex-

ceed the antacid capabilities of the leading ethical antacid suspensions as well as tablets. In addition, the manufacturing process contributes importantly to the flavor and to the texture of the tablets. Patients can take Camalox Tablets in full dosage day after day without tiring of the taste.

Inactive Ingredients: Citric acid, colloidal silicon dioxide, flavors, light mineral oil, magnesium stearate, mannitol, microcrystalline cellulose, silica, saccharin sodium, sorbitol solution, starch.

Acid Neutralizing Capacity
Camalox Suspension—36.9 mEq/10 mL
Camalox Tablets—36.7 mEq/2 tablets
Sodium Content
Camalox Suspension—1.2 mg (0.05 mEq)/5 mL
Camalox Tablets—1.0 mg (0.04 mEq)/tablet

Indications: A high potency antacid for the symptomatic relief of hyperacidity associated with the diagnosis of peptic ulcer, gastritis, peptic esophagitis, gastric hyperacidity, heartburn, or hiatal hernia.

Directions for Use: Camalox Suspension—two to four teaspoonfuls, four times a day, taken 30 minutes to 1 hour after meals and at bedtime, or as directed by a physician.
Camalox Tablets—each Camalox Tablet is equivalent to one teaspoonful of Camalox Suspension. Two to four tablets, well-chewed, 30 minutes to one hour after meals and at bedtime, or as directed by a physician.

Patient Warnings: Do not take more than 16 teaspoonfuls or tablets in a 24-hour period or use the maximum dosage for more than two weeks or use if you have kidney disease except under the advice and supervision of a physician. Keep this and all drugs out of the reach of children.

Drug Interaction Precaution: Do not use with patients taking a prescription antibiotic drug containing any form of tetracycline. As with all aluminum-containing antacids, Camalox may prevent the proper absorption of tetracycline.

How Supplied: Camalox Suspension—white liquid in convenient 12 fluid ounce (355 mL) plastic bottles (NDC 0067-0180-71).
Camalox Tablets—Bottles of 50 tablets (NDC 0067-0185-50).

Rationale: Studies reveal that clinical symptoms of gastroesophageal reflux correlate with lower esophageal sphincter (LES) incompetency. Although the mechanism of action is unknown, gastric alkalinization has been shown to increase LES pressure.
Camalox is an ideal antacid for the treatment of reflux esophagitis. The balanced formulation of Camalox exerts its neutralizing effect faster and longer than the leading ethical antacids providing prompt symptomatic relief.

Continued on next page

Rorer Consumer—Cont.

Camalox has been shown to produce significant increases in LES pressure providing a physiological barrier against reflux.*

Because Camalox is a high potency antacid with excellent acid neutralizing capacity, fewer and smaller doses are possible.

The refreshing vanilla-mint flavor and smooth texture of Camalox have earned a high level of patient acceptance and wearability. Available in equally effective dosage forms . . . physician-preferred suspension and convenient tablets.

*Higgs, R.H., Smyth, R.D., and Castell, D.O., Gastric Alkalinization—Effect on Lower-Esophageal-Sphincter Pressure and Serum Gastrin, *N. Engl. J. Med.* 291:486-490, 1974.

Shown in Product Identification Section, page 426

FERMALOX®
[fĕr 'mă-lŏx ″]
Hematinic

Formula: Each *uncoated* tablet contains: Ferrous Sulfate 200 mg; Maalox® (magnesium-aluminum hydroxide) 200 mg.

Inactive Ingredients: Confectioners' sugar, ethylcellulose, flavors, iron oxides, magnesium stearate, starch, talc.

Advantages: "A less irritating, more easily tolerated medicinal iron compound (Fermalox) fills an important need in the treatment of iron-deficiency states. The demonstration of effective absorption by means of the radioactive iron tracer, plus thousands of clinical cases showing satisfactory rise of hemoglobin level, fully establishes the efficacy of this medicament. In addition, the almost complete absence of the common adverse reactions to ordinary iron medicaments enables the physician to continue use of the drug until a satisfactory therapeutic result is obtained."[1]

Indications: For use as a hematinic in iron-deficiency conditions as may occur with: rapid growth, pregnancy, blood loss, menorrhagia, post-surgical convalescence, pathologic bleeding.

Usual Adult Dose: Two tablets daily; in mild cases dosage may be reduced to one tablet daily.

Warning: As with any drug, if you are pregnant or nursing a baby, seek the advice of a health professional before using this product. Keep this and all drugs out of the reach of children. In case of accidental overdose, seek professional assistance or contact a poison control center immediately.

How Supplied: Bottles of 100 tablets (NDC 0067-0260-68) with child-resistant caps.

1. Price, A.H., Erf, L., and Bierly, J.: *J.A.M.A.* 167:1612 (July 26), 1958.

MAALOX®
[mā 'lŏx ″]
Magnesia and Alumina Oral Suspension and Tablets, Rorer Antacid
A Balanced Formulation of Magnesium and Aluminum Hydroxides

Description: Maalox® Suspension is a balanced combination of magnesium and aluminum hydroxides. . . first in order of preference for all routine purposes of antacid medication. The high neutralizing power of magnesium hydroxide and the established acid binding capacity of aluminum hydroxide support the reputation of Maalox® for reliable antacid action.

Maalox® Suspension: 225 mg Aluminum Hydroxide Equivalent to Dried Gel, USP, and 200 mg Magnesium Hydroxide per 5 mL.

Inactive Ingredients: Citric acid, methylparaben, natural flavor, propylparaben, saccharin sodium, sorbitol, purified water, and other ingredients.

Maalox® Tablets: (200 mg Magnesium Hydroxide, 200 mg Dried Aluminum Hydroxide Gel) per tablet

Inactive Ingredients: Citric acid, flavors, magnesium stearate, mannitol, microcrystalline cellulose, saccharin sodium, sorbitol solution, starch.

Extra Strength Maalox® Tablets: (400 mg Magnesium Hydroxide, 400 mg Dried Aluminum Hydroxide Gel) per tablet

Inactive Ingredients: Confectioner's sugar, flavors, glycerin, magnesium stearate, mannitol, saccharin sodium, sorbitol, sucrose, talc.

Acid Neutralizing Capacity
Maalox® Suspension—26.6 mEq/10 ml
Maalox® Tablets—19.4 mEq/2 tablets
Extra Strength Maalox® Tablets—23.4 mEq/tablet

Sodium Content
Maalox® Suspension and Tablets are dietetically sodium-free*. Each teaspoonful (5 mL) of Maalox® Suspension contains approximately 0.06 mEq sodium (1.4 mg) and Maalox® and Extra Strength Maalox® Tablets contain approximately 0.03 mEq (0.7 mg) and 0.06 mEq (1.4 mg) sodium respectively per tablet.

*Dietetically insignificant.

Indications: As an antacid for symptomatic relief of hyperacidity associated with the diagnosis of peptic ulcer, gastritis, peptic esophagitis, gastric hyperacidity, heartburn or hiatal hernia.

Advantages: Many patients prefer Maalox® whether they are taking it for occasional heartburn or routinely on an ulcer therapy regimen. Once started on Maalox®, patients tend to stay on Maalox® because of effectiveness, taste, and non-constipating characteristics . . . three important reasons for Maalox® when prolonged therapy is necessary. In addition, Maalox® Suspension and Tablets are sodium-free.

Directions for Use:
Maalox® Suspension: Two to four teaspoonfuls, four times a day, taken twenty minutes to one hour after meals and at bedtime, or as directed by a physician.
Maalox® Tablets: Two to four tablets, well chewed, twenty minutes to one hour after meals and at bedtime, or as directed by a physician.
Extra Strength Maalox® Tablets: One or two tablets, well chewed, four times a day, taken twenty minutes to one hour after meals and at bedtime, or as directed by a physician. May be followed with milk or water.
Patient Warnings: Do not take more than 16 teaspoonfuls of Maalox® Suspension, 16 Maalox® Tablets, or 8 Extra Strength Maalox® Tablets in a 24-hour period or use the maximum dosage for more than 2 weeks or use if you have kidney disease, except under the supervision of a physician.

Drug Interaction Precaution: Do not use with patients taking a prescription antibiotic drug containing any form of tetracycline. As with all aluminum-containing antacids, Maalox® may prevent the proper absorption of the tetracycline. Keep this and all drugs out of the reach of children.

How Supplied:
Maalox® Suspension is available in plastic bottles of 12 fluid ounces (355 mL) (NDC 0067-0330-71), 5 fluid ounces (148 mL) (NDC 0067-0330-62), and 26 fluid ounces (769 mL) (NDC 0067-0330-44).
Maalox® Tablets (400 mg) available in bottles of 100 tablets (NDC 0067-0335-68).
Extra Strength Maalox® Tablets (800 mg) available in bottles of 50 (NDC 0067-0340-50). Also available in boxes of 24 (NDC 0067-0340-24) and 100 tablets (NDC 0067-0340-67) in easy-to-carry strips.
V.A. Stock #6505-00-993-3507A [boxes of 100 tablets (in cellophane strips)].
Shown in Product Identification Section, page 426

EXTRA STRENGTH
MAALOX® Plus (Reformulated Maalox Plus)
Alumina, Magnesia and Simethicone Oral Suspension and Tablets, Rorer Antacid/Anti-Gas

☐ Lemon Swiss creme
  Cherry creme
  Mint creme
  . . . the flavors preferred by the physician and patient.
☐ Physician-proven Maalox® formula for antacid effectiveness.
☐ Simethicone, at a recognized clinical dose, for antiflatulent action.

Description: Extra Strength Maalox® Plus, a balanced combination of magnesium and aluminum hydroxides plus simethicone, is a non-constipating, lemon swiss-creme flavored, antacid/anti-gas.

Composition: To provide symptomatic relief of hyperacidity plus alleviation of gas symptoms, each teaspoonful/tablet contains:

Active Ingredients	Extra Strength Maalox® Plus Per Tsp. (5 mL)	Maalox® Plus Per Tablet
Magnesium Hydroxide	450 mg	200 mg
Aluminum Hydroxide (equivalent to dried gel, USP)	500 mg	200 mg
Simethicone	40 mg	25 mg

Inactive Ingredients: Extra Strength Maalox® Plus Suspension: Citric acid, flavors, methylparaben, propylparaben, purified water, saccharin sodium, sorbitol, and other ingredients.
Maalox® Plus Tablets: Citric acid, confectioners' sugar, D&C red No. 30, D&C yellow No. 10, dextrose, flavors, glycerin, magnesium stearate, mannitol, saccharin sodium, sorbitol solution, starch, talc. To aid in establishing proper dosage schedules, the following information is provided:

Minimum Recommended Dosage:		
	Per 2 Tsp. (10 mL)	Per Tablet
Acid neutralizing capacity	58.1 mEq	11.4 mEq
Sodium content*	2.3 mg	0.8 mg
Sugar content	None	0.55 g
Lactose content	None	None

Indications: As an antacid for symptomatic relief of hyperacidity associated with the diagnosis of peptic ulcer, gastritis, peptic esophagitis, gastric hyperacidity, heartburn, or hiatal hernia. As an antiflatulent to alleviate the symptoms of gas, including postoperative gas pain.

Advantages: Among antacids, Extra Strength Maalox® Plus Suspension and Maalox® Plus Tablets are uniquely palatable—an important feature which encourages patients to follow your dosage directions. Extra Strength Maalox® Plus Suspension and Maalox® Plus Tablets have the time-proven, nonconstipating, sodium-free* Maalox® formula —useful for those patients suffering

*Dietetically insignificant. Contains approximately 0.05 mEq sodium per teaspoonful of Suspension. Each Maalox® Plus Tablet contains approximately 0.03 mEq sodium per Tablet.

from the problems associated with hyperacidity. Additionally, Extra Strength Maalox® Plus Suspension and Maalox® Plus Tablets contain simethicone to alleviate discomfort associated with entrapped gas.

Directions for Use:
Extra Strength Maalox® Plus Suspension: Two to four teaspoonfuls, four times a day, taken twenty minutes to one hour after meals and at bedtime, or as directed by a physician.

Patient Warnings: Do not take more than 12 teaspoonfuls in a 24-hour period or use the maximum dosage for more than 2 weeks or use if you have kidney disease except under the advice and supervision of a physician.

Maalox® Plus Tablets: One to four tablets, well chewed, four times a day, taken twenty minutes to one hour after meals and at bedtime, or as directed by a physician.

Patient Warnings: Do not take more than 16 tablets in a 24-hour period or use the maximum dosage for more than two weeks or use if you have kidney disease except under the advice and supervision of a physician.

Drug Interaction Precaution: Do not use with patients taking a prescription antibiotic containing any form of tetracycline. As with all aluminum-containing antacids, Maalox® Plus may prevent the proper absorption of the tetracycline. Keep this and all drugs out of the reach of children.

How Supplied:
Extra Strength Maalox® Plus Suspension is available in plastic bottles of 5 fl oz (148 mL) (NDC 0067-0333-62), 12 fl oz (355 mL) (NDC 0067-0333-71), and 26 fl oz (769 mL) (NDC 0067-0333-44) in lemon Swiss creme; 12 fl oz in cherry creme (NDC 0067-0336-71); and 12 fl oz in mint creme (NDC 0067-0338-71).
Maalox® Plus Tablets are available in bottles of 50 tablets (NDC 0067-0339-50) and 100 tablets (NDC 0067-0339-67), convenience packs of 12 tablets (NDC 0067-0339-19), Roll Packs of 12 tablets (NDC 0067-0339-23), and 36 tablets (NDC 0067-0339-33).

Shown in Product Identification Section, page 426

MAALOX® TC Suspension and Tablets
Therapeutic Concentrate
(Magnesium & Aluminum Hydroxides Oral Suspension and Tablets, Rorer)

Description: Maalox® TC Suspension is a potent, concentrated, balanced formulation of 300 mg magnesium hydroxide and 600 mg aluminum hydroxide (equivalent to dried gel, USP) per teaspoonful (5 mL). This formulation produces a therapeutically concentrated antacid that exceeds standard antacids in acid neutralizing capacity. Maalox® TC Suspension is formulated to reduce the need to alter therapy due to treatment-induced changes in bowel habits.

Palatability is enhanced by a pleasant-tasting peppermint flavor.

Inactive Ingredients: Citric acid, flavor, guar gum, methylparaben, propylparaben, sorbitol solution, purified water.
Maalox® TC Tablets contain 300 mg magnesium hydroxide and 600 mg dried aluminum hydroxide gel per tablet, with a pleasant-tasting peppermint-lemon-creme flavor. *In vivo* testing demonstrates a longer duration of action for the tablets when compared with equivalent doses of suspension. Maalox® TC tablets thus overcome the usual deficiencies of antacid tablets.

Inactive Ingredients: Confectioners' sugar, flavors, glycerin, magnesium stearate, mannitol, sorbitol solution, sucrose, talc.
Acid Neutralizing Capacity
Maalox® TC Suspension—27.2 mEq/ 5 mL
Maalox® TC Tablets—28.0 mEq/tablet
Sodium Content:
Maalox® TC Suspension—0.8 mg/ 5 mL (0.03 mEq)*
Maalox® TC Tablets—0.5 mg/tablet (0.02 mEq)*

* Dietetically insignificant.

Indications: Maalox® TC Suspension and Tablets are indicated for the symptomatic relief of hyperacidity associated with the diagnosis of peptic ulcer and other gastrointestinal conditions where a high degree of acid neutralization is desired.

Directions for Use: Maalox® TC Suspension—one or two teaspoonfuls 20 minutes to one hour after meals and at bedtime. Higher dosage regimens may be employed under the direct supervision of a physician in the treatment of active peptic ulcer disease.
Maalox® TC Tablets—each Maalox® tablet is equivalent to one teaspoon of Maalox® TC Suspension. One or two Maalox® TC tablets, well chewed one hour after meals and at bedtime. Higher dosage regimens may be employed under the direct supervision of a physician in the treatment of active peptic ulcer disease.

Patient Warning: Do not take more than 8 teaspoonfuls of the suspension or 8 tablets in a 24-hour period, or use the maximum dosage of this product for more than two weeks except under the advice and supervision of a physician. Also, if you have kidney disease, do not use except under the advice and supervision of a physician.

Drug Interaction Precaution: Do not use with patients taking a prescription antibiotic drug containing any form of tetracycline. As with all aluminum-containing antacids, Maalox® TC may prevent the proper absorption of the tetracycline. Keep this and all drugs out of the reach of children.

Continued on next page

Rorer Consumer—Cont.

Professional Labeling

Indications: Maalox® TC is indicated for the prevention of stress-induced upper gastrointestinal hemorrhage. As an antacid, for the symptomatic relief of hyperacidity associated with the diagnosis of peptic ulcer and other gastrointestinal conditions where a high degree of acid neutralization is desired.

Directions for Use: PREVENTION OF STRESS-INDUCED UPPER GASTRO-INTESTINAL HEMORRHAGE: 1) Aspirate stomach via nasogastric tube* and record pH. 2) Instill 10 mL of Maalox® TC followed by 30 mL of water via nasogastric tube. Clamp tube. 3) Wait one hour. Aspirate stomach and record pH. 4a) If pH equals or exceeds 4.0, apply drainage or intermittent suction for one hour, then repeat the cycle. 4b) If pH is less than 4.0, instill double (20 mL) Maalox® TC followed by 30 mL of water. Clamp tube. 5) Wait one hour. If pH equals or exceeds 4.0, see number 7. If pH is still less than 4.0, instill double (40 mL) Maalox® TC followed by 30 mL of water. Clamp tube. 6) Wait one hour. If pH equals or exceeds 4.0, see number 7. If pH is still less than 4.0, instill double (80 mL)** Maalox® TC followed by 30 mL of water. 7) Drain for one hour and repeat cycle with the effective dosage of Maalox® TC. IN HYPERACID STATES FOR SYMPTOMATIC RELIEF: One or two teaspoonfuls as needed between meals and at bedtime or as directed by a physician. Higher dosage regimens may be employed under the direct supervision of a physician in the treatment of active peptic ulcer disease.

---

*If nasogastric tube is not in place, administer 20 mL of Maalox® TC orally q2h.

**In a recent clinical study,[1] 20 mL of Maalox® TC, q2h, was sufficient in more than 85 percent of the patients. No patient studied required more than 80 mL of Maalox® TC q2h.

Precaution: Aluminum-magnesium hydroxide containing antacids should be used with caution in patients with renal impairment.

Adverse Effects: Occasional regurgitation and mild diarrhea have been reported with the dosage recommended for the prevention of stress-induced upper gastrointestinal hemorrhage.

References: 1. Zinner MJ, Zuidema GD, Smith PL, Mignosa M: The prevention of upper gastrointestinal tract bleeding in patients in an intensive care unit. *Surg Gynec & Obstet* 153:214–220, 1981. 2. Lucas CE, Sugawa C, Riddle J et al.: Natural history and surgical dilemma of "stress" gastric bleeding. *Arch Surg* 102:266–273, 1971. 3. Hastings PR, Skillman JJ, Bushnell LS, Silen W: Antacid titration in the prevention of acute gastrointestinal bleeding: a controlled, randomized trial in 100 critically ill pa-

tients. *New England J Med* 298:1042–1045, 1978. 4. Day SB, MacMillan BG, Altemeier WA: Curling's Ulcer, An Experiment of Nature. Springfield, IL, Charles C. Thomas Co., 1972, p 205. 5. Skillman JJ, Bushnell LS, Goldman H, Silen W: Respiratory failure, hypotension, sepsis, and jaundice. A clinical syndrome associated with lethal hemorrhage from acute stress ulceration of the stomach. *Am J Surg* 117:523–530, 1969. 6. Priebe HJ, Skillman JJ, Bushnell LS et al.: Antacid versus cimetidine in preventing acute gastrointestinal bleeding. *New England J Med* 302:426–430, 1980. 7. Silen W: The prevention and management of stress ulcers. *Hospital Practice* 15:93–97, 1980. 8. Herrmann V, Kaminski DL: Evaluation of intragastric pH in acutely ill patients. *Arch Surg* 114:511–514, 1979. 9. Martin LF, Staloch DK, Simonowitz DA et al.: Failure of cimetidine prophylaxis in the critically ill. *Arch Surg* 114:492–496, 1979. 10. Zinner MJ, Turtinen L, Gurll N, Reynolds DG: The effect of metiamide on gastric mucosal injury in rat restraint. *Clin Res* 23:484A, 1975. 11. Zinner M, Turtinen BA, Gurll NJ: The role of acid and ischemia in production of stress ulcers during canine hemorrhagic shock. *Surgery* 77:807–816, 1975. 12. Winans CS: Prevention and treatment of stress ulcer bleeding: Antacids or cimetidine? *Drug Therapy* (hospital) 12:37–45, 1981.

How Supplied: Maalox® TC Suspension is available in a 12-fluid ounce (355 mL) plastic bottle (NDC 0067-0334-71). Maalox® TC Tablets are available in plastic bottles of 48 tablets (NDC 0067-0344-48).

Shown in Product Identification Section, page 426

MYOFLEX® CREME
[mī'ō-flex]
(Trolamine Salicylate)

Indications: MYOFLEX is indicated as a topical analgesic for the temporary relief of minor aches and pains of muscles and joints due to backache, muscle strains, sprains and bruises, or overexertion. It is a useful topical adjunct in arthritis and rheumatism as a cream for patients with minor rheumatic stiffness or sore hands and feet.

Contraindications: MYOFLEX is contraindicated in patients sensitive to its ingredients.

Description: Myoflex contains as its active ingredient 10% Trolamine (formerly Triethanolamine) salicylate in a nongreasy base. It is a nonirritating, nonburning, odorless, stainless, readily absorbed cream. Trolamine salicylate is a topical analgesic. The empirical formula of trolamine salicylate is $C_6H_{15}NO_3 \cdot C_7H_6O_3$, molecular weight 287.31. Its chemical structure is:

$$COOH \cdot N(C_2H_4OH)_3$$

Trolamine salicylate is a light reddish viscous liquid with a faint odor. It is miscible in all proportions with water, glycerin, propylene glycol, and ethyl alcohol.

Clinical Pharmacology: Salicylic acid is the active moiety of MYOFLEX. Salicylic acid is enzymatically biotransformed to salicyluric acid and salicylphenolic glucuronide and eliminated in the urine. Salicylic acid is rapidly distributed throughout all body tissues, mainly by pH-dependent passive processes. It can be detected in synovial, spinal and peritoneal fluids, in saliva and in milk. It readily crosses the placental barrier. About 50% to 90% of salicylic acid is bound to plasma proteins, mainly to albumin.

The urinary excretion of salicylic acid equivalents was studied in 12 normal, healthy male subjects after MYOFLEX application. Salicylic acid was absorbed from MYOFLEX in 11 of 12 normal subjects over the 24-hour period post-application with a mean salicylic acid excretion of 13.5%.

Trolamine salicylate does not block neuronal membranes as do topical anesthetics. Some degree of percutaneous absorption occurs through the skin and blood levels have been demonstrated following topical application in animals and humans. Trolamine salicylate is not a counterirritant analgesic.

Warnings: For external use only. Avoid contact with eyes or mucous membranes. Keep out of the reach of children. If condition worsens, or if symptoms persist for more than 7 days, or clear up and occur again within a few days, discontinue use and consult a doctor.

As with any drug, if you are pregnant or nursing a baby, seek the advice of a health professional before using this product.

Precautions: General—Apply to affected parts only. Do not apply to broken or irritated skin.

Appropriate precautions should be taken by persons known to be sensitive to salicylates. If a reaction develops, the drug should be discontinued.

Drug Interactions—There are no known drug interactions with MYOFLEX. However, salicylates may counteract the effects of uricosuric agents such as probenecid and enhance the effects of oral anticoagulants such as coumadin. Therefore, they must be used with caution in patients on anticoagulants that affect the prothrombin time. Caution should also be exercised in patients concurrently treated with a sulfonylurea hypoglycemic agent, methotrexate, barbiturates and diphenylhydantoin, because these drugs may be displaced from plasma protein binding sites by salicylate resulting in an enhanced effect. Diphenylhydantoin intoxication has been precipitated by concomitant use of aspirin. The diuretic action of spironolactone is inhibited by salicylates.

Usage in Pregnancy (Category C)—Studies have not been performed in animals or humans to determine whether this drug affects fertility in males or females, has mutagenic, carcinogenic or teratogenic potential or other adverse effects on the fetus. Aspirin causes testicular atrophy and inhibition of spermatogenesis in animals and has been shown to be teratogenic in animals and to increase the incidence of still births and neonatal deaths in pregnant women. As with other salicylates, MYOFLEX should be used during pregnancy only if the potential benefit justifies the potential risk to the fetus.

Chronic, high dose salicylate therapy of pregnant women increases the length of gestation and the frequency of post-maturity and prolongs spontaneous labor. It is, therefore, recommended that MYOFLEX be used during the last three months of pregnancy only under the close supervision of a physician.

Nursing Mothers—Salicylates are excreted in the breast milk of nursing mothers. Caution should be therefore exercised when MYOFLEX is administered to a nursing woman.

Pediatric Use—Safety and effectiveness of MYOFLEX in children have not been established.

Adverse Reactions: If applied to large skin areas, the absorbed salicylate may cause typical salicylate side effects such as tinnitus, nausea, or vomiting.

Overdosage: Acute overdosage with MYOFLEX is unlikely. A 2 oz. MYOFLEX tube contains the salicylate equivalent of about 56 grains of aspirin. Early signs and symptoms from repeated large doses consist of headache, dizziness, tinnitus (which may be absent in children or the elderly), difficulty in hearing, dimness of vision, mental confusion, lassitude, drowsiness, sweating, thirst, hyperventilation, nausea, vomiting and occasionally diarrhea. Treatment of acute salicylate poisoning is a medical emergency and should be undertaken in a hospital.

Directions for Use: Adults —Rub into painful or sore area two or three times daily. Wrists, elbows, knees or ankles may be wrapped loosely with 2″ or 3″ elastic bandage after application.

How Supplied:
NDC 0067-1170-02 Tubes, 2 oz.
NDC 0067-1170-04 Tubes, 4 oz.
NDC 0013-5404-62 Pump Dispenser, 3 oz.
NDC 0067-1170-08 Jars, 8 oz.
NDC 0067-1170-16 Jars, 16 oz.
Store at controlled room temperature 15–30°C (59–86°F) (jars).
Protect from freezing or excessive heat (tubes and pump).

Shown in Product Identification Section, page 426

PERDIEM®
[pĕr ″dē ′ŭm]

Indication: For relief of constipation.

Actions: Perdiem®, with its 100% natural, gentle action provides comfortable relief from constipation. Perdiem® is a unique combination of bulk-forming fiber and natural stimulant. The vegetable mucilages of Perdiem® soften the stool and provide pain-free evacuation of the bowel with no chemical stimulants. Perdiem® is effective as an aid to elimination for the hemorrhoid or fissure patient prior to and following surgery.

Composition: Perdiem® contains as its active ingredients, 82% psyllium (Plantago Hydrocolloid) and 18% senna (Cassia Pod Concentrate) which are natural vegetable derivatives. Each rounded teaspoonful (6.0 g) contains 3.25 g psyllium, 0.74 g senna, 1.8 mg of sodium, 35.5 mg of potassium, and 4 calories. Perdiem® is "Dye-Free" and contains no artificial sweeteners.

Inactive Ingredients: Acacia, iron oxides, natural flavors, paraffin, sucrose, talc.

Patient Warning: Should not be used in the presence of undiagnosed abdominal pain. Frequent or prolonged use without the direction of a physician is not recommended, as it may lead to laxative dependence. Do not use in patients with a history of psyllium allergy. Psyllium allergy is rare but can be severe. If an allergic reaction occurs, discontinue use.

Bulk-forming agents have the potential to obstruct the esophagus, particularly in the presence of esophageal narrowing or when consumed with insufficient fluid. Patients should be made aware of the symptoms of esophageal obstruction, including chest pain/pressure, regurgitation, and difficulty swallowing. Patients experiencing these symptoms should seek immediate medical attention. Patients with esophageal narrowing or dysphagia should not use Perdiem®.

As with any drug, if you are pregnant or nursing a baby, seek the advice of a health professional before using this product. Keep this and all drugs out of the reach of children. In case of accidental overdose, seek professional assistance or contact a poison control center immediately.

Directions for Use—Adults: In the evening and/or before breakfast, 1–2 rounded teaspoonfuls of Perdiem® granules (in single or partial teaspoon doses) should be placed in the mouth and swallowed with at least 8 fl oz of cool beverage after the dose. Additional liquid would be helpful. Perdiem® granules should not be chewed.

Perdiem® generally takes effect within 12 hours. Subsequent doses may be adjusted after adequate laxation is obtained.

Note: It is extremely important that Perdiem® be taken with at least 8 fl oz of cool liquid.

In Severe Cases of Constipation: Perdiem® may be taken more frequently, up to 2 rounded teaspoonfuls every 6 hours not to exceed 5 teaspoonfuls in a 24-hour period. In severe cases, 24 to 72 hours may be required for optimal relief.

For Patients Habituated to Strong Purgatives: Two rounded teaspoonfuls of Perdiem® in the morning and evening may be required along with half the usual dose of the purgative being used. The purgative should be discontinued as soon as possible and the dosage of Perdiem® granules reduced when and if bowel tone shows lessened laxative dependence.

For Colostomy Patients: To ensure formed stools, give one to two rounded teaspoonfuls of Perdiem® in the evening.

For Clinical Regulation: For patients confined to bed, for those of inactive habits, and in the presence of cardiovascular disease where straining must be avoided, one rounded teaspoonful of Perdiem® taken once or twice daily will provide regular bowel habits.

For Children: From age 7–11 years, give one rounded teaspoonful one to two times daily. From age 12 and older, give adult dosage.

How Supplied: Granules: 100-gram (3.5 oz) (NDC 0067-0690-68) and 250-gram (8.8 oz) (NDC 0067-0690-70) canisters, Hospital Unit Dose 50 6-gram packets in a gravity feed dispenser (NDC 0067-0690-08).

Shown in Product Identification Section, page 426

PERDIEM® FIBER
[pĕr ″dē ′ŭm]

Indications: Perdiem® Fiber provides gentle relief from simple, chronic, and spastic constipation. In addition, it relieves constipation associated with convalescence, pregnancy, and advanced age. Perdiem® Fiber is also indicated for use in special diets lacking in residue fiber to aid regularity and in the management of constipation associated with irritable bowel syndrome, diverticular disease, hemorrhoids, and anal fissures.

Action: Perdiem® Fiber, is a 100% natural bulk-forming fiber that gently helps maintain regularity and prevents constipation. Perdiem® Fiber's unique form is easy to swallow and requires no mixing but must be followed by at least 8 ounces of cool liquid. Perdiem® Fiber's 100% natural psyllium formulation can safely be taken for prolonged periods as a source of fiber under the direction of a physician.

Composition: Perdiem® Fiber contains as its active ingredient 100% psyllium (Plantago Hydrocolloid), a natural vegetable derivative. Each rounded teaspoonful (6.0 g) contains 4.03 g of psyllium, 1.8 mg of sodium, 36.1 mg of potassium and 4 calories. Perdiem® Fiber is "Dye-Free" and contains no artificial sweeteners.

Inactive Ingredients: Acacia, iron oxides, natural flavors, paraffin, sucrose, talc, titanium dioxide.

Patient Warning: Should not be used in the presence of undiagnosed abdominal pain. Frequent or prolonged use without the direction of a physician is not recommended.

Continued on next page

Rorer Consumer—Cont.

Do not use in patients with a history of psyllium allergy. Psyllium allergy is rare but can be severe. If an allergic reaction occurs, discontinue use.

Bulk-forming agents have the potential to obstruct the esophagus, particularly in the presence of esophageal narrowing or when consumed with insufficient fluid. Patients should be made aware of the symptoms of esophageal obstruction, including chest pain/pressure, regurgitation, and difficulty swallowing. Patients experiencing these symptoms should seek immediate medical attention. Patients with esophageal narrowing or dysphagia should not use Perdiem® Fiber. Keep this and all drugs out of the reach of children. In case of accidental overdose, seek professional assistance or contact a poison control center immediately.

Directions for Use—Adults: In the evening and/or before breakfast, 1 to 2 rounded teaspoonfuls (6.0 to 12.0 g) of Perdiem® Fiber granules (in full or partial teaspoon doses) should be placed in the mouth and swallowed with at least 8 fl oz of cool beverage after the dose. Additional liquid would be helpful. Perdiem® Fiber granules should not be chewed. Children: For children age 7–11, give 1 rounded teaspoonful 1–2 times daily. Age 12 and older, give adult dosage.

Note: It is extremely important that Perdiem® Fiber be taken with at least 8 fl oz of cool liquid.

In Severe Cases of Constipation: Perdiem® Fiber may be taken more frequently, up to 2 rounded teaspoonfuls every 6 hours depending upon need and response not to exceed 5 teaspoonfuls in a 24-hour period. In obstinate cases, 48 to 72 hours may be required to provide optimal benefit.

After Rectal Surgery: The vegetable mucilages of Perdiem® Fiber soften the stool and ensure pain-free evacuation of the bowel. Perdiem® Fiber is effective as an aid to elimination for the hemorrhoid or fissure patient prior to and following surgery.

For Clinical Regulation: For patients confined to bed—after an operation for example—and for those of inactive habits, 1 rounded teaspoonful of Perdiem® Fiber taken 1–2 times daily will ensure regular bowel habits.

During Pregnancy: Because of its natural ingredient and bulking action, Perdiem® Fiber is effective for expectant mothers when used under a physician's care. In most cases 1–2 rounded teaspoonfuls taken each evening is sufficient.

How Supplied: Granules: 100-gram (3.5 oz) (NDC 0067-0795-68) and 250-gram (8.8 oz) (NDC 0067-0795-70) canisters, Hospital Unit Dose 50 6-gram packets in a gravity feed dispenser (NDC 0067-0795-08).

Shown in Product Identification Section, page 426

Ross Laboratories
COLUMBUS, OH 43216

ADVANCE®
[ad-vans']
Nutritional Beverage With Iron

Usage: As a fortified milk/soy-based feeding more appropriate than 2% low-fat milk for older babies and toddlers.

Features:
- A more appropriate distribution of calories from protein, fat and carbohydrate than in 2% lowfat milk.
- Recommended levels of vitamins and minerals to complement the solid-food diet of older infants.
- 1.8 mg of iron (as ferrous sulfate) per 100 Calories to help avoid iron deficiency.
- A combination of heat-treated soy and cow's-milk proteins to help reduce the risk of cow's-milk-induced enteric blood loss.
- 16 Calories per fluid ounce.

Availability:
Concentrated Liquid: 13-fl-oz cans; 12 per case; No. 3313.
Ready To Feed: (Prediluted, 16 Cal/fl oz) 32-fl-oz cans; 6 per case; No. 3301. For hospital use, Ready To Feed ADVANCE in disposable nursing bottles is available in the Ross Hospital Formula System.

Preparation:
Concentrated Liquid: Standard dilution (16 Cal/fl oz) is one part Concentrated Liquid to one part water.
Ready To Feed: Do not dilute.

Composition: Ready To Feed (Concentrated Liquid at standard dilution has similar composition and nutrient values. For specific information, refer to product label.)

Ingredients: Ⓤ-D Water, corn syrup, nonfat milk, soy oil, soy protein isolate, corn oil, calcium phosphate tribasic, mono- and diglycerides, soy lecithin, magnesium chloride, ascorbic acid, carrageenan, potassium citrate, choline chloride, taurine, ferrous sulfate, m-inositol, alpha-tocopheryl acetate, zinc sulfate, niacinamide, calcium pantothenate, cupric sulfate, thiamine chloride hydrochloride, vitamin A palmitate, riboflavin, pyridoxine hydrochloride, folic acid, manganese sulfate, phylloquinone, biotin, vitamin D3 and cyanocobalamin. 6.3 fl oz provides 100 Cal; 1 liter provides 540 Cal.

Nutrients:	Per 100 Cal	
Protein	3.7	g
Fat	5.0	g
Carbohydrate	10.2	g
Water	170	g
Linoleic Acid	2300	mg
Vitamins:		
Vitamin A	300	IU
Vitamin D	60	IU
Vitamin E	3.0	IU
Vitamin K	8	mcg
Thiamine (Vit. B_1)	120	mcg
Riboflavin (Vit. B_2)	170	mcg
Vitamin B_6	75	mcg
Vitamin B_{12}	0.3	mcg
Niacin	1300	mcg
Folic Acid (Folacin)	19	mcg
Pantothenic Acid	560	mcg
Biotin	4.4	mcg
Vitamin C (Ascorbic Acid)	10	mg
Choline	16	mg
Inositol	4.7	mg
Minerals:		
Calcium	94	mg
Phosphorus	72	mg
Magnesium	7.6	mg
Iron	1.8	mg*
Zinc	0.9	mg
Manganese	6	mcg
Copper	110	mcg
Iodine	18	mcg
Sodium	35	mg
Potassium	146	mg
Chloride	88	mg

*The addition of iron to this beverage conforms to the recommendation of the Committee on Nutrition of the American Academy of Pediatrics. (FAN 615-04)

ALIMENTUM®
[al "ah-men 'tum]
Protein Hydrolysate Formula With Iron

Usage: As a protein hydrolysate formula designed for the dietary management of infants with sensitivity to cow's-milk protein or other intact proteins, or with pancreatic insufficiency. Alimentum is a hypoallergenic feeding that may also be useful in the dietary management of infants with chronic diarrhea, multiple food allergies, protein-energy malnutrition and carbohydrate or fat malabsorption and galactosemia.

Features:
- Caloric distribution similar to that of breast milk (11% protein equivalent, 41% carbohydrate, 48% fat).
- Hydrolyzed casein supplemented with free amino acids for infants who are sensitive to or unable to digest intact protein.
- Fifty percent of the fat as medium-chain triglycerides, an easily digested and absorbed fat source.
- A dual-carbohydrate system of tapioca starch and sucrose to maximize the use of available digestive enzymes and absorptive pathways.
- Lactose-free carbohydrate to avoid lactose-associated diarrhea.
- Corn-free formulation to eliminate potential causes of corn allergy.

Availability:
Ready To Feed only: (Prediluted, 20 Cal/fl oz)
32-fl-oz cans; 6 per case; No. 237. For hospital use, prebottled ALIMENTUM is available in the Ross Hospital Formula System.

Preparation:
Ready To Feed: Do not dilute.

Composition: Ready To Feed

Ingredients: 87% water, 4.5% sucrose, 2.3% casein hydrolysate (enzymatically hydrolyzed and charcoal treated), 2.2% modified tapioca starch, 1.9% fractionated coconut oil (medium-chain triglycerides), 1.5% safflower oil, minerals (calcium citrate, calcium phosphate dibasic, potassium phosphate dibasic, calcium hydroxide, magnesium chloride, potassium chloride, sodium chloride, potassium citrate, ferrous sulfate, zinc sulfate, cupric sulfate, manganese sulfate, potassium iodide), soy oil, carrageenan, vitamins (ascorbic acid, choline chloride, m-inositol, alpha-tocopheryl acetate, niacinamide, calcium pantothenate, vitamin A palmitate, thiamine chloride hydrochloride, riboflavin, pyridoxine hydrochloride, folic acid, phylloquinone, biotin, vitamin D₃, cyanocobalamin), L-cystine dihydrochloride, L-tyrosine, L-tryptophan, taurine and L-carnitine.

5 fl oz provides 100 Cal; 1 liter provides 676 Cal.

Nutrients:	Per 100 Cal	
Protein Equivalent	2.75	g
Fat	5.54	g
Carbohydrate	10.2	g
Water	133	g
Linoleic Acid	1600	mg
Vitamins:		
Vitamin A	300	IU
Vitamin D	60	IU
Vitamin E	3.0	IU
Vitamin K	15	mcg
Thiamine (Vit. B₁)	60	mcg
Riboflavin (Vit. B₂)	90	mcg
Vitamin B₆	60	mcg
Vitamin B₁₂	0.45	mcg
Niacin	1350	mcg
Folic Acid (Folacin)	15	mcg
Pantothenic Acid	750	mcg
Biotin	4.5	mcg
Vitamin C		
(Ascorbic Acid)	9.0	mg
Choline	8	mg
Inositol	5	mg
Minerals:		
Calcium	105	mg
Phosphorus	75	mg
Magnesium	7.5	mg
Iron	1.8	mg
Zinc	0.75	mg
Manganese	30	mcg
Copper	75	mcg
Iodine	15	mcg
Sodium	44	mg
Potassium	118	mg
Chloride	80	mg

The addition of iron to this formula conforms to the recommendation of the Committee on Nutrition of the American Academy of Pediatrics.
(FAN 549-01)

CLEAR® EYES
[klēr īz]
Lubricating Eye Redness Reliever

Description: Clear Eyes is a sterile, isotonic buffered solution containing the active ingredients naphazoline hydrochloride 0.012% and glycerin 0.2%, as well as boric acid, purified water and sodium borate. Edetate disodium 0.1% and benzalkonium chloride 0.01% are added as preservatives. (Contains vasoconstrictor.)

Clear Eyes contains laboratory tested and scientifically blended ingredients, including an effective vasoconstrictor that narrows swollen blood vessels and rapidly whitens reddened eyes in a formulation that produces a refreshing, soothing effect. Clear Eyes is a sterile, isotonic solution compatible with the natural fluids of the eye.

Indications: Clear Eyes is a decongestant ophthalmic solution specially designed for temporary relief of redness due to minor eye irritation and to protect against further irritation or dryness of the eye.

Warnings: To avoid contamination, do not touch tip of container to any surface. Replace cap after using. If you experience eye pain, changes in vision, continued redness or irritation of the eye, or if the condition worsens or persists for more than 72 hours, discontinue use and consult a physician. If you have glaucoma, do not use this product except under the advice and supervision of a physician. Overuse of this product may produce increased redness of the eye. If solution changes color or becomes cloudy, do not use. KEEP THIS AND ALL MEDICINES OUT OF THE REACH OF CHILDREN. REMOVE CONTACT LENSES BEFORE USING.

Directions: Instill one or two drops in the affected eye(s), up to four times daily.

How Supplied: In 0.2-fl-oz, 0.5-fl-oz and 1.0-fl-oz plastic dropper bottles.
Shown in Product Identification Section, page 426
(FAN 2222-03)

EAR DROPS BY MURINE®
[myūr'ēn]
See Murine Ear Wax Removal System/Murine Ear Drops

ISOMIL®
[ī'sō-mil]
Soy Protein Formula With Iron

Usage: As a beverage for infants, children and adults with an allergy or sensitivity to cow's milk. A feeding following diarrhea. A feeding for patients with disorders for which lactose should be avoided: lactase deficiency, lactose intolerance and galactosemia.

Availability:
Powder: 14-oz cans, measuring scoop enclosed; 6 per case; No. 00107.
Concentrated Liquid: 13-fl-oz cans; 24 per case; No. 02110.
Ready To Feed: (Prediluted, 20 Cal/fl oz)
32-fl-oz cans; 6 per case; No. 00230.
8-fl-oz cans; 4 six-packs per case; No. 00173.
For hospital use, Ready To Feed Isomil in disposable nursing bottles is available in the Ross Hospital Formula System.

Preparation:
Powder: Standard dilution (20 Cal/fl oz) is one level, unpacked scoop of Powder (8.7g) for each 2 fl oz of warm water.

Concentrated Liquid: Standard dilution (20 Cal/fl oz) is one part Concentrated Liquid to one part water.
Ready To Feed: Do not dilute.
Note: All forms of Isomil should be shaken well before opening and before feeding.

Composition: Ready To Feed (Concentrated Liquid and Powder at standard dilution have similar composition and nutrient values. For specific information, refer to product labels.)

Ingredients: (Pareve, Ⓤ) 86% water, 4.8% corn syrup, 2.5% sucrose, 2.1% soy oil, 2.0% soy protein isolate, 1.4% coconut oil, 0.14% calcium citrate, 0.13% calcium phosphate tribasic, potassium citrate, potassium phosphate monobasic, potassium chloride, mono- and diglycerides, soy lecithin, magnesium chloride, carrageenan, ascorbic acid, L-methionine, potassium phosphate dibasic, sodium chloride, choline chloride, taurine, m-inositol, ferrous sulfate, alpha-tocopheryl acetate, zinc sulfate, L-carnitine, niacinamide, calcium pantothenate, cupric sulfate, vitamin A palmitate, thiamine chloride hydrochloride, riboflavin, pyridoxine hydrochloride, folic acid, manganese sulfate, potassium iodide, phylloquinone, biotin, vitamin D₃ and cyanocobalamin.

5 fl oz provides 100 Cal. 1 liter provides 676 Cal.

Nutrients:	Per 100 Cal	
Protein	2.66	g
Fat	5.46	g
Carbohydrate	10.1	g
Water	133	g
Linoleic Acid	1300	mg
Vitamins:		
Vitamin A	300	IU
Vitamin D	60	IU
Vitamin E	3.0	IU
Vitamin K	15	mcg
Thiamine (Vit. B₁)	60	mcg
Riboflavin (Vit. B₂)	90	mcg
Vitamin B₆	60	mcg
Vitamin B₁₂	0.45	mcg
Niacin	1350	mcg
Folic Acid (Folacin)	15	mcg
Pantothenic Acid	750	mcg
Biotin	4.5	mcg
Vitamin C		
(Ascorbic Acid)	9	mg
Choline	8	mg
Inositol	5	mg
Minerals:		
Calcium	105	mg
Phosphorus	75	mg
Magnesium	7.5	mg
Iron	1.8	mg*
Zinc	0.75	mg
Manganese	30	mcg
Copper	75	mcg
Iodine	15	mcg
Sodium	44	mg

Continued on next page

If desired, additional information on any Ross Product will be provided upon request to Ross Laboratories.

Ross—Cont.

Potassium	108	mg
Chloride	62	mg

*The addition of iron to this formula conforms to the recommendation of the Committee on Nutrition of the American Academy of Pediatrics.
(FAN 579-05)

ISOMIL® SF
[ī'sō-mil]
Sucrose–Free Soy Protein Formula With Iron

Usage: As a beverage for infants, children and adults with an allergy or sensitivity to cow's-milk protein or an intolerance to sucrose. A feeding following acute diarrhea. A feeding for patients with disorders for which lactose and sucrose should be avoided.

Availability:
Concentrated Liquid: 13-fl-oz cans; 12 per case; No. 00119.
Ready To Feed: (Prediluted, 20 Cal/fl oz) 32-fl-oz cans; 6 per case; No. 00128.
For hospital use, Ready To Feed Isomil SF in disposable nursing bottles is available in the Ross Hospital Formula System.

Preparation:
Concentrated Liquid: Standard dilution (20 Cal/fl oz) is one part Concentrated Liquid to one part water.
Ready To Feed: Do not dilute.
Note: All forms of Isomil SF should be shaken well before opening and before feeding.

Composition: Ready To Feed (Concentrated Liquid at standard dilution has similar composition and nutrient values. For specific information, refer to product label.)

Ingredients: (Pareve, Ⓤ) 87.4% water, 6.4% hydrolyzed cornstarch, 2.1% soy oil, 2.0% soy protein isolate, 1.4% coconut oil, minerals (calcium citrate, calcium phosphate tribasic, potassium citrate, potassium phosphate monobasic, potassium chloride, magnesium chloride, potassium phosphate dibasic, sodium chloride, ferrous sulfate, zinc sulfate, cupric sulfate, manganese sulfate, potassium iodide), mono- and diglycerides, soy lecithin, vitamins (ascorbic acid, choline chloride, m-inositol, alpha-tocopheryl acetate, niacinamide, calcium pantothenate, vitamin A palmitate, thiamine chloride hydrochloride, riboflavin, pyridoxine hydrochloride, folic acid, phylloquinone, biotin, vitamin D_3, cyanocobalamin), carrageenan, L-methionine, taurine and L-carnitine.
5 fl oz provides 100 Cal; 1 liter provides 676 Cal.

Nutrients:	Per 100 Cal	
Protein	2.66	g
Fat	5.46	g
Carbohydrate	10.1	g
Water	133	g
Linoleic Acid	1300	mg

Vitamins:		
Vitamin A	300	IU
Vitamin D	60	IU
Vitamin E	3.0	IU
Vitamin K	15	mcg
Thiamine (Vit. B_1)	60	mcg
Riboflavin (Vit. B_2)	90	mcg
Vitamin B_6	60	mcg
Vitamin B_{12}	0.45	mcg
Niacin	1350	mcg
Folic Acid (Folacin)	15	mcg
Pantothenic Acid	750	mcg
Biotin	4.5	mcg
Vitamin C (Ascorbic Acid)	9	mg
Choline	8	mg
Inositol	5	mg

Minerals:		
Calcium	105	mg
Phosphorus	75	mg
Magnesium	7.5	mg
Iron	1.8	mg*
Zinc	0.75	mg
Manganese	30	mcg
Copper	75	mcg
Iodine	15	mcg
Sodium	44	mg
Potassium	108	mg
Chloride	62	mg

*The addition of iron to this formula conforms to the recommendation of the Committee on Nutrition of the American Academy of Pediatrics.
(FAN 503-03)

MURINE® EAR WAX REMOVAL SYSTEM/MURINE® EAR DROPS
[myūr'ēn]
Carbamide Peroxide
Ear Wax Removal Aid

Description: MURINE EAR DROPS contains the active ingredient carbamide peroxide, 6.5%. It also contains alcohol (6.3%), glycerin, polysorbate 20 and other ingredients. The MURINE EAR WAX REMOVAL SYSTEM includes a 1.0-fl-oz soft bulb ear washer. This system is the only complete medically approved system to safely remove ear wax. Application of carbamide peroxide drops followed by warm-water irrigation is an effective, medically recommended way to help loosen excessive and/or hardened ear wax.

Actions: The carbamide peroxide formula in MURINE EAR DROPS is an aid in the removal of wax from the ear canal. Anhydrous glycerin penetrates and softens wax while the release of oxygen from carbamide peroxide provides a mechanical action resulting in the loosening of the softened wax accumulation. It is usually necessary to remove the loosened wax by gently flushing the ear with warm water using the soft bulb ear washer provided.

Indications: The MURINE EAR WAX REMOVAL SYSTEM is indicated for occasional use as an aid to soften, loosen and remove excessive ear wax.

Warning: DO NOT USE if you have ear drainage or discharge, ear pain, irritation, or rash in the ear or are dizzy; consult a doctor. DO NOT USE if you have

an injury or perforation (hole) of the eardrum or after ear surgery, unless directed by a doctor.
Do not use for more than 4 days; if excessive ear wax remains after use of this product, consult a doctor. Avoid contact with the eyes. KEEP THIS AND ALL MEDICINES OUT OF THE REACH OF CHILDREN.

Directions: FOR USE IN THE EAR ONLY. Adults and children over 12 years, tilt head sideways and place 5 to 10 drops in ear. Tip of applicator should not enter ear canal. Keep drops in ear for several minutes by keeping head tilted or placing cotton in ear. Use twice daily for up to 4 days if needed, or as directed by a doctor. Any wax remaining after treatment may be removed by gently flushing the ear with warm water, using a soft bulb ear washer. Children under 12 years, consult a doctor.
Used regularly, the Murine Ear Wax Removal System helps keep the ear canal free from blockage due to accumulated ear wax.
Note: When the ear canal is irrigated, the tip of the ear washer should not obstruct the flow of water leaving the ear canal.

How Supplied: The MURINE EAR WAX REMOVAL SYSTEM contains 0.5-fl-oz drops and a 1.0-fl-oz soft bulb ear washer.
Also available in 0.5-fl-oz drops only, MURINE EAR DROPS.
Shown in Product Identification Section, page 426
(FAN 2223)

MURINE®
[myūr'ēn]
Eye Lubricant

Description: Murine eye lubricant is a sterile, isotonic buffered solution containing the active ingredients 1.4% polyvinyl alcohol and 0.6% povidone. Also contains benzalkonium chloride, dextrose, disodium edetate, potassium chloride, purified water, sodium bicarbonate, sodium chloride, sodium citrate and sodium phosphate (mono- and dibasic). (No vasoconstrictor.)
Murine is a clear solution formulated to more closely match the natural tear fluid of the eye for gentle, soothing relief from minor eye irritation while moisturizing and preventing dryness. Use as desired to temporarily relieve minor eye irritation, dryness and burning due to conditions such as dust, smoke, smog, sun glare, wearing contact lenses, colds, allergies, swimming, reading, driving, TV or close work.

Indications: For the temporary relief or prevention of further discomfort due to minor eye irritations and symptoms related to dry eyes.

Warning: To avoid contamination, do not touch tip of container to any other surface. Replace cap after using. If you experience eye pain, changes in vision, continued redness or irritation of the eye, or if the condition worsens or persists for more than 72 hours, discontinue use and consult a physician. If solution changes color or becomes cloudy, do not use. KEEP THIS AND ALL MEDICINES OUT OF THE REACH OF CHILDREN. REMOVE CONTACT LENSES BEFORE USING.

Directions: Instill one or two drops in the affected eye(s) as needed.

How Supplied: In 0.2-fl-oz, 0.5-fl-oz and 1.0-fl-oz plastic dropper bottles.
Shown in Product Identification Section, page 426
(FAN 2202-04)

MURINE® PLUS
[*myūr ′ēn*]
Lubricating Eye Redness Reliever

Description: Murine Plus is a sterile, non-staining buffered solution containing the active ingredients 1.4% polyvinyl alcohol, 0.6% povidone and 0.05% tetrahydrozoline hydrochloride. Also contains benzalkonium chloride, dextrose, disodium edetate, potassium chloride, purified water, sodium bicarbonate, sodium chloride, sodium citrate and sodium phosphate (mono- and dibasic).
Murine Plus is an isotonic, sterile ophthalmic solution, formulated to more closely match the natural tear fluid of the eye. Its contains demulcents for gentle, soothing relief from minor eye irritation as well as the sympathomimetic agent, tetrahydrozoline hydrochloride, which produces local vasoconstriction in the eye. Thus, the drug effectively narrows swollen blood vessels locally and provides symptomatic relief of edema and hyperemia of conjunctival tissues due to eye allergies, minor local irritations and conjunctivitis. Use up to 4 times daily, to remove redness due to minor eye irritation caused by conditions such as dust, smoke, smog, sun glare, wearing contact lenses, colds, allergies, swimming, reading, driving, TV or close work. The effect of Murine Plus is prompt (apparent within minutes) and sustained.

Indications: For the temporary relief or prevention of further discomfort due to minor eye irritations and symptoms related to dry eyes plus removal of redness.

Warning: To avoid contamination, do not touch tip of container to any surface. Replace cap after using. If you experience eye pain, changes in vision, continued redness or irritation of the eye, or if the condition worsens or persists for more than 72 hours, discontinue use and consult a physician. If you have glaucoma, do not use this product except under the advice and supervision of a physician. Overuse of this product may produce increased redness of the eye. If solution changes color or becomes cloudy, do not use. KEEP THIS AND ALL MEDICINES OUT OF THE REACH OF CHILDREN. REMOVE CONTACT LENSES BEFORE USING.

Directions: Instill one or two drops in the affected eye(s), up to four times daily.

How Supplied: In 0.5-fl-oz and 1.0-fl-oz plastic dropper bottle.
Shown in Product Identification Section, page 426
(FAN 2202-04)

PEDIALYTE®
[*pē ′dē-ah-līt ″*]
Oral Electrolyte Maintenance Solution

Usage: For maintenance of water and electrolytes during mild or moderate diarrhea in infants and children; for maintenance of water and electrolytes following corrective parenteral therapy for severe diarrhea.
Features:
- Ready To Use—no mixing or dilution necessary.
- Balanced electrolytes to replace stool losses and provide maintenance requirements.
- Provides glucose to promote sodium and water absorption.
- Fruit-flavored form available to enhance compliance in older infants and children.
- Plastic quart bottles are resealable, easy to pour and easy to measure.
- No coloring added.
- Widely available in grocery, drug and convenience stores.

Availability:
32-fl-oz plastic bottles; 8 per case; Unflavored, No. 336—NDC 0074-6470-32; Fruit-flavored, No. 365—NDC 0074-6471-32.
8-fl-oz bottles; 4 six-packs per case; Unflavored, No. 160—NDC 0074-6470-08. For hospital use, Pedialyte is available in the Ross Hospital Formula System.

Dosage: See Administration Guide for maintenance of body water and electrolytes in mild or moderate diarrhea (Pedialyte Unflavored or Fruit-Flavored) and management of mild to moderate dehydration secondary to moderate to severe diarrhea (Rehydralyte® Oral Electrolyte Rehydration Solution).
Pedialyte (Unflavored or Fruit-Flavored) or Rehydralyte should be offered frequently in amounts tolerated. Total daily intake should be adjusted to meet individual needs, based on thirst and response to therapy. The suggested intakes for maintenance are based on water requirements for ordinary energy expenditure.[1] The suggested intakes for replacement are based on fluid losses of 5% or 10% of body weight, including maintenance requirement.
[See table on next page].

Composition: Unflavored Pedialyte (Fruit-Flavored Pedialyte has similar composition and nutrient value. For specific information, see product label.)

Ingredients: (Pareve, Ⓤ) Water, dextrose, potassium citrate, sodium chloride and sodium citrate.

Provides:	Per 8 Fl Oz	Per Liter	Per 32 Fl Oz
Sodium (mEq)	10.6	45	42.4
Potassium (mEq)	4.7	20	18.8
Chloride (mEq)	8.3	35	33.2
Citrate (mEq)	7.1	30	28.4
Dextrose (g)	5.9	25	23.6
Calories	24	100	96

(FAN 387-01)

RCF®
Ross Carbohydrate Free
Low-Iron Soy Protein Formula Base

Usage: For use in the dietary management of persons unable to tolerate the type or amount of carbohydrate in milk or conventional infant formulas; many of these patients have intractable diarrhea and are not able to tolerate other formulas. This product has been formulated to contain no carbohydrate, which must be added before feeding.

Availability:
Concentrated Liquid only: 13-fl-oz cans; 12 per case; No. 108.

Preparation:
RCF is for use only under the supervision of a physician. Physician's instructions must include the amount and type of carbohydrate and the amount of water to be added to RCF. Standard dilution is one part Formula Base to one part prescribed carbohydrate and water solution. If a physician specifies other types or amounts of carbohydrate, or other amounts of water, to be added to RCF, those instructions should be followed completely.
A full-strength formula, 20 Calories per fluid ounce, may be prepared with one of the following typical carbohydrates:
[See table on next page].

Composition: Concentrated Liquid

Ingredients: (Pareve, Ⓤ) 87% water, 4.4% soy protein isolate, 4.2% soy oil, 2.8% coconut oil, minerals (calcium phosphates [mono- and tribasic], potassium citrate, potassium chloride, magnesium chloride, calcium carbonate, sodium chloride, zinc sulfate, ferrous sulfate, cupric sulfate, manganese sulfate, potassium iodide), carrageenan, mono- and diglycerides, soy lecithin, vitamins (ascorbic acid, choline chloride, m-inositol, alpha-tocopheryl acetate, niacinamide, calcium pantothenate, vitamin A palmitate, thiamine chloride hydrochloride, riboflavin, pyridoxine hydrochloride, folic acid, phylloquinone, biotin, vitamin D_3, cyanocobalamin), L-methionine, taurine and L-carnitine.
4.2 fl oz of RCF, without added carbohydrate or water, provides 100 Cal (81 Cal/100 mL). 5 fl oz of 20 Cal/fl oz formula provides 100 Cal; see directions.
[See table on page 673].
(FAN 523-04)

Continued on next page

If desired, additional information on any Ross Product will be provided upon request to Ross Laboratories.

Ross—Cont.

REHYDRALYTE®
[rē-hī′drə-līt″]
Oral Electrolyte Rehydration Solution

Usage: For replacement of water and electrolytes lost during moderate to severe diarrhea.

Features:
- Ready To Use—no mixing or dilution necessary.
- Safe, economical alternative to IV therapy.
- 75 mEq of sodium per liter for effective replacement of fluid deficits.
- 2½% glucose solution to promote sodium and water absorption and provide energy.
- Widely available in pharmacies.

Availability: 8-fl-oz bottles; 4 six-packs per case; No. 162; NDC 0074-0162-01.

Dosage: (See Administration Guide under Pedialyte.)

Ingredients: (Pareve, Ⓤ) Water, dextrose, sodium chloride, potassium citrate and sodium citrate.

Type of Carbohydrate	Amount of Carbohydrate*	Water	RCF Formula Base
Table Sugar (sucrose)	4 level tablespoonfuls	12 fl oz	13 fl oz
Dextrose Powder (hydrous)	6 level tablespoonfuls	12 fl oz	13 fl oz
Polycose® Glucose Polymers Powder	9 level tablespoonfuls	12 fl oz	13 fl oz

* Approximately 52 grams needed for 20 Cal/fl oz formula.

Provides:	Per 8 Fl Oz	Per Liter
Sodium (mEq)	17.7	75
Potassium (mEq)	4.7	20
Chloride (mEq)	15.4	65
Citrate (mEq)	7.1	30
Dextrose (g)	5.9	25
Calories	24	100
(FAN 437-01)		

SELSUN BLUE®
[sel′sən blü]
Dandruff Shampoo (selenium sulfide lotion, 1%)

Selsun Blue is a non-prescription antidandruff shampoo containing the active ingredient selenium sulfide, 1%, in a freshly scented, pH balanced formula to leave hair clean and manageable. Available in Dry, Oily, Normal, Extra Conditioning and Extra Medicated formulas (also contains 0.5% menthol).

Inactive ingredients:
Dry formula —Acetylated lanolin alcohol, ammonium laureth sulfate, ammonium lauryl sulfate, cetyl acetate, citric acid, cocamide DEA, cocamidopropyl betaine, DMDM hydantoin, FD&C blue No. 1, fragrance, hydroxypropyl methylcellulose, magnesium aluminum silicate, polysorbate 80, sodium chloride, titanium dioxide, water and other ingredients.

Normal formula —Ammonium laureth sulfate, ammonium lauryl sulfate, citric acid, cocamide DEA, cocamidopropyl betaine, DMDM hydantoin, FD&C blue No. 1, fragrance, hydroxypropyl methylcellulose, magnesium aluminum silicate, sodium chloride, titanium dioxide, water and other ingredients.

Oily formula —Ammonium laureth sulfate, ammonium lauryl sulfate, citric acid, cocamide DEA, cocamidopropyl betaine, DMDM hydantoin, FD&C blue No. 1, fragrance, hydroxypropyl methylcellulose, magnesium aluminum silicate, sodium chloride, titanium dioxide, water and other ingredients.

Extra Conditioning formula —Acetylated lanolin alcohol, aloe, ammonium laureth sulfate, ammonium lauryl sulfate, cetyl acetate, citric acid, cocamide DEA, cocamidopropyl betaine, DMDM hydantoin, FD&C blue No. 1, fragrance, glycol distearate, hydroxypropyl methylcellulose, magnesium aluminum silicate, polysorbate 80, propylene glycol, sodium chloride, TEA-lauryl sulfate, titanium dioxide, water and other ingredients.

Extra Medicated formula —Ammonium laureth sulfate, ammonium lauryl sulfate, citric acid, cocamide DEA, cocamidopropyl betaine, DMDM hydantoin, D&C red No. 33, FD&C blue No. 1, fragrance, hydroxypropyl methylcellulose, magnesium aluminum silicate, sodium chloride, TEA-lauryl sulfate, water and other ingredients.

Clinical testing has shown Selsun Blue to be as safe and effective as other leading shampoos in helping control dandruff symptoms with regular use.

Directions: Shake well before using. Lather, rinse thoroughly and repeat. For best results, use at least twice a week for effective dandruff control.

Warnings: For external use only. Keep out of eyes—if this happens, rinse thoroughly with water. If used just before or after bleaching, tinting or permanent

Pedialyte, Rehydralyte Administration Guide

For Infants and Young Children

Age	2 Weeks	3 Months	6 Months	9	1	1½	2	2½ Years	3	3½	4
Approximate Weight[2]											
(lb)	7	13	17	20	23	25	28	30	32	35	38
(kg)	3.2	6.0	7.8	9.2	10.2	11.4	12.6	13.6	14.6	16.0	17.0
PEDIALYTE UNFLAVORED or FRUIT-FLAVORED fl oz/day for maintenance*	13 to 16	28 to 32	34 to 40	38 to 44	41 to 46	45 to 50	48 to 53	51 to 56	54 to 58	56 to 60	57 to 62
REHYDRALYTE fl oz/day for Replacement for 5% Dehydration (including maintenance)*	18 to 21	38 to 42	47 to 53	53 to 59	58 to 63	64 to 69	69 to 74	74 to 79	78 to 82	83 to 87	85 to 90
REHYDRALYTE fl oz/day for Replacement for 10% Dehydration (including maintenance)*	23 to 26	48 to 52	60 to 66	68 to 74	75 to 80	83 to 88	90 to 95	97 to 102	102 to 106	110 to 114	113 to 118

Administration Guide does not apply to infants less than 1 week of age. For children over 4 years, maintenance intakes may exceed 2 qt daily.

1. Extrapolated from Barness L: Nutrition and nutritional disorders, in Behrman RE, Vaughan VC III: *Nelson Textbook of Pediatrics*, ed 12. Philadelphia, WB Saunders Co, 1983, pp 136-138.
2. Weight based on the 50th percentile of weight for age of the National Center for Health Statistics (NCHS) reference data. Hamill PVV, Drizd TA, Johnson CL, et al: Physical growth: National Center for Health Statistics percentiles. *Am J Clin Nutr* 1979; 32:607-629.
* Fluid intakes do not take into account ongoing stool losses. Fluid loss in the stool should be replaced by consumption of an extra amount of Pedialyte or Rehydralyte equal to stool losses in addition to the amounts given in this Administration Guide.

waving, rinse hair for at least five minutes in cool running water. If irritation occurs, discontinue use. Keep out of the reach of children.

How Supplied: 4-, 7- and 11-fl-oz plastic bottles.

Shown in Product Identification Section, page 426

(FAN 2137-02)

SIMILAC®
[*sim 'ə-lak*]
Low-Iron Infant Formula

Usage: When an infant formula is needed: if the decision is made to discontinue breastfeeding before age 1 year, if a supplement to breastfeeding is needed or as a routine feeding if breastfeeding is not adopted.

Availability:
Powder: 1-lb cans, measuring scoop enclosed; 6 per case; No. 03139.
Concentrated Liquid: 13-fl-oz cans; 24 per case; No. 00264.
Ready To Feed: (Prediluted, 20 Cal/fl oz)
32-fl-oz cans; 6 per case; No. 00232.
8-fl-oz cans; 4 six-packs per case; No. 00177.
4-fl-oz nursing bottles; 6 per carry-home carton, 8 cartons per case; No. 00480.
8-fl-oz nursing bottles; 6 per carry-home carton, 4 cartons per case; No. 00880.
For hospital use, Ready To Feed Similac in disposable nursing bottles is available in the Ross Hospital Formula System.

Preparation:
Powder: Standard dilution (20 Cal/fl oz) is one level, unpacked scoop Powder (8.7 g) for each 2 fl oz of warm water.
Concentrated Liquid: Standard dilution (20 Cal/fl oz) is one part Concentrated Liquid to one part water.
Ready To Feed: Do not dilute.

Composition: Ready To Feed (Concentrated Liquid and Powder at standard dilution have similar composition and nutrient values. For specific information, refer to product labels.)

Ingredients: Ⓓ-D Water, nonfat milk, lactose, soy oil, coconut oil, mono- and diglycerides, soy lecithin, vitamins (ascorbic acid, choline chloride, m-inositol, alpha-tocopheryl acetate, niacinamide, calcium pantothenate, vitamin A palmitate, thiamine chloride hydrochloride, riboflavin, pyridoxine hydrochloride, folic acid, phylloquinone, biotin, vitamin D_3, cyanocobalamin), carrageenan, minerals (zinc sulfate, ferrous sulfate, cupric sulfate, manganese sulfate) and taurine.

5 fl oz provides 100 Cal; 1 liter provides 676 Cal.

Nutrients:	Per 100 Cal	
Protein	2.22	g
Fat	5.37	g
Carbohydrate	10.7	g
Water	133	g
Linoleic Acid	1300	mg
Vitamins:		
Vitamin A	300	IU
Vitamin D	60	IU
Vitamin E	3.0	IU
Vitamin K	8	mcg
Thiamine (Vit. B_1)	100	mcg
Riboflavin (Vit. B_2)	150	mcg
Vitamin B_6	60	mcg
Vitamin B_{12}	0.25	mcg
Niacin	1050	mcg
Folic Acid (Folacin)	15	mcg
Pantothenic Acid	450	mcg
Biotin	4.4	mcg
Vitamin C (Ascorbic Acid)	9	mg
Choline	16	mg
Inositol	4.7	mg
Minerals:		
Calcium	75	mg
Phosphorus	58	mg
Magnesium	6	mg
Iron	0.22	mg*
Zinc	0.75	mg
Manganese	5	mcg
Copper	90	mcg
Iodine	15	mcg
Sodium	28	mg
Potassium	108	mg
Chloride	66	mg

*This product, like milk, is deficient in iron; additional iron should be supplied from other sources.

(FAN 503-02)

Nutrients:	Without Carbohydrate Per 100 Cal		With Carbohydrate + Water Per 100 Cal*	
Protein	4.95	g	2.96	g
Fat	8.91	g	5.33	g
Carbohydrate	0.01	g	10.1	g
Water	110	g	133	g
Linoleic Acid	2170	mg	1300	mg
Vitamins:				
Vitamin A	500	IU	300	IU
Vitamin D	100	IU	60	IU
Vitamin E	5	IU	3.0	IU
Vitamin K	25	mcg	15	mcg
Thiamine (Vit. B_1)	100	mcg	60	mcg
Riboflavin (Vit. B_2)	150	mcg	90	mcg
Vitamin B_6	100	mcg	60	mcg
Vitamin B_{12}	0.75	mcg	0.45	mcg
Niacin	2230	mcg	1350	mcg
Folic Acid (Folacin)	25	mcg	15	mcg
Pantothenic Acid	1240	mcg	750	mcg
Biotin	7.5	mcg	4.5	mcg
Vitamin C (Ascorbic Acid)	13.6	mg	9	mg
Choline	13	mg	8	mg
Inositol	8	mg	5	mg
Minerals:				
Calcium	173	mg	105	mg
Phosphorus	124	mg	75	mg
Magnesium	12.4	mg	7.5	mg
Iron	0.37	mg†	0.22	mg†
Zinc	1.24	mg	0.75	mg
Manganese	50	mcg	30	mcg
Copper	124	mcg	75	mcg
Iodine	25	mcg	15	mcg
Sodium	73	mg	44	mg
Potassium	180	mg	108	mg
Chloride	103	mg	62	mg

* When 52 g of carbohydrate and 12 fl oz of water are mixed with 13 fl oz of RCF. Composition will vary depending on quantity of carbohydrate and water used. If carbohydrate is not added to this product, a 1:1 dilution with water provides approximately 12 Cal/fl oz (40.6 Cal/100 mL).
† This product is deficient in iron; additional iron should be supplied from other sources.

SIMILAC® PM 60/40
[*sim 'ə-lak*]
Low-Iron Infant Formula

Usage: For infants in the lower range of homeostatic capacity; those who are predisposed to hypocalcemia; and those whose renal, digestive or cardiovascular functions would benefit from lowered mineral levels. Similac PM 60/40 should be used as directed by a physician.

Availability: Powder only: 1-lb cans, measuring scoop enclosed; 6 per case; No. 00850. For hospital use, Ready To Feed Similac PM 60/40 in disposable nursing bottles is available in the Ross Hospital Formula System. (Ready To Feed has composition and nutrient values similar to Powder. For specific information see bottle tray.)

Preparation: Standard dilution (20 Cal/fl oz) is one level, unpacked scoop (8.6 g) of Powder for each 2 fl oz of warm water.

Continued on next page

If desired, additional information on any Ross Product will be provided upon request to Ross Laboratories.

Ross—Cont.

Higher caloric feedings may be prepared by adding 8.56 g (one level, unpacked scoop) of Similac PM 60/40 to the following amounts of water:

For:	Water:	Yields:
24 Cal/fl oz	48 mL	55 mL (1.8 fl oz)
27 Cal/fl oz	42 mL	49 mL (1.6 fl oz)
30 Cal/fl oz	37 mL	44 mL (1.5 fl oz)

Composition: Powder. (Ready To Feed has composition and nutrient values similar to Powder. For specific information see bottle tray.)

Ingredients: ⑪-D Lactose, corn oil, coconut oil, whey protein concentrate, sodium caseinate, minerals (calcium phosphate tribasic, potassium citrate, potassium chloride, magnesium chloride, sodium chloride, calcium carbonate, zinc sulfate, ferrous sulfate, cupric sulfate, manganese sulfate, potassium iodide), vitamins (m-inositol, ascorbic acid, choline chloride, alpha-tocopheryl acetate, niacinamide, calcium pantothenate, vitamin A palmitate, thiamine chloride hydrochloride, riboflavin, pyridoxine hydrochloride, folic acid, phylloquinone, vitamin D_3, biotin, cyanocobalamin), taurine and L-carnitine.

5 fl oz provides 100 Cal when prepared as directed.

1 liter of prepared formula provides 676 Cal.

Nutrients:	Per 100 Cal	
Protein	2.22	g
Fat	5.59	g
Carbohydrate	10.2	g
Water	134	g
Linoleic Acid	1300	mg
Vitamins:		
Vitamin A	300	IU
Vitamin D	60	IU
Vitamin E	2.5	IU
Vitamin K	8	mcg
Thiamine (Vit. B_1)	100	mcg
Riboflavin (Vit. B_2)	150	mcg
Vitamin B_6	60	mcg
Vitamin B_{12}	0.25	mcg
Niacin	1050	mcg
Folic Acid (Folacin)	15	mcg
Pantothenic Acid	450	mcg
Biotin	4.5	mcg
Vitamin C		
(Ascorbic Acid)	9	mg
Choline	12	mg
Inositol	24	mg
Minerals:		
Calcium	56	mg
Phosphorus	28	mg
Magnesium	6	mg
Iron	0.22	mg*
Zinc	0.75	mg
Manganese	5	mcg
Copper	90	mcg
Iodine	6	mcg
Sodium	24	mg
Potassium	86	mg
Chloride	59	mg

*This product, like milk, is deficient in iron; additional iron should be supplied from other sources.

Precautions: In conditions where the infant is losing abnormal quantities of one or more electrolytes, it may be necessary to supply electrolytes from sources other than the formula. It may be necessary to supply low-birth-weight infants weighing less than 1500 g at birth additional calcium, phosphorus and sodium during periods of rapid growth.
(FAN 475-03)

SIMILAC® SPECIAL CARE® WITH IRON 24
[sim 'ə-lak]
Premature Infant Formula

Usage: When a 24 Cal/fl oz iron-fortified feeding is desired for growing, low-birth-weight infants and premature infants before switching to a standard term feeding (20 Cal/fl oz). Similac Special Care With Iron is intended for feeding these infants until they reach a weight of 3600 g (approx. 8 lb).

Availability: Ready To Feed only: 4-fl-oz nursing bottles; 6 per carry-home carton, 8 cartons per case; No. 00214.
For hospital use, Ready To Feed Similac Special Care With Iron 24 in disposable nursing bottles is available in the Ross Hospital Formula System.

Preparation: Ready To Feed: Add water only if directed by a physician.

Composition: Ready To Feed

Ingredients: ⑪-D Water, nonfat milk, hydrolyzed cornstarch, lactose, fractionated coconut oil (medium-chain triglycerides), whey protein concentrate, soy oil, coconut oil, minerals (calcium phosphate tribasic, sodium citrate, magnesium chloride, calcium carbonate, potassium citrate, potassium chloride, ferrous sulfate, zinc sulfate, cupric sulfate, manganese sulfate), vitamins (ascorbic acid, choline chloride, m-inositol, niacinamide, alpha-tocopheryl acetate, calcium pantothenate, riboflavin, Vitamin A palmitate, thiamine chloride hydrochloride, pyridoxine hydrochloride, biotin, folic acid, phylloquinone, vitamin D_3, cyanocobalamin), mono- and diglycerides, soy lecithin, carrageenan, taurine and L-carnitine.

4.2 fl oz provides 100 Cal; 1 liter provides 812 Cal.

Nutrients:	Per 100 Cal	
Protein	2.71	g
Fat	5.43	g
Carbohydrate	10.6	g
Water	109	g
Linoleic Acid	700	mg
Vitamins:		
Vitamin A	680	IU
Vitamin D	150	IU
Vitamin E	4.0	IU
Vitamin K	12	mcg
Thiamine (Vit. B_1)	250	mcg
Riboflavin (Vit. B_2)	620	mcg
Vitamin B_6	250	mcg
Vitamin B_{12}	0.55	mcg
Niacin	5000	mcg
Folic Acid (Folacin)	37	mcg
Pantothenic Acid	1900	mcg
Biotin	37	mcg

Vitamin C		
(Ascorbic Acid)	37	mg
Choline	10	mg
Inositol	5.5	mg
Minerals:		
Calcium	180	mg
Phosphorus	90	mg
Magnesium	12	mg
Iron	1.8	mg
Zinc	1.5	mg
Manganese	12	mcg
Copper	250	mcg
Iodine	6	mcg
Sodium	43	mg
Potassium	129	mg
Chloride	81	mg

*The addition of iron to this formula conforms to the recommendation of the Committee on Nutrition of the American Academy of Pediatrics.
Shake well before feeding.
(FAN 523-01)

SIMILAC® WITH IRON
[sim 'ə-lak]
Infant Formula

Usage: When an iron-fortified infant formula is needed: if the decision is made to discontinue breastfeeding before age 1 year, if a supplement to breastfeeding is needed or as a routine feeding if breastfeeding is not adopted.

Availability:
Powder: 1-lb cans, measuring scoop enclosed; 6 per case; No. 03360.
Concentrated Liquid: 13-fl-oz cans; 24 cans per case; No. 00414.
Ready To Feed: (Prediluted, 20 Cal/fl oz) 32-fl-oz cans; 6 per case; No. 00241. 8-fl-oz cans; 4 six-packs per case; No. 00179.
4-fl-oz nursing bottles; 6 per carry-home carton, 8 cartons per case; No. 06201.
8-fl-oz nursing bottles; 6 per carry-home carton, 4 cartons per case; No. 06202.
For hospital use, Ready To Feed Similac With Iron in disposable nursing bottles is available in the Ross Hospital Formula System.

Preparation:
Powder: Standard dilution (20 Cal/fl oz) is one level, unpacked scoop Powder (8.7 g) for each 2 fl oz of warm water.
Concentrated Liquid: Standard dilution (20 Cal/fl oz) is one part Concentrated Liquid to one part water.
Ready To Feed: Do not dilute.

Composition: Ready To Feed (Concentrated Liquid and Powder at standard dilution have similar composition and nutrient values. For specific information, refer to product labels.)

Ingredients: ⑪-D Water, nonfat milk, lactose, soy oil, coconut oil, mono- and diglycerides, soy lecithin, vitamins (ascorbic acid, choline chloride, m-inositol, alpha-tocopheryl acetate, niacinamide, calcium pantothenate, vitamin A palmitate, thiamine chloride hydrochloride, riboflavin, pyridoxine hydrochloride, folic acid, phylloquinone, biotin, vitamin D_3, cyanocobalamin), carrageenan, minerals (ferrous sulfate, zinc sulfate, cupric sulfate, manganese sulfate) and taurine.

5 fl oz provides 100 Cal; 1 liter provides 676 Cal.

Nutrients:	Per 100 Cal	
Protein	2.22	g
Fat	5.37	g
Carbohydrate	10.7	g
Water	133	g
Linoleic Acid	1300	mg
Vitamins:		
Vitamin A	300	IU
Vitamin D	60	IU
Vitamin E	3.0	IU
Vitamin K	8	mcg
Thiamine (Vit. B$_1$)	100	mcg
Riboflavin (Vit. B$_2$)	150	mcg
Vitamin B$_6$	60	mcg
Vitamin B$_{12}$	0.25	mcg
Niacin	1050	mcg
Folic Acid (Folacin)	15	mcg
Pantothenic Acid	450	mcg
Biotin	4.4	mcg
Vitamin C		
(Ascorbic Acid)	9	mg
Choline	16	mg
Inositol	4.7	mg
Minerals:		
Calcium	75	mg
Phosphorus	58	mg
Magnesium	6	mg
Iron	1.8	mg*
Zinc	0.75	mg
Manganese	5	mcg
Copper	90	mcg
Iodine	15	mcg
Sodium	28	mg
Potassium	108	mg
Chloride	66	mg

*The addition of iron to this formula conforms to the recommendation of the Committee on Nutrition of the American Academy of Pediatrics.
(FAN 526-02)

TRONOLANE®
[*tron 'ə-lān*]
Anesthetic Cream for Hemorrhoids
Anesthetic Suppositories for Hemorrhoids

Description: The active ingredient in Tronolane is a topical anesthetic agent (Cream: pramoxine hydrochloride 1%; Suppositories: pramoxine 1% as pramoxine and pramoxine HCl), chemically unrelated to the benzoate esters of the "caine" type, which is chemically designated as a 4-n-butoxyphenyl gammamorpholinopropyl-ether hydrochloride. The cream contains the following inactive ingredients: A nongreasy zinc oxide cream base containing beeswax, cetyl alcohol, cetyl esters wax, glycerin, methylparaben, propylparaben, sodium lauryl sulfate, water and zinc oxide. The suppository contains the following inactive ingredients: A base containing hydrogenated cocoa glycerides and zinc oxide.

Indications: Tronolane is a topical anesthetic indicated for the temporary relief of the pain, burning, itching and discomfort that accompany hemorrhoids. It has a soothing, lubricating action on mucous membranes.

Tronolane contains a rapidly acting topical anesthetic producing analgesia that lasts up to 5 hours. Because the drug is chemically unrelated to other anesthetics, cross-sensitization is unlikely. Patients who are already sensitized to the "caine" anesthetics can generally use Tronolane.

The emollient/emulsion base of Tronolane cream provides soothing lubrication, making bowel movements more comfortable. Tronolane cream is in a nondrying base that is nongreasy and nonstaining to undergarments.

Warnings: If bleeding is present, consult physician. Certain persons can develop allergic reactions to ingredients in this product. During treatment, if condition worsens or persists 7 days, consult physician. For children under 12 years, use only as directed by physician. Keep out of the reach of children. As with any drug, if you are pregnant or nursing a baby, we recommend that you seek the advice of a health care professional before using this product.

Dosage and Administration: CREAM: Apply up to five times daily, especially morning, night, and after bowel movements, or as directed by physician. *External*—Apply liberally to affected area. *Intrarectal*—Remove cap from tube and attach clean applicator. Remove protective cover from clean applicator. Squeeze tube to fill applicator and lubricate tip with cream. Gently insert applicator into rectum and squeeze tube again. Thoroughly cleanse applicator after use.

Dosage and Administration: SUPPOSITORIES: Use up to five times daily, especially morning, night, and after bowel movements, or as directed by physician. Detach one suppository from pack. Separate foil at rounded end and peel apart until suppository is exposed. Insert suppository into the rectum, pointed end first.

How Supplied: Tronolane is available in 1-oz and 2-oz cream tubes and 10- and 20-count suppository boxes.

Shown in Product Identification Section, pages 426 & 427
(FAN 2093-03)

Rydelle Laboratories, Inc.
Subsidiary of S. C. Johnson & Son, Inc.
1525 HOWE STREET
RACINE, WI 53403

AVEENO® BATH TREATMENTS
[*ah-ve 'no*]
REGULAR FORMULA AND OILATED FOR DRY SKIN

AVEENO® BATH TREATMENTS contain colloidal oatmeal, a natural oat derivative developed especially for soothing and cleaning itchy, sore, sensitive skin.
AVEENO® BATH TREATMENTS contain no soaps or synthetic detergents that may be harmful to the skin. They cleanse naturally because of their unique adsorptive properties.
AVEENO BATH TREATMENTS can be used in the care of itch due to dry skin, rashes, psoriasis, hemorrhoidal and genital irritations, poison ivy/oak, and sunburn. They are safe for use on children and can be used in the treatment of chicken pox, diaper rash, prickly heat and hives.

Ingredients: Aveeno Bath Regular: 100% colloidal oatmeal; Aveeno Bath Oilated: 43% colloidal oatmeal, mineral oil, and a specially selected emollient.
Shown in Product Identification Section, page 427

AVEENO® CLEANSING BAR
[*ah-ve 'no*]
FOR NORMAL TO OILY SKIN

AVEENO® Cleansing Bar For Normal To Oily Skin is made especially for itchy, sensitive skin that is irritated by ordinary soaps.
More than 50% of this mild skin cleanser is colloidal oatmeal, noted for its soothing and protective qualities.
Aveeno® Cleansing Bar is completely soap-free. It leaves no harsh alkaline film to irritate delicate skin, and it leaves skin feeling soft and comfortable.

Ingredients: Aveeno® Colloidal Oatmeal, 51%; in a sudsing soap-free base containing a mild surfactant.
Shown in Product Identification Section, page 427

AVEENO® CLEANSING BAR
[*ah-ve 'no*]
FOR ACNE

AVEENO® Cleansing Bar For Acne is a unique soap-free cleanser. It combines colloidal oatmeal, a long recognized, natural anti-itch treatment and gentle adsorbing cleanser, with special medication to eliminate most blackheads or acne pimples.

Ingredients: Aveeno® Colloidal Oatmeal, 51%; salicylic acid 2%; in a sudsing soap-free base containing a mild surfactant.
Shown in Product Identification Section, page 427

AVEENO® CLEANSING BAR
[*ah-ve 'no*]
FOR DRY SKIN

AVEENO® Cleansing Bar For Dry Skin is a unique, soap-free cleanser for itchy, dry, sensitive skin that is irritated by ordinary soaps. It contains over 15% skin-softening emollients to help replace natural skin oils and 51% colloidal oatmeal, recommended for its soothing and protective qualities.

Ingredients: Aveeno® Colloidal Oatmeal, 51%, in a sudsing soap-free base containing vegetable oils, glycerine, and a mild surfactant.
Shown in Product Identification Section, page 427

Continued on next page

Rydelle—Cont.

AVEENO® LOTION
[ah-ve'no]
FOR RELIEF OF DRY, ITCHY SKIN

AVEENO® Lotion has been clinically proven to relieve dry skin. It contains natural colloidal oatmeal to relieve the itch often associated with dry skin. It is noncomedogenic and contains no fragrance, parabens, or lanolin which can cause allergic reactions.

Active Ingredients: Colloidal oatmeal 1%, allantoin 0.5%.
Also Contains: Water, glycerin, distearyldimonium chloride, petrolatum, isopropyl palmitate, cetyl alcohol, dimethicone, sodium chloride, benzyl alcohol.

Shown in Product Identification Section, page 427

AVEENO® SHOWER AND BATH OIL
[ah-ve'no]
FOR RELIEF OF DRY ITCHY SKIN

AVEENO® Shower and Bath Oil combines the lubricating properties of mineral oil with the natural anti-itch benefits of colloidal oatmeal for the relief of dry, itchy skin. It contains no fragrance, parabens or lanolin which can cause allergic reactions.

Active Ingredient: Colloidal oatmeal 5%
Also contains: Mineral oil, glyceryl stearate and PEG 100 stearate, laureth-4, benzyl alcohol, silica, benzaldehyde.

Shown in Product Identification Section, page 427

RHULICREAM®
(External analgesic/Skin protectant)

Rhulicream® works on contact to provide fast, soothing, temporary relief of the itching and pain associated with many minor skin irritations. Apply this non-greasy calamine formula after exposure to poison ivy/oak/sumac to dry oozing and weeping, help to control further spreading and promote healing.

Directions: Adults and children 2 years and older: Apply to affected area no more than 4 times daily. Children under 2: Consult a physician.

Warnings: For external use only. Avoid contact with eyes. If condition does not improve or recurs within 7 days, discontinue use and consult a physician. Keep out of children's reach. If ingested contact a physician or poison control center. Store at 59°–86°F.

Active Ingredients: Benzocaine 5.0%, Calamine 3.0%, Camphor 0.3% in a base of Water, Glycerin, Distearyldimonium Chloride, Petrolatum, Isopropyl Palmitate, Cetyl Alcohol, Dimethicone, Sodium Chloride.

How Supplied: 2 oz. tube.
Shown in Product Identification Section, page 427

RHULIGEL®
(External analgesic)

Rhuligel® provides fast, cooling, temporary relief of the itching and pain associated with many minor skin irritations, including poison ivy/oak/sumac, insect bites, and sunburn. Clear Rhuligel is non-greasy and invisible on the skin. Won't stain clothing.

Directions: Adults and children 2 years and older: Apply to affected area no more than 4 times daily. Children under 2: Consult a physician.

Warnings: For external use only. Avoid contact with eyes. If condition does not improve or recurs within 7 days, discontinue use and consult a physician. Keep out of children's reach. If ingested contact a physician or poison control center. Store at 59°–86°F.

Active Ingredients: Benzyl Alcohol 2%, Menthol 0.3%, Camphor 0.3% in a base of SD Alcohol 23A 31% w/w, Purified Water, Propylene Glycol, Carbomer 940, Triethanolamine, Benzophenone-4, EDTA.

How Supplied: 2 oz. tube.
Shown in Product Identification Section, page 427

RHULISPRAY®
(External analgesic/Skin protectant)

Rhulispray® works on contact to provide fast, cooling, temporary relief of the itching and pain associated with many minor skin irritations. Calamine-based formula dries the oozing and weeping of poison ivy/oak/sumac. Convenient spray action eliminates the need to touch delicate inflamed skin.

Directions: Shake well before use. Adults and children 2 years and older: Apply to affected area no more than 4 times daily. Children under 2: Consult a physician.

Warnings: For external use only. Avoid contact with eyes. If condition does not improve or recurs within 7 days, discontinue use and consult a physician. Keep out of children's reach. If ingested contact a physician or poison control center. Store at 59°–86°F.

Caution: Flammable. Contents under pressure. Do not puncture or incinerate. Intentional misuse by deliberately concentrating and inhaling the contents can be harmful or fatal. Do not use near an open flame. May burst at temperatures above 120°F.

Active Ingredients (in concentrate): Calamine 13.8%, Benzocaine 5.0%, Camphor 0.7% in a base of Benzyl Alcohol, Hydrated Silica, Isobutane, Isopropyl Alcohol 70% w/w (concentrate), Oleyl Alcohol, Sorbitan Trioleate.

How Supplied: 4 oz. aerosol.
Shown in Product Identification Section, page 427

Sandoz Pharmaceuticals/ Consumer Division
59 ROUTE 10
EAST HANOVER, NJ 07936

ACID MANTLE® CREME
[ă'sĭd-mănt'l]

Description: A greaseless, water-miscible preparation containing buffered aluminum acetate. Other ingredients: aluminum sulfate, calcium acetate, cetearyl alcohol, glycerin, light mineral oil, methylparaben, purified water, sodium lauryl sulfate, synthetic beeswax, white petrolatum, white potato dextrin. May also contain: ammonium hydroxide, citric acid.

Indications: A vehicle for compatible topical drugs. Restores and maintains protective acidity of the skin. Provides relief of mildly irritated skin due to exposure to soaps, detergents, chemicals, alkalis. Aids in the treatment of diaper rash, bath dermatitis, athlete's foot, anogenital pruritis, acne, winter eczema and dry, rough, scaly skin of varied causes.

Caution: Limited compatibility and stability with Vitamin A, neomycin and other water-sensitive antibiotics. For external use only. Not for ophthalmic use.

Warnings: Keep this and all drugs out of the reach of children. In case of accidental ingestion, seek professional assistance or contact a Poison Control Center immediately.

Directions: Apply several times daily, especially after wet work.

How Supplied: 1 oz tubes; 4 oz and 1 lb jars.

BiCOZENE® Creme External Analgesic
[bī-cō-zēn]

Active Ingredients: Benzocaine 6%, resorcinol 1.67% in a specially prepared cream base.

Inactive Ingredients: Castor Oil, Chlorothymol, Ethanolamine Stearates, Glycerin, Glyceryl Borate, Glyceryl Stearates, Parachlorometaxylenol, Polysorbate 80, Sodium Stearate, Triglycerol Diisostearate, Perfume.

Indications: For the temporary relief of pain and itching associated with minor burns, sunburn, minor cuts, scrapes, insect bites or minor skin irritations.

Actions: Benzocaine is a topical anesthetic and resorcinol is a topical antipruritic, at the concentrations used in BiCozene Creme. Both exert their actions by depressing cutaneous sensory receptors.

Warnings: Do not apply over large areas of the body. Caution: Use only as directed. Keep away from the eyes. Not for prolonged use. If the symptoms persist for more than seven days or clear up and reoccur within a few days, or if a rash or irritation develops, discontinue use and consult a physician. For external use only. **KEEP ALL MEDICINES OUT OF THE REACH OF CHILDREN.** In case of accidental ingestion, seek professional assistance or contact a Poison Control Center immediately.

Drug Interaction Precautions: No known drug interaction.

Dosage and Administration: Apply liberally to affected area as needed, several times a day.

How Supplied: BiCozene Creme is available in 1-ounce tubes.

Shown in Product Identification Section, page 427

CAMA® ARTHRITIS PAIN RELIEVER
[kă 'măh]

Description: Each CAMA Inlay-Tab® contains: Active ingredients: aspirin, USP, 500 mg (7.7 grains); magnesium oxide, USP, 150 mg; dried aluminum hydroxide gel, USP, 150 mg. Other ingredients: colloidal silicon dioxide, croscarmellose sodium, hydrogenated vegetable oil, methylcellulose, methylparaben, microcrystalline cellulose, polyethylene glycol, povidone, pregelatinized starch, starch, Yellow 6, Yellow 10.

Indications: For the temporary relief of minor arthritic pain.

Warnings: If redness or swelling is present, consult a doctor because these could be signs of a serious condition. Do not take this drug if you have asthma unless directed by a doctor. Do not take this product if you have stomach problems (such as heartburn, upset stomach, or stomach pain) that persists or recurs, or if you have ulcers or bleeding problems, unless directed by a doctor. Children and teenagers should not use this medicine for chicken pox or flu symptoms before a doctor is consulted about Reye syndrome, a rare but serious illness reported to be associated with aspirin. If pain persists for more than 10 days, consult a physician immediately. As with any drug, if you are pregnant or nursing a baby, seek the advice of a health professional before using this product. **IMPORTANT:** Do not take this product during the last 3 months of pregnancy unless directed by a doctor. Aspirin taken near the time of delivery may cause bleeding problems in both mother and child. If ringing in the ears or a loss of hearing occurs, consult a doctor before taking any more of this product. Stop taking this product if dizziness occurs. Do not take this product if you are presently taking a prescription drug for anticoagulation (thinning the blood), gout or if you have an aspirin allergy. Do not take this product if you are taking a prescription drug for diabetes unless directed by a doctor. **Keep this and all medicines out of the reach of children. In case of accidental overdose, contact a physician immediately.**

Directions For Use: Adults—2 tablets with a full glass of water every 6 hours. Not to exceed 8 tablets in 24 hours unless

directed by a physician. Do not use in children under 12 years of age except under the advice and supervision of a physician.

How Supplied: CAMA Arthritis Pain Reliever Tablets (white with salmon inlay), imprinted "Cama 500" on one side, "Dorsey" on the other, in bottles of 100.

DORCOL® CHILDREN'S COUGH SYRUP
[door 'call]

Description: Each teaspoonful (5 ml) of DORCOL Children's Cough Syrup contains pseudoephedrine hydrochloride 15 mg, guaifenesin 50 mg, dextromethorphan hydrobromide 5 mg. Other ingredients: benzoic acid, Blue 1, edetate disodium, flavors, glycerin, propylene glycol, purified water, Red 40, sodium hydroxide, sucrose, tartaric acid.

Indications: Temporarily relieves your child's cough due to minor throat and bronchial irritation as may occur with the common cold. Helps loosen phlegm (mucus) and thin bronchial secretions to rid the bronchial passageways of bothersome mucus. Helps drain bronchial tubes and makes coughs more productive. Temporarily relieves nasal stuffiness due to the common cold and promotes nasal and/or sinus drainage.

Warnings: Do Not give your child more than the recommended dosage because at higher doses nervousness, dizziness or sleeplessness may occur. Do Not give this preparation if your child has high blood pressure, heart disease, diabetes or thyroid disease. Do Not give this product for persistent or chronic cough such as occurs with asthma or where cough is accompanied by excessive secretions. Keep this and all drugs out of the reach of children. In case of accidental overdose, seek professional assistance or contact a Poison Control Center immediately. A persistent cough may be a sign of a serious condition. If cough or other symptoms persist for more than one week, tend to recur or are accompanied by high fever, rash or persistent headache, consult a physician before continuing use. *Drug Interaction Precaution:* Do not give this product if your child is presently taking a prescription antihypertensive or antidepressant drug containing a monoamine oxidase inhibitor except under the advice and supervision of a physician.

Directions For Use: Children under 2 years—consult physician.
By age:
Children 2 to under 6 years: 1 teaspoonful every 4 hours.
Children 6 to under 12 years: 2 teaspoonfuls every 4 hours.
By weight:
Children 25 to 45 pounds: 1 teaspoonful every 4 hours.
Children 46 to 85 pounds: 2 teaspoonfuls every 4 hours.
Unless directed by a physician, do not exceed 4 doses in 24 hours.

Professional Labeling: The suggested dosage for pediatric patients is:

3–12 months	3 drops/Kg of body weight every 4 hours	
12–24 months	7 drops (0.2 ml)/Kg of body weight every 4 hours	

Maximum 4 doses in 24 hours.

How Supplied: DORCOL Children's Cough Syrup (grape colored), in 4 fl oz and 8 fl oz plastic bottles with tamper-evident band around child-resistant cap.

Shown in Product Identification Section, page 427

DORCOL® CHILDREN'S DECONGESTANT LIQUID
[door 'call]

Description: Each teaspoonful (5 ml) of DORCOL Children's Decongestant Liquid contains pseudoephedrine hydrochloride 15 mg. Other ingredients: benzoic acid, edetate disodium, flavors, purified water, sodium hydroxide, sorbitol, sucrose, Yellow 6, Yellow 10.

Indications: Provides temporary relief of nasal congestion due to the common cold, hay fever or other upper respiratory allergies, or associated with sinusitis. Reduces swelling of nasal passages; to restore freer breathing through the nose. Promotes nasal and sinus drainage; relieves sinus pressure.

Directions For Use: Children under 2 years—consult physician.
By age:
Children 2 to under 6 years: 1 teaspoonful every 4 to 6 hours.
Children 6 years and older: 2 teaspoonfuls every 4 to 6 hours.
By weight:
Children 25 to 45 pounds: 1 teaspoonful every 4 to 6 hours.
Children 46 to 85 pounds: 2 teaspoonfuls every 4 to 6 hours.
Unless directed by a physician, do not exceed 4 doses in 24 hours.

Professional Labeling: The suggested dosage for pediatric patients is:

3–12 months	3 drops/Kg of body weight every 4–6 hours	
12–24 months	7 drops (0.2 ml)/Kg of body weight every 4–6 hours	

Maximum of 4 doses in 24 hours.

Warnings: Do not give your child more than the recommended dosage because at higher doses nervousness, dizziness, or sleeplessness may occur. If symptoms do not improve within seven days or are accompanied by high fever, consult a physician before continuing use. Do not give this preparation if your child has high blood pressure, heart disease, diabetes, or thyroid disease except under the advice and supervision of a physician. Keep this and all drugs out of the reach of children. In case of accidental overdose, seek professional assistance or contact a Poison Control Center immediately. *Drug Interaction Precaution:* Do

Continued on next page

Sandoz Pharm.—Cont.

not give this product if your child is presently taking a prescription antihypertensive or antidepressant drug containing a monoamine oxidase inhibitor except under the advice and supervision of a physician.

How Supplied: DORCOL Children's Decongestant Liquid (pale orange), in 4 fl oz bottles with tamper-evident band around child-resistant cap.

Shown in Product Identification Section, page 427

DORCOL® CHILDREN'S FEVER & PAIN REDUCER
[*door 'call*]

Description: Each teaspoonful (5 ml) of DORCOL Children's Fever & Pain Reducer contains acetaminophen 160 mg. Other ingredients: benzoic acid, edetate disodium, flavors, glycerin, polyethylene glycol, purified water, Red 40, sodium chloride, sucrose.

Indications: For temporary relief of your child's fever and occasional minor aches, pains and headache.

Directions For Use: Children under 2 years—consult physician.
By age:
Children 2 to under 4 years: 1 teaspoonful
Children 4 to under 6 years: 1½ teaspoonfuls
Children 6 years of age and older: 2 teaspoonfuls
By weight:
Children 25 to 35 pounds: 1 teaspoonful
Children 36 to 45 pounds: 1½ teaspoonfuls
Children 46 to 60 pounds: 2 teaspoonfuls
Give every 4 hours while symptoms persist or as directed by a physician. Unless directed by a physician do not exceed 5 doses in 24 hours.

Professional Labeling: The suggested dosage for pediatric patients is:
3–12 months   3 drops/Kg of body weight every 4 hours
12–24 months 7 drops (0.2 ml)/Kg of body weight every 4 hours
Maximum of 5 doses in 24 hours.

Warnings: Do not give this product to your child for more than 5 days. Consult your physician if symptoms persist, new ones occur, or if fever persists for more than 3 days (72 hours) or recurs. Do not exceed recommended dosage. Keep this and all drugs out of the reach of children. In case of accidental overdose, seek professional assistance or contact a Poison Control Center immediately.

How Supplied: DORCOL Children's Fever & Pain Reducer (red), in 4 fl oz bottles with tamper-evident band around child-resistant cap.

Shown in Product Identification Section, page 427

DORCOL® CHILDREN'S LIQUID COLD FORMULA
[*door 'call*]

Description: Each teaspoonful (5 ml) of DORCOL Children's Liquid Cold Formula contains: pseudoephedrine hydrochloride 15 mg and chlorpheniramine maleate 1 mg. Other ingredients: benzoic acid, Blue 1, flavors, purified water, Red 40, sorbitol, sucrose, Yellow 10. May also contain sodium hydroxide.

Indications: Provides temporary relief of nasal congestion, sneezing and rhinorrhea due to the common cold, hay fever or other upper respiratory allergies or associated with sinusitis. Reduces swelling of nasal passages and restores freer breathing. Promotes nasal and sinus drainage; relieves sinus pressure.

Directions For Use: Children under 6 years—consult physician.
By age:
Children 6 to under 12 years: 2 teaspoonfuls every 4 to 6 hours.
By weight:
Children 45 to 85 pounds: 2 teaspoonfuls every 4 to 6 hours.
Unless directed by a physician, do not exceed 4 doses in 24 hours.

Professional Labeling: The suggested dosage for pediatric patients is:
3–12 months   2 drops/Kg of body weight every 4–6 hours
12–24 months   5 drops (0.2 ml)/Kg of body weight every 4–6 hours
2–6 years   1 teaspoonful every 4–6 hours
Maximum of 4 doses in 24 hours.

Warnings: Do not give your child more than the recommended dosage because at higher doses nervousness, dizziness, or sleeplessness may occur. Do not give this preparation if your child has high blood pressure, heart disease, diabetes, thyroid disease, asthma, glaucoma, or difficulty in urination due to enlargement of the prostate gland except under the advice and supervision of a physician. If symptoms do not improve within 7 days or are accompanied by high fever, consult a physician before continuing use. May cause drowsiness. May cause excitability especially in children. Keep this and all drugs out of the reach of children. In case of accidental overdose, seek professional assistance or contact a Poison Control Center immediately. *Drug Interaction Precaution:* Do not give this product if your child is presently taking a prescription antihypertensive or antidepressant drug containing a monoamine oxidase inhibitor except under the advice and supervision of a physician.

Caution: Avoid alcoholic beverages or operating a motor vehicle or heavy machinery while taking this product.

How Supplied: DORCOL Children's Liquid Cold Formula (light brown), in 4 fl oz bottles with tamper-evident band around child-resistant cap.

Shown in Product Identification Section, page 427

EX–LAX® Chocolated Laxative

Active Ingredient: Yellow phenolphthalein, 90 mg phenolphthalein per tablet.

Inactive Ingredients: Cocoa, Confectioners' Sugar, Hydrogenated Palm Kernel Oil, Lecithin, Nonfat Dry Milk, Vanillin.

Indication: For relief of occasional constipation (irregularity).

Caution: Do not take any laxative when abdominal pain, nausea, or vomiting are present. Frequent or prolonged use of this or any other laxative may result in dependence on laxatives. If skin rash appears, do not use this or any other preparation containing phenolphthalein.

Warnings: Keep this and all drugs out of the reach of children. In case of accidental overdose, seek professional assistance or contact a poison control center immediately. As with any drug, if you are pregnant or nursing a baby, seek the advice of a health care professional before using this product.

Drug Interaction Precautions: No known drug interaction.

Dosage and Administration: Adults: Chew 1 to 2 tablets, preferably at bedtime. Children over 6 years: Chew ½ to 1 tablet.

How Supplied: Available in boxes of 6, 18, 48, and 72 chewable chocolate-flavored tablets.

Shown in Product Identification Section, page 427

EX–LAX® Unflavored Laxative Pills

Active Ingredient: Yellow phenolphthalein, 90 mg phenolphthalein per pill.

Inactive Ingredients: Acacia, Alginic Acid, Carnauba Wax, Colloidal Silicon Dioxide, Dibasic Calcium Phosphate, Iron Oxides, Magnesium Stearate, Microcrystalline Cellulose, Sodium Benzoate, Sodium Lauryl Sulfate, Starch, Stearic Acid, Sucrose, Talc, Titanium Dioxide.

Indication: For relief of occasional constipation (irregularity).

Caution: Do not take any laxative when abdominal pain, nausea, or vomiting are present. Frequent or prolonged use of this or any other laxative may result in dependence on laxatives. If skin rash appears, do not use this or any other preparation containing phenolphthalein.

Warnings: Keep this and all drugs out of the reach of children. In case of accidental overdose, seek professional assistance or contact a poison control center immediately. As with any drug, if you are pregnant or nursing a baby, seek the advice of a health care professional before using this product.

Drug Interaction Precautions: No known drug interaction.

Dosage and Administration: Adults take 1 to 2 pills with a glass of water, preferably at bedtime. Children over 6 years: 1 pill.

How Supplied: Available in boxes of 8, 30, and 60 unflavored pills.

Shown in Product Identification Section, page 427

EXTRA GENTLE EX-LAX®

Active Ingredients: Docusate Sodium, 75 mg. and Yellow Phenolphthalein 65 mg. per tablet.

Inactive Ingredients: Acacia, Croscarmellose Sodium, Dibasic Calcium Phosphate, Colloidal Silicon Dioxide, Magnesium Stearate, Microcrystalline Cellulose, Red 7, Stearic Acid, Sucrose, Talc, Titanium Dioxide.

Indication: For relief of occasional constipation (irregularity).

Caution: Do not take any laxative when abdominal pain, nausea or vomiting are present. Frequent or prolonged use of this or any other laxative may result in dependence on laxatives. If skin rash appears, do not use this or any other preparation containing phenolphthalein.

Warnings: Keep this and all drugs out of the reach of children. In case of accidental overdose, seek professional assistance or contact a poison control center immediately. As with any drug, if you are pregnant or nursing a baby, seek the advice of a health care professional before using this product.

Drug Interaction Precautions: No known drug interaction.

Dosage and Administration: Adults take 1 or 2 pills with water, preferably at bedtime, or as directed by physician. Children over 6 years: 1 pill, as needed.

How Supplied: Available in boxes of 24 pills.

Shown in Product Identification Section, page 427

GAS–X® AND EXTRA STRENGTH GAS-X®
High–Capacity Antiflatulent

Active Ingredients: GAS-X®—Each tablet contains 80 mg. simethicone. EXTRA STRENGTH GAS-X®—Each tablet contains 125 mg. simethicone.

Inactive Ingredients: calcium phosphates dibasic and tribasic, colloidal silicon dioxide, calcium silicate, microcrystalline cellulose, flavors, compressible sugar and talc. Extra strength Gas-X also contains Red 30 and Yellow 10.

Indications: For relief of the pain and pressure symptoms of excess gas in the digestive tract, which is often accompanied by complaints of bloating, distention, fullness, pressure, pain, cramps or excess anal flatus.

Actions: GAS-X acts in the stomach and intestines to disperse and reduce the formation of mucus-trapped gas bubbles. The GAS-X defoaming action reduces the surface tension of gas bubbles so that they are more easily eliminated.

Warning: Keep this and all medicines out of the reach of children.

Drug Interaction Precautions: No known drug interaction.

Dosage and Administration: Adults: Chew thoroughly and swallow one or two tablets as needed after meals and at bedtime. Do not exceed six GAS-X tablets or four EXTRA STRENGTH GAS-X tablets in 24 hours, except under the advice and supervision of a physician.

Professional Labeling: GAS-X may be useful in the alleviation of postoperative gas pain, and for use in endoscopic examination.

How Supplied: GAS-X is available in white, chewable, scored tablets in boxes of 36 tablets and convenience packages of 12 tablets.
EXTRA STRENGTH GAS-X is available in yellow, chewable, scored tablets in boxes of 18 tablets.

Shown in Product Identification Section, page 427

GENTLE NATURE®
NATURAL VEGETABLE LAXATIVE

Active Ingredients: 20 mg. Sennosides per tablet.

Inactive Ingredients: Alginic Acid, Calcium Phosphate Dibasic, Magnesium Stearate, Microcrystalline Cellulose, Silicon Dioxide, Sodium Lauryl Sulfate, Starch, Stearic Acid.

Indications: For short-term relief of constipation.

Actions: Sennosides is a highly purified form of senna. The purification process removes components found in senna concentrate which may cause griping and cramps.
Sennosides has no laxative effect until they are carried to the lower part of the alimentary system by the regular working of the digestive process. In the bowel, the active glycosides are freed by the natural bowel micro-organisms. The freed laxative agent then gently encourages the muscle wave action of elimination. The gentle, predictable working of the laxative in the bowel, usually in 8–10 hours, or overnight if taken at bedtime, is apt to produce a well-formed stool in a natural-feeling way.

Caution: Not to be used when abdominal pain, nausea, or vomiting are present. Take only as needed. Frequent or prolonged use may result in dependence on laxatives. Keep this and all medications out of reach of children.

Drug Interaction Precautions: No known drug interaction.

Dosage and Administration: Adults— Take 1 or 2 tablets daily with water, preferably at bedtime, or as directed by your physician. Children over 6 years—1 tablet daily as required.

How Supplied: Available in boxes of 16 blister packed uncoated pills.

Shown in Product Identification Section, page 427

THERAFLU®
Flu and Cold Medicine
Flu, Cold & Cough Medicine

Description: Each packet of TheraFlu Flu and Cold Medicine contains: acetaminophen 500 mg, pseudoephedrine hydrochloride 60 mg, and chlorpheniramine maleate 4 mg. Each packet of TheraFlu Flu, Cold & Cough Medicine also contains dextromethorphan hydrobromide 20 mg. Other ingredients: ascorbic acid, citric acid, natural lemon flavors, sodium citrate, sucrose, titanium dioxide, tribasic calcium phosphate, pregelatinized starch, Yellow 6, and Yellow 10.

Indications: Provides temporary relief of the symptoms associated with flu, common cold and other upper respiratory infections including: headache, body-aches, fever, minor sore throat pain, nasal and sinus congestion, runny nose and sneezing. TheraFlu Flu, Cold & Cough Medicine also suppresses coughs due to minor throat and bronchial irritation.

Warnings: Keep this and all drugs out of the reach of children. In case of accidental overdose, seek professional assistance or contact a Poison Control Center immediately. Unless directed by a doctor, do not take this product if you have heart disease, high blood pressure, thyroid disease, diabetes, asthma, glaucoma, difficulty in breathing, or difficulty in urination due to enlargement of the prostate gland or are taking a prescription drug for high blood pressure or depression or are taking sedatives or tranquilizers without first consulting your doctor. Do not exceed recommended dosage or take for more than 7 days. If symptoms persist or new ones occur, or if fever persists for more than 3 days or recurs, consult a doctor. May cause excitability, especially in children. May cause drowsiness. Avoid drinking alcohol, driving or operating machinery while taking this product. As with any drug, if you are pregnant or nursing a baby, seek the advice of a health professional before using this product. Do not take the cough formula if cough is accompanied by excessive secretions, for persistent cough such as occurs with smoking, asthma, or emphysema. A persistent cough may be sign of a serious condition. If cough recurs, or is accompanied by fever, rash or persistent headache, consult a doctor.

Dosage and Administration: Adults and children 12 years and over—dissolve one packet in 6 oz. cup of hot water. Sip while hot. Sweeten to taste, if desired. May repeat every 4 hours, but not to exceed 4 doses in 24 hours.

How Supplied: TheraFlu Flu and Cold Medicine powder in foil packets, 6 packets per carton. TheraFlu Flu, Cold & Cough Medicine powder in foil packets, 6 packets per carton.

Shown in Product Identification Section, page 427

Continued on next page

Sandoz Pharm.—Cont.

TRIAMINIC® ALLERGY TABLETS
[trī"ah-mǐn'ǐc]

Description: Each TRIAMINIC Allergy Tablet contains: phenylpropanolamine hydrochloride 25 mg, chlorpheniramine maleate 4.0 mg. Other ingredients: calcium stearate, calcium sulfate, colloidal silicon dioxide, methylcellulose, methylparaben, microcrystalline cellulose, polyethylene glycol, povidone, pregelatinized starch, titanium dioxide, Yellow 10.

Indications: For the temporary relief of runny nose, nasal congestion, sneezing, itching of the eyes, nose or throat and watery eyes as may occur in hay fever or other upper respiratory allergies (allergic rhinitis).

Warnings: Do not exceed the recommended dosage because at higher doses nervousness, dizziness or sleeplessness may occur. This preparation may cause drowsiness; this preparation may cause excitability especially in children. Do not take this preparation if you have high blood pressure, heart disease, diabetes, thyroid disease or are presently taking a prescription antihypertensive or antidepressant drug containing a monoamine oxidase inhibitor except under the advice and supervision of a physician. Do not give this preparation to children under 6 years except under the advice and supervision of a physician. Do not take this preparation if you have asthma, glaucoma or difficulty in urination due to enlargement of the prostate gland except under the advice and supervision of a physician. If symptoms do not improve within 7 days or are accompanied by high fever, consult a physician before continuing use. As with any drug, if you are pregnant or nursing a baby, seek the advice of a health professional before using this product. Keep this and all drugs out of the reach of children. In case of accidental overdose, seek professional assistance or contact a Poison Control Center immediately.

Caution: Avoid alcoholic beverages, operating a motor vehicle or heavy machinery while taking this product.

Dosage: Adults and children 12 and over—1 tablet every 4 hours. Children 6 to under 12 years—½ tablet every 4 hours. Unless directed by physician, do not exceed 6 doses in 24 hours or give to children under 6 years.

How Supplied: TRIAMINIC Allergy Tablets (yellow), scored, in blister packs of 24.

TRIAMINIC® CHEWABLES
[trī"ah-mǐn'ǐc]

Description: Each TRIAMINIC Chewable contains: phenylpropanolamine hydrochloride 6.25 mg, chlorpheniramine maleate 0.5 mg. Other ingredients: calcium stearate, citric acid, flavors, magnesium trisilicate, mannitol, microcrystalline cellulose, saccharin sodium, sucrose, Yellow 6, Yellow 10.

Indications: For the temporary relief of children's nasal congestion, runny nose, and sneezing due to the common cold or hay fever.

Warnings: Do not exceed recommended dosage because at higher doses nervousness, dizziness, or sleeplessness may occur Do not give this product to children for more than 7 days. If symptoms do not improve or are accompanied by fever, consult a doctor. Do not give this product to children who have heart disease, high blood pressure, thyroid disease, diabetes, asthma or glaucoma unless directed by a doctor. May cause drowsiness. May cause excitability. *Drug Interaction Precaution:* Do not give this product to a child who is taking a prescription drug for high blood pressure or depression, without first consulting the child's doctor. Keep this and all drugs out of the reach of children. In case of accidental overdose, seek professional assistance or contact a Poison Control Center immediately.

Dosage: Children 6 to 12 years—2 tablets every 4 hours. Children under 6, consult your physician.

Professional Labeling: The suggested dosage for children 2 to 6 years is 1 tablet every 4 hours.

How Supplied: TRIAMINIC Chewables (hexagonal, yellow), in blister packs of 24.

TRIAMINIC® COLD TABLETS
[trī"ah-mǐn'ǐc]

Description: Each TRIAMINIC Cold Tablet contains: phenylpropanolamine hydrochloride 12.5 mg and chlorpheniramine maleate 2 mg. Other ingredients: calcium stearate, colloidal silicon dioxide, flavor, lactose, methylcellulose, methylparaben, microcrystalline cellulose, polyethylene glycol, povidone, pregelatinized starch, Red 40, saccharin sodium, titanium dioxide, Yellow 6.

Indications: Temporarily relieves runny nose, nasal congestion and sneezing due to colds and allergies. Also relieves itching nose or throat and itchy, watery eyes associated with allergies.

Warnings: Unless directed by a doctor, do not take this product if you have heart disease, high blood pressure, thyroid disease, diabetes, asthma, glaucoma, difficulty in breathing, difficulty in urination due to enlargement of the prostate gland or are taking a prescription drug for high blood pressure or depression. Do not exceed recommended dosage or take for more than 7 days. If symptoms persist or are accompanied by fever, consult a doctor. May cause excitability especially in children. May cause drowsiness. Avoid drinking alcohol, driving or operating machinery while taking this product. As with any drug, if you are pregnant or nursing a baby, seek the advice of a health professional before using this product. Keep this and all drugs out of the reach of children. In case of accidental overdose, seek professional assistance or contact a Poison Control Center immediately.

Caution: Avoid alcoholic beverages, operating a motor vehicle or heavy machinery while taking this product.

Dosage and Administration: Adults and children 12 and over—2 tablets every 4 hours. Children 6 to under 12 years—1 tablet every 4 hours. Unless directed by physician, do not exceed 6 doses in 24 hours.

How Supplied: TRIAMINIC Cold Tablets (orange), imprinted "DORSEY" on one side, "TRIAMINIC" on the other, in blister packs of 24.

Shown in Product Identification Section, page 427

TRIAMINIC® EXPECTORANT
[trī"ah-mǐn'ǐc]

Description: Each teaspoonful (5 ml) of TRIAMINIC Expectorant contains: phenylpropanolamine hydrochloride 12.5 mg and guaifenesin 100 mg. Other ingredients: alcohol (5%), benzoic acid, edetate disodium, flavors, purified water, saccharin, saccharin sodium, sodium hydroxide, sorbitol, sucrose, Yellow 6, Yellow 10.

Indications: Provides prompt relief of cough and nasal congestion due to the common cold. The expectorant component helps loosen bronchial secretions and rid the bronchial passageways of bothersome mucus. The decongestant and expectorant are provided in an antihistamine-free formula.

Warnings: Do not take this product: 1) if cough is accompanied by excessive secretions, 2) for persistent cough such as occurs with smoking, asthma or emphysema, or 3) if you have heart disease, high blood pressure, thyroid disease, diabetes, difficulty in urination due to enlargement of the prostate gland, or are taking a prescription drug for high blood pressure or depression, unless directed by a doctor. Do not: 1) give this product to children under two years of age, 2) exceed recommended dosage, or 3) take for more than 7 days, unless directed by a doctor. If symptoms persist, are accompanied by a fever, rash or persistent headache or if cough recurs, consult a doctor. As with any drug, if you are pregnant or nursing a baby, seek advice from a health professional before using this product. Keep this and all drugs out of the reach of children. In case of accidental overdose, seek professional assistance or contact a Poison Control Center immediately.

Dosage and Administration: Adults and children 12 and over (96+ lbs)—2 teaspoonfuls every 4 hours. Children 6 to under 12 years (48–95 lbs)—1 teaspoonful every 4 hours. Children 2 to under 6 years (24–47 lbs)—½ teaspoonful every 4 hours. Unless directed by physician, do not exceed 6 doses in 24 hours or give to children under 2 years of age.

Professional Labeling: The suggested dosage for pediatric patients is:

3–12 months .75 ml (⅛ tsp)*
(12–17 lbs) every 4 hours
12–24 months 1.25 ml (¼ tsp)
(18–23 lbs) every 4 hours

*(⅛ tsp is approximately .75 ml)

How Supplied: TRIAMINIC Expectorant (yellow), in 4 fl oz and 8 fl oz plastic bottles with tamper-evident band around child-resistant cap.

Shown in Product Identification Section, page 427

TRIAMINIC® NITE LIGHT™
Nighttime Cough and Cold Medicine for Children
[tri"ah-min'ic]

Description: Each teaspoonful (5 ml) of Triaminic® Nite Light™ contains: Pseudoephedrine hydrochloride 15 mg, chlorpheniramine maleate 1 mg, dextromethorphan hydrobromide 7.5 mg in a palatable non-alcoholic vehicle. Other ingredients: benzoic acid, Blue 1, citric acid, flavors, propylene glycol, purified water, Red 33, dibasic sodium phosphate, sorbitol, sucrose.

Indications: Temporarily quiets your child's cough associated with the common cold. Also, provides temporary relief of nasal stuffiness, sneezing, runny nose, and itchy watery eyes caused by the common cold, hay fever or other upper respiratory allergies.

Warnings: Do not exceed recommended dosage or take for more than 7 days. A persistent cough may be a sign of a serious condition. If symptoms persist for more than one week, tend to recur, or are accompanied by fever, rash, or persistent headache, consult a physician. May cause excitability especially in children. Unless directed by a physician, do not take this product: 1) if cough is accompanied by excessive phlegm (mucus), 2) for persistent or chronic cough such as occurs with smoking, asthma or emphysema, or 3) if you or your child has heart disease, high blood pressure, thyroid disease, diabetes, asthma, glaucoma, difficulty in breathing, or difficulty in urination due to enlargement of the prostate gland. May cause marked drowsiness. Alcohol, sedatives, and tranquilizers may increase the drowsiness effect. Avoid alcoholic beverages while taking this product. Use caution when driving a motor vehicle or operating machinery. As with any drug, if you are pregnant or nursing a baby, seek the advice of a health professional before using this product. Keep this and all drugs out of the reach of children. In case of accidental overdose, seek professional assistance, or call a Poison Control Center immediately. **DRUG INTERACTION PRECAUTION:** Do not take this product if you are taking a prescription drug for high blood pressure or depression, or if you are taking sedatives or

tranquilizers, without first consulting your physician.

Dosage and Administration: Children 12 and over (96+ lbs.)—4 teaspoonfuls every 6–8 hours. Children 6 to under 12 years (48–95 lbs.)—2 teaspoonfuls every 6–8 hours. Unless directed by physician, do not exceed 4 doses in 24 hours. For convenience, a True-Dose™ dosage cup is provided with each 4 fl. oz. and 8 fl. oz. bottle.

Professional Labeling: The suggested dosage for pediatric patients is:

3 to under ¼ teaspoon or 1.25 ml
12 months
(12–17 lbs.)
12 months to ½ teaspoon or 2.5 ml
under 2 years
(18–23 lbs.)
2 to under 1 teaspoonful or 5 ml
6 years

How Supplied: Triaminic® Nite Light™ Nighttime Cough and Cold Medicine for Children, in 4 fl. oz. and 8 fl. oz. plastic bottles packaged in cartons with tamper-evident band around child-resistant cap.

Shown in Product Identification Section, page 428

TRIAMINIC® SYRUP
[trī"ah-mĭn'ĭc]

Description: Each teaspoonful (5 ml) of TRIAMINIC Syrup contains: phenylpropanolamine hydrochloride 12.5 mg and chlorpheniramine maleate 2 mg in a nonalcoholic vehicle. Other ingredients: benzoic acid, edetate disodium, flavors, purified water, sodium hydroxide, sorbitol, sucrose. Contains FD&C Yellow No. 6 as a color additive.

Indications: Provides temporary relief of nasal congestion, runny nose and sneezing that may occur with the common cold or with hay fever or other upper respiratory allergies. Relieves itching of the nose or throat and itchy, watery eyes.

Warnings: Do not take this product: 1) if you have heart disease, high blood pressure, thyroid disease, diabetes, asthma, glaucoma, difficulty in breathing, difficulty in urination due to enlargement of the prostate gland, or 2) if you are taking a prescription drug for high blood pressure or depression, or 3) if you are taking sedatives or tranquilizers, unless directed by a doctor. Do not exceed recommended dosage or take for more than 7 days. If symptoms persist or are accompanied by fever, consult a doctor. May cause excitability especially in children. May cause drowsiness. Alcohol, sedatives, or tranquilizers may increase drowsiness. Avoid driving or operating machinery while taking this product. As with any drug, if you are pregnant or nursing a baby, seek the advice of a health professional before using this product. Keep this and all drugs out of the reach of children. In case of accidental overdose, seek professional assistance or contact a Poison Control Center immediately.

Dosage and Administration: Adults and children 12 and over (96+ lbs)—2 teaspoonfuls every 4 hours. Children 6 to under 12 years (48–95 lbs)—1 teaspoonful every 4 hours. Unless directed by physician, do not exceed 6 doses in 24 hours. Consult physician for dosage under 6 years of age.

Professional Labeling: The suggested dosage for pediatric patients is:

3–12 months .75 ml (⅛ tsp)*
(12–17 lbs) every 4 hours

*(⅛ tsp is approximately .75 ml)
12–24 months 1.25 ml (¼ tsp)
(18–23 lbs) every 4 hours
2–6 years 2.5 ml (½ tsp)
(24–47 lbs) every 4 hours

How Supplied: TRIAMINIC Syrup (orange), in 4 fl oz and 8 fl oz plastic bottles with tamper-evident band around child-resistant cap.

Shown in Product Identification Section, page 427

TRIAMINIC–DM® SYRUP
[trī"ah-mĭn'ĭc]

Description: Each teaspoonful (5 ml) of TRIAMINIC-DM Syrup contains: phenylpropanolamine hydrochloride 12.5 mg and dextromethorphan hydrobromide 10 mg in a nonalcoholic vehicle. Other ingredients: benzoic acid, Blue 1, flavors, propylene glycol, purified water, Red 40, sodium chloride, sorbitol, sucrose.

Indications: Provides relief of cough due to minor throat and bronchial irritation as may occur with the common cold or inhaled irritants. Promotes nasal and sinus drainage. The decongestant and antitussive are provided in an alcohol-free and antihistamine-free formula.

Warnings: Do not take this product: 1) if cough is accompanied by excessive secretions, 2) for persistent cough such as occurs with smoking, asthma or emphysema, or 3) if you have heart disease, high blood pressure, thyroid disease, diabetes, difficulty in urination due to enlargement of the prostate gland, or are taking a prescription drug for high blood pressure or depression, unless directed by a doctor. Do not exceed recommended dosage or take for more than 7 days. If symptoms persist, are accompanied by a fever, rash or persistent headache or if cough recurs, consult a doctor. As with any drug, if you are pregnant or nursing a baby, seek the advice from a health professional before using this product. Keep this and all drugs out of the reach of children. In case of accidental overdose, seek professional assistance or contact a Poison Control Center immediately.

Dosage and Administration: Adults and children 12 and over (96+ lbs)—2 teaspoonfuls every 4 hours. Children 6 to under 12 years (48–95 lbs)—1 teaspoonful every 4 hours. Children 2 to under 6 years (24–47 lbs)—½ teaspoonful every

Continued on next page

682   PDR For Nonprescription Drugs®

Sandoz Pharm.—Cont.

4 hours. Unless directed by physician, do not exceed 6 doses in 24 hours or give to children under 2 years of age.

Professional Labeling: The suggested dosage for pediatric patients is:
3–12 months .75 ml (⅛ tsp)*
(12–17 lbs) every 4 hours
12–24 months 1.25 ml (¼ tsp)
(18–23 lbs) every 4 hours

*(⅛ tsp is approximately .75 ml)

How Supplied: TRIAMINIC-DM Syrup (dark red), in 4 fl oz and 8 fl oz plastic bottles with tamper-evident band around child-resistant cap.
Shown in Product Identification Section, page 427

TRIAMINIC–12® TABLETS
[trī"ah-mĭn'ĭc]

Description: Each TRIAMINIC - 12 Tablet contains: phenylpropanolamine hydrochloride 75 mg and chlorpheniramine maleate 12 mg. Other ingredients: carnauba wax, colloidal silicon dioxide, lactose, methylcellulose, polyethylene glycol, povidone, Red 30, stearic acid, titanium dioxide, Yellow 6.
TRIAMINIC-12 Tablets contain the nasal decongestant phenylpropanolamine, and the antihistamine chlorpheniramine, in a formulation providing 12 hours of symptomatic relief.

Indications: For the temporary relief of nasal congestion due to the common cold, hay fever or other upper respiratory allergies and associated with sinusitis. Helps decongest sinus openings, sinus passages; promotes nasal and/or sinus drainage; temporarily restores freer breathing through the nose. For temporary relief of running nose, sneezing, itching of the nose or throat and itchy and watery eyes as may occur in allergic rhinitis (such as hay fever).

Warnings: Do not give this product to children under 12 years except under the advice and supervision of a physician. Do not take this preparation if you have high blood pressure, heart disease, diabetes, thyroid disease, asthma, glaucoma or difficulty in urination due to enlargement of the prostate gland except under the advice and supervision of a physician. Do not exceed the recommended dosage because at higher doses nervousness, dizziness, or sleeplessness may occur. This preparation may cause drowsiness; this preparation may cause excitability, especially in children. If symptoms do not improve within seven days or are accompanied by high fever, consult a physician before continuing use. As with any drug, if you are pregnant or nursing a baby, seek the advice of a health professional before using this product. Keep this and all drugs out of the reach of children. In case of accidental overdose, seek professional assistance or contact a Poison Control Center immediately.

Caution: Avoid driving a motor vehicle or operating heavy machinery. Avoid alcoholic beverages while taking this product.

Drug Interaction Precaution: Do not take this product if you are presently taking a prescription antihypertensive or antidepressant drug containing a monoamine oxidase inhibitor except under the advice and supervision of a physician.

Directions: Adults and children over 12 years of age—1 tablet swallowed whole every 12 hours. Unless directed by physician, do not exceed 2 tablets in 24 hours.

Note: The nonactive portion of the tablet that supplies the active ingredients may occasionally appear in your stool as a soft mass.

How Supplied: TRIAMINIC-12 Tablets (orange), imprinted "DORSEY" on one side, "TRIAMINIC 12" on the other, in blister packs of 10 and 20.
Shown in Product Identification Section, page 427

TRIAMINICIN® TABLETS
[trī"ah-mĭn'ĭ-sĭn]

Description: Each TRIAMINICIN Tablet contains: phenylpropanolamine hydrochloride 25 mg, chlorpheniramine maleate 4 mg and acetaminophen 650 mg. Other ingredients: calcium stearate, colloidal silicon dioxide, croscarmellose sodium, lactose, methylcellulose, methylparaben, polyethylene glycol, povidone, pregelatinized starch, Red 40, titanium dioxide, Yellow 10.

Indications: Temporarily relieves runny nose, sneezing, itching of the nose or throat, and itchy, watery eyes due to hay fever (allergic rhinitis) or other upper respiratory allergies. For the temporary relief of nasal congestion due to hay fever or other upper respiratory allergies or associated with sinusitis. Temporarily relieves nasal congestion, runny nose and sneezing associated with the common cold. For the temporary relief of occasional minor aches, pains and headache associated with the common cold.

Warnings: Do not take this product if you have heart disease, high blood pressure, thyroid disease, diabetes, asthma, glaucoma, emphysema, chronic pulmonary disease, shortness of breath, difficulty in breathing, or difficulty in urination due to enlargement of the prostate gland unless directed by a doctor. Do not exceed recommended dosage because at higher doses nervousness, dizziness, or sleeplessness may occur. Do not take this product for more than 7 days. If symptoms do not improve, new ones occur, or if fever persists for more than three days (72 hours) or recurs, consult a doctor. May cause drowsiness; alcohol, sedatives and tranquilizers may increase the drowsiness effect. Avoid alcoholic beverages while taking this product. Do not take this product if you are taking sedatives or tranquilizers without first consulting

your doctor. Use caution when driving a motor vehicle or operating machinery. May cause excitability especially in children. As with any drug, if you are pregnant or nursing a baby, seek the advice of a health professional before using this product. *Drug Interaction Precaution:* Do not take this product if you are presently taking a prescription drug for high blood pressure or depression or are taking sedatives or tranquilizers, without first consulting your doctor. Keep this and all drugs out of the reach of children. In case of accidental overdose, seek professional assistance or contact a Poison Control Center immediately. Prompt medical attention is critical for adults as well as for children even if you do not notice any signs or symptoms.

Dosage and Administration: Adults and children 12 years and older: Take 1 tablet every 4 hours while symptoms persist or as directed by a physician. Unless directed by a physician, do not exceed 6 doses in 24 hours or give to children under 12 years.

How Supplied: TRIAMINICIN Tablets (yellow), imprinted "DORSEY" on one side, "TRIAMINICIN" on the other, in blister packs of 12, 24 and 48, and bottles of 100 tablets.
Shown in Product Identification Section, page 428

TRIAMINICOL® MULTI-SYMPTOM COLD TABLETS
[trī"ah-mĭn'ĭ-call]

Description: Each TRIAMINICOL Multi-Symptom Cold Tablet contains: phenylpropanolamine hydrochloride 12.5 mg, chlorpheniramine maleate 2 mg, dextromethorphan hydrobromide 10 mg. Other ingredients: calcium stearate, colloidal silicon dioxide, lactose, methylcellulose, methylparaben, microcrystalline cellulose, polyethylene glycol, povidone, pregelatinized starch, Red 40, titanium dioxide.

Indications: Temporarily relieves coughs due to minor throat and bronchial irritation. Temporarily relieves runny nose, nasal congestion and sneezing due to colds and allergies. Also relieves itching nose or throat and itchy, watery eyes associated with allergies.

Warnings: Unless directed by a doctor, **DO NOT** take this product: **1)** if cough is accompanied by excessive secretions, **2)** for persistent cough such as occurs with smoking, asthma or emphysema, or **3)** if you have heart disease, high blood pressure, thyroid disease, diabetes, asthma, glaucoma, difficulty in breathing, difficulty in urination due to enlargement of the prostate gland or are taking a prescription drug for high blood pressure or depression. Do not exceed recommended dosage or take for more than 7 days. If symtoms persist, are accompanied by fever, rash or persistent headache or if cough recurs, consult a doctor. May cause excitability especially in children. May cause drowsiness. Avoid drinking alcohol, driving or operating machinery while taking this product. As with any drug, if you are pregnant or nursing a baby, seek the advice of a health professional before using this product. Keep this and all drugs out of the reach of children. In case of accidental overdose, seek professional assistance or contact a Poison Control Center immediately.

Dosage and Administration: Adults and children 12 and over—2 tablets every 4 hours. Children 6 to under 12 years—1 tablet every 4 hours. For nighttime cough relief, give the last dose at bedtime. Unless directed by physician, do not exceed 6 doses in 24 hours or give to children under 6 years.

How Supplied: TRIAMINICOL Multi-Symptom Cold Tablets (cherry pink), imprinted "DORSEY" on one side, "TRIAMINICOL" on the other, in blister packs of 24.
Shown in Product Identification Section, page 428

TRIAMINICOL® MULTI-SYMPTOM RELIEF
[trī "ah-mĭn 'ĭ-call]

Description: Each teaspoonful (5 ml) of TRIAMINICOL Multi-Symptom Relief contains: phenylpropanolamine hydrochloride 12.5 mg, chlorpheniramine maleate 2 mg, dextromethorphan hydrobromide 10 mg in a palatable nonalcoholic vehicle. Other ingredients: benzoic acid, flavors, propylene glycol, purified water, Red 40, saccharin sodium, sodium chloride, sorbitol, sucrose.

Indications: Provides relief of runny nose, nasal congestion and sneezing that may occur with the common cold. Suppresses cough due to minor throat and bronchial irritation. Promotes nasal and sinus drainage.

Warnings: Do not take this product: 1) if cough is accompanied by excessive secretions, 2) for persistent cough such as occurs with smoking, asthma or emphysema, or 3) if you have heart disease, high blood pressure, thyroid disease, diabetes, asthma, glaucoma, difficulty in breathing, difficulty in urination due to enlargement of the prostate gland, or 4) if you are taking a prescription drug for high blood pressure or depression, or are taking sedatives or tranquilizers, unless directed by a doctor. Do not exceed recommended dosage or take for more than 7 days. If symptoms persist, are accompanied by a fever, rash or persistent headache, or if cough recurs, consult a doctor. May cause excitability especially in children. May cause marked drowsiness. Alcohol, sedatives or tranquilizers may increase drowsiness. Avoid driving or operating machinery while taking this product. As with any drug, if you are pregnant or nursing a baby, seek advice of a health professional before using this product. Keep this and all drugs out of the reach of children. In case of accidental overdose, seek professional assistance or contact a Poison Control Center immediately.

Dosage and Administration: Adults and children 12 and over (96+ lbs)—2 teaspoonfuls every 4 hours. Children 6 to under 12 years (48–95 lbs)—1 teaspoonful every 4 hours. Unless directed by physician, do not exceed 6 doses in 24 hours or give to children under 6 years of age.

Professional Labeling: The suggested dosage for pediatric patients is:

3–12 months	.75 ml (⅛ tsp)*	
(12–17 lbs)	every 4 hours	
12–24 months	1.25 ml (¼ tsp)	
(18–23 lbs)	every 4 hours	
2–6 years	2.5 ml (½ tsp)	
(24–47 lbs)	every 4 hours	

*(⅛ tsp is approximately .75 ml)

How Supplied: TRIAMINICOL Multi-Symptom Relief (red), in 4 fl oz and 8 fl oz plastic bottles with tamper-evident band around child-resistant cap.
Shown in Product Identification Section, page 428

URSINUS® INLAY–TABS®
[yur "sĭgn 'us]

Description: Each URSINUS INLAY-TAB contains: pseudoephedrine hydrochloride 30 mg and aspirin 325 mg. Other ingredients: calcium stearate, lactose, microcrystalline cellulose, pregelatinized starch, sodium starch glycolate, starch, Yellow 6, Yellow 10.

Indications: For the temporary relief of nasal congestion due to the common cold, hay fever or associated with sinusitis. For the temporary relief of occasional minor aches, pains and headache.

Warnings: Children and teenagers should not use this medicine for chicken pox or flu symptoms before a doctor is consulted about Reye syndrome, a rare but serious illness reported to be associated with aspirin. Unless directed by a doctor: 1) Do not take this product if you are allergic to aspirin or if you have asthma; or if you have stomach distress, ulcers or bleeding problems; 2) Do not take this product if you have heart disease, high blood pressure, thyroid disease, diabetes, or difficulty in urination due to enlargement of the prostate gland, and 3) As with any drug, if you are pregnant or nursing a baby, seek the advice of a health professional before using this product. **IMPORTANT:** Do not take this product during the last 3 months of pregnancy unless directed by a doctor. Aspirin taken near the time of delivery may cause bleeding problems in both mother and child. Do not exceed recommended dosage because at higher doses nervousness, dizziness, or sleeplessness may occur. Do not take this product for more than 7 days. If symptoms do not improve, are accompanied by fever, or new symptoms occur, consult a doctor. Stop taking this product if ringing in the ears or other symptoms occur. *Drug Interaction Precaution:* Do not take this product if you are presently taking a prescription drug for high blood pressure or depression. Do not take this product if you are presently taking a prescription drug for anticoagulation (thinning the blood), diabetes, gout or arthritis without first consulting your doctor.
Keep this and all medicines out of the reach of children. In case of accidental overdose, contact a physician immediately.

Directions: Adults and children 12 years and older: 2 tablets every 4 hours while symptoms persist or as directed by a physician. Drink a full glass of water with each dose. Do not take more than 4 doses in 24 hours. For chicken pox or flu see Warnings.

How Supplied: URSINUS INLAY-TABS (white with yellow inlay), in bottles of 24 and 100.

Schering Corporation
a wholly owned subsidiary of
Schering-Plough Corporation
GALLOPING HILL ROAD
KENILWORTH, NJ 07033

A and D Ointment
REG. T.M.

Description: An ointment containing the emollients, anhydrous lanolin and petrolatum. Also contains: Fragrance, Mineral Oil, Fish Liver Oil and Cholecalciferol.

Indications: *Diaper rash—A and D Ointment* provides prompt, soothing relief for diaper rash and helps heal baby's tender skin; forms a moisture-proof shield that helps protect against urine and detergent irritants; comforts baby's skin and helps prevent chafing.
Chafed Skin—A and D Ointment helps skin retain its vital natural moisture; quickly soothes chafed skin in adults and children and helps prevent abnormal dryness.
Abrasions and Minor Burns—A and D Ointment soothes and helps relieve the smarting and pain of abrasions and minor burns, encourages healing and prevents dressings from sticking to the injured area.

Warning: Keep this and all drugs out of the reach of children.

Overdosage: In case of accidental ingestion, seek professional assistance or contact a poison control center immediately.

Dosage and Administration: *Diaper Rash*—Simply apply a thin coating of **A and D Ointment** at each diaper change. A modest amount is all that is needed to provide protective and healing action.
Chafed Skin—Gently smooth a small quantity of **A and D Ointment** over the area to be treated.
Abrasions, Minor Burns—Wash with lukewarm water and mild soap. When

Continued on next page

Information on Schering products appearing on these pages is effective as of November 1, 1989.

Schering—Cont.

dry, apply **A and D Ointment** liberally. When a sterile dressing is used, change the dressing daily and apply fresh **A and D Ointment.** If no improvement occurs after 48 to 72 hours or if condition worsens, consult your physician.

How Supplied: A and D Ointment is available in 1½-ounce (42.5 g) and 4-ounce (113 g) tubes and 1-pound (454 g) jars.
Store away from heat.
Copyright© 1973, 1977, Schering Corporation. All rights reserved.
Shown in Product Identification
Section, page 428

AFRIN®
[a 'frin]
Nasal Spray 0.05%
Nasal Spray Pump 0.05%
Cherry Scented Nasal Spray 0.05%
Menthol Nasal Spray 0.05%
Nose Drops 0.05%
Children's Strength Nose Drops
0.025%

Description: AFRIN products contain oxymetazoline hydrochloride, the longest acting topical nasal decongestant available. Each ml of AFRIN Nasal Spray, Nasal Spray Pump, and Nose Drops contains Oxymetazoline Hydrochloride, USP 0.5 mg (0.05%); Benzalkonium Chloride, Glycine, Phenylmercuric Acetate (0.02 mg/ml), Sorbitol, and Water.
Each ml of AFRIN Children's Strength Nose Drops contains Oxymetazoline Hydrochloride, USP 0.25 mg (0.025%); Benzalkonium Chloride, Glycine, Phenylmercuric Acetate (0.02 mg/ml), Sorbitol, and Water.
AFRIN Menthol Nasal Spray contains cooling aromatic vapors of menthol, eucalyptol and camphor and polysorbate, in addition to the ingredients of AFRIN Nasal Spray.
AFRIN Cherry Scented Nasal Spray contains artificial cherry flavor in addition to the ingredients in regular AFRIN.

Indications: For temporary relief of nasal congestion "associated with" colds, hay fever and sinusitis.

Actions: The sympathomimetic action of AFRIN products constricts the smaller arterioles of the nasal passages, producing a prolonged, gentle and predictable decongesting effect. In just a few minutes a single dose, as directed, provides prompt, temporary relief of nasal congestion that lasts up to 12 hours. AFRIN products last up to 3 or 4 times longer than most ordinary nasal sprays. AFRIN products used at bedtime help restore freer nasal breathing through the night.

Warnings: Do not exceed recommended dosage because burning, stinging, sneezing or increase of nasal discharge may occur. Do not use these products for more than 3 days. If nasal congestion persists, consult a physician. The use of the dispensers by more than one

person may spread infection. Keep these and all medicines out of the reach of children.

Overdosage: In case of accidental ingestion, seek professional assistance or contact a Poison Control Center immediately.

Dosage and Administration: Because AFRIN has a long duration of action, twice-a-day administration—in the morning and at bedtime—is usually adequate.
AFRIN Nasal Spray, Cherry Scented Nasal Spray and Menthol Nasal Spray, 0.05%—For adults and children 6 years of age and over: With head upright, spray 2 or 3 times into each nostril twice daily—morning and evening. To spray, squeeze bottle quickly and firmly. Do not tilt head backward while spraying. Wipe nozzle clean after use. Not recommended for children under six.
Afrin Nasal Spray Pump, 0.05%—For adults and children 6 years of age and over: Two or three sprays in each nostril twice daily—morning and bedtime. Remove protective cap. Hold bottle with thumb at base and nozzle between first and second fingers. With head upright, insert metered pump spray nozzle in nostril. Depress pump 2 or 3 times, all the way down, with a firm even stroke and sniff deeply. Repeat in other nostril. Do not tilt head backward while spraying. Wipe tip clean after each use. Before using the first time, remove the protective cap from the tip and prime the metered pump by depressing pump firmly several times.
AFRIN Nose Drops—For adults and children 6 years of age and over: Tilt head back, apply 2 or 3 drops into each nostril twice daily—morning and evening. Immediately bend head forward toward knees. Hold a few seconds, then return to upright position. Wipe dropper clean after each use. Not recommended for children under six.
AFRIN Children's Strength Nose Drops—Children 2 through 5 years of age: Tilt head back, apply 2 or 3 drops into each nostril twice daily—morning and evening. Promptly move head forward toward knees. Hold a few seconds, then return child to upright position. Wipe dropper clean after each use. For children under 2 years, use only as directed by a physician.

How Supplied: AFRIN Nasal Spray 0.05% (1:2000), 15 ml and 30 ml plastic squeeze bottles.
AFRIN Nasal Spray Pump 0.05% (1:2000), 15 ml spray pump bottles.
AFRIN Cherry Scented Nasal Spray 0.05% (1:2000), 15 ml plastic squeeze bottle.
AFRIN Menthol Nasal Spray 0.05% (1:2000), 15 ml plastic squeeze bottle.
AFRIN Nose Drops, 0.05% (1:2000), 20 ml dropper bottle.
AFRIN Children's Strength Nose Drops, 0.025% (1:4000), 20 ml dropper bottle.
Store all nasal sprays and nose drops between 2° and 30°C (36° and 86°F).
Shown in Product Identification
Section, page 428

AFRINOL®
[a 'frin-ol]
Extended Release Tablets
Long-Acting Nasal Decongestant

Active Ingredients: Each Extended Release Tablet contains: 120 mg pseudoephedrine sulfate. Each tablet also contains: Acacia, Butylparaben, Calcium Sulfate, Carnauba Wax, Corn Starch, FD&C Blue No. 1, Gelatin, Lactose, Magnesium Stearate, Neutral Soap, Oleic Acid, Povidone, Rosin, Sugar, Talc, White Wax, Zein. Half the dose (60 mg) is released after the tablet is swallowed and the other half is released hours later; continuous relief is provided for up to 12 hours . . . without drowsiness.

Indications: For temporary relief of nasal congestion due to the common cold, hay fever or other upper respiratory allergies, and nasal congestion associated with sinusitis.

Actions: Promotes nasal and/or sinus drainage, helps decongest sinus openings, sinus passages.

Warnings: Do not exceed recommended dosage because at higher doses nervousness, dizziness or sleeplessness may occur. Do not take this preparation if you have high blood pressure, heart disease, diabetes, or thyroid disease, except under the advice and supervision of a physician. If symptoms do not improve within 7 days or are accompanied by fever, consult a physician before continuing use. Keep this and all drugs out of the reach of children.
As with any drug, if you are pregnant or nursing a baby, seek the advice of a health professional before using this product.

Drug Interactions: Do not take this product if you are presently taking a prescription drug for high blood pressure or depression, without first consulting your physician.

Overdosage: In case of accidental overdose, seek professional assistance or contact a poison control center immediately.

Dosage and Administration: Adults and children 12 years and over—One tablet every 12 hours. AFRINOL is not recommended for children under 12 years of age.

How Supplied: AFRINOL Extended Release Tablets—Boxes of 12 and bottles of 100.
Store between 2° and 30°C (36° and 86°F). Protect from excessive moisture.
Shown in Product Identification
Section, page 428

CHLOR–TRIMETON®
[klor-tri 'mĕ-ton]
Allergy Syrup
Allergy Tablets 4 mg
Long Acting Allergy REPETABS®
Tablets 8 mg and 12 mg

Active Ingredients: Each Allergy Tablet contains: 4 mg CHLOR-TRIMETON (brand of chlorpheniramine maleate, USP); also contains: Corn Starch, D&C

Yellow No. 10 Al Lake, Lactose, Magnesium Stearate. Each REPE-TABS® Tablet contains: 8 mg or 12 mg CHLOR-TRIMETON (brand of chlorpheniramine maleate); 8 mg Repetabs also contains: Acacia, Butylparaben, Calcium Phosphate, Calcium Sulfate, Carnauba Wax, Corn Starch, D&C Yellow No. 10 Al Lake, FD&C Yellow No.6 Al Lake, Lactose, Magnesium Stearate, Neutral Soap, Oleic Acid, Povidone, Rosin, Sugar, Talc, White Wax, Zein.

12 mg Repetabs also contains: Acacia, Butylparaben, Calcium Phosphate, Calcium Sulfate, Carnauba Wax, Corn Starch, D&C Yellow No. 10 Al Lake, FD&C Blue No. 2 Al Lake, FD&C Yellow No. 6, FD&C Yellow No. 6 Al Lake, Lactose, Magnesium Stearate, Neutral Soap, Oleic Acid, Potato Starch, Rosin, Sugar, Talc, White Wax, Zein. Half the dose is released after the tablet is swallowed, and the other half is released hours later; continuous relief is provided for up to 12 hours.

Each teaspoonful (5 ml) of Allergy Syrup contains: 2 mg CHLOR-TRIMETON (brand of chlorpheniramine maleate) in a pleasant-tasting syrup containing approximately 7% alcohol. Also contains: Benzaldehyde, FD&C Green No. 3, FD&C Yellow No. 6, Flavor, Glycerin, Menthol, Methylparaben, Propylene Glycol, Propylparaben, Sugar, Vanillin, Water.

Indications: For temporary relief of hay fever symptoms: sneezing; runny nose; watery, itchy eyes, itching of the nose or throat.

Actions: The active ingredient in CHLOR-TRIMETON is an antihistamine with anticholinergic (drying) and sedative side effects. Antihistamines appear to compete with histamine for cell receptor sites on effector cells.

Warnings: May cause excitability especially in children. Do not give the REPE-TABS Tablets to children under 12 years, or the Allergy Syrup and Tablets to children under 6 years except under the advice and supervision of a physician. Do not take this product if you have asthma, glaucoma, emphysema, chronic pulmonary disease, shortness of breath, difficulty in breathing, or difficulty in urination due to enlargement of the prostate gland unless directed by a physician. May cause drowsiness; alcohol may increase the drowsiness effect. Avoid alcoholic beverages while driving a motor vehicle or operating machinery. As with any drug, if you are pregnant or nursing a baby, seek the advice of a health professional before using this product. Keep this and all drugs out of the reach of children. In case of accidental overdose, seek professional assistance or contact a Poison Control Center immediately.

Dosage and Administration: Allergy Syrup—Adults and Children 12 years and over: Two teaspoonfuls (4 mg) every 4 to 6 hours, not to exceed 12 teaspoonfuls in 24 hours. Children 6 through 11 years: one teaspoonful (2 mg) every 4 to 6 hours, not to exceed 6 teaspoonfuls in 24

hours. For children under 6 years, consult a physician.

Allergy Tablets—Adults and Children 12 years and over: One tablet (4 mg) every 4 to 6 hours, not to exceed 6 tablets in 24 hours. Children 6 through 11 years: One half the adult dose (break tablet in half) every 4 to 6 hours, not to exceed 3 whole tablets in 24 hours. For children under 6 years, consult a physician.

Allergy REPETABS Tablets—Adults and Children 12 years and over: One tablet in the morning and one tablet in the evening, not to exceed 24 mg (3 tablets of 8 mg; 2 tablets of 12 mg) in 24 hours. For children under 12 years, consult a physician.

Professional Labeling: Dosage—Allergy Syrup: Children 2 through 5 years: ½ teaspoonful (1 mg) every 4 to 6 hours; Allergy Tablets: Children 2 through 5 years: one-quarter tablet (1 mg) every 4 to 6 hours.

Allergy REPETABS Tablets—Children 6 to 12 years: One tablet (8 mg) at bedtime or during the day, as indicated.

How Supplied: CHLOR-TRIMETON Allergy Tablets, 4 mg, yellow compressed, scored tablets impressed with the Schering trademark and product identification letters, TW or numbers, 080; box of 24, bottles of 100.

CHLOR-TRIMETON Allergy Syrup: 2 mg per 5 ml, blue-green-colored liquid; 4-fluid ounce (118 ml). Protect from light; however, if color fades potency will not be affected.

CHLOR-TRIMETON Allergy REPE-TABS Tablets, 8 mg, sugar-coated, yellow tablets branded in red with the Schering trademark and product identification letters, CC or numbers, 374; boxes of 24, 48, bottles of 100.

CHLOR-TRIMETON REPETABS Tablets, 12 mg, sugar coated orange tablets branded in black with Schering trademark and product identification letters AAE or numbers 009; boxes of 12 and 24, bottles of 100.

Store the tablets and syrup between 2° and 30°C (36° and 86°F).

Shown in Product Identification Section, page 428

CHLOR-TRIMETON®

[*klor 'tri 'mĕ-ton*]
Decongestant Tablets
Long Acting CHLOR-TRIMETON®
Decongestant REPETABS® Tablets

Active Ingredients: Each tablet contains: 4 mg CHLOR-TRIMETON (brand of chlorpheniramine maleate, USP) and 60 mg pseudoephedrine sulfate. Each tablet also contains: Corn Starch, FD&C Blue No. 1, Lactose, Magnesium Stearate, Povidone.

Each REPETABS Tablet contains: 8 mg CHLOR-TRIMETON (brand of chlorpheniramine maleate) and 120 mg pseudoephedrine sulfate. Each repetab also contains: Acacia, Butylparaben, Calcium Sulfate, Carnauba Wax, Corn Starch, D&C Yellow No. 10 Al Lake, FD&C Blue No. 1 Al Lake, FD&C Yellow No. 6 Al Lake, Gelatin, Lactose, Magnesium Stea-

rate, Neutral Soap, Oleic Acid, Povidone, Rosin, Sugar, Talc, White Wax, Zein. Half the dose of each ingredient is released after the tablet is swallowed and the other half is released hours later providing continuous long-lasting relief up to 12 hours.

Indications: For temporary relief of hay fever symptoms (sneezing; running nose; watery, itchy eyes, itching of the nose or throat) and nasal congestion due to hay fever and associated with sinusitis.

Actions: The antihistamine, chlorpheniramine maleate, provides temporary relief of running nose, sneezing, itching of the nose or throat, and itchy and watery eyes as may occur in allergic rhinitis (such as hayfever). The decongestant, pseudoephedrine sulfate reduces swelling of nasal passages; shrinks swollen membranes; and temporarily restores freer breathing through the nose.

Warnings: If symptoms do not improve within 7 days or are accompanied by fever, consult a physician before continuing use. May cause excitability especially in children. Do not exceed recommended dosage because at higher doses nervousness, dizziness or sleeplessness may occur. Do not take this product if you have asthma, glaucoma, emphysema, chronic pulmonary disease, shortness of breath, difficulty in breathing, heart disease, high blood pressure, thyroid disease, diabetes, or difficulty in urination due to enlargement of the prostate gland. Do not give the Decongestant Tablets to children under 6 years or the REPETABS Tablets to children under 12 years unless directed by a physician. May cause drowsiness; alcohol may increase the drowsiness effect. Avoid alcoholic beverages while taking this product. Use caution when driving a motor vehicle or operating machinery. Keep this and all drugs out of the reach of children. In case of accidental overdose, seek professional assistance or contact a Poison Control Center immediately. As with any drug, if you are pregnant or nursing a baby, seek the advice of a health professional before using this product.

Drug Interaction Precaution: Do not take this product if you are presently taking a prescription drug for high blood pressure or depression, without first consulting your doctor.

Dosage and Administration: Tablets—ADULTS AND CHILDREN 12 YEARS AND OVER: One tablet every 4 to 6 hours, not to exceed 4 tablets in 24 hours. CHILDREN 6 THROUGH 11 YEARS—One half the adult dose (break tablet in half) every 4 to 6 hours not to exceed 2 whole tablets in 24 hours. For children under 6 years, consult a physician.

Continued on next page

Information on Schering products appearing on these pages is effective as of November 1, 1989.

Schering—Cont.

REPETABS Tablets—ADULTS AND CHILDREN 12 YEARS AND OVER: one tablet every 12 hours.

Professional Labeling: Tablets—Children 2-5 years—one quarter the adult dose every 4 hours, not to exceed 1 tablet in 24 hours.

How Supplied: CHLOR-TRIMETON Decongestant Tablets—boxes of 24 and 48. Long Acting CHLOR-TRIMETON Decongestant REPETABS Tablets boxes of 12 and 36.
Store these CHLOR-TRIMETON Products between 2° and 30°C (36°and 86°F); and protect from excessive moisture.
Shown in Product Identification Section, page 428

COD LIVER OIL CONCENTRATE
[kod liv'er oyl kon-sen-trāt]
Tablets
Capsules
Tablets with Vitamin C

Active Ingredients: Tablets—A pleasantly flavored concentrate of cod liver oil with Vitamins A & D added. Each tasty, chewable tablet provides: 4000 IU of vitamin A and 200 IU of cholecalciferol (vitamin D).
Capsules—A concentrate of cod liver oil with Vitamins A and D added. Each capsule provides: 10,000 IU of vitamin A and 400 IU of cholecalciferol (vitamin D).
Tablets with Vitamin C—A pleasantly-flavored concentrate of cod liver oil with Vitamins A, D and C added. Each tablet provides, 4000 IU of Vitamin A, 200 IU of cholecalciferol (vitamin D) and 50 mg of Vitamin C.
Tablets may be chewed or swallowed.

Inactive Ingredients: Capsules—Corn oil, gelatin, glycerin, vitamin E.
Tablets with Vitamin C—Acacia, Butylparaben, Carnauba Wax, Confectioners Glaze, FD&C Yellow No. 5 Aluminum Lake, FD&C Yellow No. 6 Aluminum Lake, Flavor, Gelatin, Magnesium Stearate, Sugar, Wheat Flour, White Wax.

Indications: Cod Liver Oil Concentrate Tablets and Capsules are recommended for prevention and treatment of diseases due to deficiencies in Vitamins A and D. The tablets with Vitamin C are recommended for prevention and treatment of diseases due to deficiencies of Vitamins A, D and C.

Warnings: Keep these and all drugs out of the reach of children.
As with any drug, if you are pregnant or nursing a baby, seek the advice of a health professional before using these products.

Precautions: Cod Liver Oil Concentrate Tablets and Tablets with Vitamin C contain FD&C Yellow No. 5 (tartrazine) as a color additive.
Persons sensitive to tartrazine or aspirin should consult a physician.

Overdosage: In case of accidental overdose, seek professional assistance or

contact a Poison Control Center immediately.

Dosage and Administration: Tablets: Two tablets daily, or as prescribed by a physician, taken preferably before meals.
Capsules: One capsule daily, or as prescribed by a physician, taken preferably before meals.
Tablets with Vitamin C: Two tablets daily, taken preferably before meals.

How Supplied: Cod Liver Oil Concentrate Tablets: bottles of 100. Cod Liver Oil Concentrate Capsules: bottles of 40 and 100. Cod Liver Oil Concentrate Tablets with Vitamin C: bottles of 100 tablets.

COMPLEX 15®
Phospholipid Hand & Body Moisturizing Cream
Formulated For Mild To˜Severe Dry Skin

Ingredients: Water, Mineral Oil, Glycerin, Squalane, Caprylic/Capric Triglyceride, Dimethicone, Glyceryl Stearate, Glycol Stearate, PEG-50 Stearate, Stearic Acid, Cetyl Alcohol, Myristyl Myristate, Lecithin, Diazolidinyl Urea, Carbomer 934, Magnesium Aluminum Silicate, C10–30 Carboxylic Acid Sterol Ester, Sodium Hydroxide, Tetrasodium EDTA, BHT

COMPLEX 15® Hand and Body Cream is formulated for mild to severe dry skin with a system modeled from nature. It contains lecithin, a phospholipid water-binding agent found naturally in the skin. Each phospholipid molecule holds 15 molecules of water, restoring the natural moisture balance. COMPLEX 15 Hand and Body Cream is nongreasy and absorbs quickly into the skin. COMPLEX 15 Hand and Body Cream is unscented, contains no parabens or lanolin. COMPLEX 15 Hand and Body Cream is proven to be hypoallergenic and noncomedogenic.

Directions: Apply to the hands and body as needed or as directed by a physician. Avoid contact with eyes.
FOR EXTERNAL USE ONLY

How Supplied: COMPLEX 15® Hand & Body Moisturizing Cream is available in 4 ounce jars (0085-4151-04).

Schering Corporation
Kenilworth, NJ 07033 USA

COMPLEX 15®
Phospholipid Hand & Body Moisturizing Lotion
Formulated For Mild To Severe Dry Skin

Ingredients: Water, Caprylic/Capric Triglyceride, Glycerin, Glyceryl Stearate, Dimethicone, PEG-50 Stearate, Squalane, Cetyl Alcohol, Glycol Stearate, Myristyl Myristate, Stearic Acid, Lecithin, C10–30 Carboxylic Acid Sterol Ester, Diazolidinyl Urea, Carbomer 934, Magnesium Aluminum Silicate, Sodium Hydroxide, BHT, Tetrasodium EDTA

COMPLEX 15® Hand and Body Lotion is formulated for mild to severe dry skin with a system modeled from nature. It contains lecithin, a phospholipid water-binding agent found naturally in the skin. Each phospholipid molecule holds 15 molecules of water, restoring the natural moisture balance. COMPLEX 15 Hand and Body Lotion is nongreasy and absorbs quickly into the skin. COMPLEX 15 Hand and Body Lotion is unscented, contains no parabens, lanolin, or mineral oil. COMPLEX 15 Hand and Body Lotion is proven to be hypoallergenic and noncomedogenic.

Directions: Apply to the hands and body as needed, or as directed by a physician. Avoid contact with eyes.
FOR EXTERNAL USE ONLY

How Supplied: COMPLEX 15® Hand and Body Moisturizing Lotion is available in 8 fluid ounce bottles (0085-4115-08).

Schering Corporation
Kenilworth, NJ 07033

COMPLEX 15®
Phospholipid Moisturizing Face Cream

Ingredients: Water, Caprylic/Capric Triglyceride, Glycerin, Squalane, Glyceryl Stearate, Propylene Glycol, PEG-50 Stearate, Cetyl Alcohol, Dimethicone, Glycol Stearate, Myristyl Myristate, Stearic Acid, Carbomer 934, Magnesium Aluminum Silicate, Diazolidinyl Urea, Lecithin, Sodium Hydroxide, C10–30 Carboxylic Acid Sterol Ester, BHT, Tetrasodium EDTA

COMPLEX 15® Face Cream is formulated for mild to severe dry skin with a system modeled from nature. It contains lecithin, a phospholipid water-binding agent found naturally in the skin. Each phospholipid molecule holds 15 molecules of water, restoring the natural moisture balance. COMPLEX 15 Face Cream is nongreasy and absorbs quickly into the skin. COMPLEX 15 Face Cream is unscented, contains no parabens, lanolin or mineral oil. COMPLEX 15 Face Cream is proven to be hypoallergenic and noncomedogenic.

Directions: Apply to the face as needed or as directed by a physician. Avoid contact with eyes.
FOR EXTERNAL USE ONLY.

How Supplied: COMPLEX 15® Moisturizing Face Cream is available in 2.5 oz. tubes (0085-4100-25).

Schering Corporation
Kenilworth, NJ 07033

CORICIDIN® Tablets
[kor-a-see'din]
CORICIDIN 'D'® Decongestant Tablets
CORICIDIN® Nasal Mist

Active Ingredients: CORICIDIN Tablets—2 mg CHLOR-TRIMETON® (brand of chlorpheniramine maleate, USP); 325 mg (5gr) acetaminophen.

CORICIDIN 'D' Decongestant Tablets—2 mg chlorpheniramine maleate, USP; 12.5 mg phenylpropanolamine hydrochloride, USP; 325 mg (5 gr) acetaminophen.
CORICIDIN Nasal Mist—.05% oxymetazoline hydrochloride.

Inactive Ingredients: CORICIDIN Tablets—Acacia, Butylparaben, Calcium Sulfate, Carnauba Wax, Cellulose, Corn Starch, FD&C Red No. 40, FD&C Yellow No. 6 Aluminum Lake, Lactose, Magnesium Stearate, Povidone, Sugar, Titanium Dioxide, and White Wax. May also contain Talc.
CORICIDIN 'D' Decongestant Tablets—Acacia, Butylparaben, Calcium Sulfate, Carnauba Wax, Cellulose, Corn Starch, Magnesium Stearate, Povidone, Sugar, Titanium Dioxide, and White Wax. May also contain Talc.
CORICIDIN Nasal Mist—Benzalkonium Chloride, Glycine, Phenylmercuric Acetate (0.02 mg/ml), Sorbitol, and Water.

Indications: CORICIDIN Tablets—For effective, temporary relief of cold and flu symptoms.
CORICIDIN 'D' Decongestant Tablets—For effective, temporary relief of congested cold, flu and sinus symptoms.
CORICIDIN Nasal Mist— For temporary relief of nasal congestion associated with the common cold, hay fever or sinusitis.

Actions: CORICIDIN Tablets relieve annoying cold and flu symptoms such as minor aches and pains, fever, sneezing, running nose and watery/itchy eyes.
CORICIDIN 'D' Tablets relieve the same annoying cold and flu symptoms as well as stuffy nose, nasal membrane swelling and sinus headache.
CORICIDIN Nasal Mist is "symptom specific" and designed to shrink swollen nasal membranes promptly and help restore freer breathing through the nose.

Warnings: CORICIDIN Tablets: Do not take this product for pain for more than 10 days (for adults) or 5 days (for children 6 years through 11 years), and do not take for fever for more than 3 days unless directed by a physician. If pain or fever persists or gets worse, if new symptoms occur, or if redness or swelling is present, consult a physician because these could be signs of a serious condition. May cause excitability especially in children. Do not take this product if you have asthma, glaucoma, emphysema, chronic pulmonary disease, shortness of breath, difficulty in breathing, difficulty in urination due to enlargement of the prostate gland, or give this product to children under 6 years, unless directed by a physician. May cause drowsiness; alcohol, sedatives, and tranquilizers may increase the drowsiness effect. Avoid alcoholic beverages while taking this product. Do not take this product if you are taking sedatives or tranquilizers, without first consulting your physician. Use caution when driving a motor vehicle or operating machinery. Keep this and all drugs out of the reach of children. In case of accidental overdose, seek professional assistance or contact a Poison Control Center immedi-

ately. Prompt medical attention is critical for adults as well as for children even if you do not notice any signs or symptoms. As with any drug, if you are pregnant or nursing a baby, seek the advice of a health professional before using this product.
CORICIDIN 'D' Decongestant Tablets: Do not take this product for pain or congestion for more than 7 days (adults) or 5 days (children 6 through 11 years), and do not take for fever for more than 3 days unless directed by a physician. If pain or fever persists or gets worse, if new symptoms occur, or if redness or swelling is present, consult your physician because these could be signs of a serious condition. May cause excitability, especially in children. Do not exceed recommended dosage because at higher doses nervousness, dizziness, or sleeplessness may occur. Do not take this product if you have asthma, glaucoma, emphysema, chronic pulmonary disease, shortness of breath, difficulty in breathing, heart disease, high blood pressure, thyroid disease, diabetes, difficulty in urination due to enlargement of the prostate gland, or give this product to children under 6 years unless directed by a physician. May cause drowsiness; alcohol, sedatives, and tranquilizers may increase the drowsiness effect. Avoid alcoholic beverages while taking this product. Use caution when driving a motor vehicle or operating machinery. Keep this and all drugs out of the reach of children. In case of accidental overdose, seek professional assistance or contact a Poison Control Center immediately. Proper medical attention is critical for adults and children even if you do not notice any signs or symptoms. As with any drug, if you are pregnant or nursing a baby, seek the advice of a health care professional before using this product. *Drug Interaction Precaution:* Do not take this product if you are presently taking a prescription drug for high blood pressure or depression, sedatives, tranquilizers or appetite-controlling medication containing phenylpropanolamine without first consulting your physician.
CORICIDIN Nasal Mist—Do not exceed recommended dosage because burning, stinging, sneezing, or increase of nasal discharge may occur. Do not use this product for more than 3 days. If nasal congestion persists, consult a physician. The use of this dispenser by more than one person may spread infection. For adult use only. Keep this and all medicines out of the reach of children.

Dosage and Administration: CORICIDIN Tablets—Adults and children 12 years and over—2 tablets every 4 hours not to exceed 12 tablets in 24 hours. Children 6 through 11 years: 1 tablet every 4 hours not to exceed 5 tablets in 24 hours.
CORICIDIN 'D' Decongestant Tablets—Adults and children 12 years and over: 2 tablets every 4 hours not to exceed 12 tablets in 24 hours. Children 6 through 11 years: 1 tablet every 4 hours not to exceed 5 tablets in 24 hours.
CORICIDIN Nasal Mist— For adults and children 6 years of age and over: With

head upright spray two or three times in each nostril twice daily—morning and evening, to spray squeeze bottle quickly and firmly. Do not tilt head backward while spraying. Wipe nozzle clean after use. Not recommended for children under six.

How Supplied: CORICIDIN Tablets—bottles of 12, 24, 48, and 100.
CORICIDIN 'D' Decongestant Tablets—bottles of 12, 24, 48, and 100.
CORICIDIN Decongestant Nasal Mist—Plastic squeeze bottles of ½ fl. oz. (15 ml.)
Store the tablets, nasal mist, and syrup between 2° and 30°C (36° and 86°F).
Shown in Product Identification Section, page 429

CORICIDIN® DEMILETS®
[*kor-a-see'din dem'ē-lets*]
Tablets for Children

CORICIDIN DEMILETS Tablets—1.0 mg chlorpheniramine maleate, USP; 80 mg acetaminophen, USP; 6.25 mg phenylpropanolamine hydrochloride, USP.

Inactive Ingredients: Corn Starch, D&C Yellow No. 10 Al Lake, FD&C Yellow No. 6 Al Lake, Flavor, Lactose, Magnesium Stearate, Mannitol, Saccharin, Stearic Acid.

Indications: CORICIDIN DEMILETS Tablets—For temporary relief of children's congested cold, flu and sinus symptoms.

Actions: CORICIDIN DEMILETS Tablets provide relief of annoying cold, flu and sinus symptoms: running nose, stuffy nose, sneezing, watery/itchy eyes, minor aches, pains and fever.

Warnings: CORICIDIN DEMILETS Tablets—Give water with each dose. Do not give this product for more than 5 days, but if fever is present, persists or recurs, limit dosage to 3 days; if symptoms persist or new ones occur, consult a physician. This product may cause drowsiness, therefore, driving a motor vehicle or operating heavy machinery must be avoided while taking it. Alcoholic beverages must also be avoided while taking this product. It may cause excitability, especially in children. Do not exceed recommended dosage because at higher doses severe liver damage, nervousness, dizziness, elevation of blood pressure or sleeplessness is more likely to occur. Do not administer this product to persons who have asthma, glaucoma, difficulty in urination due to enlargement of the prostate gland, high blood pressure, heart disease, diabetes or thyroid disease, or give this product to children less than 6 years old, except under the advice and supervision of a physician. Keep this and all drugs out of the reach of children. As with any drug, if you are pregnant or nursing a baby, seek the advice of a

Continued on next page

Information on Schering products appearing on these pages is effective as of November 1, 1989.

Schering—Cont.

health professional before using this product.

Drug Interactions: CORICIDIN DEMILETS Tablets—Do not give this product to persons who are presently taking a prescription antihypertensive or antidepressant medication containing a monoamine oxidase inhibitor or an appetite-controlling medication containing phenylpropanolamine except under the advice and supervision of a physician.

Overdosage: In case of accidental overdose, seek professional assistance or contact a Poison Control Center immediately.

Dosage and Administration: CORICIDIN DEMILETS Tablets—Under 6 years: As directed by a physician. 6 through 11 years: Two DEMILETS Tablets every 4 hours not to exceed 12 tablets in a 24-hour period, or as directed by a physician.

How Supplied: CORICIDIN DEMILETS Tablets—boxes of 36, individually wrapped in a child's protective pack. Store the tablets between 2° and 30°C (36° and 86°F). Protect from excessive moisture.

Shown in Product Identification Section, page 429

CORICIDIN® Maximum Strength Sinus Headache Caplets
[kor-a-see 'din]

Active Ingredients: Each caplet contains: acetaminophen 500 mg (500 mg is a non-standard extra strength dosage of acetaminophen, as compared to the standard of 325 mg); CHLOR-TRIMETON® (brand of chlorpheniramine maleate) 2 mg; phenylpropanolamine hydrochloride 12.5 mg.

Inactive Ingredients: Each caplet also contains Carnauba Wax, Cellulose, FD&C Yellow No. 6 Al Lake, Hydroxypropyl Methylcellulose, Magnesium Stearate, Povidone.

Indications: For temporary relief of sinus headache and congestion.

Actions: CORICIDIN Sinus Headache Caplets have been formulated with an antihistamine for temporary relief of the running nose that often accompanies upper respiratory allergies and sinusitis; a non-aspirin pain reliever for temporary relief of sinus headache pain and a decongestant for temporary relief of nasal membrane swelling, thus promoting freer breathing.

Warnings: Do not take this product for pain or congestion for more than 7 days, and do not take for fever for more than 3 days unless directed by a physician. If pain or fever persists or gets worse, if new symptoms occur, or if redness or swelling is present, consult your physician because these could be signs of a serious condition. May cause excitability especially in children. Do not exceed recommended dosage because at higher

doses nervousness, dizziness, or sleeplessness may occur. Do not take this product if you have asthma, glaucoma, emphysema, chronic pulmonary disease, shortness of breath, difficulty in breathing, heart disease, high blood pressure, thyroid disease, diabetes, difficulty in urination due to enlargement of the prostate gland, or give this product to children under 12 years, unless directed by a physician. May cause drowsiness; alcohol, sedatives, and tranquilizers may increase the drowsiness effect. Avoid alcoholic beverages while taking this product. Use caution when driving a motor vehicle or operating machinery. Keep this and all drugs out of the reach of children. In case of accidental overdose, seek professional assistance or contact a Poison Control Center Immediately. Prompt medical attention is critical for adults as well as for children even if you do not notice any signs or symptoms. As with any drug, if you are pregnant or nursing a baby, seek the advice of a health care professional before using this product.

Drug Interaction Precaution: Do not take this product if you are presently taking a prescription drug for high blood pressure or depression, sedatives, tranquilizers, or appetite-controlling medication containing phenylpropanolamine without first consulting your physician.

Dosage and Administration: Adults and children 12 years and older: 2 caplets every 6 hours not to exceed 8 caplets in a 24-hour period, or as directed by a physician. Swallow one caplet at a time. Store between 2° and 30°C (36° and 86°F). Protect from excessive moisture.

How Supplied: Box of 24 coated caplets.
Shown in Product Identification Section, page 429

DEMAZIN®
[dem 'a-zin]
Nasal Decongestant/Antihistamine TIMED-RELEASE Tablets Syrup

Description: Each **TIMED-RELEASE Tablet** contains: 25 mg phenylpropanolamine hydrochloride and 4 mg CHLOR-TRIMETON® (brand of chlorpheniramine maleate, USP). Half the dose is released after the tablet is swallowed and the other half is released hours later; continuous relief is provided for up to 8 hours.

Each **TIMED-RELEASE Tablet** also contains: Acacia, Butylparaben, Calcium Phosphate, Calcium Sulfate, Carnauba Wax, Corn Starch, Diatomaceous Earth, FD&C Blue No. 1, FD&C Blue No. 2 Al Lake, Kaolin, Lactose, Magnesium Stearate, Neutral Soap, Oleic Acid, Stearic Acid, Sugar, Talc, White Wax, and Zein.

Each teaspoonful (5 ml) of **Syrup** contains 12.5 mg phenylpropanolamine hydrochloride, USP and 2 mg CHLOR-TRIMETON® (brand of chlorpheniramine maleate, USP) in a pleasant-tasting syrup containing approximately 7.5% alcohol.

Each teaspoonful of **Syrup** also contains: Benzaldehyde, FD&C Blue No. 1, FD&C

Green No. 3, FD&C Yellow No. 6, Flavor, Glycerin, Menthol, Methylparaben, Propylene Glycol, Propylparaben, Sugar, Vanillin, and Water.

Indications: For temporary relief of running nose, sneezing, itching of the nose or throat, and itchy and watery eyes as may occur in allergic rhinitis (such as hay fever); nasal congestion due to the common cold (cold), hay fever or other upper respiratory allergies, or associated with sinusitis.

Actions: Phenylpropanolamine hydrochloride is a sympathomimetic agent which acts as an upper respiratory and pulmonary decongestant and mild bronchodilator. It exerts desirable sympathomimetic action with relatively little central nervous system excitation, so that wakefulness and nervousness are reduced to a minimum. Chlorpheniramine maleate antagonizes many of the characteristic effects of histamine. It is of value clinically in the prevention and relief of many allergic manifestations.

The oral administration of phenylpropanolamine hydrochloride with chlorpheniramine maleate produces a complementary action on congestive conditions of the upper respiratory tract, thus often obviating the need for topical nasal therapy.

Warnings: If symptoms do not improve within 7 days or are accompanied by high fever, consult a physician before continuing use. May cause excitability especially in children. Do not exceed recommended dosage because at higher doses nervousness, dizziness, or sleeplessness may occur. Do not take this product if you have asthma, glaucoma, emphysema, chronic pulmonary disease, shortness of breath, difficulty in breathing, heart disease, high blood pressure, thyroid disease, diabetes, or difficulty in urination due to enlargement of the prostate gland or give this product to children under 6 years, unless directed by a physician. May cause drowsiness; alcohol may increase the drowsiness effect. Avoid alcoholic beverages while taking this product. Use caution when driving a motor vehicle or operating machinery. Keep this and all drugs out of reach of children. In case of accidental overdose, seek professional assistance or contact a Poison Control Center immediately. As with any drug, if you are pregnant or nursing a baby, seek the advice of a health professional before using this product.

Drug Interaction Precaution: Do not take this product if you are presently taking a prescription drug for high blood pressure or depression or an appetite-controlling medication containing phenylpropanolamine without first consulting your doctor.

Dosage and Administration: TIMED-RELEASE Tablets—**Adults and children 12 years and older:** 2 tablets every 8 hours not to exceed 6 tablets in 24 hours. **Children 6 through 11 years:** 1 tablet every 8 hours not to exceed 3 tablets in 24 hours. For children under 6 years, consult a physician. **Syrup**

—**Adults and children 12 years and older:** Two teaspoonfuls every 4–6 hours not to exceed 12 teaspoonfuls in 24 hours, or as directed by a physician. **Children 6 through 11 years:** One teaspoonful every 4 hours not to exceed 6 teaspoonfuls in 24 hours or as directed by a physician. For children under 6 years, consult a physician.

How Supplied: DEMAZIN TIMED-RELEASE Tablets, blue, sugar-coated tablets branded in red with the Schering trademark and product identification number 751; box of 24 and bottle of 100. DEMAZIN Syrup, blue-colored liquid, bottles of 4 fluid ounces (118 ml). **Store DEMAZIN TIMED-RELEASE Tablets and Syrup between 2° and 30°C (36° and 86°F).**
Copyright © 1983, 1985 Schering Corporation.
All rights reserved.

DERMOLATE® Anti-Itch Cream
[*dur'mō-lāt*]

Active Ingredients: DERMOLATE Anti-Itch Cream contains hydrocortisone 0.5% in a greaseless, vanishing cream. It also contains: Ceteareth-30, Cetearyl Alcohol, Mineral Oil, Petrolatum, Propylene Glycol, Sodium Phosphate, Water.

Indications: For the temporary relief of minor skin irritations, itching and rashes due to eczema, dermatitis, insect bites, poison ivy, poison oak, poison sumac, soaps, detergents, cosmetics and jewelry.

Actions: DERMOLATE Anti-Itch Cream provides temporary relief of itching and minor skin irritation.

Warnings: DERMOLATE Anti-Itch Cream is for external use only. Avoid contact with the eyes. Discontinue use and consult a physician if condition worsens or if symptoms persist for more than seven days.
Do not use on children under 2 years of age except under the advice and supervision of physician. Keep these and all drugs out of the reach of children.

Overdosage: In case of accidental ingestion, seek professional assistance or contact a Poison Control Center immediately.

Dosage and Administration: *For adults and children 2 years of age and older:* Gently massage into affected skin area not more than 3 or 4 times daily. *For children under 2 years of age,* there is no recommended dosage except under the advice and supervision of a physician.

How Supplied: DERMOLATE Anti-Itch Cream—30 g (1.0 oz.) tube, and 15 g (½ oz) tubes.
Store between 2° and 30°C (36° and 86°F).

DISOPHROL® Chronotab®
[*dĭ'sō-frōl*]
Sustained–Action Tablets

Description: EACH DISOPHROL® Chronotab® SUSTAINED-ACTION TABLET CONTAINS: 120 mg of pseu-

doephedrine sulfate and 6 mg of dexbrompheniramine maleate. Half of the medication is released after the tablet is swallowed and the remaining amount of medication is released hours later providing continuous long-lasting relief for 12 hours. Also contains: Acacia, Butylparaben, Calcium Sulfate, Carnauba Wax, Corn Starch, FD&C Yellow No. 6 Al Lake, FD&C Red No. 40 Al Lake, Gelatin, Lactose, Magnesium Stearate, Neutral Soap, Oleic Acid, Povidone, Rosin, Sugar, Talc, White Wax, Zein.

Indications: For temporary relief of nasal congestion due to the common cold, hay fever, or other upper respiratory allergies, and associated with sinusitis. Helps decongest sinus openings, sinus passages. Reduces swelling of nasal passages; shrinks swollen membranes; and temporarily restores freer breathing through the nose. Alleviates running nose, sneezing, itching of the nose or throat, and itchy and watery eyes as may occur in allergic rhinitis (such as hay fever).

Warnings: If symptoms do not improve within 7 days or are accompanied by fever, consult a physician before continuing use. May cause excitability especially in children. Do not exceed recommended dosage because at higher doses nervousness, dizziness, or sleeplessness may occur. Do not take this product if you have asthma, glaucoma, emphysema, chronic pulmonary disease, shortness of breath, difficulty in breathing, heart disease, high blood pressure, thyroid disease, diabetes, or difficulty in urination due to enlargement of the prostate gland or give this product to children under 12 years, unless directed by a physician. May cause drowsiness; alcohol may increase the drowsiness effect. Avoid alcoholic beverages while taking this product. Use caution when driving a motor vehicle or operating machinery. Keep this and all drugs out of the reach of children. In case of accidental overdose, seek professional assistance or contact a Poison Control Center immediately. As with any drug, if you are pregnant or nursing a baby, seek the advice of a health professional before using this product.

Drug Interaction Precaution: Do not take this product if you are presently taking a prescription drug for high blood pressure or depression, without first consulting your physician.

Dosage and Administration: ADULTS AND CHILDREN 12 YEARS AND OVER—one tablet every 12 hours. Do not exceed two tablets in 24 hours.

How Supplied: DISOPHROL Chronotab Sustained-Action Tablets, sugarcoated, cherry-red tablets branded in black with either the product identification code 85-WMH or one of the Schering trademarks and the numbers, 231; bottle of 100.
Store between 2° and 30°C (36° and 86°F).
© 1982, 1985, Schering Corporation.

DRIXORAL®
[*dricks-or'al*]
Antihistamine/Nasal Decongestant Syrup

Description: Each 5 ml (1 teaspoonful) of DRIXORAL Syrup contains 2 mg brompheniramine maleate and 30 mg pseudoephedrine sulfate; also contains Citric Acid, D&C Red No. 33, FD&C Yellow No. 6, Flavor, Propylene Glycol, Sodium Benzoate, Sodium Citrate, Sorbitol, Sugar, Water. Drixoral Syrup is alcohol-free.

Indications: DRIXORAL Syrup contains a nasal decongestant with an antihistamine in a pleasant-tasting wild cherry flavor to provide temporary relief of nasal congestion due to the common cold, hay fever or other upper respiratory allergies. Helps decongest sinus openings, sinus passages. Alleviates running nose, sneezing, itching of the nose or throat, and itchy and watery eyes due to hay fever. DRIXORAL Syrup is ideal for adults and children who prefer a syrup instead of tablets or capsules.

Warnings: If symptoms do not improve within 7 days or are accompanied by fever, consult a physician before continuing use. May cause drowsiness. May cause excitability especially in children. Do not exceed recommended dosage because at higher doses nervousness, dizziness, or sleeplessness may occur. Do not give this product to children under 6 years except under the advice and supervision of a physician. Do not take this product if you have asthma, glaucoma, emphysema, chronic pulmonary disease, shortness of breath, difficulty in breathing, difficulty in urination due to enlargement of the prostate gland, high blood pressure, heart disease, diabetes, or thyroid disease except under the advice and supervision of a physician. As with any drug, if you are pregnant or nursing a baby, seek the advice of a health professional before using this product. CAUTION: Avoid driving a motor vehicle or operating heavy machinery. Avoid alcoholic beverages while taking this product. Keep this and all drugs out of the reach of children. In case of accidental overdose, seek professional assistance or contact a Poison Control Center immediately.

Drug Interaction Precaution: Do not take this product if you are presently taking a prescription drug for high blood pressure or depression, without first consulting your doctor.

Directions: Adults and children 12 years of age and over: two teaspoonfuls every 4–6 hours. Children 6 to under 12 years of age: 1 teaspoonful every 4–6 hours. Do not exceed 4 doses in 24 hours. Children under 6 years of age, consult a physician.

Continued on next page

Schering—Cont.

Store between 2° and 30°C (36° and 86°F).

Overdosage: In case of accidental overdose, seek professional assistance or contact a Poison Control Center immediately.

How Supplied: DRIXORAL Syrup is available in 4 fl. oz. (118 ml) bottles. Copyright © 1984, 1985, Schering Corporation, Kenilworth, NJ, USA 07033. All rights reserved.

Shown in Product Identification Section, page 429

DRIXORAL®
[*dricks-or'al*]
Sustained-Action Tablets

Description: EACH DRIXORAL SUSTAINED-ACTION TABLET CONTAINS: 120 mg of pseudoephedrine sulfate and 6 mg of dexbrompheniramine maleate. Half of the medication is released after the tablet is swallowed and the remaining amount of medication is released hours later providing continuous long-lasting relief for 12 hours. Also contains: Acacia, Butylparaben, Calcium Sulfate, Carnauba Wax, Corn Starch, D&C Yellow No. 10 Al Lake, FD&C Blue No. 1 Al Lake, FD&C Yellow No. 6 Al Lake, Gelatin, Lactose, Magnesium Stearate, Neutral Soap, Oleic Acid, Povidone, Rosin, Sugar, Talc, White Wax, Zein.

Indications: For temporary relief of nasal congestion due to the common cold, hay fever, or other upper respiratory allergies, and associated with sinusitis. Helps decongest sinus openings, sinus passages. Reduces swelling of nasal passages; shrinks swollen membranes; and temporarily restores freer breathing through the nose. Alleviates running nose, sneezing, itching of the nose or throat, and itchy and watery eyes as may occur in allergic rhinitis (such as hay fever).

Actions: The antihistamine, dexbrompheniramine maleate, provides temporary relief of sneezing; watery, itchy eyes; running nose due to hay fever and other upper respiratory allergies. The decongestant, pseudoephedrine sulfate, temporarily restores freer breathing through the nose and promotes sinus drainage.

Warnings: If symptoms do not improve within 7 days or are accompanied by fever, consult a physician before continuing use. May cause excitability especially in children. Do not exceed recommended dosage because at higher doses nervousness, dizziness, or sleeplessness may occur. Do not take this product if you have asthma, glaucoma, emphysema, chronic pulmonary disease, high blood pressure, thyroid disease, diabetes, or difficulty in urination due to enlargement of the prostate gland or give this product to children under 12 years, unless directed by a physician. May cause drowsiness; alcohol may increase the drowsiness effect.

Avoid alcoholic beverages while taking this product. Use caution when driving a motor vehicle or operating machinery. Keep this and all drugs out of the reach of children. In case of accidental overdose, seek professional assistance or contact a Poison Control Center immediately. As with any drug, if you are pregnant or nursing a baby, seek the advice of a health professional before using this product.

Drug Interaction Precaution: Do not take this product if you are presently taking a prescription drug for high blood pressure or depression, without first consulting your physician.

Dosage and Administration: ADULTS AND CHILDREN 12 YEARS AND OVER—one tablet every 12 hours. Do not exceed two tablets in 24 hours.

How Supplied: DRIXORAL Sustained-Action Tablets, green, sugar-coated tablets branded in black with the product name, boxes of 10, 20, and 40, bottle of 100.

Store between 2° and 30°C (36° and 86°F).
© 1982, 1985, Schering Corporation.
Shown in Product Identification Section, page 429

DRIXORAL® PLUS
[*dricks-or'al*]
Extended-Release Tablets

Active Ingredients: Acetaminophen, Dexbrompheniramine Maleate, Pseudoephedrine Sulfate.

Also Contains: Calcium Phosphate, Carnauba Wax, D&C Yellow No. 10 Al Lake, FD&C Blue No. 1 Al Lake, FD&C Yellow No. 6 Al Lake, Hydroxypropyl Methylcellulose, Magnesium Stearate, Methylparaben, PEG, Propylparaben, Stearic Acid.
DRIXORAL® PLUS Extended-Release Tablets combine a nasal decongestant and an antihistamine with a nonaspirin analgesic in a special 12-hour continuous-acting timed-release tablet.

Indications: The *decongestant* temporarily relieves nasal congestion due to the common cold, hay fever or other upper respiratory allergies, and associated with sinusitis. Reduces swelling of nasal passages; shrinks swollen membranes; and temporarily restores freer breathing through the nose. Also helps decongest sinus openings, sinus passages. The *nonaspirin analgesic* temporarily relieves occasional minor aches, pains, and headache and reduces fever due to the common cold. The *antihistamine* alleviates running nose, sneezing, itching of the nose or throat, and itchy and watery eyes as may occur in allergic rhinitis (such as hay fever).

EACH DRIXORAL PLUS EXTENDED-RELEASE TABLET CONTAINS: 60 mg of pseudoephedrine sulfate, 3 mg of dexbrompheniramine maleate and 500 mg of acetaminophen. These ingredients are released continuously, providing long-lasting relief for 12 hours.

Directions: ADULTS AND CHILDREN 12 YEARS AND OVER—two tablets every 12 hours. Do not exceed four tablets in 24 hours. Children under 12 years of age: consult a doctor.

Warnings: Do not take this product for more than 7 days. If symptoms do not improve, or are accompanied by fever that lasts for more than three days (72 hours) or recurs, or if new symptoms occur, consult a physician before continuing use. If pain or fever persists or gets worse, or if redness or swelling is present, consult a physician because these could be signs of a serious condition. May cause excitability especially in children. Do not exceed recommended dosage because at higher doses nervousness, dizziness, or sleeplessness may occur. Do not take this product if you have asthma, glaucoma, emphysema, chronic pulmonary disease, shortness of breath, difficulty in breathing, heart disease, high blood pressure, thyroid disease, difficulty in urination due to enlargement of the prostate gland, or give this product to children under 12 years unless directed by a physician. May cause drowsiness; alcohol, sedatives, and tranquilizers may increase the drowsiness effect. Avoid alcoholic beverages while taking this product. Use caution when driving a motor vehicle or operating machinery. Keep this and all drugs out of the reach of children. In case of accidental overdose, seek professional assistance or contact a Poison Control Center immediately. Prompt medical attention is critical for adults as well as for children even if you do not notice any signs or symptoms. As with any drug, if you are pregnant or nursing a baby, seek the advice of a health professional before using this product.

Drug Interaction Precaution: Do not take this product if you are presently taking a prescription drug for high blood pressure or depression, sedatives or tranquilizers, without first consulting your physician.

How Supplied: DRIXORAL PLUS Extended-Release Tablets are available in boxes of 12's and 24's and bottles of 48.
Store between 2° and 30°C (36° and 86°F).
Protect from excessive moisture.
Shown in Product Identification Section, page 429

EMKO® BECAUSE®
[*em'ko bē-koz'*]
Vaginal Contraceptive Foam

Description: A non-hormonal, non-scented aerosol foam contraceptive in a portable applicator/foam unit containing six applications of an 8.0% concentration of the spermicide nonoxynol-9. Also contains: Benzethonium Chloride, Glyceryl Monostearate, PEG, Pluronic F-68 (Poloxamer 188), Quaternium-15, Stearic Acid, Triethanolamine, and Water.

Indications: Vaginal contraceptive intended for the prevention of pregnancy.

BECAUSE Foam provides effective protection alone or it may be used instead of spermicidal jelly or cream to give added protection with a diaphragm.

BECAUSE Foam also may be used to give added protection to other methods of contraception: with a condom; as a backup to the IUD or oral contraceptives during the first month of use; in the event more than one oral contraceptive pill is forgotten and extra protection is needed during that menstrual cycle.

Actions: Each applicatorful of BECAUSE Foam provides the correct amount of nonoxynol-9, the most widely used spermicide, to prevent pregnancy effectively. The foam covers the inside of the vagina and forms a layer of spermicidal material between the sperm and the cervix. The powerful spermicide prevents pregnancy by killing sperm after contact. BECAUSE Foam is effective immediately upon insertion. No waiting period is needed for effervescing or melting to take place since BECAUSE is introduced into the vagina as a foam.

Warnings: If vaginal or penile irritation occurs and continues, a physician should be consulted. Not effective orally. Where pregnancy is contraindicated, further individualization of the contraceptive program may be needed. Do not burn, incinerate or puncture container. Keep this and all drugs out of the reach of children and in case of accidental ingestion, call a Poison Control Center, emergency medical facility, or a doctor.

Dosage and Administration: Although no contraceptive can guarantee 100% effectiveness, for reliable protection against pregnancy follow directions. One applicatorful of BECAUSE Contraceptive Foam must be inserted before each act of sexual intercourse. BECAUSE Foam can be inserted immediately or up to one hour before intercourse. If more than one hour has passed before intercourse or if intercourse is repeated, another applicatorful of BECAUSE Foam must be inserted.

Directions for Use: The BECAUSE CONTRACEPTOR has a foam container attached to an applicator barrel.

With the container pushed all the way into the barrel, shake well. Pull the container upward until it stops. Tilt container to side to release foam into barrel. Allow foam to fill barrel to about one inch from end and return container to straight position. Foam will expand to fill remainder of barrel.

Hold contraceptor at top of the barrel part and gently insert applicator barrel deep into the vagina (close to the cervix). For ease of insertion, lie on your back with knees bent. With applicator barrel in place, push container all the way into the barrel. This deposits the foam properly. Remove the Contraceptor with the container still pushed all the way in the applicator barrel to avoid withdrawing any of the foam. No waiting period is needed before intercourse. BECAUSE Contraceptive Foam is effective immediately after proper insertion.

As with other vaginal contraceptive foam, cream and jelly products, douching is *not* recommended after using BECAUSE Foam. However, if douching is desired for cleansing purposes, you *must* wait at least six hours following your last act of sexual intercourse to allow BECAUSE Foam's full spermicidal activity to take place. Refer to package insert directions and diagrams for further details and applicator cleansing instructions.

How to Use the BECAUSE CONTRACEPTOR with a Diaphragm.

Insert one applicatorful of BECAUSE Foam directly into the vagina according to above directions and then insert diaphragm. After insertion, BECAUSE Foam is effective immediately and remains effective up to one hour before intercourse. If more than one hour has passed or you are going to repeat intercourse, insert another applicatorful of BECAUSE Foam *without removing your diaphragm.*

Storage: Contents under pressure. Do not burn, incinerate, or puncture the applicator. Store at normal room temperature. Do not expose to extreme heat or open flame or store at temperatures above 120°F. If stored at temperatures below 60°F, warm to room temperature before using.

How Supplied: Disposable 10 gm CONTRACEPTOR containing six applications of BECAUSE Contraceptive Foam. This foam is also available in the original form of EMKO® Foam with the regular applicator.

Copyright © 1985, Schering Corporation

Shown in Product Identification Section, page 429

EMKO®
[em 'kō]
Vaginal Contraceptive Foam

Description: A non-hormonal, non-scented aerosol foam contraceptive containing an 8.0% concentration of the spermicide nonoxynol-9. Also contains: Benzethonium Chloride, Glyceryl Monostearate, PEG, Pluronic F-68 (Poloxamer 188), Quaternium-15, Stearic Acid, Triethanolamine, and Water.

Indications: Vaginal contraceptive intended for the prevention of pregnancy. EMKO Foam provides effective protection alone or it may be used instead of spermicidal jelly or cream to give added protection with a diaphragm.

EMKO Foam also may be used to give added protection to other methods of contraception: with a condom; as a backup to the IUD or oral contraceptives during the first month of use; in the event more than one oral contraceptive pill is forgotten and extra protection is needed during that menstrual cycle.

Actions: Each applicatorful of EMKO Foam provides the correct amount of nonoxynol-9, the most widely used spermicide, to prevent pregnancy effectively. The foam covers the inside of the vagina and forms a layer of spermicidal material between the sperm and the cervix.

The powerful spermicide prevents pregnancy by killing sperm after contact. EMKO Foam is effective immediately upon insertion. No waiting period is needed for effervescing or melting to take place since EMKO is introduced into the vagina as a foam.

Warnings: If vaginal or penile irritation occurs and continues, a physician should be consulted. Where pregnancy is contraindicated, further individualization of the contraceptive program may be needed. Do not burn, incinerate or puncture can. Keep this and all drugs out of the reach of children and in case of accidental ingestion, call a Poison Control Center, emergency medical facility, or a doctor.

Dosage and Administration: Although no contraceptive can guarantee 100% effectiveness, for reliable protection against pregnancy read and follow directions carefully. One applicatorful of EMKO Contraceptive Foam must be inserted before each act of sexual intercourse. EMKO Foam can be inserted immediately or up to one hour before intercourse. If more than one hour has passed before intercourse or if intercourse is repeated, another applicatorful of EMKO Foam must be inserted.

Directions for Use:
Check Foam Supply with Weigh Cap.
With the cap on the can, hold the can in midair by the white button. As long as the black is showing, a full dose of foam is available. When the black begins to disappear, purchase a new can of EMKO Foam. USE *only if black is showing* to assure a full application. SHAKE CAN WELL before filling applicator. *Remove cap and place the can in an upright position on a level surface.* Place the EMKO regular applicator in an upright position over valve on top of can. Press down on the applicator gently. Allow foam to fill to the ridge in applicator barrel. The plunger will rise up as the foam fills the applicator. Remove the filled applicator from the can to stop flow. Hold the filled applicator by the barrel and gently insert deep into the vagina (close to the cervix). For ease of insertion, lie on your back with knees bent. With the applicator in place, push plunger into applicator until it stops. This deposits the foam properly. Remove the applicator with the plunger still pushed all the way in to avoid withdrawing any of the foam. No waiting period is needed before intercourse. EMKO Contraceptive Foam is effective immediately after proper insertion. As with other vaginal contraceptive foam, cream, and jelly products, douching is *not* recommended after using EMKO Foam. However, if douching is desired for cleansing purposes, you *must* wait at least six hours following your last act of sexual intercourse to allow EMKO

Continued on next page

Information on Schering products appearing on these pages is effective as of November 1, 1989.

Schering—Cont.

Foam's full spermicidal activity to take place. Refer to package insert directions and diagrams for further details and applicator cleansing instructions.

How to Use EMKO with a Diaphragm. Insert one applicatorful of EMKO Foam directly into the vagina according to above directions and then insert your diaphragm. After insertion, EMKO Foam is effective immediately and remains effective up to one hour before intercourse. If more than one hour has passed or you are going to repeat intercourse, insert another applicatorful of EMKO Foam *without removing your diaphragm.*

Storage: Contents under pressure. Do not burn, incinerate or puncture can. Store at normal room temperature. Do not expose to extreme heat or open flame or store at temperatures above 120°F. If stored at temperatures below 60°F, warm to room temperature before using.

How Supplied: EMKO Contraceptive Foam, 40 gm can with applicator and storage purse. Refill cans without applicator and purse available in 40 gm and 90 gm sizes. All sizes feature a unique weighing cap that indicates when a new foam supply is needed. EMKO Foam also comes in the convenient BECAUSE® CONTRACEPTOR®, a portable six-use, combination foam/applicator unit.
Copyright © 1985, Schering Corporation
Shown in Product Identification Section, page 429

MOL–IRON®
[mōl-i ′ern]
Tablets
Tablets with Vitamin C

Active Ingredients: MOL-IRON products are highly effective and unusually well tolerated even by children and pregnant women.
Tablets: Each tablet contains 195 mg ferrous sulfate, USP (39 mg elemental iron). Tablets with Vitamin C: Each tablet contains 195 mg ferrous sulfate (39 mg elemental iron) and 75 mg ascorbic acid.

Inactive Ingredients: Each MOL-IRON Tablet contains Acacia, Butylparaben, Calcium Sulfate, Carnauba Wax, FD&C Blue No. 1 Aluminum Lake, FD&C Red No. 40 Aluminum Lake, Magnesium Stearate, Povidone, Stearic Acid, Sugar, Talc, Titanium Dioxide, White Wax.
In addition to the above ingredients, MOL-IRON Tablets with Vitamin C contain confectioners glaze.

Indications: For the prevention and treatment of iron-deficiency anemias.

Warnings: Keep these and all drugs out of the reach of children. In case of accidental overdose, seek professional assistance or contact a Poison Control Center immediately. As with any drug, if you are pregnant or nursing a baby, seek the advice of a health professional before using this product.

Dosage and Administration: Tablets—(Taken preferably after meals): Adults and Children 12 years and older—1 or 2 tablets 3 times daily; Children 6 through 11 years—1 tablet 3 times daily; or as prescribed by a physician. Tablets with Vitamin C—(Taken preferably after meals): Adults and Children 12 years and older—1 or 2 tablets 3 times daily; Children 6 through 11 years—1 tablet 3 times daily; or as prescribed by a physician.

How Supplied: MOL-IRON Tablets—brownish colored tablets, bottles of 100; MOL-IRON Tablets with Vitamin C—bottles of 100.
Store between 2° and 30°C (36° and 86°F).

TINACTIN® Antifungal
[tin-ak ′tin]
Cream 1%
Solution 1%
Powder 1%
Powder (1%) Aerosol
Liquid (1%) Aerosol
Jock Itch Cream 1%
Jock Itch Spray Powder 1%

Description: TINACTIN Cream 1% is a white homogeneous, nonaqueous preparation containing the highly active synthetic fungicidal agent, tolnaftate. Each gram contains 10 mg tolnaftate solubilized in BHT, Carbomer 934 P, Monoamylamine, PEG, Propylene Glycol, and Titanium Dioxide.
TINACTIN Jock Itch Cream 1% is a smooth white homogeneous cream containing the highly active synthetic fungicidal agent, tolnaftate. Each gram contains 10 mg tolnaftate finely dispersed in a water-washable emulsion containing: Cetearyl Alcohol, Ceteareth-30, Chlorocresol, Mineral Oil, Petrolatum, Propylene Glycol, Sodium Phosphate and Water. Phosphoric acid and sodium hydroxide used to adjust pH.
TINACTIN Solution 1% contains in each ml tolnaftate 10 mg, BHT, and PEG. The solution solidifies at low temperatures but liquefies readily when warmed, retaining its potency.
TINACTIN Liquid Aerosol contains 91 mg tolnaftate in a vehicle of Alcohol SD-40-2 (36% w/w), BHT and PPG-12 Buteth-16. The spray deposits solution containing a concentration of 1% tolnaftate.
Each gram of **TINACTIN Powder 1%** contains tolnaftate 10 mg in a vehicle of corn starch and talc.
TINACTIN Powder Aerosol contains 91 mg tolnaftate in a vehicle of Alcohol SD-40-2 (14% w/w), BHT, Hydrocarbon Propellant, PPG-12 Buteth-16 and Talc. The spray deposits a white clinging powder containing a concentration of 1% tolnaftate.
TINACTIN Jock Itch Spray Powder contains 91 mg tolnaftate in a vehicle of Alcohol SD-40-2 (14% w/w), BHT, Hydrocarbon Propellant, PPG-12 Buteth-16, Talc. The spray deposits a white clinging powder containing a concentration of 1% tolnaftate.

Indications: TINACTIN Cream, Solution, Liquid Aerosol and TINACTIN Jock Itch Cream are highly active antifungal agents that are effective in killing superficial fungi of the skin which cause tinea pedis (athlete's foot), tinea cruris (jock itch) and tinea corporis (body ringworm).
TINACTIN Powder, Powder Aerosol and TINACTIN Jock Itch Spray Powder are effective in killing superficial fungi of the skin which cause tinea cruris (jock itch) and tinea pedis (athlete's foot). All forms begin to relieve burning, itching and soreness within 24 hours. The powder and powder aerosol forms aid the drying of naturally moist areas.

Actions: The active ingredient in TINACTIN, tolnaftate, is a highly active synthetic fungicidal agent that is effective in the treatment of superficial fungous infections of the skin. It is inactive systemically, virtually nonsensitizing, and does not ordinarily sting or irritate intact or broken skin, even in the presence of acute inflammatory reactions. TINACTIN products are odorless, greaseless, and do not stain or discolor the skin, hair, or nails.

Warnings: Keep these and all drugs out of the reach of children. Do not use in children under 2 years of age except under the advice and supervision of a physician.
TINACTIN Powder Aerosol and **Liquid Aerosol:** Avoid spraying in eyes. Contents under pressure. Do not puncture or incinerate. Flammable mixture, do not use or store near heat or open flame. Exposure to temperatures above 120°F may cause bursting. Never throw container into fire or incinerator. Use only as directed. Intentional misuse by deliberately concentrating and inhaling the contents can be harmful or fatal.

Precautions: If irritation occurs or symptoms do not improve within 10 days, discontinue use and consult your physician or podiatrist.
TINACTIN products are for external use only. Keep out of eyes.
TINACTIN is not effective on nail or scalp infections.

Overdosage: In case of accidental ingestion, seek professional assistance or contact a Poison Control Center immediately.

Dosage and Administration: Children under 12 years of age should be supervised in the use of TINACTIN.
TINACTIN Cream and TINACTIN Jock Itch Cream—Wash and dry infected area. Then apply one-half inch ribbon of cream and rub gently on infected area morning and evening or as directed by a doctor. Spread evenly. Best results in athlete's foot and body ringworm are usually obtained with 4 weeks' use of this product and in jock itch, with 2 weeks' use. To help prevent recurrence of athlete's foot, continue treatment for two weeks after disappearance of all symptoms.

TINACTIN Solution—Wash and dry infected area. Then apply two or three drops morning and evening or as directed by a doctor, and massage gently to cover the infected area. Best results in athlete's foot and body ringworm are usually obtained with 4 weeks' use of this product and in jock itch, with 2 weeks' use. To help prevent recurrence of athlete's foot, continue treatment for two weeks after disappearance of all symptoms.

TINACTIN Liquid Aerosol—Wash and dry infected area. Spray from a distance of 6 to 10 inches morning and evening or as directed by a doctor. For athlete's foot, spray between toes and on feet. For jock itch, spray infected area. Best results in athlete's foot are usually obtained with 4 weeks' use of this product and in jock itch, with 2 weeks' use. Continue treatment for two weeks after symptoms disappear. To help prevent reinfection of athlete's foot, bathe daily, dry carefully and apply **TINACTIN Powder** daily.

TINACTIN Powder—Wash and dry infected area. Sprinkle powder liberally on all areas of infection and in shoes or socks morning and evening or as directed by a doctor. Best results in athlete's foot are usually obtained with 4 weeks' use of this product and in jock itch, with 2 weeks' use. Continue treatment for two weeks after symptoms disappear. To prevent recurrence of athlete's foot, bathe daily, dry carefully and apply **TINACTIN Powder.**

TINACTIN Powder Aerosol and **TINACTIN Jock Itch Spray Powder**—Wash and dry infected area. Shake container well before using. Spray liberally from a distance of 6 to 10 inches onto affected area morning and night or as directed by a doctor. Best results in athlete's foot are usually obtained with 4 weeks' use of this product and in jock itch, with 2 weeks' use. To help prevent recurrence of athlete's foot, bathe daily, dry carefully and apply **TINACTIN Powder Aerosol.**

How Supplied: TINACTIN Antifungal Cream 1%, 15 g (½ oz) and 30 g (1 oz) collapsible tube with dispensing tip. **TINACTIN Antifungal Solution 1%,** 10 ml (⅓ oz) plastic squeeze bottle. **TINACTIN Antifungal Liquid (1%) Aerosol,** 113 g (4 oz) spray can. **TINACTIN Antifungal Powder 1%,** 45 g (1.5 oz) and 90 g (3.0 oz) plastic containers. **TINACTIN Antifungal Powder (1%) Aerosol,** 100 g (3.5 oz) and 150 g (5.0 oz) spray containers. **TINACTIN Antifungal Jock Itch Cream 1%,** 15 g (½ oz) collapsible tube with dispensing tip. **TINACTIN Antifungal Jock Itch Spray Powder (1%),** 100 g (3.5 oz) spray can.

Store TINACTIN products between 36° and 86°F (2° and 30°C).

© 1984, 1985, 1987 Schering Corporation, Kenilworth NJ 07033
Shown in Product Identification Section, page 429

Schwarz Pharma
Kremers Urban Company
P.O. BOX 2038
MILWAUKEE, WI 53201

FEDAHIST® Decongestant Syrup
FEDAHIST® Tablets
[*fed 'a-hist "*]

Description: Decongestant Syrup: Each 5 mL (teaspoonful) of FEDAHIST® Decongestant Syrup contains 30 mg of pseudoephedrine hydrochloride USP and 2 mg of chlorpheniramine maleate USP.
Tablets: Each FEDAHIST® Tablet contains 60 mg of pseudoephedrine hydrochloride USP and 4 mg of chlorpheniramine maleate USP.
Inactive Ingredients: Decongestant Syrup: citric acid, FD&C blue No. 1, FD&C red No. 40, flavors, glycerin, methylparaben, purified water, saccharin sodium, sodium benzoate, sorbitol solution, sucrose and other ingredients.
Tablets: colloidal silicon dioxide, lactose, magnesium stearate, microcrystalline cellulose, stearic acid, and talc.

Indications: For the temporary relief of nasal congestion, runny nose, sneezing, itching of the nose or throat, and itchy, watery eyes due to the common cold, hay fever, sinusitis, or other upper respiratory allergies.

Warnings: May cause excitability, especially in children. May cause drowsiness; alcohol, sedatives, and tranquilizers may increase the drowsiness effect. Avoid alcoholic beverages while taking this product. Do not take this product if you are taking sedatives or tranquilizers without first consulting your doctor. Use caution when driving a motor vehicle or operating machinery. Do not exceed recommended dosage because at higher doses nervousness, dizziness or sleeplessness may occur. If symptoms do not improve within 7 days, or are accompanied by high fever, consult a doctor before continuing use. Do not take this product if you have high blood pressure, heart disease, diabetes, thyroid disease, asthma, glaucoma, emphysema, chronic pulmonary disease, shortness of breath, difficulty in breathing or difficulty in urination due to enlargement of the prostate gland unless directed by a doctor. As with any drug, if you are pregnant or nursing a baby, seek the advice of a health professional before using this product.
Keep this and all medications out of children's reach. In case of accidental overdose contact a doctor or poison control center immediately.
Drug Interaction Precaution: Do not take this product if you are presently taking a prescription drug for high blood pressure or depression without first consulting your doctor.

Directions: Decongestant Syrup: *Adults and children 12 years of age and older:* 2 teaspoonfuls every 4 to 6 hours not to exceed 8 teaspoonfuls in 24 hours.
Children 6 to under 12 years of age: 1 teaspoonful every 4 to 6 hours not to exceed 4 teaspoonfuls in 24 hours.
Children under 6 years of age: consult a doctor.
Professional Labeling: *Children 2 to under 6 years of age:* ½ teaspoonful every 4 to 6 hours not to exceed 2 teaspoonfuls in 24 hours.
Tablets: *Adults and children 12 years of age and older:* 1 tablet every 4 to 6 hours not to exceed 4 tablets in 24 hours.
Children 6 to under 12 years of age: ½ tablet every 4 to 6 hours not to exceed 2 tablets in 24 hours.
Children under 6 years of age: consult a doctor.

How Supplied: FEDAHIST Decongestant Syrup is a grape-colored and flavored syrup in 4 oz bottles (NDC 0091-0052-04).
FEDAHIST Tablets are white, scored and imprinted with "KU" on one side and "050" on the other. Bottles of 100 tablets (NDC 0091-0050-01) and blister packs of 24 tablets (NDC 0091-0050-24). Store at controlled room temperature 15°–30° C (59°–86° F).
Shown in Product Identification Section, page 430

FEDAHIST® Expectorant Syrup
FEDAHIST® Expectorant Pediatric Drops
[*fed 'a-hist "*]

Description: Expectorant Syrup: Each 5 mL (teaspoonful) of FEDAHIST® Expectorant Syrup contains 30 mg of pseudoephedrine hydrochloride USP and 200 mg of guaifenesin USP.
Expectorant Pediatric Drops: Each mL of FEDAHIST® Expectorant Pediatric Drops contains 7.5 mg of pseudoephedrine hydrochloride USP and 40 mg of guaifenesin USP.
Inactive Ingredients: Expectorant Syrup: benzoic acid, citric acid, FD&C red No. 40, flavors, glycerin, polyethylene glycol, povidone, purified water, saccharin sodium, sodium citrate, sorbitol solution, and other ingredients.
Expectorant Pediatric Drops: benzoic acid, citric acid, FD&C yellow No. 6, flavors, glycerin, polyethylene glycol, povidone, purified water, saccharin sodium, sodium citrate, sorbitol solution, and other ingredients.

Indications: Helps loosen phlegm (sputum) and thin bronchial secretions to rid the bronchial passageways of bothersome mucus, and makes coughs more productive. For the temporary relief of nasal and bronchial congestion due to the common cold, sinusitis, hay fever, or other upper respiratory allergies.

Warnings: Do not take this product for persistent or chronic cough such as occurs with smoking, asthma, chronic bronchitis, or emphysema, or where cough is accompanied by excessive phlegm (sputum) unless directed by a doctor. A persistent cough may be a sign of a serious condition. If cough persists

Continued on next page

Schwarz Pharma—Cont.

for more than 1 week, tends to recur, or is accompanied by fever, rash, or persistent headache, consult a doctor.

Do not exceed recommended dosage because at higher doses nervousness, dizziness, or sleeplessness may occur. Do not take this product for more than 7 days. If symptoms do not improve or are accompanied by fever, consult a doctor. Do not take this product if you have heart disease, high blood pressure, thyroid disease, diabetes, or difficulty in urination due to enlargement of the prostate gland unless directed by a doctor.

As with any drug, if you are pregnant or nursing a baby, seek the advice of a health professional before using this product.

Keep this and all medications out of children's reach. In case of accidental overdose, contact a doctor or poison control center immediately.

Drug Interaction Precaution: Do not take this product if you are presently taking a prescription drug for high blood pressure or depression without first consulting your doctor.

Directions: Expectorant Syrup: *Adults and children 12 years of age and older:* 2 teaspoonfuls every 4 to 6 hours not to exceed 8 teaspoonfuls in 24 hours.
Children 6 to under 12 years of age: 1 teaspoonful every 4 to 6 hours not to exceed 4 teaspoonfuls in 24 hours.
Children 2 to under 6 years of age: ½ teaspoonful every 4 to 6 hours not to exceed 2 teaspoonfuls in 24 hours.
Children under 2 years of age: consult a doctor.

Expectorant Pediatric Drops: Take by mouth only.
Children 6 to under 12 years of age: 4 mL every 4 to 6 hours not to exceed 4 doses (16 mL) in 24 hours.
Children 2 to under 6 years of age: 2 mL every 4 to 6 hours not to exceed 4 doses (8 mL) in 24 hours.
Professional Labeling: *Children under 2 years of age:* The dose should be adjusted to age or weight and be given every 4 to 6 hours not to exceed 4 doses in 24 hours.

Age or Weight	Starting Dose
1–3 months (8–12 lb)	¼ mL
4–6 months (13–17 lb)	½ mL
7–9 months (18–20 lb)	¾ mL
10–23 months (21–30 lb)	1 mL

How Supplied: FEDAHIST Expectorant Syrup is a red-colored and fruit-flavored syrup in 4 oz bottles (NDC 0091-0057-04).
FEDAHIST Expectorant Pediatric Drops is an orange-colored and fruit-flavored solution in 1 oz bottles (NDC 0091-0051-30).
Store at controlled room temperature 15°–30°C (59°–86°F).

Shown in Product Identification Section, page 430

LACTRASE® Capsules
[lăk 'trās]
(lactase)

Description: Each LACTRASE® Capsule contains 250 mg of standardized lactase dispersed in a lactose-free base.
Inactive Ingredients: gelatin, magnesium stearate, maltodextrin, red iron oxide, titanium dioxide, yellow iron oxide, and other ingredients.

Indications: LACTRASE is indicated for individuals exhibiting symptoms of lactose intolerance or lactase insufficiency as identified by a lactose tolerance test or by exhibiting gastrointestinal disturbances after consumption of milk or dairy products.

Action: Though lactase is normally present in adequate quantities in infants, in many populations its concentration naturally declines starting at about 4–5 years of age and is low in a substantial number of individuals by their teens or early 20s. Within certain geographic and ethnic groups, especially in adult Blacks, Orientals, American Indians, and Eastern European Jews, the lactase activity may be even lower earlier. Although many of them can easily digest smaller quantities of lactose in milk, after consumption of an excessive volume of milk or dairy products, they may exhibit symptoms of lactose intolerance.
Lactose is a nonabsorbable disaccharide found as a common constituent in most dairy products. Under normal conditions, dietary lactose is hydrolyzed in the jejunum and proximal ileum by beta-D-galactosidase or lactase. Lactase is produced in the brush border of the columnar epithelial cells of the intestinal villi. Lactase hydrolyzes lactose into two monosaccharides, glucose and galactose, that are readily absorbed by the intestine.
When available lactase is insufficient to split the lactose, the unabsorbable sugar remains in the small intestine for an extended period, presenting an osmotic load that increases and retains intraluminal fluid and intensifies intestinal motility; thus the individual reports a bloated feeling and cramps. The undigested lactose is decomposed by the intestinal flora in the lower intestine and excessive carbon dioxide and hydrogen is produced. These gases contribute to flatulence and increased abdominal discomfort. The lactic acid and other short-chain acids raise the osmolality, hinder fluid reabsorption and decrease transit time of the contents of the colon, leading to diarrhea. Often hydrogen is noticed in the expired breath of a lactase-deficient patient.

Precautions: It should be noted that in diabetic persons who use LACTRASE, the milk sugar will be metabolically available and may result in increased blood glucose levels. Individuals with galactosemia may not have milk in any form, lactose enzyme modified or not.

Directions: Generally, one or two LACTRASE Capsules swallowed **with**

milk or dairy products is all that is necessary to digest the milk sugar contained in a normal serving. If the individual is severely intolerant to lactose, additional capsules may be taken until a satisfactory response is achieved as recognized by resolution of the symptoms. LACTRASE Capsules are safe to take and higher quantities in severe cases will be well-tolerated.
If the individual cannot swallow capsules, the contents of the capsules may be sprinkled onto dairy products before consuming. LACTRASE will not alter the taste of the dairy product when used in this manner.
Milk may also be pretreated with LACTRASE; simply add the contents from one or two capsules to each quart of milk, shake gently, and store the milk in the refrigerator for 24 hours. LACTRASE will break down milk sugars to digestible simple sugars. LACTRASE powder will not alter the appearance of milk; however the taste may be slightly sweeter than untreated milk.

How Supplied: LACTRASE Capsules are opaque orange and opaque white and are imprinted "KREMERS URBAN" and "505". They are supplied in blister packs containing 10 capsules (NDC 0091-3505-10) or 30 capsules (NDC 0091-3505-03) and in bottles containing 100 capsules (NDC 0091-3505-01).
Store at controlled room temperature 15°–30°C (59°–86°F).

Shown in Product Identification Section, page 430

EDUCATIONAL MATERIAL

Good News For People Who Can't Digest Milk.
For people who cannot digest dairy products because they lack the enzyme necessary for the digestion of milk sugar, this pamphlet explains how the problem comes about, its symptoms and how it can be treated with Lactrase®, an enzyme supplement. A table addressing the lactose content of food is included.

Scot-Tussin Pharmacal Co., Inc.
**50 CLEMENCE STREET
CRANSTON, RI 02920-0217**

SCOT–TUSSIN® Sugar-Free DM
No Sugar, Alcohol, Sorbitol, Sodium, Cholesterol or Decongestant
COUGH & COLD MEDICINE

Composition: Each 5 ml (1 teaspoonful) contains:
Dextromethorphan
HBr., USP .... 15 mg.
Chlorpheniramine
Maleate, USP .... 2 mg.
Recommended for use by diabetics and others on sugar restricted diets.

How Supplied: Bottles of 4 fl. oz. (NDC 0372-0036-04)

**SCOT–TUSSIN® Sugar-Free
Expectorant
No Sugar, Sodium, Dye, Cholesterol**

Composition: Each 5 ml (1 teaspoonful) contains:
Guaifenesin, USP......................... 100 mg
Alcohol 3.5 per cent
Recommended for use by diabetics and others on sugar restricted diets.

How Supplied: Bottles of 4 fl. oz. (NDC 0372-0006-04).

SmithKline Beecham Consumer Brands
**Unit of SmithKline Beecham Inc.
POST OFFICE BOX 1467
PITTSBURGH, PA 15230**

**A–200® Pediculicide Shampoo
Concentrate
A–200® Pediculicide Gel
Concentrate**

Description: Active ingredients: Pyrethrins 0.33%, piperonyl butoxide technical 4% (equivalent to 3.2% butylcarbityl (6-propylpiperonyl) ether) and 0.8% related compounds. **Inactive Ingredients:** Shampoo—Benzyl alcohol, Butyl Stearate, Fragrance, Mineral Spirits, Octoxynol 9, Oleic Acid, Oleoresin Parsley Seed and Water. Gel—Benzyl alcohol, Butyl Stearate, Carbomer 940, Fragrance, Mineral Spirits, Octoxynol 9, Oleic Acid, Oleoresin Parsley Seed, Triisopropanolamine, and Water.

Inert ingredients: 95.67%.

Indications: A-200 is indicated for the treatment of human pediculosis—head lice, body lice and pubic lice, and their eggs. A-200 Gel is specially formulated for pubic lice and head lice in children, where control of application is desirable.

Actions: A-200 is an effective pediculicide for control of head lice (*Pediculus humanus capitis*), pubic lice (*Phthirus pubis*) and body lice (*Pediculus humanus corporis*), and their nits.

Warnings: May cause eye injury. Do not get in eyes or permit contact with mucous membranes. Harmful if swallowed. Wash thoroughly after handling. Do not leave children unattended with product on their heads.

Drug Interaction: NOT TO BE USED BY PERSONS ALLERGIC TO RAGWEED. If skin irritation or infection is present or develops, discontinue use and consult a physician.

Precaution: If in Eyes: Flush with plenty of water. Get medical attention.

Symptoms and Treatment of Oral Overdosage: If swallowed: Call a physician, local Poison Control Center, or the Rocky Mountain Poison Control Center at 303-592-1710 (Collect) 24 hours a day. Drink 1 or 2 glasses of water and induce vomiting by touching the back of throat with finger. Do not induce vomiting or give anything by mouth to an unconscious person.

Dosage and Administration: It is a violation of Federal law to use this product in a manner inconsistent with its labeling.

Directions for Use: 1. Apply A-200 Shampoo to **dry** hair and scalp or other infested areas. Use enough to completely wet area being treated. Massage in. (For head lice, avoid getting product into eyes. Helpful hint: When shampooing a child's head, place towel across forehead.) 2. Allow product to remain for 10 minutes, but no longer. 3. Add small quantities of water, and work rich lather into hair and scalp. 4. Rinse thoroughly with warm water. Towel dry. 5. Comb hair with special A-200 precision comb to remove dead lice and eggs. (See left side panel for combing suggestions.) Repeat treatment in 7–10 days or earlier if reinfestation has occurred. Do not use more than 2 applications of A-200 Shampoo in 24 hours. When used on children, adult supervision is recommended.

Additional Control Measures: At time of shampoo treatment, all infested clothing, bed linen and other articles should be laundered in hot water or dry cleaned. Carpets, upholstery and mattresses should be vacuumed thoroughly. Combs and brushes should be soaked in hot water (above 130°) for 5 to 10 minutes.

Storage and Disposal: Store at room temperature. Do not reuse empty bottle. Wrap and put in trash.
How Supplied: A-200 Shampoo Concentrate in 2 and 4 fl. oz. unbreakable plastic bottles and A-200 Gel Concentrate in 1 oz. tubes, all with special comb and bilingual patient insert.

Literature Available: Additional patient literature available upon request.
Shown in Product Identification Section, page 430

**ASTHMAHALER® Mist
epinephrine bitartrate bronchodilator
Alcohol Free Formula**

Active Ingredients: Contains epinephrine bitartrate 7 mg per ml in inert propellant.

Inactive Ingredients: Cetylpyridinium Chloride, Propellants 11, 12, & 114, Sorbitan Trioleate.

Indications: For temporary relief of shortness of breath, tightness of chest, and wheezing due to bronchial asthma.

Warnings: Do not use this product unless a diagnosis of asthma has been made by a doctor. Do not use this product if you have heart disease, high blood pressure, thyroid disease, diabetes, or difficulty in urination due to enlargement of the prostate gland unless directed by a doctor. Do not use this product if you have ever been hospitalized for asthma or if you are taking any prescription drug for asthma unless directed by a doctor.
DO NOT USE THIS PRODUCT MORE FREQUENTLY OR AT HIGHER DOSES THAN RECOMMENDED UNLESS DIRECTED BY A DOCTOR. Ex-

cessive use may cause nervousness and rapid heart beat, and possibly, adverse effects on the heart.
DO NOT CONTINUE TO USE THIS PRODUCT, BUT SEEK MEDICAL ASSISTANCE IMMEDIATELY IF SYMPTOMS ARE NOT RELIEVED WITHIN 20 MINUTES OR BECOME WORSE.

Drug Interaction Precaution: Do not use this product if you are presently taking a prescription drug for high blood pressure or depression, without first consulting your doctor.
As with any drug, if you are pregnant or nursing a baby, seek the advice of a health professional before using this product.
Keep this and all medication out of the reach of children. In case of accidental overdose, consult a physician immediately.
Contents under pressure. Do not puncture or incinerate container. Do not expose to heat or store at temperature above 120°F.

Dosage and Administration: For oral inhalation only. Each inhalation contains the equivalent of 0.16 milligram of epinephrine base.
Dosage: Inhalation dosage for adults and children 4 years of age and older: Start with one inhalation, then wait at least 1 minute. If not relieved, use once more. Do not use again for at least 3 hours. Use of this product by children should be supervised by an adult. Children under 4 years of age: consult a doctor.

Directions: Shake well before each use.
1. Remove plastic dust cap, take mouthpiece off metal vial and fit other end of mouthpiece onto top of vial, turn vial upside down. Shake well.
2. Breathe out fully and place mouthpiece well into mouth, aimed at the back of the throat.
3. As you begin to breathe in deeply, press the vial firmly down into the adapter with the index finger. This releases one dose.
4. Release pressure on vial and remove unit from mouth. Hold the breath as long as possible, then breathe out slowly.
The plastic mouthpiece should be cleaned daily. Remove metal vial and wash adapter with soap and hot water and rinse thoroughly. Dry and replace with vial.

How Supplied: ½ fl. oz. (15 ml). Available as combination package metal vial plus plastic mouthpiece, or as refill metal vial only.

**ASTHMANEFRIN®
Solution "A" Bronchodilator**

Active Ingredients: Racepinephrine hydrochloride equivalent to 2.25% epinephrine base.

Inactive Ingredients: Benzoic acid, Chlorobutanol, Glycerin, Hydrochloric

Continued on next page

SmithKline Beecham—Cont.

Acid, Sodium Bisulfite, Sodium Chloride, Water.

Indications: For temporary relief of shortness of breath, tightness of chest, and wheezing due to bronchial asthma.

Warnings: Do not use this product unless a diagnosis of asthma has been made by a doctor. Do not use this product if you have heart disease, high blood pressure, thyroid disease, diabetes, or difficulty in urination due to enlargement of the prostate gland unless directed by a doctor. Do not use this product if you have ever been hospitalized for asthma or if you are taking any prescription drug for asthma unless directed by a doctor. **DO NOT USE THIS PRODUCT MORE FREQUENTLY OR AT HIGHER DOSES THAN RECOMMENDED UNLESS DIRECTED BY A DOCTOR.** Excessive use may cause nervousness and rapid heart beat, and possibly, adverse effects on the heart. **DO NOT CONTINUE TO USE THIS PRODUCT, BUT SEEK MEDICAL ASSISTANCE IMMEDIATELY IF SYMPTOMS ARE NOT RELIEVED WITHIN 20 MINUTES OR BECOME WORSE.** Do not use this product if it is brown in color or cloudy.

Drug Interaction Precaution: Do not use this product if you are presently taking a prescription drug for high blood pressure or depression, without first consulting your doctor.
As with any drug, if you are pregnant or nursing a baby, seek the advice of a physician before using this product.
Keep this and all medication out of the reach of children.
Store at room temperature; avoid excessive heat.

Dosage and Administration: Inhalation dosage for adults and children 4 years of age and older: 1 to 3 inhalations not more often than every 3 hours. The use of this product by children should be supervised by an adult. Children under 4 years of age: consult a doctor.

Directions: For use in hand-held rubber bulb nebulizer. Pour at least 8 drops of solution into AsthmaNefrin Nebulizer.
Care of Solution: Refrigerate once bottle has been opened.

How Supplied: ½ fl. oz. (15 ml) and 1 fl. oz. (30 ml) Solutions. FOR USE WITH ASTHMANEFRIN® NEBULIZER.

ESOTÉRICA® MEDICATED FADE CREAM
Regular
Sunscreen Formula
Facial with Sunscreens and Moisturizers
Sensitive Skin Formula—Unscented

Description:
Regular:
Active Ingredient: Hydroquinone 2%.
Inactive Ingredients: BHA, ceresin, citric acid, dimethicone, fragrance, glyc-

eryl stearate, isopropyl palmitate, laureth-23, methylparaben, mineral oil, PEG 6-32 stearate, poloxamer 188, propylene glycol, propylene glycol stearate, propylparaben, sodium bisulfite, sodium lauryl sulfate, steareth-20, stearyl alcohol, trisodium EDTA, water.
Sunscreen Formula:
Active Ingredients: Octyl dimethyl PABA 3.3%, benzophenone-3 2.5%, hydroquinone 2%. **Inactive Ingredients:** Allantoin ascorbate, BHA, ceresin, dimethicone, fragrance, glyceryl stearate, isopropyl palmitate, laureth-23, methylparaben, mineral oil, PEG 6-32 stearate, poloxamer 188, propylene glycol, propylparaben, sodium bisulfite, sodium lauryl sulfate, steareth-10, steareth-20, stearyl alcohol, trisodium EDTA, water.
Facial—With Sunscreens and Moisturizers:
Active Ingredients: Octyl dimethyl PABA 3.3%, benzophenone-3 2.5%, hydroquinone 2%. **Inactive Ingredients:** BHA, ceresin, ceteareth-3, citric acid, dimethicone, fragrance, glyceryl stearate, isopropyl myristate, methylparaben, poloxamer 188, propylene glycol, propylparaben, sodium bisulfite, sodium lauryl sulfate, steareth-20, stearyl alcohol, trisodium EDTA, water.
Sensitive Skin Formula—Unscented:
Active Ingredient: Hydroquinone 1.5%.
Inactive Ingredients: BHA, ceresin, citric acid, dimethicone, glyceryl stearate, isopropyl palmitate, laureth-23, methylparaben, mineral oil, PEG 6-32 stearate, poloxamer 188, propylene glycol , propylene glycol stearate, propylparaben, sodium bisulfite, sodium lauryl sulfate, steareth-20, stearyl alcohol, trisodium EDTA, water.
Fragrance in all except Sensitive Skin Formula.

Indications: Regular, Sunscreen Formula and Sensitive Skin Formula: Indicated for helping fade darkened skin areas including age spots, liver spots, freckles and melasma on the face, hands, legs and body and when used as directed helps prevent their recurrence. Facial with Sunscreen: Specially designed to help fade darkened skin areas including age spots, liver spots, freckles and melasma on the face and when used as directed helps prevent their recurrence. It has emollients to help moisturize while it lightens, so it makes an excellent night cream as well.

Actions: Esotérica Medicated helps bleach and lighten hyperpigmented skin.

Contraindications: Should not be used by persons with known sensitivity to hydroquinone.

Warnings: Do not use if skin is irritated. Some individuals may be sensitive to the active ingredient(s) in this cream. Discontinue use if irritation appears. Avoid contact with eyes. Excessive exposure to the sun should be avoided. For external use only.
Facial and Sunscreen Formula: Not for use in the prevention of sunburn.

Directions: Apply Esotérica to areas you wish to lighten and rub in well. Use

cream in the morning and at bedtime for at least six weeks for maximum results. Esotérica is greaseless and may be used under makeup.

How Supplied: 3 oz. plastic jars.

FEMIRON® Multi-Vitamins and Iron
[fem 'i 'ern]

Active Ingredients: Iron (from ferrous fumarate) 20 mg; Vitamin A 5,000 I.U.; Vitamin D 400 I.U.; Thiamine (Vitamin B$_1$) 1.5 mg; Riboflavin (Vitamin B$_2$) 1.7 mg; Niacinamide 20 mg; Ascorbic Acid (Vitamin C) 60 mg; Pyridoxine (Vitamin B$_6$) 2 mg; Cyanocobalamin (Vitamin B$_{12}$) 6 mcg; Calcium Pantothenate 10 mg; Folic Acid .4 mg; and Tocopherol Acetate (Vitamin E) 15 I.U.

Indications: For use as an iron and vitamin supplement.

Actions: Helps ensure adequate intake of iron and vitamins.

Warning: Keep out of reach of children.

Precaution: Alcoholics and individuals with chronic liver or pancreatic disease may have enhanced iron absorption with the potential for iron overload. NOTE: Unabsorbed iron may cause some darkening of the stool.

Symptoms and Treatment of Oral Overdosage: Toxicity and symptoms are primarily due to iron overdose. Abdominal pain, nausea, vomiting and diarrhea may occur, with possible subsequent acidosis and cardiovascular collapse with severe poisoning. **Treatment:** Induce vomiting immediately. Administer milk, eggs to reduce gastric irritation. Contact a physician immediately.

Dosage and Administration: Women: One tablet daily.

How Supplied: Bottles of 35, 60, and 90 tablets. Femiron Iron Supplement (no added vitamins) is also available.

GERITOL COMPLETE™ Tablets
[jer 'e-tol]
The High Iron Multi-Vitamin/Mineral

Active Ingredients (Per Tablet): Vitamin A (5000 IU, including 1,250 IU from Beta Carotene); Vitamin E (30 IU); Vitamin C (60 mg.); Folic Acid (400 mcg.); Vitamin B$_1$ (1.5 mg.); Vitamin B$_2$ (1.7 mg.); Niacin (20 mg.); Vitamin B$_6$ (2 mg.); Vitamin B$_{12}$ (6 mcg.); Vitamin D (400 IU); Biotin (300 mcg.); Pantothenic Acid (10 mg.); Vitamin K (50 mcg.); Calcium (162 mg.); Phosphorus (125 mg.); Iodine (150 mcg.); Iron (50 mg.); Magnesium (100 mg.); Copper (2 mg.); Manganese (7.5 mg.); Potassium (37.5 mg.); Chloride (34.1 mg.); Chromium (15 mcg.); Molybdenum (15 mcg.); Selenium (15 mcg.); Zinc (15 mg.); Nickel (5 mcg.); Silicon (80 mcg.).

Inactive Ingredients: Carnauba wax, Crospovidone, Flavors, Gelatin, Glycerides of Stearic and Palmitic acids, Hydroxypropyl cellulose, Hydroxypropyl methylcellulose, Magnesium stearate, Microcrystalline cellulose, Polyethylene glycol, Silicon dioxide, Stearic acid, White wax, FD&C Red #40, FD&C Blue #2, FD&C Yellow #6, Titanium dioxide.

Indications: For use as a dietary supplement.

Actions: Help treat and prevent iron deficiency.

Warnings: Keep out of reach of children.

Precaution: Alcoholics and individuals with chronic liver or pancreatic disease may have enhanced iron absorption with the potential for iron overload. NOTE: Unabsorbed iron may cause some darkening of the stool.

Symptoms and Treatment of Oral Overdose: Toxicity and symptoms are primarily due to iron overdose. Abdominal pain, nausea, vomiting and diarrhea may occur, with possible subsequent acidosis and cardiovascular collapse with severe poisoning. If an overdose is suspected, immediately seek professional assistance by contacting your physician, the local poison control center, or the Rocky Mt. Poison Control Center at 303-592-1710 (Collect), 24 hours a day.

Dosage and Administration (Adults): One (1) tablet daily after mealtime.

How Supplied: Bottles of 14, 40, 100, and 180 tablets.

GERITOL® Liquid
[*jer'e-tol*]
High Potency Iron & Vitamin Tonic

Active Ingredients Per Dose (½ fluid ounce): Iron (as ferric ammonium citrate) 50 mg; Thiamine (B$_1$) 2.5 mg; Riboflavin (B$_2$) 2.5 mg; Niacinamide 50 mg; Panthenol 2 mg; Pyridoxine (B$_6$) 0.5 mg; Cyanocobalamin (B$_{12}$) 0.75 mcg; Methionine 25 mg; Choline Bitartrate 50 mg.

Inactive Ingredients: Alcohol, Benzoic acid, Caramel color, Citric acid, Invert sugar, Sucrose, Water, Flavors.

Indications: For use as a dietary supplement.

Actions: Help treat and prevent iron deficiency.

Warnings: Keep out of reach of children.

Precaution: Alcohol accelerates absorption of ferric iron. Alcoholics and individuals with chronic liver or pancreatic disease may have enhanced iron absorption with the potential for iron overload. NOTE: Unabsorbed iron may cause some darkening of the stool.

Symptoms and Treatment of Oral Overdose: Toxicity and symptoms are primarily due to iron overdose. Abdominal pain, nausea, vomiting and diarrhea may occur, with possible subsequent acidosis and cardiovascular collapse with severe poisoning. If an overdose is suspected, immediately seek professional assistance by contacting your physician, the local poison control center, or the

Rocky Mt. Poison Control Center at 303-592-1710 (Collect), 24 hours a day.

Dosage and Administration (Adults): As an iron supplement and for normal menstrual needs: One (1) tablespoonful (0.5 fl. oz.) daily at mealtime. For iron deficiency: One (1) tablespoonful (0.5 fl. oz.) three times daily at mealtime or as directed by a physician.

How Supplied: Bottles of 4 oz., and 12 oz.

7001M
11/14/83

HOLD®
4 Hour Cough Suppressant Lozenge

Active Ingredient: 5.0 mg. dextromethorphan HBr per lozenge. **Inactive Ingredients:** Corn syrup, flavors, magnesium trisilicate, sucrose, vegetable oil, Yellow 10.

Indications: Suppresses coughs for up to 4 hours.

Actions: Dextromethorphan is the most widely used, non-narcotic/non-habit forming antitussive. A 10-20 mg. dose has been recognized as being effective in relieving the discomfort of coughs up to 4 hours by reducing cough intensity and frequency.

Warnings: If cough persists or is accompanied by high fever, consult a physician promptly. Do not administer to children under 6. Do not exceed recommended dose. Keep this and all other medications out of reach of children.

Drug Interaction: No known drug interaction. As with any drug, if you are pregnant or nursing a baby, seek the advice of a health professional before using this product.

Symptoms and Treatment of Oral Overdosage: The principal symptom of overdose with dextromethorphan HBr is slowing of respiration. Should a large overdose be suspected seek professional assistance by contacting your physician, the local poison control center, or The Rocky Mt. Poison Control Center at 303-592-1710 (Collect) 24 hours a day.

Dosage and Administration: Adults (12 years and older): Take 2 suppressants one after the other, every 4 hours as needed. Children (6-12 years): One suppressant every 4 hours as needed. Let dissolve fully.

How Supplied: 10 individually wrapped suppressants come packaged in a plastic tube container. Children's Hold (Cherry Flavor) also available.

LIQUIPRIN®
Infants' Drops and Children's Elixir (acetaminophen)

Description: Liquiprin is a nonsalicylate analgesic and antipyretic particularly suitable for infants and children. Liquiprin Drops is a raspberry-flavored, reddish pink solution. Liquiprin Elixir is

a cherry-flavored, reddish solution. Neither contain alcohol.

Active Ingredient:
Liquiprin Drops: Acetaminophen 80 mg per 1.66 ml (top mark on dropper). Liquiprin Elixir: Acetaminophen 80 mg per ½ teaspoon.

Inactive Ingredients: Liquiprin Elixir: Citric acid, dextrose, flavors, fructose, glycerin, high-fructose corn syrup, methylparaben, PEG-600, propylparaben, Red 33, Red 40, sodium citrate, sodium gluconate, sucrose, water.
Liquiprin Drops: Citric acid, dextrose, flavors, fructose, glycerin, high-fructose corn syrup, methylparaben, PEG-600, propylene glycol, propylparaben, Red 33, Red 40, sodium citrate, sodium gluconate, sucrose, water.

Actions: Liquiprin Children's Elixir and Infants' Drops safely and effectively reduces fever and pain in infants and children without the hazards of salicylate therapy (e.g., gastric mucosal irritation).

Warnings: Do not give this product for pain for more than 5 days or for fever for more than 3 days unless directed by a doctor. If pain or fever persists or gets worse, if new symptoms occur, or if redness or swelling is present, consult a doctor because these could be signs of a serious condition.

Indications: Liquiprin is indicated for use in the treatment of infants and children with conditions requiring reduction of fever and/or relief of pain such as mild upper respiratory infections (tonsillitis, common cold, flu), teething, headache, myalgia, postimmunization reactions, posttonsillectomy discomfort and gastroenteritis. As adjunctive therapy with antibiotics or sulfonamides, Liquiprin may be useful as an analgesic and antipyretic in bacterial or viral infections, such as bronchitis, pharyngitis, tracheobronchitis, sinusitis, pneumonia, otitis media and cervical adenitis.

Precautions and Adverse Reactions: If a sensitivity reaction occurs, the drug should be discontinued. Liquiprin has rarely been found to produce side effects. It is usually well tolerated by patients who are sensitive to products containing aspirin.

Usual Dosage:
Liquiprin Drops and Elixir may be given alone or mixed with milk, juices, applesauce or other beverages and foods. All dosages may be repeated every 4 hours, if pain and fever persist, but not to exceed 5 times daily or as directed by physician.
Liquiprin Drops should be administered in the following dosages:
Under 2 years, under 24 lbs.: Consult physician
2–3 years, 24–35 lbs.: 160 mg—2 dropperfuls
4–5 years, 36–47 lbs.: 240 mg—3 dropperfuls

Continued on next page

SmithKline Beecham—Cont.

Liquiprin Elixir should be administered in the following dosages:
Under 2 years, under 24 lbs.: Consult physician
2–3 years, 24–35 lbs.: 1 teaspoonful
4–5 years, 36–47 lbs.: 1½ teaspoonfuls
6–8 years, 48–59 lbs.: 2 teaspoonfuls
9–10 years, 60–71 lbs.: 2½ teaspoonfuls
11–12 years, 72–95 lbs.: 3 teaspoonfuls
How Supplied: Liquiprin Drops is available in a 1.16 fl. oz. (35 ml) plastic bottle with a calibrated dropper and child-resistant cap, and safety-sealed package.
Liquiprin Elixir is available in a 4 fl. oz. plastic bottle with a pre-marked measuring cup and child-resistant cap, and safety sealed package.

Shown in Product Identification Section, page 430

MASSENGILL®
Baby Powder Soft Cloth Towelette
Unscented Soft Cloth Towelette

Inactive Ingredients: Baby Powder: Water, Lactic Acid, Sodium Lactate, Potassium Sorbate, Octoxynol-9, Disodium EDTA, Cetylpyridinium Chloride, and Fragrance. Unscented: Water, Octoxynol-9, Lactic Acid, Sodium Lactate, Potassium Sorbate, Disodium EDTA, and Cetylpyridinium Chloride.

Indications: For cleansing and refreshing the external vaginal area.

Actions: Massengill Soft Cloth Towelettes safely cleanse the external vaginal area. The towelette delivery system makes the application soft and gentle.

Warnings: For external use only. Avoid contact with eyes.

Directions: Remove towelette from foil packet, unfold, and gently wipe. Throw away towelette after it has been used once.

How Supplied: Sixteen individually wrapped, disposable towelettes per carton.

MASSENGILL®
Disposable Douches
MASSENGILL®
Liquid Concentrate
MASSENGILL® Powder

Ingredients:
DISPOSABLES: Vinegar & Water-Extra Mild—Water and Vinegar.
Vinegar & Water-Extra Cleansing—Water, Vinegar, Cetylpyridinium Chloride, Diazolidinyl Urea, Disodium EDTA.
Belle-Mai—Water, SD Alcohol 40, Lactic Acid, Sodium Lactate, Octoxynol-9, Cetylpyridinium Chloride, Propylene Glycol (and) Diazolidinyl Urea (and) Methyl Paraben (and) Propyl Paraben, Disodium EDTA, Fragrance, FD&C Blue #1.
Country Flowers—Water, SD Alcohol 40, Lactic Acid, Sodium Lactate, Octoxynol-9, Cetylpyridinium Chloride, Propylene Glycol (and) Diazolidinyl Urea (and) Methyl Paraben (and) Propyl Paraben,

Disodium EDTA, Fragrance, D&C Red #28, FD&C Blue #1.
Fresh Mountain Breeze—Water, SD Alcohol 40, Lactic Acid, Sodium Lactate, Octoxynol-9, Cetylpyridinium Chloride, Propylene Glycol (and) Diazolidinyl Urea (and) Methyl Paraben (and) Propyl Paraben, Disodium EDTA, Fragrance, D&C Yellow #10, FD&C Blue #1.
Unscented—Water, SD Alcohol 40, Lactic Acid, Sodium Lactate, Octoxynol-9, Cetylpyridinium Chloride, Propylene Glycol (and) Diazolidinyl Urea (and) Methyl Paraben (and) Propyl Paraben, Disodium EDTA.
Baking Soda & Water—Sanitized Water, Sodium Bicarbonate (Baking Soda).
LIQUID CONCENTRATE: Water, SD Alcohol 40, Lactic Acid, Sodium Lactate, Octoxynol-9, Methyl Salicylate, Eucalyptol, Menthol, Thymol, D&C Yellow #10, FD&C Yellow #6.
POWDER: Sodium Chloride, Ammonium alum, PEG-8, Phenol, Methyl Salicylate, Eucalyptus Oil, Menthol, Thymol, D&C Yellow #10, FD&C Yellow #6.
FLORAL POWDER: Sodium Chloride, Ammonium Alum, Octoxynol-9, SD Alcohol 23-A, Fragrance, FD&C Yellow #6 (Sunset Yellow).

Indications: Recommended for routine cleansing at the end of menstruation, after use of contraceptive creams or jellies (check the contraceptive package instructions first) or to rinse out the residue of prescribed vaginal medication (as directed by physician).

Actions: The buffered acid solutions of Massengill Douches are valuable adjuncts to specific vaginal therapy following the prescribed use of vaginal medication or contraceptives and in feminine hygiene.

Directions:
DISPOSABLES: Twist off flat, wing-shaped tab from bottle containing pre-mixed solution, attach nozzle supplied and use. After douching, simply throw away bottle and nozzle.
LIQUID CONCENTRATE: Fill cap ¾ full and pour contents into douche bag containing 1 quart of warm water. Mix thoroughly.
POWDER: Dissolve two rounded teaspoonfuls in a douche bag containing 1 quart of warm water. Mix thoroughly.

Warning: Vaginal cleansing douches should not be used more than twice weekly except on the advice of a physician. If irritation occurs, discontinue use. Do not douche during pregnancy except under the advice and supervision of your physician. Douching does not prevent pregnancy.
Keep out of reach of children. In case of accidental ingestion, seek professional assistance by contacting your physician, the local poison control center, or the Rocky Mt. Poison Control Center at 303-592-1710 (Collect), 24 hours a day.

How Supplied: Disposable—6 oz. disposable plastic bottle.
Liquid Concentrate—4 oz., 8 oz., plastic bottles.

Powder—4 oz., 8 oz., 16 oz., 22 oz. Packettes—10's, 12's.

MASSENGILL® Medicated
Disposable Douche
MASSENGILL® Medicated Liquid
Concentrate

Active Ingredient: Cepticin™ (0.30% povidone-iodine).

Indications: For symptomatic relief of minor irritation and itching associated with vaginitis due to *Candida albicans*, *Trichomonas vaginalis* and *Gardnerella vaginalis*.

Action: Povidone-iodine is widely recognized as an effective broad spectrum microbicide against both gram-negative and gram-positive bacteria, fungi, yeasts and protozoa. While remaining active in the presence of blood, serum or bodily secretions, it possesses virtually none of the irritating properties of iodine.

Warnings: If symptoms persist after seven days of use, or if redness, swelling or pain develop during treatment, consult a physician. Women with iodine-sensitivity should not use this product. Women may douche during menstruation if they douche gently. Do not douche during pregnancy, or while nursing, unless directed by a physician. Douching does not prevent pregnancy. Keep out of reach of children. In case of accidental ingestion, seek professional assistance by contacting your physician, the local poison control center, or the Rocky Mt. Poison Control Center at 303-592-1710 (Collect), 24 hours a day.

Dosage and Administration: Disposables: Dosage is provided as a single-unit concentrate to be added to 6 oz. of sanitized water supplied in a disposable bottle. A specially designed nozzle is provided. After use, the unit is discarded. Use one bottle daily for seven days. Even if symptoms are relieved earlier, treatment should be continued for the full seven days. Liquid Concentrate: The product is provided in concentrate form, to be mixed with water and administered using a douche bag or bulb syringe.
Fill cap and pour contents into 1 quart of warm water. Mix thoroughly. Use once daily for five days, even though symptoms may be relieved earlier. For maximum relief, use for seven days.

How Supplied: Disposables: 6 oz. bottle of sanitized water with 0.17 oz. vial of povidone-iodine and nozzle. Liquid Concentrate: 4 oz., 8 oz., plastic bottles.

MASSENGILL®
Medicated Soft Cloth Towelette

Active Ingredient: Hydrocortisone 0.5%.

Inactive Ingredients: Diazolidinyl Urea, DMDM Hydantoin, Isopropyl Myristate, Methylparaben, Polysorbate 60, Propylene Glycol, Propylparaben, Sorbitan Stearate, Steareth-2, Water.

Indications: For temporary, soothing relief of minor external feminine itching or other itching associated with minor skin irritations, inflammation, and rashes.

Actions: Adults and Children two years of age and older—apply to the affected area not more than three to four times daily. Children under two years of age—consult a physician before using.

Warning: For external use only. Avoid contact with eyes. If condition worsens, symptoms persist for more than seven days, or symptoms recur within a few days, discontinue use and consult a physician. If experiencing a vaginal discharge, see a physician. Keep this and all drugs out of the reach of children. As with any drug, if you are pregnant or nursing a baby, seek the advice of a health professional before using this product. In case of accidental ingestion, seek professional assistance or contact a Poison Control Center immediately.

Directions: Remove towelette from foil packet, unfold, and gently wipe. Throw away towelette after it has been used once.

How Supplied: Ten individually wrapped, disposable towelettes per carton.

NATURE'S REMEDY®
Natural Vegetable Laxative

Active Ingredients: Cascara sagrada 150 mg, aloe 100 mg.

Inactive Ingredients: Calcium stearate, cellulose, lactose, coating, colors (contains FD&C Yellow No. 6).

Indications: For gentle, overnight relief of constipation.

Actions: Nature's Remedy has two natural active ingredients that give gentle, overnight relief of constipation. These ingredients, cascara sagrada and aloe, gently stimulate the body's natural function.

Warnings: Do not take any laxative when nausea, vomiting, abdominal pain, or other symptoms of appendicitis are present. Frequent or prolonged use of laxatives may result in dependence on them. If pregnant or nursing, consult your physician before using this or any medicine.

Symptoms and Treatment of Oral Overdosage: If an overdose is suspected, immediately seek professional assistance by contacting your physician, local poison control center, or the Rocky Mountain Poison Control Center at 303-592-1710 (Collect) 24 hours a day.

Dosage and Administration: Adults, swallow two tablets daily along with a full glass of water; children (8–15 yrs.), one tablet daily; or as directed by a physician.

How Supplied: Beige, film-coated tablets with foil-backed blister packaging in boxes of 12s, 30s and 60s.

Shown in Product Identification Section, page 430

N'ICE® Medicated Sugarless Sore Throat and Cough Lozenges
[ni 'ce]

Active Ingredient: <u>Cherry</u>—Each lozenge contains 5.0 mg. menthol in a sorbitol base. <u>Citrus</u>—Each lozenge contains 5.0 mg. menthol in a sorbitol base. <u>Menthol Eucalyptus</u>—Each lozenge contains 5.0 mg. menthol in a sorbitol base. <u>Menthol Mint</u>—Each lozenge contains 5.0 mg. menthol in a sorbitol base. <u>Children's Berry</u>—Each lozenge contains 3.0 mg. menthol in a sorbitol base.

Inactive Ingredients: <u>Cherry</u>—Blue 1, Flavors, Red 40, Sorbitol, Tartaric Acid. <u>Citrus</u>—Citric Acid, Flavors, Saccharin Sodium, Sodium Citrate, Sorbitol, Yellow 10. <u>Menthol Eucalyptus</u>—Citric Acid, Flavors, Sorbitol. <u>Menthol Mint</u>—Blue 1, Flavor, Hydrogenated Glucose Syrup, Sorbitol, Yellow 10. <u>Children's Berry</u>—Citric Acid, Flavor, Red 33, Sodium Citrate, Sorbitol.

Indications: Temporarily relieves occasional minor sore throat pain and coughs as may occur with a cold.

Actions: Menthol in a sorbitol base soothes irritated throat tissue and leaves the throat feeling cool.

Warnings: Do not administer to children under six years of age unless directed by a physician. A persistent cough may be a sign of a serious condition. If cough or sore throat is severe, persists for more than 2 days, is accompanied or followed by fever, headache, rash, nausea, or vomiting, consult a doctor promptly. Do not take this product for persistent or chronic cough such as occurs with smoking, asthma, emphysema, or if cough is accompanied by excessive phlegm (mucus) unless directed by a doctor. **Keep this and all medicines out of the reach of children.**

Drug Interaction: No known drug interaction.

Symptoms and Treatment of Oral Overdosage: Should a large overdose of N'ICE (Cherry, Citrus, Menthol Eucalyptus, Menthol Mint, or Children's Berry) be suspected, with symptoms of nausea, vomiting and diarrhea, seek professional assistance. Contact your physician, the local poison control center, or the Rocky Mountain Poison Control Center at 303-592-1710 (Collect) 24 hours a day.

Dosage and Administration: <u>Cherry, Citrus, Menthol Eucalyptus, Menthol Mint</u>—Let lozenge dissolve slowly in the mouth. Repeat as needed, up to 10 lozenges per day. <u>Children's Berry</u>—Take two lozenges. Let lozenges dissolve slowly in the mouth. Repeat as needed, up to 10 lozenges per day.

Professional Labeling: For the temporary relief of pain associated with tonsillitis, pharyngitis, throat infections or stomatitis.

How Supplied: Available in packages of 2, 8 and 16 lozenges.

N'ICE® Sore Throat Spray
[ni 'ce]

Active Ingredients: Menthol 0.12%, Glycerin 25%.

Inactive Ingredients: Alcohol, Blue 1, Flavor, Hydrogenated Glucose Syrup, Phosphoric Acid, Poloxamer 338, Saccharin Sodium, Sodium Phosphate Dibasic, Sorbitol, Water.

Indications: For temporary relief of minor pain and protection of irritated areas in sore throat and mouth.

Actions: Menthol in a sugarless spray/gargle soothes irritated throat tissue and leaves the throat feeling cool.

Warnings: If sore throat is severe, persists for more than 2 days, is accompanied by or followed by fever, headache, rash, nausea or vomiting, consult a doctor promptly. If sore mouth symptoms do not improve in 7 days, see your dentist or doctor promptly. KEEP THIS AND ALL MEDICINES OUT OF THE REACH OF CHILDREN.

Drug Interaction: No known drug interaction.

Symptoms and Treatment of Oral Overdosage: Should a large overdose of N'ICE Sore Throat Spray be suspected, with symptoms of nausea, vomiting and diarrhea, seek professional assistance. Contact your physician, the local poison control center, or the Rocky Mountain Poison Control Center at 303-592-1710 (Collect) 24 hours a day.

Directions: Adults and children 2 years and older: Spray affected area four times. Repeat as needed or as directed by a doctor. Children under 12 should be supervised in the use of this product. Children under 2: consult a doctor.

Professional Labeling: For the temporary relief of pain associated with tonsillitis, pharyngitis, throat infections or stomatitis.

How Supplied: In 6 fl. oz. plastic bottles with sprayer, and 12 fl. oz. plastic bottles.

OXY ACNE MEDICATIONS
OXY-5® and OXY-10®
with SORBOXYL®
Benzoyl peroxide lotion 5% and 10%
with silica oil absorber
Vanishing and Tinted Formulas

Description: Active Ingredient: Oxy-5: Benzoyl peroxide 5%. Oxy-10: Benzoyl peroxide 10%.

Inactive Ingredients: Oxy-5 Vanishing: Water, sodium PCA, cetyl alcohol, silica (Sorboxyl®), propylene glycol, citric acid, sodium lauryl sulfate, methylparaben, propylparaben.
Oxy-5 Tinted: Water, titanium dioxide, sodium PCA, cetyl alcohol, silica (Sorboxyl®), iron oxides, propylene glycol, citric acid, sodium lauryl sulfate, stearyl alcohol, methylparaben, propylparaben.

Continued on next page

SmithKline Beecham—Cont.

Oxy-10 Vanishing: Water, silica (Sorboxyl®), cetyl alcohol, propylene glycol, citric acid, sodium citrate, sodium lauryl sulfate, methylparaben and propylparaben.

Oxy-10 Tinted: Water, titanium dioxide, silica (Sorboxyl®), cetyl alcohol, glyceryl stearate, propylene glycol, stearic acid, iron oxides, sodium lauryl sulfate, citric acid, sodium citrate, methylparaben, propylparaben.

Indications: Topical medications for the treatment of acne vulgaris.

Action: Provides antibacterial activity against Propionibacterium acnes.

Additional Benefits: Absorbs excess skin oil up to 12 hours. Vanishing formulas are colorless, odorless, greaseless lotions that vanish upon application. Tinted formulas are flesh tone, odorless, greaseless lotions that cover up acne pimples while they treat them.

Directions for Use: Wash skin thoroughly and dry well. Shake well before using. Dab on smoothing into oily acne pimple areas of face, neck and body (see Warning). Apply once a day initially, then two or three times a day, or as directed by a physician.

Warning: Those with known sensitivity to benzoyl peroxide or especially sensitive skin should not use this medication. Before using, determine if you are sensitive by applying to a small affected area once a day for two days. Follow label instructions and continue use if no discomfort occurs. If, during treatment, irritation, redness, burning, itching or excessive drying and peeling occur, reduce dosage or frequency of use. Discontinue if irritation is severe and if it persists, consult a doctor. Keep away from eyes, lips, and mouth. Using other topical acne medications at the same time or immediately following use of this product may increase dryness or irritation of the skin. If this occurs, only one medication should be used unless directed by a doctor. Keep this and all drugs out of the reach of children. This product may bleach hair or dyed fabrics. Keep tightly closed. Store at room temperature, avoid excessive heat. For external use only.

Symptoms and Treatment of Ingestion: These symptoms are based upon medical judgment, not on actual experience. Theoretically, ingestion of very large amounts may cause nausea, vomiting, abdominal discomfort, and diarrhea. If an oral overdose is suspected, contact a physician, the local poison control center, or the Rocky Mountain Poison Control Center at 303-592-1710 (Collect) 24 hours a day.

How Supplied: 1 fl. oz. plastic bottles.
Shown in Product Identification Section, page 430

OXY CLEAN®
Medicated Cleanser, Medicated Soap, and Lathering Facial Scrub

Active Ingredient: Oxy Clean® Medicated Cleanser: Salicylic Acid* 0.5%, SD Alcohol 40B 40%.
Oxy Clean® Medicated Soap: Salicylic Acid* 3.5%.
Oxy Clean® Lathering Facial Scrub: None.
*Salicylic Acid (2-Hydroxybenzoic Acid).

Inactive Ingredients:
Oxy Clean® Medicated Cleanser: Water, propylene glycol, sodium lauryl sulfate, citric acid, menthol.
Oxy Clean® Lathering Facial Scrub: Water, sodium borate, sodium methyl cocoyl taurate, sodium lauryl sulfoacetate, glyceryl stearate (and) PEG-100 stearate, sodium laureth sulfate, silica, fragrance, Oleth-20, potassium undecylenoyl hydrolyzed animal protein, potassium sorbate, triclosan.

Other Ingredients:
Oxy Clean® Medicated Soap: Sodium tallowate, sodium cocoate, water, triethanolamine, fragrance, iron oxides, trisodium HEDTA, sodium borate, D&C Green No. 5.

Indications: These skin care products are useful for opening plugged pores and for removing excess dirt and oil. Also helps remove and prevent blackheads.

Additional Benefits: When used regularly cleanses acne-prone skin and removes dirt, grime and excess skin oil. For a complete anti-acne program, after using Oxy Clean® follow use with Oxy-5® Tinted and Vanishing, or Oxy-10® Tinted and Vanishing acne pimple medications.

Warning (Oxy Clean® Medicated Cleanser and Soap): For external use only. If skin irritation develops, discontinue use and consult a physician. May be irritating to eyes or mucous membranes. If contact occurs, flush thoroughly with water. Using other topical acne medications at the same time or immediately following use of this product may increase dryness or irritation of the skin. If this occurs, only one medication should be used unless directed by a doctor. Keep this and all drugs out of reach of children. Store at room temperature. Keep away from flame, fire and heat.

Warning (Oxy Clean® Lathering Facial Scrub): Avoid contact with eyes. If particles get into eyes, flush thoroughly with water and avoid rubbing eyes. Discontinue use if skin irritation or excessive dryness develops. Not to be used on infants or children under 3 years of age. Do not use on inflamed skin. Keep out of reach of children.

Symptoms and Treatment of Ingestion: If large amounts are ingested, nausea, vomiting, or gastrointestinal irritation may develop. If an oral overdose is suspected, contact a physician, the local poison control center, or the Rocky Mountain Poison Control Center at 303-592-1710 (Collect) 24 hours a day.

Dosage and Administration: See labeling instructions for use.

How Supplied:
Medicated Liquid Cleanser—4 fl. oz.
Medicated Soap—3.25 oz. soap bar.
Lathering Facial Scrub—2.65 oz. Plastic Tube.
Shown in Product Identification Section, page 430

OXY CLEAN® MEDICATED PADS
Regular, Sensitive Skin, and Maximum Strength

Active Ingredient:
Oxy Clean® Medicated Pads Regular Strength: Salicylic Acid* 0.5%, SD Alcohol 40B 40%.
Oxy Clean® Medicated Pads Sensitive Skin: Salicylic Acid* 0.5%, SD Alcohol 40B 16%.
Oxy Clean® Medicated Pads Maximum Strength: Salicylic Acid* 2.0%, SD Alcohol 40B 50%.
*Salicylic Acid (2-Hydroxybenzoic Acid).

Inactive Ingredients:
Oxy Clean® Medicated Pads Regular Strength: Water, propylene glycol, sodium lauryl sulfate, citric acid, fragrance, menthol.
Oxy Clean® Medicated Pads Sensitive Skin: Water, disodium lauryl sulfosuccinate, dimethicone copolyol, PEG-4, sodium lauroyl sarcosinate, sodium PCA, fragrance, menthol, sodium carbonate, trisodium EDTA.
Oxy Clean® Medicated Pads Maximum Strength: Water, PEG-8, propylene glycol, sodium lauryl sulfate, citric acid, fragrance, menthol.

Indications: These medicated pad products are useful for opening plugged pores and for removing excess dirt and oil. Also helps remove and prevent blackheads.

Additional Benefits: When used regularly cleanses acne-prone skin and removes dirt, grime and excess skin oil. For a complete anti-acne program, after using Oxy Clean® follow use with Oxy-5® Tinted and Vanishing, or Oxy-10® Tinted and Vanishing acne pimple medications.

Warning: For external use only. If skin irritation develops, discontinue use and consult a physician. May be irritating to eyes or mucous membranes. If contact occurs, flush thoroughly with water. Using other topical acne medications at the same time or immediately following use of this product may increase dryness or irritation of the skin. If this occurs, only one medication should be used unless directed by a doctor. Keep this and all drugs out of reach of children. Store at room temperature. Keep away from flame, fire and heat.

Symptoms and Treatment of Ingestion: If large amounts are ingested, nausea, vomiting, or gastrointestinal irritation may develop. If an oral overdose is suspected, contact a physician, the local poison control center, or the Rocky

Mountain Poison Control Center at 303-592-1710 (Collect) 24 hours a day.

Dosage and Administration: See labeling instructions for use.

How Supplied:
Medicated Pads Regular Strength—Plastic Jar/50 pads or 90 pads
Medicated Pads Sensitive Skin—Plastic Jar/50 pads or 90 pads
Medicated Pads Maximum Strength—Plastic Jar/50 pads or 90 pads
Shown in Product Identification Section, page 430

OXY NIGHT WATCH™
Maximum Strength and Sensitive Skin Formulas

Active Ingredient:
Oxy Night Watch™ Maximum Strength: Salicylic Acid (2-Hydroxybenzoic Acid) 2.0%.
Oxy Night Watch™ Sensitive Skin: Salicylic Acid (2-Hydroxybenzoic Acid) 1.0%.

Inactive Ingredients:
Water, cetyl alcohol, silica (Sorboxyl®), propylene glycol, sodium lauryl sulfate, stearyl alcohol, methylparaben, disodium EDTA and propylparaben.

Indications: These medicated skin products help unplug clogged pores and penetrate pores to treat pimples and blackheads before they form.

Additional Benefits: Absorbs excess skin oil up to 12 hours. Stays on all night to treat and prevent pimples and blackheads.

Directions for Use: At bedtime, wash face gently using a non-abrasive soap. Rinse thoroughly and pat dry. Shake tube well. Squeeze out a small amount of lotion. Smooth a thin layer evenly over entire face, avoiding eyes, lips and mouth. Do not wash off. Oxy Night Watch™ works best when left on overnight. The next morning, wash face and pat dry. If you have dry skin, apply a non-oily moisturizer.

Warning: For external use only. If skin irritation develops, discontinue use and consult a physician. Using other topical acne medications at the same time or immediately following use of this product may increase dryness or irritation of the skin. If this occurs, only one medication should be used unless directed by a doctor.

How Supplied: 2.0 oz. plastic tubes.
Shown in Product Identification Section, page 430

OXY 10® DAILY FACE WASH

Active Ingredient: Benzoyl peroxide 10%.

Inactive Ingredients: Water, sodium cocoyl isethionate, cocamidopropyl betaine, xanthan gum, sodium lauroyl sarcosinate, sodium citrate, citric acid, diazolidinyl urea, methylparaben, propylparaben.

Indications: Antibacterial skin wash used as an aid in the treatment of acne vulgaris.

Actions: Promotes antibacterial activity against Propionibacterium acnes.

Additional Benefits: When used instead of regular soap, cleanses acne-prone skin and removes dirt, grime and excess skin oil.
For a complete anti-acne program, follow Oxy 10® Daily Face Wash with Oxy-5® acne-pimple medication. Or for stubborn acne, use Oxy-10® maximum strength acne-pimple medication.

Contraindications: Should not be used by persons with known sensitivity to benzoyl peroxide.

Warning: Persons with sensitive skin or known allergy to benzoyl peroxide should not use this medication. First test on a small affected area by applying this product as directed once a day for two days. If discomforting irritation or undue dryness occurs during treatment, reduce frequency of use or dosage. If excessive itching, redness, burning, swelling, irritation or dryness occurs, discontinue use and consult a physician. Using other topical acne medications at the same time or immediately following use of this product may increase dryness or irritation of the skin. If this occurs, only one medication should be used unless directed by a doctor. Avoid contact with eyes, lips and mouth. May bleach hair or dyed fabrics.
For external use only.

Directions: Shake well. Wet area to be washed. Apply Oxy 10® Daily Face Wash massaging gently for 1 to 2 minutes. Rinse thoroughly. Use 2 to 3 times daily or as directed by physician.

Symptoms and Treatment of Ingestion: These symptoms are based upon medical judgment, not on actual experience. Theoretically, ingestion of very large amounts may cause nausea, vomiting, abdominal discomfort, and diarrhea. If an oral overdose is suspected, contact a physician, the local poison control center, or the Rocky Mountain Poison Control Center at 303-592-1710 (Collect) 24 hours a day.

How supplied: 4 fl. oz. plastic bottles.
Shown in Product Identification Section, page 430

SERUTAN®
[sĕr 'u-tan]
Natural-Fiber Laxative Toasted Granules

Active Ingredient: Psyllium (2.5 gm. per teaspoon).

Indications: For relief of occasional constipation (irregularity). This product generally produces bowel movement in 12 to 72 hours.

Actions: Softens stools, increases bulk volume and water content.

Warnings: Do not use laxative products when abdominal pain, nausea, or vomiting are present unless directed by a doctor.
If you have noticed a sudden change in bowel habits that persists over a period of two weeks, consult a doctor before using a laxative.
Laxative products should not be used for a period longer than one week unless directed by a doctor.
Rectal bleeding or failure to have a bowel movement after use of a laxative may indicate a serious condition. Discontinue use and consult your doctor.

Dosage and Administration: Serutan Toasted Granules may be sprinkled on cereals, soups, casseroles, ice cream, or other foods, or eaten directly from the container.
Adults should take one to three teaspoonfuls at any one time accompanied by a full glass (8 oz.) of liquid. A total of up to 12 teaspoonsful per day may be taken.

How Supplied: Available in 6 oz. and 18 oz. plastic containers.

SOMINEX®
[som 'in-ex]

Active Ingredients: Each tablet contains Diphenhydramine HCl, 25 mg.

Inactive Ingredients: Corn starch, dibasic calcium phosphate, magnesium stearate, microcrystalline cellulose, silicon dioxide, FD&C Blue #1.

Indications: Helps to reduce difficulty falling asleep.

Action: An antihistamine with anticholinergic and sedative effects.

Warnings: Do not give to children under 12 years of age. If sleeplessness persists continuously for more than two weeks, consult your doctor. Insomnia may be a symptom of serious underlying medical illness. Avoid alcoholic beverages while taking this product. Do not take this product if you are taking sedatives or tranquilizers, without first consulting your doctor. Do not take this product if you have asthma, glaucoma, emphysema, chronic pulmonary disease, shortness of breath, difficulty in breathing, or difficulty in urination due to enlargement of the prostate gland unless directed by a doctor. As with any drug, if you are pregnant or nursing a baby, seek the advice of a health professional before using this product. Keep this and all drugs out of the reach of children. In case of accidental overdose, seek professional assistance or contact a poison control center immediately or the Rocky Mountain Poison Control Center at 303-592-1710 (Collect) 24 hours a day.

Drug Interaction: Monoamine oxidase (MAO) inhibitors prolong and intensify the anticholinergic effects of antihistamines. The CNS depressant effect is heightened by alcohol and other CNS depressant drugs.

Symptoms and Treatment of Oral Overdosage: Antihistamine overdos-

Continued on next page

SmithKline Beecham—Cont.

age reactions may vary from central nervous system depression to stimulation. Stimulation is particularly likely in children. Atropine-like signs and symptoms, such as dry mouth, fixed and dilated pupils, flushing, and gastrointestinal symptoms, may also occur.

Dosage and Administration: Take 2 tablets thirty minutes before bedtime, or as directed by a physician.

How Supplied: Available in blister packs of 16, 32, and 72 tablets.

SOMINEX® Liquid
[som 'in-ex]

Active Ingredients: Each fluid ounce (30 ml.) contains 50 mg. Diphenhydramine HCl. Also contains Alcohol, 10% by volume.

Inactive Ingredients: Citric Acid, Dibasic Sodium Phosphate, Flavors, FD&C Blue No. 1, Glycerin, Polyethylene Glycol, Sodium Saccharin, Sorbitol, Water, Xanthan Gum.

Indications: Helps to reduce difficulty falling asleep.

Actions: An antihistamine with anticholinergic and sedative effects.

Warnings: Do not give to children under 12 years of age. If sleeplessness persists continuously for more than two weeks, consult your doctor. Insomnia may be a symptom of serious underlying medical illness. Avoid alcoholic beverages while taking this product. Do not take this product if you are taking sedatives or tranquilizers, without first consulting your doctor. Do not take this product if you have asthma, glaucoma, emphysema, chronic pulmonary disease, shortness of breath, difficulty in breathing, or difficulty in urination due to enlargement of the prostate gland unless directed by a doctor. As with any drug, if you are pregnant or nursing a baby, seek the advice of a health professional before using this product. Keep this and all drugs out of the reach of children. In case of accidental overdose, seek professional assistance or contact a poison control center immediately or the Rocky Mountain Poison Control Center at 303-592-1710 (Collect) 24 hours a day.

Drug Interaction: Monoamine oxidase (MAO) inhibitors prolong and intensify the anticholinergic effects of antihistamines. The CNS depressant effect is heightened by alcohol and other CNS depressant drugs.

Symptoms and Treatment of Oral Overdosage: Antihistamine overdosage reactions may vary from central nervous system depression to stimulation. Stimulation is particularly likely in children. Atropine-like signs and symptoms, such as dry mouth, fixed and dilated pupils, flushing, and gastrointestinal symptoms, may also occur.

Dosage and Administration: Dosage is one fluid ounce (30 ml.) thirty minutes before bedtime, or as directed by a physician. Use dosage cup provided, or two (2) measured tablespoons.

How Supplied: Available in 6 oz. bottles.

SOMINEX® Pain Relief Formula
[som 'in-ex]

Active Ingredients: Each tablet contains 25 mg. diphenhydramine HCl and 500 mg. acetaminophen.

Inactive Ingredients: Corn starch, crospovidone, povidone, silicon dioxide, stearic acid, FD&C Blue #1.

Indications: For sleeplessness with accompanying occasional minor aches, pains, or headache.

Action: An antihistamine with sedative effects combined with an internal analgesic.

Warnings: Do not give to children under 12 years of age. If symptoms persist continuously for more than 10 days, or if new ones occur, consult your physician. Do not exceed recommended dosage because severe liver damage may occur. Insomnia may be a symptom of serious underlying medical illness. Take this product with caution if alcohol is being consumed. Do not take this product for the treatment of arthritis, except under the advice and supervision of a physician. As with any drug, if you are pregnant or nursing a baby, seek the advice of a health professional before using this product. Keep this and all drugs out of the reach of children. In case of accidental overdose, seek professional assistance by contacting your physician, the local poison control center, or the Rocky Mountain Poison Control Center at 303-592-1710 (Collect), 24 hours a day. DO NOT TAKE THIS PRODUCT IF YOU HAVE ASTHMA, GLAUCOMA OR ENLARGEMENT OF THE PROSTATE GLAND, EXCEPT UNDER THE ADVICE AND SUPERVISION OF A PHYSICIAN.

Drug Interaction: Monoamine oxidase (MAO) inhibitors prolong and intensify the anticholinergic effects of antihistamines. The CNS depressant effect is heightened by alcohol and other CNS depressant drugs.

Symptoms and Treatment of Oral Overdosage: Antihistamine overdosage reactions may vary from central nervous system depression to stimulation. Stimulation is particularly likely in children. Atropine-like signs and symptoms, such as dry mouth, fixed and dilated pupils, flushing, and gastrointestinal symptoms, may also occur.

Dosage and Administration: Take two tablets thirty minutes before bedtime, or as directed by a physician.

How Supplied: Available in blister packs of 16 tablets and bottles of 32 tablets.

S.T.37®
Antiseptic Solution

Active Ingredients: Hexylresorcinol (0.1%), Glycerin (28.2%).

Inactive Ingredients: Sodium bisulfite; Water.

Indications: For use on cuts, abrasions, burns, scalds, sunburn and the hygienic care of the mouth.

Actions: S.T.37 is a non-stinging, non-staining antiseptic solution that provides soothing protection and helps relieve pain of burns, cuts, abrasions and mouth irritations.

Warnings: If redness, irritation, swelling or pain persists or increases or if infection occurs, discontinue use and consult physician. In case of deep or puncture wounds or serious burns, consult physician. Keep out of reach of children.

Dosage and Administration: For cuts, burns, scalds and abrasions apply undiluted, bandage lightly keeping bandage wet with S.T.37 antiseptic solution. For hygienic care of the mouth, dilute with 1 or 2 parts of warm water. To be used as a rinse and gargle.

How Supplied: 5.5 and 12 fl. oz. bottles.

SUCRETS® (Regular and Mentholated)
Sore Throat Lozenges
[su 'krets]

Active Ingredient: Hexylresorcinol, 2.4 mg. per lozenge.

Inactive Ingredients: Citric acid (Mentholated only), Blue 1, Corn Syrup, Flavors, Sucrose, Yellow 10.

Indications: For temporary relief of occasional minor sore throat pain and mouth irritations.

Actions: Hexylresorcinol's soothing anesthetic action quickly relieves minor throat irritations.

Warnings: If sore throat is severe, persists more than 2 days, is accompanied or followed by fever, rash, nausea or vomiting, see a doctor promptly. If sore mouth symptoms do not improve in 7 days, see a doctor or dentist promptly. KEEP THIS AND ALL MEDICINES OUT OF THE REACH OF CHILDREN.

Drug Interaction: No known drug interaction.

Symptoms and Treatment of Oral Overdosage: Should a large overdose of Sucrets (Regular or Mentholated) be suspected, with symptoms of profuse sweating, nausea, vomiting and diarrhea, seek professional assistance. Call your physician, local poison control center or the Rocky Mountain Poison Control Center at 303-592-1710 (Collect) 24 hours a day.

Dosage and Administration: Adults and children 2 years of age and older: Dissolve slowly in the mouth. Repeat as needed.

Professional Labeling: For the temporary relief of pain associated with tonsillitis, pharyngitis, throat infections or stomatitis.

How Supplied: Sucrets-Regular: Available in tins of 24 and 48 individually wrapped lozenges. Sucrets-Mentholated: Available in tins of 24 lozenges.

SUCRETS® Cold Relief Formula
[su'krets]
Lozenges

Active Ingredients: Each lozenge contains Hexylresorcinol 2.4 mg., Menthol 10 mg.

Inactive Ingredients: Blue 1, Corn Syrup, Flavors, Silicon Dioxide, Sucrose.

Indications: For temporary relief of occasional minor sore throat pain, cough, and nasal congestion associated with a cold.

Warnings: A persistent cough may be a sign of a serious condition. If sore throat, cough or congestion is severe, lasts more than 2 days, is accompanied or followed by fever, rash, nausea, vomiting or persistent headache, see a doctor promptly. Do not take this product for chronic cough such as occurs with smoking, asthma, emphysema, or if cough is accompanied by excessive phlegm, unless directed by a doctor. KEEP THIS AND ALL MEDICINES OUT OF THE REACH OF CHILDREN.

Drug Interaction: No known drug interaction.

Symptoms and Treatment of Oral Overdosage: Should a large overdose of Sucrets Cold Relief Formula be suspected, with symptoms of profuse sweating, nausea, vomiting and diarrhea, seek professional assistance. Call your doctor, local poison control center, or the Rocky Mountain Poison Control Center at 303-592-1710 (collect) 24 hours a day.

Dosage and Administration: Adults and children 2 years of age and older: Dissolve slowly in the mouth. Repeat every two hours as needed. Do not administer to children under 2 years of age, unless directed by a doctor.

Professional Labeling: For the temporary relief of pain associated with tonsillitis, pharyngitis, throat infections or stomatitis.

How Supplied: Available in tins of 24 individually wrapped lozenges.

SUCRETS® Cough Control Formula
[su'krets]
Cough Control Lozenges

Active Ingredient: Dextromethorphan hydrobromide, 5.0 mg. per lozenge.

Inactive Ingredients: Blue 1, Corn Syrup, Flavors, Red 40, Sucrose, Vegetable Oil, Yellow 10, and other ingredients.

Indications: For temporary suppression of cough due to minor throat and bronchial irritation associated with a cold or inhaled irritants.

Actions: Dextromethorphan is the most widely used non-narcotic/non-habit

forming antitussive. A 10-20 mg. dose in adults (5–10 mg. in children over 6, and 2.5–5 mg. in children 2–5) has been recognized as being effective in relieving the frequency and intensity of cough for up to 4 hours.

Warnings: A persistent cough may be a sign of a serious condition. If cough persists for more than 1 week, tends to recur, or is accompanied by fever, rash or persistent headache, consult a doctor. Do not take this product for persistent or chronic cough such as occurs with smoking, asthma, emphysema or if cough is accompanied by excessive phlegm unless directed by a doctor. As with any drug, if you are pregnant or nursing a baby, seek the advice of a health professional before using this product.
KEEP THIS AND ALL MEDICINES OUT OF THE REACH OF CHILDREN.

Drug Interaction: No known drug interaction.

Symptoms and Treatment of Oral Overdosage: Slowing of respiration is the principal symptom of dextromethorphan HBr overdose. Should a large overdose be suspected, seek professional assistance. Call your physician, the local poison control center, or the Rocky Mt. Poison Control Center at 303-592-1710 (Collect), 24 hours a day.

Dosage and Administration: Adults and children 12 years and older: Take 2 lozenges. Children 2 to under 12 years: Take 1 lozenge. Repeat every 4 hours as needed. Do not administer to children under 2 years of age unless directed by a doctor.

Professional Labeling: Same as those outlined under Indications.

How Supplied: Available in tins of 24 lozenges.

SUCRETS® Maximum Strength
SUCRETS® Wild Cherry, Regular Strength
SUCRETS® Children's Cherry Flavored
Sore Throat Lozenges
[su'krets]

Active Ingredient: Maximum Strength: Dyclonine Hydrochloride 3.0 mg. per lozenge. Wild Cherry, Regular Strength: Dyclonine Hydrochloride 2.0 mg. per lozenge. Children's Cherry: Dyclonine Hydrochloride 1.2 mg. per lozenge.

Inactive Ingredients: Maximum Strength: Citric Acid, Corn Syrup, Silicon Dioxide, Sucrose, Yellow 10. Wild Cherry, Regular Strength: Blue 1, Corn Syrup, Flavor, Red 40, Silicon Dioxide, Sucrose, Tartaric Acid. Children's Cherry: Blue 1, Citric Acid, Corn Syrup, Red 40, Silicon Dioxide, Sucrose.

Indications: For temporary relief of occasional minor sore throat pain and mouth irritations.

Actions: Dyclonine Hydrochloride's soothing anesthetic action relieves minor throat irritations.

Warnings: If sore throat is severe, persists more than 2 days, is accompanied or followed by fever, headache, rash, nausea, or vomiting, consult a doctor promptly. If sore mouth symptoms do not improve in 7 days, see your dentist or doctor promptly. KEEP THIS AND ALL MEDICINES OUT OF THE REACH OF CHILDREN.

Drug Interaction: No known drug interaction.

Symptoms and Treatment of Oral Overdosage: Reactions due to large overdosage are systemic and involve the central nervous system and cardiovascular system. Central nervous system reactions are characterized by excitation and/or depression. Nervousness, dizziness, blurred vision or tremors may occur. Reactions involving the cardiovascular system include depression of the myocardium, hypotension or bradycardia. Should a large overdose be suspected seek professional assistance. Call your physician, local poison control center or the Rocky Mountain Poison Control Center at 303-592-1710 (Collect), 24 hours a day.

Dosage and Administration: Adults and children 2 years of age or older: Allow to dissolve slowly in the mouth. Repeat every two hours as needed. Do not administer to children under 2 years of age unless directed by a doctor.

Professional Labeling: For the temporary relief of pain associated with tonsillitis, pharyngitis, throat infections or stomatitis.

How Supplied: Available in tins of 24 lozenges.

SUCRETS MAXIMUM STRENGTH SPRAYS
[su'krets]

Active Ingredient: Dyclonine Hydrochloride 0.1%.

Inactive Ingredients: Cherry: Alcohol (12.5%), Dibasic Sodium Phosphate, Flavor, Glycerin, Monobasic Sodium Phosphate, Phosphoric Acid, Potassium Sorbate, Red 33, Sorbitol, Water, Yellow 6. Mint: Alcohol (11%), Blue 1, Flavor, Glycerin, Monobasic Sodium Phosphate, Phosphoric Acid, Sodium Benzoate, Sorbitol, Water, Yellow 10.

Indications: Temporary relief of occasional minor sore throat pain due to colds, throat irritations, and mouth and gum irritations.

Actions: Dyclonine Hydrochloride's soothing anesthetic action quickly relieves minor throat irritations.

Warnings: If sore throat is severe, persists for more than 2 days, is accompanied or followed by fever, headache, rash, nausea or vomiting, consult a doctor promptly. If sore mouth symptoms do not improve in 7 days, see your dentist or doctor promptly. KEEP THIS AND ALL

Continued on next page

SmithKline Beecham—Cont.

MEDICINES OUT OF THE REACH OF CHILDREN.

Drug Interaction: No known drug interaction.

Symptoms and Treatment of Oral Overdosage: Reactions due to large overdosage are systemic and involve the central nervous system and cardiovascular system. Central nervous system reactions are characterized by excitation and/or depression. Nervousness, dizziness, blurred vision or tremors may occur. Reactions involving the cardiovascular system include depression of the myocardium, hypotension or bradycardia. Should a large overdose be suspected seek professional assistance. Call your physician, local poison control center or the Rocky Mountain Poison Control Center at 303-592-1710 (Collect), 24 hours a day.

THERMOTABS®
[*ther'mo-tabs*]
Buffered Salt Tablets

Active Ingredients: Per tablet—sodium chloride—450 mg.; potassium chloride—30 mg.

Inactive Ingredients: Acacia, Calcium carbonate, Calcium stearate, Dextrose.

Indications: To minimize fatigue and prevent muscle cramps and heat prostration due to excessive perspiration.

Actions: Thermotabs are designed for tennis players, joggers, golfers and other athletes who experience excessive perspiration. Also for use in steel mills, industrial plants, kitchens, stores, or other locations where high temperatures cause heat fatigue, cramps or heat prostration.

Warnings: Keep out of reach of children.

Precaution: Individuals on a salt-restricted diet should use THERMOTABS only under the advice and supervision of a physician.

Symptoms and Treatment of Oral Overdosage: Signs of salt overdose include diarrhea and muscular twitching. If an overdose is suspected, contact a physician, the local poison control center, or call the Rocky Mt. Poison Control Center at 303-592-1710 (Collect), 24 hours a day.

Dosage and Administration: One tablet with a full glass of water, 5 to 10 times a day depending on temperature and conditions.

How Supplied: 100 tablet bottles.

TUMS® Antacid Tablets
TUMS E–X® Antacid Tablets

Description: Tums: Active Ingredient: Calcium Carbonate, precipitated U.S.P. 500 mg.
Tums Original Flavor: Inactive Ingredients: Flavor, mineral oil, sodium polyphosphate, starch, sucrose, talc.

Tums Assorted Flavors: Inactive Ingredients: Adipic acid, colors (contains FD&C Yellow No. 6), flavors, mineral oil, sodium polyphosphate, starch, sucrose, talc.

An antacid composition providing liquid effectiveness in a low-cost, pleasant-tasting tablet. Tums tablets are free of the chalky aftertaste usually associated with calcium carbonate therapy and remain pleasant tasting even during long-term therapy. Each TUMS tablet contains not more than 2 mg of sodium and is considered to be dietetically sodium free. Non-laxative/non-constipating.

Tums E-X: Active Ingredient: Calcium Carbonate, 750 mg.

Tums E-X Wintergreen Flavor Inactive Ingredients: Colors (contains FD&C Yellow No. 6), flavor, mineral oil, sodium polyphosphate, starch, sucrose, talc.

Tums E-X Cherry Flavor Inactive Ingredients: Adipic acid, color, flavor, mineral oil, sodium polyphosphate, starch, sucrose, talc.

Tums E-X Peppermint Flavor Inactive Ingredients: Flavor, mineral oil, sodium polyphosphate, starch, sucrose, talc.

Tums E-X Assorted Flavors Inactive Ingredients: Adipic acid, colors (contains FD&C Yellow No. 6), flavors, mineral oil, sodium polyphosphate, starch, sucrose, talc.

Each tablet contains not more than 2 mg of sodium and is considered to be dietetically sodium free. Non-laxative/non-constipating.

Indications: For fast relief of acid indigestion, heartburn, sour stomach and upset stomach associated with these symptoms.

Actions: Tums lowers the upper limit of the pH range without affecting the innate antacid efficiency of calcium carbonate. One tablet, when tested *in vitro* according to the *Federal Register* procedure (*Fed. Reg.* 39-19862, June 4, 1974), neutralizes 10 mEq of 0.1N HCl. This high neutralization capacity combined with a rapid rate of reaction makes Tums an ideal antacid for management of conditions associated with hyperacidity. It effectively neutralizes free acid yet does not cause systemic alkalosis in the presence of normal renal function. A double-blind placebo-controlled clinical study demonstrated that calcium carbonate taken at a dosage of 16 Tums tablets daily for a two-week period was non-constipating/non-laxative.

Warnings: Tums: Do not take more than 16 tablets in a 24-hour period or use the maximum dosage of this product for more than 2 weeks, except under the advice and supervision of a physician.
Tums E-X: Do not take more than 10 tablets in a 24-hour period or use the maximum dosage of this product for more than two weeks, except under the advice and supervision of a physician. Keep this and all drugs out of the reach of children.

Dosage and Administration: Chew 1 or 2 TUMS tablets as symptoms occur.

Repeat hourly if symptoms return, or as directed by a physician. No water is required. Simulated Drip Method: The pleasant-tasting TUMS tablet may be kept between the gum and cheek and allowed to dissolve gradually by continuous sucking to prolong the effective relief time.

Important Dietary Information—As a Source of Extra Calcium—Chew 1 or 2 tablets after meals or as directed by a physician.
Tums Original and Assorted Flavors: The 500 mg of calcium carbonate in each tablet provide 200 mg of elemental calcium which is 20% of the adult U.S. RDA for calcium. Five tablets provide 100% of the daily calcium needs for adults.
Tums E-X: The 750 mg of calcium carbonate in each tablet provide 300 mg of elemental calcium which is 30% of the adult U.S. RDA for calcium. Four tablets provide 120% of the daily calcium needs for adults.

Professional Labeling: Indicated for the symptomatic relief of hyperacidity associated with the diagnosis of peptic ulcer, gastritis, peptic esophagitis, gastric hyperacidity, and hiatal hernia.

How Supplied: Tums: Peppermint and Assorted Flavors of Cherry, Lemon, Orange and Lime are available in 12-tablet rolls, 3-roll wraps, and bottles of 75 and 150 tablets. **Tums E-X Wintergreen, E-X Cherry, E-X Peppermint, and Assorted Flavors of Cherry, Lemon, Lime and Orange:** 8-tablet rolls, 3-roll wraps and bottles of 48 and 96 tablets.

Shown in Product Identification Section, page 430

TUMS® Liquid Extra-Strength Antacid
TUMS® Liquid Extra-Strength Antacid with Simethicone

Description: Tums Liquid and Tums Liquid with Simethicone is an extra-strength antacid with a fresh, minty flavor.

Tums Liquid Extra-Strength Antacid

Active Ingredient: 1,000 mg Calcium Carbonate per teaspoon.

Inactive Ingredients: Carboxymethylcellulose Sodium, Citric Acid, Glycerin, Magnesium Aluminum Silicate, Methylparaben, Peppermint Oil, Potassium Pyrophosphate, Propylparaben, Sorbitol, Sucrose, Water.

Indications: For the relief of acid indigestion, heartburn, sour stomach and the symptoms of upset stomach associated with these conditions.

Tums Liquid Extra-Strength Antacid with Simethicone

Active Ingredients: 1,000 mg Calcium Carbonate and 30 mg Simethicone per teaspoon.

Inactive Ingredients: Carboxymethylcellulose Sodium, Citric Acid, Glycerin, Magnesium Aluminum Silicate, Methylparaben, Peppermint Oil, Potassium Pyrophosphate, Propylparaben, Sorbitol, Sucrose, Water.

Indications: For the relief of acid indigestion, heartburn, sour stomach and the symptoms of upset stomach and gas associated with these conditions.

Sodium Content: Tums Liquid and Tums Liquid with Simethicone: Each teaspoonful contains less than 5 mg of sodium which is considered dietetically sodium free.

Calcium Rich: Tums Liquid and Tums Liquid with Simethicone: Each teaspoonful contains 400 mg of elemental calcium which is 40% of the adult U.S. RDA for calcium.

Acid Neutralizing Capacity: Tums Liquid and Tums Liquid with Simethicone: 20.0 mEq/5 ml.

Directions: Tums Liquid and Tums Liquid with Simethicone: Take one or two teaspoonfuls as symptoms occur. Repeat hourly if symptoms return, or as directed by a physician.

Warnings: Tums Liquid and Tums Liquid with Simethicone: Do not take more than 8 teaspoonfuls in a 24-hour period or the maximum dosage of this product for more than 2 weeks except under the advice and supervision of a physician. Store at room temperature. Keep this and all drugs out of the reach of children.

How Supplied: Tums Liquid and Tums Liquid with Simethicone are available in 12 oz. bottles.
Shown in Product Identification Section, page 430

VIVARIN® Stimulant Tablets
[*vi 'va-rin*]

Active Ingredient: Each tablet contains 200 mg. caffeine alkaloid.

Inactive Ingredients: Dextrose, magnesium stearate, microcrystalline cellulose, silicon dioxide, Starch, Yellow #6, Yellow #10.

Indications: Helps restore mental alertness or wakefulness when experiencing fatigue or drowsiness.

Actions: Stimulates cerebrocortical areas involved with active mental processes.

Warnings: The recommended dose of this product contains about as much caffeine as two cups of coffee. Limit the use of caffeine containing medications, foods, or beverages while taking this product because too much caffeine may cause nervousness, irritability, sleeplessness, and, occasionally, rapid heart beat. For occasional use only. Not intended for use as a substitute for sleep. If fatigue or drowsiness persists or continues to recur, consult a doctor. Do not give to children under 12 years of age. As with any drug, if you are pregnant or nursing a baby, seek the advice of a health professional before using this product. In case of accidental overdose, seek professional assistance or contact a poison control center

immediately. Keep this and all drugs out of the reach of children.

Drug Interaction: Use of caffeine should be lowered or avoided if drugs are being used to treat cardiovascular ailments, psychological problems, or kidney trouble.

Precaution: Higher blood glucose levels may result from caffeine use.

Symptoms and Treatment of Oral Overdosage: Convulsions may occur if caffeine is consumed in doses larger than 10 g. Emesis should be induced to empty the stomach. In case of accidental overdose, seek professional assistance by contacting your physician, the local poison control center, or the Rocky Mt. Poison Control Center at 303-592-1710 (Collect), 24 hours a day.

Dosage and Administration: Adults and children 12 years of age and over: Oral dosage is 1 tablet (200 mg.) not more than every 3 to 4 hours.

How Supplied: Available in packages of 16, 40 and 80 tablets.

EDUCATIONAL MATERIAL

Feminine Hygiene and You (Film, Video)
This 14-minute color film begins with a simple explanation of how a woman's body works (reproductive system, menstrual cycle, and vaginal secretions), then explains douching. Free loan to physicians, pharmacists and clinics. Available in 16mm and VHS.

A Personal Guide to Feminine Freshness
A 16-page illustrated booklet on vaginal infections, feminine hygiene and douching. Free to physicians, pharmacists and patients in limited quantities. These items are available by writing SmithKline Beecham Consumer Brands or by calling 800-245-1040. PA residents call 800-242-1718.

SmithKline Consumer Products
A SmithKline Beckman Company
ONE FRANKLIN PLAZA
P. O. BOX 8082
PHILADELPHIA, PA 19101

A.R.M.® Allergy Relief Medicine Maximum Strength Caplets

Product Information: A.R.M. combines two important medicines in one safe, fast-acting caplet:
- The highest level of antihistamine available without prescription—for better relief of sneezing, runny nose and itchy, weepy eyes.
- A clinically proven sinus decongestant to help ease breathing and drain sinus congestion for hours.

Directions: One caplet every 4 hours, not to exceed 6 caplets daily.

Children (6–12 years): one-half the adult dose. Children under 6 years use only as directed by physician.

TAMPER-RESISTANT PACKAGE FEATURES FOR YOUR PROTECTION:
- The carton has been sealed at the factory with a clear overwrap printed with "safety sealed."
- Each caplet is encased in a clear plastic cell with a foil back.
- The name A.R.M. appears on each caplet (see product illustration on front of carton).
- **DO NOT USE THIS PRODUCT IF ANY OF THESE TAMPER-RESISTANT FEATURES ARE MISSING OR BROKEN. IF YOU HAVE ANY QUESTIONS, PLEASE CALL 1-800-543-3434 TOLL FREE.**

Warning: Do not exceed recommended dosage. If symptoms do not improve within 7 days, or are accompanied by high fever, consult a physician before continuing use. Stop use if dizziness, sleeplessness or nervousness occurs. If you have or are being treated for depression, high blood pressure, glaucoma, diabetes, asthma, difficulty in urination due to enlarged prostate, heart disease or thyroid disease, use only as directed by physician. Do not take this product if you are taking another medication containing phenylpropanolamine.
Avoid alcoholic beverages while taking this product. Do not drive or operate heavy machinery. May cause drowsiness. May cause excitability, especially in children. Keep this and all drugs out of reach of children. In case of accidental overdose, seek professional assistance or contact a poison control center immediately. As with any drug, if you are pregnant or nursing a baby, seek the advice of a health professional before using this product. Store at controlled room temperature (59°–86°F.).

Formula: Active Ingredients: Each caplet contains Chlorpheniramine Maleate, 4 mg., Phenylpropanolamine Hydrochloride, 25 mg. **Inactive Ingredients (listed for individuals with specific allergies):** Carnauba Wax, D&C Yellow 10, FD&C Yellow 6 (Sunset Yellow) as a color additive, Gelatin, Hydroxypropyl Methylcellulose, Lactose, Magnesium Stearate, Polyethylene Glycol, Sodium Starch Glycolate, Starch.

How Supplied: Consumer packages of 20 and 40 caplets.
Shown in Product Identification Section, page 431

ACNOMEL® CREAM acne therapy

Description: Cream—sulfur, 8%; resorcinol, 2%; alcohol, 11% (w/w); nongreasy, dries oily skin, easy to apply.

Indications: Acnomel Cream is highly effective in the treatment of pimples and blemishes due to acne.

Continued on next page

SmithKline Consumer—Cont.

Directions: Wash and dry affected areas thoroughly. Apply a thin coating of Acnomel Cream once or twice daily, making sure it does not get into the eyes or on eyelids. Do not rub in. If a marked chapping effect occurs, discontinue use temporarily.

Warning: Acnomel should not be applied to acutely inflamed area. If undue skin irritation develops or increases, discontinue use and consult physician. Keep this and all drugs out of reach of children. In case of accidental ingestion, seek professional assistance or contact a poison control center immediately. Keep tube tightly closed to prevent drying. Store at controlled room temperature (59°–86°F.).

Inactive Ingredients: Bentonite, Fragrance, Iron Oxides, Potassium Hydroxide, Propylene Glycol, Titanium Dioxide, Purified Water.

How Supplied: Cream—in specially lined 1 oz. tubes.
Shown in Product Identification Section, page 430

AQUA CARE® CREAM
With 10% Urea
Effective Medication for Dry Skin Relief

Product Information: AQUA CARE, with 10% urea, is a topical cream formulated to restore nature's moisture balance to rough, dry skin. The special urea ingredient penetrates the surface of the skin to both restore lost moisture and soften dry, rough skin.

Directions: Apply two or three times daily to affected area or as your physician directs.

Warning: Discontinue use if irritation occurs.
Store at controlled room temperature (59°–86°F.).
FOR EXTERNAL USE ONLY

Formula: Purified water, urea 10%, cetyl esters wax, DEA-oleth-3 phosphate, petrolatum, trolamine, glycerin, carbomer 934, mineral oil and lanolin alcohol, lanolin oil, benzyl alcohol, and fragrance.

How Supplied: Available in 2.5 oz. tubes.
Shown in Product Identification Section, page 431

AQUA CARE® LOTION
With 10% Urea
Effective Medication for Dry Skin Relief

Product Information: AQUA CARE, with 10% urea, is a topical lotion formulated to restore nature's moisture balance to rough, dry skin. The special urea ingredient penetrates the surface of the skin to both restore lost moisture and soften dry, rough skin.

Directions: Apply two or three times daily to affected area or as your physician directs.

Warning: Discontinue use if irritation occurs.
Store at controlled room temperature (59°–86°F.).
FOR EXTERNAL USE ONLY

Formula: 10% urea with purified water, mineral oil, petrolatum, propylene glycol stearate, sorbitan stearate, cetyl alcohol, lactic acid, magnesium aluminum silicate, sodium lauryl sulfate, methylparaben and propylparaben.

How Supplied: Available in 8 oz. and 16 oz. bottles.
Shown in Product Identification Section, page 431

BENZEDREX® INHALER
Nasal Decongestant

Description: Each inhaler packed with propylhexedrine, 250 mg. Inactive ingredients: Lavender Oil, Menthol.

Indications: For temporary relief of nasal congestion in colds and hay fever; also for ear block and pressure pain during air travel.

Directions: Insert in nostril. Close other nostril. Inhale twice. Treat other nostril the same way. Avoid excessive use.
Inhaler loses potency after 2 or 3 months' use but some aroma may linger.

Warning: Ill effects may result if taken internally. In the case of accidental overdose or ingestion of contents, seek professional assistance or contact a poison control center immediately. Keep this and all drugs out of reach of children.
TAMPER-RESISTANT PACKAGE FEATURES FOR YOUR PROTECTION:
- The carton has been sealed at the factory with a clear overwrap printed with "safety sealed."
- Inhaler sealed with imprinted cellophane.
- DO NOT USE THIS PRODUCT IF ANY OF THESE TAMPER-RESISTANT FEATURES ARE MISSING OR BROKEN. IF YOU HAVE ANY QUESTIONS, PLEASE CALL 1-800-543-3434 TOLL FREE.

How Supplied: In single plastic tubes.
Shown in Product Identification Section, page 431

CLEAR BY DESIGN®
Medicated Acne Gel for Sensitive Skin

Product Information: CLEAR BY DESIGN contains benzoyl peroxide, an effective anti-acne agent available without a prescription in a lower 2.5% strength. CLEAR BY DESIGN is as effective as 10% benzoyl peroxide but with less of the irritation and redness that you may get with the higher strengths. Greaseless, colorless CLEAR BY DESIGN is invisible while it works fast. Helps prevent new acne pimples and blackheads from forming.

Directions: Wash problem areas thoroughly but gently and dry well. Using fingertip, apply CLEAR BY DESIGN to all affected and surrounding areas of face, neck, and body. Apply one or two times a day as directed by a physician.

Warning: Persons with a known allergy to benzoyl peroxide should not use this medication. To test for an allergy, apply CLEAR BY DESIGN on a small affected area once a day for two days. If discomforting irritation or undue dryness occurs during treatment, reduce frequency of use or amount. If excessive itching, redness, burning, swelling, irritation or dryness occurs, discontinue use and consult a physician. Avoid contact with eyes, lips and mouth. May bleach hair or dyed fabrics. Keep tightly closed. Keep this and all drugs out of reach of children. Store at controlled room temperature (59°–86°F.); avoid excessive heat.
FOR EXTERNAL USE ONLY

Formula: Benzoyl Peroxide, 2.5% in a gel base. Also contains: Purified water, carbomer 940, dioctyl sodium sulfosuccinate, sodium hydroxide, and edetate disodium.

How Supplied: Available in 1.5 oz. tubes.
Shown in Product Identification Section, page 431

CLEAR BY DESIGN®
Medicated Cleansing Pads
for Sensitive Skin

Product Information: CLEAR BY DESIGN Medicated Pads for sensitive skin are specially formulated to be less irritating. The pads clean deep down to remove the dirt and oil that can clog pores, clear up existing pimples and blackheads and prevent new acne pimples and blackheads from forming.

Directions: Cleanse the skin thoroughly. Use the pad to wipe face and neck thoroughly. Use one to three times daily. Do not rinse.

Warnings: Persons with a known allergy to salicylic acid should not use this medication. If discomforting irritation or undue dryness occurs during treatment, reduce frequency of use. If excessive itching, redness, burning, swelling, irritation, or dryness occurs, discontinue use and consult a physician promptly. Using other topical acne medications at the same time or immediately following use of this product may increase dryness or irritation of the skin. If this occurs, only one medication should be used unless directed by a doctor. Avoid contact with eyes, lips and mouth. Keep jar tightly closed. Keep this and all drugs out of reach of children. In case of accidental ingestion, seek professional assistance or contact a poison control center immediately. Store at controlled room temperature (59°–86°F.). Avoid excessive heat.

FOR EXTERNAL USE ONLY

Contains: Active Ingredient: Salicylic Acid 1%. **Inactive Ingredients:** Water, SD Alcohol 40B 16% (w/w), Disodium Laurethsulfosuccinate, Dimethicone Copolyol, Citric Acid, Fragrance, Cocoamphodiacetate, Sodium Carbonate.

How Supplied: Available in Jars containing 60 pads.
Shown in Product Identification Section, page 431

CONGESTAC®
Congestion Relief Medicine
Decongestant/Expectorant
Caplets

Product Information: Helps you breathe easier by temporarily relieving nasal congestion associated with the common cold, sinusitis, hay fever and allergies. Also helps relieve chest congestion by loosening phlegm and clearing bronchial passages of excess mucus. Contains no antihistamines which may overdry or make you drowsy.

Directions: One caplet every 4 hours not to exceed 4 caplets in 24 hours. Children (6 to 12 years): one-half the adult dose (break caplet in half). Children under 6 years use only as directed by physician.

TAMPER-RESISTANT PACKAGE FEATURES FOR YOUR PROTECTION:
• The carton has been sealed at the factory with a clear overwrap printed with "safety sealed."
• Each caplet is encased in a clear plastic cell with a foil back.
• The letter "C" appears on each caplet (see product illustration on front of carton).
• DO NOT USE THIS PRODUCT IF ANY OF THESE TAMPER-RESISTANT FEATURES ARE MISSING OR BROKEN. IF YOU HAVE ANY QUESTIONS, PLEASE CALL 1-800-543-3434 TOLL FREE.

Warning: Do not exceed recommended dosage. If symptoms do not improve within 7 days or are accompanied by high fever, rash, shortness of breath or persistent headache, consult a physician before continuing use. Do not use if you have high blood pressure, heart disease, diabetes, thyroid disease or a persistent or chronic cough, except under the advice and supervision of a physician. Keep this and all drugs out of reach of children. In case of accidental overdose, seek professional assistance or contact a poison control center immediately. As with any drug, if you are pregnant or nursing a baby, seek the advice of a health professional before using this product.

Drug Interaction Precaution: Do not take this product if you are presently taking a prescription antihypertensive or antidepressant drug containing a monoamine oxidase inhibitor except under the advice and supervision of a physician.

Formula: Active Ingredients: Each caplet contains Pseudoephedrine Hydrochloride 60 mg., Guaifenesin 400 mg. **Inactive Ingredients (listed for individuals with specific allergies):** Cellulose, Croscarmellose Sodium, Hydroxypropyl Methylcellulose, Magnesium Stearate, Polyethylene Glycol, Povidone, Silica Gel, Starch.

Store at controlled room temperature (59°–86°F.).
The Congestac horizontal color bar is a trademark.

How Supplied: In consumer packages of 12 and 24 caplets.
Shown in Product Identification Section, page 431

CONTAC®
MAXIMUM STRENGTH
Continuous Action Nasal
Decongestant/Antihistamine
Caplets

Composition: [See table page 709]

Product Information: Each CONTAC Maximum Strength continuous action caplet provides up to 12 hours of relief. Part of the caplet goes to work right away for fast relief; the rest is released gradually to provide up to 12 hours of prolonged relief. With just *one* caplet in the morning and *one* at bedtime, you feel better all day, sleep better at night, breathing freely without congestion. CONTAC Maximum Strength provides:
• A NASAL DECONGESTANT which helps clear nasal passages, shrinks swollen membranes and helps decongest sinus openings.
• AN ANTIHISTAMINE at the maximum level to help relieve itchy, watery eyes, sneezing, and runny nose.

Indications: For temporary relief of nasal congestion due to the common cold, hay fever or other upper respiratory allergies, and nasal congestion associated with sinusitis.

Directions: One caplet every 12 hours. Do not exceed 2 caplets in 24 hours.

NOTE: The nonactive portion of the caplet that supplies the active ingredients may occasionally appear in your stool as a soft mass.

TAMPER-RESISTANT PACKAGING FEATURES FOR YOUR PROTECTION:
• The carton is protected by a clear overwrap printed with "safety sealed"; do not use if overwrap is missing or broken.
• Each caplet is encased in a plastic cell with a foil back; do not use if cell or foil is broken.
• The name CONTAC appears on each caplet; do not use this product if the CONTAC name is missing.
• A package insert is provided for information on tamper-resistant packaging.

Warnings: Do not give this product to children under 12 years except under the advice and supervision of a physician. Do not exceed recommended dosage because at higher doses nervousness, dizziness, or

sleeplessness may occur. Do not take this product if you have high blood pressure, heart disease, diabetes or thyroid disease except under the advice and supervision of a physician. If symptoms do not improve within 7 days or are accompanied by high fever, consult a physician before continuing use. Do not take this product if you have asthma, glaucoma or difficulty in urination due to enlargement of the prostate gland except under the advice and supervision of a physician. Do not take this product if you are taking another medication containing phenylpropanolamine. Avoid alcoholic beverages while taking this product. Do not drive or operate heavy machinery. May cause drowsiness. May cause excitability, especially in children. Keep this and all drugs out of reach of children. In case of accidental overdose, seek professional assistance or contact a poison control center immediately. As with any drug, if you are pregnant or nursing a baby, seek the advice of a health professional before using this product. Store at controlled room temperature (59°–86°F.).

Drug Interaction Precaution: Do not take this product if you are presently taking a prescription antihypertensive or antidepressant drug containing monoamine oxidase inhibitor except under the advice and supervision of a physician.

Formula: Active Ingredients: Each Maximum Strength caplet contains Phenylpropanolamine Hydrochloride 75 mg.; Chlorpheniramine Maleate 12 mg. (which is a higher dose of antihistamine than CONTAC capsules). **Inactive Ingredients (listed for individuals with specific allergies):** Acetylated Monoglycerides, Carnauba Wax, Colloidal Silicon Dioxide, Ethylcellulose, Hydroxypropyl Methylcellulose, Lactose, Stearic Acid, Titanium Dioxide.

How Supplied: Consumer packages of 10, 20 and 40 caplets.
Note: There are other CONTAC products. Make sure this is the one you are interested in.
Shown in Product Identification Section, page 431

CONTAC®
MAXIMUM STRENGTH SINUS
Caplets
Non-Drowsy Formula
Decongestant • Analgesic

[See table page 709]

Product Information: Two caplets every 6 hours to help relieve the discomforts of sinusitis symptoms.

Product Benefits: CONTAC SINUS contains a decongestant and a non-aspirin analgesic. These safe and effective ingredients provide temporary relief from these major sinusitis symptoms: sinus pressure, nasal congestion, headache and pain.

Continued on next page

SmithKline Consumer—Cont.

NO ANTIHISTAMINE DROWSINESS

Directions: Two caplets every 6 hours, not to exceed 8 caplets in any 24-hour period. Children under 12 should use only as directed by physician.

TAMPER-RESISTANT PACKAGING FEATURES FOR YOUR PROTECTION:

- The carton is protected by a clear overwrap printed with "safety sealed"; do not use if overwrap is missing or broken.

- Two caplets (one dose) are encased in a clear plastic cell with a foil back; do not use if cell or foil is broken.

- The name CONTAC-S appears on each caplet; do not use this product if the CONTAC-S name is missing.

- A package insert is provided for information on tamper-resistant packaging.

Warnings: Do not exceed recommended dosage. If symptoms do not improve within 7 days, or worsen, consult a physician before continuing use. Individuals being treated for depression, high blood pressure, heart disease, diabetes, thyroid disease, or difficulty in urination due to enlargement of the prostate gland should use only as directed by a physician. Stop use if dizziness, sleeplessness or nervousness occurs. Keep this and all drugs out of reach of children. In case of accidental overdose, seek professional assistance or contact a poison control center immediately. As with any drug, if you are pregnant or nursing a baby, seek the advice of a health professional before using this product. Store at controlled room temperature (59°–86°F.).

Formula: Active Ingredients: Each caplet contains Decongestant—Pseudoephedrine Hydrochloride 30 mg., Analgesic and Fever Reducer—Acetaminophen 500 mg. (500 mg. is a non-standard dosage of acetaminophen, as compared to the standard of 325 mg.). **Inactive Ingredients (listed for individuals with specific allergies):** Cellulose, Crospovidone, FD&C Red 3, Hydroxypropyl Methylcellulose, Magnesium Stearate, Polyethylene Glycol, Polysorbate 80, Povidone, Starch, Titanium Dioxide and trace amounts of other inactive ingredients.

How Supplied: Consumer packages of 24 caplets.

Note: There are other CONTAC products. Make sure this is the one you are interested in.

Shown in Product Identification Section, page 431

CONTAC®
MAXIMUM STRENGTH SINUS
Tablets

Non-Drowsy Formula
Decongestant • Analgesic

[See table on next page]

Product Information: Two tablets every 6 hours to help relieve the discomforts of sinusitis symptoms.

Product Benefits: CONTAC SINUS contains a decongestant and a non-aspirin analgesic. These safe and effective ingredients provide temporary relief from these major sinusitis symptoms: sinus pressure, nasal congestion, headache and pain.

NO ANTIHISTAMINE DROWSINESS

Directions: Two tablets every 6 hours, not to exceed 8 tablets in any 24-hour period. Children under 12 should use only as directed by physician.

TAMPER-RESISTANT PACKAGING FEATURES FOR YOUR PROTECTION:

- The carton is protected by a clear overwrap printed with "safety sealed"; do not use if overwrap is missing or broken.

- Two tablets (one dose) are encased in a clear plastic cell with a foil back; do not use if cell or foil is broken.

- The letters C-S appear on each tablet; do not use this product if these letters are missing.

- A package insert is provided for information on tamper-resistant packaging.

Warnings: Do not exceed recommended dosage. If symptoms do not improve within 7 days, or worsen, consult a physician before continuing use. Individuals being treated for depression, high blood pressure, heart disease, diabetes, thyroid disease, or difficulty in urination due to enlargement of the prostate gland should use only as directed by a physician. Stop use if dizziness, sleeplessness or nervousness occurs. Keep this and all drugs out of reach of children. In case of accidental overdose, seek professional assistance or contact a poison control center immediately. As with any drug, if you are pregnant or nursing a baby, seek the advice of a health professional before using this product.

Formula: Active Ingredients: Each tablet contains Decongestant—Pseudoephedrine Hydrochloride 30 mg., Analgesic and Fever Reducer—Acetaminophen 500 mg. (500 mg. is a non-standard dosage of acetaminophen, as compared to the standard of 325 mg.). **Inactive Ingredients (listed for individuals with specific allergies):** Cellulose, Crospovidone, FD&C Red 3, Hydroxypropyl Methylcellulose, Magnesium Stearate, Polyethylene Glycol, Polysorbate 80, Povidone, Starch, Titanium Dioxide and trace amounts of other inactive ingredients.

How Supplied: Consumer packages of 24 tablets.

Note: There are other CONTAC products. Make sure this is the one you are interested in.

Shown in Product Identification Section, page 431

CONTAC®
Continuous Action Nasal
Decongestant/Antihistamine
Capsules

Composition:
[See table on next page]

Product Information: Each CONTAC continuous action capsule contains over 600 "tiny time pills." Some go to work right away. The rest are scientifically timed to dissolve slowly to give up to 12 hours of relief. With just *one* capsule in the morning and *one* at bedtime, you feel better all day, sleep better at night, breathing freely without congestion. CONTAC provides:

- A NASAL DECONGESTANT which helps clear nasal passages, shrinks swollen membranes and helps decongest sinus openings.

- AN ANTIHISTAMINE to help relieve itchy, watery eyes, sneezing, and runny nose.

Indications: For temporary relief of nasal congestion due to the common cold, hay fever or other upper respiratory allergies, and nasal congestion associated with sinusitis.

Directions: One capsule every 12 hours. Do not exceed 2 capsules in 24 hours.

TAMPER-RESISTANT PACKAGING FEATURES FOR YOUR PROTECTION:

- The carton is protected by a clear overwrap printed with "safety sealed"; do not use if overwrap is missing or broken.

- Each capsule is encased in a plastic cell with a foil back; do not use if cell or foil is broken.

- Each CONTAC capsule is protected by a red Perma-Seal™ band which bonds the two capsule halves together; do not use if capsule or band is broken.

- A package insert is provided for information on tamper-resistant packaging.

Warnings: Do not give this product to children under 12 years except under the advice and supervision of a physician. Do not exceed recommended dosage because at higher doses nervousness, dizziness, or sleeplessness may occur. Do not take this product if you have high blood pressure, heart disease, diabetes or thyroid disease except under the advice and supervision of a physician. If symptoms do not improve within 7 days or are accompanied by a high fever, consult a physician be-

CONTAC	CONTAC Maximum Strength Continuous Action Decongestant Caplets	CONTAC Continuous Action Decongestant Capsules	CONTAC Severe Cold Formula Caplets (each 2 caplet dose)	CONTAC Sinus Non-Drowsy Formula Caplets (each 2 caplet dose)	CONTAC Sinus Non-Drowsy Formula Tablets (each 2 tablet dose)
Phenylpropanolamine HCl	75.0 mg	75.0 mg	25.0 mg	—	—
Chlorpheniramine Maleate	12.0 mg	8.0 mg	4.0 mg	—	—
Pseudoephedrine HCl				60.0 mg	60.0 mg
Acetaminophen	—	—	1000.0 mg	1000.0 mg	1000.0 mg
Dextromethorphan Hydrobromide	—	—	30.0 mg	—	—

fore continuing use. Do not take this product if you have asthma, glaucoma or difficulty in urination due to enlargement of the prostate gland except under the advice and supervision of a physician. Do not take this product if you are taking another medication containing phenylpropanolamine. Avoid alcoholic beverages while taking this product. Do not drive or operate heavy machinery. May cause drowsiness. May cause excitability, especially in children. Keep this and all drugs out of reach of children. In case of accidental overdose, seek professional assistance or contact a poison control center immediately. As with any drug, if you are pregnant or nursing a baby, seek the advice of a health professional before using this product. Store at controlled room temperature (59°–86°F.).

Drug Interaction Precaution: Do not take this product if you are presently taking a prescription antihypertensive or antidepressant drug containing monoamine oxidase inhibitor except under the advice and supervision of a physician.

Formula: Active Ingredients: Each capsule contains Phenylpropanolamine Hydrochloride 75 mg.; Chlorpheniramine Maleate 8 mg. **Inactive Ingredients (listed for individuals with specific allergies):** Benzyl Alcohol, Cetylpyridinium Chloride, D&C Red 33, Yellow 10, FD&C Red 3, Yellow 6 (Sunset Yellow) as a color additive, Gelatin, Glyceryl Distearate, Microcrystalline Wax, Silicon Dioxide, Sodium Lauryl Sulfate, Starch, Sucrose, and trace amounts of other inactive ingredients.

How Supplied: Consumer packages of 10, 20 and 40 capsules.
Note: There are other CONTAC products. Make sure this is the one you are interested in.
Shown in Product Identification Section, page 431

CONTAC®
Severe Cold Formula
Caplets
Analgesic • Decongestant
Antihistamine • Cough Suppressant

Composition: [See table above]

Product Information: Two caplets every 6 hours to help relieve the discomforts of severe colds with flu-like symptoms.

Product Benefits: CONTAC Severe Cold Formula contains a non-aspirin an-

algesic, a decongestant, an antihistamine and a cough suppressant. These safe and effective ingredients provide temporary relief from these major cold symptoms: fever, body aches and pains, minor sore throat pain, headache, runny nose, postnasal drip, sneezing, itchy, watery eyes, nasal and sinus congestion, and temporarily relieves cough due to the common cold.

Directions: Two caplets every 6 hours, not to exceed 8 caplets in any 24 hour period. Children under 12 should use only as directed by physician.
TAMPER-RESISTANT PACKAGING FEATURES FOR YOUR PROTECTION:
- The carton is protected by a clear overwrap printed with "safety sealed"; do not use if overwrap is missing or broken.
- Each caplet is encased in a plastic cell with a foil back; do not use if cell or foil is broken.
- The letters SCF appear on each caplet; do not use this product if these letters are missing.
- A package insert is provided for information on tamper-resistant packaging.

Warnings: Do not exceed recommended dosage. If symptoms do not improve within 7 days, or worsen, consult a physician before continuing use. Individuals being treated for depression, high blood pressure, asthma, heart disease, diabetes, thyroid disease, glaucoma or difficulty in urinating due to an enlarged prostate should use only as directed by a physician. Do not take this product if you are taking another medication containing phenylpropanolamine. Avoid alcoholic beverages while taking this product. Do not drive or operate heavy machinery. May cause drowsiness. Stop use if dizziness, sleeplessness or nervousness occurs. A persistent cough may be a sign of a serious condition. If cough persists for more than 1 week, tends to recur, or is accompanied by fever, rash or persistent headache, consult a doctor. Do not take this product for persistent or chronic cough such as occurs with smoking, asthma, emphysema, or if cough is accompanied by excessive phlegm (mucus), unless directed by a doctor. May cause excitability, especially in children. Keep this and all drugs out of reach of children. In case of accidental overdose, seek professional assistance or contact a poison control center immediately. As with any drug, if you are pregnant or nursing a baby, seek the advice of a health professional before using this product.

Store at controlled room temperature (59°–86°F.).

Drug Interaction Precaution: Do not take if you are presently taking a prescription antihypertensive or antidepressant drug containing monoamine oxidase inhibitor except under the advice and supervision of a physician.

Formula: Active Ingredients: Each caplet contains Acetaminophen, 500 mg. *(500 mg. is a non-standard dose of acetaminophen, as compared to the standard of 325 mg.);* Dextromethorphan Hydrobromide, 15 mg.; Phenylpropanolamine Hydrochloride, 12.5 mg.; Chlorpheniramine Maleate, 2 mg. **Inactive Ingredients (listed for individuals with specific allergies):** Cellulose, FD&C Blue 1, Hydroxypropyl Methylcellulose, Polyethylene Glycol, Polysorbate 80, Povidone, Sodium Starch Glycolate, Starch, Stearic Acid, Titanium Dioxide.

How Supplied: Consumer packages of 10, 20 and 40 caplets.

Note: There are other CONTAC products. Make sure this is the one you are interested in.
Shown in Product Identification Section, page 431

CONTAC® Cough Formula
Cough Suppressant and Expectorant
With 6–8 Hour Cough Control

Composition: [See table on next page]

Product Information: ALCOHOL-FREE, cherry flavored CONTAC Cough Formula provides temporary relief of coughs due to the common cold and chest congestion. It contains:
- A non-narcotic cough suppressant **to temporarily relieve your cough for 6–8 hours.**
- An expectorant to **help loosen phlegm (sputum)** and thin bronchial secretions to rid the bronchial passageways of bothersome mucus, drain bronchial tubes, and make coughs more productive.

Directions: Take every 6–8 hours.
ADULTS: Fill medicine cup provided to "ADULT DOSE" line (3 teaspoons). Do not exceed 4 doses (12 teaspoons) in 24 hours. CHILDREN 6–12: Fill medicine cup provided to "CHILDREN 6–12 DOSE" line (1½ teaspoons). Do not exceed 4 doses (6 teaspoons) in 24 hours.

Continued on next page

SmithKline Consumer—Cont.

TAMPER-RESISTANT PACKAGING FEATURES FOR YOUR PROTECTION:
- The carton has been sealed at the factory with a clear overwrap printed with "Safety Sealed."
- Imprinted seal around bottle cap. Seal is printed with "SKCP."
- DO NOT USE THIS PRODUCT IF ANY OF THESE TAMPER-RESISTANT FEATURES ARE MISSING OR BROKEN. IF YOU HAVE ANY QUESTIONS ABOUT CONTAC COUGH FORMULA OR OUR PACKAGING, PLEASE CALL TOLL FREE 1-800-543-3434.

Warnings: Do not take this product for persistent or chronic cough such as occurs with smoking, asthma, chronic bronchitis, or emphysema, or where cough is accompanied by excessive phlegm (sputum), unless directed by a doctor. A persistent cough may be a sign of a serious condition. If cough persists for more than 1 week, tends to recur, or is accompanied by fever, rash or persistent headache, consult a doctor. Do not give this product to children under 6 years of age unless directed by a doctor. As with any drug, if you are pregnant or nursing a baby, seek the advice of a health professional before using this product. Keep this and all drugs out of the reach of children. In case of accidental overdose, seek professional assistance or contact a poison control center immediately.

Formula: Active Ingredients: Each Adult Dose Contains Dextromethorphan Hydrobromide 30 mg. (Cough Suppressant), Guaifenesin 200 mg. (Expectorant). **Inactive Ingredients (listed for individuals with specific allergies):** Citric Acid, FD&C Red 40, Natural & Artificial Flavors, Menthol, Methylparaben, Polyethylene Glycol, Propylene Glycol, Propylparaben, Sodium Benzoate, Sodium Citrate, Saccharin Sodium, Sugar and Water.

Store at controlled room temperature (59°–86°F.).

How Supplied: In 4 fl. oz. bottles.
Note: There are other CONTAC products. Make sure this is the one you are interested in.
Shown in Product Identification Section, page 431

CONTAC® Cough & Sore Throat Formula

Cough Suppressant • Expectorant and Non-Aspirin Analgesic

Composition: [See table below]

Product Information: ALCOHOL FREE, cherry flavored CONTAC Cough & Sore Throat Formula provides temporary relief of coughs due to the common cold, and chest congestion and minor sore throat pain and irritation. It contains:
- A non-narcotic cough suppressant to **temporarily relieve your cough,**
- An expectorant to **help loosen phlegm (sputum)** and thin bronchial secretions to rid the bronchial passageways of bothersome mucus, drain bronchial tubes, and make coughs more productive,
- A non-aspirin analgesic to **temporarily relieve minor aches and pains associated with a sore throat,** and
- A soothing liquid formulation to **coat a raw and irritated throat.**

Directions: Take every 4 hours as needed. ADULTS: Fill medicine cup provided to "ADULT DOSE" line (3 teaspoons). Do not exceed 6 doses (18 teaspoons) in 24 hours. CHILDREN 6–12: Fill medicine cup provided to "CHILDREN 6–12 DOSE" line (1½ teaspoons). Do not exceed 5 doses (7½ teaspoons) in 24 hours.

TAMPER-RESISTANT PACKAGING FEATURES FOR YOUR PROTECTION:
- The carton has been sealed at the factory with a clear overwrap printed with "Safety Sealed."
- Imprinted seal around bottle cap. Seal is printed with "SKCP."
- DO NOT USE THIS PRODUCT IF ANY OF THESE TAMPER-RESISTANT FEATURES ARE MISSING OR BROKEN. IF YOU HAVE ANY QUESTIONS ABOUT CONTAC COUGH & SORE THROAT FORMULA OR OUR PACKAGING, PLEASE CALL TOLL FREE 1-800-543-3434.

Warnings: Do not take this product for persistent or chronic cough such as occurs with smoking, asthma, chronic bronchitis, or emphysema, or where cough is accompanied by excessive phlegm (sputum), unless directed by a doctor. A persistent cough may be a sign of a serious condition. If cough persists for more than 1 week, tends to recur, or is accompanied by fever, rash or persistent

headache, consult a doctor. Do not give this product to children under 6 years of age unless directed by a doctor. Do not take this product for pain for more than 10 days (for adults) or 5 days (for children), and do not take for fever for more than 3 days unless directed by a doctor. If pain or fever persists or gets worse, if new symptoms occur, or if redness or swelling is present, consult a doctor because these could be signs of a serious condition. Do not give this product to children for the pain of arthritis unless directed by a doctor. If sore throat is severe, persists for more than 2 days, is accompanied or followed by fever, headache, rash, nausea, or vomiting, consult a doctor promptly. Do not exceed recommended dosage because severe liver damage may occur. Do not take additional pain relievers/fever reducers while using this product. As with any drug, if you are pregnant or nursing a baby, seek the advice of a health professional before using this product. Keep this and all drugs out of the reach of children. In case of accidental overdose, seek professional assistance or contact a poison control center immediately. Prompt medical attention is critical for adults as well as for children even if you do not notice any signs or symptoms.

Formula: Active Ingredients: Each Adult Dose Contains Acetaminophen 650 mg. (Analgesic/Fever Reducer), Dextromethorphan Hydrobromide 20 mg. (Cough Suppressant), Guaifenesin 200 mg. (Expectorant). **Inactive Ingredients (listed for individuals with specific allergies):** Citric Acid, D&C Red 33, FD&C Red 40, Menthol, Methylparaben, Natural & Artificial Flavors, Polyethylene Glycol, Propylene Glycol, Propylparaben, Sodium Benzoate, Sodium Citrate, Saccharin Sodium, Sugar and Water.

Store at controlled room temperature (59°–86°F.).

How Supplied: In 4 fl. oz. bottles.
Note: There are other CONTAC products. Make sure this is the one you are interested in.
Shown in Product Identification Section, page 431

CONTAC Liquid	CONTAC Cough Formula (each adult dose)	CONTAC Cough & Sore Throat Formula (each adult dose)	CONTAC JR. (each 5cc)	CONTAC Nighttime Cold Medicine (each fluid ounce)
Pseudoephedrine Hydrochloride	—	—	15.0 mg	60.0 mg
Acetaminophen	—	650.0 mg	160.0 mg	1000.0 mg
Dextromethorphan Hydrobromide	30.0 mg	20.0 mg	5.0 mg	30.0 mg
Doxylamine Succinate	—	—	—	7.5 mg
Guaifenesin	200.0 mg	200.0 mg	—	—
Alcohol	—	—	—	25%

CONTAC JR.®
Non-Drowsy Cold Liquid
Analgesic • Decongestant
Cough Suppressant

Composition:
[See table on preceding page]

Product Information: For nasal and sinus congestion, coughing and body aches and pains due to colds. Relieves symptoms with these reliable medicines. A gentle decongestant. For temporary relief of nasal and sinus congestion. Helps your child breathe more freely. A safe, sensible, non-narcotic cough quieter. Calms worrisome coughs due to colds.
A trusted, aspirin-free pain reliever and fever reducer. Provides temporary relief of muscular aches and pains, headaches and discomforts of fever due to colds and "flu."

Product Benefits: The good medicines in CONTAC Jr. were specially chosen to help gently relieve your child's nasal and sinus congestion, coughing, body aches and pains due to colds. DOES NOT CONTAIN ANTIHISTAMINES WHICH MAY CAUSE DROWSINESS.
Medical authorities know that for children, dose by weight—not age—means the dose you give is right for consistent, controlled relief. Use the CONTAC Jr. Accu-Measure Cup to select the right dose for your child's body weight.

Directions: Shake well before using. One dose every 4 to 6 hours, not to exceed 4 times daily. Use the CONTAC Jr. Accu-Measure Cup to measure the right dose for your child. For dose by teaspoon see bottle label.
TAMPER-RESISTANT PACKAGING FEATURES FOR YOUR PROTECTION:
• The carton has been sealed at the factory with a clear overwrap printed with "Safety Sealed."
• Imprinted seal around bottle-cap. Seal is printed with "SKCP."
• DO NOT USE THIS PRODUCT IF ANY OF THESE TAMPER-RESISTANT FEATURES ARE MISSING OR BROKEN. IF YOU HAVE ANY QUESTIONS ABOUT CONTAC JR. OR OUR PACKAGING, PLEASE CALL TOLL FREE 1-800-543-3434.

Warning: Do not exceed recommended dosage for your child's body weight. For children under 31 lbs. or under 3 years of age, consult a physician. If symptoms persist for 7 days or are accompanied by high fever, severe or recurrent pain, or if child is being treated for depression, high blood pressure, diabetes, heart disease or thyroid disease, consult a physician. Stop use if dizziness, sleeplessness or nervousness occurs. Do not give this product for persistent or chronic cough such as occurs with asthma or if cough is accompanied by excessive phlegm (mucus) unless directed by a doctor. Keep this and all drugs out of reach of children. In case of accidental overdose, seek professional assistance or contact a poison control center immediately.

Formula: Active Ingredients: Each 5 cc. (average teaspoon) contains Pseudoephedrine Hydrochloride 15.0 mg. (nasal decongestant); Acetaminophen 160.0 mg. (analgesic/antipyretic); Dextromethorphan Hydrobromide 5.0 mg. (anti-tussive). **Inactive Ingredients (listed for individuals with specific allergies):** Citric Acid, D&C Red 33, FD&C Yellow 6 (Sunset Yellow) as a color additive, Flavors, Methyl and Propyl Paraben, Polyethylene Glycol, Propylene Glycol, Saccharin Sodium, Sodium Benzoate, Sodium Citrate, Sorbitol, Purified Water.

Store at controlled room temperature (59°–86°F.).

How Supplied: A clear red liquid in 4 oz. size bottle.
Note: There are other CONTAC products. Make sure this is the one you are interested in.
Shown in Product Identification Section, page 431

CONTAC®
Nighttime Cold Medicine
Antihistamine • Analgesic
Cough Suppressant • Nasal
Decongestant

Composition:
[See table on preceding page]

Product Information: CONTAC Nighttime Cold Medicine:
• Provides temporary relief from nasal and sinus congestion, runny nose, coughing, postnasal drip, sneezing, itchy, watery eyes and minor aches and pains associated with the common cold, sore throat, and flu, so you can get the rest you need.
• Contains a non-aspirin analgesic and fever reducer, a cough suppressant, a nasal decongestant and an antihistamine.
In consumer testing, the soothing mint taste of CONTAC Nighttime Cold Medicine was preferred over the taste of original NYQUIL* Nighttime Colds Medicine.

Directions: ADULTS—Take 1 fluid ounce at bedtime in dosage cup provided. May be repeated every 6 hours as needed, not to exceed 4 fluid ounces in 24 hours. Children under 12 should use only as directed by physician.

TAMPER-RESISTANT PACKAGING FEATURES FOR YOUR PROTECTION:
• The carton has been sealed at the factory with a clear overwrap printed with "safety sealed."
• Imprinted seal around bottle cap. Seal is printed with "SKCP."
• DO NOT USE THIS PRODUCT IF ANY OF THESE TAMPER-RESISTANT FEATURES ARE MISSING OR BROKEN. IF YOU HAVE ANY QUESTIONS ABOUT CONTAC NIGHTTIME COLD MEDICINE OR PACKAGING, PLEASE CALL 1-800-543-3434 TOLL FREE.

Warnings: Do not exceed recommended dosage. If symptoms do not im-

prove or worsen within 7 days, or are accompanied by high fever, or difficulty in breathing, consult a doctor before continuing use. Do not take this product for pain for more than 10 days or for fever for more than 3 days unless directed by a doctor. If pain or fever persists or gets worse, if new symptoms occur, or if redness or swelling is present, consult a doctor because these could be signs of a serious condition. If sore throat is severe, persists for more than 2 days, is accompanied or followed by fever, headache, rash, nausea, or vomiting, consult a doctor promptly. A persistent cough may be a sign of a serious condition. If cough persists for more than one week, tends to recur or is accompanied by a high fever, a fever lasting more than 3 days, a rash, a persistent headache, shortness of breath or chest pain when breathing, consult a doctor. Stop use if dizziness, sleeplessness, or nervousness occurs. Individuals who have been or are being treated for depression, high blood pressure, glaucoma, diabetes, asthma, difficulty in urination due to enlarged prostate, heart disease or thyroid disease should use only as directed by a doctor. Avoid alcoholic beverages while taking this product. Do not drive or operate heavy machinery. May cause marked drowsiness. May cause excitability, especially in children. Keep this and all drugs out of reach of children. In case of accidental overdose, seek professional assistance or contact a poison control center immediately. Prompt medical attention is critical for adults as well as children even if you do not notice any signs or symptoms. As with any drug, if you are pregnant or nursing a baby, seek the advice of a health professional before using this product.

Formula: Active Ingredients: Each 1 oz. Dose Contains: Acetaminophen 1000 mg. (Analgesic/Fever Reducer), Dextromethorphan Hydrobromide 30 mg. (Cough Suppressant), Pseudoephedrine Hydrochloride 60 mg. (Nasal Decongestant), Doxylamine Succinate 7.5 mg. (Antihistamine), Alcohol 25%. **Inactive Ingredients (listed for individuals with specific allergies):** Citric Acid, FD&C Green 3, Yellow 6 (Sunset Yellow) as a color additive, Flavor, Polyethylene Glycol, Sodium Benzoate, Sodium Citrate, Saccharin Sodium, Sorbitol, Sugar and Water.

Store at controlled room temperature (59°–86°F.).

How Supplied: In 6 fl. oz. bottles.
Note: There are other CONTAC products. Make sure this is the one you are interested in.
*NYQUIL is a registered trademark of Richardson-Vicks Inc.
Shown in Product Identification Section, page 431

Continued on next page

SmithKline Consumer—Cont.

ECOTRIN®
Enteric-Coated Aspirin
Antiarthritic, Antiplatelet

Description: 'Ecotrin' is enteric-coated aspirin (acetylsalicylic acid, ASA) available in tablet and caplet forms in 325 mg. and 500 mg. dosage units. *(500 mg. is a non-standard, maximum strength dosage of aspirin, as compared to the standard of 325 mg.)*
The enteric coating covers a core of aspirin and is designed to resist disintegration in the stomach, dissolving in the more neutral-to-alkaline environment of the duodenum. Such action helps to protect the stomach from damage that may result from ingestion of plain, buffered or highly buffered aspirin (see SAFETY).

Indications: 'Ecotrin' is indicated for:
• conditions requiring chronic or long-term aspirin therapy for pain and/or inflammation, e.g., rheumatoid arthritis, juvenile rheumatoid arthritis, systemic lupus erythematosus, osteoarthritis (degenerative joint disease), ankylosing spondylitis, psoriatic arthritis, Reiter's syndrome and fibrositis,
• antiplatelet indications of aspirin (see the ANTIPLATELET-EFFECT section) and
• situations in which compliance with aspirin therapy may be affected because of the gastrointestinal side effects of plain, i.e., non-enteric-coated, or buffered aspirin.

Dosage: For analgesic or anti-inflammatory indications, the OTC maximum dosage for aspirin is 4000 mg. per day in divided doses, i.e., 2 325 mg. tablets or caplets q4h or 3 325 mg. tablets or caplets or 2 500 mg. tablets or caplets q6h.
For antiplatelet effect dosage: see the ANTIPLATELET EFFECT section.
Under a physician's direction, the dosage can be increased or otherwise modified as appropriate to the clinical situation. When 'Ecotrin' is used for anti-inflammatory effect, the physician should be attentive to plasma salicylate levels, and may also caution the patient to be alert to the development of tinnitus as an indicator of elevated salicylate levels. It should be noted that patients with a high frequency hearing loss (such as may occur in older individuals) may have difficulty perceiving the tinnitus. Tinnitus would then not be a reliable indicator in such individuals.

Inactive Ingredients: Inactive ingredients (listed for individuals with specific allergies): Cellulose, Cellulose Acetate Phthalate, D&C Yellow 10, Diethyl Phthalate, FD&C Yellow 6 (Sunset Yellow) as a color additive, Silicon Dioxide, Sodium Starch Glycolate, Starch, Stearic Acid, Titanium Dioxide, and trace amounts of other inactive ingredients.

Bioavailability: The bioavailability of aspirin from 'Ecotrin' has been demonstrated in a number of salicylate excretion studies. The studies show levels of salicylate (and metabolites) in urine ex-

creted over 48 hours for 'Ecotrin' do not differ statistically from plain, i.e., non-enteric-coated, aspirin.
Plasma studies, in which 'Ecotrin' has been compared with plain aspirin in steady-state studies over eight days, also demonstrate that 'Ecotrin' provides plasma salicylate levels not statistically different from plain aspirin.
Information regarding salicylate levels over a range of doses was generated in a study in which 24 healthy volunteers (12 male and 12 female) took daily (divided) doses of either 2600 mg., 3900 mg., or 5200 mg. of 'Ecotrin'. Plasma salicylate levels generally acknowledged to be anti-inflammatory (15 mg./dL.) were attained at daily doses of 5200 mg., on Day 2 by females and Day 3 by males. At 3900 mg., anti-inflammatory levels were attained at Day 3 by females and Day 4 by males. Dissolution of the enteric coating occurs at a neutral-to-basic pH and is therefore dependent on gastric emptying into the duodenum. With continued dosing, appropriate plasma levels are maintained.

Safety: The safety of 'Ecotrin' has been demonstrated in a number of endoscopic studies comparing 'Ecotrin', plain aspirin, as well as plain buffered and "arthritis-strength" buffered preparations. In these studies, all forms of aspirin were dosed to the OTC maximum (3900–4000 mg. per day) for up to 14 days. The normal healthy volunteers participating in these studies were gastroscoped before and after the courses of treatment, and 14-day drug-free periods followed active drug. Compared to all the other preparations, there was statistically significantly less gastric damage during the 'Ecotrin' courses. There was also statistically less duodenal damage when compared with the plain, i.e., non-enteric-coated, aspirin.
Details of studies demonstrating the safety and bioavailability of 'Ecotrin' are available to health care professionals. Write: Medical Affairs Department, SmithKline Consumer Products, P.O. Box 8082, Philadelphia, PA 19101.

Warning:
Consumer Warning: Children and teenagers should not use this medicine for chicken pox or flu symptoms before a doctor is consulted about Reye syndrome, a rare but serious illness reported to be associated with aspirin. If pain persists for more than 10 days, or if redness is present, or in arthritic or rheumatic conditions affecting children under 12, consult a physician immediately. Discontinue use if dizziness, ringing in ears, or impaired hearing occurs. If you experience persistent or unexplained stomach upset, consult a physician. Keep this and all drugs out of children's reach. In case of accidental overdose, seek professional assistance or contact a poison control center immediately. As with any medicine, if you are pregnant or nursing a baby, seek the advice of a health professional before using this product. Store at controlled room temperature (59°–86°F.).
Professional Warning: There have been occasional reports in the literature

concerning individuals with impaired gastric emptying in whom there may be retention of one or more 'Ecotrin' tablets over time. This unusual phenomenon may occur as a result of outlet obstruction from ulcer disease alone or combined with hypotonic gastric peristalsis. Because of the integrity of the enteric coating in an acidic environment, these tablets may accumulate and form a bezoar in the stomach. Individuals with this condition may present with complaints of early satiety or of vague upper abdominal distress. Diagnosis may be made by endoscopy or by abdominal films which show opacities suggestive of a mass of small tablets *(Ref.: Bogacz, K. and Caldron, P.: Enteric-coated Aspirin Bezoar: Elevation of Serum Salicylate Level by Barium Study. Amer. J. Med. 1987:83, 783–6.).* Management may vary according to the condition of the patient. Options include: gastrotomy and alternating slightly basic and neutral lavage *(Ref.: Baum, J.: Enteric-Coated Aspirin and the Problem of Gastric Retention. J. Rheum., 1984:11, 250–1.).* While there have been no clinical reports, it has been suggested that such individuals may also be treated with parenteral cimetidine (to reduce acid secretion) and then given sips of slightly basic liquids to effect gradual dissolution of the enteric coating. Progress may be followed with plasma salicylate levels or via recognition of tinnitus by the patient.
It should be kept in mind that individuals with a history of partial or complete gastrectomy may produce reduced amounts of acid and therefore have less acidic gastric pH. Under these circumstances, the benefits offered by the acid-resistant enteric coating may not exist.

Antiplatelet Effect: FDA has approved the professional labeling of aspirin to reduce the risk of death and/or nonfatal myocardial infarction (MI) in patients with a previous infarction or unstable angina pectoris. Previously, wording was added to the professional labeling of aspirin approving its use in reducing the risk of transient ischemic attacks in men.
Labeling for both indications follows:
Aspirin for Myocardial Infarction
Indication: Aspirin is indicated to reduce the risk of death and/or nonfatal myocardial infarction in patients with a previous infarction or unstable angina pectoris.
Clinical Trials: The indication is supported by the results of six, large, randomized multicenter, placebo-controlled studies involving 10,816 predominantly male, post-myocardial infarction (MI) patients and one randomized placebo-controlled study of 1,266 men with unstable angina.[1–7] Therapy with aspirin was begun at intervals after the onset of acute MI varying from less than three days to more than five years and continued for periods of from less than one year to four years. In the unstable angina study, treatment was started within one month after the onset of unstable angina and continued for 12 weeks, and patients with complicating conditions such as

congestive heart failure were not included in the study.

Aspirin therapy in MI patients was associated with about a 20 percent reduction in the risk of subsequent death and/or nonfatal reinfarction, a median absolute decrease of 3 percent from the 12 to 22 percent event rates in the placebo groups. In aspirin-treated unstable angina patients, the reduction in risk was about 50 percent, a reduction in event rate in the placebo group over the 12 weeks of the study.

Daily dosage of aspirin in the post-myocardial infarction studies was 300 mg. in one study and 900 to 1500 mg. in five studies. A dose of 325 mg. was used in the study of unstable angina.

Adverse Reactions

Gastrointestinal Reactions: Doses of 1000 mg. per day of aspirin caused gastrointestinal symptoms and bleeding that in some cases were clinically significant. In the largest postinfarction study (the Aspirin Myocardial Infarction Study [AMIS] with 4,500 people), the percentage incidences of gastrointestinal symptoms of a standard, solid-tablet formulation and placebo-treated subjects, respectively, were: stomach pain (14.5%; 4.4%); heartburn (11.9%; 4.8%); nausea and/or vomiting (7.6%; 2.1%); hospitalization for gastrointestinal disorder (4.9%; 3.5%). In the AMIS and other trials, aspirin-treated patients had increased rates of gross gastrointestinal bleeding. Symptoms and signs of gastrointestinal irritation were not significantly increased in subjects treated for unstable angina with buffered aspirin in solution.

Cardiovascular and Biochemical: In the AMIS trial, the dosage of 1000 mg. per day of aspirin was associated with small increases in systolic blood pressure (BP) (average 1.5 to 2.1 mmHg) and diastolic BP (0.5 to 0.6 mmHg), depending upon whether maximal or last available readings were used. Blood urea nitrogen and uric acid levels were also increased, but by less than 1.0 mg.%. Subjects with marked hypertension or renal insufficiency had been excluded from the trial so that the clinical importance of these observations for such subjects or for any subjects treated over more prolonged periods is not known. It is recommended that patients placed on long-term aspirin treatment, even at doses of 300 mg. per day, be seen at regular intervals to assess changes in these measurements.

Sodium in Buffered Aspirin for Solution Formulations: One tablet daily of buffered aspirin in solution adds 553 mg. of sodium to that in the diet and may not be tolerated by patients with active sodium-retaining states such as congestive heart or renal failure. This amount of sodium adds about 30 percent to the 70 to 90 meq. intake suggested as appropriate for dietary treatment of essential hypertension in the 1984 Report of the Joint National Committee on Detection, Evaluation, and Treatment of High Blood Pressure.[8]

Dosage and Administration: Although most of the studies used dosages exceeding 300 mg. daily, two trials used only 300 mg. and pharmacologic data indicate that this dose inhibits platelet function fully. Therefore, 300 mg. or a conventional 325 mg. aspirin dose daily is a reasonable, routine dose that would minimize gastrointestinal adverse reactions for both solid, oral dosage forms (buffered and plain aspirin) and buffered aspirin in solution.

References:

1. Elwood, P.C., et al.: A Randomized Controlled Trial of Acetylsalicylic Acid in the Secondary Prevention of Mortality from Myocardial Infarction, *Br. Med. J.* 1:436–440, 1974.
2. The Coronary Drug Project Research Group: Aspirin in Coronary Heart Disease, *J. Chronic Dis.* 29:625–642, 1976.
3. Breddin, K., et al.: Secondary Prevention of Myocardial Infarction: A Comparison of Acetylsalicylic Acid, Phenprocoumon or Placebo, *Homeostasis* 470:263–268, 1979.
4. Aspirin Myocardial Infarction Study Research Group: A Randomized Controlled Trial of Aspirin in Persons Recovered from Myocardial Infarction, *J.A.M.A.* 243:661–669, 1980.
5. Elwood, P.C., and Sweetnam, P.M.: Aspirin and Secondary Mortality After Myocardial Infarction, *Lancet* pp. 1313–1315, Dec. 22–29, 1979.
6. The Persantine-Aspirin Reinfarction Study Research Group, Persantine and Aspirin in Coronary Heart Disease, *Circulation* 62: 449–469, 1980.
7. Lewis, H.D., et al.: Protective Effects of Aspirin Against Acute Myocardial Infarction and Death in Men with Unstable Angina, Results of a Veterans Administration Cooperative Study, *N. Engl. J. Med.* 309:396–403, 1983.
8. 1984 Report of the Joint National Committee on Detection, Evaluation, and Treatment of High Blood Pressure, U.S. Department of Health and Human Services and U.S. Public Health Service, National Institutes of Health. NIH Pub. No. 84–1088.

Aspirin for Transient Ischemic Attacks

Indication: For reducing the risk of recurrent transient ischemic attacks (TIAs) or stroke in men who have had transient ischemia of the brain due to fibrin platelet emboli. There is inadequate evidence that aspirin or buffered aspirin is effective in reducing TIAs in women at the recommended dosage. There is no evidence that aspirin or buffered aspirin is of benefit in the treatment of completed strokes in men or women.

Clinical Trials: The indication is supported by the results of a Canadian study[1] in which 585 patients with threatened stroke were followed in a randomized clinical trial for an average of 26 months to determine whether aspirin or sulfinpyrazone, singly or in combination, was superior to placebo in preventing transient ischemic attacks, stroke or death. The study showed that, although sulfinpyrazone had no statistically significant effect, aspirin reduced the risk of continuing transient ischemic attacks, stroke or death by 19 percent and reduced the risk of stroke or death by 31 percent. Another aspirin study carried out in the United States with 178 patients showed a statistically significant number of "favorable outcomes," including reduced transient ischemic attacks, stroke and death.[2]

Precautions: Patients presenting with signs and symptoms of TIAs should have a complete medical and neurologic evaluation. Consideration should be given to other disorders that resemble TIAs. Attention should be given to risk factors: it is important to evaluate and treat, if appropriate, other diseases associated with TIAs and stroke, such as hypertension and diabetes.

Concurrent administration of absorbable antacids at therapeutic doses may increase the clearance of salicylates in some individuals. The concurrent administration of nonabsorbable antacids may alter the rate of absorption of aspirin, thereby resulting in a decreased acetylsalicylic acid/salicylate ratio in plasma. The clinical significance of these decreases in available aspirin is unknown. Aspirin at dosages of 1,000 mg. per day has been associated with small increases in blood pressure, blood urea nitrogen, and serum uric acid levels. It is recommended that patients placed on long-term aspirin treatment be seen at regular intervals to assess changes in these measurements.

Adverse Reactions: At dosages of 1,000 mg. or higher of aspirin per day, gastrointestinal side effects include stomach pain, heartburn, nausea and/or vomiting, as well as increased rates of gross gastrointestinal bleeding.

Dosage and Administration: Adult dosage for men is 1,300 mg. a day, in divided doses of 650 mg. twice a day or 325 mg. four times a day.

References:

1. The Canadian Cooperative Study Group: Randomized Trial of Aspirin and Sulfinpyrazone in Threatened Stroke, *N. Engl. J. Med.* 299:53, 1978.
2. Fields, W. S., et al.: Controlled Trial of Aspirin in Cerebral Ischemia, *Stroke* 8:301–316, 1980.

Store at controlled room temperature (59°–86°F.).

Supplied:

'Ecotrin' Tablets
325 mg. in bottles of 100, 250 and 1000.
500 mg. in bottles of 60 and 150.

'Ecotrin' Caplets
325 mg. in bottles of 75.
500 mg. in bottles of 50.

TAMPER-RESISTANT PACKAGE FEATURES:

- The carton has been sealed at the factory with a clear overwrap printed with "safety sealed."
- Bottle has imprinted "SKCP" seal under cap.
- The words ECOTRIN REG or ECOTRIN MAX appear on each tablet or caplet (see product illustration printed on carton).

Continued on next page

SmithKline Consumer—Cont.

- DO NOT USE THIS PRODUCT IF ANY OF THESE TAMPER-RESIST-ANT FEATURES ARE MISSING OR BROKEN. IF YOU HAVE ANY QUESTIONS, PLEASE CALL 1-800-543-3434 TOLL FREE.

Shown in Product Identification Section, page 432

FEOSOL® CAPSULES
Hematinic

Product Information: FEOSOL capsules provide the body with ferrous sulfate, iron in its most efficient form, for iron deficiency and iron-deficiency anemia when the need for such therapy has been determined by a physician.

The special targeted-release capsule is formulated to reduce stomach upset, a common problem with iron.

Directions: *Adults:* 1 or 2 capsules daily or as directed by a physician. *Children:* As directed by a physician.

TAMPER-RESISTANT PACKAGING FEATURES FOR YOUR PROTECTION:

- The carton is protected by a clear overwrap printed with "safety sealed"; do not use if overwrap is missing or broken.
- Each capsule is encased in a plastic cell with a foil back; do not use if cell or foil is broken.
- Each FEOSOL capsule is protected by a red Perma-Seal™ band which bonds the two capsule halves together; do not use if capsule is broken or band is missing or broken.
- A package insert is provided for information on tamper-resistant packaging.

Warnings: Do not exceed recommended dosage. The treatment of any anemic condition should be under the advice and supervision of a physician. Iron-containing medication may occasionally cause constipation or diarrhea. Since oral iron products interfere with absorption of oral tetracycline antibiotics, these products should not be taken within two hours of each other. This package is child-safe; however, keep this and all drugs out of reach of children. In case of accidental overdose, seek professional assistance or contact a poison control center immediately. As with any drug, if you are pregnant or nursing a baby, seek the advice of a health professional before using this product. Store at controlled room temperature (59°–86°F.).

Formula: Active Ingredients: Each capsule contains 159 mg. of dried ferrous sulfate USP (50 mg. of elemental iron), equivalent to 250 mg. of ferrous sulfate USP. **Inactive Ingredients (listed for individuals with specific allergies):** Benzyl Alcohol, Cetylpyridinium Chloride, D&C Red 33, Yellow 10, FD&C Blue 1, Red 3, Red 40, Gelatin, Glyceryl Stearates, Iron Oxide, Polyethylene Glycol, Povidone, Sodium Lauryl Sulfate, Starch, Sucrose, White Wax and trace amounts of other inactive ingredients.

How Supplied: Packages of 30 and 60 capsules, bottles of 500; in Single Unit Packages of 100 capsules (intended for institutional use only).

Also available in Tablets and Elixir.

Note: There are other FEOSOL products. Make sure this is the one you are interested in.

Shown in Product Identification Section, page 432

FEOSOL® ELIXIR
Hematinic

Product Information: FEOSOL Elixir, an unusually palatable iron elixir, provides the body with ferrous sulfate—iron in its most efficient form. The standard elixir for simple iron deficiency and iron-deficiency anemia when the need for such therapy has been determined by a physician.

Directions: Adults: 1 to 2 teaspoonfuls three times daily. Children: ½ to 1 teaspoonful three times daily preferably between meals. Infants: as directed by physician. Mix with water or fruit juice to avoid temporary staining of teeth; do not mix with milk or wine-based vehicles.

TAMPER-RESISTANT PACKAGE FEATURE: Imprinted seal around top of bottle; do not use if seal is missing.

Warning: The treatment of any anemic condition should be under the advice and supervision of a physician. Since oral iron products interfere with absorption of oral tetracycline antibiotics, these products should not be taken within two hours of each other. Occasional gastrointestinal discomfort (such as nausea) may be minimized by taking with meals and by beginning with one teaspoonful the first day, two the second, etc. until the recommended dosage is reached. Iron-containing medication may occasionally cause constipation or diarrhea, and liquids may cause temporary staining of the teeth (this is less likely when diluted). Keep this and all drugs out of reach of children. In case of accidental overdose, seek professional assistance or contact a poison control center immediately. As with any drug, if you are pregnant or nursing a baby, seek the advice of a health professional before using this product.

Store at controlled room temperature (59°–86°F.).

Formula: Each 5 ml. (1 teaspoonful) contains ferrous sulfate USP, 220 mg. (44 mg. of elemental iron); alcohol, 5%. **Inactive Ingredients (listed for individuals with specific allergies):** Citric Acid, FD&C Yellow 6 (Sunset Yellow) as a color additive, Flavors, Glucose, Saccharin Sodium, Sucrose, Purified Water.

How Supplied: A clear orange liquid in 16 fl. oz. bottles.

Also available in Tablets and Capsules.

Note: There are other FEOSOL products. Make sure this is the one you are interested in.

Shown in Product Identification Section, page 432

FEOSOL® TABLETS
Hematinic

Product Information: FEOSOL Tablets provide the body with ferrous sulfate, iron in its most efficient form, for iron deficiency and iron-deficiency anemia when the need for such therapy has been determined by a physician. The distinctive triangular-shaped tablet has a coating to prevent oxidation and improve palatability.

Directions: *Adults* —one tablet 3 to 4 times daily after meals and upon retiring or as directed by a physician. *Children 6 to 12 years* —one tablet three times a day after meals. *Children under 6 and infants* —use Feosol® Elixir.

TAMPER-RESISTANT PACKAGE FEATURES FOR YOUR PROTECTION:

- The carton has been sealed at the factory with a clear overwrap printed with "safety sealed."
- Bottle has imprinted "SKCP" seal under cap.
- FEOSOL Tablets are triangular shaped (see product illustration printed on carton).
- DO NOT USE THIS PRODUCT IF ANY OF THESE TAMPER-RESIST-ANT FEATURES ARE MISSING OR BROKEN. IF YOU HAVE ANY QUESTIONS, PLEASE CALL 1-800-543-3434 TOLL FREE.

Warning: Do not exceed recommended dosage. The treatment of any anemic condition should be under the advice and supervision of a physician. Since oral iron products interfere with absorption of oral tetracycline antibiotics, these products should not be taken within two hours of each other.

Occasional gastrointestinal discomfort (such as nausea) may be minimized by taking with meals and by beginning with one tablet the first day, two the second, etc. until the recommended dosage is reached. Iron-containing medication may occasionally cause constipation or diarrhea.

Keep this and all drugs out of reach of children. In case of accidental overdose, seek professional assistance or contact a poison control center immediately.

As with any drug, if you are pregnant or nursing a baby, seek the advice of a health professional before using this product.

Store at controlled room temperature (59°–86°F.).

Formula: Active Ingredients: Each tablet contains 200 mg. of dried ferrous sulfate USP (65 mg. of elemental iron), equivalent to 325 mg. (5 grains) of ferrous sulfate USP. **Inactive Ingredients (listed for individuals with specific allergies):** Calcium Sulfate, D&C Yellow 10, FD&C Blue 2, Glucose, Hydroxypropyl Methylcellulose, Mineral Oil, Polyethylene Glycol, Sodium Lauryl Sulfate, Starch, Stearic Acid, Talc, Titanium Di-

Each tablet/ caplet contains:	SINE-OFF Tablets-Aspirin Formula	SINE-OFF Maximum Strength Allergy/Sinus Formula Caplets	SINE-OFF Maximum Strength No Drowsiness Formula Caplets
Chlorpheniramine maleate	2.0 mg	2.0 mg	—
Phenylpropanolamine HCl	12.5 mg	—	—
Aspirin	325.0 mg	—	—
Acetaminophen	—	500.0 mg	500.0 mg
Pseudoephedrine HCl	—	30.0 mg	30.0 mg

oxide, and trace amounts of other inactive ingredients.

How Supplied: Bottles of 100 and 1000 tablets; in Single Unit Packages of 100 tablets (intended for institutional use only).

Also available in Capsules and Elixir.

Note: There are other FEOSOL products. Make sure this is the one you are interested in.

Shown in Product Identification Section, page 432

ORNEX®
decongestant/analgesic Caplets

Product Information: For temporary relief of nasal congestion, headache, aches, pains and fever due to colds, sinusitis and flu.

NO ANTIHISTAMINE DROWSINESS

Directions: Adults—TWO CAPLETS every 4 hours, not to exceed 8 caplets in any 24-hour period. Children (6 to 12 years)—ONE CAPLET every 4 hours, not to exceed 4 caplets in 24 hours.

TAMPER-RESISTANT PACKAGE FEATURES FOR YOUR PROTECTION:

- The carton has been sealed at the factory with a clear overwrap printed with "safety sealed."
- Each caplet is encased in a clear plastic cell with a foil back.
- The name ORNEX appears on each caplet (see product illustration on front of carton).
- **DO NOT USE THIS PRODUCT IF ANY OF THESE TAMPER-RESISTANT FEATURES ARE MISSING OR BROKEN. IF YOU HAVE ANY QUESTIONS, PLEASE CALL 1-800-543-3434 TOLL FREE.**

Warnings: Do not exceed recommended dosage. Do not give to children under 6 or use for more than 10 days, unless directed by physician. If you have or are being treated for depression, high blood pressure, diabetes, heart disease or thyroid disease, use only as directed by physician. Stop use if dizziness, sleeplessness or nervousness occurs. This package is for households without young children. Keep this and all medicines out of reach of children. In case of accidental overdose, seek professional assistance or contact a poison control center immediately. As with any drug, if you are pregnant or nursing a baby, seek the advice of a health professional before using this product. Store at controlled room temperature (59°–86°F.).

Formula: Active Ingredients: Each caplet contains Pseudoephedrine Hydrochloride 30 mg., Acetaminophen 325 mg.
Inactive Ingredients (listed for individuals with specific allergies): Cellulose, Crospovidone, FD&C Blue 1, Hydroxypropyl Methylcellulose, Magnesium Stearate, Polyethylene Glycol, Polysorbate 80, Povidone, Starch, Titanium Dioxide, and trace amounts of other inactive ingredients.

How Supplied: In consumer packages of 24 and 48 caplets. Also, Dispensary Packages of 792 caplets for industrial dispensaries and student health clinics only.

Shown in Product Identification Section, page 432

SINE–OFF® Maximum Strength Allergy/Sinus Formula Caplets

Composition: [See table above]

Product Information: SINE-OFF Maximum Strength Allergy/Sinus Formula provides maximum strength relief from upper respiratory allergy, hay fever and sinusitis symptoms. This formula contains acetaminophen, a non-aspirin pain reliever.

Product Benefits: Relieves itchy, watery eyes, sneezing, runny nose and postnasal drip • Eases headache pain and pressure • Promotes sinus drainage • Shrinks swollen membranes to relieve congestion.

Directions: Adults and children over 12 years of age: 2 caplets every 6 hours, not to exceed 8 caplets in any 24-hour period. Children under 12 should use only as directed by a physician.

TAMPER-RESISTANT PACKAGING FEATURES FOR YOUR PROTECTION:

- The carton has been sealed at the factory with a clear overwrap printed with "safety sealed."
- Each caplet is encased in a clear plastic cell with a foil back.
- The name SINE-OFF appears on each caplet (see product illustration on front of carton).
- **DO NOT USE THIS PRODUCT IF ANY OF THESE TAMPER-RESISTANT FEATURES ARE MISSING OR BROKEN. IF YOU HAVE ANY QUESTIONS, PLEASE CALL 1-800-543-3434 TOLL FREE.**

Warnings: Do not exceed recommended dosage. If symptoms do not improve within 7 days, consult a physician before continuing use. Individuals being treated for depression, high blood pressure, asthma, heart disease, diabetes, thyroid disease, glaucoma or difficulty urinating due to an enlarged prostate gland should use only as directed by a physician. Do not take this product if you are taking sedatives or tranquilizers. Avoid alcoholic beverages while taking this product. Do not drive or operate heavy machinery. May cause drowsiness. Stop use if dizziness, sleeplessness or nervousness occurs. May cause excitability, especially in children. **This package is child-safe;** however, keep this and all drugs out of reach of children. In case of accidental overdose, seek professional assistance or contact a poison control center immediately. As with any drug, if you are pregnant or nursing a baby, seek the advice of a health professional before using this product.

Store at controlled room temperature (59°–86°F.).

Formula: Active Ingredients: Each caplet contains Chlorpheniramine Maleate 2 mg., Pseudoephedrine Hydrochloride 30 mg., Acetaminophen 500 mg. *(500 mg. is a non-standard dosage of acetaminophen as compared to the standard of 325 mg.).* **Inactive Ingredients (listed for individuals with specific allergies):** Cellulose, Crospovidone, D&C Red 30, D&C Yellow 10, FD&C Blue 2, Hydroxypropyl Methylcellulose, Magnesium Stearate, Polyethylene Glycol, Povidone, Starch, Titanium Dioxide, and trace amounts of other inactive ingredients.

How Supplied: Consumer packages of 24 caplets.

Note: There are other SINE-OFF products. Make sure this is the one you are interested in.

Also Available: SINE-OFF® Sinus Medicine Tablets with Aspirin in 24's, 48's, 100's. SINE-OFF® Maximum Strength No Drowsiness Formula Caplets 24's.

Shown in Product Identification Section, page 432

SINE–OFF® Maximum Strength No Drowsiness Formula Caplets

Composition: [See table above]

Product Information: SINE-OFF Maximum Strength No Drowsiness Formula provides maximum strength relief from headache and sinus pain. Relieves pressure and congestion due to sinusitis, allergic sinusitis or the common cold. This

Continued on next page

SmithKline Consumer—Cont.

formula contains acetaminophen, a non-aspirin pain reliever.

NO ANTIHISTAMINE DROWSINESS

Product Benefits: Eases headache, pain and pressure • Promotes sinus drainage • Shrinks swollen membranes to relieve congestion.

Directions: Adults and children over 12 years of age: 2 caplets every 6 hours, not to exceed 8 caplets in any 24-hour period. Children under 12 should use only as directed by physician.

TAMPER-RESISTANT PACKAGE FEATURES FOR YOUR PROTECTION:

• The carton has been sealed at the factory with a clear overwrap printed with "safety sealed."
• Each caplet is encased in a clear plastic cell with a foil back.
• The name SINE-OFF appears on each caplet (see product illustration on front of carton).
• **DO NOT USE THIS PRODUCT IF ANY OF THESE TAMPER-RESIST-ANT FEATURES ARE MISSING OR BROKEN. IF YOU HAVE ANY QUESTIONS, PLEASE CALL 1-800-543-3434 TOLL FREE.**

Warnings: Do not exceed recommended dosage. If symptoms do not improve within 7 days, consult a physician before continuing use. Individuals being treated for depression, high blood pressure, heart disease, thyroid disease, or difficulty in urination due to enlargement of the prostate gland should use only as directed by a physician. Stop use if dizziness, sleeplessness or nervousness occurs. This package is child-safe; however, keep this and all drugs out of reach of children. In case of accidental overdose, seek professional assistance or contact a poison control center immediately. As with any drug, if you are pregnant or nursing a baby, seek the advice of a health professional before using this product.

Store at controlled room temperature (59°–86°F.).

Formula: Active Ingredients: Each caplet contains: 30 mg. Pseudoephedrine Hydrochloride, 500 mg. Acetaminophen (*500 mg. is a non-standard dosage of acetaminophen, as compared to the standard of 325 mg.*). **Inactive Ingredients (listed for individuals with specific allergies):** Cellulose, Crospovidone, FD&C Red 3, FD&C Yellow 6 (Sunset Yellow) as a color additive, Hydroxypropyl Methylcellulose, Magnesium Stearate, Polyethylene Glycol, Polysorbate 80, Povidone, Starch, Titanium Dioxide, and trace amounts of other inactive ingredients.

How Supplied: Consumer packages of 24 caplets.

Note: There are other SINE-OFF products. Make sure this is the one you are interested in.

Also Available:
SINE-OFF® Tablets with Aspirin
SINE-OFF® Maximum Strength Allergy/Sinus Formula Caplets
Shown in Product Identification Section, page 432

SINE–OFF® Sinus Medicine Tablets–Aspirin Formula
Relieves sinus headache and congestion.

Composition:

[See table on preceding page]

Product Information: SINE-OFF relieves headache, pain, pressure and congestion due to sinusitis, allergic sinusitis, or the common cold.

Product Benefits: Eases headache, pain and pressure • Promotes sinus drainage • Shrinks swollen membranes to relieve congestion • Relieves postnasal drip.

Directions: Adults: 2 tablets every 4 hours, not to exceed 8 tablets in any 24-hour period. Children (6–12) one-half the adult dosage. Children under 6 years should use only as directed by a physician.

TAMPER-RESISTANT PACKAGE FEATURES FOR YOUR PROTECTION:

• The carton has been sealed at the factory with a clear overwrap printed with "safety sealed."
• Each tablet is encased in a clear plastic cell with a foil back.
• The name SINE-OFF appears on each tablet (see product illustration on front of carton).
• **DO NOT USE THIS PRODUCT IF ANY OF THESE TAMPER-RESIST-ANT FEATURES ARE MISSING OR BROKEN. IF YOU HAVE ANY QUESTIONS, PLEASE CALL 1-800-543-3434 TOLL FREE.**

Warning: Children and teenagers should not use this medicine for chicken pox or flu symptoms before a doctor is consulted about Reye syndrome, a rare but serious illness reported to be associated with aspirin. Do not exceed recommended dosage. If symptoms do not improve within 7 days, consult a physician before continuing use. Individuals being treated for depression, high blood pressure, asthma, heart disease, diabetes, thyroid disease, glaucoma or enlarged prostate should use only as directed by a physician. Do not take this product if you are taking another medication containing phenylpropanolamine. ☐ Avoid alcoholic beverages while taking this product. Do not drive or operate heavy machinery as this preparation may cause drowsiness. ☐ Stop use if dizziness, sleeplessness or nervousness occurs. ☐ May cause excitability, especially in children. Keep this and all drugs out of reach of children. In case of accidental overdose, seek professional assistance or contact a poison control center immediately. As with any drug, if you are pregnant or nursing a baby, seek the advice of a health professional before using this product.

Store at controlled room temperature (59°–86°F.).

Formula: Active Ingredients: Chlorpheniramine Maleate 2 mg.; Phenylpropanolamine Hydrochloride 12.5 mg. Aspirin 325 mg. **Inactive Ingredients (listed for individuals with specific allergies):** Acacia, Calcium Sulfate, D&C Yellow 10, Ethylcellulose, FD&C Yellow 6 (Sunset Yellow) as a color additive, Gelatin, Guar Gum, Polysorbate 80, Silicon Dioxide, Starch, Sucrose, Titanium Dioxide, and trace amounts of other inactive ingredients.

How Supplied: Consumer packages of 24, 48 and 100 tablets.

Note: There are other SINE-OFF products. Make sure this is the one you are interested in.

Also Available: SINE-OFF® Maximum Strength Allergy/Sinus Formula Caplets 24's. SINE-OFF® Maximum Strength No Drowsiness Formula Caplets 24's.
Shown in Product Identification Section, page 432

TELDRIN®
Chlorpheniramine Maleate
Timed-Release Allergy Capsules
Maximum Strength 12 mg.

Product Information: Hay fever and allergies are caused by grass and tree pollen, dust and pollution. TELDRIN provides up to 12 hours of relief from hay fever/upper respiratory allergy symptoms: sneezing, runny nose, itchy, watery eyes. TELDRIN is formulated to release some medication initially and the rest gradually over a prolonged period.

Directions: Adults and children over 12: Just one capsule in the morning, and one in the evening. Do not give to children under 12 without the advice and consent of a physician. Not to exceed 24 mg. (2 capsules) in 24 hours.

TAMPER-RESISTANT PACKAGING FEATURES FOR YOUR PROTECTION:

• The carton is protected by a clear overwrap printed with "safety sealed"; do not use if overwrap is missing or broken.
• Each capsule is encased in a plastic cell with a foil back; do not use if the cell or foil is broken.
• Each TELDRIN capsule is protected by a green PERMA-SEAL™ band which bonds the two capsule halves together; do not use if capsule or band is broken.
• A package insert is provided for information on tamper-resistant packaging.

Warning: Do not take this product if you have asthma, glaucoma, or difficulty in urination due to enlargement of the prostate gland, except under the advice and supervision of a physician. Do not drive or operate heavy machinery. May cause drowsiness. Avoid alcoholic beverages while taking this product. May cause excitability, especially in children. Keep this and all drugs out of the reach of children. In case of accidental overdose, seek professional assistance or contact a poison control center immediately. As with any drug, if you are pregnant or nursing a baby, seek the advice of a health professional before using this product.

Formula: Active Ingredient: Each capsule contains Chlorpheniramine Maleate, 12 mg. **Inactive Ingredients (listed for individuals with specific allergies):** Benzyl Alcohol, Cetylpyridinium Chloride, D&C Red 33, Ethylcellulose, FD&C Green 3, Red 3, Red 40, Yellow 6 (Sunset Yellow) as a color additive, Gelatin, Hydrogenated Castor Oil, Silicon Dioxide, Sodium Lauryl Sulfate, Starch, Sucrose, and trace amounts of other inactive ingredients.
Store at controlled room temperature (59°–86°F.).

How Supplied: Maximum Strength 12 mg. Timed-Release capsules in packages of 12, 24 and 48 capsules.
Shown in Product Identification Section, page 432

TROPH–IRON®
Vitamins B₁, B₁₂ and Iron

Indications: For deficiencies of vitamins B₁, B₁₂ and iron.

Directions: Liquid—One teaspoonful daily, or as directed by physician. While its effectiveness is in no way affected, TROPH-IRON Liquid may darken as it ages.

TAMPER-RESISTANT PACKAGE FEATURE: Sealed, imprinted bottle cap; do not use if broken.

Warning: The treatment of any anemic condition should be under the advice and supervision of a physician. Since oral iron products interfere with absorption of oral tetracycline antibiotics, these products should not be taken within two hours of each other.
Iron-containing medications may occasionally cause gastrointestinal discomfort, such as nausea, constipation or diarrhea.
Keep this and all drugs out of reach of children. In case of accidental overdose, seek professional assistance or contact a poison control center immediately.
As with any drug, if you are pregnant or nursing a baby, seek the advice of a health professional before using this product.
Store at room temperature (59°–86°F).

Formula: Each 5 ml. (1 teaspoonful) contains Thiamine Hydrochloride (vitamin B₁), 10 mg.; Cyanocobalamin (vitamin B₁₂), 25 mcg.; Iron, 20 mg., present as soluble ferric pyrophosphate. **Inactive Ingredients (listed for individuals with specific allergies):** Citric Acid, FD&C Red 40, Flavor, Glucose, Glycerin, Methyl and Propyl Paraben, Saccharin Sodium, Sodium Citrate, Purified Water.

How Supplied: Liquid—in 4 fl. oz. (118 ml) bottles.
Shown in Product Identification Section, page 432

TROPHITE®
Vitamins B₁ and B₁₂

Indications: For deficiencies of vitamins B₁ and B₁₂.

Directions: One 5 ml. teaspoonful or as directed by physician.

Important: Dispense liquid only in original bottle or an amber bottle. This product is light-sensitive. Never dispense in a flint, green, or blue bottle.
Trophite Liquid may be mixed with water, milk, or fruit or vegetable juices immediately before taking.
Store at controlled room temperature (59°–86°F.).

TAMPER-RESISTANT PACKAGE FEATURE: Liquid—Sealed, imprinted bottle cap; do not use if broken.

Warning: Keep this and all drugs out of reach of children. In case of accidental overdose, seek professional assistance or contact a poison control center immediately.
As with any drug, if you are pregnant or nursing a baby, seek the advice of a health professional before using this product.

Formula: Each 5 ml. (1 teaspoonful) contains Thiamine Hydrochloride (vitamin B₁), 10 mg.; and Cyanocobalamin (vitamin B₁₂), 25 mcg. **Inactive Ingredients (listed for individuals with specific allergies):** LIQUID—D&C Red 33, Yellow 10, Dextrose, FD&C Blue 1, Flavor, Glycerin, Methyl and Propyl Paraben, Sodium Tartrate, Tartaric Acid, Purified Water.

How Supplied: Liquid—4 fl. oz. (118 ml.) bottles.
Shown in Product Identification Section, page 432

E. R. Squibb & Sons, Inc.
GENERAL OFFICES
P.O. BOX 4000
PRINCETON, NJ 08540

THERAGRAN® LIQUID
High Potency Vitamin Supplement

Each 5 ml. teaspoonful contains:

		Percent US RDA*
Vitamin A	10,000 IU	200
Vitamin D	400 IU	100
Vitamin C	200 mg	333
Thiamine	10 mg	667
Riboflavin	10 mg	588
Niacin	100 mg	500
Vitamin B₆	4.1 mg	205
Vitamin B₁₂	5 mcg	83
Pantothenic Acid	21.4 mg	214

*US Recommended Daily Allowance

Ingredients: water, sugar, glycerin, propylene glycol, sodium ascorbate, niacinamide, polysorbate 80, ascorbic acid, carboxymethylcellulose sodium, d-panthenol, riboflavin-5-phosphate sodium, thiamine hydrochloride, vitamin A palmitate, pyridoxine hydrochloride, (sodium benzoate and methylparaben as preservatives), ferric ammonium citrate, artificial and natural flavors, cholecalciferol, cyanocobalamin

Usage: For 12 year olds and older—1 teaspoonful daily.

How Supplied: In bottles of 4 fl. oz.

Storage: Store at room temperature; avoid excessive heat.
(C0262D)
Shown in Product Identification Section, page 433

ADVANCED FORMULA THERAGRAN® TABLETS
(High Potency Multivitamin Formula)

TABLET CONTENTS: For Adults—Percentage of US recommended daily allowance

Vitamins	Quantity	US RDA
Vitamin A	5000 IU	100%
(plus 1250 IU from Beta-Carotene)		
Vitamin B₁	3 mg	200%
Vitamin B₂	3.4 mg	200%
Vitamin B₆	3 mg	150%
Vitamin B₁₂	9 mcg	150%
Vitamin C	90 mg	150%
Vitamin D	400 IU	100%
Vitamin E	30 IU	100%
Niacin	30 mg	150%
Folic Acid	0.4 mg	100%
Pantothenic Acid	10.0 mg	100%
Biotin	35 mcg	12%

Ingredients: Lactose, ascorbic acid, microcrystalline cellulose, gelatin, sucrose, *dl*-alpha-tocopheryl acetate, niacinamide, starch, calcium pantothenate, sodium caseinate, hydroxypropyl methylcellulose, povidone, pyridoxine hydrochloride, riboflavin, silicon dioxide, magnesium stearate, thiamine mononitrate, vitamin A acetate, polyethylene glycol, triacetin, stearic acid, titanium dioxide, annatto, beta-carotene, Red 40, folic acid, biotin, ergocalciferol, cyanocobalamin.

Warning: KEEP OUT OF REACH OF CHILDREN.

Usage: 1 tablet daily.

How Supplied: Bottles of 1000; Packs of 30, 100, and 180; and Unimatic® cartons of 100.

Storage: Store at room temperature; avoid excessive heat; keep tightly closed. UNIMATIC® is a trademark of E.R. Squibb & Sons, Inc.
Shown in Product Identification Section, page 433

ADVANCED FORMULA THERAGRAN-M® TABLETS
(High Potency Multivitamin Formula with Minerals)

TABLET CONTENTS: For Adults—Percentage of US Recommended Daily Allowance

Vitamins	Quantity	US RDA
Vitamin A	5000 IU	100%
(plus 1250 IU from beta-carotene)		
Vitamin B₁	3 mg	200%
Vitamin B₂	3.4 mg	200%
Vitamin B₆	3 mg	150%
Vitamin B₁₂	9 mcg	150%

Continued on next page

Squibb—Cont.

Vitamin C	90 mg	150%
Vitamin D	400 IU	100%
Vitamin E	30 IU	100%
Niacin	30 mg	150%
Folic Acid	0.4 mg	100%
Pantothenic Acid	10.0 mg	100%
Biotin	35 mcg	12%
Minerals		
Iron	27.0 mg	150%
Copper	2.0 mg	100%
Iodine	150.0 mcg	100%
Zinc	15.0 mg	100%
Magnesium	100.0 mg	25%
Calcium	40.0 mg	4%
Phosphorus	31.0 mg	3%
Chromium	15.0 mcg	*
Molybdenum	15.0 mcg	*
Selenium	10.0 mcg	*
Manganese	5.0 mcg	*
Electrolytes		
Chloride	7.5 mg	*
Potassium	7.5 mg	*

*US RDA not established.

Ingredients: Dibasic calcium phosphate, lactose, magnesium oxide, ascorbic acid, ferrous fumarate, gelatin, sucrose, dl-alpha-tocopheryl acetate, niacinamide, crospovidone, zinc oxide, povidone, starch, manganese sulfate, hydroxypropyl methylcellulose, potassium chloride, calcium pantothenate, sodium caseinate, cupric sulfate, magnesium stearate, silicon dioxide, pyridoxine hydrochloride, stearic acid, riboflavin, thiamine mononitrate, polyethylene glycol, triacetin, vitamin A acetate, beta-carotene, potassium citrate, Red 40, folic acid, titanium dioxide, potassium iodide, chromic chloride, Blue 2, sodium molybdate, biotin, sodium selenate, ergocalciferol, cyanocobalamin.

Usage: 1 tablet daily.

How Supplied: Bottles of 1000; Packs of 30, 60, 100, and 180; and Unimatic® cartons of 100.

Storage: Store at room temperature; avoid excessive heat; keep tightly closed. UNIMATIC® is a trademark of E.R. Squibb & Sons, Inc.

Shown in Product Identification Section, page 433

THERAGRAN® STRESS FORMULA
High Potency Multivitamin Formula with Iron and Biotin

TABLET CONTENTS: For Adults— Percentage of US Recommended Daily Allowance

Ingredients	Quantity	US RDA
Vitamin B₁	15 mg	1000%
Vitamin B₂	15 mg	882%
Vitamin B₆	25 mg	1250%
Vitamin B₁₂	12 mcg	200%
Vitamin C	600 mg	1000%
Vitamin E	30 IU	100%
Niacin	100 mg	500%
Pantothenic Acid	20 mg	200%
Iron	27 mg	150%

Folic Acid	400 mcg	100%
Biotin	45 mcg	15%

Ingredients: Ascorbic acid, niacinamide, ferrous fumarate, microcrystalline cellulose, lactose, pyridoxine hydrochloride, starch, dl-alpha-tocopheryl acetate, gelatin, calcium pantothenate, croscarmellose sodium, hydroxypropyl methylcellulose, povidone, riboflavin, thiamine mononitrate, sodium caseinate, magnesium stearate, silicon dioxide, stearic acid, titanium dioxide, Red 40, Yellow 6, polyethylene glycol, triacetin, folic acid, biotin, cyanocobalamin.

Usage: For adults—1 tablet daily or as directed by physician.

How Supplied: Bottles of 75.

Storage: Store at room temperature; avoid excessive heat. (C0584)

Shown in Product Identification Section, page 433

Standard Homeopathic Company
**210 WEST 131st STREET
BOX 61067
LOS ANGELES, CA 90061**

HYLAND'S BED WETTING TABLETS

Active Ingredients: *Equisetum hyemale* (Scouring Rush) 2X HPUS, *Rhus aromatica* (Fragrant Sumac) 3X HPUS, *Belladonna* 3X HPUS (0.0003% Alkaloids).

Inactive Ingredients: Lactose USP.

Indications: A homeopathic combination for the temporary relief of involuntary urination (common bed wetting) in children.

Directions: Children 3 to 12 years: 2 to 3 tablets before meals and at bedtime, or as directed by a licensed health care practitioner. Children over 12 years: double the above recommended dose.

Warnings: If symptoms persist for more than seven days or worsen, consult a Health Care Professional. As with any drug, if you are pregnant or nursing a baby, seek the advice of a health professional before using this product. Keep this and all medication out of the reach of children.

How Supplied: Bottles of 125—one grain sublingual tablets (NDC 54973-7501-01). Store at room temperature.

HYLAND'S CALMS FORTÉ TABLETS

Active Ingredients: *Passiflora* (Passion Flower) 1X triple strength HPUS, *Avena sativa* (Oat) 1X triple strength HPUS, *Humulus lupulus* (Hops) 1X double strength HPUS, *Chamomilla* (Chamomile) 2X HPUS, *Calcarea Phosphorica* (Calcium Phosphate) 3X HPUS, *Ferrum Phosphorica* (Iron Phosphate) 3X HPUS, *Kali Phosphoricum* (Potassium Phosphate) 3X HPUS, *Natrum Phosphoricum*

(Sodium Phosphate) 3X HPUS, *Magnesia Phosphoricum* (Magnesium Phosphate) 3X HPUS.

Inactive Ingredients: Lactose USP.

Indications: Temporary symptomatic relief of simple nervous tension and insomnia.

Directions: Adults, As a relaxant: 1 to 2 tablets as needed or 3 times daily between meals. In insomnia: 1 to 3 tablets ½ to 1 hour before retiring. Repeat as needed without danger of side effects. Children, As a relaxant: 1 tablet as needed or 3 times daily before meals. In insomnia: 1 to 2 tablets 1 hour before retiring. Non-habit-forming.

Warnings: If symptoms persist for more than seven days or worsen, consult a Health Care Professional. As with any drug, if you are pregnant or nursing a baby, seek the advice of a health professional before using this product. Keep this and all medication out of the reach of children.

How Supplied: Bottles of 100 four grain tablets (NDC 54973-1121-02). Store at room temperature. Bottles of 50 four grain tablets (NDC 54973-1121-01). Store at room temperature.

HYLAND'S COLIC TABLETS

Active Ingredients: *Disocorea* (Wild Yam) 2X HPUS, *Chamomilla* (Chamomile) 3X HPUS, *Colocynth* (Bitter Apple) 3X HPUS.

Inactive Ingredients: Lactose USP.

Indications: A homeopathic combination for the temporary relief of colic and gas pains caused by irritating food, feeding too quickly, swallowing air and similar conditions during teething, colds and other minor upset periods in children.

Directions: For children to 2 years of age: administer 2 tablets dissolved in a teaspoon of water or on the tongue every 15 minutes until relieved; then every 2 hours as required. Children over 2 years: 3 tablets dissolved on the tongue as above; or as recommended by a licensed health care practitioner.

Warnings: If symptoms persist for more than seven days or worsen, consult a Health Care Professional. Keep this and all medication out of the reach of children.

How Supplied: Bottles of 125—one grain sublingual tablets (NDC 54973-7502-01). Store at room temperature.

HYLAND'S COUGH SYRUP WITH HONEY™

Active Ingredients: Each fluid ounce contains: *Ipecacuanha* (Ipecac) 3X HPUS, *Aconitum napellus* (Aconite) 3X HPUS, *Spongia Tosta* (Sponge) 3X HPUS, *Antimonium Tartaricum* (Potassium Antimony Tartrate) 6X HPUS.

Inactive Ingredients: Simple syrup and honey.

Indications: A homeopathic combination for the temporary relief of symptoms of simple, dry, tight or tickling coughs due to colds in children.

Directions: Children 1 to 12 years: 1 to 3 teaspoonfuls as required. Children over 12 years and adults: 3 to 4 teaspoonfuls as required. May be taken with or without water. Repeat as often as necessary to relieve symptoms. For children under 1 year of age, consult a licensed health care practitioner.

Warnings: Do not use this product for persistent or chronic cough such as occurs with asthma, smoking or emphysema; or if cough is accompanied with excessive mucus, unless directed by a licensed health care practitioner. If symptoms persist for more than seven days, tend to recur, or are accompanied by a high fever, rash, or persistent headache, consult a Health Care Professional. As with any drug, if you are pregnant or nursing a baby, seek the advice of a health professional before using this product. Keep this and all medication out of the reach of children.

How Supplied: Bottles of 4 fluid ounces (120 ml) (NDC 54973-7503-02). Store at room temperature.

HYLAND'S C–PLUS™COLD TABLETS

Active Ingredients: *Eupatorium perfoliatum* (Boneset) 2X HPUS, *Euphrasia officinalis* (Eyebright) 2X HPUS, *Gelsemium sempervirens* (Yellow Jasmine) 3X HPUS, *Kali Iodatum* (Potassium Iodide) 3X HPUS.

Inactive Ingredients: Lactose USP, Natural Raspberry Flavor.

Indications: A homeopathic combination for the temporary relief of symptoms of runny nose and sneezing due to common head colds in children.

Directions: Children 1 to 3 years: 2 tablets every 15 minutes for 4 doses, then hourly until relieved. For children 3 to 6 years: 3 tablets as above; for children 6 and older: 6 tablets as above or as directed by a licensed health care practitioner.

Warnings: If symptoms persist for more than seven days or worsen, consult a Health Care Professional. As with any drug, if you are pregnant or nursing a baby, seek the advice of a health professional before using this product. Keep this and all medication out of the reach of children.

How Supplied: Bottles of 125—one grain sublingual tablets (NDC 54973-7505-01). Store at room temperature.

HYLAND'S TEETHING TABLETS

Active Ingredients: *Calcarea Phosphorica* (Calcium Phosphate) 3X HPUS, *Chamomilla* (Chamomile) 3X HPUS, *Coffea Cruda* (Coffee) 3X HPUS, *Belladonna* 3X HPUS (Alkaloids 0.0003%).

Inactive Ingredients: Lactose USP.

Indications: A homeopathic combination for the temporary relief of symptoms of simple restlessness and wakeful irritability due to cutting of teeth.

Directions: 2 to 3 tablets in a teaspoon of water or on the tongue, 4 times per day. If the child is restless or wakeful, 2 tablets every hour for 6 doses or as directed by a licensed health care practitioner.

Warnings: If symptoms persist for more than seven days or worsen, consult a Health Care Professional. As with any drug, if you are pregnant or nursing a baby, seek the advice of a health professional before using this product. Keep this and all medication out of the reach of children.

How Supplied: Bottles of 125—one grain sublingual tablets (NDC 54973-7504-01). Store at room temperature.

HYLAND'S VITAMIN C FOR CHILDREN™

Active Ingredients: 25 mg Vitamin C as Sodium Ascorbate (30 mg).

Inactive Ingredients: Lactose USP, Natural Lemon Flavor.

Indications: Each tablet provides children with 55% of the daily recommended requirement of Vitamin C. Sodium Ascorbate is preferred to Ascorbic Acid when gastric irritation may result from free acid.

Directions: Children 2 years and older: 1 to 2 tablets on the tongue or as directed by a licensed health care practitioner.

Warning: Keep this and all medication out of the reach of children.

How Supplied: Bottles of 125—one grain sublingual tablets (NDC 54973-7506-01). Store at room temperature. Tablets may turn brown in color with exposure to light. Color change does not affect potency.

Stellar Pharmacal Corp.
Div./Star Pharmaceuticals, Inc.
**1990 N.W. 44TH STREET
POMPANO BEACH, FL
33064-8712**

STAR-OTIC®
**Antibacterial, Antifungal, Nonaqueous Ear Solution
For Prevention of "Swimmer's Ear"**

Active Ingredients: Acetic acid nonaqueous, Burow's solution, Boric acid, in a propylene glycol vehicle, with an acid pH and a low surface tension.

Indications: For the prevention of otitis externa, commonly called "Swimmer's Ear".

Actions: Star-Otic is antibacterial, antifungal, hydrophilic, has an acid pH and a low surface tension. Acetic acid and boric acid inhibit the rapid multiplication of microorganisms and help maintain the lining mantle of the ear canal in its normal acid state. Burow's solution (aluminum acetate) is a mild astringent. Propylene glycol reduces moisture in the ear canal.

Warning: Do not use in ear if tympanic membrane (ear drum) is perforated or punctured.

Symptoms and Treatment of Overdosage: Discontinue use if undue irritation or sensitivity occurs.

Dosage and Administration: Adults and Children: For the prevention of otitis externa (Swimmer's Ear). In susceptible persons, instill 2–3 drops of Star-Otic in each ear before and after swimming or bathing, or as directed by physician.

Professional Labeling: Same as those outlined under Indications.

How Supplied: Available in ½ oz measured drop, safety tip, plastic bottle.
Shown in Product Identification Section, page 433

EDUCATIONAL MATERIAL

First Aid Prevention for Swimmer's Ear
Public health information on cause and care of preventing swimmer's ear.
Star-Otic Patient Instruction Pads
Instructions for patients on use of Star-Otic to prevent swimmer's ear.

Stuart Pharmaceuticals
**a business unit of
ICI Americas Inc.
WILMINGTON, DE 19897 USA**

ALternaGEL®
[al-tern 'a-jel]
**Liquid
High-Potency Aluminum Hydroxide Antacid**

Description: ALternaGEL is available as a white, pleasant-tasting, high-potency aluminum hydroxide liquid antacid.

Ingredients: Each 5 mL teaspoonful contains: Active: 600 mg aluminum hydroxide (equivalent to dried gel, USP) providing 16 milliequivalents (mEq) of acid-neutralizing capacity (ANC), and less than 2.5 mg (0.109 mEq) of sodium and no sugar. Inactive: butylparaben, flavors, propylparaben, purified water, simethicone, and other ingredients.

Indications: ALternaGEL is indicated for the symptomatic relief of hyperacidity associated with peptic ulcer, gastritis, peptic esophagitis, gastric hyperacidity, hiatal hernia, and heartburn. ALternaGEL will be of special value to those patients for whom magnesium-containing antacids are undesirable, such as

Continued on next page

Stuart—Cont.

patients with renal insufficiency, patients requiring control of attendant G.I. complications resulting from steroid or other drug therapy, and patients experiencing the laxation which may result from magnesium or combination antacid regimens.

Directions: One to two teaspoonfuls, as needed, between meals and at bedtime, or as directed by a physician: May be followed by a sip of water if desired. Concentrated product. Shake well before using. Keep tightly closed.

Warnings: As with all medications, ALternaGEL should be kept out of the reach of children. ALternaGEL may cause constipation.
Except under the advice and supervision of a physician: do not take more than 18 teaspoonfuls in a 24-hour period, or use the maximum dose of ALternaGEL for more than two weeks.

Drug Interaction Precaution:
ALternaGEL should not be taken concurrently with an antibiotic containing any form of tetracycline.

How Supplied: ALternaGEL is available in bottles of 12 fluid ounces and 5 fluid ounces, and 1 fluid ounce hospital unit doses. NDC 0038-0860.
Shown in Product Identification Section, page 433

DIALOSE® Capsules
[di 'a-lose]
Stool Softener Laxative

Description: DIALOSE is a sodium-free, nonhabit forming, stool softener containing docusate potassium in capsules of 100 mg.
The docusate in DIALOSE is a highly efficient surfactant which facilitates absorption of water by the stool to form a soft, easily evacuated mass. Unlike stimulant laxatives, DIALOSE does not interfere with normal peristalsis, neither does it cause griping nor sensations of urgency.

Ingredients: Each capsule contains: Active: docusate potassium. Inactive: Blue 1, gelatin, lactose, magnesium stearate, Red 28, Red 40, silicon dioxide, titanium dioxide.

Indications: DIALOSE is an effective aid to soften or prevent formation of hard stools in a wide range of conditions that may lead to constipation. DIALOSE helps to eliminate straining associated with obstetric, geriatric, cardiac, surgical, anorectal, or proctologic conditions. In cases of mild constipation, the fecal softening action of DIALOSE can prevent constipation from progressing and relieve painful defecation.

Directions: *Adults:* Adjust dosage as needed, one capsule one to three times daily. *Children:* 6 years and over—One capsule at bedtime, or as directed by physician. *Children:* under 6 years—As directed by physician. It is helpful to in-

crease the daily intake of fluids by taking a glass of water with each dose.

Warnings: As with any drug, if you are pregnant or nursing a baby, seek the advice of a health professional before using this product. Keep out of the reach of children.

How Supplied: Bottles of 36 and 100 pink capsules, identified "STUART 470". Also available in 100 capsule unit dose boxes (10 strips of 10 capsules each). NDC 0038-0470
Shown in Product Identification Section, page 433

DIALOSE® PLUS Capsules
[di 'a-lose Plus]
Stool Softener/Stimulant Laxative

Description: DIALOSE PLUS provides a sodium-free formulation of docusate potassium in capsules of 100 mg and casanthranol, 30 mg.

Ingredients: Each capsule contains: Active: docusate potassium, casanthranol. Inactive: gelatin, lactose, magnesium stearate, Red 33, silicon dioxide, titanium dioxide, Yellow 10.

Indications: DIALOSE PLUS is indicated for the treatment of constipation characterized by lack of moisture in the intestinal contents, resulting in hardness of stool and decreased intestinal motility. DIALOSE PLUS combines the advantages of the stool softener, docusate potassium, with the peristaltic activating effect of casanthranol.

Directions: *Adults:* Initially, one capsule two times a day. *Children:* As directed by physician. When adequate bowel function is restored, the dose may be adjusted to meet individual needs. It is helpful to increase the daily intake of fluids by taking a glass of water with each dose.

Warnings: As with any drug, if you are pregnant or nursing a baby, seek the advice of a health professional before using this product. And, as with any laxative, DIALOSE PLUS should not be used when abdominal pain, nausea, or vomiting are present. Frequent or prolonged use may result in dependence on laxatives. Keep out of the reach of children.

How Supplied: Bottles of 36, 100, and 500 yellow capsules, identified "STUART 475". Also available in 100 capsule unit dose boxes (10 strips of 10 capsules each). NDC 0038-0475
Shown in Product Identification Section, page 433

EFFER-SYLLIUM®
[ef'fer-sil 'lium]
Natural Fiber Bulking Agent

Description: EFFER-SYLLIUM is a tan, granular powder. Each rounded teaspoonful, or individual packet (7 g) contains psyllium hydrocolloid, 3 g.

Ingredients: Active: psyllium hydrocolloid. Inactive: citric acid, ethyl vanillin, lemon and lime flavors, potassium

bicarbonate, potassium citrate, saccharin calcium, starch, sucrose.
EFFER-SYLLIUM contains less than 5 mg sodium per rounded teaspoonful and is considered dietetically sodium free.

Indications: EFFER-SYLLIUM is indicated to restore normal bowel habits in chronic constipation, to promote normal elimination in irritable bowel syndrome, and to ease passage of stools in presence of anorectal disorders. EFFER-SYLLIUM produces a soft, lubricating bulk which promotes natural elimination.
EFFER-SYLLIUM is not a one-dose, fast-acting bowel regulator. Administration for several days may be needed to establish regularity.

Directions:
Adults: One rounded teaspoonful, or one packet, in a glass of water one to three times a day, or as directed by physician. *Children, 6 years and over:* One level teaspoonful, or one-half packet (3.5 g) in one-half glass of water at bedtime, or as directed by physician. *Children, under 6 years:* As directed by physician.

Instructions: Pour EFFER-SYLLIUM into a *dry* glass, add water and stir briskly. Drink immediately. To avoid caking, always use a *dry* spoon to remove EFFER-SYLLIUM from its container. Replace cap tightly. Keep in a dry place.

Caution: People sensitive to psyllium powder should avoid inhalation as it may cause an allergic reaction such as wheezing.

Warning: As with all medications, keep out of the reach of children.

How Supplied: Bottles of 9 oz and 16 oz, and individual convenience packets (7 g each) packaged in boxes of 12 and 24. NDC 0038-0440.
Shown in Product Identification Section, page 433

FERANCEE®
[fer 'an-see]
Chewable Hematinic

Two Tablets Daily Provide:

	US RDA*	
Iron	744%	134 mg
Vitamin C	500%	300 mg

*Percentage of US Recommended Daily Allowances for adults and children 4 or more years of age.

Ingredients: Active: ferrous fumarate, sodium ascorbate, ascorbic acid. Inactive: confectioner's sugar, flavors, magnesium stearate, mannitol, povidone, saccharin calcium, starch, Yellow 5 (tartrazine), Yellow 6.

Indications: A pleasant-tasting hematinic for iron deficiency anemias, well-tolerated FERANCEE is particularly useful when chronic blood loss, onset of menses, or pregnancy create additional demands for iron supplementation. Available information indicates a low incidence of staining of the teeth by ferrous fumarate, alone or in combination with ascorbic acid. The peach-cherry flavored chewable tablets dissolve quickly in the mouth and may be either chewed or swallowed.

Directions:
Adults: Two tablets daily, or as directed by physician.
Chidren over 6 years of age: One tablet daily, or as directed by physician.
Children under 6 years of age: As directed by physician.

Warnings: As with any drug, if you are pregnant or nursing a baby, seek the advice of a health professional before using this product. Keep out of the reach of children. In case of accidental overdose, seek professional assistance or contact a Poison Control Center immediately.

How Supplied: Bottles of 100 brown and yellow, two-layer tablets identified "STUART 650" on brown layer. A child-resistant cap is standard on each bottle as a safeguard against accidental ingestion by children. Keep in a dry place. Replace cap tightly.
NDC 0038-0650.

FERANCEE®–HP Tablets
[fer-an-see hp]
High Potency Hematinic
One Tablet Daily Provides:
US RDA*

Iron	611%	110 mg
Vitamin C	1000%	600 mg

*Percentage of US Recommended Daily Allowances for adults and children 4 or more years of age.

Ingredients: Active: ferrous fumarate, sodium ascorbate, ascorbic acid. Inactive: flavor, hydrogenated vegetable oil, microcrystalline cellulose, povidone, Red 40, and other ingredients.

Indications: FERANCEE-HP is a high potency formulation of iron and vitamin C and is intended for use as either:
(1) a maintenance hematinic for those patients needing a daily iron supplement to maintain normal hemoglobin levels, or
(2) intensive therapy for the acute and/or severe iron deficiency anemia where a high intake of elemental iron is required.
The use of well-tolerated ferrous fumarate provides high levels of elemental iron with a low incidence of gastric distress. The inclusion of 600 mg of vitamin C per tablet serves to maintain more of the iron in the absorbable ferrous state.

Precautions: Because FERANCEE-HP contains 110 mg of elemental iron per tablet, it is recommended that its use be limited to adults, ie over 12 years of age.

Directions: One tablet per day after a meal or as directed by a physician. Should be sufficient to maintain normal hemoglobin levels in most patients with a history of recurring iron deficiency anemia. Not recommended for children under 12 years of age.
For acute and/or severe iron deficiency anemia, two or three tablets per day taken one tablet per dose after meals. (Each tablet provides 110 mg elemental iron).

Warnings: As with all medications, keep out of the reach of children. In case of accidental overdose, seek professional assistance or contact a Poison Control Center immediately.

How Supplied: FERANCEE-HP is supplied in bottles of 60 red, film coated, oval shaped tablets.
NDC 0038-0863.
Note: A child-resistant safety cap is standard on each bottle of 60 tablets as a safeguard against accidental ingestion by children.
Shown in Product Identification Section, page 433

HIBICLENS® Antiseptic
Antimicrobial
[hibi-klenz]
Skin Cleanser
(chlorhexidine gluconate)

Description: HIBICLENS is an antiseptic antimicrobial skin cleanser possessing bactericidal activities. HIBICLENS contains 4% w/v HIBITANE® (chlorhexidine gluconate), a chemically unique hexamethylenebis biguanide with inactive ingredients: fragrance, isopropyl alcohol 4%, purified water, Red 40, and other ingredients, in a mild, sudsing base adjusted to pH 5.0–6.5 for optimal activity and stability as well as compatability with the normal pH of the skin.

Action: HIBICLENS is bactericidal on contact. It has antiseptic activity and a persistent antimicrobial effect with rapid bactericidal activity against a wide range of microorganisms, including gram-positive bacteria, and gram-negative bacteria such as *Pseudomonas aeruginosa*. The effectiveness of HIBICLENS is not significantly reduced by the presence of organic matter, such as blood.[1]
In a study[2] simulating surgical use, the immediate bactericidal effect of HIBICLENS after a single six-minute scrub resulted in a 99.9% reduction in resident bacterial flora, with a reduction of 99.98% after the eleventh scrub. Reductions on surgically gloved hands were maintained over the six-hour test period.
HIBICLENS displays persistent antimicrobial action. In one study,[2] 93% of a radiolabeled formulation of HIBICLENS remained present on uncovered skin after five hours.
HIBICLENS prevents skin infection thereby reducing the risk of cross-infection.

Indications: HIBICLENS is indicated for use as a surgical scrub, as a healthcare personnel handwash, for patient preoperative showering and bathing, as a patient preoperative skin preparation, and as a skin wound cleanser and general skin cleanser.

Safety: The extensive use of chlorhexidine gluconate for over 20 years outside the United States has produced no evidence of absorption of the compound through intact skin. The potential for producing skin reactions is extremely low. HIBICLENS can be used many times a day without causing irritation, dryness, or discomfort. Experimental studies indicate that when used for cleaning superficial wounds, HIBICLENS will neither cause additional tissue injury nor delay healing.

Warnings: FOR EXTERNAL USE ONLY. KEEP OUT OF EYES, EARS AND MOUTH. HIBICLENS SHOULD NOT BE USED AS A PREOPERATIVE SKIN PREPARATION OF THE FACE OR HEAD. MISUSE OF HIBICLENS HAS BEEN REPORTED TO CAUSE SERIOUS AND PERMANENT EYE INJURY WHEN IT HAS BEEN PERMITTED TO ENTER AND REMAIN IN THE EYE DURING SURGICAL PROCEDURES. IF HIBICLENS SHOULD CONTACT THESE AREAS, RINSE OUT PROMPTLY AND THOROUGHLY WITH WATER. Avoid contact with meninges. HIBICLENS should not be used by persons who have a sensitivity to it or its components. Chlorhexidine gluconate has been reported to cause deafness when instilled in the middle ear through perforated ear drums. Irritation, sensitization and generalized allergic reactions have been reported with chlorhexidine-containing products, especially in the genital areas. If adverse reactions occur, discontinue use immediately and if severe, contact a physician. Keep this and all drugs out of the reach of children. In case of accidental ingestion, seek professional assistance or contact a Poison Control Center immediately.
Accidental ingestion: Chlorhexidine gluconate taken orally is poorly absorbed. Treat with gastric lavage using milk, egg white, gelatin or mild soap. Employ supportive measures as appropriate. Avoid excessive heat (above 104°F).

Directions for Use:
Patient preoperative skin preparation
Apply HIBICLENS liberally to surgical site and swab for at least two minutes. Dry with a sterile towel. Repeat procedure for an additional two minutes and dry with a sterile towel.
Preoperative showering and whole-body bathing
The patient should be instructed to wash the entire body, including the scalp, on two consecutive occasions immediately prior to surgery. Each procedure should consist of two consecutive thorough applications of HIBICLENS followed by thorough rinsing. If the patient's condition allows, showering is recommended for whole-body bathing. The recommended procedure is: Wet the body, including hair. Wash the hair using 25 mL of HIBICLENS and the body with another 25 mL of HIBICLENS. Rinse. Repeat. Rinse thoroughly after second application.
Skin wound and general skin cleansing
Wounds which involve more than the superficial layers of the skin should not be routinely treated with HIBICLENS. HIBICLENS should not be used for repeated general skin cleansing of large

Continued on next page

Stuart—Cont.

body areas except in those patients whose underlying condition makes it necessary to reduce the bacterial population of the skin. To use, thoroughly rinse the area to be cleansed with water. Apply the minimum amount of HIBICLENS necessary to cover the skin or wound area and wash gently. Rinse again thoroughly.

Health-care personnel use

SURGICAL HAND SCRUB

Directions for use of HIBICLENS Liquid: Wet hands and forearms to the elbows with warm water. (Avoid using very cold or very hot water.) Dispense about 5 mL of HIBICLENS into cupped hands. Spread over both hands. Scrub hands and forearms for 3 minutes without adding water, using a brush or sponge. (Avoid using extremely hard-bristled brushes.) While scrubbing, pay particular attention to fingernails, cuticles, and interdigital spaces. (Do not use excessive pressure to produce additional lather.) Rinse thoroughly with warm water. Dispense about 5 mL of HIBICLENS into cupped hands. Wash for an additional 3 minutes. (No need to use brush or sponge.) Then rinse thoroughly. Dry thoroughly.

HAND WASH

Wet hands with water. (Avoid using very cold or very hot water.) Dispense about 5 mL of HIBICLENS into cupped hands. Wash for 15 seconds. (Do not use excessive pressure to produce additional lather.) Rinse thoroughly with warm water. Dry thoroughly.

Directions for use of HIBICLENS® Sponge/Brush: Open package and remove nail cleaner. Wet hands. Use nail cleaner under fingernails and to clean cuticles. Wet hands and forearms to the elbow with warm water. (Avoid using very cold or very hot water.) Wet sponge side of sponge/brush. Squeeze and pump immediately to work up adequate lather. Apply lather to hands and forearms using *sponge* side of the product. *Start 3 minute scrub* by using the brush side of the product to scrub *only* nails, cuticles, and interdigital areas. Use sponge side for scrubbing hands and forearms. (Avoid using brush on these more sensitive areas.) Rinse thoroughly with warm water. Scrub for an additional 3 minutes *using sponge side* only. To produce additional lather, add a small amount of water and pump the sponge. (While scrub-

bing, do not use excessive pressure to produce lather—a small amount of lather is all that is required to adequately cleanse skin with HIBICLENS.) Rinse and dry thoroughly, blotting hands and forearms with a soft sterile towel.

IMPORTANT LAUNDERING ADVICE FOR HOSPITAL STAFF AND OTHER USERS OF ANTISEPTIC PATIENT SKIN PREPARATIONS CONTAINING CHLORHEXIDINE GLUCONATE

Chlorhexidine gluconate is a unique agent that most closely fits the definition of an ideal antimicrobial agent, having (among others) one of the most important characteristics of persistent activity. This persistence is due to chlorhexidine gluconate binding to the protein of the skin and, thus, being available for residual activity over a relatively long period of time.

Chlorhexidine gluconate, however, binds not only to protein of the skin, but also to many fabrics, particularly cotton. Thus, special laundering procedures should be considered when such products contact these fabrics. As a result of such contact, chlorhexidine gluconate may become adsorbed onto the fabric and not be removed by washing. If sufficient available chlorine is present during the washing procedure, a fast brown stain may develop due to a chemical reaction between chlorhexidine gluconate and chlorine.

SUGGESTED LAUNDERING PROCEDURES TO LIMIT STAINING

1. Not Aging. Avoid allowing the product to age (set) on unwashed linens.

2. Flushing and Washing. A flush operation as the initial step in the wash process is helpful in the laundering of linen exposed to chlorhexidine gluconate. Such flushing is also important in the laundering of linen which contains organic materials such as blood or pus. For best results, warm water flushes (90°–100°F) are recommended. After a number of initial flushings followed by a washing with a low alkaline/nonchlorine detergent, most articles which come in contact with chlorhexidine gluconate should have an acceptable level of whiteness. If a rewash process using bleach is necessary to achieve a greater degree of whiteness, the bleach used should be a nonchlorine bleach.

3. Not Using Chlorine Bleach. Modern laundering methods often make

the use of chlorine bleach unnecessary. It is worthwhile trying to wash without chlorine to ascertain if the resulting degree of whiteness is acceptable. Omission of chlorine from the laundering process can extend the useful life of cotton articles since oxidizing bleaches such as chlorine may cause some damage to cellulose even when used in low concentration.

4. Changing to a Peroxide-Type Bleach, Such as Sodium Perborate, Sodium Percarbonate or Hydrogen Peroxide. This should eliminate the reaction which could occur with the use of chlorine bleaches. If a chlorine bleach must be used, a concentration of less than 7 ppm available chlorine ($\frac{1}{10}$ the normal bleach level) is suggested to minimize possible staining.

A NOTE ON LAUNDERING OF PERSONAL CLOTHING

The laundering procedures set forth above using low alkaline, nonchlorinated laundry detergents are also applicable to laundering of uniforms and lab coats. Commerically available laundry detergents which do not contain chlorine include Borax, Borateem, Dreft, Oxydol, and Ivory Snow. These products, however, will not remove stains previously set into the fabric.

RECLAMATION OF STAINED LINENS

For those linens which previously have been stained due to the chemical reaction between chlorhexidine gluconate and chlorine, the following laundering procedure may be helpful in reducing the visible stain:

[See table below].

How Supplied: *For general handwashing locations:* pocket-size, 15 mL foil Packettes; plastic disposable bottles of 4 oz and 8 oz with dispenser caps; and 16 oz filled globes. *For surgical scrub areas:* disposable, unit-of-use 22 mL impregnated Sponge/Brushes with nail cleaner; plastic disposable bottles of 32 oz and 1 gal. The 32-oz bottle is designed for a special foot-operated wall dispenser. A hand-operated wall dispenser is available for the 16-oz globe. Hand pumps are available for 16 oz, 32 oz, and 1 gal sizes.
NDC 0038-0575 (liquid).
NDC 0038-0577 (sponge/brush).

References:
1. Lowbury EJL, and Lilly HA: The effect of blood on disinfection of surgeons' hands, Brit. J. Surg. 61:19–21 (Jan.) 1974.
2. Peterson AF, Rosenberg A, Alatary SD: Comparative evaluation of surgical scrub preparations, Surg. Gynecol. Obstet. 146:63–65 (Jan.) 1978.
Shown in Product Identification Section, page 433

Operation	Water Level	Temperature	Time (Min)	Supplies/ 100 lb
Break	Low	180°F	20	1.5 lb oxalic acid
Flush	High	Cold	1	—
Emulsify	Low	160°F	5	18 oz emulsifier
Flush	High	Cold	1	—
Bleach	Low	180°F	20	2 lb alkali builder and 1 lb organic bleach
Rinse	High	Cold	1	
Antichlor	High	Cold	2	4 oz antichlor
Rinse	High	Cold	1	
Rinse	High	Cold	1	—
Sour	Low	Cold	4	2 oz rust removing sour

HIBISTAT®
Germicidal Hand Rinse
HIBISTAT® TOWELETTE
Germicidal Hand Wipe
[*hi-bi-stat*]
(chlorhexidine gluconate)

Description: HIBISTAT is a germicidal hand rinse which provides rapid bactericidal action and has a persistent antimicrobial effect against a wide range of microorganisms. HIBISTAT is a clear, colorless liquid containing 0.5% w/w HIBITANE® (chlorhexidine gluconate) with inactive ingredients: emollients, isopropyl alcohol 70%, purified water.

Indications: HIBISTAT is indicated for health-care personnel use as a germicidal hand rinse. HIBISTAT is for hand hygiene on physically clean hands. It is used in those situations where hands are physically clean, but in need of degerming, when routine handwashing is not convenient or desirable. HIBISTAT provides rapid germicidal action and has a persistent effect.
HIBISTAT should be used in-between patients and procedures where there are no sinks available or continued return to the sink area is inconvenient. HIBISTAT can be used as an alternative to detergent-based products when hands are physically clean. Also, HIBISTAT is an effective germicidal hand rinse following a soap and water handwash.

Warnings: Flammable. This product is alcohol based. Alcohol is extremely flammable. It should be kept away from flame or devices which may generate an electrical spark.
FOR EXTERNAL USE ONLY. KEEP OUT OF EYES, EARS AND MOUTH. HIBISTAT SHOULD NOT BE USED AS A PREOPERATIVE SKIN PREPARATION OF THE FACE OR HEAD. MISUSE OF CHLORHEXIDINE-CONTAINING PRODUCTS HAS BEEN REPORTED TO CAUSE SERIOUS AND PERMANENT EYE INJURY WHEN IT HAS BEEN PERMITTED TO ENTER AND REMAIN IN THE EYE DURING SURGICAL PROCEDURES. IF HIBISTAT SHOULD CONTACT THESE AREAS, RINSE OUT PROMPTLY AND THOROUGHLY WITH WATER. Avoid contact with meninges. HIBISTAT should not be used by persons who have a sensitivity to it or its components. Chlorhexidine gluconate has been reported to cause deafness when instilled in the middle ear through perforated ear drums. Irritation, sensitization and generalized allergic reactions have been reported with chlorhexidine-containing products, especially in the genital areas. If adverse reactions occur, discontinue use immediately and if severe, contact a physician. Keep this and all drugs out of the reach of children. In case of accidental ingestion, seek professional assistance or contact a Poison Control Center immediately.
Avoid excessive heat (above 104°F).
Accidental ingestion: Chlorhexidine gluconate taken orally is poorly absorbed. Treat with gastric lavage using milk, egg white, gelatin or mild soap avoiding pulmonary aspiration. Do not use apomorphine. Assist respiration if necessary and keep patient warm. Intravenous levulose can accelerate alcohol metabolism. In severe cases, hemodialysis or peritoneal dialysis may be appropriate.

Directions for Use: HIBISTAT Towelette: Rub hands vigorously with the HIBISTAT Towelette for approximately 15 seconds, paying particular attention to nails and interdigital spaces. HIBISTAT dries rapidly in use. No water or towel drying is necessary. The emollients contained in the HIBISTAT Towelette protect the hands from the potential drying effect of alcohol.
HIBISTAT Liquid: Dispense about 5 mL of HIBISTAT into cupped hands and rub vigorously until dry (about 15 seconds), paying particular attention to nails and interdigital spaces. HIBISTAT dries rapidly in use, No water or toweling is necessary. The emollients contained in HIBISTAT protect the hands from the potential drying effect of alcohol.

Laundering: Chlorhexidine gluconate chemically reacts with chlorine to form a brown stain on fabric. Fabric which has come in contact with chlorhexidine gluconate should be rinsed well and washed without the addition of chlorine products. If bleach is desired, only non-chlorine bleach should be used. Full laundering instructions are packed with each case of HIBISTAT. (Please see HIBICLENS for full laundering instructions.)

How Supplied: In plastic disposable bottles of 4 oz and 8 oz with flip-top cap, and in disposable towelettes containing 5 mL, packaged 50 towelettes to a carton.
NDC 0038-0585 (bottles)
NDC 0038-0587 (towelettes)

KASOF® Capsules
[*kay'sof*]
High Strength Stool Softener
Laxative

Ingredients: Each capsule contains: Active: docusate potassium, 240 mg. Inactive: Blue 1, gelatin, glycerin, methylparaben, polyethylene glycol, propylparaben, purified water, Red 40, sorbitol, Yellow 10.

Indications: KASOF provides a highly efficient wetting action to restore moisture to the bowel, thus softening the stool to prevent straining. The action of KASOF does not interfere with normal peristalsis and generally does not cause griping or extreme sensation of urgency. KASOF is sodium-free, containing a unique potassium formulation, without the problems associated with sodium intake. KASOF is especially valuable for the severely constipated, as well as patients with anorectal disorders, such as hemorrhoids and anal fissures. KASOF is ideal for patients with any condition that can be complicated by straining at stool, for example, cardiac patients. The simple, one-a-day dosage helps assure patient compliance in maintaining normal bowel function.

Directions: Adults: One KASOF capsule daily for several days, or until bowel movements are normal and gentle. It is helpful to increase the daily intake of fluids by drinking a glass of water with each dose.
Store in a closed container, protect from freezing and avoid excessive heat (104°F).

Warnings: As with any drug, if you are pregnant or nursing a baby, seek the advice of a health professional before using this product. Keep out of the reach of children.

How Supplied: KASOF is available in bottles of 30 and 60 brown, gelatin capsules, identified "Stuart 380".
NDC 0038-0380.
Shown in Product Identification Section, page 433

MYLANTA®
[*my-lan'ta*]
Liquid and Tablets
Antacid/Anti-Gas

Ingredients: Each chewable tablet or each 5 mL (one teaspoonful) of liquid contains: Active: Aluminum hydroxide (Dried Gel, USP in tablet and equiv. to Dried Gel, USP in liquid) 200 mg, Magnesium hydroxide 200 mg, Simethicone 20 mg. Inactive: Tablets: dextrates, flavors, magnesium stearate, mannitol, sorbitol, starch, Yellow 10. Liquid: butylparaben, carboxymethylcellulose sodium, flavors, hydroxypropyl methylcellulose, microcrystalline cellulose, propylparaben, purified water, sorbitol solution with no added sugar.

Sodium Content: MYLANTA contains an insignificant amount of sodium per daily dose and is considered dietetically sodium free. Typical values are 0.68 mg (0.03 mEq) sodium per 5 mL teaspoonful of liquid and 0.77 mg (0.03 mEq) per tablet.

Acid Neutralizing Capacity: Two teaspoonfuls of MYLANTA liquid will neutralize 25.4 mEq of acid. Two MYLANTA tablets will neutralize 23.0 mEq.

Indications: MYLANTA, a well-balanced combination of two antacids and simethicone, provides consistently dependable relief of symptoms associated with gastric hyperacidity, and mucus-entrapped air or "gas". These indications include:
    Common heartburn (pyrosis)
    Hiatal hernia
    Peptic esophagitis
    Gastritis
    Peptic ulcer
The exceptionally pleasant tasting liquid and soft, easy-to-chew tablets encourage patients' acceptance, thereby minimizing the skipping of prescribed doses. MYLANTA is appropriate whenever there is a need for effective relief of temporary gastric hyperacidity and mucus-entrapped gas.

Continued on next page

Stuart—Cont.

Directions: *Liquid:* Shake well, 2–4 teaspoonfuls between meals and at bedtime or as directed by a physician. *Tablets:* 2–4 tablets, well chewed, between meals and at bedtime or as directed by a physician.

Warnings: Keep this and all drugs out of the reach of children.
Except under the advice and supervision of a physician: Do not take more than 24 teaspoonfuls or 24 tablets in a 24 hour period or use the maximum dose for more than two weeks. Do not use this product if you have kidney disease. Magnesium hydroxide and other magnesium salts, in the presence of renal insufficiency, may cause central nervous system depression and other symptoms of hypermagnesemia.

Drug Interaction Precaution: Do not use this product for any patient receiving a prescription antibiotic containing any form of tetracycline.

How Supplied: MYLANTA is available as a white, pleasant tasting liquid suspension, and as a two-layer yellow and white chewable tablet, identified on yellow layer "STUART 620". Liquid supplied in 5 oz, 12 oz and 24 oz bottles. Tablets supplied in boxes of individually wrapped 40's and 100's, economy size bottles of 180, consumer convenience pocket packs of 48 and roll packs of 12 tablets each. Also available for hospital use in liquid unit doses of 1 oz, and bottles of 5 oz.
NDC 0038-0610 (liquid). NDC 0038-0620 (tablets).
Shown in Product Identification Section, page 433

MYLANTA®-II
[*my-lan'ta*]
Liquid and Tablets
Double Strength Antacid/Anti-Gas

Ingredients: Each chewable tablet or each 5 mL (one teaspoonful) of liquid contains: Active: Aluminum hydroxide (Dried Gel, USP in tablet and equiv. to Dried Gel, USP in liquid)   400 mg
Magnesium hydroxide   400 mg
Simethicone   40 mg
Tablets: Blue 1, cereal solids, confectioner's sugar, flavors, glycerin, lactose, mannitol, starch, Yellow 10. Liquid: butylparaben, carboxymethylcellulose sodium, flavors, hydroxypropyl methylcellulose, microcrystalline cellulose, potassium citrate, propylparaben, purified water, sorbitol solution with no added sugar.
Sodium Content: MYLANTA-II contains an insignificant amount of sodium per daily dose. Typical values are 1.14 mg (0.05 mEq) sodium per 5 mL teaspoonful of liquid and 1.3 mg (0.06 mEq) per tablet.
Acid Neutralizing Capacity: Two teaspoonfuls of MYLANTA-II liquid will neutralize 50.8 mEq of acid. Two MYLANTA-II tablets will neutralize 46.0 mEq.

Indications: MYLANTA-II is a double strength antacid with an anti-gas ingredient for the relief of heartburn, acid indigestion, sour stomach and accompanying gas.The exceptionally pleasant tasting liquid and soft, easy-to-chew tablets encourage patient acceptance, thereby minimizing the skipping of prescribed doses. MYLANTA-II provides consistently dependable relief of the symptoms of peptic ulcer and other problems related to acid hypersecretion. The high potency of MYLANTA-II is achieved through its concentration of noncalcium antacid ingredients. Thus MYLANTA-II can produce both rapid and long lasting neutralization without the acid rebound associated with calcium carbonate. The balanced formula of aluminum and magnesium hydroxides minimizes undesirable bowel effects. Simethicone is effective for the relief of concomitant distress caused by mucus-entrapped gas and swallowed air.

Directions: Liquid: Shake well, 2–4 teaspoonfuls between meals and at bedtime, or as directed by a physician. Tablets: 2–4 tablets, well-chewed, between meals and at bedtime, or as directed by a physician.
Because patients with peptic ulcer vary greatly in both acid output and gastric emptying time, the amount and schedule of dosages should be varied accordingly.

Warnings: Keep this and all drugs out of the reach of children.
Except under the advice and supervision of a physician: Do not take more than 12 teaspoonfuls or 12 tablets in a 24 hour period or use the maximum dose for more than two weeks. Do not use this product if you have kidney disease. Magnesium hydroxide and other magnesium salts, in the presence of renal insufficiency, may cause central nervous system depression and other symptoms of hypermagnesemia.

Drug Interaction Precaution: Do not use this product for any patient receiving a prescription antibiotic containing any form of tetracycline.

How Supplied: MYLANTA-II is available as a white, pleasant tasting liquid suspension, and a two-layer green and white chewable tablet, identified on green layer "STUART 651". Liquid supplied in 5 oz, 12 oz and 24 oz bottles. Tablets supplied in boxes of 60 individually wrapped chewable tablets, consumer convenience pocket packs of 24, and roll packs of 8 tablets each. Also available for hospital use in liquid unit dose bottles of 1 oz, and bottles of 5 oz.
NDC 0038-0652 (liquid). NDC 0038-0651 (tablets).
Shown in Product Identification Section, page 433

MYLICON® Tablets and Drops
[*my'li-con*]
Antiflatulent

Ingredients: Each tablet or 0.6 mL of drops contains: Active: simethicone, 40 mg. Inactive: Tablets: calcium silicate, lactose, povidone, saccharin calcium. Drops: carbomer 934P, citric acid, flavors, hydroxypropyl methylcellulose, purified water, Red 3, saccharin calcium, sodium benzoate, sodium citrate.

Indications: For relief of the painful symptoms of excess gas in the digestive tract. Such gas is frequently caused by excessive swallowing of air or by eating foods that disagree. If condition persists consult your physician. MYLICON is a valuable adjunct in the treatment of many conditions in which the retention of gas may be a problem, such as: postoperative gaseous distention, air swallowing, functional dyspepsia, peptic ulcer, spastic or irritable colon, diverticulosis. The defoaming action of MYLICON relieves flatulence by dispersing and preventing the formation of mucus-surrounded gas pockets in the gastrointestinal tract. MYLICON acts in the stomach and intestines to change the surface tension of gas bubbles enabling them to coalesce; thus the gas is freed and is eliminated more easily by belching or passing flatus.
Infants: MYLICON drops are also useful for relief of the painful symptoms of excess gas associated with such conditions as colic, lactose intolerance, or air swallowing.

Directions:
Tablets—One or two tablets four times daily after meals and at bedtime. May also be taken as needed up to 12 tablets daily or as directed by a physician. TABLETS SHOULD BE CHEWED THOROUGHLY.
Drops—Adults and Children 0.6 mL four times daily after meals and at bedtime or as directed by a physician. Shake well before using.
Infants (under 2 years): Initially, 0.3 mL four times daily, after meals and at bedtime, or as directed by a physician. The dosage can also be mixed with 1 oz of cool water, infant formula, or other suitable liquids to ease administration. Dosage should not exceed 12 doses per day.

Warnings: Keep this and all drugs out of the reach of children.

How Supplied: Bottles of 100 and 500 white, scored, chewable tablets, identified front "STUART", reverse "450," and dropper bottles of 30 mL (1 fl oz) pink, pleasant tasting liquid. Also available in 100 tablet unit dose boxes (10 strips of 10 tablets each).
NDC 0038-0450 (tablets).
NDC 0038-0630 (drops).
Shown in Product Identification Section, page 433

MYLICON®-80 Tablets
[*my'li-con*]
High-Capacity Antiflatulent

Ingredients: Each tablet contains: Active: simethicone, 80 mg. Inactive: flavor, cereal solids, lactose, mannitol, povidone, Red 3, talc.

Indications: For relief of the painful symptoms of excess gas in the digestive tract. Such gas is frequently caused by excessive swallowing of air or by eating foods that disagree. If condition persists, consult your physician. MYLICON-80 is a high capacity antiflatulent for adjunctive treatment of many conditions in which the retention of gas may be a problem, such as the following: air swallowing, functional dyspepsia, postoperative gaseous distention, peptic ulcer, spastic or irritable colon, diverticulosis. MYLICON-80 has a defoaming action that relieves flatulence by dispersing and preventing the formation of mucus-surrounded gas pockets in the gastrointestinal tract. MYLICON-80 acts in the stomach and intestines to change the surface tension of gas bubbles enabling them to coalesce; thus, the gas is freed and is eliminated more easily by belching or passing flatus.

Directions: One tablet four times daily after meals and at bedtime. May also be taken as needed up to 6 tablets daily or as directed by a physician. TABLETS SHOULD BE CHEWED THOROUGHLY.

Warnings: Keep this and all drugs out of the reach of children.

How Supplied: Economical bottles of 100 and convenience packages of individually wrapped 12 and 48 pink, scored, chewable tablets identified "STUART 858". Also available in 100 tablet unit dose boxes (10 strips of 10 tablets each). NDC 0038-0858.

Shown in Product Identification Section, page 433

MYLICON®-125 Tablets
[*my'li-con*]
Maximum Strength Antiflatulent

Ingredients: Each tablet contains: Active: simethicone, 125 mg. Inactive: cereal solids, flavor, lactose, mannitol, povidone, Red 3, talc.

Indications: MYLICON-125 is useful for relief of the painful symptoms of excess gas in the digestive tract. Such gas is frequently caused by excessive swallowing of air or by eating foods that disagree. If condition persists, consult your physician. MYLICON-125 is the strongest possible antiflatulent for adjunctive treatment of many conditions in which the retention of gas may be a problem, such as the following: air swallowing, functional dyspepsia, postoperative gaseous distention, peptic ulcer, spastic or irritable colon, diverticulosis. MYLICON-125 has a defoaming action that relieves flatulence by dispersing and preventing the formation of mucus-surrounded gas pockets in the gastrointestinal tract. MYLICON-125 acts in the stomach and intestines to change the surface tension of gas bubbles enabling them to coalesce; thus, the gas is freed and is eliminated more easily by belching or passing flatus.

Directions: One tablet four times daily after meals and at bedtime or as directed by physician. TABLETS SHOULD BE CHEWED THOROUGHLY.

Warnings: Keep this and all drugs out of the reach of children.

How Supplied: Convenience packages of individually wrapped 12 and 60 dark pink, scored chewable tablets identified "STUART 455". Also available in 100 tablet unit dose boxes (10 strips of 10 tablets each). NDC 0038-0455.

Shown in Product Identification Section, page 434

OREXIN® SOFTAB® Tablets
[*or'ex-in*]
High Potency Vitamin Supplement

One Tablet Daily Provides:

VITAMINS:	US RDA*	
B₁	540%	8.1 mg
(thiamin)		
B₆	205%	4.1 mg
(pyridoxine hydrochloride)		
B₁₂	417%	25 mcg
(cyanocobalamin)		

*Percentage of US Recommended Daily Allowances for adults and children 4 or more years of age.

Ingredients: Active: thiamin mononitrate, pyridoxine hydrochloride, cyanocobalamin. Inactive: flavor, mannitol, saccharin calcium, sodium chloride, starch.

Indications: OREXIN is a high-potency vitamin supplement providing vitamins B₁, B₆, and B₁₂.
OREXIN SOFTAB tablets are specially formulated to dissolve quickly in the mouth. They may be chewed or swallowed. Dissolve tablet in a teaspoonful of water or fruit juice if liquid is preferred.

Directions: One tablet daily or as directed by a physician.

Warnings: Keep this and all drugs out of the reach of children.

How Supplied: Bottles of 100 pale pink SOFTAB tablets, identified "STUART".
NDC 0038-0280.

Shown in Product Identification Section, page 434

PROBEC®-T Tablets
[*pro'bec-t*]
Vitamin B Complex Supplement

One Tablet Daily Provides:

VITAMINS:	US RDA*	
C	1000%	600 mg
B₁	813%	12.2 mg
(thiamin)		
B₂	588%	10 mg
(riboflavin)		
Niacin	500%	100 mg
B₆	205%	4.1 mg
(pyridoxine hydrochloride)		
B₁₂	83%	5 mcg
(cyanocobalamin)		
Pantothenic Acid	184%	18.4 mg

*Percentage of US Recommended Daily Allowances for adults and children 4 or more years of age.

DOSAGE: One tablet a day with a meal or as directed by physician.

Ingredients: Active: sodium ascorbate, niacinamide, calcium pantothenate, ascorbic acid, thiamin mononitrate, riboflavin, pyridoxine hydrochloride, cyanocobalamin. Inactive: calcium sulfate, carnauba wax, magnesium oxide, pharmaceutical glaze, povidone, Red 30, sucrose, titanium dioxide, white wax, Yellow 10.

Indications: PROBEC-T is a high-potency B complex supplement with 600 mg of vitamin C in easy to swallow odorless tablets.

Directions: One tablet a day with a meal or as directed by physician.

Warnings: As with all medications, keep out of the reach of children.

How Supplied: Bottles of 60, peach colored, capsule-shaped tablets. NDC 0038-0840.

Shown in Product Identification Section, page 434

THE STUART FORMULA® Tablets
Multivitamin/Multimineral Supplement

One Tablet Daily Provides:

VITAMINS:	US RDA*	
A	100%	5,000 IU
D	100%	400 IU
E	50%	15 IU
C	100%	60 mg
Folic Acid	100%	0.4 mg
B₁	80%	1.2 mg
(thiamin)		
B₂	100%	1.7 mg
(riboflavin)		
Niacin	100%	20 mg
B₆	100%	2 mg
(pyridoxine hydrochloride)		
B₁₂	100%	6 mcg
(cyanocobalamin)		
MINERALS:	**US RDA**	
Calcium	16%	160 mg
Phosphorus	12%	125 mg
Iodine	100%	150 mcg
Iron	100%	18 mg
Magnesium	25%	100 mg

*Percentage of US Recommended Daily Allowances for adults and children 4 or more years of age.

Ingredients: Each tablet contains: Active: dibasic calcium phosphate, magnesium oxide, ascorbic acid, ferrous fumarate, dl-alpha tocopheryl acetate, folic acid, niacinamide, vitamin A palmitate, cyanocobalamin, pyridoxine hydrochloride, riboflavin, thiamin mononitrate, ergocalciferol, potassium iodide. Inactive: calcium sulfate, carnauba wax, pharmaceutical glaze, povidone, sodium starch glycolate, starch, sucrose, titanium dioxide, white wax.

Indications: The STUART FORMULA tablet provides a well-balanced multivitamin/multimineral formula intended for use as a daily dietary supplement for adults and children over age four.

Directions: One tablet daily or as directed by physician.

Continued on next page

Stuart—Cont.

Warnings: Keep this and all drugs out of the reach of children. In case of accidental overdose, seek professional assistance or contact a Poison Control Center immediately.

How Supplied: Bottles of 100 and 250 white round tablets. Child-resistant safety caps are standard on both bottles as a safeguard against accidental ingestion by children.
NDC 0038-0866.

Shown in Product Identification Section, page 434

STUART PRENATAL® Tablets
Multivitamin/Multimineral
Supplement

One Tablet Daily Provides:

VITAMINS	RDA*	
A	100%	4,000 IU
D	100%	400 IU
E	100%	11 mg
C	100%	100 mg
Folic Acid	100%	0.8 mg
B₁	100%	1.5 mg
(thiamin)		
B₂	100%	1.7 mg
(riboflavin)		
Niacin	100%	18 mg
B₆	100%	2.6 mg
(pyridoxine hydrochloride)		
B₁₂	100%	4 mcg
(cyanocobalamin)		
MINERALS	RDA*	
Calcium	17%	200 mg
Iron	330%**	60 mg
Zinc	100%	25 mg

*Recommended Dietary Allowances (Food and Nutrition Board, NAS/NRC-1980) for pregnant and lactating women.
**Recommended Dietary Allowances (Food and Nutrition Board, NAS/NRC-1980) for adults, not pregnant and lactating women.

Ingredients
Active: calcium sulfate, ferrous fumarate, ascorbic acid, dl-alpha tocopheryl acetate, zinc oxide, niacinamide, vitamin A acetate, pyridoxine hydrochloride, riboflavin, thiamin mononitrate, folic acid, cholecalciferol, cyanocobalamin. Inactive: croscarmellose sodium, hydroxypropyl methylcellulose, microcrystalline cellulose, pregelatinized starch, red iron oxide, titanium dioxide.

Indications: STUART PRENATAL is a nonprescription multivitamin/multimineral supplement for use before, during, and after pregnancy. It provides vitamins equal to 100% or more of the RDA for pregnant and lactating women, plus essential minerals, including 60 mg of elemental iron as well-tolerated ferrous fumarate, and 200 mg of elemental calcium (nonalkalizing and phosphorus-free), and 25 mg zinc. STUART PRENATAL also contains 0.8 mg folic acid.

Directions: Before, during and after pregnancy, one tablet daily, or as directed by a physician.

Warning: In case of accidental overdose, seek professional assistance or contact a Poison Control Center immediately.

How Supplied: Bottles of 100 light pink tablets imprinted "STUART 071". A child-resistant safety cap is standard on 100 tablet bottles as a safeguard against accidental ingestion by children.
NDC-0038-0071.

Shown in Product Identification Section, page 434

STUARTINIC® Tablets
[stu "are-tin 'ic]
Hematinic

One Tablet Daily Provides:

	US RDA*	
Iron	556%	100 mg
VITAMINS:		
C	833%	500 mg
B₁	327%	4.9 mg
(thiamin)		
B₂	353%	6 mg
(riboflavin)		
Niacin	100%	20 mg
B₆	40%	0.8 mg
(pyridoxine hydrochloride)		
B₁₂	417%	25 mcg
(cyanocobalamin)		
Pantothenic		
Acid	92%	9.2 mg

*Percentage of US Recommended Daily Allowances for adults and children 4 or more years of age.

Ingredients: Active: ferrous fumarate, ascorbic acid, sodium ascorbate, niacinamide, calcium pantothenate, thiamin mononitrate, riboflavin, pyridoxine hydrochloride, cyanocobalamin. Inactive: flavor, hydrogenated vegetable oil, microcrystalline cellulose, povidone, Yellow 6, Yellow 10, and other ingredients.

Indications: STUARTINIC is a complete hematinic for patients with history of iron deficiency anemia who also lack proper amounts of vitamin C and B-complex vitamins due to inadequate diet. The use of well-tolerated ferrous fumarate in STUARTINIC provides a high level of elemental iron with a low incidence of gastric distress. The inclusion of 500 mg of Vitamin C per tablet serves to maintain more of the iron in the absorbable ferrous state. The B-complex vitamins improve nutrition where B-complex deficient diets contribute to the anemia.

Warnings: As with any drug, if you are pregnant or nursing a baby, seek the advice of a health professional before using this product. Keep out of the reach of children. In case of accidental overdose, seek professional assistance or contact a Poison Control Center immediately.

Dosage: One tablet daily taken after a meal or as directed by physician. Because of the high amount of iron per tablet, STUARTINIC is not recommended for children under 12 years of age.

How Supplied: STUARTINIC is supplied in bottles of 60 yellow, film coated, oval shaped tablets. NDC 0038-0862.

Note: A child-resistant safety cap is standard on each 60 tablet bottle as a safeguard against accidental ingestion by children.

Shown in Product Identification Section, page 434

Syntex Laboratories, Inc
3401 HILLVIEW AVENUE
PALO ALTO, CA 94304

CARMOL® 10
10% urea lotion
for total body
dry skin care.

Active Ingredient: Urea 10% in a scented lotion of purified water, carbomer 940, cetyl alcohol, isopropyl palmitate, PEG-8 dioleate, PEG-8 distearate, propylene glycol, propylene glycol dipelargonate, stearic acid, sodium laureth sulfate, trolamine, and xanthan gum.

Indications: For total body dry skin care.

Actions: Keratolytic CARMOL 10 is non-occlusive, contains no mineral oil or petrolatum. CARMOL 10 is hypoallergenic; contains no lanolin, parabens or other preservatives.

Precautions: For external use only. Discontinue use if irritation occurs. Keep out of the reach of children. In case of accidental ingestion, seek professional assistance or contact a poison control center immediately.

Dosage and Administration: Rub in gently on hands, face or body. Repeat as necessary.

How Supplied: 6 fl. oz. bottle.

CARMOL® 20
20% Urea Cream
Extra strength for
rough, dry skin

Active Ingredients: Urea 20% in a non-lipid vanishing cream containing carbomer 940, hypoallergenic fragrance, isopropyl myristate, isopropyl palmitate, propylene glycol, purified water, sodium laureth sulfate, stearic acid, trolamine, xanthan gum.

Indications: Especially useful on rough, dry skin of hands, elbows, knees and feet.

Actions: Keratolytic. Contains no parabens, lanolin or mineral oil.

Precautions: For external use only. Keep away from eyes. Use with caution on face or broken or inflamed skin; transient stinging may occur. Discontinue use if irritation occurs. Keep out of the reach of children. In case of accidental ingestion, seek professional assistance or contact a poison control center immediately.

Dosage and Administration: Apply once or twice daily or as directed. Rub in well.

How Supplied: 3 oz. tubes, 1 lb. jars.

Thompson Medical Company, Inc.
919 THIRD AVENUE
NEW YORK, NY 10022

ASPERCREME®
[ăs-per-crēme]
External Analgesic Rub

Description: ASPERCREME® is available as an odor-free creme and lotion for use as a topical massage rub that temporarily relieves minor muscle aches and pains without stomach upset. Aspercreme does not contain aspirin.

Active Ingredients: Salycin® 10% (Thompson Medical's brand of Trolamine Salicylate).

Other Ingredients: Creme: Cetyl Alcohol, Glycerin, Methylparaben, Mineral Oil, Potassium Phosphate, Propylparaben, Stearic Acid, Triethanolamine, Water. Lotion: Cetyl Alcohol, Fragrance, Glyceryl Stearate, Isopropyl Palmitate, Lanolin, Methylparaben, Potassium Phosphate, Propylene Glycol, Propylparaben, Sodium Lauryl Sulfate, Stearic Acid, Water.

Actions: External analgesic rub.

Indications: Analgesic rub for temporary relief of minor aches and pains of muscles associated with simple backaches, strains and sprains. Aspercreme is aspirin free.

Warnings: Use only as directed. If prone to allergic reaction from aspirin or salicylate, consult your doctor before using. If redness is present or condition worsens, or if pain persists for more than 7 days or clears up and occurs again within a few days, discontinue use and consult a doctor. Do not use on children under 10 years of age. Do not apply if skin is irritated or if irritation develops. As with any drug, if you are pregnant or nursing a baby, seek the advice of a health professional before using this product. For external use only. Avoid contact with eyes. Keep this and all medicines out of the reach of children. In case of accidental ingestion seek professional assistance or contact a Poison Control Center immediately.

Dosage and Administration: Apply generously directly to affected area. Massage into painful area until thoroughly absorbed into skin, repeat as necessary, especially before retiring but not more than 4 times daily.

How to Store: Protect from freezing and temperatures above 100°F. Close cap tightly after use.

How Supplied: Creme: 1¼ oz., 3 oz. and 5 oz. tubes. Lotion: 6 oz. bottle.

CORTIZONE–5
Creme and Ointment
Anti-itch
(hydrocortisone)

Description: CORTIZONE-5 creme and ointment are topical anti-itch preparations.

Active Ingredient: Hydrocortisone 0.5%.

Other Ingredients: Creme: Aluminum Sulfate, Calcium Acetate, Glycerin, Light Mineral Oil, Methylparaben, Potato Dextrin, Purified Water, Sodium Lauryl Sulfate, White Petroleum. May Also Contain: Cetearyl Alcohol, Propylparaben, Sodium C_{12-15} Alcohols Sulfate, Synthetic Beeswax, White Wax. Ointment: White Petrolatum.

Indications: CORTIZONE-5 is recommended for the temporary relief of itching associated with minor skin irritations, inflammations and rashes due to: eczema, dermatitis, psoriasis, insect bites, poison ivy, oak, sumac, detergents, soaps, cosmetics, jewelry, external anal and genital itching.

Warnings: For external use only. Avoid contact with the eyes. In case of accidental ingestion get professional assistance or contact a poison control center immediately. Do not use on children under two years of age unless under the advice and supervision of a doctor. If condition worsens, or symptoms persist for more than seven days, discontinue use and consult a doctor. Do not use for external genital itching if vaginal discharge is present; consult a physician.
KEEP THIS AND ALL MEDICINES OUT OF THE REACH OF CHILDREN.

Dosage and Administration: For use by adults and children 2 years of age and older. Apply to affected area, not more than three or four times daily.

How to Store: Store at room temperature.

How Supplied: CORTIZONE-5 creme: 1 oz, and 2 oz. tubes. CORTIZONE-5 ointment: 1 oz tube.

Shown in Product Identification Section, page 434

DEXATRIM® Capsules
[dĕx-a-trĭm]
Prolonged action anorectic for weight control contains
phenylpropanolamine HCl   50mg
(time release)

DEXATRIM® Maximum Strength Plus Vitamin C/Caffeine-Free Capsules
phenylpropanolamine HCl   75mg
(time release)
Vitamin C   180mg
(immediate release)

DEXATRIM® Maximum Strength Caffeine-Free Capsules
phenylpropanolamine HCl   75mg
(time release)

DEXATRIM® Maximum Strength Plus Vitamin C/Caffeine-Free Caplets
phenylpropanolamine HCl   75mg
(time release)
Vitamin C   180mg
(immediate release)

DEXATRIM® Maximum Strength Caffeine-Free Caplets
phenylpropanolamine HCl   75mg
(time release)

DEXATRIM® Maximum Strength Pre-Meal Caplets
phenylpropanolamine HCl   25mg
(immediate release)

Indication: DEXATRIM® is an appetite suppressant for use in conjunction with a calorie-restricted diet for fast weight loss. It is available in time release and immediate release dosage forms.

Caution: READ BEFORE USING. For adult use only. Do not give this product to children under 12 years of age. Persons between the ages of 12 and 18 or over 60 are advised to consult their doctor or pharmacist before using this or any drug. If nervousness, dizziness, headaches, rapid pulse, palpitations, sleeplessness, or other symptoms occur, stop using and consult your physician.

Warning: DO NOT EXCEED RECOMMENDED DOSAGE. Taking more of this or any drug than is recommended can cause untoward health complications. It is sensible to check your blood pressure regularly. Do not use if you have high blood pressure, diabetes, heart, thyroid, kidney, or other disease or are being treated for high blood pressure or depression except under the advice and supervision of a doctor. As with any drug if you are pregnant or nursing a baby, seek the advice of a health professional before using this product. Do not use continuously for more than 3 months. When you have reached your desired weight or are able to control your appetite by yourself, use DEXATRIM only as needed.

Drug Interaction Precaution: Do not take if you are presently taking another medication containing phenylpropanolamine, or any type of nasal decongestant, or a prescription drug for high blood pressure or depression, or any other type

Continued on next page

Thompson—Cont.

of prescription medication except under the advice and supervision of a doctor. KEEP THIS AND ALL MEDICATION OUT OF THE REACH OF CHILDREN. In case of accidental overdose seek professional assistance or contact a Poison Control Center immediately.

Dosage and Administration:
Capsule Dosage Forms: DEXATRIM®, DEXATRIM® Maximum Strength Plus Vitamin C, DEXATRIM® Maximum Strength/Caffeine-Free.
Caplet Dosage Forms: DEXATRIM® Maximum Strength Plus Vitamin C, DEXATRIM® Maximum Strength/Caffeine-Free.
Administration: One capsule or caplet at midmorning (10 am) with a full glass of water.
Immediate Release Caplet Dosage Form: DEXATRIM® Maximum Strength Pre-Meal Caplets:
Administration: One caplet 30 minutes before each meal with one or two full glasses of water. Do not exceed 3 caplets in 24 hours.

How Supplied: All Dexatrim products are supplied in tamper-evident blister packages. Do not use if individual seals are broken.
DEXATRIM® Capsules: Packages of 28 with 1250 calorie DEXATRIM Diet Plan.
DEXATRIM® Maximum Strength Plus Vitamin C/Caffeine-Free Capsules: Packages of 10, 20 and 40 with 1250 calorie DEXATRIM Diet Plan.
DEXATRIM® Maximum Strength Capsules/Caffeine-Free: Packages of 10, 20 and 40 with 1250 calorie DEXATRIM Diet Plan.
DEXATRIM® Maximum Strength Plus Vitamin C/Caffeine-Free Caplets: Packages of 10, 20 and 40 with 1250 calorie DEXATRIM Diet Plan.
DEXATRIM® Maximum Strength Caplets/Caffeine-Free: Packages of 10, 20 and 40 with 1250 calorie DEXATRIM Diet Plan.
DEXATRIM® Maximum Strength Pre-Meal Caplets: Packages of 30 and 60 with 1250 calorie DEXATRIM Diet Plan.

References: Altschuler, S., and Frazer, D.L., Double-Blind Clinical Evaluation of the Anorectic Activity of Phenylpropanolamine Hydrochloride Drops and Placebo Drops in the Treatment of Exogenous Obesity. *Current Therapeutic Research*, 40(1), 211–217, July 1986.
Altschuler, S., et. al., Three Controlled Trials of Weight Loss with Phenylpropanolamine, *Int J Obesity*, 1982;6:549–556.
Blackburn, G.L., et. al., Determinants of the Pressor Effect of Phenylpropanolamine in Healthy Subjects. *JAMA*, 1989; 261:3267–3272.
Morgan, J.P., et. al., Subjective Profile of Phenylpropanolamine: Absence of Stimulant or Euphorigenic Effects at Recommended Dose Levels. *J Clin Psychopharm*, 1989;9(1):33–38.
Lasagna, L., *Phenylpropanolamine—A Review*, New York, John Wiley and Sons, 1988.

All referenced materials available on request.
Shown in Product Identification Section, page 434

ENCARE®
[en 'kar]
Vaginal Contraceptive Suppositories

Description: Encare is an effective contraceptive in vaginal suppository form available without a prescription. Encare is reliable because it offers two-way protection: (1) Encare kills sperm on contact by releasing a precise dose of nonoxynol 9, the spermicide most recommended by doctors. (2) Encare gently disperses a physical barrier of protection against the cervix to help prevent pregnancy.
Encare is an effective contraceptive in vaginal suppository form.

Active Ingredient: Each Suppository contains 2.27% Nonoxynol 9.

Other Ingredients: Fragrance, Lactalbumin, Polyethylene Glycols, Potassium Coco-Hydrolyzed Animal Protein, Sodium Bicarbonate, Sodium Lauryl Sulfate, Sodium Tartrate, Tartaric Acid.

Indications: Encare is effective in the prevention of pregnancy.

Action: Encare is 100% free of hormones and free of the serious side effects associated with oral contraceptives.
Encare is convenient and easy to use. Women like Encare because each insert is individually wrapped and can be easily carried in a pocket or purse. There are other reasons why women use Encare. It is approximately as effective as vaginal foam contraceptives in actual use, yet there is no applicator, so there is nothing to fill, remove, or clean. In addition, women may find Encare convenient to use in place of a second application of jelly or cream in conjunction with a diaphragm.
Because Encare can be inserted as much as an hour before intercourse, it does not interfere with spontaneity or ruin the mood. Many men are not even aware a woman is using Encare. Encare has been used successfully by millions of women throughout Europe and America.

Special Warning: Spermicidal contraceptives should not be used during pregnancy. Some experts believe that there may be an increased risk of birth defects occurring in children whose mothers used a spermicidal contraceptive at the time of conception or during pregnancy. If you believe you may be pregnant, have a pregnancy test before using a spermicidal contraceptive. If you have used a spermicidal contraceptive after becoming pregnant, or used a spermicidal contraceptive when you became pregnant, discuss this issue with your physician.

Cautions: If your doctor has told you that you should not become pregnant, consult him as to which method, including Encare, is best for you.

If vaginal irritation occurs and continues, contact your physician.
Do not take orally. **KEEP THIS AND ALL DRUGS OUT OF THE REACH OF CHILDREN.** In case of accidental ingestion, call a Poison Control Center, emergency medical facility or a doctor immediately.
Encare should be kept away from excessive heat. Store at room temperature. Should the product inadvertently be exposed to higher temperatures, hold under cold water for two minutes before removing protective wrap.

Dosage and Administration: For best protection against pregnancy, it is essential to follow package instructions. At least 10 minutes before intercourse, place one Encare insert with your fingertip as far as possible into the vagina, towards the small of your back. Best protection will occur when Encare is placed deep into the vagina. You may feel a pleasant sensation of warmth as Encare effervesces and distributes the spermicide, nonoxynol 9, within the vagina. This is a natural attribute to the product.
IMPORTANT: It is essential to insert Encare at least 10 minutes before intercourse. If one chooses, Encare can be inserted up to one hour before intercourse. If intercourse has not taken place within one hour after insertion, use a new Encare insert. Use a new Encare insert each time intercourse is repeated. Encare can be used safely as frequently as needed. Douching after use of Encare is not required; however, should you desire to do so, wait at least six hours after intercourse.

How Supplied: Boxes of 12 and 24 inserts.

References: Barwin, B., Encare Oval: A Clinical Study, *Contraceptive Delivery System*, 4, 331–334, 1983. Masters, W., In Vivo Evaluation of an Effervescent Intravaginal Contraceptive Inserted by Simulated Coital Activity, *Fertility and Sterility*, 32, 161–165, 1979.

NP-27®
Cream, Solution, Spray Powder and Powder
Antifungal
(tolnaftate)

Description: NP-27 contains the maximum strength available without a prescription of tolnaftate, a clinically proven ingredient which kills athlete's foot fungus and jock itch fungus on contact. It is available as a cream, solution, spray powder and powder.

Active Ingredients: Cream, Solution and Powder: Tolnaftate 1%.
Spray Powder: Tolnaftate 1%, contains: SD Alcohol 40 14.9%.

Other Ingredients: Cream: BHT, Polyethylene Glycol 400, Propylene Glycol, Titanium Dioxide. May also contain: *n*-Amylamine, Carbomer 934P, Carbomer 940, Diisopropanolamine. Solution: BHT, Polyethylene Glycol 400. May also contain: Propylene Glycol. Spray Powder:

Isobutane, Isopropyl Myristate, Talc. Powder: Cornstarch, Talc.

Indications: An effective antifungal agent that kills athlete's foot fungus and jock itch fungus on contact and helps prevent reinfection. Provides quick relief of the itching, burning, scaling and discomfort that can accompany these conditions.

Warnings: For external use only. Do not use on children under 2 years of age except under the advice and supervision of a doctor. Children under 12 years of age should be supervised in the use of the product. If irritation occurs or if there is no improvement within 2 weeks, discontinue use and consult a doctor or pharmacist. Keep this and all medications out of the reach of children. In case of accidental ingestion, seek professional assistance or contact a Poison Control Center immediately. Avoid eye contact. Not effective on scalp or nails.

Dosage and Administration: Cleanse skin with soap and water and dry thoroughly. Apply a thin layer over affected area morning and night or as directed by a doctor. To help prevent recurrence, continue treatment for 2 weeks after disappearance of all symptoms. For athlete's foot pay special attention to the spaces between the toes.

How Supplied: Available in 0.5 oz. and 1 oz. cream; 0.5 oz. solution; 3.5 oz. spray powder; 1.5 oz powder.

How to Store: Store at room temperature.

Shown in Product Identification Section, page 434

SLEEPINAL®
Night-time Sleep Aid Capsules
(Diphenhydramine HCl)

Description: SLEEPINAL is a night-time sleep aid. When taken prior to bedtime, it helps to increase drowsiness and aids in falling asleep.

Active Ingredient: Diphenhydramine HCl 50 mg.

Other Ingredients: FD&C Blue No. 1, Gelatin, Lactose, Magnesium Stearate, Povidone, Talc.

Indications: For relief of occasional sleeplessness.

Action: SLEEPINAL is an antihistamine with anticholinergic and sedative action.

Warnings: **Read before using.** Do not exceed recommended dosage. Do not give to children under 12 years of age. If sleeplessness persists continuously for more than 2 weeks, consult a doctor. Insomnia may be a symptom of serious underlying medical illness. Do not take this product if you have asthma, glaucoma, emphysema, chronic pulmonary disease, shortness of breath, difficulty in breathing, or difficulty in urination due to enlargement of the prostate gland unless directed by a doctor. Avoid alcoholic beverages while taking this product. Do not

take this product if you are taking sedatives or tranquilizers, without first consulting your doctor. As with any drug, if you are pregnant or nursing a baby, seek the advice of a health professional before using this product.
KEEP THIS AND ALL MEDICATIONS OUT OF THE REACH OF CHILDREN. In the case of accidental overdose, seek professional assistance or contact a Poison Control Center immediately.

Dosage and Administration: Adults and children 12 years of age and over: Oral dosage, one capsule at bedtime if needed, or as directed by a doctor.

How to Store: Store in a dry place at controlled room temperature 15° C–30° C (59° F–86° F).

How Supplied: Sleepinal is supplied in tamper-evident blister packages. Do not use if individual seals are broken. Packages of 16 and 32 capsules.
Shown in Product Identification Section, page 434

ULTRA SLIM·FAST®
Nutritional Meal Replacement Drink—Part of the Ultra Slim·Fast Program

Description: A precisely portioned, nutritionally balanced liquid meal replacement to be used in conjunction with whole-food meals for weight loss or weight-loss maintenance. Unlike "fasting" diets, the ULTRA Slim·Fast program provides a combination of convenient, palatable meal replacements and whole-food meals in an integrated program that makes it pleasant to lose weight and keep it off. The delicious,

thick ULTRA Slim·Fast "milkshake" provides a nutritious, low-calorie answer to cravings for "sweet" or "forbidden" food, while the high fiber content promotes feelings of satiety. The ULTRA Slim·Fast Program, scientifically developed with the help of physicians and dietitians, includes a complete diet plan with menu suggestions. The Program teaches behavior modification to aid in the eating-pattern and life-style changes that can make weight reduction succeed permanently.

Uses: The ULTRA Slim·Fast program is recommended to help the moderately obese patient (up to 50 pounds overweight) to achieve safe, rapid weight loss. It is also indicated for the patient who wishes to maintain weight loss, or to control or reverse modest weight gains.

Professional Supplementary Materials: Physicians and dietitians may also send for patient samples and free support materials. Write to Ultra SlimFast Medical Program, Slim·Fast Foods, PO Box 5047, FDR Station, NY, NY 10150.

Nutritional Information: ULTRA Slim·Fast provides an exceptionally safe, nutritious weight-loss regimen. One ULTRA Slim·Fast "shake" made with 1% low-fat milk includes 33% of the U.S. RDA of 18 essential nutrients. It is an excellent source of dietary fiber (5 grams in chocolate flavor, 4 grams in vanilla or strawberry), calcium (50% of adult RDA), and protein (15 grams, largely from casein, providing 27% of total calories). And it is low in fat (just 3 or 4 grams—depending on flavor, 12% or 16% of calories).
[See table]

Serving Size: 1.16 oz. Servings per container: 13		One Serving with 8 Fl. Oz. Vitamin A&D Protein-Fortified 1% Low Fat-Milk
Each Serving Provides:	**One Serving**	
Calories	100	220
Protein	5 grams	15 grams
Carbohydrate	20 grams	34 grams
Fat	less than 1 gram	3 grams
Sodium	130 mg.	270 mg.
Potassium	220 mg.	660 mg.
Fiber (Dietary)	4 grams	4 grams
Percentage of Adult U.S. Recommended Daily Allowance (U.S. RDA):		
Protein	10%	35%
Vitamin A	25%	35%
Vitamin C (Ascorbic Acid)	30%	35%
Thiamine (Vitamin B$_1$)	30%	35%
Riboflavin (Vitamin B$_2$)	10%	35%
Niacin	35%	35%
Calcium	15%	50%
Iron	35%	35%
Vitamin D	10%	35%
Vitamin E	35%	35%
Vitamin B$_6$	30%	35%
Folic Acid	25%	30%
Vitamin B$_{12}$	20%	35%
Phosphorus	15%	40%
Iodine	10%	35%
Magnesium	25%	35%
Zinc	30%	35%
Copper	35%	35%
Biotin	35%	35%
Pantothenic Acid	25%	35%
Manganese	1 mg.*	1 mg.*

*No U.S. RDA established.

Continued on next page

Thompson—Cont.

Ingredients: Sucrose, Nonfat Dry Milk, Whey Powder, Corn Bran, Calcium Caseinate, Soy Protein Isolate, Purified Cellulose; Maltodextrin, Cellulose Gum, Fructose, Guar Gum, Carrageenan, Hydrogenated Soybean Oil, Natural and Artificial Flavors, Lecithin, Citric Acid, DL-Methionine, Artificial Colors, **Aspartame, and the following Vitamins and Minerals: Magnesium Oxide, Calcium Phosphate, Potassium Chloride, Ferric Orthophosphate, Vitamin E Acetate, Ascorbic Acid, Niacinamide, Zinc Oxide, Vitamin A Palmitate, Manganese Sulfate, Calcium Pantothenate, Copper Sulfate, Pyridoxine Hydrochloride, Thiamine Mononitrate, Vitamin D_3, Riboflavin, Biotin, Folic Acid, Potassium Iodide, Vitamin B_{12}.
Nutritional information and ingredient disclosure may vary slightly in Chocolate Royale and French Vanilla flavors.
**Phenylketonurics: Contains phenylalanine.

Directions: FOR FAST WEIGHT LOSS: Enjoy a rich, delicious and satisfying Ultra Slim·Fast shake for breakfast, one for lunch and another in the afternoon as a snack; then have a sensible, low-fat, well-balanced dinner. Three highly nutritious Ultra Slim·Fast shakes provide 12 or 15 grams of healthy dietary fiber and 100% of the U.S. recommended daily allowance of natural protein plus 18 essential vitamins and minerals, including iron and calcium. The Ultra Slim·Fast program is nutritionally balanced so you feel great as you lose weight fast.

IMPORTANT, USE A SHAKER OR BLENDER. Simply add 1 rounded measuring scoop (inside can) of ULTRA Slim·Fast to 8 oz. of protein-fortified 1% low-fat milk. (For best taste, add ice.) SHAKE or BLEND for 30 seconds.
FOR WEIGHT MAINTENANCE AND GOOD HEALTH: Enjoy ULTRA Slim·Fast daily in place of EITHER breakfast OR lunch (and a second time, as needed, in place of snacks). For the other two regular meals, follow a nutritionally balanced eating program.

Warnings: Phenylketonurics—Contains phenylalanine.
IMPORTANT: Anyone who is pregnant or nursing, has a health problem, or wants to lose more than 50 pounds or more than 20% of their starting body weight should consult a physician before starting any weight-loss program.
Ultra Slim·Fast should not be used as your sole source of nutrition; eat at least one well-balanced meal daily.

How Supplied: Flavors: Chocolate Royale, French Vanilla, Strawberry Supreme. Available in 15 oz. cans (425 grams, 13 servings)—including measuring scoop and diet plan suggestions.
[See table above]
Shown in Product Identification Section, page 434

The Ultra Slim·Fast®
Medical Program . . .

. . . is NOT . . .

● **A fasting program** requiring abstinence from solid foods.
● **A fad diet** with questionable nutritional balance.
● **An inconvenient diet** requiring complex preparation.
● **An unappealing diet** with unappetizing ingredients.
● **A "miracle" diet** promising unhealthy, overly rapid weight loss, with no follow-through.
● **Expensive** (as some clinic- or hospital-based programs are)

. . . IS . . .

● **A combination** of meal replacements and "real" foods.
● **A precisely proportioned, highly nutritious food** low in calories and fat.
● **Convenient and readily available** (without prescription).
● **Palatable, delicious** "milkshake" meals plus tasty solid-food meals.
● **An aid to behavior modification** vital for achieving and maintaining weight loss.
● **Economical** (usually less costly than the meal or snack it replaces).

Triton Consumer Products, Inc.
**5105-190 TOLLVIEW DRIVE
ROLLING MEADOWS, IL 60008**

MG 217® PSORIASIS MEDICATION
**Skin Care: Ointment and Lotion
Hair/Scalp Care: Shampoo and Conditioner**

Active Ingredients: OINTMENT —Coal Tar Solution USP 2%, Salicylic Acid 1.5% and Colloidal Sulfur 1.1%. **LOTION**—Coal Tar Solution USP 5% with Jojoba. **SHAMPOO**—Coal Tar Solution USP 5%, Salicylic Acid 2% and Colloidal Sulfur 1.5%. **CONDITIONER**—Coal Tar Solution USP 2%.

Action/Uses: Effective relief for itching, scaling and flaking of Psoriasis or Seborrhea.

Caution: For external use only. Keep out of the reach of children. Avoid contact with eyes. If undue skin irritation occurs, discontinue use. For shampoo/conditioner, in isolated cases, temporary discoloration of blond, bleached or tinted hair may occur.

Administration: OINTMENT or LOTION—Wash affected areas of skin with mild soap/water and dry. Rub MG 217 in well. Apply twice daily or as needed. Not for use on the scalp. **SHAMPOO**—Shake well before using. Wet hair, then massage liberal amount of MG 217 into scalp and leave on for 5–10 minutes. Use daily or as needed. **CONDITIONER**—After shampooing, massage liberal amount of MG 217 into scalp and leave on for several minutes. Rinse thoroughly. Use daily or as needed.

How Supplied: OINTMENT—3.8 oz. and 15.3 oz. plastic jars. **LOTION**—4 oz. plastic bottles. **SHAMPOO**—4 oz., 8 oz. and 16 oz. plastic bottles. **CONDITIONER**—4 oz. plastic bottles.

Products are cross-indexed by generic and chemical names in the **YELLOW SECTION**

UAS Laboratories
**9201 PENN AVENUE SOUTH
#10
MINNEAPOLIS, MN 55431**

DDS–ACIDOPHILUS
Capsule, Tablet & Powder free of dairy products, corn, soy, and preservatives

Description: DDS-Acidophilus is the source of a special strain of Lactobacillus acidophilus free of dairy products, corn, soy and preservatives. Each capsule or tablet contain one billion viable DDS-1 L.acidophilus at the time of manufacturing. One gram of powder contains two billion viable DDS-1 L.acidophilus.

Indications and Usages: An aid in implanting the gut with beneficial Lactobacillus acidophilus under conditions of digestive disorders, acne, yeast infections, and following antibiotic therapy.

Administration: One to two capsules or tablets twice daily before meals. One-fourth teaspoon powder can be substituted for two capsules or tablets.

How Supplied: Bottles of 100 capsules or tablets. 12 bottles per case. Powder is available in 2 oz. bottle; 12 bottles per case.

Storage: Keep refrigerated under 40°F.

EDUCATIONAL MATERIAL

DDS-Acidophilus
Booklet describing superior-strain Acidophilus without dairy products, corn, soy, or preservatives. Two billion viable DDS-L. acidophilus per gram.

Products are cross-indexed by product category in the **BLUE SECTION**

UltraBalance Products
5800 SOUNDVIEW DRIVE
GIG HARBOR, WA 98335

ULTRABALANCE WEIGHT MANAGEMENT PRODUCT

ULTRABALANCE PROTEIN FORMULA

Description: UltraBalance Protein Formula is a partially predigested, lactalbumin-based formula that is vitamin/mineral enriched and contains no common allergen-derived materials. Contains no corn, wheat, soy, egg, milk casein, lactose, yeast, sweetener, artificial flavoring/coloring or stimulants.

Composition: Hydrolyzed lactalbumin, rice protein concentrate, potassium citrate, tricalcium phosphate, natural vanilla flavors, magnesium oxide, beta carotene, high oleic safflower oil, potassium chloride, calcium carbonate, ascorbic acid, iron amino acid chelate, zinc amino acid chelate, dl alpha tocopheryl acetate, ChromeMate-GTF™, molybdenum amino acid chelate, selenium amino acid chelate, manganese amino acid chelate, copper amino acid chelate, niacinamide, pyridoxine hydrochloride, calcium pantothenate, riboflavin, thiamine hydrochloride, folic acid, potassium iodide, vitamin D3 (cholecalciferol), biotin and cyanocobalamin.

Actions/Uses: Used for weight management as well as food allergy testing/treatment. Provides 100% RDA for all vitamins and minerals except calcium.

Preparation: 1 level scoop of Protein mixed with 8 oz diluted fruit juice either 2 or 3 times per day depending on patient's needs.

ULTRABALANCE HERBULK

Description: Used as a part of the UltraBalance Program for weight management or separately as a soluble fiber supplement. Completely natural, contains no narcotics or stimulants.

Composition: Psyllium seed powder, rice flour, guar gum, Mezotrace™ (dolomite-limestone), prune fiber concentrate, cellulose gum, ascorbic acid.

Actions/Uses: Provides fiber for the digestive system without contributing excessive calories.

Preparation: 1 level scoop of Herbulk mixed with 8 oz diluted juice either 2 or 3 times per day depending on patient's needs.

How Supplied: UltraBalance Weight Management "Kit" consists of one can Protein, one can Herbulk, Program Description Booklet. Also available are Patient Workbook, Recipe Book/Menu Planner, Lifestyle Modification Tapes. Available through licensed health practitioners.

The Upjohn Company
KALAMAZOO, MI 49001

BACIGUENT® Antibiotic Ointment

Active Ingredient: Each gram contains 500 units of bacitracin. Also contains anhydrous lanolin, mineral oil, and white petrolatum.

Indications: *Baciguent* is a first aid ointment to help prevent infection and aid in the healing of minor cuts, burns and abrasions.

How Supplied: Available in ½ oz and 1 oz tubes.

CHERACOL D® Cough Formula
Maximum Strength Cough Relief

Active Ingredients: Each teaspoonful (5 ml) contains dextromethorphan hydrobromide, 10 mg; guaifenesin, 100 mg; alcohol, 4.75%. Also contains benzoic acid, FD&C Red #40, flavors, fragrances, fructose, glycerin, propylene glycol, sodium chloride, sucrose, and purified water.

Indications: *Cheracol D* Cough Formula helps quiet dry, hacking coughs, and helps loosen phlegm and mucus. Recommended for adults and children 2 years of age and older.

Dosage and Administration: Adults and children 12 years of age and over: 2 teaspoonfuls. Children 6 to 12 years: 1 teaspoonful. Children 2 to 6 years: ½ teaspoonful. These doses may be repeated every four hours if necessary.

How Supplied: Available in 2 oz, 4 oz and 6 oz bottles.
Shown in Product Identification Section, page 434

CHERACOL PLUS®
Head Cold/Cough Formula

Active Ingredients: Each tablespoonful (15 ml) contains phenylpropanolamine hydrochloride, 25 mg; dextromethorphan hydrobromide, 20 mg; chlorpheniramine maleate, 4 mg; and alcohol, 8%. Also contains flavors, glycerin, methylparaben, propylene glycol, propylparaben, FD&C Red #40, sodium chloride, sorbitol solution, and purified water.

Indications: *Cheracol Plus* syrup is an effective 3-ingredient, maximum strength formula for the temporary relief of head cold symptoms and cough (without narcotic side effects).

Dosage and Administration: Adults and children over 12 years of age: 1 tablespoonful every 4 hours or as directed by a physician. Do not take more than 6 tablespoonfuls in a 24-hour period. Do not administer to children under 12 years of age.

How Supplied: Available in 4 oz and 6 oz bottles.
Shown in Product Identification Section, page 434

CITROCARBONATE® Antacid

Active Ingredients: When dissolved, each 3.9 grams (1 teaspoonful) contains approximately: sodium bicarbonate, 0.78 gram and sodium citrate, 1.82 grams. **As derived from (per teaspoonful):** Sodium bicarbonate 2.34 gram; citric acid anhydrous, 1.19 gram; sodium citrate hydrous, 254 mg; calcium lactate pentahydrate, 151 mg; sodium chloride, 79 mg; monobasic sodium phosphate anhydrous, 44 mg; and magnesium sulfate dried, 42 mg. Each 3.9 grams (teaspoonful) contains 30.46 mEq (700.6 mg) of sodium.

Indications: For the relief of heartburn, acid indigestion, and sour stomach; and upset stomach associated with these symptoms.

Dosage and Administration: Adults: 1 to 2 teaspoonfuls (not to exceed 5 level teaspoonfuls per day) in a glass of cold water after meals. Persons 60 years or older: ½ to 1 teaspoonful after meals. Children 6 to 12 years: ¼ to ½ teaspoonful. For children under 6 years: Consult physician.

How Supplied: Available in 5 oz and 10 oz bottles.

CORTAID® Cream with Aloe
CORTAID® Ointment with Aloe
CORTAID® Lotion
(hydrocortisone acetate)
CORTAID® Spray
(hydrocortisone)

Antipruritic

Description: *Cortaid* Cream with Aloe contains hydrocortisone acetate (equivalent to 0.5% hydrocortisone) in a greaseless, odorless, vanishing cream that leaves no residue. Also contains aloe vera, butylparaben, cetyl palmitate, glyceryl stearate, methylparaben, polyethylene glycol, stearamidoethyl diethylamine, and purified water.
Cortaid Ointment with Aloe contains hydrocortisone acetate (equivalent to 0.5% hydrocortisone) in a soothing, lubricating ointment. Also contains aloe vera, butylparaben, cholesterol, methylparaben, mineral oil, white petrolatum, and microcrystalline wax.
Cortaid Lotion contains hydrocortisone acetate (equivalent to 0.5% hydrocortisone) in a greaseless, odorless, vanishing lotion. Also contains butylparaben, cetyl palmitate, glyceryl monostearate, methylparaben, polysorbate 80, propylene glycol, stearamidoethyl diethylamine, and purified water.
Cortaid Spray contains 0.5% hydrocortisone in a quick-drying, nonstaining, nonaerosol, vanishing liquid spray. Also contains alcohol (46%), glycerin, methylparaben, and purified water.

Indications: Formulations of *Cortaid* are indicated for the temporary relief of minor skin irritations, inflammation, itches and rashes due to dermatitis, insect bites, eczema, psoriasis, poison ivy, poison oak, poison sumac, soaps, deter-

Continued on next page

Upjohn—Cont.

gents, cosmetics, jewelry, and external genital and anal itching.

Uses: The vanishing action of *Cortaid* Cream with Aloe makes it cosmetically acceptable when the skin rash treated is on an exposed part of the body such as the hands or arms. *Cortaid* Ointment with Aloe is best used where protection, lubrication and soothing of dry and scaly lesions is required; the ointment is also preferred for treating itchy genital and anal areas. *Cortaid* Lotion is thinner than the cream and is especially suitable for hairy body areas such as the scalp or arms. *Cortaid* Spray is a quick-drying, nonstaining formulation suitable for covering hard-to-reach areas of the skin.

Warnings: All formulations of *Cortaid* are for external use only. Avoid contact with the eyes. If condition worsens or if symptoms persist for more than 7 days, discontinue use of this product and consult a physician. Do not use on children under 2 years of age except under the advice and supervision of a physician. Keep this and all drugs out of the reach of children. In case of accidental ingestion, seek professional assistance or contact a poison control center immediately.

Dosage and Administration: For adults and children 2 years of age and older, apply as follows: *Cortaid* Cream with Aloe, *Cortaid* Ointment with Aloe or *Cortaid* Lotion: gently massage into the affected area not more than 3 to 4 times daily. *Cortaid* Spray: spray on affected area not more than 3 to 4 times daily.

How Supplied: Formulations of *Cortaid* (hydrocortisone acetate) are available in: Cream with Aloe ½ oz and 1 oz tubes; Ointment with Aloe ½ oz and 1 oz tubes; Lotion 1 oz bottle. *Cortaid* Spray (hydrocortisone) is available in 1.5 fluid oz pump spray bottles.

Shown in Product Identification Section, page 434

CORTEF® Feminine Itch Cream
(hydrocortisone acetate)
Antipruritic

Description: *Cortef* Feminine Itch Cream contains hydrocortisone acetate (equivalent to hydrocortisone 0.5%) in an odorless, vanishing cream base that quickly disappears into the skin to avoid staining of clothing. Also contains aloe vera, butylparaben, cetyl palmitate, glyceryl monostearate, methylparaben, polyethylene glycol, stearamidoethyl diethylamine, and purified water.

Indications: For effective temporary relief of minor skin irritations and external genital itching. It relieves the itch and takes the redness out of the skin to break the annoying itch/scratch cycle.

Warnings: For external use only. Avoid contact with the eyes. If condition worsens, or if symptoms persist for more than 7 days, discontinue use of this product and consult a physician. Do not use

on children under 2 years of age except under the advice and supervision of a physician. Keep this and all drugs out of the reach of children. In case of accidental ingestion, seek professional assistance or contact a poison control center immediately.

Dosage and Administration: Apply to affected area not more than 3 to 4 times daily.

How Supplied: *Cortef* Feminine Itch Cream (hydrocortisone acetate) is available in ½ oz tubes.

HALTRAN® Tablets
Ibuprofen/Analgesic
MENSTRUAL CRAMP RELIEVER

WARNING: ASPIRIN SENSITIVE PATIENTS. Do not take this product if you have had a severe allergic reaction to aspirin, eg—asthma, swelling, shock or hives, because even though this product contains no aspirin or salicylates cross-reactions may occur in patients allergic to aspirin.

Indications: For the pain of menstrual cramps and also the temporary relief of minor aches and pains associated with the common cold, headache, toothache, muscular aches, backache, for the minor pain of arthritis and for reduction of fever.

Directions: *Adults:* Take 1 tablet every 4 to 6 hours while symptoms persist. If pain or fever does not respond to 1 tablet, 2 tablets may be used, but do not exceed 6 tablets in 24 hours, unless directed by a doctor. The smallest effective dose should be used. Take with food or milk if occasional and mild heartburn, upset stomach, or stomach pain occurs with use. Consult a doctor if these symptoms are more than mild or if they persist. *Children:* Do not give this product to children under 12 except under the advice and supervision of a doctor.

Warnings: Do not take for pain for more than 10 days or for fever for more than 3 days unless directed by a doctor. If pain or fever persists or gets worse, if new symptoms occur, or if the painful area is red or swollen, consult a doctor. These could be signs of serious illness. If you are under a doctor's care for any serious condition, consult a doctor before taking this product. As with aspirin and acetaminophen, if you have any condition which requires you to take prescription drugs or if you have had any problems or serious side effects from taking any non-prescription pain reliever, do not take HALTRAN Tablets (ibuprofen) without first discussing it with your doctor. If you experience any symptoms which are unusual or seem unrelated to the condition for which you took ibuprofen, consult a doctor before taking any more of it. Although ibuprofen is indicated for the same conditions as aspirin and acetaminophen, it should not be taken with them except under a doctor's direction. Before using any drug, including HALTRAN, you should seek the advice of a health professional if you are

pregnant or nursing a baby. IT IS ESPECIALLY IMPORTANT NOT TO USE IBUPROFEN DURING THE LAST 3 MONTHS OF PREGNANCY UNLESS SPECIFICALLY DIRECTED TO DO SO BY A DOCTOR BECAUSE IT MAY CAUSE PROBLEMS IN THE UNBORN CHILD OR COMPLICATIONS DURING DELIVERY. Keep this and all drugs out of the reach of children. In case of accidental overdose, seek professional assistance or contact a poison control center immediately.

Active Ingredient: Each tablet contains ibuprofen USP 200 mg.

Other Ingredients: Carnauba wax, cornstarch, hydroxypropyl methylcellulose, propylene glycol, silicon dioxide, pregelatinized starch, stearic acid, and titanium dioxide.
Store at room temperature. Avoid excessive heat 40°C (104°F).

How Supplied: Blister package of 12; bottles of 30 and 50.
Shown in Product Identification Section, page 434

Advanced Formula
KAOPECTATE®
Concentrated Anti-Diarrheal

Active Ingredient: Each tablespoon contains 600 mg attapulgite.

Inactive Ingredients: Flavors, glucono-delta-lactone, magnesium aluminum silicate, methylparaben, sorbic acid, sucrose, titanium dioxide, xanthan gum and purified water; Peppermint flavor contains FD&C Red #40.

Indications: For the relief of diarrhea and cramps. Relieves diarrhea within 24 hours.

Dosage and Administration: For best results, take full recommended dose at first sign of diarrhea and after each subsequent bowel movement. (Maximum 7 times in 24 hours.) Adults and children 12 years of age and over: 2 tablespoons. Children 6 to under 12 years of age: 1 tablespoon. Children 3 to under 6 years of age: ½ tablespoon.

How Supplied: Regular flavor available in 3 oz, 8 oz, 12 oz and 16 oz bottles. Peppermint flavor available in 3 oz, 8 oz and 12 oz bottles.
Shown in Product Identification Section, page 434

KAOPECTATE® Chewable Tablets
Anti-Diarrheal

Active Ingredient: Each tablet contains 300 mg attapulgite.

Inactive Ingredients: Cornstarch, dextrins, dextrose, FD&C Red #3, FD&C Red #40, flavor, magnesium stearate, sucrose, titanium dioxide.

Indications: For the fast relief of diarrhea and cramps; in a good-tasting, easy-to-take form especially suitable for children aged 3 and up.

Dosage and Administration: Chew tablets thoroughly and swallow. For best results, take full recommended dose at first sign of diarrhea and after each subsequent bowel movement (maximum 7 times in 24 hours). Children 3 to under 6 years of age: 1 tablet; Children 6 to under 12 years of age: 2 tablets; Adults and children 12 years of age and over: 4 tablets.

Warnings: Unless directed by a physician, do not use in infants and children under 3 years of age or for more than two days or in the presence of high fever. Keep this and all drugs out of the reach of children. In case of accidental overdose, seek professional assistance or contact a poison control center immediately.

How Supplied: Blister packs of 16 chewable tablets.
Shown in Product Identification Section, page 434

Maximum Strength
KAOPECTATE® Tablets
Anti-Diarrheal

Active Ingredient: Each tablet contains 750 mg attapulgite.

Inactive Ingredients: Croscarmellose sodium, pectin, sucrose and zinc stearate.

Indications: For the relief of diarrhea and cramps. Relieves diarrhea within 24 hours.

Dosage and Administration: Swallow whole tablets with water; do not chew. For best results, take full recommended dose.
Adults: Take 2 tablets after the initial bowel movement and 2 tablets after each subsequent bowel movement, not to exceed 12 tablets in 24 hours. Children 6 to 12 years of age: Take 1 tablet after the initial bowel movement and 1 tablet after each subsequent bowel movement, not to exceed 6 tablets in 24 hours.
Children 3 to under 6 years of age: Use Advanced Formula *Kaopectate* Liquid Anti-Diarrheal (Regular or Peppermint Flavor), or *Kaopectate* Chewable Tablets.

How Supplied: Available in blister packs of 12 and 20 tablets.
Shown in Product Identification Section, page 434

MOTRIN® IB
Caplets or Tablets
(ibuprofen, USP)
Pain Reliever/Fever Reducer
WARNING: ASPIRIN-SENSITIVE PATIENTS. Do not take this product if you have had a severe allergic reaction to aspirin, eg—asthma, swelling, shock or hives because even though this product contains no aspirin or salicylates, cross-reactions may occur in patients allergic to aspirin.

Indications: For the temporary relief of minor aches and pains associated with the common cold, headache, toothache, muscular aches, backache, for the minor pain of arthritis, for the pain of menstrual cramps, and for reduction of fever.

Directions: Adults: Take 1 caplet or tablet every 4 to 6 hours while symptoms persist. If pain or fever does not respond to 1 caplet or tablet, 2 caplets or tablets may be used, but do not exceed 6 caplets or tablets in 24 hours, unless directed by a doctor. The smallest effective dose should be used. Take with food or milk, if occasional and mild heartburn, upset stomach or stomach pain occurs with use. Consult a doctor if these symptoms are more than mild or if they persist. Children: Do not give this product to children under 12 except under the advice and supervision of a doctor.

Warnings: Do not take for pain for more than 10 days or for fever for more than 3 days unless directed by a doctor. If pain or fever persists or gets worse, if new symptoms occur, or if the painful area is red or swollen, consult a doctor. These could be signs of serious illness. If you are under a doctor's care for any serious condition, consult a doctor before taking this product. As with aspirin and acetaminophen, if you have any condition which requires you to take prescription drugs or if you have had any problems or serious side effects from taking any nonprescription pain reliever, do not take MOTRIN® IB without first discussing it with your doctor. If you experience any symptoms which are unusual or seem unrelated to the condition for which you took ibuprofen, consult a doctor before taking any more of it. Although ibuprofen is indicated for the same conditions as aspirin and acetaminophen, it should not be taken with them except under a doctor's direction. Do not combine this product with any other ibuprofen-containing product. As with any drug, if you are pregnant or nursing a baby, seek the advice of a health professional before using this product. IT IS ESPECIALLY IMPORTANT NOT TO USE IBUPROFEN DURING THE LAST 3 MONTHS OF PREGNANCY UNLESS SPECIFICALLY DIRECTED TO DO SO BY A DOCTOR BECAUSE IT MAY CAUSE PROBLEMS IN THE UNBORN CHILD OR COMPLICATIONS DURING DELIVERY. Keep this and all drugs out of the reach of children. In case of accidental overdose, seek professional assistance or contact a poison control center immediately. **Store at room temperature. Avoid excessive heat 40°C (104°F).**
Active Ingredient: Each caplet or tablet contains ibuprofen 200 mg.
Other Ingredients: Carnauba wax, cornstarch, hydroxypropyl methylcellulose, propylene glycol, silicon dioxide, pregelatinized starch, stearic acid, titanium dioxide.

How Supplied: Bottles of 24, 50, 100, and 165 Caplets or Tablets.
Shown in Product Identification Section, page 434

MYCIGUENT® Antibiotic Ointment

Active Ingredient: Each gram contains 5 mg of neomycin sulfate (equivalent to 3.5 mg neomycin). Also contains anhy-

drous lanolin, mineral oil, and white petrolatum.

Indications: *Myciguent* is a first aid ointment to help prevent infection and aid in the healing of minor cuts, burns and abrasions.

How Supplied: Available in ½ oz, 1 oz and 4 oz tubes.

MYCITRACIN® Triple Antibiotic Ointment

Active Ingredients: Each gram contains 500 units of bacitracin, 5 mg of neomycin sulfate (equivalent to 3.5 mg neomycin) and 5000 units of polymyxin B sulfate. Also contains butylparaben, cholesterol, methylparaben, microcrystalline wax, mineral oil, and white petrolatum.

Indications: *Mycitracin* is a first aid ointment to help prevent infection and aid in the healing of minor cuts, burns and abrasions.

How Supplied: Available in $\frac{1}{32}$ oz unit-dose, ½ oz and 1 oz tubes.
Shown in Product Identification Section, page 435

PYRROXATE® Capsules
Extra Strength
Decongestant/Antihistamine/
Analgesic Capsules

Description: *Pyrroxate* provides single-capsule, multisymptom relief for colds, allergies, nasal/sinus congestion, runny nose, sneezing, and watery eyes. Because it contains the non-aspirin analgesic **acetaminophen,** *Pyrroxate* gives temporary relief of occasional minor aches, pains, headache, and helps in the reduction of fever. *Pyrroxate* is caffeine and aspirin-free.

Ingredients: Each *Pyrroxate* Capsule contains: chlorpheniramine maleate, 4 mg; phenylpropanolamine HCl, 25 mg; acetaminophen, 500 mg. The 500 mg (7.69 gr) strength of acetaminophen per capsule is non-standard, as compared to the established standard of 325 mg (5 gr) acetaminophen per capsule. Also contains benzyl alcohol, butylparaben, D & C yellow No. 10, erythrosine sodium, FD & C blue No. 1, FD & C yellow No. 6 (sunset yellow) as a color additive, gelatin, glycerin, magnesium stearate, methylparaben, propylparaben, sodium lauryl sulfate, sodium propionate, starch, and talc.

Indications: *Pyrroxate* Capsules are for the temporary relief of runny nose, sneezing, itching of the nose or throat; for the temporary relief of nasal congestion due to the common cold, allergies (hay fever), and sinus congestion; for the temporary relief of occasional minor aches, pains, headache, and for the reduction of fever.

Actions: Chlorpheniramine maleate is an antihistamine effective in controlling runny nose, sneezing, watery eyes, and

Continued on next page

Upjohn—Cont.

itching of the nose and throat. Phenylpropanolamine HCl is an oral nasal decongestant effective in relieving nasal/sinus congestion due to the common cold or allergies (hay fever). Acetaminophen is a clinically effective analgesic and antipyretic without aspirin side effects.

Warnings: Do not take this product for more than 7 days. If symptoms persist, do not improve, or new ones occur, or if fever persists for more than 3 days, discontinue use and consult your physician. Do not take this product if you have asthma, glaucoma, difficulty in urination due to the enlargement of the prostate gland, high blood pressure, diabetes, thyroid disease, or if you are presently taking a prescription antihypertensive or antidepressant drug containing a monamine oxidase inhibitor, except under the advice and supervision of a physician. As with any drug, if you are pregnant or nursing a baby, seek the advice of a health professional before using this product. Do not exceed recommended dosage because severe liver damage may occur and at higher doses, nervousness, dizziness or sleeplessness may occur. Do not take this product for the treatment of arthritis except under the advice and supervision of a physician.

Cautions: Avoid alcoholic beverages, driving a motor vehicle, or operating heavy machinery while taking this product. This product may cause drowsiness or excitability, especially in children. Keep this and all drugs out of the reach of children. In case of accidental overdose, seek professional assistance or contact a poison control center immediately.

Dosage and Administration: Take 1 capsule every 4 hours or as directed by a physician. Do not take more than 6 capsules in a 24-hour period. Do not administer to children under 12 years of age.

How Supplied: Black/yellow capsules available in blister packages of 24 and bottles of 500.

Shown in Product Identification Section, page 435

SIGTAB® Tablets
High Potency Vitamin Supplement

Each tablet contains:		% U.S. RDA*
Vitamin A	5000 IU	100
Vitamin D	400 IU	100
Vitamin E	15 IU	50
Vitamin C	333 mg	555
Folic Acid	0.4 mg	100
Thiamine	10.3 mg	686
Riboflavin	10 mg	588
Niacin	100 mg	500
Vitamin B$_6$	6 mg	300
Vitamin B$_{12}$	18 mcg	300
Pantothenic Acid	20 mg	200

*Percentage of U.S. Recommended Daily Allowance.

Recommended Dosage: 1 tablet daily

Ingredient List: Sucrose, Sodium Ascorbate (Vit. C), Calcium Sulfate, Nia-

cinamide, Vitamin E Acetate, Calcium Pantothenate, Vitamin A Acetate, Thiamine Mononitrate (B-1), Riboflavin (B-2), Gelatin, Pyridoxine HCl (B-6), Povidone, Lacca, Magnesium Stearate, Silica, Artificial Color, Sodium Benzoate, Folic Acid, Polyethylene Glycol, Cholecalciferol (Vit. D), Carnauba Wax, Cyanocobalamin (B-12), Medical Antifoam.

How Supplied: Available in bottles of 90 and 500 tablets.

UNICAP® Capsules/Tablets
Multivitamin Supplement
100% RDA of Essential Vitamins in Easy to Swallow Capsule
Sugar and Sodium Free Tablet

Indications: Dietary multivitamin supplement of ten essential vitamins for health-conscious families (adults and children 4 or more years of age).
Each capsule contains:

		% U.S. RDA*
Vitamin A	5000 Int. Units	100
Vitamin D	400 Int. Units	100
Vitamin E	30 Int. Units	100
Vitamin C	60 mg	100
Folic Acid	400 mcg	100
Thiamine	1.5 mg	100
Riboflavin	1.7 mg	100
Niacin	20 mg	100
Vitamin B$_6$	2 mg	100
Vitamin B$_{12}$	6 mcg	100

Each tablet has same content except:

Vitamin E	15 Int. Units	50

*Percentage of U.S. Recommended Daily Allowance.

Ingredient List:
Capsules: Gelatin, Ascorbic Acid (Vit. C), Soybean Oil, Glycerin, Vitamin E Acetate, Niacinamide, Yellow Wax, Lecithin, Pyridoxine Hydrochloride (B-6), Thiamine Mononitrate (B-1), Riboflavin (B-2), Vitamin A Palmitate, Titanium Dioxide, Corn Oil, Folic Acid, FD&C Yellow No. 5, Ethyl Vanillin, Vanilla Enhancer, FD&C Yellow No. 6, Cholecalciferol (Vit. D), Cyanocobalamin (B-12).
Tablets: Calcium Phosphate, Ascorbic Acid (Vit. C), Vitamin E Acetate, Hydroxypropyl Methylcellulose, Niacinamide Ascorbate, Artificial Color, Vitamin A Acetate, Magnesium Stearate, Pyridoxine Hydrochloride (B-6), Riboflavin (B-2), Silica Gel, Thiamine Mononitrate (B-1), FD&C Yellow No. 5, Folic Acid, Artificial Flavor, Cholecalciferol (Vit. D), Carnauba Wax, Cyanocobalamin (B-12).

Recommended Dosage: 1 capsule or tablet daily.

How Supplied: Available in bottles of 120 capsules or tablets.

UNICAP Jr™ Chewable Tablets
Good-tasting, Orange-flavored Chewable Tablet

Indications: Dietary multivitamin supplement providing up to 100% of the RDA of essential vitamins. For **children** 4 or more years of age.

Each tablet contains:		% U.S. RDA*
Vitamin A	5000 Int. Units	100
Vitamin D	400 Int. Units	100
Vitamin E	15 Int. Units	50
Vitamin C	60 mg	100
Folic Acid	400 mcg	100
Thiamine	1.5 mg	100
Riboflavin	1.7 mg	100
Niacin	20 mg	100
Vitamin B$_6$	2 mg	100
Vitamin B$_{12}$	6 mcg	100

*Percentage of U.S. Recommended Daily Allowance.

Ingredient List: Sucrose, Mannitol, Sodium Ascorbate (Vit C), Lactose, Cornstarch, Niacinamide, Citric Acid, Vitamin E Acetate, Povidone, Artificial Flavor, Dextrins, Silica, Calcium Stearate, Pyridoxine HCl (B-6), Artificial Color, Vitamin A Acetate, Thiamine Mononitrate (B-1), Riboflavin (B-2), Folic Acid, Cyanocobalamin (B-12), Cholecalciferol (Vit D).

Recommended Dosage: 1 tablet daily.

How Supplied: Available in bottles of 120 tablets.

UNICAP M® Tablets
Multivitamins and Minerals
Sugar Free and Sodium Free

Indications: Dietary supplement providing up to 100% of the RDA for essential vitamins and minerals, including vitamin C and B-complex vitamins for persons 12 or more years of age.

Each tablet contains:		% U.S. RDA
Vitamin A	5000 Int. Units	100
Vitamin D	400 Int. Units	100
Vitamin E	30 Int. Units	100
Vitamin C	60 mg	100
Folic Acid	400 mcg	100
Thiamine	1.5 mg	100
Riboflavin	1.7 mg	100
Niacin	20 mg	100
Vitamin B$_6$	2 mg	100
Vitamin B$_{12}$	6 mcg	100
Pantothenic Acid	10 mg	100
Iodine	150 mcg	100
Iron	18 mg	100
Copper	2 mg	100
Zinc	15 mg	100
Calcium	60 mg	6
Phosphorus	45 mg	5
Manganese	1 mg	+
Potassium	5 mg	+

+ Recognized as essential in human nutrition, but no U.S. Recommended Daily Allowance (U.S. RDA) has been established.

Ingredient List: Calcium Phosphate, Ascorbic Acid (Vit C) Vitamin E Acetate, Ferrous Fumarate, Cellulose, Niacinamide Ascorbate, Artificial Color, Zinc Oxide, Calcium Pantothenate, Vitamin A Acetate, Potassium Sulfate, Magnesium Stearate, Cupric Sulfate, Silica Gel, Manganese Sulfate, Pyridoxine Hydrochloride, Riboflavin (B-2), Thiamine Mononitrate (B-1), FD&C Yellow No. 5, Folic Acid, Artificial Flavor, Cholecalciferol (Vit D), Potassium Iodide, Carnauba Wax, Cyanocobalamin (B-12).

Recommended Dosage: 1 tablet daily.

How Supplied: Available in bottles of 120 and 500 tablets.

Shown in Product Identification Section, page 435

UNICAP® Plus Iron Tablets
Multivitamin Supplement With 100% of the U.S. RDA of Essential Vitamins Plus Calcium and Extra Iron
Sugar Free and Sodium Free

Indications: Dietary multivitamin supplement providing essential vitamins. 125% of the RDA of Iron plus Calcium for women 12 or more years of age.

Each tablet contains:		% U.S. RDA*
Vitamins		
Vitamin A	5000 Int. Units	100
Vitamin D	400 Int. Units	100
Vitamin E	30 Int. Units	100
Vitamin C	60 mg	100
Folic Acid	400 mcg	100
Thiamine	1.5 mg	100
Riboflavin	1.7 mg	100
Niacin	20 mg	100
Vitamin B₆	2 mg	100
Vitamin B₁₂	6 mcg	100
Pantothenic Acid	10 mg	100
Minerals		
Iron	22.5 mg	125
Calcium	100 mg	10

*Percentage of U.S. Recommended Daily Allowance.

Ingredient List: Calcium Phosphate, Cellulose, Ascorbic Acid (Vit C), Ferrous Fumarate, Vitamin E Acetate, Artificial Color, Niacinamide, Vitamin A Acetate, Calcium Pantothenate, Magnesium Stearate, Silica Gel, Pyridoxine HCl (B-6), Riboflavin (B-2), Thiamine Mononitrate (B-1), Folic Acid, Artificial Flavor, Cholecalciferol (Vit D), Carnauba Wax, Cyanocobalamin (B-12).

Recommended Dosage: 1 tablet daily.

How Supplied: Available in bottles of 120 tablets.

UNICAP Sr.™ Tablets
Vitamins and Minerals for Mature Adults Based on the National Academy of Sciences–National Research Council Recommendations for People Over 50
Sugar Free and Sodium Free

Indications: Dietary supplement of essential vitamins and minerals formulated for the nutritional needs of mature adults.

Each tablet contains:		% RDDA*
Vitamin A	5000 Int. Units	100
(includes 200 IU Beta-Carotene)		
Vitamin D	200 Int. Units	100
Vitamin E	15 Int. Units	50
Vitamin C	60 mg	100
Folic Acid	400 mcg	100
Thiamine	1.2 mg	100
Riboflavin	1.4 mg	100
Niacin	16 mg	100
Vitamin B₆	2.2 mg	100

Vitamin B₁₂	3 mcg	100
Pantothenic Acid	10 mg	100
Iodine	150 mcg	100
Iron	10 mg	100
Copper	2 mg	100
Zinc	15 mg	100
Calcium	100 mg	12
Phosphorus	77 mg	10
Magnesium	30 mg	9
Manganese	1 mg	+
Potassium	5 mg	+

*Percentage of Recommended Daily Dietary Allowance for Adults 51 years and over, National Academy of Sciences–National Research Council.

+Recognized as essential in human nutrition, but no U.S. Recommended Daily Allowance (U.S. RDA) has been established.

Ingredient List: Calcium Phosphate, Cellulose, Ascorbic Acid (Vit C), Magnesium Oxide, Vitamin E Acetate, Ferrous Fumarate, Artificial Color, Zinc Oxide, Niacinamide, Calcium Pantothenate, Vitamin A Acetate, Magnesium Stearate, Potassium Sulfate, Cupric Sulfate, Silica Gel, Beta-Carotene, Manganese Sulfate, Pyridoxine Hydrochloride (B-6), Riboflavin (B-2), Thiamine Mononitrate (B-1), Folic Acid, Artificial Flavor, Cholecalciferol (Vit D), Potassium Iodide, Carnauba Wax, Cyanocobalamin (B-12).

Recommended Dosage: 1 tablet daily.

How Supplied: Available in bottles of 120 tablets.

Shown in Product Identification Section, page 435

UNICAP T® Tablets
Therapeutic Potency Vitamin and Mineral Formula
Sugar Free and Sodium Free

Indications: Dietary supplement providing higher levels of vitamin C and B-complex vitamins essential for the return to, and maintenance of good health. For persons 12 or more years of age.

Each tablet contains:		% U.S. RDA
Vitamin A	5000 Int. Units	100
Vitamin D	400 Int. Units	100
Vitamin E	30 Int. Units	100
Vitamin C	500 mg	833
Folic Acid	400 mcg	100
Thiamine	10 mg	667
Riboflavin	10 mg	588
Niacin	100 mg	500
Vitamin B₆	6 mg	300
Vitamin B₁₂	18 mcg	300
Pantothenic Acid	25 mg	250
Iodine	150 mcg	100
Iron	18 mg	100
Copper	2 mg	100
Zinc	15 mg	100
Manganese	1 mg	+
Potassium	5 mg	+
Selenium	10 mcg	+

+ Recognized as essential in human nutrition, but no U.S. Recommended Daily Allowance (U.S. RDA) has been established.

Ingredient List: Ascorbic Acid (Vit C), Niacinamide Ascorbate, Cellulose, Hydroxypropyl Methylcellulose, Vitamin E Acetate, Ferrous Fumarate, Artificial Color, Calcium Pantothenate, Calcium Phosphate, Zinc Oxide, Vitamin A Acetate, Magnesium Stearate, Potassium Sulfate, Thiamine Mononitrate (B-1), Riboflavin (B-2), Selenium Yeast, Pyridoxine Hydrochloride (B-6), Cupric Sulfate, Silica Gel, Manganese Sulfate, FD&C Yellow No. 5, Folic Acid, Artificial Flavor, Cholecalciferol (Vit D), Potassium Iodide, Carnauba Wax, Cyanocobalamin (B-12).

Recommended Dosage: 1 tablet daily.

How Supplied: Available in bottles of 60 tablets.

Shown in Product Identification Section, page 435

Wakunaga of America Co., Ltd.
Subsidiary of Wakunaga Pharmaceutical Co., Ltd.
23501 MADERO
MISSION VIEJO, CA 92691

KYOLIC®
Odor Modified Garlic

Active Ingredient: Aged Garlic Extract.

Indications: Dietary Supplement.

Suggested Use: Average serving, four capsules or tablets a day during or after meals.

How Supplied: Liquid—Kyolic-Aged Garlic Extract Flavor and Odor Modified Enriched with Vitamin B₁ and B₁₂ (and empty gelatine capsules) 2 fl oz (62 capsules) and 4 fl oz (124 capsules). Kyolic-Aged Garlic Extract Flavor and Odor Modified Plain (and empty gelatine capsules) 2 fl oz (62 capsules) and 4 fl oz (124 capsules).

Tablets and Capsules—Ingredients per Tablet or Capsule:
Kyolic—Super Formula 100 Tablets: Aged Garlic Extract Powder (300 mg), Whey (168 mg) blended with natural vegetable sources: Cellulose and Algin, bottles of 100 and 200 tablets.
Kyolic—Super Formula 100 Capsules: Aged Garlic Extract Powder (300 mg), Whey (168 mg), bottles of 100 and 200 capsules.
Kyolic—Super Formula 101 Garlic Plus® Tablets: Aged Garlic Extract Powder (270 mg) blended with Brewer's Yeast (27 mg), Kelp (9 mg), bottles of 100 and 200 tablets.
Kyolic—Super Formula 101 Garlic Plus® Capsules: Aged Garlic Extract Powder (270 mg) blended with Brewer's Yeast (27 mg), Kelp (9 mg), bottles of 50, 100 and 200 capsules.
Kyolic—Super Formula 102 Tablets: Aged Garlic Extract Powder (350 mg), "Kyolic Enzyme Complex™" [Amylase, Protease, Cellulase and Lipase] (30 mg), bottles of 100 and 200 tablets.

Continued on next page

Wakunaga—Cont.

Kyolic—Super Formula 102 Capsules: Aged Garlic Extract Powder (350 mg), "Kyolic Enzyme Complex™" [Amylase, Protease, Cellulase and Lipase] (30 mg), bottles of 100 and 200 tablets.
Kyolic—Super Formula 103 Capsules: Aged Garlic Extract Powder (220 mg), Ester C® [Calcium Ascorbate] (150 mg), Astragulus membranaceous (100 mg), Calcium lactate (80 mg), bottles of 100 and 200 capsules.
Kyolic—Super Formula 104 Capsules: Aged Garlic Extract Powder (300 mg), Lecithin (200 mg), bottles of 100 and 200 capsules.
Kyolic—Super Formula 105 Capsules: Aged Garlic Extract Powder (250 mg), Beta-Carotene (37.5 mg) d-Alpha-Tocopheryl Acid Succinate [Vitamin E] (50 mg) in a base of Alfalfa and Parsley, bottles of 100 capsules.
Kyolic—Super Formula 106 Capsules: Aged Garlic Extract Powder (300 mg), d-Alpha Tocopheryl Succinate [Vitamin E] (90 mg), Hawthorn Berry (50 mg), Cayenne Pepper (10 mg), bottles of 50 and 100 capsules.
Professional label "SGP" is available in liquid and Aged Garlic Extract powder forms.

Shown in Product Identification Section, page 435

EDUCATIONAL MATERIAL

From Soil to Shelf
Brochure describing our company, garlic fields, aging tanks and factory, plus our product line.

Walker, Corp & Co., Inc.
P.O. BOX 1320
EASTHAMPTON PL. &
N. COLLINGWOOD AVE.
SYRACUSE, NY 13201

EVAC–U–GEN®
[e-vak-ū-jen]

Description: Evac-U-Gen® is available as purple scored tablets, each containing 97.2 mg of yellow phenolphthalein. Also contains anise oil, corn syrup solids, D&C red 7, FD&C blue 1, lactose, magnesium stearate, saccharin sodium and sugar.

Action and Uses: For temporary relief of occasional constipation and to help restore a normal pattern of evacuation. A mild, non-griping, stimulant laxative in chewable, anise-flavored form, Evac-U-Gen provides gentle, overnight relief by softening of the feces through selective action on the intramural nerve plexus of intestinal smooth muscle, and increases the propulsive peristaltic activity of the colon. It is frequently helpful in preparing the bowel for diagnostic procedures.

Indications: Because of its gentle and non-toxic nature, Evac-U-Gen is especially recommended for persons over 55, and in the presence of hemorrhoids. It is also suitable in pregnancy and for children. Safe for nursing mothers, Evac-U-Gen does not affect the infant. It may be useful when straining at the stool is a hazard, as in hernia, cardiac or hypertensive patients.

Contraindications: Contraindicated in patients with a history of sensitivity to phenolphthalein. Evac-U-Gen should not be used when abdominal pain, nausea, vomiting, or other symptoms of appendicitis are present.

Side Effects: If skin rash appears, use of Evac-U-Gen or other preparations containing phenolphthalein should be discontinued. May cause coloration of feces or urine if such are sufficiently alkaline.

Warning: Frequent or prolonged use may result in dependence on laxatives. Keep this and all medication out of reach of children.

Administration and Dosage: Adults: chew one or two tablets night or morning. **Children:** Over 6, chew ½ tablet daily. Intensity of action is proportional to dosage, but individually effective doses vary. Evac-U-Gen is usually active 6 to 8 hours after administration, but residual action may last 3 to 4 days.

How Supplied: Evac-U-Gen is available in bottles of 35, 100, 500, 1000 and 6000 tablets.

Shown in Product Identification Section, page 435

Walker Pharmacal Company
4200 LACLEDE AVENUE
ST. LOUIS, MO 63108

PRID SALVE
(Smile's PRID Salve)
Drawing Salve and Anti-infectant

Active Ingredients: Ichthammol (Ammonium Ichthosulfonate) Phenol (Carbolic Acid) Lead Oleate, Rosin, Bees Wax, Lard.

Description: PRID has a very stiff consistency and is almost black in color.

Indication: PRID is an anti-infective salve, which also serves as a skin protective ointment. As a drawing salve, PRID softens the skin around the foreign body, and assists the natural rejection. PRID also helps to prevent the spread of infection. PRID aids in relieving the discomfort of minor skin irritations, superficial cuts, scratches and wounds. PRID is also helpful in the treatment of boils and carbuncles. PRID has been used with some success in the treatment of acne and furunculosis as well as other skin disorders.

Warning: When applied to fingers or toes, do not use a bandage; use loose gauze so as to not interfere with circulation. Apply according to directions for use and in no case to large areas of the body without a physician's direction. Keep out of eyes.

Caution: If PRID salve is not effective in 10 days, see your physician.

Directions For Use: Wash affected parts thoroughly with hot water; dry and apply PRID at least twice daily on a clean bandage or gauze. After irritation subsides, repeat application once a day for several days. DO NOT irritate by squeezing or pressing skin area.

How Supplied: PRID is packaged in a telescoping orange metal can containing 20 grams of PRID salve.

Wallace Laboratories
P.O. BOX 1001
HALF ACRE ROAD
CRANBURY, NJ 08512

MALTSUPEX®
(malt soup extract)
Powder, Liquid, Tablets

Composition: 'Maltsupex' is a nondiastatic extract from barley malt, which is available in powder, liquid, and tablet form. 'Maltsupex' has a gentle laxative action and promotes soft, easily passed stools. Each **Tablet** contains 750 mg of 'Maltsupex' and approximately 0.15 to 0.25 mEq of potassium. Tablet Ingredients: acetylated monoglycerides, FD&C Yellow #5, FD&C Yellow #6, flavor (artificial), hydroxypropyl methylcellulose, polyethylene glycol, povidone, stearic acid, talc, titanium dioxide. Each tablespoonful (½ fl oz) of **Liquid** and each heaping tablespoonful of **Powder** contains the equivalent of 16 g of Malt Soup Extract Powder and 3.1 to 5.5 mEq of potassium. Other Ingredients: none.

Indications: 'Maltsupex' is indicated for the dietary management and treatment of functional constipation in infants and children. It is also useful in treating constipation in adults, including those with laxative dependence.

Warnings: Do not use when abdominal pain, nausea or vomiting are present. If constipation persists, consult a physician. Keep this and all medications out of the reach of children.
'Maltsupex' Powder and Liquid only—Do not use these products except under the advice and supervision of a physician if you have kidney disease.
As with any drug, if you are pregnant or nursing a baby, seek the advice of a health professional before using this product.

Precautions: In patients with diabetes, allow for carbohydrate content of approximately 14 grams per tablespoonful of **Liquid** (56 calories), 13 grams per tablespoonful of **Powder** (52 calories), and 0.6 grams per Tablet (3 calories).
Tablets only: This product contains FD&C Yellow No. 5 (tartrazine) which may cause allergic-type reactions (including bronchial asthma) in certain sus-

ceptible individuals. Although the overall incidence of FD&C Yellow No. 5 (tartrazine) sensitivity in the general population is low, it is frequently seen in patients who also have aspirin hypersensitivity.

Dosage and Administration: General—The recommended daily dosage of 'Maltsupex' may vary from 6 to 32 grams for infants (2 years or less) and 12 to 64 grams for children and adults, accompanied by adequate fluid intake with each dose. Use the smallest dose that is effective and lower dosage as improvement occurs. Use heaping measures of the **Powder. 'Maltsupex' Liquid** mixes more easily if stirred first in one or two ounces of warm water.

Powder and Liquid (Usual Dosage)— **Adults:** 2 tablespoonfuls (32 g) twice daily for 3 or 4 days, or until relief is noted, then 1 to 2 tablespoonfuls at bedtime for maintenance, as needed. Drink a full glass (8 oz) of liquid with each dose. **Children:** 1 or 2 tablespoonfuls in 8 ounces of liquid once or twice daily (with cereal, milk or preferred beverage). **Bottle-Fed Infants (over 1 month):** ½ to 2 tablespoonfuls in the day's total formula, or 1 to 2 teaspoonfuls in a single feeding to correct constipation. To prevent constipation (as when switching to whole milk) add 1 to 2 teaspoonfuls to the day's formula or 1 teaspoonful to every second feeding. **Breast-Fed Infants (over one month):** 1 to 2 teaspoonfuls in 2 to 4 ounces of water or fruit juice once or twice daily.

Tablets—**Adults:** Start with 4 tablets (3 g) four times daily (with meals and bedtime) and adjust dosage according to response. Drink a full glass (8 oz) of liquid with each dose.

How Supplied: 'Maltsupex' is supplied in 8 ounce (NDC 0037-9101-12) and 16 ounce (NDC 0037-9101-08) jars of 'Maltsupex' Powder; 8 fluid ounce (NDC 0037-9001-12) and 1 pint (NDC 0037-9001-08) bottles of 'Maltsupex' Liquid; and in bottles of 100 'Maltsupex' Tablets (NDC 0037-9201-01).

'Maltsupex' **Powder** and **Liquid** are Distributed by

WALLACE LABORATORIES
Division of
CARTER-WALLACE, INC.
Cranbury, New Jersey 08512

'Maltsupex' **Tablets** are Manufactured by

WALLACE LABORATORIES
Division of
CARTER-WALLACE, INC.
Cranbury, New Jersey 08512
Rev. 10/85

Shown in Product Identification Section, page 435

RYNA™
(Liquid)
RYNA–C® ℃
(Liquid)
RYNA–CX® ℃
(Liquid)

Description:
RYNA Liquid—Each 5 mL (one teaspoonful) contains:
Chlorpheniramine maleate ....2 mg
Pseudoephedrine hydrochloride....30 mg
Other ingredients: flavor (artificial), glycerin, malic acid, sodium benzoate, sorbitol, purified water, in a clear, slightly yellow colored, lemon-vanilla flavored demulcent base containing no sugar, dyes, or alcohol.
RYNA-C Liquid—Each 5 mL (one teaspoonful) contains, in addition:
Codeine phosphate...........................10 mg
  (WARNING: May be habit-forming)
Other ingredients: flavor (artificial), glycerin, malic acid, purified water, saccharin sodium, sodium benzoate, sorbitol, in a clear, colorless to slightly yellow, cinnamon-flavored, demulcent base containing no sugar, dyes, or alcohol.
RYNA-CX Liquid—Each 5 mL (one teaspoonful) contains:
Codeine phosphate...........................10 mg
  (WARNING: May be habit-forming)
Pseudoephedrine hydrochloride....30 mg
Guaifenesin ....100 mg
Other ingredients: flavors (artificial), glycerin, glycine, malic acid, povidone, propylene glycol, purified water, saccharin sodium, sorbitol, in a clear, colorless, cherry-vanilla-menthol flavored demulcent base containing no sugar, dyes, or alcohol.

Actions:
Chlorpheniramine maleate in RYNA and RYNA-C is an antihistamine that antagonizes the effects of histamine.
Codeine phosphate in RYNA-C and RYNA-CX is a centrally-acting antitussive that relieves cough.
Pseudoephedrine hydrochloride in RYNA, RYNA-C and RYNA-CX is a sympathomimetic nasal decongestant that acts to shrink swollen mucosa of the respiratory tract.
Guaifenesin in RYNA-CX is an expectorant that increases mucus flow to help prevent dryness and relieve irritated respiratory tract membranes.

Indications:
RYNA: For the temporary relief of the concurrent symptoms of nasal congestion, sneezing, itchy and watery eyes, and running nose as occur with the common cold or allergic rhinitis.
RYNA-C: Temporarily relieves cough, nasal congestion, runny nose and sneezing as may occur with the common cold.
RYNA-CX: Temporarily relieves cough and nasal congestion as may occur with the common cold. Relieves irritated membranes in the respiratory passageways by preventing dryness through increased mucus flow.

Warnings:
For RYNA:
Do not give this product to children taking other medication or to children un-

der 6 years except under the advice and supervision of a physician. Do not exceed recommended dosage unless directed by a physician because nervousness, dizziness, or sleeplessness may occur at higher doses. If symptoms do not improve within 3 days or are accompanied by high fever, discontinue use and consult a physician. Do not take this product except under the advice and supervision of a physician if you have any of the following symptoms or conditions: high blood pressure; heart disease; thyroid disease; diabetes; asthma; glaucoma; or difficulty in urination due to enlargement of the prostate.

For RYNA-C and RYNA-CX:
Adults and children who have a chronic pulmonary disease or shortness of breath, or children who are taking other drugs, should not take these products unless directed by a physician. Do not give these products to children under 6 years of age except under the advice and supervision of a physician. A persistent cough may be a sign of a serious condition. If cough persists for more than one week, tends to recur, or is accompanied by fever, rash or persistent headache, consult a physician. Do not take these products for persistent or chronic cough such as occurs with smoking, asthma, emphysema, or if cough is accompanied by excessive phlegm (mucus) unless directed by a physician. Do not take these products if you have glaucoma, asthma, emphysema, difficulty in breathing, difficulty in urination due to enlargement of the prostate gland, heart disease, high blood pressure, thyroid disease, or diabetes unless directed by a physician. May cause or aggravate constipation.
Do not take these products or give to children for more than 7 days. If symptoms do not improve or are accompanied by fever, consult a physician. Unless directed by a physician, do not exceed recommended dosage because nervousness, dizziness or sleeplessness may occur at higher doses.

For RYNA and RYNA-C:
These products contain an antihistamine which may cause excitability, especially in children, or drowsiness or may impair mental alertness. Combined use with alcohol, sedatives, or other depressants may have an additive effect. Do not drive motor vehicles, operate machinery, or drink alcoholic beverages while taking these products.
As with any drug, if you are pregnant or nursing a baby, seek the advice of a health professional before using these products.

Drug Interaction Precaution: Persons who are presently taking a prescription drug for high blood pressure or depression should not use these products without consulting a physician.

Dosage and Administration:
Adults: 2 teaspoonfuls every 6 hours
Children 6 to under 12 years: 1 teaspoonful every 6 hours.

Continued on next page

Shown in Product Identification Section, page 435

Wallace—Cont.

Children under 6 years: consult a physician.
DO NOT EXCEED 4 DOSES IN 24 HOURS.

Ryna-C and Ryna-CX:

A special measuring device should be used to give an accurate dose of these products to children under 6 years of age. Giving a higher dose than recommended by a physician could result in serious side effects for the child.

How Supplied:
RYNA: bottles of 4 fl oz (NDC 0037-0638-66) and one pint (NDC 0037-0638-68).
RYNA-C: bottles of 4 fl oz (NDC 0037-0522-66) and one pint (NDC 0037-0522-68).
RYNA-CX: bottles of 4 fl oz (NDC 0037-0801-66) and one pint (NDC 0037-0801-68).
TAMPER-RESISTANT BAND ON CAP, PRINTED "WALLACE LABORATORIES". DO NOT USE IF BAND IS MISSING OR BROKEN.

Storage:
RYNA: Store below 30° (86°F).
RYNA-C and RYNA-CX: Store at controlled room temperature. Protect from excessive heat and freezing.
KEEP THESE AND ALL DRUGS OUT OF THE REACH OF CHILDREN. IN CASE OF ACCIDENTAL OVERDOSE, SEEK PROFESSIONAL ASSISTANCE OR CONTACT A POISON CONTROL CENTER IMMEDIATELY.

WALLACE LABORATORIES
Division of
CARTER-WALLACE, Inc.
Cranbury, New Jersey 08512
Rev. 8/88
*Shown in Product Identification
Section, page 435*

SYLLACT®
(Powdered Psyllium Seed Husks)

Description: Each rounded teaspoonful of fruit-flavored **'Syllact'** contains approximately 3.3 g of powdered psyllium seed husks and an equal amount of dextrose as a dispersing agent, and provides about 14 calories. Potassium sorbate, methyl and propylparaben are added as preservatives. Other ingredients: citric acid, dextrose, FD&C Red #40, flavor (artificial), and saccharin sodium.

Actions: The active ingredient in 'Syllact' is hydrophilic mucilloid, non-absorbable dietary fiber derived from the powdered husks of natural psyllium seed, which acts by increasing the water content and bulk volume of stools. It gives 'Syllact' a bland, non-irritating, laxative action and promotes physiologic evacuation of the bowel.

Indications: 'Syllact' is indicated for the treatment of constipation and, when recommended by a physician, in other disorders where the effect of additional bulk and fiber is desired.

Warnings: Do not swallow dry. Drink a full glass (8 oz) of water or other liquid with each dose. If constipation persists, consult a physician. Do not use if fecal impaction, intestinal obstruction, or abdominal pain, nausea or vomiting are present. Keep this and all medications out of the reach of children.
As with any drug, if you are pregnant or nursing a baby, seek the advice of a health professional before using this product.

Dosage and Administration: The actual daily dosage depends on the need and response of the patient. Adults may take up to 9 teaspoonfuls daily, in divided doses, for several days to provide optimum benefit when constipation is chronic or severe. Lower the dosage as improvement occurs. Use a dry spoon to measure powder. Tighten lid to keep out moisture.
Usual Adult Dosage—One rounded teaspoonful of 'Syllact' in a full glass (8 oz) of cool water or other beverage taken orally one to three times daily. If desired, an additional glass of liquid may be taken after each dose.
Children's Dosage—6 years and older—Half the adult dosage with the same fluid intake requirement.

How Supplied: 'Syllact' Powder—in 10 oz jars (NDC 0037-9501-13).
Rev. 10/85
WALLACE LABORATORIES
Division of
CARTER-WALLACE, INC.
Cranbury, New Jersey 08512
*Shown in Product Identification
Section, page 435*

Warner-Lambert Company
Consumer Health Products Group
201 TABOR ROAD
MORRIS PLAINS, NJ 07950

PROFESSIONAL STRENGTH EFFERDENT
Denture Cleanser

Cleansing Ingredients: Potassium monopersulfate, sodium perborate, sodium carbonate, sodium tripolyphosphate, EDTA and surfactants.

Other Ingredients: Sodium bicarbonate, citric acid, colors and flavors.

Indications: For effective and convenient daily denture cleaning to remove plaque and stains and to inhibit bacterial growth on dentures and removable orthodontic appliances.

Actions: Efferdent's effervescent cleansing action removes stubborn stains between teeth, whitens and brightens, fights plaque and leaves dentures and removable orthodontic appliances fresh tasting and odor free.

Warnings: Keep out of the reach of children. DO NOT PUT TABLETS IN MOUTH.

Dosage and Administration: For best results, use at least once daily. Dentures may be soaked safely in Efferdent overnight.

How Supplied: Available in boxes of 20, 40, 60 and 96 tablets.
*Shown in Product Identification
Section, page 435*

HALLS® MENTHO–LYPTUS®
Cough Suppressant Tablets

Active Ingredients: Each tablet contains eucalyptus oil and menthol.

Inactive Ingredients: Corn Syrup, Flavoring, Sugar and Artificial Colors.

Indications: For temporary relief of minor throat irritation and coughs due to colds or inhaled irritants. Makes nasal passages feel clearer.

Warning: A persistent cough or sore throat may be a sign of a serious condition. If cough persists for more than 1 week, tends to recur, or is accompanied by fever, rash or persistent headache, or if sore throat is severe, persistent or accompanied by high fever, headache, nausea, and vomiting, consult a doctor. Do not take this product for sore throat lasting more than 2 days or persistent or chronic cough such as occurs with smoking, asthma, emphysema, or if cough is accompanied by excessive phlegm (mucus) unless directed by a doctor. Keep this and all drugs out of the reach of children.

Dosage and Administration: Adults and children 3 years and over dissolve one tablet slowly in mouth. Repeat every hour as needed or as directed by a doctor. Children under 3 years: consult a doctor.

How Supplied: Halls Mentho-Lyptus Cough Suppressant Tablets are available in single sticks of 9 tablets each, in 3-stick packs, and in bags of 30 tablets. They are available in five flavors: Regular, Cherry, Honey-Lemon, Ice Blue, and Spearmint.
*Shown in Product Identification
Section, page 435*

HALLS® Vitamin C Drops

Description: Halls Vitamin C Drops are a delicious way to get 100% of the U.S. Recommended Daily Allowance of Vitamin C. Each drop provides 60 mg. of Vitamin C (100% U.S. RDA)

Ingredients: Sugar, Glucose Syrup, Sodium Ascorbate, Citric Acid, Ascorbic Acid, Natural Flavoring and Artificial Color (Including Yellow 5 and Yellow 6).

Indication: Dietary Supplementation.

How Supplied: Halls Vitamin C Drops are available in single sticks of 9 drops each and in bags of 30 drops. They are available in 5 great-tasting all-natural citrus flavors: tangerine, lemon, sweet grapefruit, lime and orange.

LISTERINE® Antiseptic

Active Ingredients: Thymol .06%, Eucalyptol .09%, Methyl Salicylate .06% and Menthol .04%. Also contains: Water, Alcohol 26.9%, Benzoic Acid, Poloxamer 407 and Caramel.

Indications: To help prevent and reduce supragingival plaque and gingivitis; for general oral hygiene and bad breath.

Actions: Listerine Antiseptic has been shown to help prevent and reduce supragingival plaque and gingivitis when used in a conscientiously applied program of daily oral hygiene and regular professional care. Its effect on periodontitis has not been determined. Listerine is the only nonprescription mouthrinse that has received the American Dental Association's Council on Dental Therapeutics Seal of Acceptance for helping to prevent and reduce plaque above the gumline and gingivitis.

Directions: Rinse full strength for 30 seconds with ⅔ ounce (4 teaspoonfuls) morning and night. If bad breath persists, see your dentist.

How Supplied: Listerine Antiseptic is supplied in 3, 6, 12, 18, 24, 32, 48 and 58 fl. oz. bottles.
Shown in Product Identification Section, page 435

LISTERINE ANTISEPTIC THROAT LOZENGES

Active Ingredients: Each lozenge contains: Hexylresorcinol.

Inactive Ingredients: Caramel, Corn Syrup, Flavoring, Glycerin and Sugar.

Indications: For fast temporary relief of minor sore throat pain.

Actions: When allowed to dissolve slowly in the mouth Listerine Lozenges bathes the throat with the soothing pain-relieving action of Hexylresorcinol, a safe and effective topical anesthetic. Listerine Lozenges provide fast temporary relief from minor sore throat pain of colds, smoking and mouth irritations.

Warnings: Severe or persistent sore throat, or sore throat accompanied by high fever, headache, nausea and vomiting, may be serious. Consult physician promptly. Do not use more than 2 days or administer to children under 3 years of age unless directed by a physician. Keep this and all drugs out of the reach of children.

Dosage: 1 lozenge every 2 hours as needed.

Storage: Store at room temperature.

How Supplied: 24 count packages.

Available in: Regular Strength (Hexylresorcinol 2.4 mg.) in Cherry, Lemon-Mint and Regular flavors and Maximum Strength (Hexylresorcinol 4.0 mg.).
Shown in Product Identification Section, page 435

LISTERMINT®
Mouthwash with Fluoride

Active Ingredient: Sodium Fluoride (0.02%). Also contains: Water, SD alcohol 38-B (6.65%), glycerin, poloxamer 407, sodium lauryl sulfate, sodium citrate, flavoring, sodium saccharin, zinc chloride, citric acid, D&C Yellow No. 10, FD&C Green No. 3.

Indications: Aids in prevention of dental cavities and freshens breath.

Directions: Adults and children 6 years of age and older: Use twice a day after brushing teeth with toothpaste. Vigorously swish 10 ml. (2 teaspoonfuls) of rinse between teeth for 1 minute and spit out. Do not swallow the rinse. Do not eat or drink for 30 minutes after rinsing.

Warnings: Children under 12 years of age should be supervised in the use of this product. Consult a dentist or physician for use in children under 6 years of age. Developing teeth of children under 6 years of age may become permanently discolored if excessive amounts of fluoride are repeatedly swallowed. This is not a dentifrice and should not be used as a substitute for regular toothbrushing. Keep this and all drugs out of reach of children.

How Supplied: Listermint with Fluoride is supplied to consumers in 6, 12, 18, 24 and 32 fl. oz. bottles.
Shown in Product Identification Section, page 436

LUBRIDERM® CREAM
Skin Lubricant Moisturizer

Composition:
Scented—Contains Water, Mineral Oil, Petrolatum, Glycerin, Glyceryl Stearate, PEG 100 Stearate, Hydrogenated Polyisobutene, Lanolin, Lanolin Alcohol, Lanolin Oil, Cetyl Alcohol, Sorbitan Laurate, Fragrance, Methylparaben, Butylparaben, Propylparaben, Quaternium-15.

Fragrance Free—Contains Water, Mineral Oil, Petrolatum, Glycerin, Glyceryl Stearate, PEG 100 Stearate, Hydrogenated Polyisobutene, Lanolin, Lanolin Alcohol, Lanolin Oil, Cetyl Alcohol, Sorbitan Laurate, Methylparaben, Butylparaben, Propylparaben, Quaternium-15.

Actions and Uses: Lubriderm Cream is an emollient-rich formula designed for extremely dry skin. Lubriderm cream relieves the roughness, dryness, and discomfort associated with dry or chapped skin and helps protect the skin from drying.
Lubriderm Cream is ideal for overnight treatment of extra dry skin. It smooths on easily and penetrates to help smooth, soften, and moisturize.

Administration and Dosage: Apply as often as needed to extra dry skin areas.

Precautions: For external use only.

How Supplied:
Scented: Available in 2.7 oz. pump container.
Fragrance Free: Available in a 2.7 oz. pump container.
Shown in Product Identification Section, page 436

LUBRIDERM® LOTION
Skin Lubricant Moisturizer

Composition:
Scented—Contains Water, Mineral Oil, Petrolatum, Sorbitol, Lanolin, Lanolin Alcohol, Stearic Acid, Triethanolamine, Cetyl Alcohol, Fragrance, Butylparaben, Methylparaben, Propylparaben, Sodium Chloride.

Fragrance Free—Contains Water, Mineral Oil, Petrolatum, Sorbitol, Lanolin, Lanolin Alcohol, Stearic Acid, Triethanolamine, Cetyl Alcohol, Butylparaben, Methylparaben, Propylparaben, Sodium Chloride.

Actions and Uses: Lubriderm Lotion is an oil-in-water emulsion indicated for use in softening, soothing and moisturizing dry chapped skin. Lubriderm relieves the roughness, tightness and discomfort associated with dry or chapped skin and helps protect the skin from further drying.
Lubriderm's extra-rich formula smoothes easily into skin without leaving a sticky film.

Administration and Dosage: Apply as often as needed to hands, face and body for skin protection.

Precautions: For external use only.

How Supplied:
Scented: Available in 1, 4, 8, 12 and 16 fl. oz. plastic bottles.
Fragrance Free: Available in 1, 8, 12 and 16 fl. oz. plastic bottles.
Shown in Product Identification Section, page 436

LUBRIDERM LUBATH®
Skin Conditioning Oil

Composition: Contains Mineral Oil, PPG-15 Stearyl Ether, Oleth-2, Nonoxynol-5, Fragrance, D&C Green No. 6.

Actions and Uses: Lubriderm Skin Conditioning Oil is a lanolin-free, mineral oil–based, bath oil designed for softening and soothing dry skin during the bath. The formula disperses into countless droplets of oil that coat the skin and help lubricate and soften. It is equally effective in hard or soft water and provides an excellent way to moisturize the skin and help counterbalance the drying effects of harsh soaps and hot water.

Administration and Dosage: Two to four capfuls in bath, or apply with moistened cloth in shower and rinse. For use as a skin cleanser, rub into wet skin and rinse.

Continued on next page

Warner-Lambert—Cont.

Precautions: Avoid getting in eyes; if this occurs, flush with clear water. When using any bath oil, take precautions against slipping. For external use only.

How Supplied: Available in 8 fl. oz. plastic bottles.

Shown in Product Identification Section, page 436

ROLAIDS®

Active Ingredient: Dihydroxyaluminum Sodium Carbonate 334 mg.

Inactive Ingredients: Corn Starch, Corn Syrup, Flavoring, Magnesium Stearate and Sugar. May also contain pregelatinized starch. Contains 53 mg. sodium per tablet.

Indications: For the relief of heartburn, sour stomach or acid indigestion and upset stomach associated with these symptoms.

Actions: Rolaids® provides rapid neutralization of stomach acid. Each tablet has acid-neutralizing capacity of 75–80 ml. of 0.1N hydrochloric acid and the ability to maintain the pH of the stomach contents close to 3.5 for a significant period of time.

Due to the relatively low solubility and other physical and chemical properties of dihydroxyaluminum sodium carbonate (DASC), it is for the most part nonabsorbed.

Although sodium is present in DASC, the sodium is available for absorption only when the antacid reacts with stomach acid. When Rolaids are consumed in excess of the amount of acid present in the stomach, this sodium is unavailable for absorption and the active ingredient is passed through the digestive system unchanged, with no sodium released.

Warnings: Keep this and all drugs out of the reach of children. Do not take more than 24 tablets in a 24-hour period, nor use the maximum dosage of this product for more than two weeks, nor use this product if you are on a sodium-restricted diet, except under the advice and supervision of a physician.

Drug Interaction Precaution: Do not take this product if you are presently taking a prescription antibiotic drug containing any form of tetracycline.

Dosage and Administration: Chew 1 or 2 tablets as symptoms occur. Repeat hourly if symptoms return or as directed by a physician.

How Supplied: Rolaids is available in Regular (Peppermint), Spearmint and Wintergreen Flavors. One roll contains 12 tablets; 3-pack contains three 12-tablet rolls; one bottle contains 75 tablets; one bottle contains 150 tablets.

Shown in Product Identification Section, page 436

CALCIUM RICH ROLAIDS®

Active Ingredient: Calcium Carbonate 550 mg. per tablet.

Inactive Ingredients:
Cherry Flavor: Corn Starch, FD&C Red No. 3, Flavoring, Magnesium Stearate, Mannitol, Polyethylene Glycol, Sugar and Titanium Dioxide.
Assorted Fruit Flavors: Colors (FD&C Blue No. 1, Red 3, Red 40, Yellow 5 [Tartrazine] and Yellow 6), Corn Starch, Flavoring, Magnesium Stearate, Mannitol, Pregelatinized Starch and Sugar.

Indications: For the relief of heartburn, sour stomach or acid indigestion and upset stomach associated with these symptoms.

Actions: Calcium Rich Rolaids provides rapid neutralization of stomach acid. Each tablet has an acid neutralizing capacity of 110 ml of 0.1N hydrochloric acid and the ability to maintain the pH of the stomach contents at 3.5 or greater for a significant period of time. Each tablet contains less than 0.4 mg of sodium and provides 22% of the Adult U.S. RDA for calcium.

Warnings: Do not take more than 14 tablets in a 24-hour period or use the maximum dosage of this product for more than 2 weeks except under the advice and supervision of a physician. Keep this and all drugs out of the reach of children.

Drug Interaction Precaution: None.

Dosage and Administration: Chew 1 or 2 tablets as symptoms occur. Repeat hourly if symptoms return or as directed by a physician.

How Supplied: Calcium Rich Rolaids is available in Cherry and Assorted Fruit Flavors. One roll contains 12 tablets: 3-pack contains three 12-tablet rolls; one bottle contains 75 tablets; one bottle contains 150 tablets.

Shown in Product Identification Section, page 436

EXTRA STRENGTH ROLAIDS®

Active Ingredient: Calcium Carbonate 1000 mg. per tablet.

Inactive Ingredients: Acesulfame Potassium, Colors (FD&C Blue No. 1, FD&C Yellow No. 5 [Tartrazine] and Titanium Dioxide), Corn Syrup, Flavoring, Magnesium Stearate, Pregelantinized Starch and Sugar.

Indications: For the relief of heartburn, sour stomach or acid indigestion and upset stomach associated with these symptoms.

Actions: Extra Strength Rolaids provides rapid neutralization of stomach acid. Each tablet has an acid-neutralizing capacity of 200 ml. of 0.1N hydrochloric acid and the ability to maintain the pH of the stomach contents at 3.5 or greater for a significant period of time. Each tablet contains less than 0.4 mg. of

sodium and provides 40% of the Adult U.S. RDA for calcium.

Warnings: Do not take more than 8 tablets in a 24-hour period or use the maximum dosage of this product for more than 2 weeks except under the advice and supervision of a physician. Keep this and all drugs out of the reach of children.

Drug Interaction Precaution: None.

Dosage and Administration: Chew 1 or 2 tablets as symptoms occur. Repeat hourly if symptoms return or as directed by a physician.

How Supplied: Extra Strength Rolaids is available in Assorted Mint Flavors. One roll contains 10 tablets: 3-pack contains three 10-tablet rolls; one bottle contains 55 tablets; one bottle contains 110 tablets.

Shown in Product Identification Section, page 436

SODIUM FREE ROLAIDS®

Active Ingredients: Calcium Carbonate 317 mg. and magnesium hydroxide 64 mg. per tablet.

Inactive Ingredients: Corn starch, corn syrup, flavoring, magnesium stearate, mannitol and sugar.

Indications: For the relief of heartburn, sour stomach or acid indigestion and upset stomach associated with these symptoms.

Actions: Rolaids Sodium Free provides rapid neutralization of stomach acid. Each tablet has an acid neutralizing capacity of 85 ml of 0.1N hydrochloric acid and the ability to maintain the pH of the stomach contents close to 3.5 for a significant period of time. Each tablet contains less than 0.4 mg. of sodium.

Warnings: Do not take more than 18 tablets in a 24-hour period or use the maximum dosage of this product for more than 2 weeks except under the advice and supervision of a physician. Keep this and all drugs out of the reach of children.

Drug Interaction Precaution: None.

Dosage and Administration: Chew 1 or 2 tablets as symptoms occur. Repeat hourly if symptoms return, or as directed by a physician.

How Supplied: One roll contains 12 tablets: 3-pack contains three 12-tablet rolls; one bottle contains 75 tablets; one bottle contains 150 tablets.

Shown in Product Identification Section, page 436

Products are cross-indexed by generic and chemical names in the
YELLOW SECTION

Westwood Pharmaceuticals Inc.
100 FOREST AVENUE
BUFFALO, NY 14213

ALPHA KERI®
Moisture Rich Body Oil

Composition: Contains mineral oil, Hydroloc™ brand of Westwood's PEG-4 dilaurate, lanolin oil, fragrance, benzophenone-3, D&C green 6.

Action and Uses: ALPHA KERI is a water-dispersible, antipruritic oil for the care of dry skin. ALPHA KERI effectively deposits a thin, uniform, emulsified film of oil over the skin. This film helps relieve itching, lubricates and softens the skin. ALPHA KERI Moisture Rich Body Oil is an all-over skin moisturizer. Only Alpha Keri contains Hydroloc™—the unique emulsifier that provides a more uniform distribution of the therapeutic oils to moisturize dry skin. ALPHA KERI is valuable as an aid in the treatment of dry, pruritic skin and mild skin irritations such as chronic atopic dermatitis; pruritus senilis and hiemalis; contact dermatitis; "bath-itch"; xerosis or asteatosis; ichthyosis; soap dermatitis; psoriasis.

Adminstration and Dosage: ALPHA KERI *should always be used with water, either added to water or rubbed on to wet skin.* Because of its inherent cleansing properties it is not necessary to use soap when ALPHA KERI is being used.
For exact dosage, label directions should be followed.
BATH: Added as directed to bathtub of water. For optimum relief: 10 to 20 minute soak.
SHOWER: Dispense a small amount into hand and rub onto wet skin. Rinse as desired and pat dry.
SPONGE BATH: Added as directed to a basin of warm water then rubbed over entire body with washcloth.
SITZ BATH: Added as directed to tub water. Soak should last for 10 to 20 minutes.
INFANT BATH: Added as directed to basin or bathinette of water.
SKIN CLEANSING OTHER THAN BATH OR SHOWER: A small amount is rubbed onto wet skin. Rinse. Pat dry.

Precaution: The patient should be warned to guard against slipping in tub or shower.

How Supplied: 4 fl. oz. (NDC 0072-3600-04), 8 fl. oz. (NDC 0072-3600-08), 12 fl. oz. (NDC 0072-3600-12) and 16 fl. oz. (NDC 0072-3600-16) plastic bottles. Also available in non-aerosol pump spray, 3.5 oz. (NDC 0072-3601-35).
Shown in Product Identification Section, page 436

ALPHA KERI®
Moisture Rich Cleansing Bar
Non-detergent Soap

Composition: Sodium tallowate, sodium cocoate, water, mineral oil, fragrance, PEG-75, glycerin, titanium diox-

ide, lanolin oil, sodium chloride, BHT, trisodium HEDTA, D&C Green 5, D&C Yellow 10.

Action and Uses: ALPHA KERI Moisture Rich Cleansing Bar, rich in emollient oils, thoroughly cleanses as it soothes and softens the skin.

Indications: Adjunctive use in dry skin care.

Administration and Dosage: To be used as any other soap.

How Supplied: 4 oz. (NDC 0072-3500-04) bar.

KERI LOTION
Skin Lubricant—Moisturizer

Available in two formulations:
KERI Original—recommended for extremely dry skin.

Composition: Contains mineral oil in water, propylene glycol, PEG-40 stearate, glyceryl stearate, PEG-100 stearate, PEG-4 dilaurate, laureth-4, lanolin oil, methylparaben, propylparaben, carbomer-934, triethanolamine, fragrance, dioctyl sodium sulfosuccinate, quaternium-15. Freshly-scented: FD&C blue 1, D&C yellow 10.
KERI-Silky Smooth—recommended for daily use on dry skin.

Composition: Water, petrolatum, glycerin, dimethicone, steareth-2, cetyl alcohol, benzyl alcohol, laureth-23, carbomer-934, MgAl silicate, fragrance, quaternium-15, sodium hydroxide.

Action and Uses: KERI Lotion lubricates and helps hydrate the skin, making it soft and smooth. It relieves itching, helps maintain a normal moisture balance and supplements the protective action of skin lipids. Indicated for generalized dryness and itching; detergent hands; chapped or chafed skin; sunburn; "winter-itch," aging, dry skin; diaper rash; heat rash.

Administration and Dosage: Apply as often as needed. Use particularly after bathing and exposure to sun, water, soaps and detergents.

How Supplied: KERI Lotion Original 6½ oz. (NDC 0072-4600-56), 13 oz. (NDC 0072-4600-63) and 20 oz. (NDC 0072-4600-70) plastic bottles. KERI Lotion Fresh Herbal Scent 6½ oz. (NDC 0072-4500-56), 13 oz. (NDC 0072-4500-63), and 20 oz. (NDC 0072-4500-70) plastic bottles. KERI Silky Smooth 6½ oz. (NDC 0072-4400-65), 13 oz. (NDC 0072-4400-13) and 20 oz. (NDC 0072-4400-20) plastic bottle.
Shown in Product Identification Section, page 436

LAC–HYDRIN® FIVE
Fragrance Free, Patented Dry Skin Lotion

Composition: Water, lactic acid buffered with ammonium hydroxide, glycerin, petrolatum, squalane, steareth-2, POE-21-stearyl ether, propylene glycol dioctanoate, cetyl alcohol, dimethicone, cetyl palmitate, magnesium aluminum

silicate, diazolidinyl urea, methylchloroisothiazolinone and methylisothiazolinone.

Action and Uses:
Dry skin care for elbows, knees, feet and hands—LAC-HYDRIN® FIVE is dermatologically tested and guaranteed to soften and smooth even the body's roughest, driest skin.
Elegant enough to use all over, it absorbs quickly without leaving a greasy feel. And it's non-comedogenic—designed not to clog pores and cause acne.
Try LAC-HYDRIN® FIVE, the dry skin product that's unlike any other. With regular use, you'll notice a definite improvement in the appearance of your skin—or your money back.

Administration and Dosage: For best results, apply to dry skin twice a day.

Warnings: Avoid contact with eyes. For external use only.

How Supplied: 8 oz. plastic bottle (NDC 0072-5760-08) and 4 oz. plastic bottle (NDC 0072-5760-04).
Shown in Product Identification Section, page 436

MOISTUREL® CREAM
Skin Lubricant—Moisturizer

Composition: Water, petrolatum, glycerin, PG dioctanoate, cetyl alcohol, steareth-2, dimethicone, PVP/hexadecene copolymer, laureth-23, Mg Al silicate, diazolidinyl urea, carbomer-934, sodium hydroxide, methylchloroisothiazolinone and methylisothiazolinone.

Actions and Uses: A highly effective concentrated formula clinically proven to relieve dry skin and designed not to cause acne or blemishes. Free of lanolins, fragrances, and parabens that can sensitize or irritate skin. Indicated for generalized dry skin, chapped or chafed skin, diaper rash, sunburn, windburn, heat rash, itching and dryness associated with eczema.

Administration and Dosage: Apply a small amount as often as needed.

How Supplied: 4 oz. (NDC 0072-9500-04) and 16 oz. (NDC 0072-9500-16) plastic jars.
Shown in Product Identification Section, page 436

MOISTUREL® LOTION
Skin Lubricant—Moisturizer

Composition: Water, petrolatum, glycerin, dimethicone, steareth-2, cetyl alcohol, benzyl alcohol, laureth-23, Mg Al silicate, carbomer-934, sodium hydroxide, quaternium-15.

Action and Uses: MOISTUREL is a non-greasy formula that leaves the skin feeling smooth and soft. Clinically proven to relieve dry skin and designed not to cause acne or blemishes. Free of parabens and fragrances that can sensitize or irritate skin. Indicated for generalized dry skin, chapped or chafed skin,

Continued on next page

Westwood—Cont.

diaper rash, sunburn, heat rash, itching and dryness associated with eczema.

Administration and Dosage: Apply liberally as often as needed.

How Supplied: 8 oz. (NDC 0072-9100-08) and 12 oz. (NDC 0072-9100-12) plastic bottles.

Shown in Product Identification Section, page 436

MOISTUREL®
SENSITIVE SKIN CLEANSER
Pure, Clear and Soap-Free

Composition: Sodium laureth sulfate and laureth-6 carboxylic acid and disodium laureth sulfosuccinate, methyl gluceth-20, cocamidopropyl betaine, water, diazolidinyl urea, and methylchloroisothiazolinone and methylisothiazolinone.

Actions and Uses: Moisturel Sensitive Skin Cleanser is a crystal clear, lathering, soap-free cleanser. It cleans thoroughly without stinging, irritating, or drying. Unlike soaps, Moisturel Sensitive Skin Cleanser rinses refreshingly clean without leaving a film or residue. Its pure and gentle formula makes it ideal for facial use. Its nondrying, non-comedogenic, and fragrance-free formula makes it ideal for cleansing:
- Sensitive skin—even a baby's
- Dry, itchy skin caused by cold and wind, or overexposure to sun
- Skin robbed of moisture by use and removal of cosmetics
- Irritated, allergic skin
- Skin that breaks out
- Skin dried by harsh acne medications

Administration and Dosage: With skin wet, gently work Moisturel Sensitive Skin Cleanser into a rich lather by massaging in a circular motion. Rinse thoroughly and pat dry with a soft cloth.

Caution: Avoid contact with eyes. For external use only.

How Supplied: 8.75 oz. (NDC 0072-6420-08) plastic bottle with pump.
Shown in Product Identification Section, page 436

PRESUN® FOR KIDS
Children's Sunscreen

Active Ingredients: Octyl methoxycinnamate, oxybenzone, octyl salicylate. Also contains: Carbomer-940, cetyl alcohol, diazolidinyl urea, dimethicone, methylchloroisothiazolinone and methylisothiazolinone, stearic acid, triethanolamine, water and other ingredients.

Actions and Uses: 29 TIMES NATURAL PROTECTION: Used as directed, PRESUN For Kids provides 29 times your child's natural sunburn protection and may help reduce the chance of premature aging and wrinkling of the skin. Clinical research indicates that regular use of a sunscreen (SPF 15) during the first 18 years of life may reduce the risk of developing the two most common forms of skin cancer by as much as 78%.
NONSTINGING: A non-PABA, fragrance-free formula that is designed not to sting sensitive skin. (Avoid contact with eyes since all sunscreens can cause irritation and stinging of the eye.)
HYPOALLERGENIC: PRESUN For Kids is hypoallergenic and, because the known sensitizers common to most sunscreens have been removed, is suitable for your child's sensitive skin.
WATERPROOF 29: PRESUN For Kids maintains its degree of protection (SPF 29) even after 80 minutes in the water.

Warnings: For external use only. Protect from freezing. *As with all sunscreens:* Apply to a small area; check after 24 hours. Discontinue use if irritation or rash appears. Avoid contact with eyes. In case of contact, flush eyes with water. Keep out of the reach of children. Use on children under six months of age only with the advice of a physician.

Administration and Dosage: For maximum protection, smooth evenly and liberally onto dry skin before sun exposure. Massage in gently. Reapplication to dry skin after prolonged swimming, excessive perspiration or towel drying is recommended for all-day protection.

How Supplied: 4 oz. (NDC 0072-9399-04) plastic bottle.

PRESUN® 8, 15 and 39 CREAMY SUNSCREENS

Active Ingredients: Octyl dimethyl PABA, oxybenzone. Also contains: Carbomer-940, cetyl alcohol, diazolidinyl urea, dimethicone, fragrance, methylchloroisothiazolinone and methylisothiazolinone, stearic acid, triethanolamine, water, and other ingredients.

Action and Uses: 8, 15 or 39 TIMES NATURAL PROTECTION: Used as directed. PRESUN Creamy Sunscreens provide 8, 15 or 39 times your natural *sunscreen* protection and may help reduce the chance of premature aging and wrinkling of the skin as well as skin cancer caused by overexposure to the sun.
UVA/UVB PROTECTION: PRESUN Sunscren is formulated to provide protection from the harmful effects of both UVA and UVB rays.
WATERPROOF PRESUN Creamy Sunscreen maintains its degree of protection even after 80 minutes in the water.

Warnings: For external use only. Protect from freezing. Do not use if sensitive to *p*-aminobenzoic acid (PABA) or related compounds. *As with all sunscreens:* Apply to a small area; check after 24 hours. Discontinue use if irritation or rash appears. Avoid contact with eyes. In case of contact, flush eyes with water. Keep out of the reach of children. Use on children under six months of age only with the advice of a physician.

Administration and Dosage: Smooth evenly onto dry skin before sun exposure. Massage in gently. Reapply to dry skin after prolonged swimming, excessive perspiration or towel drying. Repeated applications during prolonged sun exposure are recommended.

How Supplied: 8 Creamy: 4 oz. (NDC 0072-8506-04) plastic bottle. 15 Creamy: 4 oz. (NDC 0072-8906-04) plastic bottle. 39 Creamy: 4 oz. (NDC 0072-9600-04) plastic bottle.

PRESUN® 15 FACIAL SUNSCREEN
Ultra Sunscreen Protection

Active Ingredients: 8% Octyl dimethyl PABA, 3% oxybenzone. Also contains: Benzyl alcohol, carbomer 934, cetyl alcohol, dimethicone, glyceryl stearate, laureth-23, magnesium aluminum silicate, petrolatum, propylene glycol dioctanoate, quaternium-15, sodium hydroxide, steareth-2 and water.

Action and Uses: 15 TIMES NATURAL PROTECTION: Used as directed, PRESUN 15 Facial Sunscreen provides 15 times your natural *sunburn* protection and may help reduce the chance of premature aging and wrinkling of the skin as well as skin cancer caused by overexposure to the sun.
UVA/UVB PROTECTION: PRESUN 15 Facial Sunscreen is formulated to provide protection from the harmful effects of both UVA and UVB rays.
MOISTURIZES: PRESUN 15 Facial Sunscreen was developed especially for use on the face. The special moisturizers soften and smooth your skin while protecting it from the drying effects of the sun.
SUITABLE UNDER MAKE-UP: A non-greasy cream made especially for daily use under facial make-up and designed not to clog pores or cause acne or blemishes.

Administration and Dosage: Gently smooth evenly onto dry skin before sun exposure. Reapply to dry skin after swimming, excessive perspiration or towel drying. Repeated applications during prolonged sun exposure are recommended.

Warnings: For external use only. Do not use if sensitive to *p*-aminobenzoic acid (PABA) or related compounds. *As with all sunscreens:* Apply to a small area; check after 24 hours. Discontinue use if irritation or rash appears. Avoid contact with eyes. In case of contact, flush eyes with water. Keep out of reach of children. Use on children under six months of age only with the advice of a physician.

How Supplied: 2 oz. (NDC 0072-9200-02) plastic tube.

PRESUN® 23 and
PRESUN® FOR KIDS
Spray Mist Sunscreens

Active Ingredients: Octyl dimethyl PABA, octyl methoxycinnamate, oxybenzone, octyl salicylate. Also contains: C_{12-15} alcohols benzoate, cyclomethicone, PG dioctanoate, PVP hexadecene, copolymer, and 19% (w/w) SD alcohol 40.

Actions and Uses: 23 TIMES NATU-RAL PROTECTION: Used as directed, PRESUN 23 and PRESUN For Kids Spray Mist Sunscreens provide 23 times your natural sunburn protection and may help reduce the chance of premature aging and wrinkling of the skin, as well as skin cancer caused by overexposure to the sun.

UVA/UVB PROTECTION: PRESUN 23 and PRESUN For Kids Spray Mist Sunscreens are formulated to provide protection from the harmful effects of both UVA and UVB rays.

WATERPROOF 23: PRESUN 23 and PRESUN For Kids Spray Mist Sunscreens maintain their degree of protection (SPF 23) even after 80 minutes in the water.

OZONE SAFE: This revolutionary new spray bottle design is non-aerosol. This patented spray system contains no fluorocarbons, gases or propellants of any kind which may contribute to the depletion of the ozone. It sprays pure product, even upside down.

Administration and Dosage: For best results, hold bottle about ten inches away from body while spraying. Massage in gently. Reapplication to dry skin after prolonged swimming, excessive perspiration or towel drying is recommended for all-day protection.

Warnings: For external use only. Do not use if sensitive to *p*-aminobenzoic acid (PABA) or related compounds. Avoid flame. Do not expose to heat or store above 86°F. As with all sunscreens: Apply to a small area; check after 24 hours. Discontinue use if irritation or rash appears. Avoid spraying in the eyes. In case of contact, flush eyes with water. Keep out of reach of children. Use on children under six months of age only with the advice of a physician.

How Supplied: 23 Spray Mist Sunscreen: 3.5 oz. (NDC 0072-9720-35) plastic bottle with non-aerosol pump. For Kids Spray Mist Sunscreen: 3.5 oz. (NDC 0072-9799-35) plastic bottle with non-aerosol pump.

PRESUN® 15 and 29 SENSITIVE SKIN SUNSCREENS
PABA-FREE Sunscreen Protection

Active Ingredients: Octyl methoxycinnamate, oxybenzone, octyl salicylate. Also contains: Carbomer-940, cetyl alcohol, diazolidinyl urea, dimethicone, methylchloroisothiazolinone and methylisothiazolinone, stearic acid, triethanolamine, water, and other ingredients.

Actions and Uses:
15 or 29 TIMES NATURAL PROTECTION: Used as directed, PRESUN 15 or 29 Sensitive Skin Sunscreen provides 15 or 29 times your natural *sunburn* protection and may help reduce the chance of premature aging and wrinkling of the skin as well as skin cancer caused by overexposure to the sun.

UVA/UVB PROTECTION: PRESUN 15 or 29 Sensitive Skin Sunscreen is formulated to provide protection from the harmful effects of both UVA and UVB rays.

PABA-FREE FORMULA: A PABA- and fragrance-free formula that provides a very high degree of sunburn protection and, because the known sensitizers common to most sunscreens have been removed, is suitable for sensitive skin.

WATERPROOF: PRESUN Sensitive Skin Sunscreen maintains its degree of protection even after 80 minutes in the water.

Administration and Dosage: For maximum protection, smooth evenly and liberally onto dry skin before sun exposure. Massage in gently. Reapplication to dry skin after prolonged swimming, excessive perspiration or towel drying is recommended for all-day protection.

Warnings: For external use only. Protect from freezing. *As with all sunscreens:* Apply to a small area; check after 24 hours. Discontinue use if irritation or rash appears. Avoid contact with eyes. In case of contact, flush eyes with water. Keep out of the reach of children. Use on children under six months of age only with the advice of a physician.

How Supplied: 29 Sensitive Skin: 4 oz. (NDC 0072-9300-04; NSN 6505-01-267-1483) plastic bottle. 15 Sensitive Skin: 4 oz. (NDC 0072-9370-04) plastic bottle.
Shown in Product Identification Section, page 436

Whitehall Laboratories Inc.
Division of American Home Products Corporation
685 THIRD AVENUE
NEW YORK, NY 10017

ADVIL®
[*ad 'vil*]
Ibuprofen Tablets, USP
Ibuprofen Caplets
Pain Reliever/Fever Reducer

Warning: ASPIRIN-SENSITIVE PATIENTS. Do not take this product if you have had a severe allergic reaction to aspirin, e.g.—asthma, swelling, shock or hives, because even though this product contains no aspirin or salicylates, cross-reactions may occur in patients allergic to aspirin.

Active Ingredient: Each tablet contains Ibuprofen 200 mg.

Inactive Ingredients: Acacia, Acetylated Monoglycerides, Beeswax or Carnauba Wax, Calcium Sulfate, Colloidal Silicon Dioxide, Dimethicone, Iron Oxide, Lecithin, Pharmaceutical Glaze, Povidone, Sodium Benzoate, Sodium Carboxymethylcellulose, Starch, Stearic Acid, Sucrose, Titanium Dioxide.

Indications: For the temporary relief of minor aches and pains associated with the common cold, headache, toothache, muscular aches, backache, for the minor pain of arthritis, for the pain of menstrual cramps and for reduction of fever.

Dosage and Administration: Adults: Take one tablet every 4 to 6 hours while symptoms persist. If pain or fever does not respond to one tablet, two tablets may be used but do not exceed six tablets in 24 hours unless directed by a doctor. The smallest effective dose should be used. Take with food or milk if occasional and mild heartburn, upset stomach, or stomach pain occurs with use. Consult a doctor if these symptoms are more than mild or if they persist. Children: Do not give this product to children under 12 except under the advice and supervision of a doctor.

Warnings: Do not take for pain for more than 10 days or for fever for more than 3 days unless directed by a doctor. If pain or fever persists or gets worse, if new symptoms occur, or if the painful area is red or swollen, consult a doctor. These could be signs of serious illness. If you are under a doctor's care for any serious condition, consult a doctor before taking this product. As with aspirin and acetaminophen, if you have any condition which requires you to take prescription drugs or if you have had any problems or serious side effects from taking any nonprescription pain reliever, do not take this product without first discussing it with your doctor. If you experience any symptoms which are unusual or seem unrelated to the condition for which you took ibuprofen, consult a doctor before taking any more of it. Although ibuprofen is indicated for the same conditions as aspirin and acetaminophen, it should not be taken with them except under a doctor's direction. Do not combine this product with any other ibuprofen-containing product. As with any drug, if you are pregnant or nursing a baby, seek the advice of a health professional before using this product. IT IS ESPECIALLY IMPORTANT NOT TO USE IBUPROFEN DURING THE LAST 3 MONTHS OF PREGNANCY UNLESS SPECIFICALLY DIRECTED TO DO SO BY A DOCTOR BECAUSE IT MAY CAUSE PROBLEMS IN THE UNBORN CHILD OR COMPLICATIONS DURING DELIVERY. Keep this and all drugs out of the reach of children. In case of accidental overdose, seek professional assistance or contact a poison control center immediately.

Professional Labeling: Same as stated under Indications.

How Supplied: Coated tablets in bottles of 8, 24, 50, 100, 165 and 250. Coated caplets in bottles of 24, 50, 100 and 165.

Storage: Store at room temperature; avoid excessive heat 40°C (104°F).
Shown in Product Identification Section, page 436

Continued on next page

Whitehall—Cont.

ANACIN®
[an'a-sin]
Analgesic Coated Tablets
Analgesic Coated Caplets

Description: Each tablet or caplet contains: Aspirin 400 mg, Caffeine 32 mg. Anacin® has a special protective coating that makes each tablet or caplet easy to swallow.

Indications and Usage: Anacin provides fast relief from the pain of headaches, neuralgia, neuritis, sprains, muscular aches, sinus pressure... discomforts and fever of colds... pain caused by tooth extraction and toothache... menstrual discomfort. Anacin also temporarily relieves the minor aches and pains of arthritis and rheumatism.

Warnings: Children and teenagers should not use this medicine for chicken pox or flu symptoms before a doctor is consulted about Reye syndrome, a rare but serious illness reported to be associated with aspirin. As with any drug, if you are pregnant or nursing a baby, seek the advice of a health professional before using this product. Keep this and all medicines out of children's reach. In case of accidental overdose, contact a physician immediately.

Precautions: If pain persists for more than 10 days, or redness is present, or in arthritic or rheumatic conditions affecting children under 12 years of age, consult a physician immediately.

Dosage and Administration: Two tablets or caplets with water every 4 hours, as needed. Do not exceed 10 tablets or 10 caplets daily. For children 6–12, administer half the adult dosage.

Professional Labeling: Same as those outlined under Indications.

Inactive Ingredients: Tablets contain Hydroxypropyl Methylcellulose, Microcrystalline Cellulose, Polyethylene Glycol, Starch, Surfactant.
Caplets contain Hydroxypropyl Methylcellulose, Iron Oxide, Microcrystalline Cellulose, Polyethylene Glycol, Starch, Surfactant.

How Supplied: Tablets: In tins of 12's and bottles of 30's, 50's, 100's, 200's and 300's. Caplets: In bottles of 30's, 50's and 100's. Professional Samples: Available upon request. Write Whitehall Laboratories, New York, New York 10017.
Shown in Product Identification Section, page 436

MAXIMUM STRENGTH ANACIN®
[an'a-sin]
Analgesic Coated Tablets

Description: Each tablet contains: Aspirin 500 mg, Caffeine 32 mg. Maximum Strength Anacin has a special protective coating that makes each tablet easy to swallow.

Indications and Actions: See Anacin Tablets.

Warnings: See Anacin Tablets.

Precautions: See Anacin Tablets.

Dosage and Administration: Adults: 2 Tablets with water 3 or 4 times a day. Do not exceed 8 tablets in any 24-hour period. Not recommended for children under 12 years of age.

Inactive Ingredients: Hydroxypropyl Methylcellulose, Microcrystalline Cellulose, Polyethylene Glycol, Starch, Surfactant.

How Supplied: Tablets: Tins of 12's and bottles of 20's, 40's, 75's, and 150's.

Children's ANACIN-3®
[an'a-sin thre]
Acetaminophen
Chewable Tablets, Alcohol-Free Liquid and Drops

Description: Chewable Tablets: Each Children's ANACIN-3 Chewable Tablet is cherry flavored and contains 80 mg acetaminophen.
Liquid: Children's ANACIN-3 Liquid is stable, cherry flavored, red in color. It contains no alcohol or saccharin. Each 5 mL contains 160 mg acetaminophen.
Infants' Drops: Infants' Anacin-3 Drops are stable, fruit flavored, red in color and contain no alcohol. Each 0.8 mL (one calibrated dropperful) contains 80 mg acetaminophen.

Actions: Children's Anacin-3 Chewable Tablets, Liquid and Infants' Drops are safe and effective 100% aspirin-free products designed for treatment of infants and children with conditions requiring reduction of fever or relief of pain.

Indications: Children's Anacin-3 is used for the treatment of fever and pain which may accompany conditions such as mild upper respiratory infections (tonsillitis, common cold, "grippe"), headache, myalgia, post-immunization reactions, post-tonsillectomy discomfort and gastroenteritis. Anacin-3 acetaminophen is useful as an analgesic and antipyretic in infections such as bronchitis, pharyngitis, tracheobronchitis, sinusitis, pneumonia, otitis media and cervical adenitis of viral origin or of bacterial origin when used in conjunction with an antibiotic.

Warnings: Keep this and all medicines out of children's reach. In case of accidental overdose contact a physician immediately.

Precautions: If fever persists for more than 3 days or recurs, or if pain continues for more than 5 days, consult your physician immediately.
If a rare sensitivity reaction occurs, the drug should be stopped. It is usually well tolerated by aspirin-sensitive patients.
Phenylketonurics: tablets contain phenylalanine 3.1 mg per tablet.

Dosage and Administration: All dosages may be repeated every 4 hours. Do not exceed 5 dosages in any 24-hour period.

Age	Wt (lb)	Tablet	Liquid
4–11 mo	12–17	—	½ teaspoon
1–2 yr	18–23	1–1½	¾ "
2–3 "	24–35	2	1 "
4–5 "	36–47	3	1½ "
6–8 "	48–59	4	2 "
9–10 "	60–71	5	2½ "
11–12 "	72–95	6	3 "

Infants' Drops: 0–3 months, 6 to 11 lbs: one-half dropperful. 4–11 months, 12 to 17 lbs: one dropperful. 12–23 months, 18 to 23 lbs: one and one-half droppersful. 2–3 years, 24 to 35 lbs: 2 droppersful. 4–5 years, 36 to 47 lbs: 3 droppersful.

Overdosage: Acetaminophen in massive overdosage may cause hepatic toxicity in some patients. In all cases of suspected overdose, immediately call your regional poison center or the Rocky Mountain Poison Center for assistance in diagnosis and for directions in the use of N-acetylcysteine as an antidote. The occurrence of acetaminophen overdose toxicity is uncommon in the pediatric age group. Even with large overdoses, children appear to be less vulnerable than adults to developing hepatotoxicity. This may be due to age-related differences that have been demonstrated in the metabolism of acetaminophen. Despite these differences, the measures outlined below should be immediately initiated in any child suspected of having ingested an overdose of acetaminophen.
Early symptoms following a potentially hepatotoxic overdose may include: nausea, vomiting, diaphoresis and general malaise. Clinical and laboratory evidence of hepatic toxicity may not be apparent until 48 to 72 hours post-ingestion. The stomach should be emptied promptly by lavage or by induction of emesis with syrup of ipecac. If an acute dose of 150 mg/kg body weight or greater was ingested, or if the dose cannot be accurately determined, a serum acetaminophen assay should be obtained as early as possible, but no sooner than four hours post-ingestion. Liver function studies should be obtained initially and repeated at 24-hour intervals. The antidote N-acetylcysteine should be administered as early as possible and within 16 hours of the overdose ingestion for optimal results. Following recovery there are no residual, structural or functional hepatic abnormalities.

Inactive Ingredients: Chewable Tablets: Aspartame, Cetyl Alcohol, Colloidal Silicon Dioxide, Dibutyl Sebacate, Ethyl Cellulose, FD&C Red No. 40 Lake, Flavor, Hydrogenated Vegetable Oil, Magnesium Stearate, Mannitol, Microcrystalline Cellulose, Simethicone, Sucrose and Surfactant.
Liquid: Citric Acid, D&C Red No. 33, Disodium Edetate, FD&C Red No. 40, Flavor, Glycerin, Methylparaben, Polyethylene Glycol, Propylene Glycol, Sorbitol, Sodium Benzoate, Sucrose and Water.
Infants' Drops: FD&C Red No. 40, FD&C Yellow No. 6, Flavors, Glycerin, Polyethylene Glycol, Propylene Glycol, Saccharin, Sodium Benzoate, Sorbitol and Water.

How Supplied: Chewable Tablets (colored pink, scored, imprinted "Children A–3")—bottles of 30. Liquid (colored red)—bottles of 2 and 4 fl. oz. Drops (colored red)—bottles of ½ oz. (15 mL) with calibrated plastic dropper.

All packages listed above have child-resistant safety caps and tamper-resistant packaging.

Maximum Strength
ANACIN-3®
[an 'a-sin thre]
Film Coated Acetaminophen Tablets
Film Coated Acetaminophen Caplets

Regular Strength
ANACIN-3®
Film Coated Acetaminophen Tablets

Description: Maximum Strength Tablets and Caplets: Each film coated tablet and caplet contains acetaminophen, 500 mg.
Regular Strength: Each film coated tablet contains acetaminophen, 325 mg.

Indications and Actions: Anacin-3 is a safe and effective 100% aspirin-free analgesic and antipyretic that acts fast to provide temporary relief from pain of headache, colds or "flu," sinusitis, muscle aches, bursitis, sprains, overexertion, backache and menstrual discomfort. Also for temporary relief of minor arthritis pain, toothaches and to reduce fever. Anacin-3 is particularly well suited in the presence of aspirin sensitivity, upper gastrointestinal disorders and anticoagulant therapy. It is usually well tolerated by aspirin-sensitive patients.

Warnings: Keep this and all medicines out of children's reach. In case of accidental overdose, contact a physician immediately. As with any drug, if you are pregnant or nursing a baby, seek the advice of a health professional before using this product.

Precautions: If pain persists for more than 10 days or redness is present or in arthritic or rheumatic conditions affecting children under 12, consult a physician immediately.

Dosage and Administration: Maximum Strength—Adults: Two tablets or caplets 3 or 4 times a day. Do not exceed 8 tablets or caplets in any 24-hour period. Regular Strength—Adults: 2 or 3 tablets every 4 hours not to exceed 12 tablets in any 24-hour period. Children (6–12): ½ to 1 tablet 3 to 4 times daily. Consult a physician for use by children under 6 or for use longer than 10 days.

Overdosage: Acetaminophen in massive overdosage may cause hepatic toxicity in some patients. In all cases of suspected overdose, immediately call your regional poison control center or the Rocky Mountain Poison Control Center for assistance in diagnosis and for directions in the use of N-acetylcysteine as an antidote. In adults, hepatic toxicity has rarely been reported with acute overdoses of less than 10 grams and fatalities with less than 15 grams. Importantly, young children seem to be more resistant than adults to the hepatotoxic effect of an acetaminophen overdose. Despite this, the measures outined below should be initiated in any adult or child suspected of having ingested an acetaminophen overdose.

Early symptoms following a potentially hepatoxic overdose may include: nausea, vomiting, diaphoresis and general malaise. Clinical and laboratory evidence of hepatic toxicity may not be apparent until 48 to 72 hours post-ingestion. The stomach should be emptied promptly by lavage or by induction of emesis with syrup of ipecac. Patients' estimates of the quantity of a drug ingested are notoriously unreliable. Therefore, if an acetaminophen overdose is suspected, a serum acetaminophen assay should be obtained as early as possible, but no sooner than four hours following ingestion. Liver function studies should be obtained initially and at 24-hour intervals. The antidote, N-acetylcysteine, should be administered as early as possible and within 16 hours of the overdose ingestion for optimal results. Following recovery, there is no residual, structural or functional hepatic abnormalities.

Professional Labeling: Same as those outlined under Indications.

Inactive Ingredients: Maximum and Regular Strength Tablets:
Calcium Stearate, Croscarmellose Sodium, FD&C Blue No. 1 Lake, Hydroxypropyl Methylcellulose, Microcrystalline Cellulose, Polyethylene Glycol, Povidone, Propylene Gylcol, Starch, Stearic Acid and Titanium Dioxide.
Maximum Strength Caplets:
Croscarmellose Sodium, D&C Red No. 7 Lake, FD&C Blue No. 1 Lake, Hydroxypropyl Methylcellulose, Polyethylene Glycol, Povidone, Propylene Glycol, Starch, Stearic Acid and Titanium Dioxide.

How Supplied: Maximum Strength Film Coated—Tablets (colored white, imprinted "A-3" and "500")—tins of 12 and bottles of 30, 60, and 100: Caplets (colored white, imprinted "Anacin-3")—bottles of 30's, 60's and 100's. Regular Strength Film Coated—Tablets (colored white, scored, imprinted "A-3") in bottles of 24, 50, and 100.
Shown in Product Identification Section, page 437

ANBESOL® Liquid and Gel
[an 'ba-sol "]
Antiseptic-Anesthetic

Description: Anbesol is an antiseptic-anesthetic which is available in a Maximum Strength and Regular Strength gel and liquid. Baby Anbesol, available in gel, is an anesthetic only and is alcohol-free.
The Maximum Strength formulations contain Benzocaine 20% and Alcohol 60%.
The Regular Strength formulations contain Benzocaine 6.3%, Alcohol 70%, and Phenol 0.5%.
The Baby Anbesol Gel contains Benzocaine 7.5%.

Indications: Maximum Strength and Regular Strength Anbesol are indicated for the fast temporary relief of pain due to toothache, braces, denture and orthodontic irritation, sore gums, cold and canker sores and fever blisters. Regular Strength Anbesol and Baby Anbesol Gel are also indicated for the fast temporary relief of teething pain.

Actions: Temporarily deadens sensations of nerve endings to provide relief of pain and discomfort; reduces oral bacterial flora temporarily as an aid in oral hygiene (Regular and Maximum Stengths only).

Warnings: Flammable. Keep away from fire or flame. Avoid smoking during application and until product has dried. Do not use near eyes. For persistent or excessive teething pain, consult a physician or dentist. Localized allergic reactions may occur after prolonged or repeated use. KEEP THIS AND ALL MEDICINES OUT OF THE REACH OF CHILDREN.

Precautions: Not for prolonged use. If the condition persists or irritation develops, discontinue use and consult your physician or dentist. NOT FOR USE UNDER DENTURES OR OTHER DENTAL WORK.

Dosage and Administration: Apply topically to the affected area on or around the lips, or within the mouth.

For Denture Irritation: Apply thin layer to affected area and do not reinsert dental work until irritation/pain is relieved. Rinse mouth before reinserting dentures. If irritation/pain persists, contact your physician.

Professional Labeling: Same as outlined under Indications.

Inactive Ingredients:
Maximum Strength Gel: Carbomer 934P, D&C Yellow #10, FD&C Red #40, Flavor, Polyethylene Glycol, Saccharin.
Maximum Strength Liquid: D&C Yellow #10, FD&C Red #40, Flavor, Polyethylene Glycol, Saccharin.
Regular Liquid: Camphor, Glycerin, Menthol, Potassium Iodide, Povidone Iodine.
Regular Gel: Carbomer 934P, D&C Red #33 and Yellow #10, FD&C Blue #1 and Yellow #6, Flavor, Glycerin.
Baby Gel: Carbomer 934, D& C Red #33, Disodium Edetate, Flavor, Glycerin, Polyethylene Glycol, Saccharin, Water.

How Supplied: Maximum Strength Gel in .25 oz (7.2 gram) tube, Maximum Strength Liquid in .31 oz (9 mL) bottle. Regular Liquid in two sizes— .31 fl. oz. (9 mL) and .74 fl. oz. (22 mL) bottles. Gel and Baby Gel in .25 oz. (7.2 gram) tubes.
Shown in Product Identification Section, page 437

Continued on next page

Whitehall—Cont.

ARTHRITIS PAIN FORMULA™
[är′thrīt-is′ pān′ for-mye-la]
By the Makers of Anacin® Analgesic Tablets and Caplets

Description: Each caplet contains 500 mg microfined aspirin and two buffers, 27 mg Aluminum Hydroxide and 100 mg Magnesium Hydroxide.
Arthritis Pain Formula is a buffered analgesic and antipyretic with microfined aspirin, which means the aspirin particles are so fine they dissolve more readily. The buffering agents help provide protection against stomach upset that could be associated with large anti-arthritic doses of aspirin.

Indications and Actions: Arthritis Pain Formula provides hours of relief from minor aches and pain of arthritis and rheumatism and low back pain. Also relieves the pain of headache, neuralgia, neuritis, sprains, muscular aches, discomforts and fever of colds, pain caused by tooth extraction and toothache, and menstrual discomfort.

Warnings: Children and teenagers should not use this medicine for chicken pox or flu symptoms before a doctor is consulted about Reye syndrome, a rare but serious illness reported to be associated with aspirin. Keep this and all medications out of children's reach. In case of accidental overdose, contact a physician immediately. As with any drug, if you are pregnant or nursing a baby, seek the advice of a health professional before using this product.

Precautions: If pain persists for more than 10 days, or redness is present, or in arthritic or rheumatic conditions affecting children under 12, consult a physician immediately.

Dosage and Administration: Adult Dosage: 2 caplets, 3 or 4 times a day. Do not exceed 8 caplets in any 24-hour period. For children under 12, consult a physician.

Professional Labeling: Same as stated under "Indications."

Inactive Ingredients: Hydrogenated Vegetable Oil, Microcrystalline Cellulose, Starch, Surfactant.

How Supplied: In plastic bottles of 40 (non-child-resistant size), 100 and 175 caplets.

Shown in Product Identification Section, page 437

BEMINAL® 500
[bē′min-awl]
Vitamin B Complex with Vitamin C

Each tablet contains: % US RDA*
Thiamine mononitrate
(vit. B₁)............ 25.0 mg 1717%
Riboflavin
(vit. B₂)............ 12.5 mg 735%
Niacinamide
(vit. B₃) as
niacinamide
ascorbate......... 100.0 mg 500%
Pyridoxine hydrochloride
(vit. B₆)............ 10.0 mg 500%
Calcium
pantothenate.. 20.0 mg 92%
Ascorbic acid
(vit. C) as
ascorbic acid
and niacinamide
ascorbate......... 500.0 mg 833%
Cyanocobalamin
(vit. B₁₂).......... 5.0 mcg....... 83%

Does not contain saccharin or other sweeteners.

---

*US Recommended Daily Allowance

Inactive Ingredients: Calcium Carboxymethylcellulose, ethylcellulose, FD&C Blue #2 Lake, FD&C Red #40 Lake, FD&C Yellow #6 Lake, Flavor, Iron Oxide, Lactose, Magnesium Stearate, Mannitol, Microcrystalline Cellulose, Pharmaceutical Glaze, Polyethylene Glycol, Starch, Talc, Titanium Dioxide.

Indication: Dietary Supplement

Uses: BEMINAL 500 can help replenish the vitamins depleted by the stress of sickness, infections, and surgery. BEMINAL 500 may also be used when the demand on the body's store of vitamins may be increased by dieting, the use of alcohol, jogging, and other strenuous physical exercise.

Recommended Intake: 12-year-olds and older, one tablet daily.

How Supplied: In bottles of 100 tablets.

CoADVIL™
Ibuprofen/Pseudoephedrine Caplets*
Pain Reliever/Fever Reducer/Nasal Decongestant

WARNING: ASPIRIN-SENSITIVE PATIENTS. Do not take this product if you have had a severe allergic reaction to aspirin, eg—asthma, swelling, shock or hives—because even though this product contains no aspirin or salicylates, cross-reactions may occur in patients allergic to aspirin.

Indications: For temporary relief of symptoms associated with the common cold, sinusitis or flu, including nasal congestion, headache, fever, body aches, and pains.

Directions: *Adults:* Take 1 caplet every 4 to 6 hours while symptoms persist. If symptoms do not respond to 1 caplet, 2

*Oval-Shaped tablets

caplets may be used, but do not exceed 6 caplets in 24 hours unless directed by a doctor. The smallest effective dose should be used.
Take with food or milk if occasional and mild heartburn, upset stomach, or stomach pain occurs with use. Consult a doctor if these symptoms are more than mild or if they persist. *Children:* Do not give this product to children under 12 years of age except under the advice and supervision of a doctor.

Warnings: Do not take for colds for more than 7 days or for fever for more than 3 days unless directed by a doctor. If the cold or fever persists or gets worse, or if new symptoms occur, consult a doctor. These could be signs of serious illness. As with aspirin and acetaminophen, if you have any condition which requires you to take prescription drugs or if you have had any problems or serious side effects from taking any nonprescription pain reliever, do not take this product without first discussing it with your doctor. IF YOU EXPERIENCE ANY SYMPTOMS WHICH ARE UNUSUAL OR SEEM UNRELATED TO THE CONDITION FOR WHICH YOU TOOK THIS PRODUCT, CONSULT A DOCTOR BEFORE TAKING ANY MORE OF IT. If you are under a doctor's care for any serious condition, consult a doctor before taking this product.
Do not exceed recommended dosage because at higher doses nervousness, dizziness or sleeplessness may occur. Do not take this product if you have high blood pressure, heart disease, diabetes, thyroid disease or difficulty in urination due to enlargement of the prostate gland, except under the advice and supervision of a doctor.

Drug Interaction Precaution: Do not take this product if you are presently taking a prescription drug for high blood pressure or depression without first consulting your doctor. Do not combine this product with other nonprescription pain relievers. Do not combine this product with any other ibuprofen-containing product. As with any drug, if you are pregnant or nursing a baby, seek the advice of a health professional before using this product.
IT IS ESPECIALLY IMPORTANT NOT TO USE THIS PRODUCT DURING THE LAST 3 MONTHS OF PREGNANCY UNLESS SPECIFICALLY DIRECTED TO DO SO BY A DOCTOR BECAUSE IT MAY CAUSE PROBLEMS IN THE UNBORN CHILD OR COMPLICATIONS DURING DELIVERY. Keep this and all drugs out of the reach of children. In case of accidental overdose, seek professional assistance or contact a poison control center immediately. Store at room temperature; avoid excessive heat (40°C, 104°F).

Active Ingredients: Each caplet contains Ibuprofen 200 mg and Pseudoephedrine HCl 30 mg.

Inactive Ingredients: Carnauba or Equivalent Wax, Croscarmellose Sodium, Iron Oxides, Methylparaben, Microcrystalline Cellulose, Propylparaben,

Silicon Dioxide, Sodium Benzoate, Sodium Lauryl Sulfate, Starch, Stearic Acid, Sucrose, Titanium Dioxide.

How Supplied: CoAdvil is an oval-shaped tan-colored caplet supplied in consumer blister packs of 20 and bottles of 48 and 100.

Shown in Product Identification Section, page 436

COMPOUND W®
['käm-pound W]
Solution and Gel

Description: Compound W is a Salicylic Acid (17% w/w) preparation available as a solution or gel.

Indication: Compound W is indicated for the removal of common warts.

Actions: Warts are common benign skin lesions which appear mainly on the back of hands and on fingers, but can also appear on other parts of the body. The common wart exhibits a rough, raised cauliflower-like surface. They are caused by an infectious virus which stimulates mitosis in the basal cell layer of the skin, resulting in the production of elevated epithelial growths. The keratolytic action of salicylic acid in a flexible collodion vehicle causes the cornified epithelium to swell, soften, macerate and then desquamate.

Warnings: Highly Flammable. Keep away from fire or flame. Avoid smoking during application and until product has dried. Do not use this product if you are a diabetic or have poor blood circulation as serious complications may result. Do not use on moles, birthmarks, warts with hair growing from them, genital warts, or warts on the face or mucous membranes (inside mouth, nose, anus, genitals, or on lips). If pain should develop or if infection is present, consult your physician. Do not use near eyes. If product accidentally comes in contact with eyes flush with water to remove film and continue to flush with water for 15 minutes. Do not inhale. Keep bottle tightly capped. For external use only. In case of accidental ingestion, contact a physician or a Poison Control Center immediately. Keep this and all medicines out of the reach of children.

Precautions: If redness or irritation occurs, discontinue product for 2 days and then reapply. Should stinging or irritation recur, discontinue use. Covering the treated wart with a bandage will increase effectiveness but may also increase the chance of irritation. If a bandage is used, first allow the solution or gel to dry thoroughly.

Dosage and Administration: Use on common warts once daily. 1. Soak affected area in hot water for 5 minutes. If any tissue has loosened, remove by rubbing with a washcloth or soft brush. Do not rub hard enough to cause bleeding. Dry thoroughly. 2. Using the plastic rod provided with the solution or by squeezing the tube to apply, completely cover the wart with solution or gel. To avoid irritating the skin surrounding the wart, confine the solution or gel to the wart only. To help achieve this, circle the wart with a ring of petroleum jelly. Allow the solution or gel to dry, then reapply. The area covered with the medicine will appear white. 3. Follow this procedure daily for the next 6 to 7 days. Most warts should clear within this time period. However, if the wart remains, continue the treatment for up to 12 weeks. If the wart shows no improvement, see your physician.

Professional Labeling: Same as those outlined under Indication.

Inactive Ingredients: Solution: Acetone Collodion, Alcohol 1.83% w/w, Camphor, Castor Oil, Ether 63.5%, Menthol, Polysorbate 80. Gel: Alcohol 67.5% by vol., Camphor, Castor Oil, Collodion, Colloidal Silicon Dioxide, Hydroxypropyl Cellulose, Hypophosphorous Acid, Polysorbate 80.

How Supplied: Compound W is available in .31 fluid oz. clear bottles with plastic applicators. Compound W Gel is available in .25 oz. tubes. Store at room temperature.

DENOREX®
[děn 'ō-reks]
Medicated Shampoo
DENOREX®
Mountain Fresh Herbal Scent
Medicated Shampoo
DENOREX®
Medicated Shampoo and Conditioner
DENOREX®
Extra Strength Medicated Shampoo
DENOREX®
Extra Strength Medicated Shampoo with Conditioners

Description: The Shampoo (Regular and Mountain Fresh Herbal) and the Shampoo with Conditioner contain Coal Tar Solution 9.0%, Menthol 1.5%. The Extra Strength Shampoo and the Extra Strength Shampoo with Conditioners contain Coal Tar Solution 12.5% and Menthol 1.5%.

Indications: Relieves scaling, itching, flaking of dandruff, seborrhea and psoriasis. Regular use promotes cleaner, healthier hair and scalp.

Actions: Denorex Shampoo is an antiseborrheic and antipruritic which loosens and softens scales and crusts. Coal tar helps correct abnormalities of keratinization by decreasing epidermal proliferation and dermal infiltration. Denorex also contains the antipruritic agent, menthol.

Warnings: For external use only. Discontinue treatment if irritation develops. Avoid contact with eyes. Keep this and all medicines out of children's reach.

Directions: For best results use regularly, but at least three times per week. For severe scalp problems use daily. Wet hair thoroughly and briskly massage until you obtain a rich lather. Rinse thoroughly and repeat. Your scalp may tingle slightly during treatment.

Professional Labeling: Same as stated under Indications.

Inactive Ingredients:
Shampoo: Also contains Chloroxylenol, Lauramide DEA, Stearic Acid, TEA-Lauryl Sulfate, Water (plus Hydroxypropyl Methylcellulose in the Mountain Fresh Herbal scent formula), Alcohol 7.5%.
Shampoo and Conditioner: Chloroxylenol, Citric Acid, Fragrance, Hydroxypropyl Methylcellulose, Lauramide DEA, PEG-27 Lanolin, Polyquaternium-11, TEA-Lauryl Sulfate, Water, Alcohol 7.5%.
Extra Strength: Chloroxylenol, FD&C Red #40, Fragrance, Glycol Distearate, Lauramide DEA, Methylcellulose, TEA-Lauryl Sulfate, Water, Alcohol 10.4%.
Extra Strength With Conditioners: Chloroxylenol, Citric Acid, Cocodimonium Hydrolyzed Protein, Dimethicone, FD&C Red #40, Fragrance, Glycol Distearate, Lauramide DEA, Methylcellulose, PEG-27 Lanolin, Polyquaternium-6, TEA-Lauryl Sulfate, Water, Alcohol 10.4%.

How Supplied:
Lotion: 4 oz., 8 oz. and 12 oz. bottles in Regular Scent, Mountain Fresh Herbal Scent, Shampoo and Conditioner, Extra Strength Shampoo, and Extra Strength Shampoo With Conditioners.

Shown in Product Identification Section, page 437

DERMOPLAST®
[der 'mō-plăst]
Anesthetic Pain Relief Lotion

Description: Dermoplast Lotion contains Benzocaine 8% and Menthol 0.5%.

Actions: Dermoplast is a topical anesthetic and antipruritic.

Indications: Dermoplast is indicated for the fast, temporary relief of skin pain and itching due to sunburn, insect bites, minor cuts, abrasions, minor burns, and minor skin irritations.

Warnings: FOR EXTERNAL USE ONLY.
In case of accidental ingestion, seek professional assistance or contact a Poison Control Center. Avoid contact with eyes. Not for prolonged use. If the condition for which this preparation is used persists or if rash or irritation develops, discontinue use and consult physician. Keep this and all drugs out of the reach of children.

Directions: Apply freely over sunburned or irritated skin. Repeat three or four times daily, as needed.

Inactive Ingredients: Aloe Vera Gel, Carbomer 934P, Ceteth-16, Glycerin, Glyceryl Stearate, Laneth-16, Methylparaben, Oleth-16, Propylparaben, Simethicone, Steareth-16, Triethanolamine, Water.

How Supplied: DERMOPLAST Anesthetic Pain Relief Lotion, in Net Wt 3 fl. oz.

Shown in Product Identification Section, page 437

Continued on next page

Whitehall—Cont.

DERMOPLAST®
[der 'mō-plăst]
Anesthetic Pain Relief Spray

Description: DERMOPLAST is an aerosol containing Benzocaine 20% and Menthol 0.5%.

Indications: DERMOPLAST is indicated for the fast, temporary relief of skin pain and itching due to sunburn, minor cuts, insect bites, abrasions, minor burns, and minor skin irritations. May be applied without touching sensitive affected areas. Widely used in hospitals for pain and itch of episiotomy, pruritus vulvae, and postpartum hemorrhoids.

Warnings: FOR EXTERNAL USE ONLY. Avoid spraying in eyes. Contents under pressure. Do not puncture or incinerate. Do not use near open flame. Use only as directed. Intentional misuse by deliberately concentrating and inhaling the contents can be harmful or fatal. Do not take orally. Not for prolonged use. If the condition for which this preparation is used persists, or if a rash or irritation develops, discontinue use and consult physician.

Directions for Use: Hold can in a comfortable position 6–12 inches away from affected area. Point spray nozzle and press button. To apply to face, spray in palm of hand. May be administered three or four times daily, or as directed by physician.

Inactive Ingredients: Acetylated Lanolin Alcohol, *Aloe vera* Oil, Butane, Cetyl Acetate, Hydrofluorocarbon, Methylparaben, PEG-8 Laurate, Polysorbate 85.

How Supplied: DERMOPLAST Anesthetic Pain Relief Spray, in Net Wt 2¾ oz (78 g). Do not expose to heat or temperatures above 120° F.
Shown in Product Identification Section, page 437

DRISTAN®
[drĭs 'tăn]
Decongestant/Antihistamine/Analgesic
Coated Tablets and Coated Caplets

Description: Each Dristan Coated Tablet or Coated Caplet contains: Phenylephrine HCl 5 mg, Chlorpheniramine Maleate 2 mg, Acetaminophen 325 mg.

Actions: Phenylephrine HCl is an oral nasal decongestant (sympathomimetic amine) effective as a vasoconstrictor to help reduce nasal/sinus congestion. Phenylephrine produces little or no central nervous system stimulation.
Chlorpheniramine Maleate is an antihistamine effective in the control of rhinorrhea, sneezing and lacrimation associated with elevated histamine levels in disorders of the respiratory tract.
Acetaminophen is both an analgesic and an antipyretic. Therapeutic doses of acetaminophen will effectively reduce an elevated body temperature. Also, acetaminophen is effective in reducing the discomfort of pain associated with headache.

Indications: Dristan is indicated for effective multi-symptom relief of colds/flu, sinusitis, hay fever, or other upper respiratory allergies: nasal congestion, sneezing, runny nose, fever, headache and minor aches and pains.

Warnings: Avoid alcoholic beverages and driving a motor vehicle or operating heavy machinery while taking this product. May cause drowsiness or excitability, especially in children. Persons with asthma, glaucoma, high blood pressure, diabetes, heart or thyroid disease, difficulty in urination due to enlarged prostate gland, or taking an antidepressant drug, should use only as directed by a physician. Do not exceed recommended dosage because at higher doses nervousness, dizziness, or sleeplessness may occur. If symptoms do not improve within 7 days or are accompanied by high fever, discontinue use and see a physician. As with any drug, if you are pregnant or nursing a baby, seek the advice of a health professional before using this product.
Do not give to children under 6. Keep this and all medication out of children's reach. In case of accidental overdose contact a physician immediately.

Professional Labeling: Same as those outlined under Indications.

Dosage and Administration: Adults: Two tablets or caplets every four hours, not to exceed 12 tablets or caplets in 24 hours. Children 6–12: One tablet or caplet every four hours, not to exceed six tablets or caplets in 24 hours.

Inactive Ingredients: Tablets and Caplets—Calcium Stearate, Croscarmellose Sodium, D&C Yellow #10 Lake, FD&C Yellow #6 Lake, Hydroxypropyl Methylcellulose, Microcrystalline Cellulose, Polyethylene Glycol, Povidone, Starch, Stearic Acid.

How Supplied: Yellow/White coated tablets in tins of 12 and blister packages of 24 and bottles of 48, and 100. Yellow/White coated caplets in blister packages of 20 and bottles of 40.
Shown in Product Identification Section, page 437

DRISTAN®
[drĭs 'tăn]
Nasal Spray
Menthol Nasal Spray

Description: Dristan Nasal Spray contains Phenylephrine HCl 0.5%, Pheniramine Maleate 0.2%.

Actions: Phenylephrine HCl is a sympathomimetic agent that constricts the smaller arterioles of the nasal passages producing a gentle and predictable decongesting effect. Pheniramine Maleate is an antihistamine that controls rhinorrhea, sneezing, and lacrimation associated with elevated histamine levels in disorders of the respiratory tract.

Indications: Dristan Nasal Spray provides prompt temporary relief of nasal congestion due to colds, sinusitis, hay fever or other upper respiratory allergies.

Warnings: Do not exceed recommended dosage because symptoms may occur such as burning, stinging, sneezing, or increase of nasal discharge. Do not use this product for more than 3 days. If symptoms persist, consult a physician. The use of the dispenser by more than one person may spread infection. For adult use only. Do not give this product to children under 12 years except under the advice and supervision of a physician. Keep these and all medicines out of children's reach. In case of accidental ingestion, seek professional assistance or contact a Poison Control Center immediately.

Dosage and Administration: Squeeze Bottle—With head upright, insert nozzle in nostril. Spray quickly, firmly and sniff deeply.
Metered Dose Pump—Prime the metered dose pump by depressing pump firmly several times. With head upright, insert nozzle in nostril. Depress pump 2 or 3 times, all the way down, with a firm, even stroke and sniff deeply.
Adults: Spray 2 or 3 times into each nostril. Repeat every 4 hours as needed. Children under 12 years: As directed by a physician.

Professional Labeling: Same as those outlined under Indications.

Inactive Ingredients: Dristan Nasal Spray: Benzalkonium Chloride 1:5000 in buffered isotonic aqueous solution, Eucalyptol, Hydroxypropyl Methylcellulose, Menthol, Sodium Chloride, Sodium Phosphate, Thimerosal 0.002%, Water, and Alcohol 0.4%.
Dristan Menthol Nasal Spray: Benzalkonium Chloride 1:5000 in buffered isotonic aqueous solution, Camphor, Eucalyptol, Hydroxypropyl Methylcellulose, Menthol, Methyl Salicylate, Polysorbate 80, Sodium Chloride, Sodium Phosphate, Thimerosal 0.002%, and Water.

How Supplied: Dristan Nasal Spray: 15 mL and 30 mL plastic squeeze bottles, and 15 mL metered dose pumps.
Dristan Menthol Nasal Spray: 15 mL and 30 mL plastic squeeze bottles.
Shown in Product Identification Section, page 437

DRISTAN®
[drĭs 'tăn]
Long Lasting Nasal Spray
Long Lasting Menthol Nasal Spray

Description: Dristan Long Lasting Nasal Spray contains Oxymetazoline HCl 0.05%.

Actions: The sympathomimetic action of Dristan Long Lasting Nasal Spray and Dristan Long Lasting Menthol Nasal Spray constricts the smaller arterioles of the nasal passages, producing a prolonged, up to 12 hours, gentle and predictable decongesting effect.

Indications: Dristan Long Lasting Nasal Spray and Dristan Long Lasting Menthol Nasal Spray provide prompt temporary relief of nasal congestion due to colds, sinusitis, hay fever, or other upper respiratory allergies for up to 12 hours.

Warnings: Do not exceed recommended dosage because symptoms may occur such as burning, stinging, sneezing, or increase of nasal discharge. Do not use this product for more than 3 days. If symptoms persist, consult a physician. The use of the dispenser by more than one person may spread infection. Keep these and all medicines out of the reach of children. In case of accidental ingestion, seek professional assistance or contact a Poison Control Center immediately.

Dosage and Administration: Squeeze Bottle—With head upright, insert nozzle in nostril. Spray quickly, firmly and sniff deeply.
Metered Dose Pump—Prime the metered dose pump by depressing pump firmly several times. With head upright, insert nozzle in nostril. Depress pump 2 or 3 times, all the way down, with a firm even stroke and sniff deeply.
Adults and children 6 years of age and over, spray 2 or 3 times into each nostril. Repeat twice daily—morning and evening. Not recommended for children under six.

Professional Labeling: Same as those outlined under Indications.

Inactive Ingredients: Dristan Long Lasting Nasal Spray—Benzalkonium Chloride 1:5000 in buffered isotonic aqueous solution, Hydroxypropyl Methylcellulose, Potassium Phosphate, Sodium Chloride, Sodium Phosphate, Thimerosal 0.002%, and Water.
Dristan Long Lasting Menthol Nasal Spray—Benzalkonium Chloride 1:5000 in buffered isotonic aqueous solution, Camphor, Eucalyptol, Hydroxypropyl Methylcellulose, Menthol, Potassium Phosphate, Sodium Chloride, Sodium Phosphate, Thimerosal 0.002%, Water, and Alcohol 0.4%.

How Supplied: Dristan Long Lasting Nasal Spray: 15 mL and 30 mL plastic squeeze bottles and 15 mL metered dose pump. Dristan Long Lasting Menthol Nasal Spray: 15 mL plastic squeeze bottle.
Shown in Product Identification Section, page 437

Maximum Strength DRISTAN®
[drĭs 'tăn]
Decongestant/Analgesic Coated Caplets

Description: Each Maximum Strength Dristan Coated Caplet contains: Pseudoephedrine HCl 30 mg and Acetaminophen 500 mg.

Actions: Pseudoephedrine HCl is an oral nasal decongestant and is effective in reducing nasal/sinus congestion. Acetaminophen is both an analgesic and an antipyretic. This maximum strength nonaspirin pain reliever effectively reduces headache pain and the pain of a

sinus cold. Acetaminophen also reduces an elevated body temperature.

Indications: Maximum Strength Dristan is indicated for effective relief without drowsiness from nasal and sinus congestion, sinus pressure and sinus pain due to colds, sinusitis, and upper respiratory allergies.

Warnings: Do not exceed recommended dosage because at higher doses nervousness, dizziness or sleeplessness may occur. Persons with high blood pressure, heart disease, diabetes, thyroid disease, difficulty in urination due to an enlarged prostate gland, or taking an antidepressant drug should use only as directed by a physician. If symptoms do not improve within 7 days, or are accompanied by high fever, discontinue use and see a physician. Do not give to children under 12. As with any drug, if you are pregnant or nursing a baby, seek the advice of a health professional before using this product. Keep this and all medication out of children's reach. In case of accidental overdose, contact a physician immediately.

Dosage and Administration: Adults and children over 12: Two caplets every 6 hours, not to exceed 8 caplets in any 24-hour period. Children under 12 should use only as directed by a physician.

Professional Labeling: Same as those outlined under Indications.

Inactive Ingredients: Calcium Stearate, Croscarmellose Sodium, D&C Yellow #10 Lake, FD&C Yellow #6 Lake, Hydrogenated Vegetable Oil, Hydroxypropyl Methylcellulose, Microcrystalline Cellulose, Polyethylene Glycol, Povidone, Starch, Stearic Acid, Titanium Dioxide.

How Supplied: Yellow coated caplets in blister packages of 24 and bottles of 48 and 100.
Shown in Product Identification Section, page 437

FREEZONE®
['frēz-ōn]
Solution

Description: Freezone is a solution which contains Salicylic Acid 13.6% w/w in a collodion vehicle.

Indications: Freezone is indicated for removal of corns and calluses.

Actions: Freezone penetrates corns and calluses painlessly, layer by layer, loosening and softening the corn or callus so that the whole corn or callus can be lifted off or peeled away in just a few days.

Warnings: DO NOT USE THIS PRODUCT IF YOU ARE A DIABETIC OR HAVE POOR BLOOD CIRCULATION BECAUSE SERIOUS COMPLICATIONS MAY RESULT. DO NOT USE ON IRRITATED SKIN OR ON ANY AREA THAT IS INFECTED OR REDDENED. IF INFECTION OR INFLAMMATION OCCURS OR IF DISCOMFORT PERSISTS, STOP USING THE

PRODUCT AND SEE YOUR PODIATRIST OR PHYSICIAN IMMEDIATELY. Care should be used to avoid contact of product with skin surrounding corn and callus. Do not use this product on soft corns (usually occurring between toes). If product gets into the eye, flush with water to remove film and continue to flush with water 15 more minutes. Avoid inhaling vapors. HIGHLY FLAMMABLE, KEEP AWAY FROM FIRE OR FLAME. AVOID SMOKING DURING USE AND UNTIL PRODUCT HAS DRIED. Keep bottle tightly capped. For external use only on the foot or toes. In case of accidental ingestion, contact a physician or call a Poison Control Center immediately. Keep this and all medicine out of children's reach.

Dosage and Administration: Cleanse feet thoroughly with soap. Soak in warm water for 15 to 30 minutes and dry feet thoroughly. Circle corn or callus with a ring of petroleum jelly to protect surrounding skin. Apply product one drop at a time using rod in cap to cover sufficiently each hard corn or callus only; let dry. Repeat this procedure daily until the corn or callus is removed or partially removed to provide comfort. Do not use medication for more than 14 days.

Professional Labeling: Same as outlined under Indications.

Inactive Ingredients: Alcohol (20.5%), Balsam Oregon, Castor Oil, Ether (64.8%), Hypophosphorous Acid and Zinc Chloride.

How Supplied: Available in a .31 fl. oz. glass bottle.
Store at room temperature away from heat.

MEDICATED CLEANSING PADS
[mĕd 'i-kāt-ĭd klĕnz-ĭng pădls]
By The Makers of Preparation H®
Hemorrhoidal Remedies

Description: Each cleansing pad contains Witch Hazel (50% w/v).

Indications: Medicated Cleansing Pads can be used for hemorrhoidal tissue irritation as an anal cleansing wipe, for everyday hygiene of the outer vaginal area, and as a final cleansing step at diaper changing time.

Actions: Medicated Cleansing Pads are scientifically developed, soft cloth pads which are impregnated with a solution specially designed to gently soothe, freshen and cleanse the anal or genital area. Medicated Cleansing Pads are superior for a multitude of types of personal hygiene uses and are especially recommended for hemorrhoid sufferers.

Warnings: In case of rectal bleeding, consult physician promptly. In case of continued irritation, discontinue use and consult a physician.

Precaution: Keep this and all medicines out of the reach of children.

Continued on next page

Whitehall—Cont.

Dosage and Administration: As a personal wipe—use as a final cleansing step after regular toilet tissue or instead of tissue, in cases of special sensitivity. As a compress—hemorrhoid sufferers will get additional relief by using Medicated Cleansing Pads as a compress. Fold pad and hold in contact with inflamed anal tissue for 10 to 15 minutes. Repeat several times daily while inflammation lasts.

Inactive Ingredients: Alcohol 7.4%, Glycerin, Methylparaben, Octoxynol-9, Water.

How Supplied: Jars of 40's and 100's.

MOMENTUM®
[mŏ-mĕn'tum]
Muscular Backache Formula

Description: Momentum contains Aspirin 500 mg, Phenyltoloxamine Citrate 15 mg, per caplet.

Indications: Momentum is indicated for the relief of pain due to stiffness and tight, inflamed muscles.

Actions: The combination of aspirin and phenyltoloxamine citrate act to relieve the pain of tense, knotted muscles. As pain subsides, muscles loosen and become less stiff, more relaxed and mobility is increased.

Warnings: Children and teenagers should not use this medicine for chicken pox or flu symptoms before a doctor is consulted about Reye syndrome, a rare but serious illness reported to be associated with aspirin. Do not drive a car or operate machinery while taking this medication as this preparation may cause drowsiness in some persons. As with any drug, if you are pregnant or nursing a baby, seek the advice of a health professional before using this product. Keep this and all medicines out of children's reach. In case of accidental overdose, contact a physician immediately.

Precaution: If pain persists for more than 10 days or redness is present as in arthritic or rheumatic conditions affecting children under 12, consult a physician immediately.

Dosage and Administration: Adults: Two caplets upon rising, then two caplets as needed at lunch, dinner, and bedtime. Dosage should not exceed 8 caplets in any 24-hour period. Not recommended for children.

Professional Labeling: Same as those outlined under Indications.

Inactive Ingredients: Alginic Acid, Citric Acid, Colloidal Silicon Dioxide, Hydrogenated Vegetable Oil, Microcrystalline Cellulose, Starch and Surfactant.

How Supplied: Bottles of 24 and 48 white, uncoated caplets.

OUTGRO®
['aut-grō]
Solution

Description: Outgro solution contains Tannic Acid 25%, Chlorobutanol 5%.

Indications: Outgro provides fast, temporary pain relief of ingrown toenails.

Actions: Outgro temporarily relieves pain, reduces swelling and eases inflammation accompanying ingrown toenails. Daily use of Outgro toughens tender skin—allowing the nail to be cut and thus preventing further pain and discomfort. Outgro does not affect the growth, shape or position of the nail.

Warnings: For external use only. Do not use Outgro solution for more than 7 days unless directed by a doctor. Consult a doctor if no improvement is seen after 7 days. IF YOU HAVE DIABETES OR POOR CIRCULATION, SEE A DOCTOR FOR TREATMENT OF INGROWN TOENAIL. DO NOT APPLY THIS PRODUCT TO OPEN SORES. IF REDNESS AND SWELLING OF YOUR TOE INCREASE, OR IF A DISCHARGE IS PRESENT AROUND THE NAIL, STOP USING THIS PRODUCT AND SEE YOUR DOCTOR IMMEDIATELY. Flammable. Keep away from fire or flame. Avoid smoking during use and until product has dried. In case of accidental ingestion, contact a physician or call a Poison Control Center immediately. KEEP THIS AND ALL MEDICINES OUT OF CHILDREN'S REACH.

Directions: Cleanse affected toes thoroughly. Using rod in cap, either apply Outgro Solution in the crevice where the nail is growing into the flesh or place a small piece of cotton in the nail groove (the side of the nail where the pain is) and wet cotton thoroughly with Outgro solution several times daily until nail discomfort is relieved. Change cotton at least once daily. Do not use product for more than 7 days unless directed by a doctor (podiatrist or physician). In some instances, temporary discoloration of the nail and surrounding skin may occur.

Professional Labeling: Same as outlined under Indications.

Inactive Ingredients: Ethylcellulose, Isopropyl Alcohol 83% (by volume).

How Supplied: Available in .31 fl. oz. glass bottles.

OXIPOR VHC®
['äk-si-pŏr VHC]
Lotion for Psoriasis

Description: OXIPOR VHC lotion for psoriasis contains Coal Tar Solution 48.5%, Salicylic Acid 1.0%, Benzocaine 2.0%.

Actions: Coal tar solution helps control cell growth and therefore prevents formation of new scales. Salicylic acid has a keratolytic action which helps peel off and dissolve away scales. Benzocaine is a local anesthetic that gives prompt relief from pain and itching. Alcohol is the solvent vehicle.

Indications: OXIPOR VHC has been clinically proven to relieve itching, redness and help dissolve and clear away the scales and crusts of psoriasis.

Warnings: For external use only. Avoid contact with eyes or mucous membranes. Use caution in exposing skin to sunlight after applying product. It may increase your tendency to sunburn for up to 24 hours after application. DO NOT USE in or around rectum or in genital area or groin except on advice of a doctor. Flammable. Keep away from fire or flame. Avoid smoking during application and until product has dried. Do not chill. Not for prolonged use. If condition persists or if rash or irritation develops, discontinue use and consult physician. Keep out of children's reach.

Dosage and Administration: Shake bottle well before each application. SKIN: Wash affected area before applying to remove loose scales. With a small wad of cotton, apply twice daily. Allow to dry before contact with clothing. SCALP: Apply to scalp with fingertips making sure to get down to the skin itself. Leave on for as long as possible, even overnight. Shampoo. Then remove all loose scales with a fine comb. This product may temporarily discolor light-colored hair. Discoloration can be prevented by reducing the time the product is left on the scalp. Also be sure to rinse product out of hair thoroughly.

Professional Labeling: Same as those outlined under Indications.

Inactive Ingredients: Alcohol 81% by volume, water.

How Supplied: Available in 1.9 oz. and 4.0 oz. bottles. Store at room temperature.

POSTURE®
[pos'tūr]
600 mg
High Potency Calcium Supplement

Description: Each film-coated tablet of POSTURE® contains Tribasic Calcium Phosphate 1565.2 mg, which provides 600 mg of elemental calcium. POSTURE® is specially formulated not to produce gas.

	For Adults—
Two tablets contain:	% U.S. RDA*
Elemental Calcium...... 1200 mg ...120% (as calcium phosphate)	

*Percentage of U.S. Recommended Daily Allowance

Indication: POSTURE® Tablets provide a daily source of calcium to help maintain healthy bones or to supplement dietary calcium intake when directed by a physician.

Directions for Use: One or two tablets daily, or as recommended by a physician. Keep Out of Reach of Children.

Inactive Ingredients: Croscarmellose Sodium, Ethylcellulose, Magnesium Stearate, Microcrystalline Cellulose,

Polyethylene Glycol, Povidone, Sodium Lauryl Sulfate.

How Supplied: In bottles of 60 scored tablets.

Shown in Product Identification Section, page 437

POSTURE®-D
600 mg
High Potency Calcium Supplement with Vitamin D

Description: Each film-coated tablet of POSTURE®-D contains Tribasic Calcium Phosphate 1565.2 mg, which provides 600 mg of elemental calcium and 125 IU of Vitamin D. POSTURE®-D is specially formulated not to produce gas.

	For Adults—
Two tablets	% U.S.
contain:	RDA*
Elemental Calcium...... 1200 mg ...120%	
(as calcium phosphate)	
Vitamin D..................... 250 IU 63%	

*Percentage of U.S. Recommended Daily Allowance.

Indication: POSTURE®-D Tablets provide a daily source of calcium and Vitamin D to help maintain healthy bones or to supplement dietary intake of calcium and Vitamin D when directed by a physician.

Directions for Use: One or two tablets daily, or as recommended by a physician. Keep Out of Reach of Children.

Inactive Ingredients: Croscarmellose Sodium, Ethylcellulose, Magnesium Stearate, Microcrystalline Cellulose, Polyethylene Glycol, Povidone, Sodium Lauryl Sulfate.

How Supplied: In bottles of 60 scored tablets.

Shown in Product Identification Section, page 437

PREPARATION H®
[prep-e 'rā-shen-āch]
Hemorrhoidal Ointment and Cream
PREPARATION H®
Hemorrhoidal Suppositories

Description: Preparation H is available in ointment, cream and suppository product forms. The **Ointment** contains Live Yeast Cell Derivative supplying 2,000 units Skin Respiratory Factor per ounce of Ointment, and Shark Liver Oil 3.0% in a specially prepared Rectal Petrolatum Base.
The **Cream** contains Live Yeast Cell Derivative supplying 2,000 units Skin Respiratory Factor per ounce of Cream and Shark Liver Oil 3.0% in a specially prepared Rectal Cream Base containing Petrolatum.
The **Suppositories** contain Live Yeast Cell Derivative, supplying 2,000 units Skin Respiratory Factor per ounce of Cocoa Butter Suppository Base and Shark Liver Oil 3.0%.

Actions: Live Yeast Cell Derivative acts by increasing the oxygen uptake of dermal tissues and facilitating collagen formation. Shark Liver Oil has been in-

corporated to act as a protectant which softens and soothes the tissues. Preparation H also lubricates inflamed, irritated surfaces to help make bowel movements less painful.

Indications: Preparation H helps shrink swelling of hemorrhoidal tissues caused by inflammation and gives prompt, temporary relief in many cases from pain and itch in tissues.

Precautions: In case of bleeding, or if your condition persists, a physician should be consulted.

Dosage and Administration: Ointment/Cream: Before applying, remove protective cover from applicator. Lubricate applicator before each application and thoroughly cleanse after use. It is recommended that Preparation H Hemorrhoidal ointment/cream be applied freely to the affected rectal area whenever symptoms occur, from three to five times per day, especially at night, in the morning, and after each bowel movement. Frequent application with Preparation H ointment/cream provides continual therapy which leads to more rapid improvement of hemorrhoidal symptoms. **Suppositories:** Whenever symptoms occur, remove wrapper, insert one suppository rectally from three to five times per day, especially at night, in the morning, and after each bowel movement. Frequent application with Preparation H suppositories provides continual therapy which leads to more rapid improvement of hemorrhoidal symptoms.

Professional Labeling: Same as those outlined under Indications.

Inactive Ingredients: Ointment— Beeswax, Glycerin, Lanolin, Lanolin Alcohol, Mineral Oil, Paraffin, Phenylmercuric Nitrate 1:10,000 (as a preservative), Thyme Oil.
Cream—Beeswax, BHA, Citric Acid, Glycerin, Glyceryl Oleate, Lanolin, Lanolin Alcohol, Magnesium Aluminum Silicate, Mineral Oil, Paraffin, Phenylmercuric Nitrate 1:10,000 (as a preservative), Polysorbate 80, Propyl Gallate, Propylene Glycol, Silica, Water. May also contain Methylparaben and Propylparaben.
Suppositories—Beeswax, Glycerin, Phenylmercuric Nitrate 1:10,000 (as a preservative), Polyethylene Glycol 600 Dilaurate.

How Supplied: Ointment: Net Wt. 1 oz. and 2 oz. **Cream:** Net wt. 0.9 oz. and 1.8 oz. **Suppositories:** 12's, 24's, 36's and 48's. Store at controlled room temperature in cool place but not over 80° F.

Shown in Product Identification Section, page 437

PRIMATENE®
[prīm 'a-tēn]
Mist
(Epinephrine Inhalation Aerosol Bronchodilator)

Description: Primatene Mist contains Epinephrine 5.5 mg/mL.

Action: Epinephrine is a sympathomimetic agent which eases breathing for asthma patients by reducing spasms of bronchial muscles.

Indications: Primatene Mist is indicated for temporary relief of shortness of breath, tightness of chest, and wheezing due to bronchial asthma.

Dosage and Administration: Inhalation dosage for adults and children 4 years of age and older: Start with one inhalation, then wait at least 1 minute. If not relieved, use once more. Do not use again for at least 3 hours. The use of this product by children should be supervised by an adult. Children under 4 years of age: Consult a physician. Each inhalation delivers 0.22 mg. of epinephrine.

Warnings: Do not use this product unless a diagnosis of asthma has been made by a physician. Do not use this product if you have heart disease, high blood pressure, thyroid disease, diabetes, or difficulty in urination due to enlargement of the prostate gland unless directed by a physician. As with any drug, if you are pregnant or nursing a baby, seek the advice of a health professional before using this product. Do not use this product if you have ever been hospitalized for asthma or if you are taking any prescription drug for asthma unless directed by a physician. Keep this and all drugs out of the reach of children. In case of accidental overdose, seek professional assistance or contact a poison control center immediately. DO NOT CONTINUE TO USE THIS PRODUCT, BUT SEEK MEDICAL ASSISTANCE IMMEDIATELY IF SYMPTOMS ARE NOT RELIEVED WITHIN 20 MINUTES OR BECOME WORSE. DO NOT USE THIS PRODUCT MORE FREQUENTLY OR AT HIGHER DOSES THAN RECOMMENDED UNLESS DIRECTED BY A PHYSICIAN. EXCESSIVE USE MAY CAUSE NERVOUSNESS AND RAPID HEART BEAT AND POSSIBLY, ADVERSE EFFECTS ON THE HEART. DRUG INTERACTION PRECAUTION: Do not use this product if you are presently taking a prescription drug for high blood pressure or depression, without first consulting your physician.

Precautions: Contents under pressure. Do not puncture or throw container into incinerator. Using or storing near open flame or heating above 120° F may cause bursting.

Directions For Use of The Mouthpiece:
The Primatene Mist mouthpiece, which is enclosed in the Primatene Mist 15mL size (not the refill size), should be used for inhalation only with Primatene Mist.
1. Take plastic cap off mouthpiece. (For refills, use mouthpiece from previous purchase.)
2. Take plastic mouthpiece off bottle.
3. Place other end of mouthpiece on bottle.

Continued on next page

Whitehall—Cont.

4. Turn bottle upside down. Place thumb on bottom of mouthpiece over circular button and forefinger on top of vial. Empty the lungs as completely as possible by exhaling.
5. Place mouthpiece in mouth with lips closed around opening. Inhale deeply while squeezing mouthpiece and bottle together. Release immediately and remove unit from mouth. Complete taking the deep breath, drawing the medication into your lungs and holding breath as long as comfortable.
6. Then exhale slowly keeping lips nearly closed. This distributes the medication in the lungs.
7. Replace plastic cap on mouthpiece.
8. The Primatene Mist mouthpiece should be washed once daily with soap and hot water, and rinsed thoroughly. Then it should be dried with a clean, lint-free cloth.

Inactive Ingredients: Alcohol 34%, Ascorbic Acid, Fluorocarbons (Propellant), Water. Contains No Sulfites.

How Supplied:
½ Fl. oz. (15mL) With Mouthpiece.
½ Fl. oz. (15mL) Refill
¾ Fl. oz. (22.5mL) Refill
Shown in Product Identification Section, page 437

PRIMATENE®
[prīm ′a-tēn]
**Mist Suspension
(Epinephrine Bitartrate Inhalation Aerosol Bronchodilator)**

Description: Primatene Mist Suspension contains Epinephrine Bitartrate 7.0 mg/mL.

Action: Epinephrine is a sympathomimetic agent which eases breathing for asthma patients by reducing spasms of bronchial muscles.

Indications: Primatene Mist Suspension is indicated for temporary relief of shortness of breath, tightness of chest, and wheezing due to bronchial asthma.

Dosage and Administration: Shake before using. Inhalation dosage for adults and children 4 years of age and older: Start with one inhalation, then wait at least 1 minute. If not relieved, use once more. Do not use again for at least 3 hours. The use of this product by children should be supervised by an adult. Children under 4 years of age: Consult a physician. Each inhalation delivers 0.3 mg. Epinephrine Bitartrate equivalent to 0.16 mg. Epinephrine Base.

Warnings: Do not use this product unless a diagnosis of asthma has been made by a physician. Do not use this product if you have heart disease, high blood pressure, thyroid disease, diabetes, or difficulty in urination due to enlargement of the prostate gland unless directed by a physician. As with any drug, if you are pregnant or nursing a baby, seek the advice of a health professional before using this product. Do not use this product if

you have ever been hospitalized for asthma or if you are taking any prescription drug for asthma unless directed by a physician. Keep this and all drugs out of the reach of children. In case of accidental overdose, seek professional assistance or contact a poison control center immediately.
DO NOT CONTINUE TO USE THIS PRODUCT, BUT SEEK MEDICAL ASSISTANCE IMMEDIATELY IF SYMPTOMS ARE NOT RELIEVED WITHIN 20 MINUTES OR BECOME WORSE. DO NOT USE THIS PRODUCT MORE FREQUENTLY OR AT HIGHER DOSES THAN RECOMMENDED UNLESS DIRECTED BY A PHYSICIAN. EXCESSIVE USE MAY CAUSE NERVOUSNESS AND RAPID HEART BEAT AND POSSIBLY, ADVERSE EFFECTS ON THE HEART. DRUG INTERACTION PRECAUTION: Do not use this product if you are presently taking a prescription drug for high blood pressure or depression, without first consulting your physician.

Precautions: Contents under pressure. Do not puncture or throw container into incinerator. Using or storing near open flame or heating above 120° F may cause bursting.

Directions For Use of The Inhaler:
1. SHAKE BEFORE USING.
2. HOLD INHALER WITH NOZZLE DOWN WHILE USING. Empty the lungs as completely as possible by exhaling.
3. Purse the lips as in saying "O" and hold the nozzle up to the lips keeping the tongue flat. As you start to take a deep breath, squeeze nozzle and can together, releasing one full application. Complete taking a deep breath, drawing medication into your lungs.
4. Hold breath for as long as comfortable. Then exhale slowly, keeping the lips nearly closed. This distributes the medication in the lungs.
5. The Primatene Mist Suspension nozzle should be washed once daily. After removing the nozzle from the vial, wash it with soap and hot water, and rinse thoroughly. Then it should be dried with a clean, lint-free cloth.

Inactive Ingredients: Fluorocarbons (Propellant), Sorbitan Trioleate. Contains No Sulfites.

How Supplied: ⅓ Fl. oz. (10mL) pocket-size aerosol inhaler.

PRIMATENE®
[prīm ′a-tēn]
Tablets

Description: Depending upon the state (see How Supplied), Primatene Tablets are available in 3 formulations:
(Regular Formula): Theophylline Anhydrous 130 mg, Ephedrine Hydrochloride 24 mg.
P Formula: Theophylline Hydrous 130 mg, Ephedrine Hydrochloride 24 mg, Phenobarbital 8 mg (⅛ gr) per tablet. (Warning: May be habit forming.)

M Formula: Theophylline Anhydrous 130 mg, Ephedrine Hydrochloride 24 mg, Pyrilamine Maleate 16.6 mg per tablet.

Actions: Primatene Tablets contain two bronchodilators, theophylline, a methylxanthine, and ephedrine, a sympathomimetic amine. The pharmacologic action of theophylline may be mediated through inhibition of phosphodiesterase with a resulting increase in intracellular cyclic AMP. The β-adrenergic ephedrine acts by a different mechanism to produce cyclic AMP. Used at the start of an asthma attack, Primatene acts to (1) open bronchial tubes so breathing is natural, (2) relax bronchial muscles, (3) reduce congestion. Primatene helps relieve the asthma spasms, thus permitting sleep at night and freedom from associated anxiety by day.

Indications: Primatene Tablets are indicated for relief and control of attacks of bronchial asthma and associated hay fever.

Warnings: If symptoms persist, consult your physician. Some people are sensitive to ephedrine and, in some cases, temporary sleeplessness and nervousness may occur. These reactions will disappear if the use of the medication is discontinued. Do not exceed recommended dosage.
People who have heart disease, high blood pressure, diabetes or thyroid trouble or difficulty in urination due to enlargement of the prostate gland should take this preparation only on the advice of a physician. Both the "M" and "P" formulae may cause drowsiness. People taking the "M" or "P" formula should not drive or operate machinery.
As with any drug, if you are pregnant or nursing a baby, seek the advice of a health professional before using this product. Keep all medicines out of reach of children.

Dosage and Administration: Adults: 1 or 2 tablets initially and then one every 4 hours, as needed, not to exceed 6 tablets in 24 hours. Children (6–12): One half adult dose. For children under 6, consult a physician.

Inactive Ingredients:
(Regular Formula): Croscarmellose Sodium, D&C Yellow No. 10 Lake, FD&C Yellow No. 6 Lake, Magnesium Stearate, Microcrystalline Cellulose, Silica, Starch, Stearic Acid.
P Formula (Phenobarbital): Colloidal Silicon Dioxide, D&C Yellow No. 10, FD&C Yellow No. 6, Magnesium Stearate, Sodium Starch Glycolate, Starch, Surfactant.
M Formula (Pyrilamine Maleate): D&C Yellow No. 10 Lake, FD&C Yellow No. 6 Lake, Hydrogenated Vegetable Oil, Magnesium Stearate, Microcrystalline Cellulose, Sodium Starch Glycolate, Surfactant.
Contains No Sulfites.

How Supplied: Available in three Primatene Tablet forms, Regular Formula, "M" Formula, and "P" Formula.

(Regular) Primatene Tablets are primarily available in the West and Southwest only. "P" Formula, containing phenobarbital, is available in most states. In those states where phenobarbital is Rx only, "M" Formula, containing pyrilamine maleate, is available. Both "M" and "P" formulas are supplied in glass bottles of 24 and 60 tablets. (Regular) Primatene Tablets are supplied in 24 and 60 tablet thermoform blister cartons.

*Shown in Product Identification
Section, page 437*

RIOPAN®
[rī'opan]
magaldrate
Antacid

Description: RIOPAN is a buffer antacid containing the unique chemical entity Magaldrate. Each teaspoonful (5 mL) of suspension contains Magaldrate, 540 mg. Each Chew Tablet or Swallow Tablet contains Magaldrate, 480 mg. RIOPAN is considered dietetically sodium-free (containing not more than 0.004 mEq, 0.1 mg sodium per teaspoonful or tablet).

Actions: Magaldrate, the active ingredient in RIOPAN, demonstrates a rapid and uniform buffering action. The acid-neutralizing capacity of RIOPAN is 15.0 mEq/5mL and 13.5 mEq/tablet. RIOPAN does not produce acid rebound or alkalinization.

Indications: Riopan is indicated for the relief of heartburn, sour stomach, and acid indigestion. For symptomatic relief of hyperacidity associated with the diagnosis of peptic ulcer, gastritis, peptic esophagitis, gastric hyperacidity, and hiatal hernia.

Dosage and Administration: RIOPAN (magaldrate) Antacid *Suspension* —Take one or two teaspoonfuls, between meals and at bedtime, or as directed by the physician. RIOPAN Antacid *Chew Tablets* —Chew one or two tablets, between meals and at bedtime, or as directed by the physician. RIOPAN Antacid *Swallow Tablets* —Take one or two tablets, between meals and at bedtime, or as directed by the physician. Take with enough water to swallow promptly.

Warnings: Patients should not take more than 18 teaspoonfuls (or 20 tablets) in a 24-hour period or use the maximum dosage for more than two weeks, or use if they have kidney disease except under the advice and supervision of a physician.

Drug Interaction Precaution: Do not use in patients taking a prescription antibiotic drug containing any form of tetracycline.

Inactive Ingredients: Chew Tablets: Flavor, Magnesium Stearate, Polyethylene Glycol, Sorbitol, Starch, Sucrose, Titanium Dioxide. Swallow Tablets: Flavor, Magnesium Stearate, Menthol, Microcrystalline Cellulose, Polyethylene Glycol, Starch, Talc, Titanium Dioxide. Suspension: Flavor, Glycerin, Potassium Citrate, Saccharin, Sorbitol, Xanthan Gum, Water.

How Supplied: RIOPAN Antacid *Suspension* —in 12 fl oz (355 mL) plastic bottles. Individual Cups, 1 fl oz (30 mL) ea., tray of 10—10 trays per packer. Store at room temperature (approximately 25℃). Avoid freezing. RIOPAN Antacid *Chew Tablets* —in bottles of 60 and 100. Also, single roll-packs of 12 tablets and 3-roll rollpacks of 36 tablets. RIOPAN Antacid *Swallow Tablets* —Boxes of 60 and 100 in individual film strips (6 x 10 and 10 x 10, respectively).

*Shown in Product Identification
Section, page 437*

RIOPAN PLUS®
[rī'opan]
magaldrate and simethicone
Antacid plus Anti-Gas

Description: RIOPAN PLUS is a buffer antacid plus anti-gas combination product containing the unique chemical entity Magaldrate. Each teaspoonful (5mL) of suspension contains Magaldrate, 540 mg and Simethicone, 20 mg. Each Chew Tablet contains Magaldrate, 480 mg and Simethicone, 20 mg. RIOPAN PLUS is considered dietetically sodium-free (containing not more than 0.004 mEq, 0.1 mg sodium per teaspoonful or tablet).

Actions: Magaldrate, the active antacid ingredient in RIOPAN PLUS, provides a rapid and uniform buffering action. The acid-neutralizing capacity of RIOPAN PLUS is 15.0 mEq/5mL and 13.5 mEq/tablet. RIOPAN PLUS does not produce acid rebound or alkalinization. Simethicone reduces the surface tension of gas bubbles so that the gas is more easily eliminated.

Indications: RIOPAN PLUS is indicated for the relief of heartburn, sour stomach and acid indigestion, accompanied by the symptoms of gas. For symptomatic relief of hyperacidity associated with the diagnosis of peptic ulcer, gastritis, peptic esophagitis, gastric hyperacidity, and hiatal hernia. For postoperative gas pain.

Dosage and Administration: RIOPAN PLUS (magaldrate and simethicone) Antacid plus Anti-Gas *Suspension* —Take one or two teaspoonfuls between meals and at bedtime, or as directed by the physician. RIOPAN PLUS Antacid plus Anti-Gas *Chew Tablets* —Chew one or two tablets, between meals and at bedtime, or as directed by the physician.

Warnings: Patients should not take more than 18 teaspoonfuls (or 20 tablets) in a 24-hour period, or use the maximum dosage for more than two weeks, or use if they have kidney disease, except under the advice and supervision of a physician.

Drug Interaction Precaution: Do not use in patients taking a prescription antibiotic drug containing any form of tetracycline.

Inactive Ingredients: Chew Tablets: Flavor, Magnesium Stearate, Methylcellulose, Polyethylene Glycol, Silica, Sorbitol, Starch, Sucrose, Titanium Dioxide. Suspension: Acacia, Flavor, Hydroxypropyl Methylcellulose, Menthol, PEG-8 Stearate, Saccharin, Sorbitan Stearate, Water.

How Supplied: RIOPAN PLUS Antacid plus Anti-Gas *Suspension* —in 12 fl oz (355 mL) plastic bottles. Individual Cups, 1 fl oz (30 mL) ea., tray of 10—10 trays per packer. Store at room temperature (approximately 25℃). Avoid freezing.
RIOPAN PLUS Antacid plus Anti-Gas *Chew Tablets* —in bottles of 60 and 100. Also, single rollpacks of 12 tablets and 3-roll rollpacks of 36 tablets.

*Shown in Product Identification
Section, page 437*

RIOPAN PLUS® 2
[rī'opan plus 2]
magaldrate and simethicone
Double Strength
Antacid plus Anti-Gas

Description: RIOPAN PLUS 2 is a double strength buffer antacid plus antigas combination product containing the unique chemical entity Magaldrate. Each teaspoonful (5mL) of suspension contains Magaldrate, 1080 mg and Simethicone, 30 mg. Each Chew Tablet contains Magaldrate, 1080 mg and Simethicone, 20 mg. RIOPAN PLUS 2 is considered dietetically sodium-free (containing not more than 0.013 mEq, 0.3 mg per teaspoonful or 0.021 mEq, 0.5 mg per tablet).

Actions: Magaldrate, the active antacid ingredient in RIOPAN PLUS 2, provides a rapid and uniform buffering action. The acid-neutralizing capacity of Double Strength RIOPAN PLUS 2 is 30 mEq/5mL and 30.0 mEq/tablet. RIOPAN PLUS 2 does not produce acid rebound or alkalinization. Simethicone reduces the surface tension of gas bubbles so that the gas is more easily eliminated.

Indications: RIOPAN PLUS 2 is indicated for the relief of heartburn, sour stomach and acid indigestion accompanied by the symptoms of gas. For symptomatic relief of hyperacidity associated with the diagnosis of peptic ulcer, gastritis, peptic esophagitis, gastric hyperacidity, and hiatal hernia. For postoperative gas pain.

Dosage and Administration: RIOPAN PLUS 2 (magaldrate and simethicone) *Suspension* —Take one or two teaspoonfuls between meals and at bedtime, or as directed by the physician.
RIOPAN PLUS 2 Chew Tablets—Chew one or two tablets, between meals and at bedtime, or as directed by the physician.

Warnings: Patients should not take more than 9 teaspoonfuls (or 9 tablets) in a 24-hour period, or use the maximum dosage for more than two weeks, or use if they have kidney disease, except under

Continued on next page

Whitehall—Cont.

the advice and supervision of a physician.

Drug Interaction Precaution: Do not use in patients taking a prescription antibiotic drug containing any form of tetracycline.

Inactive Ingredients: Chew Tablets: Flavor, Magnesium Stearate, Methylcellulose, Polyethylene Glycol, Saccharin, Silica, Sorbitol, Starch, Sucrose, Titanium Dioxide. Supension: Flavor, Glycerin, PEG-8 Stearate, Potassium Citrate, Saccharin, Sorbitan Stearate, Sorbitol, Xanthan Gum, Water.

How Supplied: RIOPAN PLUS 2 *Suspension* —in 12 fl oz (355 mL) plastic bottles. RIOPAN PLUS 2 Chew Tablets—in bottles of 60.

Shown in Product Identification Section, page 438

SEMICID®
[sĕm′ē-sĭd]
Vaginal Contraceptive Inserts

Description: Semicid is a safe and effective, nonsystemic, reversible method of birth control. Each vaginal contraceptive insert contains 100 mg of the spermicide nonoxynol-9. It contains no hormones and is odorless and nonmessy.
When used consistently and according to directions, the effectiveness of Semicid is approximately equal to other vaginal spermicides, but is less than oral contraceptives.

Actions: Semicid dissolves in the vagina and blends with natural vaginal secretions to provide double birth control protection: a physical barrier, plus an effective sperm killing barrier that covers the cervical opening and adjoining vaginal walls.
Semicid requires no applicator and has no unpleasant taste. Unlike foams, creams and jellies, Semicid does not drip or run, and Semicid inserts are easier to use than the diaphragm. Also, Semicid does not effervesce like some inserts, so it is not as likely to cause a burning feeling. Semicid provides effective contraceptive protection when used properly. However, no contraceptive method or product can provide an absolute guarantee against becoming pregnant.

Indication: For the prevention of pregnancy.

Warnings: **Do not insert in urinary opening (urethra).** Do not take orally. If irritation occurs, discontinue use. If irritation persists, consult your physician. Keep this and all contraceptives out of the reach of children.

Precautions: If douching is desired, one should wait at least six hours after intercourse before douching. If either partner experiences irritation, discontinue use. If irritation persists, consult a physician.

If your doctor has told you that it is dangerous to become pregnant, ask your doctor if you can use Semicid.
If menstrual period is missed, a physician should be consulted.

Dosage and Administration: To use, unwrap one insert and insert it deeply into the vagina. It is essential that Semicid be inserted at least <u>15 minutes</u> before intercourse; however, Semicid is also effective when inserted up to 1 hour before intercourse. If intercourse is delayed for more than 1 hour after Semicid is inserted, or if intercourse is repeated, then another insert must be inserted. Semicid can be used as frequently as needed.

Inactive Ingredients: Benzethonium Chloride, Citric Acid, D&C Red #21 Lake, D&C Red #33 Lake, Methylparaben, Polyethylene Glycol, Water.

How Supplied: Strip Packaging of 10's and 20's.
Keep Semicid at room temperature (not over 86°F or 30°C).
Shown in Product Identification Section, page 438

SLEEP–EZE 3®
[slēp-ēz]
Nighttime Sleep Aid Tablets
Diphenhydramine Hydrochloride

Description: Sleep-eze 3 is a nighttime sleep-aid that contains Diphenhydramine Hydrochloride, 25 mg per tablet.

Indication: Sleep-eze 3 helps to reduce difficulty in falling asleep.

Action: Sleep-eze 3 contains diphenhydramine, an antihistamine with anticholinergic and sedative action.

Warnings: Do not give to children under 12 years of age. Insomnia may be a symptom of serious underlying medical illness. If sleeplessness persists continuously for more than 2 weeks, consult your physician. As with any drug, if you are pregnant or nursing a baby, seek the advice of a health professional before using this product.
Do not take this product if you have asthma, glaucoma, emphysema, chronic pulmonary disease, shortness of breath, difficulty breathing or difficulty in urination due to enlargement of the prostate gland except under the advice and supervision of a physician.
In case of accidental ingestion or overdose, contact a physician or Poison Control Center immediately. Keep this and all medicines out of children's reach.

Drug Interaction: Avoid alcoholic beverages while taking this product. Do not take this product if you are taking sedatives or tranquilizers, without first consulting your doctor.

Precaution: This product contains an antihistamine and will cause drowsiness. It should be used only at bedtime.

Dosage and Administration: Take 2 tablets 20 minutes before going to bed.

Professional Labeling: Same as outlined under Indication.

Inactive Ingredients: Croscarmellose Sodium, Dicalcium Phosphate, D&C Yellow No. 10, FD&C Yellow No. 6, Magnesium Stearate, Microcrystalline Cellulose, Stearic Acid.

How Supplied: Packages of 12's, 24's, and 48's.

TODAY®
[tū-dā]
Vaginal Contraceptive Sponge

Description: Today Vaginal Contraceptive Sponge is a soft polyurethane foam sponge containing nonoxynol-9, a spermicide used by millions of women for over 25 years.
Today Sponge is Effective, Safe, and Convenient. Today Sponge provides 24-hour contraceptive protection without hormones, allowing spontaneity. Today Sponge is easy to use, nonmessy and disposable.

Active Ingredient: Each Today Sponge contains nonoxynol-9, one gram.

Inactive Ingredients: Benzoic acid, citric acid, sodium dihydrogen citrate, sodium metabisulfite, sorbic acid, water in a polyurethane foam sponge.

Indication: For the prevention of pregnancy.

Actions: Used as directed, Today Vaginal Contraceptive Sponge prevents pregnancy in three ways: 1) the spermicide nonoxynol-9 kills sperm before they can reach the egg; 2) Today Sponge traps and absorbs sperm; 3) Today Sponge blocks the cervix so that sperm cannot enter.
Today Sponge is designed for easy insertion into the vagina. It is positioned against the cervix, and while in place provides protection against pregnancy for 24 hours. The soft polyurethane foam sponge is formulated to feel like normal vaginal tissue and has a specially designed ribbon loop attached to an interior web for maximum strength.
In clinical trials of Today Sponge in over 1,800 women worldwide who completed over 12,000 cycles of use, the method-effectiveness, i.e., the level of effectiveness seen in women who followed the printed instructions exactly and who used Today Sponge every time that they had intercourse, was 89 to 91%.

Instructions: Remove one Today Sponge from airtight inner pack, wet thoroughly with clean tap water, and squeeze gently until it becomes very sudsy. The water activates the spermicide. Fold the sides of Today Sponge upward until it looks long and narrow and then insert it deeply into the vagina with the string loop dangling below. Protection begins immediately and continues for 24 hours. It is <u>not</u> necessary to add creams, jellies, foams, or any other additional spermicide as long as Today Sponge is in place, no matter how many acts of intercourse may occur during a 24-hour period. Always wait 6 hours after your last act of intercourse before removing Today Sponge. If you have intercourse when Today Sponge has been in place for 24 hours, it must be left in place an additional 6 hours after intercourse before removing it.

To remove Today Sponge, place a finger in the vagina and reach up and back to find the string loop. Hook a finger around the loop. Slowly and gently pull the Sponge out. Some women, especially first-time users, may have difficulty removing the Sponge. This situation may be due to tension or unusually strong muscular pressure. Simple relaxation of the vaginal muscles and bearing down should make it possible to remove the Sponge without difficulty. See User Instruction Booklet (Section 7) for details on removing Today Sponge or call the Today TalkLine 1-800-223-2329.

Warnings: For best protection against pregnancy, follow instructions exactly. Any delay in your menstrual period may be an early sign of pregnancy. If this happens, consult your physician or clinic as soon as possible. A small number of men and women may be sensitive to the spermicide in this product (nonoxynol-9) or any of its other components and should not use this product if irritation occurs and persists. If genital burning or itching occurs in either partner, stop using Today Sponge and contact your physician. If you have ever had Toxic Shock Syndrome, do not use Today Sponge. If you experience two or more of the warning signs of Toxic Shock Syndrome (TSS), including fever, vomiting, diarrhea, muscular pain, dizziness, and rash similar to sunburn, consult your physician or clinic immediately. Today Sponge should not be used during the menstrual period. After childbirth, miscarriage, other termination of pregnancy, or if you are nursing a baby, it is important to consult your physician or clinic before using this product. Today Sponge should be removed within the specified time limit (maximum wear time is 30 hours). In clinical trials, approximately one-half of all unintended pregnancies occurred during the first three months of Today Sponge use. A back-up contraceptive, such as Today Condom, is recommended for additional contraceptive protection during this time, until the user becomes familiar with Today Sponge.

Keep this and all drugs out of the reach of children. In case of accidental ingestion of Today Sponge, call a poison control center, emergency medical facility or doctor.

How To Store: Store at normal room temperature.

How Supplied: Packages of 3s, 6s, and 12s.

Shown in Product Indentification Section, page 438

TRENDAR®
Ibuprofen Tablets, USP
Menstrual Pain & Cramp Reliever

Warning: ASPIRIN SENSITIVE PATIENTS. Do not take this product if you have had a severe allergic reaction to aspirin, e.g. asthma, swelling, shock or hives, because even though

this product contains no aspirin or salicylates cross-reactions may occur in patients allergic to aspirin.

Indications: For the temporary relief of painful menstrual cramps (dysmenorrhea); also headaches, backaches and muscular aches and pains associated with premenstrual syndrome.

Dosage and Administration: Adults: Take 1 tablet every 4 to 6 hours at the onset of menstrual symptoms and while pain persists. If pain does not respond to 1 tablet, 2 tablets may be used but do not exceed 6 tablets in 24 hours, unless directed by a doctor. The smallest effective dose should be used. Take with food or milk if occasional and mild heartburn, upset stomach, or stomach pain occurs with use. Consult a doctor if these symptoms are more than mild or if they persist. Children: Do not give this product to children under 12 except under the advice or supervision of a doctor.

Warnings: Do not take for pain for more than 10 days unless directed by a doctor. If pain persists or gets worse, or if new symptoms occur, consult a doctor. These could be signs of serious illness. If you are under a doctor's care for any serious condition, consult a doctor before taking this product. As with aspirin and acetaminophen, if you have any condition which requires you to take prescription drugs or if you have had any problems or serious side effects from taking any nonprescription pain reliever, do not take this product without first discussing it with your doctor. If you experience any symptoms which are unusual or seem unrelated to the condition for which you took ibuprofen, consult a doctor before taking any more of it. Although ibuprofen is indicated for the same conditions as aspirin and acetaminophen, it should not be taken with them except under a doctor's direction. Do not combine this product with any other ibuprofen-containing product. As with any drug, if you are pregnant or nursing a baby, seek the advice of a health professional before using this product. IT IS ESPECIALLY IMPORTANT NOT TO USE IBUPROFEN DURING THE LAST 3 MONTHS OF PREGNANCY UNLESS SPECIFICALLY DIRECTED TO DO SO BY A DOCTOR BECAUSE IT MAY CAUSE PROBLEMS IN THE UNBORN CHILD OR COMPLICATIONS DURING DELIVERY. Keep this and all drugs out of the reach of children. In case of accidental overdose, seek professional assistance or contact a poison control center immediately.

Active Ingredient: Each tablet contains Ibuprofen 200 mg.

Inactive Ingredients: Acacia, Acetylated Monoglycerides, Beeswax, Calcium Sulfate, Colloidal Silicon Dioxide, Dimethicone, Iron Oxide, Lecithin, Pharmaceutical Glaze, Povidone, Sodium Benzoate, Sodium Carboxymethylcellulose, Starch, Stearic Acid, Sucrose, Titanium Dioxide.

Professional Labeling: Same as stated under Indications.

How Supplied: Coated tablets in bottles of 20's & 40's.

Storage: Store at room temperature; avoid excessive heat 40°C (104°F).

Winthrop Consumer Products
Division of Sterling Drug Inc.
90 PARK AVENUE
NEW YORK, NY 10016

BRONKAID® Mist
(Epinephrine)

Description: BRONKAID Mist, brand of epinephrine inhalation aerosol. Contains: Epinephrine, USP, 0.5% (w/w) (as nitrate and hydrochloric salts). Also contains: Alcohol 33% (w/w), ascorbic acid dichlorodifluoromethane, dichlorotetrafluroethane, purified water. Each spray delivers 0.25 mg epinephrine. Contains no sulfites.

Indication: For temporary relief of shortness of breath, tightness of chest and wheezing due to bronchial asthma.

Warnings: FOR ORAL INHALATION ONLY. Do not use this product unless a diagnosis of asthma has been made by a doctor, or if you have heart disease, high blood pressure, thyroid disease, diabetes, or difficulty in urination due to enlargement of the prostate gland, if you have ever been hospitalized for asthma or if you are taking any prescription drug for asthma. **Do not use this product more frequently or at higher doses than recommended, unless directed by a doctor.** Keep this and all drugs out of the reach of children. In case of accidental overdose, seek professional assistance or contact a poison control center immediately. As with any drug, if you are pregnant or nursing a baby, seek the advice of a health professional before using this product.

Excessive use may cause nervousness and rapid heart beat, and, possibly, adverse effects on the heart. **Do not continue to use this product, but seek medical assistance immediately if symptoms are not relieved within 20 minutes or become worse.**

Drug Interaction Precaution: Do not use this product if you are presently taking a prescription drug for high blood pressure or depression, without first consulting your doctor.

Continued on next page

This product information was effective as of November 1, 1989. Current information may be obtained directly from Winthrop Consumer Products, Division of Sterling Drug Inc., by writing to 90 Park Avenue, New York, NY 10016.

Winthrop Consumer—Cont.

Warnings: Avoid spraying in eyes. Contents under pressure. Do not break or incinerate. Using or storing near open flame or heating above 120°F may cause bursting.

Dosage: Inhalation dosage for adults and children 4 years of age and older. Start with one inhalation, then wait at least one (1) minute. If not relieved, use once more. Do not use again for at least 3 hours. The use of this product by children should be supervised by an adult. Children under 4 years of age, consult a doctor.

Directions for Use:
1. Remove cap and mouthpiece from bottle.
2. Remove cap from mouthpiece.
3. Turn mouthpiece sideways and fit metal stem of nebulizer into hole in flattened end of mouthpiece.
4. Exhale, as completely as possible. Now, hold bottle **upside down** between thumb and forefinger and close lips loosely around end of mouthpiece.
5. Inhale deeply while pressing down firmly on bottle, once only.
6. Remove mouthpiece and hold your breath a moment to allow for maximum absorption of medication. Then exhale slowly through nearly closed lips.

After use, remove mouthpiece from bottle and replace cap. Slide mouthpiece over bottle for protection. When possible rinse mouthpiece with tap water immediately after use. Soap and water will not hurt it. A clean mouthpiece always works better.

How Supplied:
Bottles of ½ fl oz (15 ml) NDC 0024-4082-15 with actuator. Also available—refills (no mouthpiece) in 15 mL (½ fl oz) NDC 0024-4083-16 and 22.5 mL (¾ fl oz) NDC 0024-4083-22.

Shown in Product Identification Section, page 438

BRONKAID® Mist Suspension (Epinephrine Bitartrate)

Active Ingredients: Each spray delivers 0.3 mg epinephrine bitartrate equivalent to 0.16 mg epinephrine base. Contains epinephrine bitartrate 7.0 mg per cc. Also contains: Cetylpyridinium chloride, dichlorodifluoromethane, dichlorotetrafluoroethane, sorbitan trioleate, trichloromonofluoromethane. Contains no sulfites.

Indication: Provides temporary relief of shortness of breath, tightness of chest, and wheezing due to bronchial asthma.

Warnings: FOR ORAL INHALATION ONLY. Do not use this product unless a diagnosis of asthma has been made by a doctor, or if you have heart disease, high blood pressure, thyroid disease, diabetes, or difficulty in urination due to enlargement of the prostate gland, if you have ever been hospitalized for asthma or if you are taking any prescription drug for

asthma. **Do not use this product more frequently or at higher doses than recommended, unless directed by a doctor.** Keep this and all drugs out of the reach of children. In case of accidental overdose, seek professional assistance or contact a poison control center immediately. As with any drug, if you are pregnant or nursing a baby, seek the advice of a health professional before using this product.

Excessive use may cause nervousness and rapid heart beat, and, possibly, adverse effects on the heart. **Do not continue to use this product, but seek medical assistance immediately if symptoms are not relieved within 20 minutes or become worse.**

Drug Interaction Precaution: Do not use this product if you are presently taking a prescription drug for high blood pressure or depression, without first consulting your doctor.

Warning: Avoid spraying in eyes. Contents under pressure. Do not break or incinerate. Using or storing near open flame or heating above 120°F may cause bursting.

Administration:
1. SHAKE WELL.
2. HOLD INHALER WITH NOZZLE DOWN WHILE USING. Empty the lungs as completely as possible by exhaling.
3. Purse the lips as in saying the letter "O" and hold the nozzle up to the lips, keeping the tongue flat. As you start to take a deep breath, squeeze nozzle and can together, releasing one full application. Complete taking deep breath, drawing medication into your lungs.
4. Hold breath for as long as comfortable. This distributes the medication in the lungs. Then exhale slowly keeping the lips nearly closed.
5. Rinse nozzle daily with soap and hot water after removing from vial. Dry with clean cloth.

Before each use, remove dust cap and inspect mouthpiece for foreign objects. Replace dust cap after each use.

Dosage: Inhalation dosage for adults and children 4 years of age and older. Start with one inhalation, then wait at least one (1) minute. If not relieved, use once more. Do not use again for at least 3 hours. The use of this product by children should be supervised by an adult. Children under 4 years of age; consult a doctor.

Professional Labeling: Same as stated under Indication.

How Supplied:
⅓ fl oz (10 cc) pocketsize aerosol inhaler, NDC 0024-4082-10 with actuator.

BRONKAID® Tablets

Description: Each tablet contains ephedrine sulfate 24 mg, guaifenesin (glyceryl guaiacolate) 100 mg, and theophylline 100 mg. Also contains: magnesium stearate, magnesium trisilicate, microcrystalline cellulose, starch.

Indication: For symptomatic control of bronchial congestion and bronchial asthma. Clears bronchial passages. Helps relieve shortness of breath, plus helps loosen phlegm.

Precautions: Do not use this product unless a diagnosis of asthma has been made by a doctor, or if you have heart disease, diabetes, difficulty in urination due to enlargement of the prostate gland, if you have ever been hospitalized for asthma or if you are taking any prescription drug for asthma unless directed by a doctor, do not continue to use this product, but seek medical assistance immediately if symptoms are not relieved within an hour or become worse. Some users of this product may experience nervousness, tremor, sleeplessness, nausea, and loss of appetite. If these symptoms persist or become worse, consult your doctor. Do not use this product if you are presently taking a prescription drug for high blood pressure or depression. Do not exceed recommended dosage unless directed by a physician.

Warnings: As with any drug, if you are pregnant or nursing a baby, seek the advice of a health professional before using this product. Keep this and all drugs out of the reach of children. In case of accidental overdose, seek professional assistance or contact a poison control center immediately.

Dosage and Administration: *Adult Dosage:* 1 tablet every four hours. Do not take more than 5 tablets in a 24-hour period. Swallow tablets whole with water. *Children under 12 years of age:* Consult a doctor. *Morning Dose:* An early dose of 1 tablet (for adults) can relieve the coughing and wheezing caused by the night's accumulation of mucus, and can help you start the day with better breathing capacity. *Before an Attack:* Many persons feel an attack of asthma coming on. One BRONKAID tablet beforehand may stop the attack before it starts. *During the Day:* The precise dose of BRONKAID tablets can be varied to meet your individual needs as you gain experience with this product. It is advisable to take 1 tablet before going to bed, for nighttime relief. However, be sure not to exceed recommended daily dosage.

How Supplied:
Boxes of 24 NDC 0024-4081-02.
Boxes of 60 NDC 0024-4081-06.

Shown in Product Identification Section, page 438

CAMPHO-PHENIQUE®
[kam 'fo-finēk]
COLD SORE GEL

Description: Contains phenol 4.7% (w/w) and camphor 10.8% (w/w). Also contains: Colloidal silicon dioxide, eucalyptus oil, glycerin, light mineral oil.

Actions: Use at the first sign of cold sore, fever blister and sun blister symptoms (tingling, pain, itching).

Indications: For relief of pain and itching due to cold sores, fever blisters and sun blisters. To combat infection from minor injuries and skin lesions.

Also effective for:

Minor skin injuries: abrasions, cuts, scrapes, burns, razor nicks and chafed or irritated skin.

Insect bites: mosquitoes, black flies, sandfleas, chiggers.

Warnings: Not for prolonged use. Not to be used on large areas. In case of deep or puncture wounds, serious burns, or persisting redness, swelling or pain, or if rash or infection develops, discontinue use and consult physician. Do not bandage if applied to fingers or toes.

Avoid using near eyes. If product gets into the eye, flush thoroughly with water and obtain medical attention. Keep this and all drugs out of the reach of children. In case of accidental ingestion, seek professional assistance or contact a poison control center immediately.

Directions for Use: For external use. Apply directly to cold sore, fever blister or injury three or four times a day.

How Supplied: Tubes of 0.23 oz (6.5 g) NDC 0024-0212-01 and 0.50 oz (14 g) NDC 0024-0212-02.

Shown in Product Identification Section, page 438

CAMPHO-PHENIQUE® Liquid
[kam'fo-finēk]

Description: Contains phenol 4.7% (w/w) and camphor 10.8% (w/w). Also contains: Eucalyptus oil, light mineral oil.

Actions: Pain-relieving antiseptic for scrapes, cuts, burns, insect bites, fever blisters, and cold sores.

Indications: For relief of pain and to combat infection from minor injuries and skin lesions.

Warnings: Not for prolonged use. Not to be used on large areas or in or near the eyes. In case of deep or puncture wounds, serious burns, or persisting redness, swelling or pain, or if rash or infection develops, discontinue use and consult physician. Do not bandage if applied to fingers or toes.

Keep this and all drugs out of the reach of children. In case of accidental ingestion, seek professional assistance or contact a poison control center immediately.

Directions for Use: For external use. Apply with cotton three or four times daily.

4 oz size only: Do not use more than ½ the contents of the 4 fl oz bottle in any 24-hour period.

How Supplied:
Bottles of ¾ fl oz   (NDC 0024-5150-05)
        1 ½ fl oz   (NDC 0024-5150-06)
        4 fl oz   (NDC 0024-5150-04)
Shown in Product Identification Section, page 438

CAMPHO-PHENIQUE™
[kam'fo-finēk]
TRIPLE ANTIBIOTIC OINTMENT PLUS PAIN RELIEVER

Description: Contains bacitracin zinc 500 units, neomycin sulfate 5 mg (equiv to 3.5 mg neomycin base), polymyxin B sulfate 5000 units, lidocaine HCl 40 mg (Pain Reliever). Also contains white petrolatum.

Actions: Pain-relieving triple antibiotic with anesthetic to help prevent infection in minor cuts, scrapes, burns and other minor wounds.

Indications: Helps prevent infections in minor cuts, burns, and other minor wounds. Provides soothing, nonstinging temporary relief of pain and itching associated with these conditions.

Warnings: For external use only. In case of deep or puncture wounds, animal bites or serious burns, consult physician. If redness, irritation, swelling or pain persists or increases, or if infection occurs, discontinue use and consult physician. Do not use in eyes or over large areas. Keep this and all drugs out of children's reach. In case of accidental ingestion seek professional assistance or contact a poison control center immediately.

Directions: Apply directly to the affected area and cover with a sterile gauze if necessary. May be applied 1 to 3 times daily as the condition indicates.

How Supplied: Tubes of 0.50 oz (NDC 0024-2015-05) and 1.0 oz (NDC 0024-2015-01).

Shown in Product Identification Section, page 438

FERGON® TABLETS
[fur-gone]
brand of ferrous gluconate
FERGON® ELIXIR

Composition: FERGON (ferrous gluconate, USP) is stabilized to maintain a minimum of ferric ions. It contains not less than 11.5 percent iron.

Each FERGON tablet contains 320 mg (5 grains) ferrous gluconate equal to approximately 36 mg ferrous iron. Also contains: acacia, carnauba wax, dextrose excipient, FD&C Red No. 40, D & C Yellow No. 10, FD & C Blue No. 1, gelatin, kaolin, magnesium stearate, parabens, povidone, precipitated calcium carbonate, sodium benzoate, starch, sucrose, talc, titanium dioxide, yellow wax. Not USP for dissolution.

FERGON Elixir contains: ferrous gluconate 6%. Also contains: alcohol 7%, flavor, glycerin, liquid glucose, purified water, saccharin sodium. Each teaspoon (5 mL) contains 300 mg (5 grains) ferrous gluconate equivalent to approximately 34 mg ferrous iron.

Action and Uses: FERGON preparations produce rapid hemoglobin regeneration in patients with iron-deficiency anemias. FERGON is better utilized and better tolerated than other forms of iron because of its low ionization constant and solubility in the entire pH range of the gastrointestinal tract. It does not precipitate proteins or have the astringency of more ionizable forms of iron, does not interfere with proteolytic or diastatic activities of the digestive system, and will not produce nausea, abdominal cramps, constipation or diarrhea in the great majority of patients.

FERGON preparations are for use in the prevention and treatment of iron deficiency. They should be taken when the need for iron supplement therapy has been determined by a physician.

Warnings: Since oral iron products interfere with absorption of oral tetracycline antibiotics, these products should not be taken within two hours of each other. Keep this and all drugs out of the reach of children. As with any drug, if you are pregnant or nursing a baby, seek the advice of a health professional before using this product. In case of accidental overdose, seek professional assistance or contact a poison control center immediately.

Dosage and Administration: *Adults* —One to two FERGON tablets or one to two teaspoonfuls of FERGON Elixir daily. *For children and infants,* as prescribed by physician.

How Supplied: FERGON Tablets of 320 mg (5 grains) bottle of 100 (NDC 0024-1015-10), bottle of 500 (NDC 0024-1015-50), and bottle of 1,000 (NDC 0024-1015-00). FERGON Elixir, 6% (5 grains per teaspoonful) bottle of 1 pint (NDC 0024-1019-16).
Shown in Product Indentification Section, page 438

NāSal™
Saline (buffered)
0.65% Sodium chloride
Nasal Spray
Nose Drops

Description: Both the nasal spray and nose drops contain sodium chloride 0.65%. Also contains: benzalkonium chloride and thimerosal 0.001% as preservative, mono- and dibasic sodium phosphates as buffers, purified water. **Contains No Alcohol.**

Actions: Immediate relief for dry nose. Formulated to match the pH of normal nasal secretions to help prevent stinging or burning.

Indications: Provides soothing relief for clogged nasal passages—without stinging or burning. Provides immediate relief for dry, inflamed nasal membranes due to colds, low humidity, allergies, minor nose bleeds, overuse of topical nasal decongestants, and other nasal irrita-

Continued on next page

This product information was effective as of November 1, 1989. Current information may be obtained directly from Winthrop Consumer Products, Division of Sterling Drug Inc., by writing to 90 Park Avenue, New York, NY 10016.

Winthrop Consumer—Cont.

tions. As an ideal nasal moisturizer, it can be used in conjunction with oral decongestants.

Adverse Reactions: No associated side effects.

Warnings: Keep this and all drugs out of the reach of children. In case of accidental ingestion seek professional assistance or contact a poison control center immediately. The use of the dispenser by more than one person may spread infection.

Dosage and Administration: *Spray* — For adults and children six years of age and over: with head upright, spray twice in each nostril as needed or as directed by physician. To spray, squeeze bottle quickly and firmly. *Nose Drops* —For infants and adults: 2 to 6 drops in each nostril as needed or as directed by physician.

How Supplied: Nasal Spray—plastic squeeze bottles of 15 mL (½ fl oz) NDC 0024-1316-01.
Nose Drops—MonoDrop® bottles of 15 mL (½ fl oz) NDC 0024-1315-01.
Shown in Product Identification Section, page 438

NEO-SYNEPHRINE®
phenylephrine hydrochloride

Description: This line of Nasal Spray, Nose Drops and Nasal Spray Pumps contains phenylephrine hydrochloride in strengths ranging from 0.125% (drops only) to 1%. Also contains: benzalkonium chloride and thimerosal 0.001% as preservatives, citric acid, purified water, sodium chloride, sodium citrate.

Action: Rapid-acting nasal decongestant.

Indications: For temporary relief of nasal congestion due to common cold, hay fever or other upper respiratory allergies, or associated with sinusitis.

Precautions: Some hypersensitive individuals may experience a mild stinging sensation. This is usually transient and often disappears after a few applications. Do not exceed recommended dosage. Follow directions for use carefully. If symptoms are not relieved after several applications, a physician should be consulted. Frequent and continued usage of the higher concentrations (especially the 1% solution) occasionally may cause a rebound congestion of the nose. Therefore, long-term or frequent use of this solution is not recommended without the advice of a physician.
Prolonged exposure to air or strong light will cause oxidation and some loss of potency. Do not use if brown in color or contains a precipitate.

Adverse Reactions: Generally very well tolerated; systemic side effects such as tremor, insomnia, or palpitation rarely occur.

Warnings: Keep these and all drugs out of the reach of children. In case of accidental ingestion seek professional assis-

tance or contact a poison control center immediately. The use of the dispenser by more than one person may spread infection.
Do not use this product if you have heart disease, high blood pressure, thyroid disease, diabetes, or difficulty in urination due to enlargement of the prostate gland unless directed by a doctor.

Dosage and Administration: *Topical* —dropper or spray. The *0.25% solution is adequate in most cases (0.125% for children 2 to 6 years)*. In resistant cases, or if more powerful decongestion is desired, the *0.5% or 1% solution* should be used. Also used as *0.5% jelly*.

How Supplied: Nasal spray 0.25%—15 mL (for children and for adults who prefer a mild nasal spray)—NDC 0024-1348-03; nasal spray 0.5%—15 mL (for adults)—NDC 0024-1353-01 and 30 mL (1 fl oz) NDC 0024-1353-05; nasal spray 1%—15 mL (extra strength for adults)—NDC 0024-1352-02; nasal spray pump 0.5%—15 mL bottle (½ fl oz) NDC 0024-1353-04; nasal solution 0.125% (for infants and small children), 15 mL bottles—NDC 0024-1345-05; nasal solution 0.25% (for children and adults who prefer a mild solution), 15 mL bottles—NDC 0024-1347-05; nasal solution 0.5% (for adults), 15 mL bottles—NDC 0024-1351-05; nasal solution 1% (extra strength for adults), 15 mL bottles—NDC 0024-1355-05; and 16 fl oz bottles—NDC 0024-1355-06; and water soluble nasal jelly 0.5%, ⅝ oz tubes—NDC 0024-1367-01.
Shown in Product Identification Section, page 438

NEO-SYNEPHRINE® 12 HOUR
oxymetazoline hydrochloride
Nasal Spray 0.05%
Vapor Nasal Spray 0.05%
Nose Drops 0.05%

Description: *Adult Strength Nasal Spray* and *Nose Drops* and *Nasal Spray Pump* contain: Oxymetazoline Hydrochloride 0.05%. Also contain: Benzalkonium Chloride and Phenylmercuric Acetate 0.002% as preservatives, Glycine, Purified Water, Sorbitol, may also contain Sodium Chloride. *Adult Strength Vapor Nasal Spray* contains Oxymetazoline Hydrochloride 0.05%. Also contains: Benzalkonium Chloride and Thimerosal 0.001% as preservatives, Camphor, Citric Acid, Eucalyptol, Menthol, Methyl Salicylate, Purified Water, Sodium Chloride, Sodium Citrate, Tyloxapol.

Action: 12 HOUR Nasal Decongestant.

Indications: Provides temporary relief, for up to 12 HOURS, of nasal congestion due to colds, hay fever, sinusitis, or allergies. NEO-SYNEPHRINE 12-HOUR Nasal Sprays, Nose Drops and Nasal Spray Pump contain oxymetazoline which provides the longest-lasting relief of nasal congestion available.

Warnings: Do not exceed recommended dosage because symptoms may occur such as burning, stinging, sneezing, or increase of nasal discharge. Nasal Spray

0.05%, Vapor Nasal Spray 0.05%, Nasal Spray Pump 0.05%, Nose Drops 0.05% not recommended for children under 6. Do not use these products for more than 3 days. If symptoms persist, consult a physician. The use of the dispenser by more than one person may spread infection.
Do not use this product if you have heart disease, high blood pressure, thyroid disease, diabetes, or difficulty in urination due to enlargement of the prostate gland unless directed by a doctor.
Keep this and all drugs out of the reach of children. In case of accidental ingestion, seek professional assistance or contact a poison control center immediately.

Dosage and Administration: *Adult Strength Nasal Spray and Vapor Nasal Spray* —For adults and children 6 years of age and over: With head upright, spray two or three times in each nostril twice daily—morning and evening. To spray, squeeze bottle quickly and firmly.
Nasal Spray Pump —For adults and children 6 to under 12 years of age (with adult supervision): spray 2 or 3 times in each nostril daily—morning and evening. Do not exceed 2 applications in any 24 hour period. Children under 6 years of age: consult a doctor. Hold bottle with thumb at base and nozzle between first and second fingers. With head upright insert spray nozzle in nostril. Depress pump 2 or 3 times, all the way down, with a firm even stroke and sniff deeply. Repeat in other nostril. Do not tilt head backward while spraying.
Adult Strength Nose Drops —For adults and children 6 years of age and over: two or three drops in each nostril twice daily—morning and evening.

How Supplied: *Nasal Spray Adult Strength* —plastic squeeze bottles of 15 ml (½ fl oz) NDC 0024-1390-03 and 30 ml (1 fl oz) NDC 0024-1394-01; Nasal Spray Pump—15 ml bottle (½ fl oz) NDC 0024-1389-01; *Vapor Nasal Spray Adult Strength* —squeeze bottles of 15 ml (½ fl oz) NDC 0024-1391-03; *Nose Drops Adult Strength* —bottles of 15 ml (½ fl oz) with dropper NDC 0024-1392-01.
Shown in Product Identification Section, page 438

NTZ®
Long Acting
Oxymetazoline hydrochloride
Nasal Spray 0.05%
Nose Drops 0.05%

Description: Both the nasal spray and nose drops contain Oxymetazoline Hydrochloride 0.05%. Also contain: Benzalkonium Chloride and Phenylmercuric Acetate 0.002% as preservatives, Glycine, Purified Water, Sorbitol, and may also contain Sodium Chloride.

Actions: 12 Hour Nasal Decongestant.

Indications: Provides temporary relief, for up to 12 hours, of nasal congestion due to colds, hay fever, sinusitis, or allergies. Oxymetazoline hydrochloride provides the longest-lasting relief of nasal congestion available. It decongests nasal passages up to 12 hours, reduces swelling of nasal passages, and temporarily restores freer breathing through the nose.

Warnings: Not recommended for children under six. Do not exceed recommended dosage because symptoms may occur such as burning, stinging, sneezing, or increase of nasal discharge. Do not use these products for more than 3 days. If symptoms persist, consult a physician. The use of the dispenser by more than one person may spread infection. Do not use this product if you have heart disease, high blood pressure, thyroid disease, diabetes, or difficulty in urination due to enlargement of the prostate gland unless directed by a doctor. Keep these and all drugs out of the reach of children. In case of accidental ingestion seek professional assistance or contact a poison control center immediately.

Dosage and Administration: Intranasally by spray and dropper. *Nasal Spray*—For adults and children 6 years of age and over: With head upright, spray 2 or 3 times in each nostril twice daily—morning and evening. To spray, squeeze bottle quickly and firmly. *Nose Drops* —For adults and children 6 years of age and over: 2 or 3 drops in each nostril twice daily—morning and evening.

How Supplied: *Nasal Spray* —plastic squeeze bottles of 15 ml (½ fl. oz.) NDC 0024-1312-02. *Nose Drops* —bottles of 15 ml (½ fl. oz.) with dropper NDC 0024-1311-03.

pHisoDerm®
[fi-zo-derm]
Skin Cleanser and Conditioner

Description: pHisoDerm, a nonsoap emollient skin cleanser, is a unique liquid emulsion containing sodium octoxynol-2 ethane sulfonate solution, water, petrolatum, octoxynol-3, mineral oil (with lanolin alcohol and oleyl alcohol), cocamide MEA, imidazolidinyl urea, sodium benzoate, tetrasodium EDTA, and methylcellulose. Adjusted to normal skin pH with hydrochloric acid. Contains no hexachlorophene. pHisoDerm contains no soap, perfumes, or irritating alkali. Its pH value, unlike that of soap, lies within the pH range of normal skin.

Actions: pHisoDerm is well tolerated and can be used frequently by those persons whose skin may be irritated by the use of soap or other alkaline cleansers, or by those who are sensitive to the fatty acids contained in soap. pHisoDerm contains an effective detergent for removing soil and acts as an active emulsifier of all types of oil—animal, vegetable, and mineral.

pHisoDerm produces suds when used with any kind of water—hard or soft, hot or cold (even cold seawater)—at any temperature and under acid, alkaline, or neutral conditions.

pHisoDerm deposits a fine film of lanolin components and petrolatum on the skin during the washing process and, thereby, helps protect against the dryness that soap can cause.

Indications: A sudsing emollient cleanser for use on skin of infants, children, and adults.

Useful for removal of ointments and cosmetics from the skin.

Directions: For external use only.
HANDS. Squeeze a few drops of pHisoDerm into the palm, add a little water, and work up a lather. Rinse thoroughly.
FACE. After washing your hands, squeeze a small amount of pHisoDerm into the palm or onto a small sponge or washcloth, and work up a lather by adding a little water. Massage the suds onto the face for approximately one minute. Rinse thoroughly. Avoid getting suds into the eyes.
BATHING. First wet the body. Work a small amount of pHisoDerm into a lather with hands or a soft wet sponge, gradually adding small amounts of water to make more lather. Rinse thoroughly.

Caution: pHisoDerm suds that get into the eyes accidentally during washing should be rinsed out promptly with a sufficient amount of water.

pHisoDerm is intended for external use only. pHisoDerm should not be poured into measuring cups, medicine bottles, or similar containers since it may be mistaken for baby formula or medications. If swallowed, pHisoDerm may cause gastrointestinal irritation.

pHisoDerm should not be used on persons with sensitivity to any of its components.

How Supplied: pHisoDerm is supplied in two formulations for regular and oily skin. It is packaged in sanitary squeeze bottles of 5 and 16 ounces. The regular formula is also supplied in squeeze bottles of 9 ounces and plastic bottles of 1 gallon.
Shown in Product Identification Section, page 438

pHisoDerm® FOR BABY
[fi'zo-derm]
Skin Cleanser

Description: pHisoDerm FOR BABY, a nonsoap emollient skin cleanser, is a unique liquid emulsion containing sodium octoxynol-2 ethane sulfonate solution, water, petrolatum, octoxynol-3, mineral oil (with lanolin alcohol and oleyl alcohol), cocamide MEA, fragrance, imidazolidinyl urea, sodium benzoate, tetrasodium EDTA, and methylcellulose. Adjusted to normal skin pH with hydrochloric acid. Contains no hexachlorophene or irritating alkali. Its pH value, unlike that of soap, lies within the pH range of normal skin.

Actions: pHisoDerm FOR BABY gently cleans babies' delicate skin without irritating. Petrolatum and lanolin leave skin soft and smooth and protect against dryness.

pHisoDerm FOR BABY rinses easily without leaving a soapy film. The powder fragrance leaves skin smelling fresh and clean.

Precautions: pHisoDerm FOR BABY suds that get into babies' eyes accidentally during washing should be rinsed out promptly with a sufficient amount of water.

pHisoDerm FOR BABY is intended for external use only. It should not be poured into measuring cups, medicine bottles, or similar containers since it may be mistaken for baby formula or medications. If swallowed, pHisoDerm FOR BABY may cause gastrointestinal irritation.

pHisoDerm FOR BABY should not be used on babies with sensitivity to any of its components.

Administration: First wet the baby's body. Work a small amount of pHisoDerm FOR BABY into a lather with hands or a soft wet sponge, gradually adding small amounts of water to make more lather. Spread the lather over all parts of the baby's body, including the head. Avoid getting suds into the baby's eyes. Wash the diaper area last. Be sure to carefully cleanse all folds and creases. Rinse thoroughly. Pat the baby dry with a soft towel.

How Supplied: pHisoDerm FOR BABY is packaged in soft plastic, sanitary, squeeze bottles of 5 and 9 ounces and can be opened and closed with one hand.
Shown in Product Identification Section, page 438

pHisoPUFF®
[fi-zo-puf]
Nonmedicated Cleansing Sponge

Description: pHisoPUFF is a nonmedicated cleansing sponge with a special dual layer construction combining a white polyester fiber side and a green sponge side.

Actions: pHisoPUFF cleanses two ways: (1) white fiber side for extra thorough cleansing to gently remove the top layer of dead skin cells, free dirt, debris, and oil trapped in this layer and reveal new, fresh skin cells and (2) green sponge side works to cleanse and rinse skin clean. Using this side will help apply your cleanser or soap more evenly. Also good for removing eye makeup.

Precautions: Do not use pHisoPUFF fiber side on skin that is irritated, sunburned, windburned, damaged, broken, or infected. Do not use on skin which is prone to rashes or itching.

Administration: For the green sponge side: Wet pHisoPUFF with warm water, apply pHisoDerm® or another skin cleanser of your choice, and develop a lather. Glide sponge over your face up and down, back and forth, or in a circle;

Continued on next page

This product information was effective as of November 1, 1989. Current information may be obtained directly from Winthrop Consumer Products, Division of Sterling Drug Inc., by writing to 90 Park Avenue, New York, NY 10016.

Winthrop Consumer—Cont.

whatever is the easiest for you. Rinse face and dry.

For the white fiber side: Wet pHisoPUFF with warm water, apply pHisoDerm or another skin cleanser of your choice, and develop a lather. Try pHisoPUFF on the back of your hand before using it on your face. Experiment by changing the pressure and speed with which you move it. Now move pHisoPUFF gently and slowly over your face. Use no more than a few seconds on each area. You can move it in any direction, whichever comes natural to you. Rinse face and dry. As you use this fiber side more often, usage and pressure may be increased to best fit your skin sensitivity. Always rinse your pHisoPUFF thoroughly each time you use it. Hold under running water, let it drain, then give it a few quick shakes.

How Supplied: Box of 1 pHisoPUFF.
Shown in Product Identification Section, page 438

WinGel®
[win 'jel]
Liquid and Tablets

Description: Each teaspoon (5 mL) of liquid contains a specially processed, short polymer, hexitol-stabilized aluminum-magnesium hydroxide equivalent to 180 mg of aluminum hydroxide and 160 mg of magnesium hydroxide. Also contains: benzoic acid, flavor, methylcellulose, purified water, red ferric oxide, saccharin sodium, sodium hypochlorite solution, sorbitol solution.

Each tablet contains a specially processed, short polymer, hexitol-stabilized aluminum-magnesium hydroxide equivalent to 180 mg of aluminum hydroxide and 160 mg of magnesium hydroxide. Also contains: D&C Red No. 28, FD&C Red No. 40, flavor, magnesium stearate, mannitol, saccharin sodium, starch. Smooth, easy-to-chew tablets.

Action: Antacid.

Indications: An antacid for the relief of acid indigestion, heartburn, and sour stomach. Nonconstipating. For the symptomatic relief of hyperacidity associated with the diagnosis of peptic ulcer, gastritis, peptic esophagitis, gastric hyperacidity, and hiatal hernia.

Warnings: *Adults and children over 6*—Patients should not take more than eight teaspoonfuls or eight tablets in a 24-hour period or use the maximum dosage of the product for more than 2 weeks, except under the advice and supervision of a physician.
Keep this and all drugs out of the reach of children. In case of accidental overdose, seek professional assistance or contact a poison control center immediately.

Drug Interaction Precautions: Antacids may react with certain prescription drugs. Do not take this product if you are presently taking a prescription antibiotic drug containing any form of tetracycline. If the patient is presently taking a pre-

scription drug, this product should not be taken without checking with the physician.

Dosage and Administration: *Adults and children over 6*—1 to 2 teaspoonfuls or 1 to 2 tablets up to four times daily, or as directed by a physician.
Acid Neutralization: The acid neutralization capacity of WinGel liquid and tablets is not less than 10 mEq/5 ml.

How Supplied:
Liquid—bottles of 6 fl oz (NDC 0024-2247-03) and 12 fl oz (NDC 0024-2247-05).
Tablets—boxes of 50 (NDC 0024-2249-05) and 100 (NDC 0024-2249-06).

Winthrop Pharmaceuticals
**90 PARK AVENUE
NEW YORK, NY 10016**

BRONKOLIXIR®
Bronchodilator • Decongestant

Description: Each 5 mL teaspoonful contains:
Ephedrine sulfate, USP ....12 mg
Guaifenesin, USP ....50 mg
Theophylline, USP ....15 mg
Phenobarbital, USP..........................4 mg
(Warning: May be habit forming.)
Also contains: Alcohol 19% (v/v), FD&C Red #40, Flavors, Glycerin, Purified Water, Saccharin Sodium, Sodium Chloride, Sodium Citrate, Sucrose.

Indications: For symptomatic control of bronchial asthma. BRONKOLIXIR is also helpful in overcoming the nonproductive cough often associated with bronchitis or colds.

Warnings: Frequent or prolonged use may cause nervousness, restlessness, or sleeplessness. Phenobarbital may cause drowsiness. Do not use if high blood pressure, heart disease, diabetes, or thyroid disease is present, unless directed by a physician. Ephedrine may cause urinary retention, especially in the presence of partial obstruction, as in prostatism. Keep this and all drugs out of the reach of children. In case of accidental overdose, seek professional assistance or contact a poison control center immediately. As with any drug, if you are pregnant or nursing a baby, seek the advice of a health professional before using this product.

Dosage: *Adults*—2 teaspoons every three or four hours, not to exceed four times daily. *Children*—over six—one half the adult dose; under six—as directed by physician.

How Supplied: Bottle of 16 fl oz (NDC 0024-1004-16)

BRONKOTABS®
Bronchodilator • Decongestant

Description: Each tablet contains ephedrine sulfate, USP, 24 mg; guaifenesin, USP, 100 mg; theophylline, USP, 100 mg; phenobarbital, USP, 8 mg. (Warning: May be habit forming.)

Also contains: Magnesium Stearate, Magnesium Trisilicate, Microcrystalline Cellulose, Starch.

Indications: For symptomatic control of bronchial asthma.

Warnings: Frequent or prolonged use may cause nervousness, restlessness, or sleeplessness. Phenobarbital may cause drowsiness. Do not use if high blood pressure, heart disease, diabetes, or thyroid disease is present unless directed by a physician. Ephedrine may cause urinary retention, especially in the presence of partial obstruction, as in prostatism. Keep this and all drugs out of the reach of children. In case of accidental overdose, seek professional assistance or contact a poison control center immediately. As with any drug, if you are pregnant or nursing a baby, seek the advice of a health professional before using this product.

Dosage: *Adults*—1 tablet every three or four hours, four to five times daily. *Children:* over six—one half the adult dose; under six—as directed by physician.

How Supplied: Bottle of 100 (NDC 0024-1006-10)
Bottle of 1000 (NDC 0024-1006-10)

DRISDOL®
**brand of ergocalciferol oral solution, USP (in propylene glycol)
Vitamin D Supplement**

Description: 200 International Units (5 μg) per drop. The dropper supplied delivers 40 drops per mL.

Indication: For the prevention of vitamin D deficiency in infants, children, and adults.

Warnings: Keep this and all drugs out of the reach of children. In case of accidental overdose, seek professional assistance or contact a poison control center immediately.

Dosage: 2 drops daily. This dose provides the US Recommended Daily Allowance for vitamin D for infants, children, and adults.

How Supplied: Bottles of 2 fl oz (NDC 0024-0391-02)

pHisoDerm
(See Winthrop Consumer Products.)

ZEPHIRAN® CHLORIDE
**brand of benzalkonium chloride
ANTISEPTIC**
AQUEOUS SOLUTION 1:750
TINTED TINCTURE 1:750
SPRAY—TINTED TINCTURE 1:750

Description: ZEPHIRAN Chloride, brand of benzalkonium chloride, NF, a mixture of alkylbenzyldimethylammonium chlorides, is a cationic quaternary ammonium surface-acting agent. It is very soluble in water, alcohol, and acetone. Aqueous solutions of ZEPHIRAN Chloride are neutral to slightly alkaline, generally colorless, and nonstaining.

They have a bitter taste, aromatic odor, and foam when shaken. ZEPHIRAN Chloride Tinted Tincture 1:750 contains alcohol 50 percent and acetone 10 percent by volume. ZEPHIRAN Chloride Spray—Tinted Tincture 1:750 contains alcohol 92 percent. The Tinted Tincture and Spray also contain an orange-red coloring agent.

Clinical Pharmacology: ZEPHIRAN Chloride solutions are rapidly acting anti-infective agents with a moderately long duration of action. They are active against bacteria and some viruses, fungi, and protozoa. Bacterial spores are considered to be resistant. Solutions are bacteriostatic or bactericidal according to their concentration. The exact mechanism of bactericidal action is unknown but is thought to be due to enzyme inactivation. Activity generally increases with increasing temperature and pH. Gram-positive bacteria are more susceptible than gram-negative bacteria (TABLE 1).

TABLE 1

Highest Dilution of ZEPHIRAN Chloride Aqueous Solution Destroying the Organism in 10 but not in 5 Minutes

Organisms	20°C
Streptococcus pyogenes	1:75,000
Staphylococcus aureus	1:52,500
Salmonella typhosa	1:37,500
Escherichia coli	1:10,500

Pseudomonas is the most resistant gram-negative genus. Using the AOAC Use-Dilution Confirmation Method, no growth was obtained when *Staphylococcus aureus*, *Salmonella choleraesuis*, and *Pseudomonas aeruginosa* (strain PRD-10) were exposed for ten minutes at 20°C to ZEPHIRAN Chloride Aqueous Solution 1:750 and Tinted Tincture 1:750. ZEPHIRAN Chloride Aqueous Solution 1:750 has been shown to retain its bactericidal activity following autoclaving for 30 minutes at 15 lb pressure, freezing, and then thawing.

The tubercle bacillus may be resistant to aqueous ZEPHIRAN Chloride solutions but is susceptible to the 1:750 tincture (AOAC Method, 10 minutes at 20°C). ZEPHIRAN Chloride solutions also demonstrate deodorant, wetting, detergent, keratolytic, and emulsifying activity.

Indications and Usage: ZEPHIRAN Chloride aqueous solutions in appropriate dilutions (see Recommended Dilutions) are indicated for the antisepsis of skin, mucous membranes, and wounds. They are used for preoperative preparation of the skin, surgeons' hand and arm soaks, treatment of wounds, preservation of ophthalmic solutions, irrigations of the eye, body cavities, bladder, urethra, and vaginal douching. ZEPHIRAN Chloride Tinted Tincture 1:750 and Spray are indicated for preoperative preparation of the skin and for treatment of minor skin wounds and abrasions.

Contraindication: The use of ZEPHIRAN Chloride solutions in occlusive dressings, casts, and anal or vaginal packs is inadvisable, as they may produce irritation or chemical burns.

Warnings: Sterile Water for Injection, USP, should be used as diluent in preparing diluted aqueous solutions intended for use on deep wounds or for irrigation of body cavities. Otherwise, freshly distilled water should be used. Tap water, containing metallic ions and organic matter, may reduce antibacterial potency. Resin deionized water should not be used since it may contain pathogenic bacteria.

Organic, inorganic, and synthetic materials and surfaces may adsorb sufficient quantities of ZEPHIRAN Chloride to significantly reduce its antibacterial potency in solutions. This has resulted in serious contamination of solutions of ZEPHIRAN Chloride with viable pathogenic bacteria. Solutions should not be stored in bottles stoppered with cork closures, but rather in those equipped with appropriate screw-caps. Cotton, wool, rayon, and other materials should not be stored in ZEPHIRAN Chloride solutions. Gauze sponges and fiber pledgets used to apply solutions of ZEPHIRAN Chloride to the skin should be sterilized and stored in separate containers. Only immediately prior to application should they be immersed in ZEPHIRAN Chloride solutions.

Since ZEPHIRAN Chloride solutions are inactivated by soaps and anionic detergents, thorough rinsing is necessary if these agents are employed prior to their use.

Antiseptics such as ZEPHIRAN Chloride solutions must not be relied upon to achieve complete sterilization, because they do not destroy bacterial spores and certain viruses, including the etiologic agent of infectious hepatitis, and may not destroy *Mycobacterium tuberculosis* and other rare bacterial strains.

ZEPHIRAN Chloride Tinted Tincture 1:750 and Spray contain flammable organic solvents and should not be used near an open flame or cautery.

If solutions stronger than 1:3000 enter the eyes, irrigate immediately and repeatedly with water. Prompt medical attention should then be obtained. Concentrations greater than 1:5000 should not be used on mucous membranes, with the exception of the vaginal mucosa (see Recommended Dilutions).

Precautions: In preoperative antisepsis of the skin, ZEPHIRAN Chloride solutions should not be permitted to remain in prolonged contact with the patient's skin. Avoid pooling of the solution on the operating table.

ZEPHIRAN Chloride solutions that are used on inflamed or irritated tissues must be more dilute than those used on normal tissues (see Recommended Dilutions). ZEPHIRAN Chloride Tinted Tincture 1:750 and Spray, which contain irritating organic solvents, should be kept away from the eyes or other mucous membranes.

Preoperative periorbital skin or head prep should be performed only before the patient, or eye, is anesthetized.

Adverse Reactions: ZEPHIRAN chloride solutions in normally used concentrations have low systemic and local toxicity and are generally well tolerated, although a rare individual may exhibit hypersensitivity.

Directions for Use:

General: For most surgical applications, the recommended concentration of ZEPHIRAN Chloride Aqueous Solution or ZEPHIRAN Chloride Tinted Tincture is 1:750 (0.13 percent). Liberal use of the solution is recommended to compensate for any adsorption of ZEPHIRAN Chloride by cotton or other materials.

To use ZEPHIRAN Chloride Spray—Tinted Tincture 1:750, remove protective cap, hold in an UPRIGHT position several inches away from the surgical field or injured area, and apply by spraying freely.

Preoperative preparation of skin: ZEPHIRAN Chloride solutions 1:750 are recommended as an antiseptic for use on unbroken skin in the preoperative preparation of the surgical field. Detergents and soaps should be thoroughly rinsed from the skin before applying ZEPHIRAN Chloride solutions. The detergent action of ZEPHIRAN Chloride solutions, particularly when used alternately with alcohol, leaves the skin smooth and clean. When ZEPHIRAN Chloride solutions are applied by friction (using several changes of sponges), dirt, skin fats, desquamating epithelium, and superficial bacteria are effectively removed, thus exposing the underlying skin to the antiseptic activity of the solutions.

The following procedure has been found satisfactory for preparation of the surgical field. On the day prior to surgery, the operative site is shaved and then scrubbed thoroughly with ZEPHIRAN Chloride Aqueous Solution 1:750. Immediately before surgery, ZEPHIRAN Chloride Tinted Tincture 1:750 or Spray is applied to the site in the usual manner (see Precautions). If the red tinted solution turns yellow during the preparation of patient's skin for surgery, it usually indicates the presence of soap (alkali) residue which is incompatible with ZEPHIRAN solutions. Therefore, rinse thoroughly and reapply the antiseptic. Because ZEPHIRAN Chloride Tinted Tincture 1:750 contains alcohol and acetone, its cleansing action on the skin is particularly effective and it dries more rapidly than the aqueous solution. The Tinted Tincture is recommended when it is desirable to outline the operative site.

Recommended Dilutions: For specific directions, see TABLES 2 and 3.

Continued on next page

This product information was effective as of September 8, 1989. Current detailed information may be obtained directly from Winthrop Pharmaceuticals, Division of Sterling Drug Inc., by writing to 90 Park Avenue, New York NY, 10016.

Winthrop Pharm.—Cont.

TABLE 2
Correct Use of ZEPHIRAN Chloride

ZEPHIRAN Chloride solutions must be prepared, stored, and used correctly to achieve and maintain their antiseptic action. Serious inactivation and contamination of ZEPHIRAN Chloride solutions may occur with misuse.

CORRECT DILUENTS	INCOMPATIBILITIES	PREFERRED FORM
Sterile Water for Injection is recommended for irrigation of body cavities. *Sterile distilled water* is recommended for irrigating traumatized tissue and in the eye. *Freshly distilled water* is recommended for skin antisepsis. *Resin deionized water* should not be used because the deionizing resins can carry pathogens (especially gram-negative bacteria); they also inactivate quaternary ammonium compounds. *Stored water* is not recommended since it may contain many organisms. *Saline* should not be used since it may decrease the antibacterial potency of ZEPHIRAN Chloride solutions.	Anionic detergents and soaps should be thoroughly rinsed from the skin or other areas prior to use of ZEPHIRAN Chloride solutions because they reduce the antibacterial activity of the solutions. Serum and protein material also decrease the activity of ZEPHIRAN Chloride solutions. Corks should not be used to stopper bottles containing ZEPHIRAN Chloride solutions. Fibers of fabrics when stored in ZEPHIRAN Chloride solutions adsorb ZEPHIRAN from the surrounding liquid. Examples are: Cotton Gauze sponges Wool Rayon Rubber materials Applicators or sponges, intended for a skin prep, should be stored separately and dipped in ZEPHIRAN Chloride solutions immediately before use. Under certain circumstances the following commonly encountered substances are incompatible with ZEPHIRAN Chloride solutions: Iodine Aluminum Silver nitrate Caramel Fluorescein Kaolin Nitrates Pine oil Peroxide Zinc sulfate Lanolin Zinc oxide Potassium Yellow oxide permanganate of mercury	ZEPHIRAN Chloride Tinted Tincture 1:750 is recommended for preoperative skin preparation because it contains alcohol and acetone which enhance its cleansing action and promote rapid drying. ZEPHIRAN Chloride Tinted Tincture 1:750, containing acetone, is recommended when it is desirable to outline the operative site. (Aqueous solutions of ZEPHIRAN Chloride used in skin preparation have a tendency to "run off" the skin.) Caution: Because of the flammable organic solvents in ZEPHIRAN Chloride Tinted Tincture 1:750 and Spray, these products should be kept away from open flame or cautery.

Surgery
Preoperative preparation of skin: Aqueous solution 1:750 and Tinted Tincture 1:750 or Spray
Surgeons' hand and arm soaks: Aqueous solution 1:750
Treatment of minor wounds and lacerations: Tinted Tincture 1:750 or Spray
Irrigation of deep infected wounds: Aqueous solution 1:3000 to 1:20,000
Denuded skin and mucous membranes: Aqueous solution 1:5000 to 1:10,000

Obstetrics and Gynecology
Preoperative preparation of skin: Aqueous solution 1:750 and Tinted Tincture 1:750 or Spray
Vaginal douche and irrigation: Aqueous solution 1:2000 to 1:5000
Postepisiotomy care: Aqueous solution 1:5000 to 1:10,000
Breast and nipple hygiene: Aqueous solution 1:1000 to 1:2000

Urology
Bladder and urethral irrigation: Aqueous solution 1:5000 to 1:20,000
Bladder retention lavage: Aqueous solution 1:20,000 to 1:40,000

Dermatology
Oozing and open infections: Aqueous solution 1:2000 to 1:5000
Wet dressings by irrigation or open dressing (Use in occlusive dressings is inadvisable.): Aqueous solution 1:5000 or less

Ophthalmology
Eye irrigation: Aqueous solution 1:5000 to 1:10,000
Preservation of ophthalmic solutions: Aqueous solution 1:5000 to 1:7500
[See table right]

Accidental Ingestion: If ZEPHIRAN Chloride solution, particularly a concentrated solution, is ingested, marked local irritation of the gastrointestinal tract, manifested by nausea and vomiting, may occur. Signs of systemic toxicity include restlessness, apprehension, weakness, confusion, dyspnea, cyanosis, collapse, convulsions, and coma. Death occurs as a result of paralysis of the respiratory muscles.

Treatment: Immediate administration of several glasses of a mild soap solution, milk, or egg whites beaten in water is recommended. This may be followed by

TABLE 3
Dilutions of ZEPHIRAN Chloride Aqueous Solution 1:750

Final Dilution	ZEPHIRAN Chloride Aqueous Solution 1:750 (parts)	Distilled Water (parts)
1:1000	3	1
1:2000	3	5
1:2500	3	7
1:3000	3	9
1:4000	3	13
1:5000	3	17
1:10,000	3	37
1:20,000	3	77
1:40,000	3	157

gastric lavage with a mild soap solution. Alcohol should be avoided as it promotes absorption.

To support respiration, the airway should be clear and oxygen should be administered, employing artificial respiration if necessary. If convulsions occur, a short-acting barbiturate may be given parenterally with caution.

How Supplied:
ZEPHIRAN Chloride Aqueous Solution
1:750
  Bottles of 8 fl oz (NDC 0024-2521-04)
  and 1 gallon (NDC 0024-2521-08)
ZEPHIRAN Chloride Tinted Tincture
1:750 (*flammable*)
  Bottles of 1 gallon (NDC 0024-2523-08)
ZEPHIRAN Chloride Spray—Tinted
Tincture 1:750 (*flammable*)
  Bottles of 1 fl oz (NDC 0024-2527-01)
  and 6 fl oz (NDC 0024-2527-03)
                                ZW-83-H

---

*This product information was effec-
tive as of January 1, 1989. Current
detailed information may be obtained
directly from Winthrop Pharmaceuticals, Division of Sterling Drug Inc., by
writing to 90 Park Avenue, New
York, NY 10016.*

Wyeth-Ayerst
Laboratories
**Division of American Home
Products Corporation
P.O. BOX 8299
PHILADELPHIA, PA 19101**

Wyeth-Ayerst
Tamper-Resistant/Evident
Packaging

Statements alerting consumers to the
specific type of Tamper-Resistant/Evi-
dent Packaging appear on the bottle labels and cartons of all Wyeth-Ayerst
over-the-counter products. This includes
plastic cap seals on bottles, individually
wrapped tablets or suppositories, and
sealed cartons. This packaging has been
developed to better protect the consumer.

ALUDROX®
[*al 'ū-drox*]
**Antacid
(alumina and magnesia)
ORAL SUSPENSION**

Composition: *Suspension* —each 5 ml
teaspoonful contains 307 mg aluminum
hydroxide [Al(OH)$_3$] as a gel and 103 mg
of magnesium hydroxide. The inactive
ingredients present are artificial and
natural flavors, benzoic acid, butylparaben, glycerin, hydroxypropyl methylcellulose, methylparaben, propylparaben, saccharin, simethicone, sorbitol solution, and water. Sodium content is
0.10 mEq per 5 ml suspension.

Indications: For temporary relief of
heartburn, upset stomach, sour stomach,
and/or acid indigestion.

Directions: *Suspension* —Two teaspoonfuls (10 ml) every 4 hours or as directed
by a physician. Medication may be followed by a sip of water if desired.

Warnings: Do not take more than 12
teaspoonfuls (60 ml) of suspension in a
24-hour period or use maximum dosage
for more than two weeks except under
the advice and supervision of a physi-

cian. As with any drug, if you are pregnant or nursing a baby, seek the advice of
a health professional before using this
product.

Drug Interaction Precautions: Do
not take this product if you are presently
taking a prescription antibiotic drug containing any form of tetracycline.
Keep at Room Temperature, Approx.
77°F (25°C).
Suspension should be kept tightly closed
and shaken well before use. Avoid freezing.
Keep this and all drugs out of the reach
of children.

How Supplied: *Oral Suspension* —bottles of 12 fluidounces.
    *Shown in Product Identification
        Section, page 438*

Professional Labeling: Consult 1990
Physicians' Desk Reference.

AMPHOJEL®
[*am 'fo-jel*]
**Antacid
(aluminum hydroxide gel)
ORAL SUSPENSION • TABLETS**

Composition: *Suspension* —Each 5 ml
teaspoonful contains 320 mg aluminum
hydroxide [Al(OH)$_3$] as a gel, and not
more than 0.10 mEq of sodium. The inactive ingredients present are artificial
and natural flavors, butylparaben, calcium benzoate, glycerin, hydroxypropyl
methylcellulose, methylparaben, propylparaben, saccharin, simethicone, sorbitol
solution, and water. *Tablets* are available
in 0.3 and 0.6 g strengths. Each contains,
respectively, the equivalent of 300 mg
and 600 mg aluminum hydroxide as a
dried gel. The 0.3 g (5 grain) tablet is
equivalent to about 1 teaspoonful of the
suspension and the 0.6 g (10 grain) tablet
is equivalent to about 2 teaspoonfuls.
Each 0.3 g tablet contains 0.08 mEq of
sodium and each 0.6 g tablet contains
0.13 mEq of sodium.

Indications: For temporary relief of
heartburn, upset stomach, sour stomach,
and/or acid indigestion.

Directions: *Suspension* —Two teaspoonfuls (10 ml) to be taken five or six times
daily, between meals and at bedtime or
as directed by a physician. Medication
may be followed by a sip of water if desired. *Tablets* —Two tablets of the 0.3 g
strength, or one tablet of the 0.6 g
strength, five or six times daily, between
meals and at bedtime or as directed by a
physician. It is unnecessary to chew the
0.3 g tablet before swallowing.

Warnings: Do not take more than 12
teaspoonfuls (60 ml) of suspension, or
more than twelve 0.3 g tablets, or more
than six 0.6 g tablets in a 24-hour period
or use this maximum dosage for more
than two weeks except under the advice
and supervision of a physician. May
cause constipation. As with any drug, if
you are pregnant or nursing a baby, seek
the advice of a health professional before
using this product.

Drug Interaction Precautions: Do
not use this product if you are presently
taking a prescription antibiotic containing any form of tetracycline.
Keep tightly closed and store at room
temperature, Approx. 77°F (25°C).
Suspension should be shaken well before
use. Avoid freezing.
Keep this and all drugs out of the reach
of children.

How Supplied: *Suspension* —Peppermint flavored; without flavor—bottles of
12 fluidounces. *Tablets* —a convenient
auxiliary dosage form—0.3 g (5 grain)
bottles of 100; 0.6 g (10 grain), boxes of
100.
    *Shown in Product Identification
        Section, page 438*

Professional Labeling: Consult 1990
Physicians' Desk Reference.

BASALJEL®
[*bā 'sel-jel*]
**(basic aluminum carbonate gel)
ORAL SUSPENSION •CAPSULES
•TABLETS**

Composition: *Suspension* —each 5 ml
teaspoonful contains basic aluminum
carbonate gel equivalent to 400 mg aluminum hydroxide [Al(OH)$_3$]. The inactive ingredients present are artificial
and natural flavors, butylparaben, calcium benzoate, glycerin, hydroxypropyl
methylcellulose, methylparaben, mineral oil, propylparaben, saccharin, simethicone, sorbitol solution, and water.
Capsule contains dried basic aluminum
carbonate gel equivalent to 608 mg of
dried aluminum hydroxide gel or 500 mg
aluminum hydroxide [Al(OH)$_3$]. The inactive ingredients present are D&C Yellow 10, FD&C Blue 1, FD&C Red 40,
FD&C Yellow 6, gelatin, polacrilin potassium, polyethylene glycol, talc, and titanium dioxide. *Tablet* contains dried basic
aluminum carbonate gel equivalent to
608 mg of dried aluminum hydroxide gel
or 500 mg aluminum hydroxide. The inactive ingredients present are cellulose,
hydrogenated vegetable oil, magnesium
stearate, polacrilin potassium, starch,
and talc.

Indications: For the symptomatic relief of hyperacidity, associated with the
diagnosis of peptic ulcer, gastritis, peptic
esophagitis, gastric hyperacidity, and
hiatal hernia.

Warnings: Do not take more than
24 tablets/capsules/teaspoonfuls of
BASALJEL in a 24-hour period, or use
this maximum dosage for more than two
weeks except under the advice and supervision of a physician. Dosage should be
carefully supervised since continued
overdosage, in conjunction with restric-
tion of dietary phosphorus and calcium,
may produce a persistently lowered
serum phosphate and a mildly elevated
alkaline phosphatase. A usually transient hypercalciuria of mild degree may
be associated with the early weeks of
therapy. As with any drug, if you are

Continued on next page

Wyeth-Ayerst—Cont.

pregnant or nursing a baby, seek the advice of a health professional before using this product.

Dosage and Administration: *Suspension* —two teaspoonfuls (10 ml) in water or fruit juice taken as often as every two hours up to twelve times daily. Two teaspoonfuls have the capacity to neutralize 23 mEq of acid. *Capsules* —two capsules as often as every two hours up to twelve times daily. Two capsules have the capacity to neutralize 24 mEq of acid. *Tablets* —two tablets as often as every two hours up to twelve times daily. Two tablets have the capacity to neutralize 25 mEq of acid. The sodium content of each dosage form is as follows: 0.13 mEq/5 ml for the suspension, 0.12 mEq per capsule, and 0.12 mEq per tablet.

Precautions: May cause constipation. Adequate fluid intake should be maintained in addition to the specific medical or surgical management indicated by the patient's condition.

Drug Interaction Precautions: Alumina-containing antacids should not be used concomitantly with any form of tetracycline therapy.

How Supplied: Suspension—bottles of 12 fluidounces.
Capsules—bottles of 100 and 500.
Tablets (scored)—bottles of 100.
Shown in Product Identification Section, page 438

Professional Labeling: Consult 1990 Physicians' Desk Reference.

CEROSE–DM®
[se-ros 'DM]
Cough/Cold Preparation with Dextromethorphan
Sugar Free • Non-Narcotic

Description: Each teaspoonful (5 mL) contains 15 mg dextromethorphan hydrobromide, 4 mg chlorpheniramine maleate, and 10 mg phenylephrine hydrochloride. Alcohol 2.4%. The inactive ingredients present are artificial flavors, citric acid, edetate disodium, FD&C Yellow 6, glycerin, saccharin sodium, sodium benzoate, sodium citrate, sodium propionate, and water.

Indications: For the symptomatic control of cough due to colds.

Dosage and Administration: Adults, and children 12 years and over, one to two teaspoonfuls 4 times daily. Children over 6 years, one teaspoonful 4 times daily. Children under 6, as directed by a physician only.

Caution: Do not exceed recommended dosage. Individuals with high blood pressure, heart disease, diabetes, or thyroid disease should consult a physician before using. If there is persistent cough or high fever which may indicate a serious condition, consult your physician. Drowsiness may occur; if so, do not drive or operate machinery or do not permit hazardous childhood activities.

Warning: As with any drug, if you are pregnant or nursing a baby, seek the advice of a health professional before using this product.
Keep this and all drugs out of the reach of children. In case of accidental overdose, seek professional assistance or contact a Poison Control Center immediately.
Keep tightly closed below 77° F (25° C).

How Supplied: Cases of 12 bottles of 4 fl. oz.; bottles of 1 pint.
Shown in Product Identification Section, page 439

COLLYRIUM for FRESH EYES
[ko-lir 'e-um]
a neutral borate solution
EYE WASH

Description: Soothing Collyrium Eye Wash for Fresh Eyes is specially formulated to soothe, refresh, and cleanse irritated eyes. Collyrium Eye Wash is a neutral borate solution that contains boric acid, sodium borate, thimerosal (not more than 0.002% as a preservative) and water.

Indications: To cleanse the eye, loosen foreign material, air pollutants or chlorinated water.

Recommended Uses:
Home—For emergency flushing of foreign bodies or whenever a soothing eye rinse is necessary.
Hospitals, dispensaries and clinics—For emergency flushing of chemicals or foreign bodies from the eye.

Directions: To open, twist off sealed, tamper-resistant top and discard. Rinse eyecup with clean water immediately before and after each use. Avoid contamination of rim and inside surfaces of cup. Fill cup one-half full with Collyrium Eye Wash. Apply cup tightly to the affected eye to prevent the escape of the liquid and tilt head backward. Open eyelid wide and rotate eyeball to thoroughly wash eye. Rinse cup with clean water after use and recap by twisting threaded eyecup on bottle.

Warnings: Do not use if solution changes color or becomes cloudy, or with a wetting solution for contact lenses or other eye care products containing polyvinyl alcohol. This product contains thimerosal (not more than 0.002% as a preservative). Do not use this product if you are sensitive to mercury.
To avoid contamination do not touch tip of container to any surface. Replace cap after using. If you experience eye pain, changes in vision, continued redness, irritation of the eye, or if the condition worsens or persists, consult a doctor. Obtain immediate medical treatment for all open wounds in or near the eye.
Keep this and all medication out of the reach of children.
Keep tightly closed at Room Temperature, Approx. 77°F (25°C).

How Supplied: Bottles of 6 fl. oz. (177 ml) with eyecup.
Shown in Product Identification Section, page 439

COLLYRIUM FRESH™
[ko-lir 'e-um]
Eye Drops
Redness Reliever
Lubricant

Description: Collyrium Fresh is a specially formulated sterile eye drop which can be used up to 4 times daily, to relieve redness and discomfort due to minor eye irritations caused by dust, smoke, smog, swimming, or sun glare.
The active ingredients are tetrahydrozoline HCl (0.05%) and glycerin (1.0%). Other ingredients include benzalkonium chloride (0.01%) and edetate disodium (0.1%) as preservatives, boric acid, hydrochloric acid and sodium borate.

Indications: For the temporary relief of redness due to minor eye irritations or discomfort due to burning or exposure to wind or sun.

Directions: Tilt head back, gently pull down lower eyelid, and instill 1 to 2 drops in the affected eye(s). Then, the lower lid should be released, the eye closed and the eye rotated once or twice before opening. This procedure can be repeated up to four times daily, or as directed by a physician.

Warnings: Do not use if solution changes color or becomes cloudy. Remove contact lenses before using. If you have glaucoma, do not use this product except under the advice and supervision of a physician. Overuse of this product may produce increased redness of the eye. To avoid contamination, do not touch tip of container to any surface. Replace cap after using. If you experience eye pain, changes in vision, continued redness or irritation of the eye, or if the condition worsens or persists for more than 72 hours, discontinue use and consult a physician.
Keep this and all medication out of the reach of children. Retain carton for complete product information.
Keep bottle tightly closed at Room Temperature, Approx. 77°F (25°C).

How Supplied: Bottles of ½ fl. oz. (15 ml) with built-in eye dropper.
Shown in Product Identification Section, page 439

NURSOY®
[nur-soy]
Soy protein isolate formula
READY–TO–FEED
CONCENTRATED LIQUID
POWDER

Breast milk is preferred feeding for newborns. NURSOY® milk-free formula is intended to meet the nutritional needs of infants and children who are not breast-fed and are allergic to cow's milk protein and/or intolerant to lactose. NURSOY Ready-to-Feed and Concentrated Liquid contain sucrose as their carbohydrate. NURSOY Powder contains corn syrup solids and sucrose as its carbohydrate. Professional advice should be followed.

Ingredients (in normal dilution supplying 20 calories per fluidounce): 87% water; 6.7% sucrose; 3.4% oleo, coconut, oleic (safflower) and soybean oils; 2.3% soy protein isolate; 0.10% potassium citrate; 0.09% monobasic sodium phosphate; 0.04% calcium carbonate; 0.04% dibasic calcium phosphate; 0.03% magnesium chloride; 0.03% calcium chloride; 0.03% soy lecithin; 0.03% calcium carrageenan; 0.03% calcium hydroxide; 0.03% L-methionine; 0.01% sodium chloride; 0.01% potassium bicarbonate; taurine; ferrous, zinc, and cupric sulfates; L-carnitine; (68 ppb) potassium iodide; ascorbic acid; choline chloride; alpha-tocopheryl acetate; niacinamide; calcium pantothenate; riboflavin; vitamin A palmitate; thiamine hydrochloride; pyridoxine hydrochloride; beta-carotene; phytonadione; folic acid; biotin; cholecalciferol; cyanocobalamin.
NURSOY Powder contains corn syrup solids and sucrose. NURSOY Ready-to-Feed and Concentrated Liquids contain only sucrose.

PROXIMATE ANALYSIS
at 20 calories per fluidounce
READY-TO-FEED, CONCENTRATED LIQUID, and POWDER

	(W/V)
Protein	2.1 %
Fat	3.6 %
Carbohydrate	6.9 %
Ash	0.35%
Water	87.0 %
Crude fiber .... not more than	0.01%
Calories/fl. oz.	20

Vitamins, Minerals: In normal dilution, each liter contains:

A	2,000	IU
D_3	400	IU
E	9.5	IU
K_1	100	mcg
C (ascorbic acid)	55	mg
B_1 (thiamine)	670	mcg
B_2 (riboflavin)	1000	mcg
B_6	420	mcg
B_{12}	2	mcg
Niacin	5000	mcg
Pantothenic acid	3000	mcg
Folic acid (folacin)	50	mcg
Choline	85	mg
Inositol	27	mg
Biotin	35	mcg
Calcium	600	mg
Phosphorus	420	mg
Sodium	200	mg
Potassium	700	mg
Chloride	375	mg
Magnesium	67	mg
Manganese	200	mcg
Iron	11.5	mg
Copper	470	mcg
Zinc	5	mg
Iodine	60	mcg

Preparation: *Ready-to-Feed* (32 fl. oz. cans of 20 calories per fluidounce formula)—shake can, open and pour into previously sterilized nursing bottle; attach nipple and feed. Cover opened can and immediately store in refrigerator. Use contents of can within 48 hours of opening.
Concentrated Liquid —For normal dilution supplying 20 calories per fluidounce, use equal amounts of NURSOY® liquid and cooled, previously boiled water. *Note: Prepared formula should be used within 24 hours.*
Powder —For normal dilution supplying 20 calories per fluidounce, add 1 scoop (8.9 grams or 1 standard tablespoonful) of NURSOY POWDER, packed and leveled, to 2 fluidounces of cooled, previously boiled water. For larger amounts of formula add ¼ standard measuring cup of powder (35.5 grams), packed and leveled, to 8 fluidounces (1 standard measuring cup) of water.
Note: Prepared formula should be used within 24 hours.

How Supplied: *Ready-to-Feed* —presterilized and premixed, 32 fluidounce (1 quart) cans, cases of 6; *Concentrated Liquid* —13 fluidounce cans, cases of 24; *Powder* —1 pound cans, cases of 6.
Shown in Product Identification Section, page 439

RESOL®
[ree 'sol]
Oral Electrolyte Rehydration and Maintenance Solution

RESOL® is intended for replacement and maintenance of water and electrolytes in diarrhea with mild to moderate dehydration in children older than 1 week. RESOL is ready to feed and presterilized, and water should not be added. Sterilized nipples should be used.

Ingredients: Water, glucose, sodium chloride, potassium citrate, citric acid, disodium phosphate, magnesium chloride, calcium chloride, and sodium citrate.

Proximate Analysis:
One fluidounce supplies about 2.5 calories.

	mEq/liter	Approximate mEq/8 fl. oz. (237 mL)
Sodium	50	12
Potassium	20	4.7
Calcium	4	0.95
Magnesium	4	0.95
Chloride	50	12
Citrate	34	8.0
Phosphate (HPO_4^{-2})	5	1.2
	gram/liter	
Glucose	20	
	mOsm/kg H_2O	
Osmolality	269	

How Supplied: Ready-to-feed—presterilized, 8 fluidounce bottles, cartons of 6 bottles (Hospital Package only); ready-to-feed—presterilized, 32 fluidounce cartons, cases of 6 cartons.
Shown in Product Identification Section, page 439

SMA®
Iron fortified
Infant formula
READY–TO–FEED
CONCENTRATED LIQUID
POWDER

Breast milk is the preferred feeding for newborns. Infant formula is intended to replace or supplement breast milk when breast-feeding is not possible or is insufficient, or when mothers elect not to breast-feed.
Good maternal nutrition is important for the preparation and maintenance of breast-feeding. Extensive or prolonged use of partial bottle feeding, before breast-feeding has been well established, could make breast-feeding difficult to maintain. A decision not to breast-feed could be difficult to reverse.
Professional advice should be followed on all matters of infant feeding. Infant formula should always be prepared and used as directed. Unnecessary or improper use of infant formula could present a health hazard. Social and financial implications should be considered when selecting the method of infant feeding.
SMA® is unique among prepared formulas for its physiologic fat blend, whey-dominated protein composition, amino acid pattern, mineral content and inclusion of beta-carotene and nucleotides.
SMA, utilizing a hybridized safflower (oleic) oil, became the first infant formula offering fat and calcium absorption equal to that of human milk, with a physiologic level of linoleic acid. Thus, the fat blend in SMA provides a ready source of energy, helps protect infants against neonatal tetany and produces a ratio of vitamin E to polyunsaturated fatty acids (linoleic acid) more than adequate to prevent hemolytic anemia and yields a serum lipid profile comparable to the breast-fed infant.
By combining reduced minerals whey with skimmed cow's milk, SMA reduces the protein content to fall within the range of human milk, adjusts the whey-protein to casein ratio to that of human milk, and subsequently reduces the mineral content to a physiologic level.
The resultant 60:40 whey-protein to casein ratio provides protein nutrition superior to a casein-dominated formula. In addition, the essential amino acids, including cystine, are present in amounts close to those of human milk. So the protein in SMA is of high biologic value.
The five nucleotides found in higher amounts in human milk have been added to SMA at the upper levels found in breast milk. Clinical studies have demonstrated that these additions allow for plasma lipid levels and gut bifido bacteria which are similar to those of human milk-fed infants. Benefits to the immunological system have also been proven.
The physiologic mineral content makes possible a low renal solute load which helps protect the functionally immature infant kidney, increases expendable water reserves and helps protect against dehydration.
Use of lactose as the carbohydrate results in a physiologic stool flora and a low stool pH, decreasing the incidence of perianal dermatitis.

Ingredients: SMA Concentrated Liquid or Ready-to-Feed. Water; nonfat milk; reduced minerals whey; oleo, coco-

Continued on next page

Wyeth-Ayerst—Cont.

nut, oleic (safflower or sunflower), and soybean oils; lactose; soy lecithin; taurine; cytidine-5'-monophosphate; calcium carrageenan; adenosine-5'-monophosphate; disodium uridine-5'-monophosphate; disodium inosine-5'-monophosphate; disodium guanosine-5'-monophosphate; *Minerals:* Potassium bicarbonate and chloride; calcium chloride and citrate; sodium bicarbonate and citrate; ferrous, zinc, cupric, and manganese sulfates. *Vitamins:* ascorbic acid, alpha-tocopheryl acetate, niacinamide, vitamin A palmitate, calcium pantothenate, thiamine hydrochloride, riboflavin, pyridoxine hydrochloride, beta-carotene, folic acid, phytonadione, biotin, cholecalciferol, cyanocobalamin.

SMA Powder. Lactose; oleo, coconut, oleic (safflower or sunflower) and soybean oils; nonfat milk; whey protein concentrate; soy lecithin; taurine; cytidine-5'-monophosphate; adenosine-5'-monophosphate; disodium uridine-5'-monophosphate; disodium inosine-5'-monophosphate; disodium guanosine-5'-monophosphate. *Minerals:* Potassium phosphate; calcium hydroxide; magnesium chloride; calcium chloride; sodium bicarbonate; ferrous sulfate; potassium hydroxide; potassium bicarbonate; zinc, cupric, and manganese sulfates; potassium iodide. *Vitamins:* Ascorbic acid, choline chloride, inositol, alpha-tocopheryl acetate, niacinamide, calcium pantothenate, vitamin A palmitate, riboflavin, thiamine hydrochloride, pyridoxine hydrochloride, beta-carotene, folic acid, phytonadione, biotin, cholecalciferol, cyanocobalamin.

PROXIMATE ANALYSIS
at 20 calories per fluidounce
READY-TO-FEED, POWDER, and CONCENTRATED LIQUID:

	(W/V)
Fat	3.6 %
Carbohydrate	7.2 %
Protein	1.5 %
60% Lactalbumin (whey protein)	0.9 %
40% Casein	0.6 %
Ash	0.25%
Crude Fiber	None
Total Solids	12.6 %
Calories/fl. oz.	20

Vitamins, Minerals: In normal dilution, each liter contains:

A	2000	IU
D₃	400	IU
E	9.5	IU
K₁	55	mcg
C (ascorbic acid)	55	mg
B₁ (thiamine)	670	mcg
B₂ (riboflavin)	1000	mcg
B₆ (pyridoxine hydrochloride)	420	mcg
B₁₂	1.3	mcg
Niacin	5000	mcg
Pantothenic Acid	2100	mcg
Folic Acid (folacin)	50	mcg
Choline	100	mg
Biotin	15	mcg
Calcium	420	mg
Phosphorus	280	mg

Sodium	150	mg
Potassium	560	mg
Chloride	375	mg
Magnesium	45	mg
Manganese	150	mcg
Iron	12	mg
Copper	470	mcg
Zinc	5	mg
Iodine	60	mcg

Preparation: *Ready-to-Feed* (8 and 32 fl. oz. cans of 20 calories per fluidounce formula)—shake can, open and pour into previously sterilized nursing bottle; attach nipple and feed immediately. Cover opened can and immediately store in refrigerator. Use contents of can within 48 hours of opening.
Powder—(1 pound can)—For normal dilution supplying 20 calories per fluidounce, use 1 scoop (or 1 standard tablespoonful) of powder, packed and leveled, to 2 fluidounces of cooled, previously boiled water. For larger amount of formula, use ¼ standard measuring cup of powder, packed and leveled, to 8 fluidounces (1 cup) of water. Three of these portions make 26 fluidounces of formula. *Concentrated Liquid*—For normal dilution supplying 20 calories per fluidounce, use equal amounts of SMA® liquid and cooled, previously boiled water.
Note: Prepared formula should be used within 24 hours.

How Supplied: *Ready-to-Feed*—presterilized and premixed, 32 fluidounce (1 quart) cans, cases of 6; 8 fluidounce cans, cases of 24 (4 carriers of 6 cans). *Powder*—1 pound cans with measuring scoop, cases of 6. *Concentrated Liquid*—13 fluidounce cans, cases of 24.
Also Available: SMA® lo-iron. For those who appreciate the particular advantages of SMA®, the infant formula closest in composition nutritionally to mother's milk, but who sometimes need or wish to recommend a formula that does not contain a high level of iron, there is SMA® lo-iron with all the benefits of regular SMA® but with a reduced level of iron of 1.4 mg per quart. Infants should receive supplemental dietary iron from an outside source to meet daily requirements.
Concentrated Liquid—13 fl. oz. cans, cases of 24. *Powder*—1 pound cans with measuring scoop, cases of 6. *Ready-to-Feed*—32 fl. oz. cans, cases of 6.
Preparation of the standard 20 calories per fluidounce formula of SMA® lo-iron is the same as SMA® iron fortified given above.
Shown in Product Identification Section, page 439

WYANOIDS® Relief Factor
[wi 'a-noids]
Hemorrhoidal Suppositories

Description: Active Ingredients: Live Yeast Cell Derivative, Supplying 2,000 units Skin Respiratory Factor Per Ounce of Cocoa Butter Suppository Base and Shark Liver Oil 3%. **Inactive Ingredients:** Beeswax, Glycerin, Phenylmercuric Nitrate 1:10,000 (as a preservative), Polyethylene Glycol 600 Dilaurate.

Indications: To help shrink swelling of hemorrhoidal tissues and provide prompt, temporary relief from pain and itching.

Usual Dosage: Use one suppository up to five times daily, especially in the morning, at night, and after bowel movements, or as directed by a physician.

Directions: Remove wrapper and insert one suppository rectally using gentle pressure. Frequent application and lubrication with Wyanoids® Relief Factor provide continual therapy which will lead to more rapid improvement of rectal conditions.

Caution: In case of bleeding or if the condition persists, the patient should consult a physician. Keep this and all medicines out of the reach of children. Do not store above 80°F.

How Supplied: Boxes of 12 and 24.
Shown in Product Identification Section, page 439

EDUCATIONAL MATERIAL

Audiovisual Programs
The ***Wyeth-Ayerst Audiovisual Catalog,*** listing audiovisual programs available through the Wyeth-Ayerst Audiovisual Library or on loan through the local Wyeth-Ayerst representative, can be obtained by writing Professional Service, Wyeth-Ayerst Laboratories, P.O. Box 8299, Philadelphia, PA 19101.

Zila Pharmaceuticals, Inc.
777 EAST THOMAS ROAD
PHOENIX, AZ 85014

ZILACTIN® Medicated Gel
ZILABRACE™ Oral Analgesic Gel
ZILADENT™ Oral Analgesic Gel

Description: ZILACTIN, ZILABRACE, and ZILADENT are patent protected* medications with fast-acting, prolonged action. Their special film-forming vehicle holds the medication in place for hours as its relieves pain.

Active Ingredients: ZILACTIN—tannic acid (7%) suspended in SD alcohol 37 (80.8% by volume); ZILABRACE—benzocaine (10%) suspended in SD alcohol 38B (71.5% by volume); ZILADENT—benzocaine (6%) suspended in SD alcohol 38B (74.9% by volume).

Indications: ZILACTIN is for fast relief from the pain, itching, or burning of canker sores, fever blisters, and cold sores. Mint-flavored ZILABRACE is for fast relief from the painful cuts and abrasions caused by dental appliances. Clove-flavored ZILADENT is for fast relief from the pain and discomfort of denture sores. Clinical studies have demonstrated that when properly applied, the gels'vehicle creates a smooth, comfortable, and very tenacious film which holds the active ingredient in place. Even inside the mouth, a single application can last six or more hours (average time 3.92 hours), providing prolonged pain relief and speeding healing. The film usually permits pain-free eating and drinking while preventing saliva, food particles, and drink from coming in contact with the sore. Even citrus beverages may be consumed without difficulty.

Application: Intraorally, the affected tissue should be dried with a gauze pad, tissue, or cotton swab before applying a thin coat of ZILACTIN, ZILABRACE, or ZILADENT. Allow 30–60 seconds for the gel to air dry into a film. Inside the mouth, ZILACTIN's film is white, ZILA-BRACE's and ZILADENT's is flesh colored. Extraorally, apply ZILACTIN directly on fever blisters and cold sores and allow to dry into a transparent film. Four applications per day the first three days may be all that is needed. For maximum effectiveness apply at first symptoms.

Warnings: A mild, but temporary stinging sensation may be experienced when applied to an open sore. As with all medication, keep out of the reach of children. DO NOT USE IN OR AROUND EYES. In the event of accidental contact with the eye, flush immediately and continuously with clear water for ten minutes. Seek immediate medical attention if pain or irritation persists.

How Supplied: ZILACTIN, ZILABRACE, and ZILADENT are available at most retail pharmacies in .25 oz. (7.1 gram) tubes. Professionals may also order ProPaks, .25 oz. (7.1 gram) professionally packed tubes, and MediPaks, .4 gram single-use foil packets, directly from Zila.

*U.S. patent numbers 4,285,934 and 4,381,296.

Distributed by:

ZILA Pharmaceuticals, Inc.

Phoenix, AZ 85014

Educational Material: Samples and literature available to physicians upon request.

Shown in Product Identification Section, page 439

SECTION 7

Diagnostics Devices and Medical Aids

This section is intended to present product information on Diagnostics, Devices and Medical Aids designed for home use by patients. The information concerning each product has been prepared, edited and approved by the manufacturer.

The Publisher has emphasized to manufacturers the necessity of describing products comprehensively so that all information essential for intelligent and informed use is available. In organizing and presenting the material in this edition the Publisher is providing all the information made available by manufacturers.

In presenting the following material to the medical profession, the Publisher is not necessarily advocating the use of any product.

Hygeia Sciences, Inc.
NEWTON, MA 02160

FIRST RESPONSE®
Home Diagnostic Test Kits
Ovulation Predictor Test

Description: This accurate, easy-to-perform and easy-to-read home ovulation predictor test gives a "Yes" or "No" result in just 10 minutes. It will help a woman find the time in her monthly cycle that she is most able to become pregnant, and it can also help her plan the timing of her pregnancy. She can do the test at home and get her results in just 10 minutes. The test is easy to read since she simply compares her result to a furnished reference color—no need for day-to-day color comparisons.

How the test works: The test measures luteinizing hormone (LH), which is always present in urine, but increases on the most fertile day of a woman's cycle. This increase or "surge" in LH triggers ovulation. FIRST RESPONSE® Ovulation Predictor Test detects this LH surge via a simple-to-read color change. Unlike other home ovulation tests, FIRST RESPONSE® Ovulation Predictor Test does not require day-to-day color comparisons since the FIRST RESPONSE® Ovulation Predictor Test result is simply compared to a reference color. If the test result is equal to or darker than the reference color, a woman knows she is about to ovulate. Most women will ovulate within 12 to 24 hours after the surge. Predicting ovulation in advance is important because the egg can only be fertilized for up to 24 hours after ovulation. Therefore, a woman is most likely to become pregnant if she has intercourse within 24 hours of her surge.

How Supplied: The FIRST RESPONSE® Ovulation Predictor Test contains all the materials needed for 5 days of testing, which is enough to detect the hormone surge for about two-thirds of ovulating women. However, since menstrual cycles can be irregular, approximately one-third of the women may need to continue testing with a 3-day refill kit. When a woman detects her surge, she may stop testing and save any unused tests to use the following month, if she does not become pregnant.

Instructions for use: The package contains simple, easy-to-follow, illustrated directions on how to perform the test. If there are any questions, a member of the FIRST RESPONSE® medical information staff is available to answer them at 1-800-367-6022, Monday through Friday, from 7 AM to 5 PM Eastern Time.
Shown in Product Identification Section, page 411

Professional Labeling
FIRST RESPONSE®
Home Diagnostic Test Kits
Pregnancy Test

Description: FIRST RESPONSE® Pregnancy Test gives a "yes" or "no" result in only 5 minutes. FIRST RESPONSE® Pregnancy Test is easy to use and takes only a few simple steps. In just 5 minutes, it turns pink for pregnant; it stays white if not pregnant. FIRST RESPONSE® Pregnancy Test is so sensitive it can be used the first day a woman misses her period. No other home pregnancy test can be used earlier. And a woman can test any time of day.

FIRST RESPONSE® Pregnancy Test is available in both single and double test kits.

How the test works: If conception occurs, a woman's body begins to produce the pregnancy hormone hCG (human chorionic gonadotropin). The FIRST RESPONSE® Pregnancy Test detects this hormone in a woman's urine. The test gives a pink color result if hCG is present in the urine. If no hCG has been detected, FIRST RESPONSE® Pregnancy Test gives a white color result, indicating that the woman is not pregnant. However, if a woman does not have her period within a few days, the test should be repeated. This is because she may have ovulated and conceived late in her cycle, resulting in a slower buildup of hCG. Also, it is possible that she may have miscalculated the day her period was due. If the result is negative in the second test and her period does not start within a week, she should consult a doctor.

Instructions for use: The package insert contains simple easy-to-follow, illustrated directions on how to perform the test. If there are any questions or additional information is needed, please call 1-800-367-6022.

FIRST RESPONSE® Pregnancy Test and Ovulation Predictor Test are manufactured by Hygeia Sciences, Inc., Newton, Mass. and distributed by Tambrands Inc., Lake Success, NY 11042. FIRST RESPONSE is a registered trademark of Tambrands® Inc. © 1989 Tambrands, Inc.
Shown in Product Identification Section, page 411

EDUCATIONAL MATERIAL

Health Information Series # 1, 2, 3, 4
Patient/Consumer Pamphlets about:
Ovulation Prediction
Detecting Pregnancy

Free to Pharmacists, Physicians and Consumers (patients).

Lavoptik Company, Inc.
661 WESTERN AVENUE N.
ST. PAUL, MN 55103

LAVOPTIK® Eye Cups

Description: Device—Sterile disposable eye cups.

How Supplied: Individually bagged eye cups are packed 12 per box, NDC 10651-01004.

LifeScan Inc.
a Johnson & Johnson company
1051 S. MILPITAS BOULEVARD
MILPITAS, CA 95035-6314

ONE TOUCH®
BLOOD GLUCOSE MONITORING SYSTEM

Description: The One Touch System provides more accurate blood glucose monitoring results for your patients with diabetes because its simple procedure reduces inaccurate readings. The One Touch System eliminates the need for user timing, wiping or blotting. Simple procedure: insert strip, press power, apply sample. Results in 45 seconds. Memory stores the most recent 250 results. Clinically proven more accurate in the hands of patients, the One Touch System helps patients achieve greater accuracy because test results are virtually technique-independent.[1] "A system such as the One Touch, which eliminates the need for the operator to start and time the test and remove the blood, results in an improvement in precision and accuracy . . . "[2]

How Supplied: One Touch® Blood Glucose System—Complete Kit—Each Complete Kit contains everything your patients need to begin blood glucose monitoring:
One Touch Blood Glucose Meter
—with 250 Test Memory and
—prompts in 7 languages, including Spanish
25 One Touch Test Strips
Carry Case
Penlet™ Blood Sampling Pen
25 Lancets
One Touch Glucose Control Solution
Instructional Audio Cassette
Owner's Booklet
4 N-Cell Batteries

For a One Touch System demonstration and a complete review of clinical data, contact your LifeScan Professional Representative. For the name of your local representative, call toll free:
In the United States: 1 800 227-8862
In Canada: 1 800 663-5521

1. *Diabetes Care*, Vol. 11, No. 10, November-December 1988, pp 791-794.
2. *Ibid.*

Ortho Pharmaceutical Corporation
Advanced Care Products
RARITAN, NJ 08869

ADVANCE®
Pregnancy Test

Active Ingredients: Human Chorionic Gonadotropin (HCG) alpha chain specific monoclonal antibody HCG, beta-chain specific antibody/enzyme conjugate, chromogenic substrate solution, and buffer solution.

Indications: An in-vitro pregnancy test for use in the home that can detect the presence of HCG in the urine as early as one (1) day past last missed period.

Actions: ADVANCE will accurately detect the presence or absence of HCG in urine in just thirty minutes. It is as accurate as pregnancy test methods used in many hospitals.

Dosage and Administration: Perform the test according to instructions. If, after thirty minutes, a blue color appears on the rounded end of the COLORSTICK, the patient can assume she is pregnant. If the rounded end of the COLORSTICK remains white, and no blue color can be seen, no pregnancy hormone has been detected and the patient is probably not pregnant. The test results may be affected by certain health conditions such as an ovarian cyst or ectopic pregnancy and by certain medications such as thiazide diuretics, plurothiazine, hormones, steroids, chemotherapeutics, and thyroid drugs. For additional reassurance, a toll-free telephone number is included in each package insert. This service is staffed by Registered Nurses who can answer any questions the patient may have about her results, or how she performed the test.

How Supplied: Each ADVANCE test contains a plastic COLORSTICK, a plastic vial containing buffer solution, a glass tube containing dried test chemicals, a glass tube containing color developing solution, a test stand with urine collection and instructions for use.

Storage: Store at room temperature (59°–86°F). Do not freeze.
Shown in Product Identification Section, page 418

DAISY 2®
Pregnancy Test

Active Ingredients: Human Chorionic Gonadotropin (HCG) antibody HCG antibody/enzyme conjugate, and chromogenic substrate solution.

Indications: An in-vitro pregnancy test for use in the home that can detect the presence of HCG in the urine as early as the first day of a missed period.

Actions: DAISY 2 will accurately check the presence or absence of HCG in urine in just 5–8 minutes. It is the same pregnancy test method used in many hospitals.

Dosage and Administration: Perform the test according to instructions. If, after 5–8 minutes, a plus (+) sign has formed in the center of the test cube, the patient is probably pregnant. If a minus (−) sign appears, no pregnancy hormone has been detected and the patient is probably not pregnant. In the unlikely event that neither sign appears, the test system has not worked properly and the patient should call the toll free number included in each package insert. This toll free number is staffed by Registered Nurses who can answer any questions the patient may have about her results, or how she performed the test. All home pregnancy test kits recommend a second test if the first test indicates that the patient is not pregnant and her period does not begin within a week. This second test may be needed because the patient may have miscalculated her period, or her body may not have accumulated enough hormone for a true reading. Many women like the reassurance that comes from double-checking the results. DAISY 2 makes this double checking easy and convenient by providing two complete and identical tests in each kit. The test results may be affected by certain health conditions such as a ovarian cyst or ectopic pregnancy and certain medications such as thiazide diuretics, plurothiazine, hormones, steroids, chemotherapeutics, and thyroid drugs.

How Supplied: Each DAISY 2 kit contains everything needed to perform two tests, two plastic test cubes, two glass tubes containing dried test chemicals, two plastic vials containing developing solution, two test stands with urine cup and urine dropper and instructions for use.

Storage: Store at room temperature (59°–86°F). Do not Freeze.
Shown in Product Identification Section, page 418

FACT PLUS™
Pregnancy Test

Active Ingredients: Human Chorionic Gonadotropin (HCG) antibody, HCG antibody/enzyme conjugate, and chromogenic substrate solution.

Indications: An in-vitro pregnancy test for use in the home that can detect the presence of HCG in the urine as early as the first day of a missed period.

Actions: FACT PLUS will accurately detect the presence or absence of HCG in urine in just 5–8 minutes. It is the same pregnancy test method used in many hospitals.

Dosage and Administration: Perform the test according to instructions. If, after 5–8 minutes, a plus (+) sign has formed in the center of the test cube, the patient is probably pregnant. If a minus (−) sign appears, no pregnancy hormone has been detected and the patient is probably not pregnant. In the unlikely event that neither sign appears the test system has not worked properly and the patient should call the toll free number included in each package insert. This toll free number is staffed by Registered Nurses who can answer any questions the patient may have about her results, or how she performed the test. The test results may be affected by various other factors and medications such as thiazide diuretics, plurothiazine, hormones, steroids, chemotherapeutics, and thyroid drugs.

How Supplied: Each FACT PLUS kit contains a plastic test cube, a glass tube containing dried test chemicals, a plastic vial containing color developing solution, a test stand with a urine collection cup and urine dropper, a test stand with urine collector and complete instructions for use.

Storage: Store at room temperature (59–86°F). Do not freeze.
Shown in Product Identification Section, page 419

Parke-Davis
Consumer Health Products Group
Division of Warner-Lambert Company
201 TABOR ROAD
MORRIS PLAINS, NJ 07950

e·p·t® plus™
Early Pregnancy Test

- Test as early as one day after your period should have started.
- Simple color change test.
- Easy to perform—just one chemical step.
- Virtually 100% accurate in laboratory tests.

How EPT PLUS works
When you're pregnant, you produce a hormone called HCG—(human chorionic gonadotropin), which is found in your urine. EPT PLUS detects the presence of this pregnancy hormone in your urine. When you perform the test, a color change in the test tube shows you whether the hormone is there. **Any color change** from the initial purplish red color means you are pregnant and should therefore see your doctor. No color change means you are not pregnant.

When to use EPT PLUS
When a woman becomes pregnant a special hormone begins to be produced and will appear in her urine. EPT PLUS measures whether this hormone is present or not. If you **are** pregnant, this hormone usually reaches a level which EPT PLUS can detect one day after your period should have started. In some cases, however, detectable levels may not be reached until several days later. EPT PLUS can be used one day after a missed period as well as any day thereafter.
EPT PLUS can tell you if you are pregnant in as fast as 10 minutes. To verify negative results the test should be rechecked at 30 minutes. During this time, you can carry the test tube with you since

EPT PLUS is completely portable, and movement will not affect the test. Any color change during this 30 minute period indicates a positive result.

Use only the first morning urine*

Use only your first urine of the morning. This is because the pregnancy hormone is most concentrated in the first urine specimen of the day. You should collect it in the clear plastic lid that covers the test kit. Be sure to rinse the lid thoroughly in clear tap water before you deposit the urine in it.

You will need only a few minutes to set up the test. If you do not have time to do the test the first thing in the morning, you can cover and store your first morning urine specimen in the refrigerator. However, be sure to do the test the same day the urine was collected. Let the urine warm to room temperature before testing.

(**Note:** After your urine has been stored for several hours a sediment may form at the bottom of the container. DO NOT mix or shake the urine. Use only the urine at the top of the container.)

*First morning urine is any urine collected after 5 hours of sleep, regardless of the time of day.

The EPT PLUS Test Kit

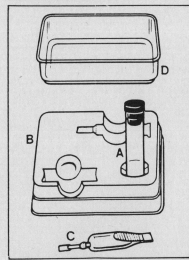

A. **Glass test tube** with rubber stopper,* which contains the special test chemicals. Leave stopper in place until you perform the test.
B. **Test holder.**
C. **Plastic vial,*** which contains the proper amount of buffer solution.
D. **Plastic lid.** Use this to collect and hold the urine for the test.

*Double Kit contains two.

EPT PLUS is simple to perform

Before you start, read all the directions and recommendations carefully.

Remove the rubber stopper from the glass test tube (A) and save it for later. Hold up the plastic vial (C) to be sure that no liquid is in the neck of the vial. Twist the top off and squeeze out entire contents into the glass test tube (A).

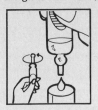

Now fill the empty plastic vial (C) with urine as you would with a medicine dropper.

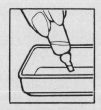

Carefully squeeze 3 drops of urine into the test tube (A).

Put the rubber stopper back on the test tube (A) and shake the tube gently to mix the contents. **Please note the color of the liquid in the tube**. In most cases, the liquid will be a deep purplish red color; however, the exact shade will vary among women.

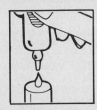

If the result is positive, the color change can begin to show as early as 10 minutes. If there is **any** change from the original purplish red color, this indicates a positive result. If the solution has not changed within that time, check the solution again at 30 minutes. (If necessary, you may carry the test tube with you.) If there is still no color change the test result is negative. Any color change during this 30-minute period indicates a positive result.

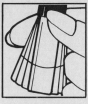

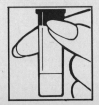

NEGATIVE (−)

If there is no color change, this means that no pregnancy hormone has been detected in your urine and you are probably not pregnant. In the unlikely event that a week passes and you still have not menstruated, you may have miscalculated your period, or the test might have been performed incorrectly. In this case, you should perform another test using a new EPT PLUS kit. If the second test still gives you a negative result—and you still have not menstruated—there could be other important reasons why your period has not begun and you should see your physician. Among other conditions, this could be a sign of ectopic pregnancy, which, unlike a usual pregnancy, is one in which the fertilized egg is implanted in a position other than the uterus (such as in the Fallopian tube). This requires immediate medical supervision.

POSITIVE (+)

If the liquid **clearly does** change color (as indicated in the color swatch shown below on right), your urine does contain the pregnancy hormone, and you can assume you are pregnant.

You should now plan to consult your physician, who is best able to advise you. (In certain rare cases HCG levels may be elevated even though you are not pregnant. Your physician can determine this. Also, use of oral contraceptives should not affect test results.)

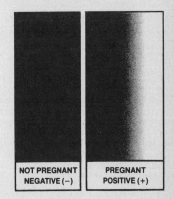

| NOT PREGNANT NEGATIVE (−) | PREGNANT POSITIVE (+) |

EPT PLUS accuracy

EPT PLUS is virtually 100% accurate in laboratory tests.

EPT PLUS is as accurate as leading hospital and lab urine tests, so you can trust the result.

INGREDIENTS*

Each test kit contains:
1. Gold sol particles coated with monoclonal HCG antibodies and a special buffer.
2. A special aqueous buffer solution.

*Not to be taken internally.
For in vitro diagnostic use.
Store at 59°–86°F.

Questions about EPT PLUS?
CALL US TOLL FREE. . . 8 AM TO 5 PM
EST WEEKDAYS AT 1-800-562-0266.

IN NEW JERSEY, CALL COLLECT AT (201) 540-2458. Registered Nurses are available to answer your calls.

e·p·t® STICK TEST
Early Pregnancy Test

- Test as early as one day after missed period.
- Easy to perform—one chemical step.
- Easy to read—a pink color at the end of the test stick signals a positive result.
- Virtually 100% accurate in laboratory tests.

EPT STICK PREGNANCY TEST

The ept stick test uses advanced technology to make home pregnancy testing simple and gives a clear and highly accurate result. The key element of this test is a stick which changes color to indicate pregnancy. **Any shade of pink that appears on the tip of the stick and remains after rinsing indicates that you are pregnant.**

HOW EPT STICK WORKS

When a woman becomes pregnant, her body produces a special hormone known as HCG (human chorionic gonadotropin), which appears in the urine. The ept stick test can detect this hormone as early as the first day after a missed period.

If you obtain a positive result, you can assume you are pregnant and should see your doctor. A negative result means that no HCG has been detected and you can assume you are not pregnant.

WHEN TO USE THE EPT STICK TEST

The ept stick test can detect HCG hormone levels in your urine as early as one day after a missed period. In some cases, however, detectable levels may not be reached until several days later. The ept stick test can be used one day after a missed period as well as any date thereafter.

BEFORE YOU BEGIN:

- Read through this entire pamphlet carefully.
- If you have any questions, call the toll free number provided on the back page of this pamphlet. Registered Nurses are available to answer your questions.

THE EPT STICK PREGNANCY TEST KIT

A. **Glass test tube** with rubber stopper,* which contains the special test chemicals. Leave stopper in place until you perform the test.

B. **Test holder.**

C. **Plastic vial,*** which contains the proper amount of buffer solution.

D. **Plastic lid.** Use this to collect and hold the urine for the test.

E. **White pouch** containing the test stick* with one end coated with test chemicals.

---

*Double Kit contains two.

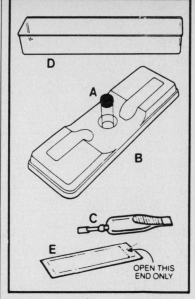

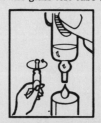

OPEN THIS END ONLY

The ept stick test is easy to perform, simply follow the pictures as indicated. (Starting below)

Urine collection

Use only first morning urine** to conduct this test. Why? Because if you are pregnant, the pregnancy hormone is most concentrated in the first urine specimen of the day. You should collect it in the clear plastic lid that covers the test kit (D). Be sure to rinse the lid thoroughly in clear tap water before you deposit the urine in it. If you do not have enough time to do the test the first thing in the morning, you can cover and store your first morning urine specimen in the refrigerator. However, be sure to do the test the same day the urine was collected. Let the urine warm to room temperature before testing.

(**NOTE:** *After your urine has been stored for several hours, a sediment may form at the bottom of the container. DO NOT mix or shake the urine. Use only the urine at the top of the container.*)

**First morning urine is any urine collected after 5 hours of sleep, regardless of the time of day.

Remove the rubber stopper from the glass test tube (A) and save it for later. Hold up the plastic vial (C) to be sure that no liquid is in the neck of the vial. Twist the top off and squeeze out entire contents into the glass test tube (A).

Now fill the empty plastic vial (C) with urine as you would with a medicine dropper.

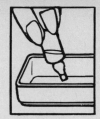

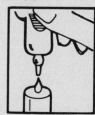

Carefully squeeze 5 drops of urine into the test tube (A).

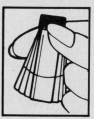

Put the rubber stopper back on the test tube (A) and shake the tube gently to mix the contents. Put the test tube back in the stand and remove the stopper.

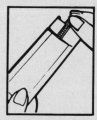

Remove the test stick from the white pouch (E) by tearing along **the line indicated.** Take out the stick handling it **only** by the thicker end. **DO NOT TOUCH THE OTHER THINNER END OF THE STICK AS THIS MAY VOID THE TEST.**

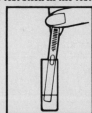

Put the test stick in the test tube (A) with the coated thinner end in the liquid. Leave the test stick in the test tube for 10 minutes.

Turn on the **cold water** faucet and allow water to run gently until water is cool. Holding the thick end of the test stick, remove it from glass tube (A). Rinse both sides of the stick under **cool, gently flowing** tap water for a slow count of 3.

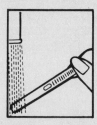

Reading your test results

If the tip of the test stick has turned any shade of *pink*, this is a positive result. You can assume you are pregnant and should consult your doctor.

If the tip of the stick is still white, and no pink color can be seen, this signals a negative result. To verify negative results, replace the test stick into the test tube and wait another 20 minutes. Remove and rinse again with tap water. If it is still white, you are probably not pregnant. If there is any shade of pink on the tip of the stick at this point it is a positive result.

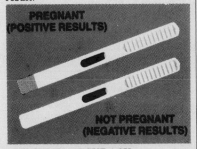

PREGNANT (POSITIVE RESULTS)

NOT PREGNANT (NEGATIVE RESULTS)

EPT STICK ACCURACY

Although the ept stick test is proven virtually 100% accurate in laboratory tests,

a low incidence of false results (positive when no pregnancy exists or negative when pregnancy is present) can occur. Check with your doctor if you get unexpected or inconsistent test results. Certain health conditions such as an ovarian cyst or an ectopic pregnancy (a pregnancy outside the uterus) can cause a false or irregular result with your test.

INGREDIENTS*

Each test kit contains:

1. Gold sol particles coated with monoclonal HCG antibodies.
2. A special aqueous buffer solution.
3. Test stick coated with monoclonal antibodies.

*Not to be taken internally. For in vitro diagnostic use.

Store at 59°–86°F.

Questions about EPT stick test?
CALL TOLL FREE 1-800-562-0266
WEEKDAYS 8 AM to 5 PM EST.
IN NEW JERSEY, CALL 1-800-338-0326.
Registered Nurses are available to answer your calls.

Marketed by
PARKE-DAVIS Consumer Health Products Division
Warner-Lambert Co.
Morris Plains, NJ 07950 USA
Shown in Product Identification Section, page 420

Products are
indexed alphabetically
in the
PINK SECTION

Warner-Lambert Company
Consumer Health Products Group
201 TABOR ROAD
MORRIS PLAINS, NJ 07950

EARLY DETECTOR™
In-Home Test for the Detection of Hidden Blood in the Stool

Description: Early Detector is an *in-vitro* diagnostic test to detect hidden blood in the stool.

Indications: There is uniform medical agreement that the earlier colorectal cancer is diagnosed and appropriate treatment instituted, the more favorable the disease prognosis. Among the early warning signs, rectal bleeding is considered the most significant symptom. The primary at-risk groups include people over the age of 40, plus those with a family history of colorectal cancer, or the presence, or family history of familial polyposis of the colon.
In-home tests such as Early Detector are considered one of the most effective methods for large-scale screening.

Actions: Early Detector is a gum guaiac–based, *in vitro* diagnostic kit that tests for occult blood in three successive bowel movements. The procedure is simple, more acceptable to patients, and easy to perform in the privacy of the home.

Directions for Use: Complete, illustrated, easy-to-follow directions are included with each test. People who are actively bleeding from other conditions such as hemorrhoids or menstruation should not take the test. Some medications such as aspirin, iron supplements, vitamin C (over 250 mg. per day), rectal ointments, and anti-inflammatory drugs can cause an error in results. For two days before and throughout the test period, patients should avoid red or rare meat, turnips, horseradish and vitamin C supplements in their diets.

How Supplied: The Early Detector In-Home Test contains 3 specimen pads with Activity Indicator® test verification spots, developer solution, a packet containing a developer tablet and an instruction booklet.

Early Detector
The Early Detector in-home test finds hidden blood in the stool. The test is fast, painless, and simple. Blood in the stool can be a sign of a number of conditions. Some of these are ulcers, diverticulosis, hemorrhoids and cancer of the colon and rectum. Early Detector can alert you and your doctor to conditions which may require medical help. Read all the instructions before you perform the test. Follow the step-by-step guide with care to get accurate results.

Why should I use Early Detector?
Blood in the stool can be a sign of various conditions, including ulcers, diverticulosis, hemorrhoids and cancer of the colon and rectum. But you may not be aware of this blood. Therefore, you may not seek

---

Warner-Lambert

Familiarize yourself with the Early Detector test kit

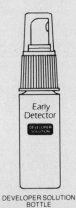

DEVELOPER SOLUTION BOTTLE

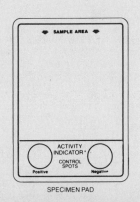

SPECIMEN PAD

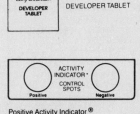

DEVELOPER TABLET

Positive Activity Indicator ®
will turn blue after you spray
with developer solution.
Negative Activity Indicator
will not change color.

the medical treatment you may need. Now there's Early Detector. The Early Detector Test is a fast, painless, and simple method of finding hidden blood in the stool. The Early Detector Test can be done in the privacy of your own home. There is nothing to mail in. You perform the test. You read the results.

How does Early Detector work?

Early Detector is a simple version of a standard laboratory test for hidden blood in the stool. The test is easy to do. After a bowel movement, you use a specimen pad to pat the anal area to get a stool specimen. The Early Detector Developer Solution is applied to the stool specimen. A chemical reaction will take place between the solution and stool specimen. If there is hidden blood in the stool, the area around the specimen will turn blue.

How often should I use Early Detector?

After age 40, when colorectal disease is most prevalent, annual screening for hidden blood in the stool with Early Detector is advisable. However, people who have a medical history of hidden blood in the stool or have a family history of gastrointestinal medical disorders should perform the test more often. The ease and convenience of Early Detector allows for more frequent and convenient screening.

What chemicals are found in Early Detector?

The final prepared Developer Solution has a stable mixture of hydrogen peroxide, gum guaiac, and denatured ethyl alcohol in water.

Each specimen pad has a positive Activity Indicator® which contains hematin, a chemical which when sprayed with Developer Solution will turn blue.

What are the precautions I should take?

The chemicals in Early Detector are not for internal use. Early Detector is made for outside the body use (FOR IN VITRO DIAGNOSTIC USE). Do not eat or drink this test.

Use the developer solution within two months after adding the tablet. (Record Date on Page 13).

EARLY DETECTOR DEVELOPER SOLUTION MAY BE IRRITATING. DO NOT GET IN EYES. IF CONTACT OCCURS, FLUSH PROMPTLY WITH WATER.

Keep the Early Detector Developer Solution away from heat and light. Keep the bottle tightly capped when not in use. CAUTION: FLAMMABLE. DO NOT USE NEAR OPEN FLAME. KEEP OUT OF REACH OF CHILDREN.

How should Early Detector be stored?

Store at room temperature (59°F–86°F)—do not refrigerate. Keep away from light and heat. Protect from direct sunlight. Keep developer solution tightly capped when not in use. Your Early Detector Test has:

  3 Individually wrapped Specimen Pads with Activity Indicator®
  1 Bottle Developer Solution
  1 Packet Containing Developer Tablet
  1 Instruction Booklet With Photographs.

How do I prepare myself to use the Early Detector Test Kit?

● Do not perform the test if you are actively bleeding from other conditions that may show up in the stool specimen. Some conditions are hemorrhoids or menstrual bleeding.

● **INTERFERING SUBSTANCES**

Some medicines such as aspirin, iron supplements and anti-inflammatory drugs for arthritis may cause the test to turn blue, even when blood due to a medical problem is not present in the stool (false positive result). Vitamin C (over 250 mg. daily) may prevent blood which may be present in the stool from turning the paper blue (false negative result). Such medicines should not be taken two (2) days prior to or during the test period. If your doctor has prescribed any of these medicines for you, check with him/her to see if it is permissible for you to stop taking your drugs for a few days. The use of rectal ointments should also be avoided while taking the test.

● Instructions for Special Diet. **FOR TWO DAYS BEFORE AND THROUGHOUT THE TEST PERIOD, FOLLOW THE SPECIAL DIET GUIDELINES BELOW.**

Do not eat:	Do eat foods such as:
Red or Rare Meat	Poultry
Turnips	Fish
Horseradish	Vegetables
Vitamin C Supplements	Fruit
(over 250 mg daily)	Peanuts
	Popcorn
	Bran Cereal

If you know that any of the above cause you discomfort, or if you are on a special diet or taking prescription medications check with your doctor before performing the test.

Instructions

Follow these with care to insure accurate results. Read all instructions before starting test.

NOTE: DEVELOPER SOLUTION SHOULD HAVE BEEN PREPARED AT LEAST 60 MINUTES PRIOR TO USE. To properly perform the test you will need to sample and test three successive bowel movements. It is important to do this test on all three bowel movements in a row. (If you miss one, continue test until three samples have been tested.) Gastrointestinal problems often bleed off and on. If you test three stool specimens in a row, you will have a better chance of finding hidden blood in the stool. You should do all three tests even if the first and second tests do not show hidden blood.

USE THESE INSTRUCTIONS FOR EACH TEST
STEP 1.
Wash hands thoroughly before using this test. Have a specimen pad and developer solution bottle close to the toilet or sink.

STEP 2.
After a bowel movement, take a specimen pad and **fold the Activity Indicator spots under to keep them free of stool.**

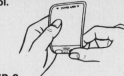

STEP 3.
Gently pat (*do not wipe*) the anal area to get a smear of stool.

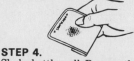

STEP 4.
Shake bottle well. Remove the clear plastic overcap from developer solution bottle. Hold bottle upright and specimen pad 1–3 inches away. Press firmly on the bottle top and spray repeatedly to wet the entire stool specimen. Be sure to spray the two Activity Indicator spots on bottom of pad. Five sprays should fully soak the pad.

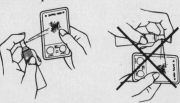

Caution: Do not spray on clothing or furniture.
STEP 5.
READ THE RESULTS IN 30–60 SECONDS. COLOR MAY FADE AFTER 60 SECONDS.
The Activity Indicator spots on the bottom of the specimen pad will show that the test is working. **The spots do not show whether there is blood in the stool.** When you spray the spots, the positive spot will turn blue and the negative spot will not change color.

NOTE: If the positive spot is blue before you spray the pad the specimen pad should not be used. If the spot does not turn blue after you have sprayed it with developer solution, do not continue test. Call toll free number (Page 11) for assistance.

Now look at the area on and around the stool specimen. **Any trace of blue color of any shade or intensity is a positive result** (except in the Activity Indicator positive spot). No trace of blue color on or around the stool specimen is a negative result. See color photo for examples of positive/negative test results (Page 12 of booklet). After reading results, flush the specimen pad in the toilet.

NOTE: If you are color blind, have someone help you read the test.

STEP 6.
Record each test result in the space provided in the Record of Early Detector Test Results (last page).

IMPORTANT: If any of the three tests show a trace of blue color, you should consult with your doctor as soon as you can. Discontinue testing and consult with your doctor if your first or second test is positive.

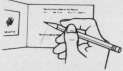

STEP 7. Wash hands thoroughly after using each test.

What do the results mean?

If a blue color (positive reading) is anywhere on the specimen pad (except in the positive circle of the Activity Indicator) this shows that there may be blood in the stool. Be sure to check edges of the smear area. If you see **ANY** blue anywhere on the specimen pad area (except in the positive circle of the Activity Indicator) within 30–60 seconds after you have sprayed the developer solution on the stool sample, the test is positive. This does not always mean that you have a serious medical problem. The blue color may be caused by the food you have eaten or the medicines you are taking or other conditions such as ulcers or hemorrhoids. As with all tests for hidden blood, the results do not give conclusive evidence of any specific disease. Early Detector is a screening tool, a diagnostic aid. It is **not** made to take the place of routine physical examinations or other tests your doctor may wish to perform. If you have a positive result from your test, you should consult with your doctor as soon as you can. Remember **only one** specimen pad of the three tests you have done has to show a blue color for you to consult with your doctor.

If your tests showed no trace of blue color this means that at the time of taking the test there was no detectable blood in the stool. However, this does not mean you are free of disease. Not all gastrointestinal disorders bleed. You may have other symptoms which led you to use this test, such as bowel habit changes (e.g., diarrhea or constipation lasting longer than 2 weeks), unexplained weight loss lasting 2 or more weeks or visually evident blood in the stool (red or black). If so, even if your tests are negative, you should consult with your doctor.

What are the limitations of the test?

As with all tests for hidden blood, results with Early Detector cannot prove the presence or absence of bleeding or illness. Early Detector is not made to replace tests that your doctor may wish to perform.

Tests to find hidden blood are being used and evaluated both in clinical practices and at leading medical centers.

Past results show that:

• In health screening surveys, the positive rate has been about 2% to 5%. Positive means any trace of blue color. However, this does not always mean that you have a serious medical prob-

lem. The blue color may be caused by the food you have eaten or the medicines you are taking.

Tests have shown that consumers can perform this test and read the results as well as a testing laboratory.

FOR ANY INFORMATION OR ASSISTANCE YOU MAY NEED CONCERNING EARLY DETECTOR YOU MAY CALL TOLL FREE 1-800-E.D. HELPS.

Shown in Product Identification Section, page 435

Whitehall Laboratories Inc.
Division of American Home Products Corporation
685 THIRD AVENUE
NEW YORK, NY 10017

CLEARBLUE EASY™
Pregnancy Test Kit

Clearblue Easy is the easiest and one of the fastest pregnancy tests available because all you have to do is hold the absorbent tip in your urine stream, replace the cap, and in 3 minutes you'll know the test is complete when a blue line appears in the small window. The large window shows the test result. If there is a blue line in the large window, you are pregnant. If there is no line, you are not pregnant.

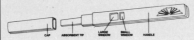

Clearblue Easy is a rapid, one-step pregnancy test for home use which detects tiny amounts of the pregnancy hormone HCG (human chorionic gonadotropin) in the urine. This hormone is produced in increasing amounts during the first part of pregnancy. Clearblue Easy uses sensitive monoclonal antibodies to detect the presence of the hormone from the first day of a missed period.

The pregnancy hormone HCG is most concentrated in the first urine specimen of the day, so you must use this urine to conduct the test.

A negative result means that no pregnancy hormone was detected and you are probably not pregnant. If your period does not start within a week, you may have miscalculated the day your period was due. Repeat the test using another Clearblue Easy test. If the second test still gives a negative result and you still have not menstruated, you should see your doctor.

Clearblue Easy is specially designed for easy use at home. However, if you do have questions about the test or results, give the Clearblue Easy TalkLine a call at 1-800-223-2329. A specially trained staff of advisors is available 24 hours a day to answer your questions.

Produced by Unipath Ltd., Bedford, U.K. Unipath, Clearblue Easy and the fan device are trademarks.

Distributed by Whitehall Laboratories, New York, NY 10017.

Shown in Product Identification Section, page 437

CLEARPLAN EASY™
One-Step Ovulation Predictor

CLEARPLAN EASY is the easiest home ovulation predictor test to use because of its unique technological design. It consists of just one piece and involves only one step to get the results. To use CLEARPLAN EASY, a woman simply urinates on the absorbent tip (a woman can test any time of day) for 5 seconds, and after 5 minutes, she can read the results. A blue line will appear in the small window to show her that the test has worked correctly. The large window indicates the presence of luteinizing hormone (LH) in her urine. If there is a line in the large window which is similar to or darker than the line in the small window, she has detected her LH surge.

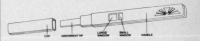

Laboratory tests confirm that CLEARPLAN EASY is over 98% accurate in detecting the LH surge as shown by radioimmunoassay (RIA).

CLEARPLAN EASY employs highly sensitive monoclonal antibody technology to accurately predict the onset of ovulation, and, consequently, the best time each month for a woman to try to become pregnant. The test monitors the amount of LH in a woman's urine. Small amounts of LH are present during most of the menstrual cycle, but the level normally rises sharply about 24 to 36 hours before ovulation (which is when an egg is released from the ovary). CLEARPLAN EASY detects this LH surge which precedes ovulation so that a woman knows 24–36 hours beforehand the time she is most able to become pregnant.

A woman will be most fertile during the 2 to 3 days after an LH surge is detected. Sperm can fertilize an egg for many hours after sexual intercourse. So, if sexual intercourse occurs during the 2–3 days after a similar or darker line appears in the large window, the chances of getting pregnant are maximized.

CLEARPLAN EASY contains 5 days of tests. If, because a woman's cycles are irregular or if for any other reason a woman does not detect her LH surge after 5 days of testing she should continue testing with a second CLEARPLAN EASY kit. CLEARPLAN EASY offers users the support of a 24-hour TalkLine (1-800-223-2329). This service is operated by trained advisors who are available to answer any questions about using the test or reading the results.

Produced by Unipath Ltd., Bedford, U.K. Unipath, CLEARPLAN EASY and the fan device are trademarks.

Distributed by Whitehall Laboratories, New York, NY 10017.

Shown in Product Identification Section, page 437

HEALTH ASSOCIATIONS

AND

ORGANIZATIONS

Organizations to contact for help with specific health problems.

HEALTH ASSOCIATIONS AND ORGANIZATIONS

AARP Pharmacy Service
500 Montgomery Street
Alexandria, VA 22314
(703) 684-0244

**Alcohol and Drug Problems
Association of North America**
444 North Capitol St., N.W.
Washington, DC 20001
(202) 737-4340

**Alcoholics Anonymous World
Services, Inc.**
P.O. Box 459
Grand Central Station
New York, NY 10163
(212) 686-1100

**Alzheimer's Disease and Related
Disorders Association, Inc.**
70 E. Lake St., Suite 600
Chicago, IL 60601
(800) 621-0379
Illinois only: (800) 572-6037

**American Anorexia Bulimia
Association, Inc.**
133 Cedar Lane
Teaneck, NJ 07666
(201) 836-1800

**American Association of Poison
Control Centers**
c/o Arizona Poison Center
Rm. 324OK
1501 N. Campbell Avenue
Tucson, AZ 85724
(602) 626-7899

American Cancer Society
1599 Clifton Road, N.E.
Atlanta, GA 30329
(404) 320-3333

**American Council on
Alcohol Problems**
3426 Bridgeland Drive
Bridgeland Drive
Bridgeton, MO 63044
(314) 739-5944

American Dental Association
211 E. Chicago Avenue
Chicago, IL 60611
(312) 440-2500

**American Diabetes
Association, Inc.**
National Service Center
1660 Duke St.
Alexandria, VA 22314
(703) 549-1500

**American Dietetic Association
Division of Practice**
216 W. Jackson Blvd. Suite 800
Chicago, IL 60606-6995
(312) 899-0040

American Foundation for the Blind
15 W. 16th Street
New York, NY 10011
(212) 620-2000
(800) 232-5463

American Heart Association
7320 Greenville Avenue
Dallas, TX 75231
(214) 706-1179

American Liver Foundation
1425 Pompton Avenue
Cedar Grove, NJ 07009
(201) 256-2550

American Lung Association
1740 Broadway
New York, NY 10019-4374
(212) 315-8700

American Medical Association
535 N. Dearborn Street
Chicago, IL 60610-4377
(312) 645-4818

American Osteopathic Association
142 E. Ohio Street
Chicago, IL 60611
(312) 280-5800

**American Osteopathic
Hospital Association**
1454 Duke Street
Alexandria, VA 22314
(703) 684-7700

**American Physical Therapy
Association**
1111 North Fairfax Street
Alexandria, VA 22314
(703) 684-2782

**American Red Cross
Blood Services Operations**
National Headquarters
1730 E. St., NW
Washington, DC 20006
(202) 639-3012

**American Society of Internal
Medicine**
1101 Vermont Ave., NW
Suite 500
Washington, DC 20005
(202) 298-1700

Arthritis Foundation
1314 Spring Street,NW
Atlanta, GA 30309
(404) 872-7100

**Asthma and Allergy Foundation
of America**
1717 Massachusetts Ave. NW
Suite 305
Washington, DC 20036
(202) 265-0265

Autism Society of America
1234 Massachusetts Ave., NW
Suite C1017
Washington, DC 20005
(202) 783-0125

Center for Sickle Cell Disease
2121 Georgia Ave., NW
Washington, DC 20059
(202) 636-7930

Citizens Alliance for VD Awareness
(312) 236-6339

Cystic Fibrosis Foundation
6931 Arlington Rd.
Bethesda, MD 20814
(301) 951-4422
1-800-FIGHTCF

**Division of STD/HIV Prevention
Center for Prevention Services
Centers for Disease Control**
Atlanta, GA 30333
(404) 639-2586

**The Epilepsy Foundation
of America**
4351 Garden City Drive
Landover, MD 20785
(301) 459-3700

**Food and Drug Administration
Press Office**
15-05
5600 Fishers Lane
Rockville, MD 20857
(301) 443-4177; (301) 443-3285

**Food and Nutrition Board
Institute of Medicine
National Academy of Sciences**
2101 Constitution Ave., NW
Washington, DC 20418
(202) 334-1732

**Huntington's Disease Society of
America**
140 W. 22nd Street
6th Floor
New York, NY 10011-2420
(212) 242-1968
(800) 345-HDSA

Joslin Diabetes Center, Inc.
One Joslin Place
Boston, MA 02215
(617) 732-2400

Juvenile Diabetes Foundation International
432 Park Ave. South
New York, NY 10016-8013
(800) 223-1138

Leukemia Society of America
733 Third Avenue
New York, NY 10017
(212) 573-8484

March of Dimes Birth Defects Foundation
1275 Mamaroneck Avenue
White Plains, NY 10605
(914) 428-7100

Medic Alert Foundation International
2323 Colorado Ave.
Turlock, CA 95381-1009
(800) IDALERT

Muscular Dystrophy Assoiciation
810 7th Avenue
New York, NY 10019
(212) 586-0808

National Association of Anorexia Nervosa & Associated Disorders- ANAD
Box 7
Highland Park, IL 60035
(708) 831-3438

National Association of the Deaf
814 Thayer Avenue
Silver Spring, MD 20910
(301) 587-1788

National Association of the Deaf
Branch Office
445 N. Pennsylvania Street
Suite 804
Indianapolis, IN 46204

National Association of Rehabilitation Facilities
Box 17675
Washington, DC 20041
(703) 648-9300

National Association for Sickle Cell Disease, Inc.
4221 Wilshire Blvd.
Suite 360
Los Angeles, CA 90010-3503
(213) 936-7205 1 (800)-421-8453

National Clearinghouse for Alcohol and Drug Information
P.O. Box 2345
Rockville, MD 20852
(301) 468-2600

National Council on Alcoholism
12 West 21st St.
New York, NY 10010
(212) 206-6770

National Federation of the Blind
1800 Johnson Street
Baltimore, MD 21230
(301) 659-9314

National Foundation for Ileitis and Colitis, Inc.
444 Park Avenue South, 11th Flr.
New York, NY 10016
(212) 685-3440
(800) 343-3637

National Health Council, Inc.
350 Fifth Avenue, Room 1118
New York, NY 10118
(212) 268-8900

National Hemophilia Foundation
The Soho Bldg
110 Greene St., Rm 406
New York, NY 10012
(212) 219-8180

HEALTH ASSOCIATIONS AND ORGANIZATIONS

National Institutes of Health
9000 Rockville Pike
Bethesda, MD 20892
(301) 496-4000

National Kidney Foundation
30 East 33rd Street
New York, NY 10016
(212) 889-2210

National Mental Health Association
1021 Prince Street
Alexandria, VA 22314-2971
(703) 684-7722

National Multiple Sclerosis Society
205 E. 42nd Street
New York, NY 10017
(212) 986-3240

National Parkinson Foundation
1501 NW 9th Avenue
Bob Hope Road
Miami, FL 33136-9990
(305) 547-6666
(800) 327-4545

**National Rehabilitation
Association**
633 S. Washington Street
Alexandria, VA 22314
(703) 836-0850

**National Society to Prevent
Blindness**
500 East Remington Road
Schaumberg, IL 60173
(708) 843-2020

**National Spinal Cord Injury
Association**
600 West Cummings Park, Suite 2000
Woburn, MA 01801
(617) 935-2722
(800) 962-9629

**Office on Smoking and Health
Technical Information Center**
5600 Fishers Lane
Park Building Room 1-16
Rockville, MD 20857
(301) 443-1690

**Planned Parenthood Federation of
America, Inc.**
810 Seventh Avenue
New York, NY 10019
Attn: Medical Division
(212) 603-4695

Psoriasis Research Institute
(formerly the International Psoriasis
Research Foundation)
600 Town & Country Village
Palo Alto, CA 94301
(415) 326-1848

**Rusk Institute of
Rehabilitation Medicine
NYU Medical Center**
400 East 34th Street
New York, NY 10016
(212) 340-6105

**United Cerebral Palsy
Associations, Inc.**
7 Penn Plaza
New York, NY 10001
(212) 268-6655

United Ostomy Association
36 Executive Park
Suite 120
Irvine, CA 92714
(714) 660-8624

**Wellness and Health Activation
Networks**
P.O. Box 923
Vienna, VA 22182-2057
(703) 281-3830

GLOSSARY

Terms commonly used in the health field

A

Abdominal aneurysm—usually due to dilatation of the aorta, the largest abdominal blood vessel, into a protruding sac caused by a weakening of its wall. May also occasionally occur in other abdominal blood vessels.

Abortion—the loss of the fetus in the course of pregnancy. Abortion may be spontaneous, induced, or done for therapeutic reasons.

Abrasion—removal of a portion of skin due to injury or a surgical procedure.

Abruptio placentae—the premature detachment of an otherwise normal placenta, the organ through which the developing fetus obtains nourishment and oxygen.

Abscess—localized collection of pus under the skin or in another part of the body, such as the ear, tooth, lung, brain or the liver; usually due to infection.

Acidosis—a condition in which the acid/base balance of body fluids is disturbed, thereby decreasing the alkaline content.

Aciduria—acid condition of the urine.

Acupuncture—ancient oriental treatment method using long fine needles in various areas of the body to reduce pain and alleviate various other disease conditions.

Acute—the quick, sharp onset of a condition such as pain, usually of limited duration.

Acute abdomen—an abdominal condition of sudden onset with severe pain and discomfort. In most instances emergency surgery is necessary.

Adenoma—a benign growth that is generally well circumscribed. It exerts pressure against surrounding tissue instead of infiltrating it as do other tumors.

Adrenal glands—two glands, each located near one of the kidneys, that secrete the hormones adrenaline and cortisone.

Adsorbent—a substance that can suck other substances to its surface, without requiring a chemical agent.

Agoraphobia—the fear of being in an open space.

AIDS—the letters stand for acquired immune deficiency syndrome, primarily a disease of homosexual men, intravenous drug abusers or people with hemophilia.

Airway—the respiratory tract, or any part of the respiratory tract that acts as a passage for air during the process of breathing.

Airway obstruction—any foreign body, or physical process that occludes the respiratory tract or any of its parts, making breathing difficult or impossible.

Albumin—a body protein present in tissue and body fluids.

Alcohol dependency—the inability to manage life's functions and responsibilities without consuming a given quantity of alcohol, or experiencing withdrawal symptoms if alcohol consumption is stopped. Alcoholism.

Alcohol poisoning—the toxic effects of excessive alchol intake.

Alkaloid—a type of chemical contained in many drugs that is made from plants or manufactured synthetically.

Allergy—an abnormal bodily reaction due to an acquired hypersensitivity on exposure to environmental substances such as dust, pollen, foods, bacteria or physical agents (heat, cold, light) that may be slight or severe. Symptoms appear in the form of respiratory symptoms (tearing, wheezing, coughing, sneezing); skin conditions (rashes, wheals or hives); or such digestive tract symptoms as belching, flatus, nausea, vomiting, abdominal pain or diarrhea.

Alopecia areata—a patchy loss of hair, usually of the scalp or beard, generally reversible.

Alzheimer's disease—mental deterioration of unknown cause, generally beginning in middle age.

Amblyopia—impaired vision, due to hereditary, structural or dietary deficiency.

Amebiasis—an infection caused by one-celled microorganisms (amebae) that mainly involves the intestine but may spread to other body organs, especially the liver.

Amenorrhea—the absence, or sudden cessation of the menstrual blood flow.

Amino acid—a substance formed during the digestive breakdown of proteins.

Amnesia—loss of memory, particularly of previous experiences.

Amniocentesis—the withdrawal, under sterile conditions, of a sample of fluid (amniotic fluid) from a thin, tough, transparent membranous sac (the amniotic sac) that surrounds, cushions and protects the developing fetus. Done to determine possible defects, and sometimes the sex of the unborn child.

Amniotic fluid—the protective fluid that is present in the amniotic sac during pregnancy to cushion the growing fetus against injury.

Amyotrophic lateral sclerosis (ALS)—a progressive disease of unknown cause of the nerves and muscles. It affects certain portions of the spinal cord with the muscles gradually wasting away (atrophy), which causes increasing weakness and eventual paralysis, especially in the muscles of the arms, shoulders, legs and those that control breathing.

Anabolism—the process of using energy to turn food taken into the body into living tissues.

Anaerobe—a microorganism that grows only when there is little, or no oxygen present.

Anal—the lowest portion of the intestinal tract.

Anal fissure—a linear ulcer extending from the sphincter up into the anal canal, which causes pain and bleeding.

Analgesic—a medication used to relieve pain.

Anaphylaxis—a severe form of allergic (hypersensitive) reaction to a substance that can be fatal if not treated immediately.

Androgens—any substance that produces masculine effects; in most instances these are male hormones.

Androsterone—a male sex hormone.

Anemia—an abnormal condition of the blood in which there is a deficiency of red blood cells, and/or a deficiency of hemoglobin, the substance which carries oxygen from the lungs to the tissues.

Aneurysm—a condition in which the wall of an artery weakens, balloons out and may burst, causing severe, possibly fatal bleeding.

Angina—a choking or suffocative type of spasmodic pain.

Angina pectoris—a severe, paroxysmal pain in the chest with a feeling of oppression or suffocation, due to an insufficient supply of blood oxygen to the heart muscle. These symptoms are usually precipitated by exertion or excitement.

Angioedema—swelling of body tissues, usually as part of an allergic reaction.

Angioneurotic edema—temporarily swollen areas of the skin or mucous membranes, and occasionally of the internal organs, which appear suddenly, often associated with hives.

Ankylosing spondylitis—an inflammation of the joints linking the vertebrae, followed by damaged joints that fuse together, resulting in pain and stiffness.

Anomaly—an abnormality or defect of a body organ or structure.

Anorectal—referring to the lowest portion of the intestinal tract, the anal canal and the rectum.

Anorexia—a loss of appetite due to illness, emotional disturbance or ingestion of certain drugs.

Anorexia nervosa—a psychological illness, mostly in adolescent girls, in which the patient eats little or no food, resulting in severe weight loss and possible death if not treated.

Anorexics—a category of drugs that suppresses the appetite, taken to enable a person to lose weight.

Antacid—an alkaline drug that neutralizes excessive stomach acids.

Anthelmintics—drugs given to destroy and expel intestinal worms.

Antibacterial—a drug that counteracts, inhibits, or destroys bacteria.

Antibiotics—chemical substances, produced by microorganisms or synthetically, that combat bacterial infections by killing other organisms or inhibiting their growth.

Antibody—a constituent of blood and body fluids that acts to protect the body against infection.

Anticaries agent—a drug that protects teeth or bones against decay or destruction.

Anticholinergics—drugs that suppress secretions from the stomach and other internal organs such as glands, dilate the pupils of the eyes, and decrease the actions of the respiratory, gastrointestinal and urinary systems.

Anticoagulant—a drug given to slow the clotting action of blood.

Antidiarrheal—an agent or substance, usually a drug, that counteracts the effects of diarrhea.

Antidote—an agent or substance, usually a drug, that counteracts a poison applied to the body externally or via ingestion, either by accident or by intention.

Antiemetic—an agent or substance, usually a drug, that counteracts nausea and/or vomiting.

Antiflatulent—an agent or substance, usually a drug, that counteracts excessive gas in the intestinal tract.

Antifungal—an agent or substance, usually a drug, that counteracts the effects of fungal organisms that cause infections of the skin, nails, hair, and of the mucous membranes.

Antigen—a substance which causes the production of antibodies when it is absorbed by the body through ingestion of food, inhalation, or application to the skin.

Antihistamine—a drug that counteracts the action of histamine, an organic compound that acts as a powerful dilator of small blood vessels. Antihistamine drugs are used to relieve symptoms of allergy and those of the common cold.

Antimicrobial (antibacterial)—an agent, usually a drug, that acts to destroy or inhibit the actions of disease-causing microorganisms, such as bacteria.

Antipruritic—an agent, usually a drug, that decreases, stops or prevents itching.

Antipyretic—an agent, usually a drug, that reduces fever.

Antiseptic—an agent, usually a drug, that inhibits the growth and development of microorganisms, such as bacteria.

Antiserum—a specially prepared liquid portion of blood that contains antibodies against a specific disease.

Antispasmodic—an agent, usually a drug, that reduces or relieves spasms in certain body tissues such as the sphincter (muscular opening) of the stomach, gallbladder or the rectum. An antispasmodic can also relieve spasms in blood vessels, or in such body parts as the bronchi.

Antitussive—an agent, usually a drug, that relieves or stops spasms of coughing.

Anxiety—a psychological condition that causes fear, apprehension and feelings of imminent danger, with accompanying physical symptoms such as difficulty in breathing, restlessness and an increase in the rate of heartbeat.

Aorta—the main artery (largest blood vessel in the body), that arises from the heart, arches through the chest down into the abdomen and carries oxygenated blood from the heart to smaller arteries, bringing oxygen to nourish the organs and tissues throughout the body.

Aortic Stenosis—narrowing of the aorta, the main blood vessel leading from the heart.

Aphasia—the inability to speak, write or communicate via appropriate signs, or to understand the writing or speaking of others, usually as a result of brain damage.

Apoplexy (stroke)—a condition caused by hemorrhage, or bleeding in the brain from a ruptured blood vessel, due to weakness in the blood vessel's wall, or blockage of the vessel from a local clot, or one that traveled from another site (embolus) in the arterial system or the heart.

Aqueous humor—fluid produced in the front portion of the eyeball. This fluid bathes the anterior structures of the eyeball. If its normal outflow is blocked, painful, dangerous pressure develops inside the eye, a condition known as glaucoma.

Arrhythmia—irregularity in the pattern of the heartbeat.

Arteriography—X-ray study of part of the arterial system to diagnose disturbance of the blood supply to any body part or area.

Arteriosclerosis—hardening of one or more arteries.

Arteritis—inflammation of one or more arteries.

Arthritis—a condition in which body joints and their supporting structures are inflamed and painful.

Ascites—an abnormal collection of fluid in the abdominal area due to disease conditions of one or more organs such as the liver, the heart or the kidneys.

Ascorbic acid (vitamin C)—a nutritional substance essential to normal body function. Deficiency causes scurvy, a condition in which the affected person suffers from bleeding and inflammation of the gums, loose teeth, and bleeding in other areas.

Aseptic—a substance that kills microorganisms, and sterilizes the area to which it is applied; sterile.

Asphyxia—state of suffocation due to some form of interference with normal breathing.

Aspirate—(noun) fluid or tissue removed from the body via suction. (verb) To suction.

Asthma—a breathing disorder caused by infection or allergy in the bronchi.

Astigmatism—an unequal curvature of the cornea, the outside front part of the eye. It distorts vision, usually is present from birth, and does not worsen with age.

Astringent—a medication that contracts blood vessels and other tissues, thereby reducing swelling, bleeding or secretions.

Atelectasis—collapse of a portion of a lung.

Athlete's foot—an infection of the foot caused by a fungal microorganism

Atopic—a type of allergy that occurs only in humans.

Atrial fibrillation—heart's upper chambers (atrium) contract irregularly at a rate of about 400 beats per minute. The result is a reduction in the efficiency of the heart's pumping action.

Atrial flutter—the atrium beats at a regular fast rate of 200-300 beats per minute.

Atrium—the upper chambers of the heart. The right atrium receives unoxygenated blood from the body on its way to the lungs to be oxygenated. The left atrium receives oxygenated blood from lungs which then is pumped out into the body.

Atrophy—the wasting of tissue, muscles or any other body part or organ.

Atypical pneumonia—inflammation of the lungs usually caused by viruses or uncommon organisms.

Auscultation—listening to various sounds, such as those produced by the heart or the lungs, with the ear or through a stethoscope.

Autism—a psychological disorder of children and some adults in which the person escapes real life by living in a world of fantasy, unable and unwilling to respond to ordinary human contact.

Autoantibody—an antibody produced by the body in reaction to its own tissues.

Autoantigen—a substance present in the body to which an individual is allergic.

Autogenous vaccine—a vaccine prepared from material taken from the body of a person who will subsequently receive the vaccine.

Autoimmune disease—a condition caused when the body produces antibodies against its own tissues.

Autoinfection—a condition in which a person becomes reinfected by microorganisms that had caused an earlier infection.

Autopsy—examination of the body after death, to increase medical knowledge or establish the cause of death.

Autosomal inheritance—inherited traits passed on by genes located in 22 pairs of autosomes, which carry all characteristics other than those of sex.

Avitaminosis—a deficiency of essential vitamins.

B

Bacillary—referring to a bacillus, a rod-shaped type of microorganism occurring in some forms that are harmless, and in others that cause disease.

Bacteremia—blood poisoning caused by the presence of bacteria in the blood.

Barium enema—a diagnostic X-ray procedure done to examine the lower intestinal tract. Barium is given in the form of an enema to make the bowel visible on the X-ray film.

Barium swallow—a liquid preparation containing barium which shows up on an X-ray. The patient swallows the liquid during X-ray examination of the stomach and intestines.

Basal cell carcinoma—a type of skin cancer in which a tumor starts in the cells just under the skin surface and develops into an ulcer.

Bell's Palsy—paralysis which distorts the face. It is caused by a lesion of the facial nerve.

Beriberi—a disease involving the heart and the nervous system, caused by a deficiency of vitamin B_1 (thiamine).

Beta blockers—drugs that reduce the rate of the heartbeat or lower the blood pressure by blocking off the effects of adrenaline-like substances.

Bile—a fluid secreted by the liver, which is carried through bile ducts into the small intestine, where it plays an important role in the digestion of fats.

Biliary—referring to the gallbladder or any portion of the gallbladder tract.

Biliary calculus—a stone in the gallbladder or in any part of the gallbladder tract.

Biopsy—removal and examination, usually under a microscope, of body tissue, to establish an exact diagnosis.

Blackhead—fatty material that has hardened into a plug inside a skin pore.

Blepharitis—an inflammation of the eyelids.

Blister—a collection of fluid formed inside a sac on or in the skin, caused by irritation, fever, a burn, or one of the various skin or infectious diseases.

Blood—the fluid that circulates through the arteries, veins and smaller blood vessels to bring nourishment to the tissues and remove wastes.

Blood brain barrier—a mechanism that prevents many substances that circulate in the blood, such as certain drugs, from getting into the circulation of the brain.

Blood component—any constituent of blood, such as red blood cells, white blood cells, platelets and others.

Blood gases—gases, such as oxygen and carbon dioxide that are dissolved in the blood.

Blood groups—also called blood types. There are four main blood groups (types) A, B, AB and O. There are also many sub-groups. Persons who have one type of blood can only receive a blood transfusion from another person who has the same blood type. The same is true for a blood donor, who can donate his blood only to a person of the same type. The exceptions are a donor of type O blood (universal donor), whose blood can be administered to any other person regardless of the other's blood type, and a person with type AB blood (universal recipient), who can receive blood from any other person, whatever his blood type. But the AB type donor can give blood only to another AB type recipient.

Blood pressure—the pressure exerted by the circulating blood against the walls of the blood vessels through which is flows.

Blood volume—the amount (volume) of blood in the body at any time, generally considered normal at 8-9% of body weight.

Boil—an area of skin filled with pus due to an infection.

Bone marrow—tissues that are contained in the cavities of bones. Red bone marrow contains developing red blood cells, white blood cells and platelets, while yellow bone marrow consists of a fatty substance.

Botulism—a type of food poisoning caused by a bacterium that grows in food that has not been properly canned or preserved. Symptoms are vomiting, abdominal pain, vision disorders, and possibly muscular paralysis.

Bowel—another term for the intestine, which consists of two parts: the small intestine and the large intestine (small bowel and large bowel).

Bowel incontinence—inability to retain or control bowel movements.

Bradycardia—a very slow heart beat, usually considered to be less than 60 beats per minute.

Breech presentation—in childbirth the baby's position in rotated so that the buttocks instead of the baby's head is presented first.

Bronchiectasis—a disease in which the bronchi [hollow tubular structures that carry inhaled air from the windpipe (trachea) to the lungs], and/or their smaller subdivisions (bronchioles) are widened due to repeated bouts of infection in the lungs. This disease is marked by foul-smelling breath and coughing spells, accompanied by spitting, and coughing up of mucus, pus-filled material from the bronchi. May also see particles of blood in mucus.

Bronchitis—inflammation of the lining of the bronchi.

Bronchodilator—a drug given to dilate the bronchial tubes when they are shut down by spasms, such as occur in asthma.

Bronchogenic—any disease or other condition that arises in the bronchi.

Bronchopneumonia—inflammation, usually due to infection, of the lower portions of the bronchi (bronchioles) and the lungs.

Bronchoscopy—visualization of the windpipe (trachea) and the bronchial structures via an endoscope, a lighted instrument passed into these passages, for examination or treatment.

Bruxism—clenching or grinding of the teeth, usually done during sleep.

Bunion—a condition, usually due to wearing improperly fitting shoes, which causes a painful deformity of the big toe.

Bursitis—inflammation of a bursa, a sac-like cavity filled with a thick fluid that lubricates areas otherwise likely to sustain damage through friction; mainly affects bursae near joints, or those underneath the tendons that move the joints.

C

Calciferol (vitamin D)—an essential nutritional substance that affects the development of bone. With insufficient intake of this vitamin bone disease may occur.

Calcium—a vital element essential to the healthy composition of bones and teeth. Insufficient intake of calcium may produce bone and teeth problems.

Callus—a hardened portion of skin, usually found on the palms of the hands or the soles, due to continual pressure and friction on these areas.

Caloric value—the measurement of heat produced by a food when it is burned (metabolized) in the body.

Calories—a calorie is the amount of heat needed to raise the temperature of 1 kilogram of water 1 degree Celsius. The amount of energy the body derives from various foods is expressed in calories.

Canals (Semicircular Ear Canals)—three connected tubes, bent into half-circles, located in the labyrinth, the part of the inner ear concerned with balance.

Cancer—a group of diseases in which the body's cells multiply and spread uncontrollably. The cells first form a tumor and later may metastasize (travel to other parts of the body) where they produce new malignancies.

Candida—a common type of yeastlike fungus. In man, Candida fungus is frequently found on the skin, in the throat, vagina, and in feces. Infection caused by this type of fungus is called candidiasis or moniliasis.

Canker sore—a small, usually ulcerated sore on the inside of the mouth, due to illness, irritation, or vitamin deficiency.

Capillary—relates to a tiny blood or lymph vessel.

Carbuncle—a skin condition caused by an infection, in which an area is filled with pus, enclosed by a hard covering that has a number of openings through which the pus may be discharged. It is bigger, and reaches down into the skin further than a boil.

Carcinogen—any substance in the environment or in food, or in some other agent, that may contribute to the development of cancer.

Cardiac—relating to the heart.

Cardiac arrest—a sudden stopping of the pumping of the heart that is fatal if not reversed within a few minutes.

Cardiac catheterization—the passing of a very fine tube into the chambers of the heart for diagnostic purposes.

Cardiac infarction—a blockage of a coronary artery (one of the arteries that supply blood to the heart muscle) by a blood clot (thrombus). The result is damage to the part of the heart muscle whose blood supply is cut off.

Cardiomiopathy—Disease of the heart muscle due to numerous causes.

Cardiopulmonary resuscitation (CPR)—the technique of resuscitating an unconscious individual when breathing or cardiac function ceases.

Cardiovascular—relating to the heart or the blood vessels.

Carditis—inflammation of the heart.

Caries—a condition that indicates decay of teeth or bones.

Carotid artery—the principal artery in the neck. There is one on each side.

Carpal tunnel syndrome—a condition due to pressure on a nerve on the palm or surface of the wrist. This causes pain, burning, tingling and numbness of the fingers and hand.

Cartilage—whitish, tough, flexible tissue situated around joints, in the spinal column, the ears, windpipe, voice box (larynx) and the tip of the nose.

Catabolism—the breakdown process of food during digestion into less complex substances.

Cataract—a condition in which the lens of the eye becomes cloudy, impairing vision. This process may be due to aging, disease, trauma, or may sometimes be found at birth as a congenital condition.

Catarrh—an inflammation of mucous membranes usually accompanied by a discharge. When it occurs only in the nose (as in the common cold), it is called rhinitis. If it affects both the nose and the throat, it is also called nasopharyngitis.

Catecholamines—chemical substances in the body that affect the actions of the involuntary nervous system.

Cathartic—a drug that speeds up the emptying action of the bowel.

Catheterization—a process in which a tube is passed into a body organ to empty it, as in urinary catheterization, or for diagnostic or treatment purposes.

CAT Scan—Computerized Axial Tomography. A complicated system using X-rays, magnetic tapes, scintillation counters and computers in order to visualize internal structures at varying levels.

Cat-scratch disease—a relatively mild infection believed to be transmitted via a virus that lives in cats, when a person is scratched by an otherwise healthy cat. Symptoms involve headache, fever and swelling of some lymph glands.

Cauterization—destruction of tissue with an electric current, some caustic substances or a hot iron.

Cellulitis—inflammation of cellular or connective tissue in various parts of the body.

Centigrade—a measurement of heat used throughout the world based on a scale that is divided into 100 degrees. Normal body temperature on this scale is 37°C, which corresponds to the Fahrenheit scale at 98.6°F.

Central nervous system—that part of the nervous system that includes the brain and the spinal cord.

Cerebral hemorrhage—bleeding from an artery or other blood vessel in the brain, caused by weakness, injury, congenital abnormality or a disease such as high blood pressure.

Cerebral palsy—a condition of weakness, poor muscular coordination and spasm caused by damage to the brain that may occur before, during, or shortly after birth.

Cerebrospinal fluid—the fluid that bathes the brain and the spinal cord.

Cerebrovascular accident—(see Stroke)

Cerumen—the wax in the ears.

Cerumenolytics—agents or drugs that dissolve ear wax.

Cervix—the neck of the womb, an important part of a woman's birth canal.

Cesarean section (C-section)—the surgical delivery of a baby through the abdomen, done when the baby is in distress during labor, when the mother is ill and not considered strong enough to cope with a normal vaginal delivery, or if the mother's birth canal is malformed, so that the baby cannot pass through safely.

Chalazion—a usually painless, slow-growing localized swelling in the margin of the eyelid due to a blockage of a small gland that is chronically inflamed.

Chancre—a symptom of syphilis, a venereal disease caused by spirochetal bacteria called treponema pallidum. The chancre is a hard skin lesion that occurs during the first stage of the disease, at the site where the spirochetes entered the body.

Chemotherapy—chemical agents or drugs used to treat various diseases, or to prevent them.

Chilblains—the swelling, reddening and itching of body parts such as the hands, fingers, nose and ears following prolonged exposure to cold.

Chlamydia trachomatis—an organism that can cause infections in the eye, urethra or genital organs.

Chloasma—brown pigmented spots or patches on the skin of the face and other parts of the body that occur with pregnancy, the menopause, or with the use of oral contraceptives.

Cholecystitis—inflammation of the gallbladder.

Cholecystokinetics—drugs that promote and affect the functioning of the gallbladder.

Cholera—an acute intestinal infection caused by bacteria that spread the disease via polluted water, food, insects and excrement.

Cholesterol—a white, crystalline substance that dissolves in fat and is present in all body tissues. It is a steroid made by the liver and the adrenal glands, and it is thought to contribute to the hardening of the arteries.

Cholinergics—drugs that act on the involuntary nervous system to increase the activity of internal organs such as the gastrointestinal tract, the heart, the lungs and produce expansion of the blood vessels.

Chorea—twitching, involuntary and irregular movement of the muscles that occurs in a number of nervous system diseases.

Chromosomes—the carriers of the genes that determine the sex and physical characteristics of each person.

Chronic—a state, or disease condition that lasts for a long period of time, without any appreciable change.

Ciliary body—a structure in the eye that holds and supports the iris (round colored portion of the eye) in place.

Circumcision—the removal of some or all of the foreskin (prepuce) of the penis, done in many infants shortly after birth, but also performed later in life if the foreskin interferes with normal function.

Cirrhosis—a degenerative disease of the liver in which liver cells are destroyed and replaced by useless fatty or fibrous tissue.

Citric acid—the acid found in citrus fruits. Useful as a scurvy preventive.

Claudication (intermittent)—lameness, limping and leg pain (chiefly in the calf muscles) on exertion. This happens when arteries narrowed by disease provide an insufficient blood supply to the muscles, often limiting the affected person to walking only a short distance at a time.

Claw toes—a deformity of the toes due to poorly fitting shoes.

Cleft lip (harelip)—a birth defect in which a baby is born with a split in the tissues below the nose extending down through the upper lip, or the lip may be absent entirely. This condition often occurs together with a cleft palate, causing feeding problems. Both conditions can be repaired by surgery.

Coagulation—the clotting of blood or other fluid into a gel or solid.

Coagulation time—a test to determine whether there is a deficiency in the blood that delays its ability to clot within a short time when it is exposed to air. The test is also done in persons who are taking certain drugs to lengthen the clotting time of the blood.

Cobalamin (vitamin B_{12})—an essential nutritive substance required for the adequate development of the red blood cells, for normal functions of the nervous system, and for various other cellular functions.

Cobalt—an essential substance which is a component of vitamin B_{12}, normally present in green, leafy vegetables. Inadequate amounts in the diet may produce anemia in children.

Coitus—the act of sexual intercourse.

Colic—abdominal pain usually caused by cramps in the intestine or stomach.

Colitis—inflammation of the lower portion of the bowel called the colon.

Collagen—the predominant protein of the white fibers in connective tissue, cartilage and bone.

Colles fracture—a break in the wrist bone that causes the hand to be displaced backward and outward.

Colonoscopy—the visualization of the inside of the colon with a lighted tube called a colonoscope that is passed into the colon through the rectum.

Color blindness—inability to distinguish between certain colors, most commonly between reds and greens, particularly when the light is dim.

Colostomy—an opening into the colon, created by abdominal surgery to relieve an intestinal obstruction or other disease of the colon. This allows the discharge of feces through the opening instead of through the rectum.

Colostrum—the fluid expressed from a new mother's breast before her milk is formed in the breast glands a process completed about three days after the baby's birth.

Coma—a level of unconsciousness from which a person cannot be aroused. Coma may be due to disease, drug abuse, other forms of poisoning or injury.

Comedone—blackhead.

Comminuted fracture—a break that occurs in such a way that the bone is broken into several pieces.

Communicable disease—a contagious disease that can be spread to other persons in a variety of ways.

Complete blood count—a laboratory examination done to determine whether a person has the normal quantity and appearance of blood constituents.

Compound fracture—a break in which the broken portion of the bone has penetrated the skin and created an open wound.

Compression fracture—a fracture in which one bony surface is driven towards another bony surface. Commonly found in fractures of the spine involving the bony segments of the spinal column.

Compulsive behavior—a psychological disturbance in which a person feels forced to behave in certain, often inappropriate ways.

Concussion—loss of consciousness produced by a blow to the head.

Congenital—a condition, deformity or disease present at the time of birth.

Congestive heart failure—a condition in which the heart fails to provide sufficient pumping action to circulate blood adequately, resulting in congestion of the lungs and other vital organs due to the accumulation of blood.

Conjunctivitis—inflammation of the mucous membrane that lines the eye balls and the inner parts of the eyelids.

Constipation—infrequent or difficult passing of hard bowel movements.

Contact dermatitis—irritation of the skin due to exposure to an irritating, or sensitizing substance such as poison ivy.

Contact lens—a very small lens made either of glass or plastic that is worn directly on the eye instead of eye glasses. It may also be worn by a person after a cataract operation, in which case the contact lens replaces the lens removed during surgery. A contact lens provides better vision for a person whose cataract has been removed because it permits peripheral vision, which eye glasses don't provide.

Contusion—a bruise; the swelling and discoloration that appear on the skin after an injury, or pressure as been applied to that area.

Convalescent serum—serum obtained from a person who has recovered from an infectious disease. It may be given to another person who is susceptible, to immunize him against the disease, or to modify its severity, if he develops it.

Conversion—a freudian term for the process by which emotions become transformed into physical (motor or sensory) manifestations.

Convulsion—seizure; the contraction of muscles in the entire body, or a body part, with resulting contortion of the affected parts. This condition may occur due to disturbances of the nervous system, as a symptom of epilepsy, during periods when an individual has a very high temperature, and in various other disease states.

Copper—an essential nutritive element present in such foods as organ meat, oysters, nuts and whole grain cereals. Its deficiency can cause anemia in children.

Corn—a thickened, often painful area on or between the toes. Usually caused by poorly fitting shoes.

Cornea—the clear, transparent portion of the eye that permits the entry of light, refracts light rays and helps focus the eye.

Coronary arteriography—a procedure used to find the place where an artery supplying blood to the heart is blocked or damaged. A dye that shows up on X-ray is injected through a catheter inserted into an artery in the arm or groin and threaded into the coronary artery.

Coronary artery—the principal artery providing the blood supply to the heart via its right and left branches.

Coronary Artery Bypass—a piece of a vein taken from the leg is grafted onto a coronary artery to bypass the blocked coronary artery, thus restoring good circulation to the heart muscle.

Coronary heart disease—a condition in which a build-up of fatty deposits narrows the arteries that supply the heart muscle with blood.

Coronary occlusion—the blockage or obstruction of the heart's blood flow; occurs as a result of heart disease in which the arteries of the heart narrow due to deposits that form on their walls, allowing formation of blood clots that cause the obstruction.

Coronary thrombosis—blockage of one of the coronary arteries by a blood clot. This cuts off the blood supply to part of the heart muscle and results in a heart attack.

Corpus luteum—a small glandular structure in the egg-forming body (ovary) of a woman's reproductive tract, which secretes estrogen and progesterone hormones and plays an important part during pregnancy.

Corticosteroids—hormonal medications, naturally or synthetically produced, derived from the adrenal glands.

Coryza—nasal discharge and inflammation of the upper respiratory tract, as occurs during a cold, or in persons who have hay fever.

Counterirritant—a substance or medication applied to the skin to irritate and mildly inflame it, in order to produce a feeling of warmth and comfort; helpful when applied to painful muscle areas during a cold, or after exertion.

Cradle cap—a fatty type of skin condition in small infants who develop yellow scaly areas and skin cracks behind the ears, crusts on the scalp, and red pimples on the face. This condition is often worse during the winter than during other seasons.

Cranium—the bony structure of the skull that contains the brain.

Crepitus—a creaking, crackling or rattling noise heard and/or felt over broken bones or joints that are subject to wear and tear. The term is also used to describe a noisy discharge of gas from the intestine.

Cretinism—a congenital lack of thyroid hormone causing arrested physical and mental development.

Crib death—also known as sudden infant death syndrome (SIDS). A baby who seems healthy or has a slight cold dies in its sleep. Usually, no cause can be found.

Crohn's disease—chronic inflammation of the intestine. Symptoms include abdominal cramps and pain, diarrhea, and sometimes fever. May recur every few months, every few years, or only once or twice in a lifetime.

Croup—a respiratory condition in young children, often due to infection, featured by a harsh, brassy cough and crowing, difficult breathing. Commonly occurs at night. If unrelieved by exposure to a warm, moist environment produced by a steam inhalator, or bathroom filled with moisture by a hot, running shower, emergency treatment must be provided, preferably in a hospital.

Culture—a process in which microorganisms in a specimen such as blood, urine or a throat swab are placed in a nutrient broth and allowed to grow, so that they can be identified, and appropriate treatment given.

Cutaneous—pertaining to the skin.

Cyanosis—a bluish discoloration of the skin and mucous membranes caused by inadequate oxygen in the blood.

Cyst—a sac of tissue anywhere in the body that contains fluid, gas, fatty or other matter.

Cystic Fibrosis—a hereditary disease of infants, children, and young adults. The inability of the pancreas to secrete digestive enzymes results in poor nutrition, abdominal cramps, and diarrhea with a typical foul odor. The lungs secrete a thick mucus, causing many respiratory infections.

Cystitis—inflammation of the urinary bladder, usually due to irritation or infection.

Cystoscopy—examination of the urinary bladder and the lower portion of the urinary tract with a lighted instrument called a cystoscope.

Cytology—the examination and study of cells.

Cytotoxic—any substance, drug, or other matter that is harmful to cells.

D

Debridement—removal of diseased, dirty or foreign matter from a wound.

Decongestant—a drug that relieves the discomfort and swelling caused by such conditions as hay fever or a cold, by shrinking the mucous membranes of the nose.

Decubitus (bed sore)—a condition caused by being bedfast, disabled, or having to lie in one position for a long time, allowing pressure on the area to break down the skin, and the underlying structures. It can be prevented by frequent change of position, exercise, good skin care, and good nutrition.

Dehydration—great loss of body fluid due to vomiting, diarrhea, loss of blood and other disease conditions. It is corrected by drinking fluids or, in serious cases, by giving fluids intravenously.

Delirium—a condition of confusion and restlessness, due to psychological or other causes, such as a high fever.

Delirium tremens—also known as the DT's; a condition of confusion and disorientation commonly associated with chronic alcoholism.

Delusion—a psychological disturbance in which a person has a false impression, belief or concept which he is convinced is true; reasonable discussion or argument will not change his belief.

Dementia—impairment of the mind; generally appears together with emotional and behavioral disturbances.

Demulcent—a substance or drug that soothes and relieves irritations of such body surfaces as the skin and mucous membranes. Internal mucous membranes, such as those lining the intestinal tract, are also relieved by demulcents when affected by certain irritating conditions.

Dengue—also known as dengue fever; an infectious disease that occurs commonly in the tropics, but may also be found in the southern U.S. It is a viral disease with symptoms that include joint pains, fever, rash, headache and weakness.

Depressant—a substance or drug that slows down excessive mental or physical activity. A tranquilizing drug, for instance, can be used to depress (reduce) excited behavior.

Depression—a state of mind in which a person feels low, has little or no hope, and may consider himself worthless. Counseling and/or treatment with an appropriate drug may relieve the condition.

Dermatitis—a skin condition caused by infection, irritation, or other disease.

Dermatologic—referring to skin, or the treatment of a skin condition.

Deviated Septum—a condition in which the wall between the nostrils (septum) is crooked, leading to obstruction of breathing.

Diabetes insipidus—a metabolic disorder due to injury of the neurohypophyseal system, which results in a deficient quantity of antidiuretic hormone being released or produced, and thus in failure of tubular reabsorption of water in the kidney. As a consequence, there is the passage of a large amount of urine of low specific gravity, and a great thirst; it is often attended by voracious appetite, loss of strength, and emaciation.

Diabetes mellitus—a disease that can be inherited, in which the pancreas doesn't secrete sufficient insulin to properly utilize body carbohydrates. In milder, adult forms of the disease weight reduction, diet or oral medication may be sufficient for treatment. In more severe cases, and in the juvenile onset form of the disease, insulin must be injected at regular intervals, and a special diet followed to control the disease and to prevent complications.

Diabetic coma—a state of unconsciousness that results when blood sugar rises to a very high level, and no effort is made to reduce it with an appropriate amount of insulin. When the blood sugar level is out of control, other metabolic disturbances follow that affect the nervous system and the level of consciousness. When this happens, treatment must be given immediately or death may result.

Diagnostic findings—findings that result from a careful physical examination, including the patient's history, laboratory tests and other special studies done to identify a condition or disease so that appropriate treatment may be started, if needed.

Diagnostic radiology—X-ray studies performed to study a complaint in order to contribute to the accurate identification of a condition or disease.

Dialysis—treatment for removal of waste from the blood, needed by patients whose kidneys no longer function properly.

Diaper rash—reddened, irritated or sore skin in the diaper region. May be caused by insufficient exposure to air, infrequent diaper changes, the composition of the baby's urine, and other factors. Frequent diaper changes, skin exposure to air, careful rinsing of diapers during laundry to remove all traces of soap or bleach help to prevent this condition.

Diaphoresis—profuse perspiration or sweat that is visible or perceptible.

Diarrhea—a condition in which a person has frequent loose bowel movements, with or without abdominal cramps, that may be caused as a result of eating certain foods, by intestinal infection or by a disease process.

Diastolic phase of blood pressure (diastole)—the lowest level noted during blood pressure measurement. It reflects the pressure within the artery and the heart's chambers as the heart muscles relax and the chambers fill with blood to prepare for the next contraction.

Diathermy—heating of the body tissues by electrical means.

Dilation and curettage—also called D&C, a procedure in which the cervix (neck of the uterus or womb) is stretched to allow insertion of an instrument called a curette, which is used to scrape the lining of the uterus. The purpose may be diagnostic, to terminate an unwanted pregnancy, or treat an incomplete abortion or miscarriage.

Disc, prolapsed—also called a slipped disc. A cartilaginous disc, which acts as a cushion between two vertebrae is displaced which results in pressure on nerves.

Dislocation—displacement of one or more bones of a joint, or other body part, from its original position. Commonly occurs during a traumatic event such as a fall.

Disorientation—a mental state in which a person is confused, may not recognize other persons he knows well, or know the time or place, or other facts he's normally well familiar with. May be due to a disease process, or to toxic states such as alcohol or drug abuse.

Dissecting aneurysm—one resulting from hemorrhage that causes longitudinal splitting of the arterial wall, producing a tear in the intima and establishing communication with the lumen; it usually affects the thoracic aorta.

Diuretic—a substance or drug that causes increased urination.

Diverticulitis—a condition in which pouches (diverticula) in the colon (lower bowel) become filled with feces and other waste material, which in turn cause inflammation and frequently infection. Often accompanied by abdominal pain.

Diverticulum—one of a number of small pouches that develop inside the colon.

Dominant inheritance—some inherited traits are dominant over others. When a fetus receives two genetic traits, and one is stronger genetically than the other, he will be born exhibiting the dominant characteristic.

Dosage—the exact quantity of a drug that has been prescribed for a given time period.

Down's Syndrome—a birth defect caused by an extra chromosome in the cells throughout the body, resulting in mental retardation and mongolian-like features.

Dropsy—a condition in which one or more body parts show swelling, usually due to a chronic disease; also called edema.

Dry socket—a condition that may follow tooth extraction. The blood clot formed after the extraction disintegrates prematurely, leaving the tooth socket empty and prone to infection. Generally occurs within two or three days after the extraction, and may last, causing considerable pain, for several weeks.

Ductus arteriosus—an opening between the pulmonary artery and the aorta, that closes shortly after birth under normal conditions.

Dumping syndrome—a condition that sometimes follows gastrointestinal surgery, particularly after removal, or partial removal of the stomach. Symptoms including sweating, dizziness, nausea, vomiting and palpitations (increased heart rate) after meals.

Duodenum—the first portion of the small intestine.

Duodenal ulcer—a lesion in the duodenum that results in the loss of tissue due to inflammation. The ulcer may penetrate the wall of the duodenum causing hemorrhage and other complications. It is caused by excessive secretion of stomach acid, intake of certain drugs, foods, or stress.

Dupuytren's Contracture—thickening and shortening of the palm of the hand causing fingers to remain in flexion.

Dwarfism—a condition in which a person remains abnormally small.

Dysentery—a severe intestinal infection that produces diarrhea; it may be caused by a variety of microorganisms.

Dyskinesia—a condition in which a person has difficulty in carrying out voluntary movements.

Dyslexia—a disorder causing reading disability.

Dysmenorrhea—pain during menstrual periods.

Dyspareunia—pain during sexual intercourse.

Dysphagia—difficulty in swallowing.

Dysphasia—difficulty in speaking, and in expressing oneself understandably to others, usually due to brain damage.

Dyspnea—difficulty in breathing; shortness of breath, usually due to disease of the heart or lungs.

Dystrophy, muscular—a disease of unknown origin in which muscles do not function normally, and eventually deteriorate.

Dysuria—difficulty or pain during urination.

E

Ecchymosis—an area of purplish discoloration on the skin, due to bleeding underneath that area.

Echocardiogram—the record made by echocardiography, which records the position and motion of the heart walls or interior structures by ultrasound.

Eclampsia—a condition in which a pregnant woman develops convulsions (seizures) shortly before, or during labor, as a result of having high blood pressure during the pregnancy, associated with kidney problems.

Ectopic pregnancy—a pregnancy which develops in one of the fallopian tubes (the tubes that conduct the fertilized egg from the ovary to the womb) instead of in the womb.

Eczema—redness, itching, weeping, oozing, and crusting of the skin, often caused by allergy or sensitivity to some material.

Eczematous—an acute or chronic inflammatory condition of the skin, due to allergy or other causes.

Edema—swelling in body tissues or in a body part, such as the legs.

Edentia—state of not having any teeth.

Electrocardiogram (ECG, EKG)—a record made by a machine called the electrocardiograph that traces the electrical activity of the heart, and indicates abnormalities if any are present.

Electroencephalogram (EEG)—a record made by a machine called an electroencephalograph that traces the electrical activity of the brain (brain waves).

Electrolyte—a substance capable of conducting an electric current when it is in solution.

Electromyogram (EMG)—a record made with a machine called an electromyograph that traces the electrical activity of muscles. It is used to diagnose muscle diseases.

Embolism—an obstruction in a blood vessel by a traveling blood clot or various other substances.

Emesis—the act of vomiting.

Emetic—a drug used to induce vomiting.

Emollient—a substance or drug that smoothes and softens irritated skin or mucous membranes.

Emphysema—a condition in which the lungs have enlarged air sacs which cause difficulty in breathing.

Empyema—the formation of pus in one of the body cavities, frequently the lung.

Encephalitis—inflammatory condition of the brain, usually due to infection.

Endocrine—refers to a gland, such as the pituitary, which secretes a hormone directly into the blood stream.

Endogenous—refers to a body process that begins, or is produced, in the body or in one of its parts.

Endometriosis—a condition in which cells that normally line the walls of the womb begin to grow on the surfaces of other organs within the pelvic structure, and sometimes also in distant areas of the body.

Endometrium—the mucous membrane that lines the womb (uterus).

Endotoxin—a toxic (poisonous) substance released by certain microorganisms inside the body when their cell walls are injured.

Enterocolitis—inflammation of the small and large intestines.

Enterovirus—a virus that lives in the intestinal tract.

Entropion—turning in of the eyelid toward the eye.

Enuresis—bedwetting during the night, a condition that occurs primarily in children. It is involuntary.

Enzyme—a body substance that reduces complex compounds such as food into simpler compounds so they can be absorbed by the body.

Epidemic—a contagious disease that spreads through a large area of a community, a country, and sometimes an entire continent.

Epidermis—the outermost portion of the skin.

Epididymitis—inflammation of the sperm duct in the testicles.

Epiglottis—a piece of cartilage behind and below the tongue that closes the top of the windpipe (trachea) when a person is about to swallow, so that the food will go down the gullet (esophagus) and not the windpipe.

Epilepsy—a disease of the nervous system in which the victim has convulsions (seizures) and lapses of unconsciousness at different intervals. Newer medications help to control this disorder.

Epiphysis—the end portion of long bone.

Epistaxis—nosebleed.

Erb's palsy—injury of the baby's upper arm muscles during birth which produces paralysis of the arm.

Eructation—the act of belching.

Erysipelas—a painful infection of the skin caused by streptococcus bacteria.

Erythema—a reddened condition of the skin, due to irritation or infection.

Erythema multiforme—a skin disease due to a variety of causes, which presents in the form of tiny elevations and small blisters.

Erythroblastosis fetalis—a blood disease of newborn infants caused by the interaction of blood factors between an Rh negative mother and an Rh positive father.

Erythrocyte—red blood cell.

Erythrocyte sedimentation rate (ESR)—a laboratory test that determines the presence of infection in the body.

Esophageal—referring to the esophagus (gullet).

Esophagoscopy—examination of the inside of the esophagus (gullet) with a lighted tube called an esophagoscope.

Essential fatty acids—fats ingested in foods that are broken down by the body into simpler fat compounds and absorbed.

Estrogen—one of the female sex hormones.

Ethanol—ethyl alcohol.

Etiology—the study of the causes of disease.

Euphoria—a feeling of happiness and well being, not necessarily based on reality, that may be caused by a drug or illness.

Exfoliation—the scaling off of dead tissue.

Exocrine—a glandular secretion delivered directly, or through a duct to the linings of body parts or to the skin.

Exophthalmos—a condition in which the eyeballs protrude, present in certain diseases.

Exotoxin—toxic substances released by bacteria or other microorganisms in the body.

Expectorant—a medication that helps in getting rid of mucus and phlegm that has accumulated in the respiratory tract.

Extremity—an arm or a leg.

F

Fahrenheit—a scale for measuring temperature in which the freezing point is 32°F, normal body temperature is 98.6°F, and boiling point is 212°F.

Fallopian tubes—the tubes that carry the egg from the ovary to the womb.

Fecal incontinence—inability to control bowel movements.

Feces—stool, bowel movement.

Fetal—pertaining to an unborn child in the mother's womb.

Fiberoptics—a process based on newer optical instruments that allows the visualization of many internal parts of the body.

Fibrillation—fast, purposeless twitching of muscles. An extremely dangerous condition when it happens to the heart muscle, and fatal if not reversed quickly.

Fibrin—a body protein essential in the clotting of blood when blood is exposed to air, such as during an injury.

Fibroid—a colloquial term for a form of benign tumor of the uterus.

Fibrosis—scar tissue that is formed after injury or surgery.

Fibrositis—an inflammation of fibrous tissue.

Fissure—a crack or fold in skin or underlying tissue.

Fistula—a passage or channel that is formed between two internal body parts, or between an interior part of the body and the surface.

Fits—convulsions or seizures, which are violent involuntary muscle contractions. They may be caused by abnormal activity in the brain, or they may be related to a fever. Epileptic seizures are convulsions that recur.

Flatus—discharge of intestinal gas.

Fluorine—an element that helps to protect teeth when it is compounded with other substances and added to drinking water, or applied directly to teeth via toothpaste or a dental treatment.

Folacin (folic acid)—an essential nutritive substance required for the proper development of red blood cells. Deficiency causes various forms of anemia.

Foreign body—any substance or material embedded in a part of the body where it doesn't belong and where it may cause injury.

Foreskin—a fold of skin that covers the tip of the penis. Also known as the prepuce.

Fowler's position—a position in which a patient's head is elevated 18-20° and the knees are raised somewhat with a pillow or other support. Helpful in case of respiratory difficulties and various other conditions.

Fracture—a break in a bone, or other body part.

Fremitus—a thrill or noise perceived through vibrations when the hand is placed on a person's chest.

Frostbite—damage done to the skin and underlying tissues when exposed to cold.

Frozen Shoulder—a stiff, painful shoulder that has lost most of its mobility.

Fumigation—disinfection of a contaminated area by means of antiseptic fumes.

Fungi—plural of fungus. A group of plants that includes mushrooms, yeasts, and molds. Many of them are parasites that cause infections, such as athlete's foot.

Furuncle—same as a boil; an infected area of skin filled with pus.

G

Gallbladder—a pear-shaped sac under the liver that stores and concentrates bile.

Gallbladder series—X-ray examination of the gallbladder to determine whether it contains gallstones, or whether there are any other abnormalities in the gallbladder or related areas.

Gallstones—solid material, usually composed of cholesterol and calcium that may accumulate in the gallbladder or bile ducts.

Gamma globulin—a body protein that contains antibodies against various infections. It may be injected into a person in danger of developing an infection, to confer temporary immunity.

Gangrene—tissue death that occurs if tissues freeze, are deprived of nourishment, after sustaining injury or with a severe infection.

Gastrectomy—the removal of the stomach by surgery.

Gastric aspiration—using suction to draw food or fluid from the stomach. Done for diagnostic purposes, after surgery of the abdomen, or in drug poisoning situations.

Gastric fluid—fluid secreted by, and present in the stomach. The stomach secretes several fluids, one of which is hydrochloric acid, which prevents the growth of bacteria and promotes digestion of food as it passes through.

Gastric lavage—a process of washing out the stomach, needed when a toxic substance has been ingested that must be removed as part of the treatment that helps the victim to survive. Lavage may also be done when a person is bleeding into the stomach. Iced fluid is injected via a tube into the stomach, removed, and new fluid is injected. The process is continued until the bleeding stops, or until a different treatment method is started.

Gastric Ulcer—a defect in the stomach lining that becomes inflamed and painful.

Gastritis—inflammation of the stomach.

Gastrointestinal—refers to the stomach and the intestines.

Gastroscopy—an examination with a lighted tube called a gastroscope that enables the physician to inspect the inside of the stomach for any abnormalities or disease conditions.

Genetic disorder—a disease or abnormality that is passed on to a member of the next generation via hereditary.

Genital wart—also known as venereal wart; caused by a virus, this type of wart is usually transmitted via sexual contact, and thrives in the warm moist areas of the genital and anal regions.

Genitourinary—refers to the genital and urinary tract areas.

Geriatric—refers to the elderly.

Germicide—any substance or drug that can kill germs.

Gestation—pregnancy.

Giardiasis—an intestinal infection caused by the organism Giardia lamblia.

Gigantism—a condition in which a person has an unusually large body, or body parts.

Gingivitis—inflammation of the gums. Symptoms include bleeding and discomfort. If untreated, infection and loss of teeth may result.

Glaucoma—an eye disease in which the fluid pressure within the eye rises, with or without accompanying pain. If the condition is not recognized, damage to eye structures and loss of vision may result.

Glucagon—a body hormone that activates sugar stored in the liver; it also affects various other body functions.

Glucose—body sugar.

Glucose Tolerance Test—a test for diabetes consisting of a series of blood tests taken at intervals after the patient swallows a dose of glucose (sugar).

Glycogen—the form in which glucose is stored in the liver.

Gonad—the sex gland, ovary in the female, and testicle in the male.

Gonococcus—the microorganism that causes gonorrhea.

Gout—a disease due to an unusually high amount of uric acid in the blood. Uric acid is deposited in the tissues, since the kidneys can't excrete the increased amount rapidly enough. Gout affects joints such as the big toe, which becomes inflamed, hot and painful.

Grand mal—the severe seizure of epilepsy.

Granulocyte—a white blood cell.

Granuloma—a nodular inflammatory lesion that contains areas of granulation. When found around the groin and genitals it is generally granuloma inguinale, a venereal disease that requires specific medical treatment.

Graves' Disease—a disease of the thyroid gland. Symptoms include bulging of the eyes, an enlarged thyroid gland, accelerated pulse, weight loss, and a tendency to perspire profusely, along with many nervous symptoms.

Gravid—pregnant.

Greenstick fracture—incomplete fracture of a long bone, usually seen in children, in which the bone is bent, but splintered only on its convex side.

Grippe—also called influenza. An acute infectious disease, caused by one of the various influenza viruses. Symptoms include chills, fever, elevated temperature, aches and pains all over the body, headache, weakness, loss of appetite and inflammation of the respiratory tract.

Growth retardation—a condition also known as "failure to thrive." It occurs as a result of genetic predisposition, certain diseases, endocrine disturbances, malnutrition and in cases where the infant does not receive enough attention and love.

Gynecologic—refers to any condition of the female, including the female anatomy and reproductive system.

H

Hallucinogen—a substance or drug that produces unrealistic perceptions in the individual who takes it.

Hallux Valgus—a deformity of the big toe, causing it to be bent toward the other toes.

Hammer toe—a congenital deformity, usually of the fourth or fifth toe at the joint that connects the toe to the foot bones (metatarsals).

Hay Fever—a popular term for seasonal allergic rhinitis; the coughing, sneezing redness and itching of the mucous membranes of the nose and eyes is due to a reaction to pollen.

Heart Murmur—abnormal heart sounds heard through the doctor's stethoscope. Some murmurs are insignificant while others can indicate an important abnormality.

Heat Exhaustion—dizziness, faintness, and rapid pulse rate caused by insufficient liquid and salt in very hot weather.

Heat Stroke—lengthy exposure to very hot conditions resulting in a dangerous rise in the body temperature and leading to unconsciousness.

Heimlich maneuver—a method used to quickly remove a chunk of food that has accidentally slipped into the respiratory tract of a person who will choke to death if the food is not recovered within a few minutes.

Hematemesis—vomiting blood.

Hematinic—an agent or drug that increases the number of red blood cells in the blood, as well as the concentration of hemoglobin.

Hematologic—referring to blood, or the study of blood.

Hematoma—a collection of blood, or of clotted blood somewhere in the body, usually caused by injury or following surgery.

Hematopoietic—the development of blood cells and other constituents.

Hematuria—blood in the urine.

Hemianopsia—partial blindness, usually due to brain damage.

Hemiplegia—paralysis of one side of the body, frequently due to a stroke.

Hemodialysis—a process of removing impurities and waste from the blood with a machine when a person's kidneys are unable to perform this essential function.

Hemoglobin—the pigment in blood that carries oxygen to the tissues, carbon dioxide (a waste product) to the lungs, and colors the blood red.

Hemolysis—destruction of red blood cells; occurs in infection, due to a toxic substance or drug, or in the laboratory after freezing, thawing, or other activities or studies involving red blood cells.

Hemolytic Anemia—destruction of the red blood cells, occuring so rapidly that the body can't make new cells fast enough. It may be hereditary, or the result of an infection or a reaction to a drug or poison.

Hemophilia—an inherited disorder in which the affected individual bleeds easily and may develop serious hemorrhage even after very minor injury, due to the presence of a clotting factor deficiency.

Hemoptysis—spitting up of blood that comes from a hemorrhage in the lungs, usually due to a disease such as tuberculosis.

Hemorrhage—severe bleeding in, or from any part of the body.

Hemorrhoid—an enlarged vein, or group of veins that develop as a result of pressure, continual irritation or disease. Most frequently occurs in the veins of the rectum, but appears in other parts of the body as well.

Hemostasis—the arrest of bleeding, either by the physiological properties of vasoconstriction and coagulation or by surgical means.

Hepatic—refers to the liver.

Hepatitis—inflammation of the liver, usually due to infection, or following ingestion of a toxic substance.

Hepatosplenomegaly—enlargement of the liver and spleen.

Hernia—a condition in which an organ inside one of the body's cavities protrudes from the cavity, usually due to a weakness of the muscles that surround it, or following disease or surgery.

Herpes Genitalis—blisters on or near the genitals that rupture, becoming painful shallow ulcers, caused by the herpes simplex virus. The virus is transmitted by sexual contact.

Herpes Simplex—a skin infection caused by the herpes simplex virus that may be triggered by many different events, such as exposure to sunlight, stress, pregnancy, or other infections. The virus appears in two forms: herpes simplex type I generally affects the face (mouths or lips); herpes simplex type II usually infects the genital area and is spread primarily through sexual contact.

Herpes Zoster (shingles)—a viral infection whose configuration follows the pathways of certain nerves. It consists of crops of blisters that break and form crusted lesions. These may be preceded, accompanied, or followed by severe pain along the course of the affected nerve segment. The condition may be particularly serious and disabling in elderly and/or debilitated persons.

Hirsutism—a condition characterized by the growth of hair in unusual places and/or excessive amounts, especially in women.

Histoplasmosis—a fungus infection caused by an organism called Histoplasma capsulatum, found in the soil and in the excrement of a number of animals in various parts of the country. The infection affects the lungs when tiny particles of the fungus are inhaled.

Hives—smooth, slightly elevated, usually itchy wheals on the skin, caused by an allergy to certain foods, infection, or emotional stress.

Hoarseness—an abnormal huskiness in the voice.

Hodgkins' Disease—malignancy of the lymph nodes and spleen, characterized by painless enlargement of the lymph nodes, weight loss, fever, night sweats, and loss of appetite.

Homeostasis—a balance within the body of its chemical and other functions and constituents, necessary for continued health.

Hormone—one of many body substances secreted by various glands, essential for normal body functioning.

Hospice—an institution which provides professional care to patients with chronic, irreversible or terminal diseases.

Humectant—an agent or substance that helps to preserve moisture in specific body areas such as the skin; or in a room, or in an oxygen tent.

Hydrocele—an abnormal sac caused by a collection of fluid.

Hydrocephalus—a condition which may be congenital or acquired, in which the head becomes abnormally large and there is increased pressure in the brain, due to excessive secretion and accumulation of cerebrospinal fluid in the ventricles (chambers in the brain).

Hyperalimentation—a process of providing food for a malnourished or debilitated person, or one unable to eat normally by infusing nourishing fluids directly into the blood stream through a central vein.

Hyperglycemia—excessive amount of sugar in the blood, as happens in uncontrolled diabetes mellitus.

Hyperkalemia—excessive amount of potassium present in the blood.

Hyperplasia—an increase in tissue, or size of an organ.

Hyperpyrexia—excessively high fever.

Hypersensitivity—excessive sensitivity to an agent or stimulus, as happens when a person is allergic.

Hypersomnia—a condition in which a person sleeps excessively at intervals, but is normal during waking periods, in contrast to being inclined to sleep continuously, as happens during periods of somnolence.

Hypertension—persistently high arterial blood pressure.

Hyperthermia—an abnormally high body temperature that may be due to a heat stroke, or is brought on by the injection of foreign protein for treatment purposes, or by other physical agents, substances or equipment.

Hyperthyroidism—a condition in which the thyroid gland, situated at the front of the neck, is enlarged, swollen and produces an excessive amount of a thyroid hormone called thyroxine. This produces weight loss, nervousness, an increased heart beat and other symptoms. Treatment is aimed at counteracting the effects of the hormone.

Hypertonic—refers to a concentration of salt (sodium chloride) greater than that present in blood.

Hypertriglyceridemia—excessive amount of fatty substances in the blood.

Hypertrophic—excessive growth of an organ or body part.

Hyperventilation—overbreathing; an increase in the depth and/or rate of breathing that may cause dizziness and occasional fainting.

Hypervitaminosis—excessive intake of vitamins, with possible toxic reactions.

Hypnotic—an agent or drug given to induce sleep.

Hypocalcemia—an insufficient amount of calcium in the blood.

Hypochondria—undue concern about health, usually caused by a mental condition such as anxiety.

Hypoglycemia—an abnormally low blood sugar level.

Hypogonadism—inadequate functioning of the sex glands.

Hypokalemia—insufficient amount of potassium in the blood.

Hypotension—abnormally low blood pressure.

Hypothermia—abnormally low body temperature, due to accidental exposure to cold, immersion in cold water, or intentionally induced as a treatment, or during surgery by using an electrically controlled hypothermia mattress.

Hypothyroidism—underactivity of the thyroid gland. Symptoms include fatigue, slowed heart rate, cold sensitivity, dry hair and skin, and weight gain.

Hypotonic—refers to a concentration of salt lower than that present in blood.

Hypoventilation—reduced ventilation of the air sacs of the lungs (alveoli), due to inadequate breathing or blockage of the airways (bronchi). Prolonged hypoventilation may lead to respiratory depression and coma.

Hypovolemic shock—a state of shock caused by a greatly reduced volume of blood, generally due to hemorrhage.

Hypoxemia—inadequate oxygenation of blood.

Hysterectomy—the operation of excising the uterus, performed either through the abdominal wall or through the vagina.

Hysteria—a psychological disturbance evidenced by inappropriate, excessively emotional behavior.

I

Iatrogenic—an effect upon the patient that results from the suggestions, treatment or prescribed activity by a doctor.

Icterus—jaundice; the yellow discoloration of the skin, due to an excess of bile in blood.

Idiopathic thrombocytopenic purpura (ITP)—a blood disease of unknown origin whose chief symptom is platelet destruction, which leaves the victim prone to bleed.

Idiosyncrasy (to drugs)—unusual sensitivity to certain drugs by some individuals.

Ileitis—inflammation of the part of the small intestine called the ileum.

Ileostomy—an opening created by surgery in the abdomen and the ileum (section of small intestine) to allow discharge of fecal material.

Ileus—acute intestinal obstruction due to various causes, accompanied by severe, colicky pain, vomiting and dehydration; a serious, potentially fatal condition, if not relieved by prompt, effective treatment.

Immune globulin—a pooled blood fraction that contains antibodies present in a large number of adults. When injected in an individual, it may confer temporary immunity against a number of infectious diseases.

Immunity, active—a person who has developed his own antibodies against a particular infectious disease is actively immune against that disease.

Immunity, passive—a person injected with immune globulin or some other type of inoculation is said to be passively (and usually only temporarily) immune against a particular infectious disease.

Immunization—the process of developing one's own antibodies against an infectious disease, or being inoculated with inactivated or killed microorganisms that cause a particular infectious disease, in order to develop antibodies and acquire protection against the infection.

Immunodeficient—every healthy individual has the capacity to fight infection with certain blood factors that fend off invading microorganisms, and prevent them from multiplying. Illness, disability and other factors may decrease a person's capacity to fend off harmful organisms, or the development of foreign cells, such as cancer cells, for instance. When that happens, the person is immunodeficient.

Immunodiffusion—a laboratory test in which the interactions of specific antigens and antibodies are observed.

Immunoglobulins—body proteins that function as antibodies to ward off infection.

Immunosuppression—suppression of the body's rejection mechanism by means of certain drugs.

Immunotherapy—treating the body in such a way as to bolster its capacity to ward off infection, or the invasion of harmful foreign cells such as cancer cells.

Impacted cerumen (ear wax)—ear wax that has hardened inside the ear, requiring special methods, such as softening and irrigation in order to remove it without damaging the delicate structures inside the ear.

Impacted feces—feces that have become too hard to leave the rectum in the process of normal elimination. Special softening agents or manual removal are required to remove the feces and prevent injury to the bowel.

Impaired consciousness—a state that occurs when a person is not fully alert, due to injury, drug abuse or for other reasons. He may be semiconscious, stuporous, or in coma.

Impetigo—an infection of the skin often seen in children, usually due to the staphylococcus bacterium. It is very contagious, and may spread all over the surface of the skin.

Impotence—the inability to complete the sex act.

Inadequate personality—a person who indicates by his behavior that he cannot cope with others, and with ordinary life responsibilities has an inadequate personality.

Inanition—a state of exhaustion due to lack of food, or the inability to assimilate (utilize) food properly.

Incontinence—the inability to control urination or the elimination of feces.

Incubation period—the period of time that elapses between exposure to an infectious disease, and showing symptoms of the disease.

Induced abortion—an abortion that is brought about by the use of drugs or other methods.

Infarction—tissue death due to deprivation of oxygen.

Infection—a disease process caused by the invasion and damaging action of microorganisms, such as bacteria or viruses.

Infectious mononucleosis—an infectious disease caused by a virus that is relatively mild and occurs mostly in young adults. Symptoms include headache, fever, sore throat, enlarged lymph glands and spleen. Also known as the "kissing disease".

Infertility—inability of an individual or a couple to have a child.

Infiltration—to pass, or inject fluid or any other material into the tissues.

Inflammation—the irritation, swelling and other harmful changes of tissue as a result of trauma, pressure, or other physical intereference in some part of the body. May also be caused by illness, infection or drugs.

Influenza—an infectious disease caused by a variety of influenza viruses, some of which cause more severe illness than others. Symptoms include headache, fever, joint pains and cough.

Inguinal hernia—protrusion of a portion of intestine through a weakened muscular wall in the groin (inguinal region).

Injection—using a needle, attached to a syringe or other sterile container, to infuse liquid material into the skin, muscles or veins to administer drugs, feed, or hydrate an individual.

Inoculation—injection of a small quantity of inactivated or killed microorganisms, or toxin produced by the organisms, to challenge an individual's body to develop antibodies against these organisms.

Intake and output (I&O)—measuring the amount of liquid a person consumes within a given period, such as 24 hours, against the amount of liquid (urine, wound drainage, vomitus, etc.) the person loses within the same time period. Done to determine whether the person receives enough liquid, and to calculate the amount of additional liquid necessary to be given to meet that person's fluid requirements.

Insomnia—inability to fall asleep, or to sleep long enough to meet the body's requirements for rest.

Insulin—a hormone produced by cell groups inside the pancreas (a gland lying across and behind the stomach) called the islets of Langerhans. Insulin converts blood sugar into body energy. When a person produces too little insulin, he develops diabetes mellitus.

Insulinoma—a tumor (growth) of the cell groups called islets of Langerans in the pancreas, which may produce excessive amounts of insulin.

Insulin shock—a condition that results if a diabetic person takes too much insulin, if his body cannot utilize the amount of insulin injected, or if he doesn't eat enough food to balance the amount of insulin injected. Symptoms include a lowered blood sugar level, tremors, cold sweat, weakness, dizziness and coma, if the condition is not reversed quickly by eating or drinking carbohydrate-containing food such as a few pieces of sugar, or a glass of orange juice. If a person develops insulin coma, he must be given glucose by injection.

Intercurrent infection—a second infectious process that occurs in a person who already has an infectious disease.

Interferon—a natural body substance formed in response to infection that defends the body against further attack by the foreign cells, organisms or viruses.

Intermittent positive pressure breathing (IPPB)—artificial respiration via a breathing machine that intermittently inflates the lungs with air or oxygen under pressure in cases where a person is unwilling, as in a case of postoperative pain, or unable to breathe normally.

Interstitial—relating to a space between cells, or inside a body organ.

Intestinal obstruction—a partial or complete blockage of the intestines.

Intestine—the portion of the digestive tract extending from the pylorus (stomach outlet) to the anus; also called bowel or gut.

Intra-articular—inside a joint.

Intracranial—inside the skull.

Intramuscular injection—an injection of fluid or a drug into muscular tissue.

Intrauterine device (IUD)—a device inserted in the womb to prevent pregnancy.

Intravenous infusion—introducing fluid, nutritive substances or drugs into a vein with a sterile needle and syringe, or other sterile apparatus.

Intravenous pyelogram (IVP)—a diagnostic procedure in which the patient is given an intravenous injection of a dye, allowing the diagnostic X-ray studies to be done of the kidneys and urinary tract.

Intubation—insertion of a tube into a body opening or passage.

Intussusception—sliding of one segment of the bowel over another. A telescope action.

Iodine—a trace element essential to health in minute (trace) quantity. Also used externally as an antiseptic.

Iritis—inflammation of the color-bearing part of the eye (the iris).

Iron—a trace element essential to certain body functions, such as the proper and adequate formation of hemoglobin. Iron deficiency results in anemia, "spoon nails," bowel disease and other symptoms.

Ischemic Heart Disease—heart disease caused by narrowing of the coronary arteries usually due to arteriosclerosis.

Irrigation—bathing a body part or cavity with fluids or medicated fluids for cleansing, healing or antiseptic purposes.

Irritant—a drug or agent that irritates the skin or other body part, either accidentally or with intent to produce tissue stimulation.

Ischemic—a body part or area that has insufficient, or no blood supply.

Isolation—placement of a patient who has an infectious disease into a separate room or area, and using various other precautions to prevent the spread of the disease to others.

J

Jaundice—yellow discoloration of the skin and the whites of the eyes caused by the presence of too much bile in the blood, usually due to liver or gallbladder disease.

Jejunum—a portion of the small intestine.

K

Karyotype—a pattern of chromosomes, lettered and numbered in pairs to perform genetic study of an individual's hereditary characteristics.

Keratitis—inflammation of the cornea, the transparent structure located at the front of the eye.

Keratoconus—a condition of unknown origin in which the eyeball becomes cone-shaped, which interferes with normal vision.

Keratolytic—refers to a drug or agent that loosens or separates the horney layer of skin.

Keratomalacia—a disease of the cornea (the transparent structure at the front of the eye) in which it becomes dry, ulcerated and may perforate. The cause is malnutrition or debilitating disease.

Kernicterus—a serious illness of the newborn in which the baby develops jaundice in certain portions of the brain.

Ketoacidosis—a state which results from the accumulation of incompletely metabolized fatty acids in the blood, upsetting the body's metabolic balance.

Kidney machine—a machine used to remove impurities and waste products from the blood of a person whose kidneys are unable to perform this vital function.

Kidney stones—lumps of solid material, that build up in the kidney. When a stone passes into one of the ureters, it causes acute pain (kidney colic).

Knee-chest position—the patient is positioned by the doctor or an assistant so that he rests on his chest and knees, in order to facilitate certain examinations.

Knock knees—when the child stands with its knees together, the ankles do not meet. This is normal in three and four year-olds and usually corrects itself.

Koplik's spots—tiny blue-and-white spots surrounded by red rings that appear inside the mouth at the points where the upper and lower teeth meet. The spots appear during the first two or three days of the onset of measles, before the rash can be seen.

Korsakoff's psychosis—a condition in which a person's memory is impaired, and he is disoriented as to time and place. He may invent facts to cover up his inability to remember certain events. Usually caused by alcoholism.

Kwashiorkor—a condition of extreme malnutrition, especially of proteins. Occurs in children who live in poor countries, or in areas of deprivation. They develop anemia, swelling of body tissues, a pot belly and other physical characteristics.

L

Labyrinthitis—inflammation of the structures of the inner ear.

Laceration—a break or tear of skin or other body tissues, usually caused by injury.

Lacrimal apparatus—the tear glands, sacs, and ducts that produce tears, and carry them down through the eyes and into the nose.

Lactation—the process following childbirth during which milk is formed in the mother's breasts to enable her to nourish her infant through suckling.

Lactic dehydrogenase (LDH)—an enzyme in the blood that rises to higher levels within several days after a person has had a heart attack. Laboratory determination of this and other enzymes helps to make a diagnosis of heart attack, and to distinguish this condition from various other diagnoses.

Lactose—milk sugar.

Laparoscopy (abdominoscopy; peritoneoscopy; ventioscopy)—a surgical procedure in which an electrically lighted tubular instrument is passed through the abdominal wall to visualize the internal organs and structures for diagnostic or treatment purposes.

Laparotomy—a surgical incision in the abdomen.

Laryngitis—inflammation of the voice box.

Laryngotracheobronchitis—a respiratory disease that occurs mostly in children as a result of infection of the respiratory tract.

Larynx—the voice box, which enables a person to speak.

Laser beam—a small, intense stream of light causing immense heat and power. Used in surgical and diagnostic procedures.

Lavage—the washing out of an organ or body cavity, such as the stomach.

Laxative—an agent that promotes emptying of the bowel.

Lead poisoning—when the salts of this chemical element are absorbed into the body, by children who eat paint chips or through the skin by workers in factories where lead is used, the result is mental retardation in children, and serious illness in adults.

Legionnaire's disease—a pneumonia-like disease caused by the organism Legionella pneumophila, which infects persons who have been exposed to it in areas where the organisms live and have become activated.

Lens—the part of the eye that enables it to focus at various distances.

Leprosy—an infectious disease, also known as Hansen's disease, caused by a mycobacterium that appears in various forms and affects nerves, the face, eyes or the extremities, depending on which type of the disease the patient has contracted. It may lead to destruction of tissue, causing various deformities in the affected body parts.

Leukopheresis—a process in which a certain amount of blood is removed from a donor, so that the white blood cells can be removed. The remaining blood is then returned to the donor. The separated white blood cells may be used to treat another person, or for various other purposes.

Leukemia—also known as cancer of the blood, leukemia is a disease of the blood-forming organs, which produces a large number of abnormal white blood cells. The disease occurs in acute and chronic form.

Leukocyte—a white blood cell.

Leukoplakia—small whitish, sometimes leathery patches on the skin that occur due to various causes.

Leukorrhea—a whitish vaginal discharge.

Levin tube—a tube that is passed into the stomach to aspirate fluid for examination, to drain fluid from the stomach postoperatively, or to perform certain treatments.

Lichen planus—a skin condition that may occur in many body areas, depending on the particular form of the disease affecting the patient.

Limbic system—that part of the nervous system that affects primarily the internal organs of the body.

Lipids—a collective term that includes body substances such as fatty acids, glycerides, and various others.

Lipoma—a benign growth composed of fatty tissues.

Lipoproteins—body compounds that contain both proteins and fatty substances.

Lithotomy position—a position in which the patient is placed on the back, with legs and knees raised for examination or treatment.

Liver—a dark-red organ in the upper right section of the abdomen. Its many functions include filtering blood, secreting bile, and converting sugars to glycogen, which is stored.

Lobar pneumonia—inflammation of one or more lobes of the lung, usually caused by a bacterium (Diplococcus pneumoniae). Symptoms are fever, rapid breathing, pain and cough.

Lobectomy—removal of a lobe of an organ—the thyroid gland, lung, liver or brain.

Lockjaw—a dangerous infectious disease caused by Clostridium tetani, an anaerobic bacterial organism. The disease is acquired when the organism invades the body through a dirty wound such as a nail puncture. The patient must be treated at once to prevent the disease, which produces spasms of all the voluntary muscles, including the jaw, which is clamped shut. Tetanus immunization, repeated at intervals, help to protect people against this disease which may be fatal if treatment is delayed.

Lues—syphilis.

Lumbago—a general term for backache in the lower part of the spine: mid- or lower back, or the lumbar and/or lumbosacral area.

Lumbar disc—a cartilaginous cushion in the low back located between vertebrae.

Lumbar puncture—the insertion of a sterile needle into the spinal canal to withdraw spinal fluid for examination, to administer spinal anesthesia during surgery, to instill medication and for various other purposes.

Lymph—a colorless fluid in the body that runs through the lymphatic channels and eventually joins the venous circulation. It consists of white blood cells and tissue fluid.

Lymphadenitis—inflammation of the lymph nodes, which are located throughout the body along the lymphatic channels.

Lymphangitis—inflammation of the lymphatic channels.

Lymphocyte—white blood cell made in lymph nodes.

Lymphocytic leukemia—a cancer of the lymphocytes (white blood cells) in which leukemic cells crowd out normal white blood cells. Symptoms are enlarged lymph glands and spleen, loss of appetite and weight, fever, and night sweats.

Lymphogranuloma venereum—an infectious disease caused by a small organism, Chlamydia, which causes genital ulcers and lymph gland enlargement in the groin.

M

Magnesium—an element present in the body that aids in muscle contraction, bone and tooth formation, nerve conduction and various other functions. Deficiency may produce irritability of muscles and nerves.

Malabsorption—inability of the intestines to absorb nutrients.

Malaise—a term that describes a general feeling of illness, headache, muscular, joint, and other pains that occur when a person has the flu or other febrile illness.

Malaria—an infectious, febrile disease transmitted (spread) through the bite of a mosquito that earlier sucked blood from another person infected by one of the several types of Plasmodium organisms that are capable of causing the disease.

Malignant—any condition that is resistant to treatment, is very severe, and may lead to death.

Mammography—X-ray examination of the breast.

Mania—a form of hyperactive behavior in which an individual becomes hyperexcitable; may be a phase of the mental disorder called manic-depressive psychosis.

Manic-depressive illness—a mental disease characterized by mood swings, in which the victim becomes alternately deeply depressed and highly excited.

Mantoux Test (PPD)—skin test done on the forearm to detect exposure to tuberculosis.

Marasmus—extreme form of malnutrition.

Masochism—a psychologic condition in which a person derives sexual gratification while being abused or hurt.

Mastectomy—surgical removal of the breast.

Mastitis—inflammation of the breast.

Mastoiditis—inflammation of the mastoid, a bone located behind the ear.

Measles—a contagious viral infection of the respiratory tract, also called rubeola. Symptoms include fever, cough, inflamed eyes, and later, a rash. German measles called rubella is a contagious disease with rash and mild fever. It can cause congenital abnormalities during early months of pregnancy.

Meconium—fecal material passed through the birth canal by the fetus if it is in distress, and by the newborn infant during the first few days of life. The stool is colored dark green, and its consistency is pasty.

Megacolon—a condition present at birth in some babies in which the nerves essential to elimination from the lower bowel are absent. This produces an accumulation of feces, and distention of the bowel and abdomen which requires surgical correction.

Melanoma—a tumor that appears on the skin. If malignant, it may spread to other parts of the body. The lesion is dark brown due to the pigment melanin.

Melasma (chloasma)—a patchy discoloration of the skin, often seen in pregnant women.

Melena—bowel movement that has a black, tarlike appearance, caused by bleeding somewhere in the intestinal tract. When such bowel movements are discovered, the individual should be promptly examined by a physician.

Menadione—a synthetic preparation of vitamin K, an essential nutrient which aids in the normal clotting process of blood. Deficiency may produce bleeding.

Menarche—the onset of the first menstrual period.

Meniere's disease—symptoms of dizziness, ringing in the ears (tinnitus), and some hearing disturbance caused by increased pressure in the labyrinth of the ear.

Meningitis—inflammation of the meninges, the covering membranes of the spinal cord and the brain.

Meningocele—a body defect in which a portion of the spinal cord membrane protrudes through the bones of the spinal column.

Menopause—cessation of monthly menstrual bleeding, usually around age 48 to 50.

Menorrhagia—excessive bleeding during the menstrual period.

Metrorrhagia—irregular menses.

Micturition—urination.

Migraine—periodic attacks of headache, often accompanied by nausea and vomiting. Usually, attacks are preceded by ocular symptoms (an aura).

Miliary tuberculosis—a form of tuberculosis that spreads throughout the body into all tissues and organs.

Minerals—metals and salts such as iron, phosphorus, calcium, and sodium chloride, important in the diet.

Minimal brain dysfunction (MBD)—a developmental or learning disorder in children, more often in boys than in girls, for which no physical basis is found, although some have slight neurological symptoms. Among the symptoms these children show are hyperactivity, poor coordination of the muscles, impulsiveness and difficulty in perception. A child with such symptoms should be carefully examined by experts to help him overcome his problems.

Mitral incompetence—distortion of the heart's mitral valve (the valve between the left atrium and the left ventricle) which prevents it from closing completely.

Mitral valve—the valve that separates the upper left chamber of the heart from the lower left chamber.

Mitral valve prolapse—the valve leafs are protruded into the atrium causing improper blood flow.

Mitral stenosis—narrowing of the mitral valve in the heart by disease. Valves leaflets cannot open and close properly which interferes with the filling and emptying of the heart's left chambers.

Mitral valvotomy—a surgical procedure to widen the narrowed mitral valve.

Molluscum contagiosum—a skin disease caused by a virus, marked by formation of small, round, elevations containing a cheesy substance.

Mongolism—an old term for Down's syndrome.

Mononucleosis—same as infectious mononucleosis, or "kissing" disease; an infectious disease caused by a virus that occurs primarily in young adults, with symptoms such as fever, sore throat, enlarged lymph nodes and spleen, and an initial decrease of white blood cells that changes to an increase as the disease runs its course.

Morbidity—state of disease, or calculated ratio of a disease state to the normal state.

Mouth-to-mouth resuscitation—a form of artificial respiration in which the rescuer breathes directly into the victim's mouth forcing air into the lungs.

Moxibustion—a popular therapeutic process first used in the Orient that produces counter-irritation on some part of the skin; done by placing a cone-shaped container filled with cotton or similar material on the skin and setting the material on fire.

Mucosa—the smooth membranous lining of the interior organs of the body. It is present in the gastrointestinal tract, the respiratory tract, the urinary tract and the genitourinary tract of men and women.

Mucus—the material secreted by the mucous membranes.

Multipara—a woman who has given birth to two or more children.

Multiple sclerosis (MS)—a degenerative disease of portions of the nervous system that results in progressive disability of muscle functions. The affected person develops difficulty in walking, using his hands, or with his vision. The disease may shown signs of improvement, then become worse again. It may progress to complete paralysis, or leave the victim partially disabled for many years without further progression of symptoms.

Mumps—a contagious viral disease; the chief symptom is swelling of the parotid glands that produce saliva. This causes swelling in front and below the ear.

Munchausen's syndrome—describes the illness of a person who has the abnormal urge to manufacture signs of illness, such as an artifically elevated temperature, apparent blood in the urine or other body part or cavity where it is not normally found, and other symptoms or signs that have no physical basis. Psychiatric treatment must be obtained to discover the reasons for the person's need for forging the illness. Such persons often move from hospital to hospital to avoid being recognized, to gain admission and treatment for their often ingeniously produced "symptoms."

Muscular atrophy—weakness and wasting of muscles due to lack of use, illness that forces a person to remain in bed for long periods, and other conditions that result in the loss of muscle mass.

Muscular dystrophy—a disease that often starts during childhood, in which muscles begin to waste away and gradually become totally useless. The cause of this disease is not yet known; heredity appears to be a factor.

Musculoskeletal—refers to the muscles and the bones of the skeleton.

Myalgia—muscular pain.

Myasthenia gravis—a disease in which muscles are chronically weak and unable to function normally. The cause of this disease is not known. It occurs more frequently in women between the ages of 20-40, and requires symptomatic, supportive treatment.

Myeloma—a cancerous, progressive disease that involves the bloodforming organs of the bone marrow, causing plasma cell tumors, weakened bone structures, anemia and kidney damage.

Myocardial infarction—gross necrosis of the myocardium, as a result of interruption of the blood supply to the area, as in coronary thrombosis.

Myocarditis—inflammation of the muscular walls of the heart (the myocardium).

Myoclonus—continuous rhythmic spasms of a muscle or group of muscles.

Myoma—excessive growth of muscular tissue into a tumor.

Myositis—inflammation of a muscle, or a group of muscles.

Myringitis—inflammation of the ear drum.

Myxedema—a disease caused by insufficient secretion of the hormone thyroxine by the thyroid gland.

N

Narcotic—a medication given to relieve pain, that often also makes a patient sleepy or stuporous, or has still other side effects. Most of these drugs can lead to addiction if they are taken indiscriminately, or for long periods of time.

Narcotic antagonist—a drug that counteracts effects of a narcotic medication.

Nasal septum—the bone that separates the two sides of the nose.

Nearsightedness—in this condition, which usually is hereditary, images of distant objects are focused in front of the retina and therefore blurred, while nearby objects are seen clearly.

Necrosis—death of cells, tissues or organs due to lack of oxygen, infection, injury, exposure to cold or burn.

Necrotizing enterocolitis—an extremely grave disease of the bowel that occurs in adults following certain types of abdominal surgery, and some other illnesses. It can also occur in newborns. The disease causes tissue death, abdominal pain, nausea, high fever and diarrhea that may be bloody. Treatment involves fluid replacement, relief of pain and antibiotics.

Neonatal—concerns the newborn period, generally the first four weeks after birth.

Neoplastic—refers to any abnormal growth in the body.

Nephritis—inflammation of the kidneys.

Neuralgia—pain that travels along nerve tracks.

Neuritis—inflammation of one or more nerves.

Neurologic—refers to an examination or study of the nervous system.

Neuroma—a tumor that arises from cells somewhere in the nervous system.

Neurosis—a behavioral disturbance with many symptoms; the most frequently apparent syndrome is anxiety.

Neurosyphilis—the third stage of syphilis which includes involvement of the nervous system.

Nevus—a mole or birthmark.

Niacin (nicotinic acid, niacinamide)—an essential nutritive substance that aids metabolism.

Nightblindness—inability to see in the dark, or in poor light, due to vitamin A deficiency.

Nits—the eggs of lice found in the hair of persons with louse infestation.

Nocturia—frequent urination during the night.

Nodule—a small swelling.

Nosocomial—refers to an infection, or other disorder picked up by a patient while he is hospitalized.

Nulliparous—refers to a woman who has never given birth.

Nystagmus—involuntary regular movements of the eyes.

O

Obstetric—refers to the care of the pregnant woman, including the prenatal period, labor, delivery and the period immediately following the delivery, as well as care in between pregnancies.

Occult blood—blood present in such small quantities and often altered in color or consistency that it can be detected only by chemical tests, or via microscopic or spectroscopic examination of the suspected material, usually the stool.

Ocular—refers to the eye.

Oligomenorrhea—abnormally infrequent or scanty menstruation.

Oligospermia—a low concentration of sperm in a man's ejaculate.

Oliguria—a small amount of urinary output in a given period of time.

Oncology—the study of cancerous diseases.

Ophthalmic—refers to the eye.

Ophthalmologist—a physician who specializes in diseases of the eye.

Opportunistic infection—an infection that occurs because an individual has lost his natural capacity to fight it, due to weakness and incompetence of his immune system, as a result of illness, malnutrition and other causes.

Optic nerve—the second cranial nerve. A sensory nerve that permits transmission of vision.

Optometrist—a person licensed to examine, measure and treat visual defects by means of corrective lenses.

Optometry—a profession whose practitioners examine eyes, determine if a person has any eye problems or disease, and prescribe, and produce corrective lenses and other optical aids.

Oral cavity—the mouth.

Orthopedics—a medical specialty whose practitioners are experts in problems or diseases of bones, joints and related structures.

Orthopnea—inability to breathe unless sitting up.

Osmosis—a process in which fluid flows from an area of a lower concentration across a semi-permeable membrane to an area of higher concentration.

Osteoarthritis—a degenerative disease that affects the joints, and often occurs as a person ages, or following injury.

Osteogenic sarcoma—a malignant bone tumor that most often occurs in the young, at ages 10-20.

Osteomalacia—a bone disease in which the bones soften and bend, with varying degrees of pain. May occur in pregnancy, metabolic disease or in vitamin D deficiency.

Osteomyelitis—inflammatory disease of the bone marrow, the surrounding bone and the end portions of bone (epiphyseal areas).

Osteoporosis—increasing weakness and fragility of the bones. Most frequently occurs in elderly, postmenopausal women and in elderly men.

OTC (over the counter, or nonprescription drug)—medicine that is available in the pharmacy or in other stores without a doctor's prescription.

Otic—refers to the ear.

Otitis media—inflammation of the middle ear.

Otorhinolaryngologic—refers to the ear, nose and throat.

Ovary—the female sex gland, present on each side in a woman's lower abdomen. Inside, egg cells (ova) are formed. It also secretes sex hormones that help the development, growth and regulation of the female reproductive system.

Oxytocic—a drug or agent that speeds up the onset of strong uterine contractions during labor. It may also be given after delivery to cause the uterus to contract and prevent uterine bleeding.

P

Pacemaker—a natural mechanism that controls the heartbeat. When it doesn't function adequately, an artificial pacemaker may be used, either temporarily or permanently. An artificial pacemaker may be external, or it may be inserted under the patient's skin. The latter technique is used when the patient requires a permanent pacemaker.

Paget's disease—there are two unrelated diseases, both called by this name. One is a chronic bone disease, also known as osteitis deformans, the other is an unusual form of breast cancer.

Palpation—using the hands to touch, feel or lightly press certain body area to determine if any abnormality is present.

Palpitation—a very rapid heart beat caused by exertion such as running, by excitement, nervousness, certain drugs and various disease conditions.

Pancreas—a glandular organ that lies across and behind the stomach. It produces pancreatic juice that aids in the digestion of food in the upper intestine. It also produces insulin.

Pancreatitis—inflammation of the pancreas.

Papanicolaou (Pap) smear—a reliable and painless test done on various body cells to determine abnormalities and detect the presence of cancer.

Papilledema—edema of the optic papilla.

Paracentesis—draining of fluid from the abdomen.

Paralysis—inability to move a body part due to loss of nerve stimulation of muscle.

Paranoid—a condition in which a person is abnormally suspicious of others, with feelings of delusion and of being persecuted by hostile people or forces.

Paraplegic—a condition in which both legs, and usually the lower portion of the trunk are paralyzed. This may happen after a stroke, an injury, and under certain other circumstances.

Parasite—an organism that lives on, and obtains its nourishment from, another organism called the host.

Parenteral drug administration—a method of administering a drug by vein or muscle.

Parkinsonism—a disease in which the victim gradually loses control of his voluntary muscles. Also known as shaking palsy and paralysis agitans.

Paronychia—inflammation or infection in the tissue surrounding a finger or a toenail.

Parotid glands—the salivary glands directly in front and below the ears.

Parturition—childbirth.

Paroxysmal tachycardia—sudden attacks of rapid heartbeat occurring spasmodically and lasting from seconds to hours.

Passive immunity—immunity temporarily conferred against a certain infectious disease by inoculating a person with a substance that contains antibodies against that disease.

Patch test—a skin test done to detect sensitivity of a person to certain substances to which he may be allergic.

Pathogen—a disease-causing microorganism.

Pathologic—refers to disease, or to the study of disease.

Pediatric—refers to the medical specialty concerned with the care of children.

Pediculosis—infestation with lice.

Pellagra—a vitamin deficiency disease that occurs when a person doesn't eat enough foods containing niacin (nicotinic acid, nicotinamide). The vitamin is present in yeast, liver, meat and whole grain enriched cereals. Pellagra symptoms include blisters, reddened areas and swelling of the skin, the gastrointestinal system and the mucous membranes of the mouth. The nervous system may also be affected.

Pelvic infections—infection of internal genital and reproductive organs, most often in women.

Peptic ulcer—an inflammation in the lining of the stomach or the small intestine. Peptic ulcer is a disease that tends to occur in people who suffer from tension and anxiety. It is treated with drugs, diet, counseling, and may require blood replacement or surgery if the ulcer penetrates the wall of the stomach or intestine, causing hemorrhage and other complications.

Pericarditis—inflammation of the sac that surrounds the heart (pericardium).

Peripheral neuritis—disease of the nerves going to the extremities.

Peristalsis—wavelike movements of the gastrointestinal tract to move its contents from one end to the other.

Peritonitis—inflammation of the lining of the abdominal cavity and its organs.

Pernicious anemia—a type of anemia that occurs mostly in elderly people when Vitamin B deficiency causes their bloodforming organs to fail to develop red blood cells normally. Treated by injections of Vitamin B_{12}, that must be continued for the remainder of the person's life.

Pertussis—whooping cough.

Petit mal—a minor seizure in which the affected person may seem to be absent-minded, day-dreaming, or twitching slightly for a few seconds, then return to his normal state.

Pharyngitis—inflammation of the back of the throat.

Phenylketonuria (PKU)—inherited metabolic abnormality in which the affected individual in unable to process a certain constituent of protein foods called phenylalanine. A toxic side product is formed that accumulates first in the blood and urine, and subsequently affects the brain and nervous system, producing mental retardation if not recognized and treated early. The condition can be diagnosed in a newborn baby's urine or blood, and corrected by providing a diet free of foods containing phenylalanine. In many parts of the country a test for this condition is required by law, so that corrective action can be taken before symptoms appear.

Pheochromocytoma—a tumor in the adrenal gland that causes high blood pressure and related symptoms. The tumor is removed by surgery.

Phimosis—a condition in which the foreskin of the penis is narrowed so that it cannot be retracted over its tip. Occurs in uncircumcised males.

Phlebitis—inflammation of a vein.

Phosphorus—an essential body element that aids in the formation of bones and teeth, the conduction of nervous impulses, in contraction of muscles and in enzyme activity.

Photophobia—sensitivity of the eyes to light.

Pin worms—small worms that settle in the rectum and are a cause of itching about the anus.

Pituitary—an important endocrine gland, also called hypophysis, that is located at the base of the brain. It secretes a number of important hormones. These include an adrenal-stimulating hormone called ACTH, a growth-stimulating hormone, a thyroid-stimulating hormone, a gonadotropic hormone which stimulates the production of sex hormones in the ovaries and testicles, a hormone that stimulates milk production in mothers who are nursing, and a hormone that stimulates the production of the pigment called melanin.

Pityriasis rosea—a common skin disease with a rose colored circular eruption and mild itching.

Placenta—a structure in the uterus of a pregnant woman attached to the umbilical cord. It supplies the growing fetus with food, oxygen, and discharges its wastes. After the birth of the baby, the placenta is expelled a short while later.

Placenta previa—the premature separation of the placenta from the womb prior to the baby's birth, a serious complication of late pregnancy causing hemorrhage and distress for the fetus.

Plasma—the liquid portion of the blood.

Plasmapheresis—a procedure in which blood is withdrawn from a donor, the red blood cells are removed, and are then retransfused into the donor; the remaining blood components separated and given to patients who need the various blood fractions or plasma.

Platelets—the blood cells that aid in clotting. Also known as thrombocytes.

Pleura—refers to a thin membrane that covers the lungs and lines the inside of the chest wall.

Pleurisy—inflammation of the membrane covering the lungs and the inside of the chest wall. It usually causes pain in breathing and the development of fluid in the pleural cavity (space between the two layers of pleura).

Pneumoencephalogram (PEG)—X-ray studies of the brain following the injection of air or gas to make thses structures visible.

Pneumonectomy—total removal of a lung.

Pneumonia—infection and inflammation of the lungs.

Pneumothorax—collapse of a lung when air or gas gets into the pleural cavity. When this happens, breathing is difficult, requiring prompt treatment.

Poison ivy or oak—itchy and blistery skin eruption due to contact with a species of ivy or oak.

Pollen—very small spores from flowering plants which are carried through the air and when inhaled can cause allergies.

Polydipsia—excessive fluid intake due to thirst.

Polyps—a protruding growth from various mucous membranes (linings). These can be benign or malignant.

Polyuria—excessive urination.

Porphyria—a condition with abnormally high amounts of pigments (porphyrins) in the blood. Symptoms are light sensitivity, stomach and intestinal pain and nerve damage.

Postpartum—the period that follows childbirth.

Postprandial—after a meal.

Potassium—an essential body element that aids in the contractions of muscles, in the transmission of nerve impulses, and in water and acid/base balance in the body. Deficiency may produce disturbances of heart functions and interfere with other vital body activities.

Premenstrual tension—occurs in some women just before a menstrual period that causes psychic tension, bloating, water-weight gain, cramps, backache and headache.

Presbyopia—decreased elasticity of the lens of the eye that occurs in the elderly and impairs light accommodation, thus interfering with accurate vision.

Preventive health care—a concept which provides for health examinations given at regular intervals to detect any beginning signs of illness, so that treatment can be provided to stop the illness before it can progress. Health counseling is also given, to help retain good health through appropriate diet, rest, exercise and other factors that promote a healthy lifestyle.

Primigravida—a woman who is pregnant for the first time.

Proctoscopy—internal examination of the rectal structures.

Prolapsed disc—displacement of cartilage between vertebra. If it presses on nerves it can cause pain and muscular weakness.

Prophylaxis—preventive treatment or health care.

Prostate—a gland in the male which surrounds the neck of the bladder and the urethra. The prostate contributes to the seminal fluid a secretion containing acid phosphatase, citric acid, and proteolytic enzymes which account for the liquefaction of the coagulated semen.

Prostatectomy—partial or complete removal of prostate gland.

Prostration—physical or mental exhaustion that may follow psychological stress, great physical exertion, exposure to very hot environmental temperatures, or severe illness.

Pruritus—itching.

Psittacosis—an infection that can be transmitted to humans from birds causing a form of pneumonia.

Psoriasis—a skin disease that produces itchy reddened patches and scales. It is not a contagious disease, but tends to run in families.

Psychiatric—pertaining to psychiatry, that branch of medicine which deals with the study, treatment and prevention of mental illness.

Psychosis—an emotional disturbance in which a person behaves irrationally, unpredictably, and may harm himself or others.

Pterygium—a disease of the eye in which a triangular piece of tissue grows out of the lining of the eyelid at its inner aspect (next to the nose) and extends toward the pupil of the eye.

Puerperium—the period of time between childbirth and the return of the womb to its normal, pre-pregnant size and shape.

Pulmonary—refers to the lungs and breathing structures.

Pulmonary edema—abnormal fluid accumulation in the lungs causing difficult breathing.

Pulmonary embolus—a blood clot lodged in the vessels of the lung.

Pupil—the circular area at the front of the eye through which light enters.

Purpura—a group of disorders characterized by purplish or brownish red discoloration, easily visible through the epidermis, caused by hemorrhage into the tissues. Bruises, black and blue marks.

Pus—a thick, yellowish liquid produced by inflammation or infection.

Pyelonephritis—inflammation of the kidneys.

Pyloric stenosis—a narrowing of the valve at the far end of the stomach. Causes food to back up.

Pyogenic—refers to an agent or organism that causes the formation of pus.

Pyorrhea—inflammation of the gums in the peridontal spaces (where the gums join the teeth), often accompanied by pus formation, and the loosening of teeth.

Pyridoxine (vitamin B₆)—an essential vitamin that aids the functions of body cells and the metabolism of amino and fatty acids. Deficiency of this vitamin may produce anemia, nervous system problems, skin lesions and seizures in small infants.

Pyuria—pus in the urine.

Q

Q fever—an infection that occurs mainly on farms, and in slaughterhouse workers. It is acquired from animals such as goats and cows through contact with their urine and feces.

Quadraplegia—complete paralysis of the upper and lower limbs.

Quinsy—a sore throat, followed by an abscess in the tissues that surround the tonsils. This condition may occur together with tonsilitis. If the abscess becomes very large, it may need to be opened and drained.

R

Rabies—a virus infection caused by an infected animal bite. The symptoms are muscle spasms, paralysis, convulsions and excitement and rage alternating with periods of calm.

Radiation therapy—the use of radioactive substances to treat a variety of diseases, but especially those which produce large numbers of abnormal cells that destroy tissues, such as cancer. The effect of radiation therapy is to destroy the cancer cells.

Radionuclide—a radioactive substance that is used to perform diagnostic and treatment procedures.

Raynaud's Disease—an intermittent condition causing spasm of the blood vessels of the fingers or toes causing pallor and/or pain. It is precipitated by cold or emotional tension.

Refraction—an examination of the eyes if needed.

Regurgitation—vomiting.

Remission—a chronic disease whose symptoms have temporarily disappeared.

Renal failure—inability of the kidneys to remove waste products from the blood and excrete them in the urine.

Respiratory arrest—the cessation of breathing.

Respiratory tract—the organs and passages concerned with breathing: the nose, pharynx, larynx, epiglottis, trachea, bronchi and the lungs.

Resuscitation—emergency procedures to restart respiratory and heart funtions that have stopped due to illness, trauma or for other reasons, to allow the victim to survive.

Retina—the light-sensitive inner layer of the eye that transmits nerve impulses to the optic nerve.

Retinol (vitamin A)—an essential vitamin that aids vision and certain cellular functions. Deficiency produces nightblindness, dry eyes and other eye problems.

Retrolental fibroplasia (RLF)—a disease of premature infants in which there is an abnormal growth of fibrous tissue behind the lens of the eye, causing blindness. The condition is caused by the excessive administration of oxygen which is toxic to his eye structures.

Reverse isolation—isolation precautions used for the protection of the patient whose immune system is weak, so that he will not be exposed to any infectious organisms carried by people in his environment.

Reye's syndrome—a virus disease usually found in children that may follow an upper respiratory infection or other virus disease. It is a dangerous disease that affects the brain and nervous system, and produces fatty accumulations in various body organs.

Rheumatic fever—a disease caused by a streptoccal infection characterized by fever, painful joint swellings, occasionally a rash and heart inflammation.

Rheumatoid arthritis—an inflammatory disease of the joints. It produces pain and swelling, destroys surrounding cartilage and decreases motion in the affected joints.

Riboflavin (vitamin B_2)—an essential vitamin that aids in protein metabolism, maintains healthy mucous membranes and helps the body convert food into energy. Deficiency may cause soreness and fissures of the lips.

Rickets—a disease of children caused by a deficiency of calcium and Vitamin D, which prevents hardening of the bones.

Ringworm—a fungus infection of the skin causing a circular rash.

Roentgen—an international unit of X- and gamma radiation.

Rubefacient—a counterirritant which reddens the skin when applied.

Rubella—German measles.

Rubeola—measles.

S

Sacroiliac joint—a joint on either side of the lower aspect of the spine.

Sadism—sexual gratification obtained by inflicting pain on another individual.

Salmonella infection—food poisoning caused by eating food contaminated by salmonella bacteria.

Salpingitis—inflammation of the fallopian tubes.

Scabies—a skin infection caused by a mite that burrows into the skin.

Scarlet fever—a streptococcal infection. Called also febris rubra and scarlatina.

Sciata—pain along the main large nerve that runs down the back of the leg.

Scurvy—a disease caused by a deficiency of vitamin C; symptoms include a tendency to bleed into the gums, inflammation of the gums, and loose teeth.

Sedative—a drug given to reduce nervousness, abnormally great excitement or irritability.

Semicircular canals—part of the inner ear containing fluid. When the head changes position the fluid shifts sending information to the brain so the person can determine their position in space.

Seminal fluid—the fluid that carries semen.

Senility—mental or physical deterioration usually due to aging.

Sepsis—infection.

Septic abortion—an abortion performed under unsanitary conditions, with the result that the woman having the abortion develops an infection of her reproductive organs that may progress to blood poisoning.

Septic shock—a sudden onset of abnormally low blood pressure, rapid pulse, fever and sometimes a skin rash caused by the absorption of toxic substances secreted by bacteria.

Septicemia—blood poisoning. The presence of harmful organisms or their toxins in the blood stream.

Serum—the liquid portion of blood that is left after the clotting components have been removed.

Sex hormones—substances produced in the body by various organs. These determine the male and female characteristics.

Shingles—(called Herpes Zoster) is a viral infection that follows the pathway of a large nerve. It causes painful skin blisters usually on one side of the body.

Shock—a group of symptoms that occur when a person's circulatory system collapses. This may happen in a severe allergic response, when a person hemorrhages, after major surgery, serious burns, or following trauma.

Sickle cell anemia—a hereditary, genetically determined hemolytic anemia occurring almost exclusively in blacks, characterized by arthralgia, acute attacks of abdominal pain, ulcerations of the lower extremities, sickle-shaped erythrocytes in the blood.

Sigmoidoscopy—examination of the portion of colon just above the rectum with a lighted instrument.

Sims position—lying with the body on its side.

Sinus—a small, hollow channel or passage inside the body, that may contain fluid or air.

Sodium—an essential element in the body that aids fluid and acid/base balance, nervous impulse transmission and muscle contractility. Deficiency may produce swelling of the tissues and other symptoms of fluid imbalance.

Spastic colon—spasms of the large bowel causing cramping pains and at times frequent bowel movements.

Spina bifida—a congenital condition characterized by defective closure of the boney encasement of the spinal cord, through which the cord and meninges may or may not protrude.

Staphylococcus—a bacterial organism that causes infection.

Stenosis—the narrowing of a channel, duct or passage in the body.

Sterile—an area that is free of germs.

Stimulant—a drug or other substance that increases mental or physical activity.

Stoma—an opening on the body's surface usually made in surgery.

Stomach ulcer—breakdown in the lining of the stomach that may or may not cause gastric bleeding.

Strabismus—an eye condition which makes it impossible for a person to focus both eyes on the same place. Treatment may include eye glasses, exercises, medication and surgery.

Streptococcus—a bacterial organism that causes a variety of infectious diseases.

Stroke—a condition with sudden onset caused by acute vascular lesions of the brain, such as hemorrhage, embolism, thrombosis, or rupturing aneurysm. It is often followed by permanent neurologic damage.

Subarachnoid hemorrhage—a hemorrhage under one of the coverings of the brain or spinal cord.

Subcutaneous injection—an injection that is given under the skin.

Subdural hemorrhage—hemorrhage into the dura mater space in the brain.

Superinfection—a new infection complicating the course of antimicrobial therapy of an existing infectious process.

Supraventricular tachycardia—a rapid heart rate that originates in the upper chambers of the heart.

Surfactant antiseptic—a specially prepared fluid that inactivates or kills certain bacteria, fungi and viruses when applied to the skin.

Sustained release dosage—a term that indicates that a drug has been manufactured so that tiny portions of each tablet or capsule are released over a period of hours at carefully calculated intervals.

Swimmer's ear—infection of the middle and/or external ear caused by moisture, allergy, a disease-causing organism or chemical irritant.

Symptom—some change in a body part, organ or function that indicates illness or a developing disorder.

Syncope—fainting.

Syndrome—a group of symptoms that occur together, suggesting the presence of a disorder or illness known to include this group of symptoms.

Synovial fluid—the fluid found in joints.

Synovitis—inflammation of the lining of a joint (synovial membrane).

Syphilis—a contagious venereal disease leading to many structural and cutaneous lesions transmitted by direct intimate contact.

Syringomyelia—a progressive disease that affects the nervous system by producing small cavities filled with fluid at the back of the spinal cord. Pain, weakness and loss of sensation occur in the victim's hand or arm, and the legs may become spastic.

Systemic—relating to the body as a whole.

Systemic lupus erythematosus—a disease that affects connective tissue (bone, tendons, cartilage) as well as other organs such as the heart, lungs and kidneys. The patient has pain in the muscles, joints, and in his abdomen. Various drugs are used to control the disease.

Systolic blood pressure (systole)—the first highest level noted during blood pressure measurement. It reflects the pressure with arteries and the heart as the heart contracts forcing blood to be pumped into the arterial circulation.

T

Tachycardia—an abnormally fast heart rate.

Tachypnea—very rapid breathing.

Talipes—clubfoot; a congenital foot deformity in which the foot is twisted inward, outward or in several other abnormal positions so that normal use of the foot for standing and walking is not possible. May be corrected, or greatly improved by surgery.

Tamponade—compression of a body part as a result of an accumulation of fluid in a surrounding body area.

Tapeworm—one of a group of long worms that lives in the intestines of man as well as in animals; may grow as long as 30 feet.

Tendinitis—inflammation of a tendon, a tough and strong band of connective tissue that connects muscles to bones.

Tennis elbow—a condition in which there is pain either on the outer or inner portion of the elbow due to an inflammation in the surrounding structures. The outer (lateral epicondylitis) form is more common than the inner (medial epicondylitis). Pain is aggravated when the hand tries to grip or grasp an object.

Teratogen—any agent that may cause a growing fetus to be born with an abnormality.

Testosterone—a male sex hormone.

Tetanus—lock jaw.

Tetany—a disorder caused by a calcium deficiency in the blood producing irritability of the nerves, muscular cramps or spasms, and sometimes convulsions.

Tetrahydrocannabinol (THC)—marijuana.

Thalassemia—a particular type of anemia that occurs in areas that border on the Mediterranean, and in Southeast Asia.

Therapeutic abortion—an abortion performed on a woman likely to develop a serious mental or physical illness if she carries the pregnancy to term and gives birth to a child.

Therapeutic dosage—the quantity of a drug calculated to improve the condition for which it is being prescribed.

Thermography—a diagnostic device that uses the temperatures in various body parts to determine the presence of abnormal conditions in these areas.

Thiamine (vitamin B_1)—an essential vitamin that aids carbohydrate metabolism, and heart and nervous functions. Deficiency causes symptoms in the circulatory and nervous systems. Deficiency disease is called beriberi.

Thoracocentesis—withdrawal of fluid from the pleural cavity (the cavity created by the membranes that line the lungs and the chest wall), to relieve pressure on the lungs and improve breathing.

Threatened abortion—spotting or vaginal bleeding that are warning signals for a pregnant woman that she may not be able to carry the pregnancy.

Thrombocytopenia—an abnormally small number of platelets in the blood.

Thrombophlebitis—swelling and inflammation of a vein often caused by a blood clot.

Thrombosis—the presence of a blood clot inside a blood vessel, blocking the vessel.

Thrush—a fungal infection of the mouth, also called Vincent's Angina.

Thyroid gland—one of the endocrine glands. It secretes, stores, and liberates as necessary the thyroid hormones which require iodine for their elaboration and which are concerned in regulating the metabolic rate.

Thyroidectomy—removal of all or part of the thyroid gland by surgery.

Thyroiditis—inflammation of the thyroid gland.

Tic douloureux—inflammation or irritation of the trigeminal nerve which branches out through the face, causing severe head and face pain.

Tinnitus—a condition in which a person hears noises or ringing in his ears. May be caused by inflammation and by certain drugs.

Tocopherol (vitamin E)—a vitamin that is believed to aid healing, and contribute to the stability of biologic membranes. Deficiency can produce destruction of red blood cells.

Tonsils—specialized lymph glands in back of the throat that keep infections in check.

Topical anesthetic—an anesthetic agent directly applied to the area where pain relief is needed.

Topical medication—a medication directly applied to the area where it is needed, rather than being taken by mouth or in some other way.

Torsion of the testicle—twisting of a testicle causing excrutiating pain. If not corrected quickly the testicle will be destroyed.

Torticollis—a contraction, often occurring in spasms, of the muscles of the neck, which causes the head to be drawn to one side. May be a congenital condition, or acquired after birth.

Toxemia of pregnancy—a condition of pregnancy causing high blood pressure and kidney failure which can lead to convulsions.

Toxicologic—refers to the study of poisonous agents and how they affect the body.

Toxin—a poisonous substance. It may be a chemical agent, or a harmful substance secreted by a microorganism.

Trachea—the windpipe.

Tracheotomy—an incision made into the windpipe to aid in breathing or to remove mucus.

Transfusion—the introduction of whole blood or blood component directly into the blood stream.

Transient ischemic attack (TIA)—temporary spasm in one of the blood vessels of the brain that is narrowed by hardening of the arteries, or because of a temporary blockage in a blood vessel. Such attacks may be the warning signals of an impending stroke.

Transplant—the transfer of tissue or an organ from one body area to another, or from one person to another, to replace a missing, diseased, or non-functioning body part or organ.

Transurethral resection—surgical removal of all or part of the prostate gland through the penis.

Tremor—trembling of one or more body part, such as the hands or the head, due to illness, weakness or inherited disorders.

Trench mouth—an infection of the gums causing painful ulcers with bleeding.

Trendelenburg position—a position in which the patient's head is at an angle of 45° below his pelvis, while he is lying on the operating table, or in bed, if he is being treated for shock.

Trichinosis—a disease caused by a roundworm called Trichinella spiralis, that lives in pigs and is transmitted when a person eats infected pork that has not been adequately cooked. When the worms' larvae enter the bloodstream, they travel to all body tissues, where they cause an inflammatory response. As cysts they can survive in muscle fibers for years. Symptoms include fever, nausea, vomiting, diarrhea and abdominal pain in the first few weeks after infection. Muscle pains and swelling in the affected areas follow the initial symptoms.

Trichomonas—a parasite that causes inflammation of the female and male genital tracts.

Tubal pregnancy—a pregnancy developed in a fallopian tube. This can rupture through the wall causing sudden severe internal bleeding.

Tube feeding—also known as gavage, is performed when a person is unable to take nourishment by eating and drinking normally. A tube is inserted through the nose or mouth and passed down into the stomach. It is anchored with adhesive tape so that it cannot move, and liquids or blended foods can then be given at prescribed intervals.

Tuberculosis—an infectious disease caused by the Mycobacterium tuberculosis. It affects primarily the lungs, but may also affect other organs, such as the stomach, skin, bones or lymph glands. A particularly severe type of the disease, called miliary tuberculosis, affects most body parts, including the brain. Infected sputum droplets passed through the air by coughing or sneezing transmit the disease to others. Treatment includes medication, adequate nourishment and sufficient rest.

Tularemia—a disease of rodents, resembling plague, which is transmitted by the bites of flies, fleas, ticks, and lice, and may be acquired by man through handling of contaminated animal products (leather) or infected animals, or the bites of fleas, ticks, and the deer fly.

Turista—travelers' diarrhea; an intestinal infection caused by bacteria, viruses, and the toxins they secrete. It is acquired by eating contaminated food, or drinking contaminated water, usually while traveling in foreign areas.

Tympanic membrane—the eardrum; a structure that transmits sounds received from the outer ear by vibrating as the sound waves hit the membrane.

Type and crossmatch—a laboratory test done prior to giving a blood transfusion to make sure the donor's blood type and other blood characteristics match those of the recipient. If this is not done, the recipient may develop a serious, and possibly fatal reaction to the donor's blood.

Typhoid fever—an infectious disease caused by a salmonella bacillus. The disease is transmitted through food, water or milk contaminated by the organism. People who have the disease may continue to act as carriers after they recover by harboring the organisms in their urine and feces. Symptoms include headache, high fever, chills, and a rash on the chest and abdomen. Antibiotics, supportive measures and urine and stool precautions are used in the treatment.

U

Ulcerative colitis—inflammation of a portion of the large bowel causing ulceration, diarrhea and bleeding.

Ultrasonography—a diagnostic technique that utilizes the reflection and transmission of ultrasonic waves to determine abnormality of disease of internal body structures.

Uremia—the presence of an abnormally high level of urea and other nitrogenous waste substances in the blood, caused by poorly or non-functioning kidneys.

Ureteritis—inflammation of the ureters.

Ureters—two tubes, each connecting a kidney to the bladder. Urine flows from the kidneys through the ureters into the bladder.

Urethra—the passageway through which urine flows from the bladder out of the body.

Uric acid—a product derived from the breakdown of protein. Accumulating in the joints it causes gout and excess amounts in the urinary system may lead to kidney stone formation.

Urinary calculus—stones formed in the urinary tract that can interfere with the flow of urine. They can cause great pain.

Urinary incontinence—failure of voluntary control of the vesical and urethral sphincters, with constant or frequent involuntary passage of urine.

Urinary urgency—frequency; a frequent urge to urinate; occurs with enlargement of the prostate that causes pressure on the bladder, with irritation, inflammation and infection of the bladder and the urethra.

Urine culture—a laboratory technique done to determine the presence and type of harmful microorganisms in the urinary tract, so that appropriate treatment can be prescribed.

Urolithiasis—the presence of a stone in the urinary tract.

Urologic—refers to the urinary tract.

Urticaria—hives; a rash usually due to an allergic reaction to food, a psychological event, a drug or some other environmental irritant.

Uterus—the womb.

V

Vaccine—a preparation that contains infectious organisms that are alive, or that have been inactivated or killed. When given to an individual in carefully prescribed amounts, his system is challenged to develop antibodies against these microorganisms and the disease they cause, so that he develops immunity against it.

Varices—varicose veins; a condition in which certain veins become dilated, knotted and weakened due to stress or disease.

Varicocele—enlarged scrotum due to varicose veins of the spermatic duct located inside the scrotum.

Varicose ulcer—an open, sore area on the skin over a varicose vein caused by erosion of the surface of the vein, or by infection.

Vascular—referring to blood vessels of the circulatory system.

Vascular fragility—a tendency of blood vessels to break down due to brittleness, weakness, infection or disease.

Vasectomy—the process of cutting the vas deferens, which normally carries sperm from the testicles to the penis, for contraceptive purposes.

Vasoconstrictor—an agent or drug that causes blood vessels to constrict or narrow.

Vasodilator—an agent or drug that dilates blood vessels.

Venereal—refers to a disease, infection or other event affecting the genital area.

Venous thrombosis—clots forming in a vein causing blockage of circulation.

Ventricle—a small cavity, such as one of the several cavities of the brain, or one of the lower chambers of the heart.

Ventricular failure—failure of the ventricles of the heart to pump blood to the body.

Ventricular fibrillation—arrhythmia characterized by fibrillary contractions of the ventricular muscle due to rapid repetitive excitation of myocardial fibers without coordinated contraction of the ventricle.

Vertebrae—the bones making up the spinal column, divided into those in the neck (cervical), chest (thoracic) and lower back (lumbar).

Vertigo—severe dizziness.

Vesicle—a bladder, or bladder-like structure, as in the case of a blister or sac-like cavity; caused by friction, inflammation or infection.

Virus—a small particle considered borderline between living and non-living matter. Viruses consist of molecules that are composed of proteins and nucleic acids. When they gain access to a living cell, they can change the cell's usual functions and reproductive capacity. Some viruses are useful, others cause disease.

Vitamin toxicity—poisoning that occurs when a person ingests excessive amounts of vitamins.

Vitamins—organic substances present in food essential for normal metabolism. Inadequate amounts lead to disease states.

Vitreous humor—the semifluid substance contained in the eyeball behind the lens.

Vocal cords—situated in the larynx, they vibrate and cause voice.

Void—the process of urination.

Volvulus—twisting of the large bowel on itself.

Vulva—the external female genitalia.

W

Wart—a benign hard growth on the skin caused by a virus, also known as verruca. May occur anywhere on the body, but appears most frequently on the sole of the foot, where it is called a plantar wart.

Wet lung—lung filled with fluid.

White blood cell—leukocyte; a constituent of blood, formed in the bone marrow and the lymph glands. White blood cells defend the body against infection.

Wilms tumor—a tumor of a kidney occurring almost exclusively in young children.

Wound culture—a laboratory procedure done to determine whether a wound is infected, and to identify the microorganism that causes the infection.

X

X-chromosome—a sex chromosome; if a fetus has two X-chromosomes in its genetic make-up, it will develop as a female.

Xeroderma—a skin condition which produces excessively dry skin.

X Ray—a form of radiation used to penetrate the body causing an exposure of a photographic film. This black and white image can then be used for diagnostic purposes.

Y

Y-chromosome—a sex chromosome; if a fetus has a Y-chromosome in its genetic make-up, it will develop as a male.

Yellow fever—an infectious disease transmitted by the bite of a mosquito that carries the causative organism. High fevers and jaundice are the main symptoms.

Z

Zinc—a trace element that aids wound healing, and acts as a component of several body enzymes.

Zoonosis—a disease of animals that may be transmitted to man (i.e. brucellosis, rabies)

First Aid for Possible Poisoning

REMEMBER: ANY NON-FOOD SUBSTANCE MAY BE POISONOUS!

1. Keep all potential poisons—household products and medicines—out of the reach of small children.
2. Use "safety caps" (child-resistant containers) as intended to avoid accidents.
3. Have 1 oz. Syrup of Ipecac in your home and in your first aid kit for camping, travel, etc.
4. Keep your Poison Center's and your physician's phone number handy.

IF YOU THINK AN ACCIDENTAL INGESTION HAS OCCURRED:

1. Keep calm—do not wait for symptoms—call for help promptly!
2. Find out if the substance is toxic—Your Poison Control Center (listed by state and city on the following pages) or your physician can tell you if a risk exists and what you should do.
3. Have the product's container or label with you at the phone.

   A. IF A POISON IS ON THE SKIN:
   Immediately remove affected clothing.
   Flood involved parts of body with water, wash with soap or detergent and rinse thoroughly.

   B. IF A POISON IS IN THE EYE:
   Immediately flush the eye with water for 10 to 15 minutes.

   C. IF A POISON IS INHALED:
   Immediately get the person to fresh air. Give mouth to mouth resuscitation if necessary.

   D. IF A POISON IS SWALLOWED:
   Medicines: Do not give anything by mouth until calling for advice.
   Chemical or Household Product: Unless patient is unconscious, having convulsions, or cannot swallow give milk or water. Then call for professional advice as to whether you should induce vomiting.
   If Vomiting is recommended: Give one tablespoon of Ipecac syrup followed by a glass (8 oz.) of clear liquid (water, juices, or pop). If the patient doesn't vomit within 15 to 20 minutes, give another tablespoon of Ipecac and more water. Do *not* use salt water. It can be dangerous.

NEVER INDUCE VOMITING IF:

1. The victim is in COMA (unconscious).
2. The victim is CONVULSING (having a fit or a seizure).
3. The victim has swallowed a CAUSTIC or CORROSIVE (e.g. LYE).

FOR REEMPHASIS:

1. Always call to be certain of possible toxicity before undertaking treatment.
2. Never induce vomiting until you are instructed to do so.
3. Do not rely on the label's antidote information—it may be out of date—call instead!
4. If you have to go to an Emergency Room, take the tablets, capsules, container, and/or label with you.
5. Don't hesitate to call your Poison Center or your doctor a second time if the victim seems to be getting worse.

Prepared by:
American Association of Poison Control Centers.

MEDICINE CABINET CHECK LIST
Prescriptions Filled

Drug dose; how often	Doctor who ordered it (Date)	Reason for taking it	Effect

Nonprescription drugs

Drug	Reason for purchase (complaint)	Date purchased	Effect

MEDICINE CABINET CHECK LIST
Prescriptions Filled

Drug dose; how often	Doctor who ordered it (Date)	Reason for taking it	Effect

Nonprescription drugs

Drug	Reason for purchase (complaint)	Date purchased	Effect

Weight Record

Check weight each month

Month	Weight

Blood Pressure Record

Take blood pressure as instructed by your doctor

Date	Blood Pressure	Date	Blood Pressure

Health aids record

Aid or equipment	date purchased	due for checkup or maintenance problems
Eye glasses		
Contact lenses		
Arch supports		
Ace bandage or Elastic stockings		
Hearing aid		
Blood pressure equipment (self-testing)		